Sickle Cell Disease

Notice

Medicine is an ever-changing science. As new research and clinical experience broaden our knowledge, changes in treatment and drug therapy are required. The authors and the publisher of this work have checked with sources believed to be reliable in their efforts to provide information that is complete and generally in accord with the standards accepted at the time of publication. However, in view of the possibility of human error or changes in medical sciences, neither the authors nor the publisher nor any other party who has been involved in the preparation or publication of this work warrants that the information contained herein is in every respect accurate or complete, and they disclaim all responsibility for any errors or omissions or for the results obtained from use of the information contained in this work. Readers are encouraged to confirm the information contained herein with other sources. For example and in particular, readers are advised to check the product information sheet included in the package of each drug they plan to administer to be certain that the information contained in this work is accurate and that changes have not been made in the recommended dose or in the contraindications for administration. This recommendation is of particular importance in connection with new or infrequently used drugs.

Sickle Cell Disease

Editors

Mark T. Gladwin, MD

Jack D. Myers Distinguished Professor and Chair
Chairman of the Department of Medicine
UPMC and the University of Pittsburgh School of Medicine
Pittsburgh, Pennsylvania

Gregory J. Kato, MD

Senior Director
CSL Behring
Clinical Research and Development
Hematology Therapeutic Area
King of Prussia, Pennsylvania

Enrico M. Novelli, MD, MS

Associate Professor of Medicine
Division of Hematology/Oncology
University of Pittsburgh
Chief, Section of Benign Hematology
Director, UPMC Adult Sickle Cell Disease Program
Pittsburgh, Pennsylvania

New York   Chicago   San Francisco   Athens   London   Madrid   Mexico City
Milan   New Delhi   Singapore   Sydney   Toronto

1 2 3 4 5 6 7 8 9 LWI 26 25 24 23 22 21

ISBN 978-1-260-45859-6
MHID 1-260-45859-8

This book was set in Minion Pro Regular by KnowledgeWorks Global Ltd.
The editors were Karen Edmonson, Jason Malley, and Kim J. Davis.
The production supervisor was Richard Ruzycka.
Project management was provided by Sarika Gupta, KnowledgeWorks Global Ltd.
Cover painting: "Ten Redefined" by Hertz Nazaire.

This book is printed on acid-free paper.

Library of Congress Cataloging-in-Publication Data

Names: Gladwin, Mark, editor. | Kato, Gregory J., editor. | Novelli, Enrico (Enrico M.), editor.
Title: Sickle cell disease / [edited by] Mark T. Gladwin, Gregory J. Kato, Enrico Novelli.
Other titles: Sickle cell disease (Gladwin)
Description: New York : McGraw Hill, [2021] | Includes bibliographical references and index. | Summary: "This book will provide students and practitioners with the most recent guidelines for patient care. Chapters include guidelines of care, diagnosis, unique cases, and cutting-edge therapies that will appeal to hematology fellows, trainees, and practicing hematologists"— Provided by publisher.
Identifiers: LCCN 2020050165 (print) | LCCN 2020050166 (ebook) | ISBN 9781260458596 (hardcover ; alk. paper) | ISBN 9781260458602 (ebook)
Subjects: MESH: Anemia, Sickle Cell
Classification: LCC RC641.7.S5 (print) | LCC RC641.7.S5 (ebook) | NLM WH 170 | DDC 616.1/527—dc23
LC record available at https://lccn.loc.gov/2020050165
LC ebook record available at https://lccn.loc.gov/2020050166

This book is dedicated to the many warriors living with sickle cell disease we editors have been honored to serve in our medical practice at Howard University, Johns Hopkins University, the National Institutes of Health, and the University of Pittsburgh. Our patients have taught us more lessons than can ever be captured in a textbook, and our medical care for them has been both humbling and rewarding. We are indebted to each one of them for sharing with us a glimpse into their daily resilience, fortitude, and grace in the face of unspeakable suffering. We are grateful for their infectious hope. Most of all, we thank them for their trust in us as we work together with them as allies to embrace the best science and medicine to advance toward a brighter future. We owe them our commitment to educate the public and medical community about this devastating disease, and to work with them to overcome the barriers to health equity engendered by poverty, systemic racism, and often inadequate medical insurance for the ultimate "pre-existing condition," an inherited genetic disease. We sincerely hope this book may contribute to worldwide excellence in care for all patients with sickle cell disease.

CONTENTS

Robert J. Adams, MS, MD
Distinguished Professor of Neurology
Medical University South Carolina
Charleston, South Carolina

Kofi Anie, PhD
Director, Psychosocial Program
Brent Sickle Cell and Thalassaemia Centre
London North West University Healthcare NHS Trust
and Imperial College London
London, United Kingdom

Kenneth I. Ataga, MD
Center for Sickle Cell Disease
Division of Hematology and Oncology
University of Tennessee Health Science Center at Memphis
Memphis, Tennessee

Sherif M. Badawy, MD
Department of Pediatrics
Northwestern University Feinberg School of Medicine
Division of Hematology, Oncology and Stem Cell
Transplantation
Ann & Robert H. Lurie Children's Hospital of Chicago
Chicago, Illinois

Samir K. Ballas, MD
Department of Medicine
Division of Hematology
Sidney Kimmel Medical College
Thomas Jefferson University
Philadelphia, Pennsylvania

John D. Belcher, PhD
Associate Professor of Medicine
Division of Hematology-Oncology-Transplantation
Department of Medicine and Vascular Biology Center
University of Minnesota Medical School
Minneapolis, Minnesota

Carlo Brugnara, MD
Department of Laboratory of Medicine
Boston Children's Hospital
Department of Pathology
Harvard Medical School
Boston, Massachusetts

Arthur L. Burnett MD, MBA, FACS
James Buchanan Brady Urological Institute
Johns Hopkins Medical Institutions
Baltimore, Maryland

Sally A. Campbell-Lee, MD
Director, Transfusion Medicine
University of Illinois at Chicago
Chicago, Illinois

Marcus Carden, MD
Assistant Professor of Pediatrics and Medicine
Divisions of Pediatric Hematology/Oncology and
Medical Hematology
Director, Pediatric Sickle Cell Program
UNC Blood Research Center
University of North Carolina School of Medicine
Chapel Hill, North Carolina

Oswaldo Castro, MD
Professor Emeritus of Medicine
Howard University College of Medicine
Washington, DC

Marina Cavazzana, MD, PhD
Professor of Paediatric Immunology
Director, Department of Biotherapy
Necker-Enfants Malades Hospital
Paris Descartes University
Paris, France

Roshan Colah, MSc, PhD
Former Director In-Charge
ICMR-National Institute of Immunohaematology
Mumbai, India

Philippe Connes, PhD
Vascular Biology and Red Blood Cell Team
University of Lyon
Lyon, France
Laboratory of Excellence GR-Ex
Paris, France

Fernando Ferreira Costa, MD, PhD
Professor of Hematology
Department of Clinical Medicine
Hemocentro da UNICAMP
School of Medical Sciences
University of Campinas
Campinas, Brazil

Michael R. DeBaun, MD, MPH
Department of Pediatrics
Vanderbilt-Meharry Center of Excellence in Sickle Cell
Disease
Vanderbilt University Medical Center
Nashville, Tennessee

Laura M. De Castro, MD, MHSc
Associate Professor of Medicine
Clinical Director, Benign Hematology Section
Division of Hematology and Oncology
University of Pittsburgh Medical Center
Pittsburgh, Pennsylvania

Vimal K. Derebail, MD, MPH
Associate Professor Medicine
Division of Nephrology and Hypertension
University of North Carolina at Chapel Hill
Chapel Hill, North Carolina

Armand Mekontso Dessap
AP-HP, Hôpitaux Universitaire Henri Mondor
DHU A-TVB, Service de Réanimation Médicale
Université Paris Est Créteil Val de Marne
Faculté de Médecine
IMRB, Groupe de Recherche Clinique CARMAS
Créteil, France

William A. Eaton, MD, PhD
NIH Distinguished Investigator
Chief, Laboratory of Chemical Physics
The National Institute of Diabetes and Digestive and
    Kidney Diseases
National Institutes of Health
Bethesda, Maryland

Paul S. Frenette, MD
Ruth L. and David S. Gottesman Institute
    for Stem Cell and Regenerative Medicine Research
Department of Cell Biology
Departments of Medicine
Albert Einstein College of Medicine
Bronx, New York

Mark T. Gladwin, MD
Jack D. Myers Distinguished Professor and Chair
Chairman of the Department of Medicine
UPMC and the University of Pittsburgh
    School of Medicine
Pittsburgh, Pennsylvania

Jeffrey Glassberg, MD
Associate Professor of Emergency Medicine
Hematology and Medical Oncology
Director of Research
The Mount Sinai Comprehensive Sickle Cell Program
Icahn School of Medicine at Mount Sinai
New York, New York

Morton F. Goldberg, MD
Director Emeritus
Wilmer Eye Institute
Johns Hopkins University School of Medicine
Baltimore, Maryland

Victor R. Gordeuk, MD
Director, Sickle Cell Center
Professor of Medicine
University of Illinois at Chicago
Chicago, Illinois

Nancy S. Green, MD
Professor of Pediatrics
Division of Hematology, Oncology and Stem Cell
    Transplantation
Associate Director
Irving Institute for Clinical Translational Research
Associate Dean for Academic Operations
Columbia University Irving Medical Center
New York, New York

Kalpna Gupta, PhD
Division of Hematology/Oncology
Department of Medicine
University of California, Irvine
Orange, California

Anoosha Habibi, MD
Sickle Cell Anemia Referral Center
Henri Mondor University Hospital
Université Paris Est (UPE)
Institut Mondor de Recherche Biomédicale (IMRB)
Institut National de la Santé et de le Recherche Médicale
    (INSERM)
Créteil, France

Jane S. Hankins, MD, MS
Associate Member
Department of Hematology
Director, Sickle Cell Program
St. Jude Children's Research Hospital
Memphis, Tennessee

Kathryn L. Hassell, MD
Professor of Medicine
Division of Hematology
Director, Colorado Sickle Cell Treatment and Research
    Center
University of Colorado Anschutz Medical Campus
Aurora, Colorado

Robert P. Hebbel, MD
Regents Professor Emeritus
Division of Hematology-Oncology-Transplantation
Department of Medicine and Vascular Biology Center
University of Minnesota Medical School
Minneapolis, Minnesota

Lewis L. Hsu, MD, PhD
Pediatric Hematology/Oncology
University of Illinois at Chicago
Chicago, Illinois

Hyacinth I. Hyacinth, MD, PhD, MPH
Aflac Cancer and Blood Disorder Center
Emory University
Department of Pediatrics and Children's Healthcare of
    Atlanta
Atlanta, Georgia

Khushnooma Italia, MSc, PhD
Product Specialist, Clinical Diagnostic Group
Bio-Rad Laboratories (India) Pvt. Ltd.
Mumbai, India

Yazdi Italia, PhD
Hon. Secretary
Valsad Raktdan Kendra
A Regional Blood Bank & Haematology Research Centre
Gujarat, India

Dipty Jain, MBBS, MD, MSc
Professor and Head
Department of Pediatrics
Government Medical College
Nagpur, India

Charles Jonassaint, PhD, MHS
Assistant Professor of Medicine
Social Work and Clinical and Translational Science
University of Pittsburgh
Pittsburgh, Pennsylvania

Ramasubramanian Kalpatthi, MD
Visiting Associate Professor of Pediatrics
Director of Sickle Cell Clinical Research
Division of Pediatric Hematology Oncology
UPMC Children's Hospital of Pittsburgh
Pittsburgh, Pennsylvania

Gregory J. Kato, MD
Senior Director
CSL Behring
Clinical Research and Development
Hematology Therapeutic Area
King of Prussia, Pennsylvania

Nigel Key, MB ChB, FRCP
Harold R. Roberts Distinguished Professor
Departments of Medicine and Pathology and Laboratory
    Medicine
Director, UNC Hemophilia and Thrombosis Center
Chief, Section of Hematology
University of North Carolina, Chapel Hill School of
    Medicine
Chapel Hill, North Carolina

Daniel B. Kim-Shapiro, MS, PhD
Department of Physics
Wake Forest University
Winston-Salem, North Carolina

Allison A. King, MD, MPH, PhD
Professor, Program in Occupational Therapy
Departments of Pediatrics, Medicine and Surgery
Washington University School of Medicine
St. Louis, Missouri

Fenella J. Kirkham, MD Research, FRCPCH
Professor of Paediatric Neurology
Developmental Neurosciences Section
UCL Great Ormond Street Institute of Child Health
London, United Kingdom
Professor of Paediatric Neurology
Clinical and Experimental Sciences
Faculty of Medicine
University of Southampton
Southampton, United Kingdom
Consultant Paediatric Neurologist
University Hospital Southampton
Southampton, United Kingdom
Consultant Paediatric Neurologist
Paediatric Neurosciences
King's College Hospital
London, United Kingdom

Elizabeth S. Klings, MD
Associate Professor of Medicine
Director of the Center for Excellence in Sickle Cell Disease
Director of the Pulmonary Hypertension
Boston University School of Medicine
Boston Medical Center
Boston, Massachusetts

Lakshmanan Krishnamurti, MD
Professor of Pediatrics
Director of Blood and Marrow Transplantation
Aflac Cancer and Blood Disorders Center
Children's Healthcare of Atlanta/Emory University
Atlanta, Georgia

Abdullah Kutlar, MD
Professor of Medicine
Director, Sickle Cell Center
Department of Medicine
Medical College of Georgia at Augusta University
Augusta, Georgia

Sophie M. Lanzkron, MD, MHS
Director, Sickle Cell Center for Adults
The Johns Hopkins Hospital
Professor of Medicine
Johns Hopkins University School of Medicine
Baltimore, Maryland

Alexis Leonard, MD
National Heart Lung and Blood Institute
Cellular and Molecular Therapeutics Branch
National Institutes of Health
Bethesda, Maryland

Huihui Li, PhD
Ruth L. and David S. Gottesman Institute
    for Stem Cell and Regenerative Medicine Research
Department of Cell Biology
Albert Einstein College of Medicine
Bronx, New York

Jane A. Little, MD
Director, Sickle Cell Disease Program
Professor of Medicine
University of North Carolina at Chapel Hill
Chapel Hill, North Carolina

Susan M. MacDonald, MD
Assistant Professor & Medical Director of Urology Practice
Division of Urology
Penn State Health Milton S. Hershey Medical Center
Hershey, Pennsylvania

Roberto Machado, MD
Division of Pulmonary, Critical Care, Sleep, and
    Occupational Medicine
Department of Medicine
Indiana University
Indianapolis, Indiana

Julie Makani, MD, PhD, FRCP, FTAAS
Muhimbili University of Health and Allied Sciences
Dar es Salaam, Tanzania

Punam Malik, MD
Director, Comprehensive Sickle Cell Program
Director, Translational Core Laboratory
Marjory J. Johnson Chair, Gene and Cell Therapy
Professor, University of Cincinnati Department of
    Pediatrics
Cincinnati, Ohio

Caterina P. Minniti, MD
Professor of Medicine and Pediatrics
Albert Einstein College of Medicine
Director, Sickle Cell Center
Division of Hematology
Montefiore Health System
Bronx, New York

Claudia R. Morris, MD
Professor of Pediatrics and Emergency Medicine
Research Director, Division of Pediatric Emergency
    Medicine
Department of Pediatrics
Co-Director of the Center for Clinical and Translational
    Research
Emory University School of Medicine
Children's Healthcare of Atlanta
Atlanta, Georgia

Rakhi P. Naik, MD, MHS
Division of Hematology
Department of Medicine
Johns Hopkins University School of Medicine
Baltimore, Maryland

Constance Tom Noguchi, PhD
Molecular Medicine Branch
National Institute of Diabetes and Digestive and Kidney
    Diseases
National Institutes of Health
Bethesda, Maryland

Enrico M. Novelli, MD, MS
Associate Professor of Medicine
Division of Hematology/Oncology
University of Pittsburgh
Chief, Section of Benign Hematology
Director, UPMC Adult Sickle Cell Disease Program
Pittsburgh, Pennsylvania

Solomon F. Ofori-Acquah, PhD
Pittsburgh Heart, Lung and Blood Vascular Medicine
    Institute
Division of Hematology and Oncology
Sickle Cell Center of Excellence
University of Pittsburgh School of Medicine
Pittsburgh, Pennsylvania
School of Biomedical and Allied Health Sciences
University of Ghana
Accra, Ghana

Kwaku Ohene-Frempong, MD
Sickle Cell Foundation of Ghana
Kumasi, Ghana

Samuel A. Oppong, MD, FWACS
Department of Obstetrics and Gynecology
University of Ghana Medical School
Accra, Ghana

Amma Twumwa Owusu-Ansah, MD
University of Pittsburgh School of Medicine
UPMC Children's Hospital of Pittsburgh
Pittsburgh, Pennsylvania

Betty S. Pace, MD
Department of Pediatrics
Georgia Cancer Center
Augusta University
Augusta, Georgia

Julie Panepinto, MD, MSPH
Professor, Pediatric Hematology
Medical College of Wisconsin/Children's Wisconsin
Milwaukee, Wisconsin

Rafal Pawlinski, PhD
Lenvil Lee Rothrock Distinguished Professor of Medicine
Division of Hematology and Oncology
University of North Carolina School of Medicine
Chapel Hill, North Carolina

David C. Rees, MA, MBBS
Professor of Paediatric Sickle Cell Disease
King's College Hospital
King's College London
London, United Kingdom

Vandana Sachdev, MD
Director, Echocardiography Laboratory
National Heart Lung and Blood Institute
NIH Clinical Center
Bethesda, Maryland

Santosh L. Saraf, MD
Associate Professor of Medicine
Sickle Cell Center
Department of Medicine
University of Illinois at Chicago
Chicago, Illinois

Alan N. Schechter, MD
Molecular Medicine Branch
National Institute of Diabetes and Digestive and Kidney
 Diseases
National Institutes of Health
Bethesda, Maryland

Adrienne W. Scott, MD
Associate Professor of Ophthalmology
Wilmer Eye Institute
Johns Hopkins University School of Medicine
Baltimore, Maryland

Beryl Serjeant, FIMLS
Sickle Cell Trust (Jamaica)
Kingston, Jamaica

Graham Serjeant, MD, FRCP
Sickle Cell Trust (Jamaica)
Kingston, Jamaica

Vivien A. Sheehan, MD, PhD
Director of Translational SCD Research
The Aflac Cancer & Blood Disorders Center
Children's Healthcare of Atlanta
Associate Professor of Pediatrics
Emory University School of Medicine
Atlanta, Georgia

Natalie R. Shilo, MD
Assistant Professor of Pediatrics
Department of Pediatrics
Division of Pulmonary Medicine
University of Connecticut Health Center
Farmington, Connecticut

Sruti Shiva, PhD
Associate Professor
Department of Pharmacology and Chemical Biology
Director of Academic Affairs, Vascular Medicine Institute
Co-Director, Center for Metabolism and Mitochondrial
 Medicine
Pittsburgh, Pennsylvania

Wally R. Smith, MD
Research, Division of General Internal Medicine
Virginia Commonwealth University
Richmond, Virginia

Martin H. Steinberg, MD
Professor of Medicine
Boston University School of Medicine
Boston, Massachusetts

Jodi-Anne Stewart, MS
Department of Pediatrics
Vanderbilt-Meharry Center for Excellence in Sickle Cell
 Disease
Meharry Medical College
Nashville, Tennessee

Hanne Stotesbury, MSc
PhD Candidate
Developmental Neurosciences Section
UCL Great Ormond Street Institute of Child Health
London, United Kingdom

John J. Strouse, MD, PhD
Associate Professor of Medicine and Pediatrics
Director, Adult Sickle Cell Program
Duke University School of Medicine
Durham, North Carolina

Prithu Sundd, PhD
Pittsburgh Heart, Lung and Blood Vascular Medicine
 Institute
Division of Pulmonary Allergy and Critical Care Medicine
Sickle Cell Center of Excellence
University of Pittsburgh School of Medicine
Pittsburgh, Pennsylvania

Marilyn J. Telen, MD
Wellcome Professor of Medicine
Director, Duke Comprehensive Sickle Cell Center
Associate Medical Director, Duke Hospital Transfusion
 Service
Duke University Medical Center
Durham, North Carolina

Swee Lay Thein, MB, BS, FRCP, FRCPath, DSc, FMedSci
Chief, Sickle Cell Branch
National Heart, Lung and Blood Institute
The National Institutes of Health
Bethesda, Maryland

John F. Tisdale, MD
Senior Investigator
National Heart Lung and Blood Institute
Cellular and Molecular Therapeutics Branch
National Institutes of Health
Bethesda, Maryland

Tim M. Townes, PhD
Professor and Chair
Department of Biochemistry & Molecular Genetics
The University of Alabama at Birmingham
Birmingham, Alabama

Marsha Treadwell, PhD
Professor of Psychiatry and Pediatrics
University of California, San Francisco
Benioff Children's Hospital Oakland
Oakland, California

Darrell J. Triulzi, MD
Director, Division of Transfusion Medicine
Department of Pathology
University of Pittsburgh Medical Center
Pittsburgh, Pennsylvania

Gregory M. Vercellotti, MD
Professor of Medicine
Division of Hematology-Oncology-Transplantation
Department of Medicine and Vascular Biology Center
University of Minnesota Medical School
Minneapolis, Minnesota

Elliott Vichinsky, MD
Professor of Pediatrics
University of California, San Francisco School of Medicine
San Francisco, California

Mark C. Walters, MD
Jordan Family Director
Blood and Marrow Transplantation Program
Professor of Pediatrics
Division of Hematology/Oncology/BMT
UCSF Benioff Children's Hospital, Oakland
Oakland, California

Winfred C. Wang, MD
Emeritus Member
Department of Hematology
St. Jude Children's Research Hospital
Memphis, Tennessee

Russell E. Ware, MD, PhD
Professor of Pediatrics
Marjory Johnson Chair of Translational Hematology
    Research
Director, Division of Hematology
Director, Global Health Center
Cincinnati Children's Hospital Medical Center
Cincinnati, Ohio

John Wood, MD
Professor of Pediatrics and Radiology
Director of Cardiovascular MRI
University of Southern California
Keck School of Medicine
Los Angeles, California

The publication of *Sickle Cell Disease* couldn't be timelier. Following Herrick's initial description of the clinical manifestations in 1910 and the discovery of sickle hemoglobin by Pauling and Itano nearly 50 years later, there has been substantial, albeit slow, progress in working out the molecular and cellular pathogenesis of the disease as well as the development of safe and effective therapies. For many decades funding both from the National Institutes of Health and the pharmaceutical industry for sickle cell disease has been disproportionately low, considering the importance of this disease, both in prevalence and severity. During this period of "slow growth," enticing enough young well-trained lab and clinical investigators to work on this disease was a challenge. Happily, during the past several years, sickle cell research has gained a robust lease on life. The impressive up-swing in scientific and clinical abstracts and presentations at recent national meetings bears this out. Importantly, Pharma is now making a major commitment, with the development of an impressive array of novel drugs that target critical sites in the pathogenesis pathway. This well-spring of enthusiasm has culminated in the realization, during the past year, that gene therapy is now in hand, with realistic prospects for disease amelioration and possible cure. With the expanding cadre of multidisciplinary scientists and clinicians entering research on sickle cell disease, this all-encompassing book will be a valuable resource.

Comparable and parallel progress in how individuals living with sickle cell disease are perceived and treated by their caregivers is paramount. In the United States, during the past century, many patients with sickle cell disease have not received proper empathy and respect from providers. Emergency rooms nationwide have often stereotyped them as "frequent flyers" and "drug-seekers." This may stem, in part, from the consequences of implicit bias and systemic racism. Unfortunately, such negative attitudes often surface in clinical settings in which caregivers are frustrated by the lack of effective therapies. In the past, emergency rooms also treated patients with severe hemophilia and painful hemarthroses in a similarly dismissive manner. However, during the last 25 years with huge advances in hemophilia care, especially self-administration of factor VIII, and now with targeted and gene therapy options, individuals living with hemophilia are now given fully appropriate respect and attention. We have every reason to hope that such a transition in attitude will occur with sickle cell caregivers.

New therapies and enlightened providers can improve the lives of people with sickle cell disease only in a setting of adequate and proper access to healthcare. Scores of years have passed since the introduction of regimens that improve and extend life such as penicillin prophylaxis, hydroxyurea, and transfusions for stroke prevention. And yet, application of these and other interventions remains distressingly suboptimal. As a result, the life expectancy of people with sickle cell disease remains shortened by decades relative to the general population. Injury from sickle cell disease begins in infancy and progresses inexorably. Access to comprehensive, multidisciplinary care beginning in childhood would extend and improve quality of life, even using currently available tools. A key to the advance in quality care for people with hemophilia was the introduction of federally supported Hemophilia Treatment Centers that are the exemplar of chronic care for an inherited illness. People with sickle cell disease deserve nothing less.

It is important that we be better educated about all aspects of sickle cell disease. This book sheds considerable light at the end of the above-mentioned dark tunnel. It covers in detail very exciting advances now underway in elucidating molecular and cellular mechanisms of pathogenesis, as well as novel and increasingly effective approaches in treatment. Let's hope that this progress leads not only to prevention of pain episodes and organ damage but also a fully supportive, unbiased attitude among physicians and nurses involved in the care of patients with sickle cell disease.

H. Franklin Bunn
Hematology Division, Brigham and Women's Hospital
Professor of Medicine, Emeritus
Harvard Medical School
Boston, Massachusetts

Kenneth R. Bridges
Vice President, Global Blood Therapeutics
San Francisco, California

Mark A. Goldberg
Hematology Division, Brigham and Women's Hospital
Associate Professor of Medicine
Harvard Medical School
Boston, Massachusetts

I sit with my 52-year-old patient with sickle cell disease and newly diagnosed pulmonary hypertension, discussing his recent decision to discontinue hydroxyurea. A pulmonary fellow in our PH clinic listens closely.

I prepare to ask him, "You know your organs will progressively fail and you will die if you do not take your hydroxyurea every day?"

I catch myself and ask, "How many times have you been told in your life that you will die?"

His expression softens and he answers, "Doc, I was told so many times as a kid that I would not live to 18, but I proved them all wrong!"

I follow up, "Did you have a brother or sister that died of sickle cell disease?"

"My older brother died of sickle cell when I was 7."

After we leave the room, I ask the fellow to reflect for a minute upon the patient's answers to these simple questions and what they explained about this person's resilience, suffering, and perhaps cynical reactions to physicians and therapeutic urgency.

This poignant exchange with a patient with sickle cell disease illustrates an important point: as physicians and scientists, it is almost impossible to understand the physical and psychological trauma of sporadic random attacks of 11-point pain on a 10-point scale ("worse than having my first child"; "like an ice pick hitting over and over on my shin bone"), missed school, headaches, strokes, fatigue, weight loss, and the traumatic loss of a sibling or loved one, that all limit sports participation, degrade school performance, and drive physical and spiritual pain. All of this is compounded by economic disparity, healthcare inequities, systemic racism, a commercially driven opioid epidemic, and in many US states an abrupt loss of comprehensive healthcare at age 18 years, when sickle cell disease becomes a "pre-existing condition."

It is impossible for most of us to understand how socioeconomic inequality compounds the already unfathomable burden of illness due to sickle cell disease. Ironically, one friend and one-time patient, who is now a chief executive in a large organization, shared his unique experience that all of his brothers who did not have sickle cell disease had either died or were incarcerated. He sincerely credits sickle cell disease with his own survival and success, as his inability to "run the streets" focused him on school and surrounded him in a protective cocoon from the violence that consumed his brothers. We can only try to imagine his resilience in the life he was given.

This book leverages the motivation from such stories to compile the collective clinical expertise of world experts and summarize the innovative, transformative, and discovery science of the field of sickle cell disease. In many ways, this book reflects a triumph of humanity over an ancient disease—cruel collateral damage in our molecular code cut by the unsparing and uncaring genetic adaptation to endemic malaria. It is a triumph, albeit far from complete, for people with sickle cell disease who as individuals, patients, participants, and partners, with families, friends, and healthcare workers, withstand this assault and partner with us to advance knowledge, science, and medicine.

This book chronicles the groundbreaking discoveries of the 20th century and almost three decades of scientific progress since the last textbook on sickle cell disease was published in 1994. The three editors share more than 80 years of collective experience working with sickle cell disease as clinicians and scientists, yet experience a sense of awe in absorbing the text, figures, and clinical images within this book, which details a remarkable collaborative journey to understand and tame this disease. More than 90 dedicated experts in the field present their combined clinical knowledge of basic mechanisms, screening, diagnosis, management, and treatment of myriad complex complications of a single base point mutation in the human genome over 34 chapters. The text covers the dizzying pace of basic and clinical discovery over 100 years from the biophysics of hemoglobin S polymerization, the transcriptional regulation of globin synthesis, the characterization of vascular inflammation and impaired redox signaling, advances in small molecule and antibody-based therapeutics, and the emergence of curative stem cell and gene editing technologies. Individual chapters have been dedicated to specific organ pathology, and the book concludes with four enlightening perspectives that exemplify the added challenges of facing sickle cell disease in resource-poor countries. The editors believe that readers will especially appreciate the case studies with "How I Treat" authoritative insights that root the text into clinical practice by providing overviews of common and rare complications by world experts in sickle cell disease, and the Key Facts, which provide at-a-glance high yield information. The text is complemented by memorable images, high-quality figures, and many original diagrams.

The editors sincerely hope that the shared clinical knowledge, cases, and expert discussions of specific complication management will support care providers and advance best practices for the many individuals living with sickle cell disease worldwide. We also hope that the gripping story of clinical and scientific discovery presented in these pages inspires new physicians, advanced practice providers, scientists, and those from every other walk of life to join this field and, together, move us closer to a world without suffering from sickle cell disease.

Mark T. Gladwin, MD

ACKNOWLEDGMENTS

We are immensely proud that this book unites a diverse authorship of more than 90 clinical and research leaders in the field of sickle cell disease. These range from senior scientific statesmen to new rising stars, drawn from at least 20 different biomedical disciplines, 40 institutions, 9 countries, and 5 continents. We thank the authors for their lifelong commitment to advancing the highest quality clinical medicine and discovery science. We would like to thank our administrator Laura Pliske and all of our colleagues who have answered the call to collaborate in the creation of this authoritative body of work.

Also, the editors would like to acknowledge the help and assistance put forth by Karen Edmonson, the Senior Content Acquisitions Editor for this book, who has provided invaluable support throughout this project, from the initial design of the book to its realization. The editors would also like to thank the many individuals at McGraw Hill responsible for bringing this book to press, including Leah Carton, Harriet Lebowitz, Kim Davis, and Sarika Gupta at KnowledgeWorks Global Ltd. for her excellent effort in coordinating the book layout and final presentation of the page layout.

Hertz Nazaire was born in Port-Au-Prince, Haiti and has been painting and sharing his love for art in Bridgeport, Connecticut for over 20 years. He works mostly with colorful oil pastels on board, often depicting subjects influenced by Haitian culture, history, and life.

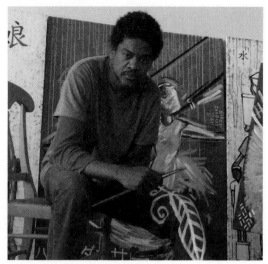

Nazaire is motivated by his life with sickle cell anemia to paint about pain and human limitations of compassion and empathy, which he explores in his art, hoping to provide inspiration. His award-winning images promoting sickle cell awareness have been published around the world in medical books and magazines.

His sickle cell disease has posed serious life challenges. Job loss due to frequent hospitalizations has made him homeless three times, and he has lived outdoors up to 18 months at a time. These difficult circumstances have led to anxiety and depression, deepening the severe pain of his disease, a scenario all too familiar to his fellow Sickle Cell Warriors. This life experience drives him to create pieces to raise awareness of these grave issues shared within his community.

He has responded to partial vision loss from his disease with increased purpose in his art. His vision limitation has changed the way he sees the world around him and the way he creates new composition.

Today he continues to seek new ways to express his art and continues to advocate and speak publicly for the much-needed awareness of sickle cell disease and science education in his community.

Hertz Nazaire's painting "Ten Redefined" is used on the cover and his painting "Hope" is shown below.

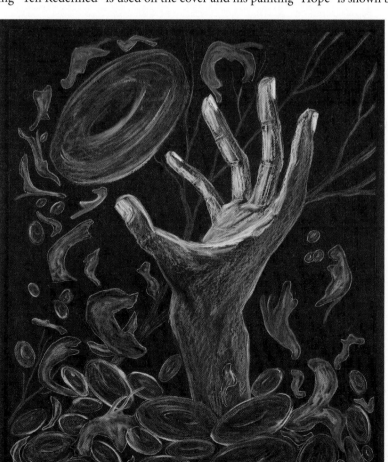

PART I
Basic Mechanisms of Disease

Overview

Authors: Betty S. Pace, Carlo Brugnara

This section highlights the pathophysiologic complexity of sickle cell disease (SCD), the prototype of single-gene molecular disorders. James Herrick published the first clinical report of SCD in 1910. However, many decades passed before Linus Pauling established SCD as the first human monogenic disorder, with an autosomal recessive inheritance pattern, in 1949. This seminal work laid the foundation for the explosion of knowledge in human molecular genetics. Over the past few decades, the pathophysiology of SCD has been explored and clarified in many aspects, but other aspects still present uncertainties and lack of detail. The molecular mechanisms of the process leading to polymerization of hemoglobin S (HbS) and sickling have been elucidated in extreme detail, and this knowledge has been critical in rationalizing the beneficial effects of several of the novel therapies developed or under development for the disease. It has also become clear that a unique feature of SCD is the pathologic involvement of multiple organs most often as a consequence of vascular/inflammatory or ischemia-reperfusion complications of the disease. The interactions of sickle cells with the endothelium and the inflammatory response associated with the disease have been examined in a variety of experimental systems, with SCD emerging as a unique model of ischemia-reperfusion (I/R) disorders. These studies have been facilitated by the development of transgenic mouse models for SCD, which recapitulate disease pathophysiology and provide a model to test therapeutic interventions.

SCD is caused by homozygous mutations at the sixth codon of the β-globin gene in the β-globin cluster (*HBB*) on chromosome 11 (Figure I-1A), resulting in the production of the single aa hemoglobin variant, β6-Glu→Val (βˢ-globin). In the *HBB* cluster, the 5 functional globin genes, including ε-Gγ-Aγ-δ-β, are arranged 5′ to 3′ along the chromosome in the order of their developmental expression. The prevalence of SCD is about 1 in 365 African Americans and about 1 in 16,300 Hispanic Americans; in addition, about 1 in 13 African Americans are sickle cell trait carriers. In the United States, approximately 2000 babies are born annually with a major hemoglobinopathy and 100,000 individuals are affected; however, the exact number of people living with SCD is unknown. Although the molecular nature of SCD is relatively simple, its distribution in affected populations is more complex. Recent whole-genome–based haplotype analysis of individuals with sickle trait in the African Genome Variation Project identified a potential single origin of the βˢ-globin allele, approximately 7300 years ago. From its point of origin, the βˢ-globin gene expanded due to a selective advantage of healthy carriers of SCD providing protection against malaria infections.

The *HBB* locus is a paradigm for tissue- and developmental stage–specific regulation. The expression of each functional globin gene relies on a direct physical interaction between the β-locus control region (β-LCR) enhancer consisting of 5 DNAse I hypersensitive sites and globin gene promoter regulatory regions. A number of key erythroid-specific and ubiquitous transcription factors, such as GATA-1, GATA-2, NF-E2, and KLF1, among others, are required to accomplish normal regulation during development. There have been at least 5 *HBB* haplotypes identified for SCD that are associated with disease severity, highlighting the role of gene modifiers for SCD, including those involved in the regulation of fetal hemoglobin (HbF) production. Several genetic point mutations in the γ-globin gene promoters upregulate transcription, whereas the β-globin-gene in *cis* is downregulated, producing nondeletion hereditary persistence of fetal hemoglobin (HPFH). Through genomic analysis, the *Xmn1-HBG2* mutation (rs7482144) on chromosome 11p, the *HBS1L-MYB* intergenic region (HMIP) on chromosome 6q23, and *BCL11A* on chromosome 2p16 were mapped as 3 major quantitative trait loci accounting for 25% to 50% of the genetic variance in HbF levels. Recent work identified multiple additional genetic modifiers for SCD that are associated with clinical severity.

HbS polymerization drives SCD pathophysiology. However, HbF is the most effective modifier of clinical phenotypes since mixed hybrid tetramers, $\alpha_2\beta^s\gamma$, are largely excluded from the HbS polymer phase. The most compelling example of the salutary effect of HbF is provided by the phenotype of compound heterozygotes for HbS and HPFH. These individuals have approximately 30% HbF "pancellularly" distributed in red blood cells (RBCs) and are mildly symptomatic. In addition, α thalassemia due to deletion of 1 or 2 α-globin genes is found in about 30% of SCD populations, which reduces intracellular concentrations of HbS and decreases polymerization to attenuate hemolysis. Other modifiers of SCD clinical phenotypes will be discussed in this section.

HbS polymerization is the central event in the pathophysiology of SCD (Figure I-1A). Two different approaches have shed light on the unique features of this process. Studies on

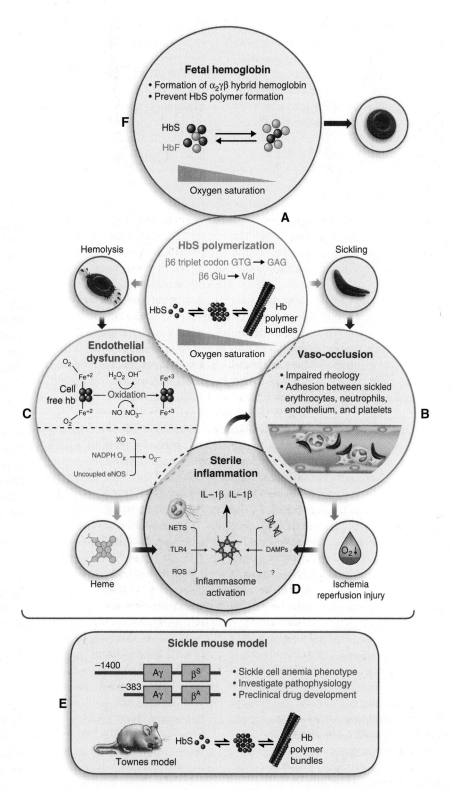

FIGURE I-1 Basic mechanisms of sickle cell disease (SCD). Shown is a summary of the mechanisms driving the clinical complications of SCD discussed in this overview. Based on current evidence, the pathophysiology of SCD is considered to be a vicious cycle of 4 major downstream processes: (**A**) hemoglobin S polymerization, (**B**) impaired red cell rheology and increased adhesion-mediated vaso-occlusion, (**C**) hemolysis-mediated endothelial dysfunction, and (**D**) concerted activation of sterile inflammation. All mechanisms are the subject of active research and provide novel therapeutic targeting. Efforts to understand globin gene regulation in the β-globin locus on chromosome 11 provided the insight required to establish SCD mouse models (**E**) and fetal hemoglobin induction (**F**), providing opportunity for preclinical animal models and discovery of molecular targets for drug development. DAMPs, damage-associated molecular patterns; HbF, fetal hemoglobin; HbS, sickle hemoglobin; IL-1β, interleukin-1β; IL-18, interleukin 18; NETs, neutrophil extracellular traps; NO, nitric oxide; ROS, reactive oxygen species; TLR4, toll-like receptor 4; XO, xanthine oxidase. Modified from Sundd P, Gladwin MT, Novelli EM. Pathophysiology of sickle cell disease. *Annu Rev Pathol.* 2019;14:263-292.

the *kinetics* of HbS polymerization have identified the presence of a delay before the onset of polymerization and an exceptionally high dependence on cellular HbS concentration (~30th power), which provides an explanation for the absence of significant clinical disease in sickle cell trait (AS). The presence of clinically significant sickling and disease in subjects double heterozygous for HbS and hemoglobin C (HbC); the beneficial effects of increased HbF values, such as in HPFH or secondary to therapeutic strategies such as hydroxyurea, decitabine, or gene therapy. The kinetics of HbS polymerization also provides a rationale for therapeutic approaches aimed at diminishing RBC dehydration or reducing HbS concentration by restricting iron availability. Therefore, any therapeutic intervention that prolongs the delay time enough for polymerization to begin in venules rather than capillaries is likely to produce significant changes in disease pathophysiology.

The *thermodynamic* approach emphasizes the steady-state concentration of polymer inside the sickle RBCs, based on the finding that presence of polymer can be demonstrated inside sickle cells even at very high oxygen saturation values. The hemoglobin desaturation measured with arterial blood gas analysis or pulse oximetry reflects the presence of polymer after transit through the lungs, which is unlikely to melt in the peripheral circulation.

Cellular heterogeneity in intracellular hemoglobin concentration is a distinguishing characteristic of SCD, which encompasses young reticulocytes with normal or low hemoglobin concentration and dense cells with exceptionally high hemoglobin concentration due to cell dehydration. Dense cells, which contain a high polymer fraction, are believed to be key contributors to the vascular complications of the disease. A subcategory of dense cells is defined as irreversibly sickled cells (ISCs), which due to abnormal cytoskeletal interactions maintain their sickled shape even when fully oxygenated or when turned into hemoglobin-free ghosts. Both dense cells and ISCs have been shown to correlate with some of the disease manifestations.

For many decades, advances in genetics and understanding of the cellular and molecular mechanisms of SCD complications resulted from studies of HbS polymerization, antisickling hemoglobin variants, and RBC membrane rheology. However, the scope of SCD research expanded beyond RBCs in the 1980s to encompass vascular biology, endothelial function, coagulation, inflammation, and chronic hemolysis, leading to accumulation of high plasma heme levels. No doubt, HbS polymerization is the primary pathophysiologic alteration with countless consequences in SCD, including the formation of sickle RBCs, cell adhesion, and the production of inflammatory molecules, which ultimately lead to vaso-occlusive crises (VOCs), a key clinical manifestation of the disease (Figure I-1B). It is established that sickle RBCs are predisposed to a number of intracellular abnormalities, and repeated HbS polymerization together with RBC dehydration and membrane oxidative damage result in alterations to the cytoskeleton composition, producing irreversibly sickled RBCs. Moreover, sickle RBCs contribute to endothelial

adhesion and activation, which are recognized as contributing to inflammation in SCD, along with the release of microparticles composed of RBC membrane components.

The pathogenesis of VOC in SCD is complex and multifactorial. Vaso-occlusion is a fundamental event in SCD pathophysiology because it not only underlies the painful clinical manifestations of the disease, but also is the origin of the most significant acute and chronic organ complications of the disease. Predisposing events to VOC such as dehydration, infection, fever, acidosis, hypoxia, and pain have been identified, in conjunction with environmental factors, such as altitude, weather, and pollution.

It has long been known that sickle erythrocytes adhere to endothelial cells much more often than normal erythrocytes. Neutrophils have subsequently emerged as key players in this interaction, due to their increased interaction with both sickle erythrocytes and the endothelium. Molecular mechanisms governing these interactions have been elucidated (eg, MAC1 integrin for RBCs/neutrophils), and complexities regarding neutrophil heterogeneity and microbiota role have emerged. Although platelets play a role in sickle cell adhesion in a variety of experimental models, clinical studies targeting platelet function have been uniformly negative. Hemolysis, nitric oxide (NO) deprivation (see later), and inflammatory cytokines further promote the vicious cycle of adhesion and sickling that underlies VOC. More basic and clinical research studies are still needed to identify reliable biomarkers of vaso-occlusion. Pharmacologic therapies aimed at interrupting the vicious cycle of VOC have shown some success, with crizanlizumab, a humanized anti–P-selectin antibody, receiving US Food and Drug Administration (FDA) approval in 2019.

The reduced survival of erythrocytes in SCD is due to chronic hemolysis. Upon intravascular lysis, RBCs, heme, and cell-free hemoglobin are released into the circulation and are normally bound by haptoglobin to prevent toxic effects, while hemopexin binds free heme (Figure I-1C). However, these systems are insufficient to buffer the exceptionally large amounts of hemoglobin and heme released from lysing sickle erythrocytes. Cell-free hemoglobin elicits the immediate consumption of NO, constitutively produced by endothelial NO synthase. Cell-free hemoglobin produces endothelial dysfunction and NO depletion along with endothelial NO synthase uncoupling and consumption of L-arginine by arginase released during hemolysis. Free heme activates neutrophils and promotes inflammation. In addition to hemoglobin and heme, RBCs contain numerous other molecules with oxidant and inflammatory potential, called damage-associated molecular patterns (DAMPs). Release of reactive oxygen species leads to substantial oxidative stress and damage in multiple organs. In patients with more severe hemolysis, the disease is characterized by a constellation of clinical symptoms including gallstones, pulmonary hypertension, leg ulcers, nephropathy, and priapism.

In SCD, VOC occurring primarily in the microcirculation reduces oxygenation, culminating in tissue damage and I/R injury to elicit inflammatory responses. Dying cells present cytosolic calcium accumulation, mitochondrial dysfunction, and cell swelling, followed by release of major inflammatory DAMPs, such as adenosine triphosphate, heme, extracellular vesicles, and heat shock proteins, among others. Other factors, including plasma histamine due to mast cell activation and degranulation, are elevated at steady state in SCD and increase further during painful VOC episodes.

The activation of inflammatory cells and their signaling pathways leads to the secretion of numerous molecules that propagate the inflammatory state in SCD (sterile inflammasome), such as cytokines, chemokines, growth factors, complement, eicosanoids, and peptides (Figure I-1D). White blood cells are key players in the inflammatory processes that trigger VOC and other complications of SCD; leukocytosis is associated with increased mortality, acute chest syndrome, and stroke. Specifically, neutrophils, monocytes, eosinophils, and mast cells respond to microorganisms and oxidative stress by releasing extracellular traps. Monocyte activation has been reported in SCD, and a role for these cells in endothelial activation has been demonstrated.

I/R is the biology of reintroduction of oxygen to an ischemic area that paradoxically exacerbates local tissue injury. The process of I/R involves 4 phases, including the triggering vascular event, local tissue injury, evolution of inflammation, and vascular wall damage. During the initial ischemic insult, oxygen depletion ensues, cell metabolism shifts to anaerobic glycolysis, and antioxidant capacity is depleted. Endothelial cell surfaces become proadhesive, proinflammatory, and procoagulant and endothelial barrier function degrades. Upon reintroduction of oxygen, superoxide radicals are produced and inducible NO synthase is upregulated in endothelial and smooth muscle cells. Complement activation leads to granulocyte recruitment to the vessel wall, vessel wall leak, and damaged endothelial cells. In response to I/R injury, local tissues manifest programmed responses including increases in HIF-1α, Nrf2, and endothelial NO synthase levels and changes that protect barrier function.

Oxidative stress and inflammation are intrinsic to SCD and tightly linked to its pathophysiology due to an imbalance between the production of oxidants and antioxidant capacity. The pathophysiology of SCD involves activation of multiple antioxidant genes to accomplish cellular protective mechanisms. Nrf2 activation is particularly important because it induces antioxidant enzymes and heme oxygenase-1 (HO-1), the products of which are protective. In I/R, activated monocytes travel and adhere to vascular endothelial cells, often followed by neutrophils, inducing endothelial inflammatory responses. Subsequently, sterile inflammation is triggered involving tumor necrosis factor, interleukin-1, and HMGB1 expression and release of other cytokines. In addition, chronic anemia promotes expression of HIF-1α, which contributes to the inflammatory response in experimental systems. Oxygenated and deoxygenated sickle RBCs adhere to the inflamed endothelium by diverse mechanisms, but $\alpha_V\beta_3$, P-selectin, and ICAM4 play major roles in this process.

Here, a discussion of various therapeutic approaches is based on the pathobiology of I/R in SCD in the context of a systems biology problem. Rationale for this strategy lies in the sequential nature of I/R pathology. For example, anti-inflammatory drugs such as allopurinol, sulfasalazine, or etanercept improve microvascular blood flow in sickle mice. Other agents that interrupt the cyclic nature of I/R by targeting multiple key steps might be more effective. Multiple drug treatment approaches have been effective in other diseases, but efficacy in SCD has not been established.

Paradigm-shifting insights into molecular mechanisms of globin gene regulation spawned by the discovery of the LCR in the 1990s heralded a new era in SCD research. The creation of mouse models of SCD profoundly improved the opportunities to understand the complex pathophysiology, drug development, and gene therapy approaches. The first mouse models were established with the human β^S-globin gene introduced into mice expressing wild-type mouse hemoglobin. To compensate for the limited production of human HbS and the continued presence of mouse globin, the polymerization tendency of HbS was enhanced by additional mutations such as $\beta^{Antilles}$ (β^{23}Ile) and HbD Punjab ($\beta1^{21}$Gln), generating the SAD mouse model. The SAD mouse was instrumental in developing therapies focused on prevention of cell dehydration. The subsequent discovery of gene targeting in mouse embryonic stem cells allowed deletion of mouse adult globin genes and integration of human homologous genes in the mouse genome. By 1997, 2 homozygous sickle cell anemia mouse models, Berkeley and Townes, expressing only human HbS and α-globin were created with a severe sickle cell anemia phenotype consisting of chronic hemolytic anemia, splenomegaly, and shortened survival. Subsequently, in 2006, the Townes group generated a site-directed knock-in SCD mouse model using a small construct containing human $^A\gamma$-globin gene with 383 bp of the 5′ flanking sequence and a human β^A- or β^S-globin gene with 815 bp of the 5′ flanking sequence (Figure I-1E).

SCD mouse models have advanced the understanding of different interacting factors in the complexity of VOC such as pain, hemolysis, vascular tone dysregulation, oxidative stress, inflammation, cell adhesion, and I/R injury. Biomarkers of the multiple pathogenic processes that lead to VOC, such as white blood cells, heme, serum amyloid P component, and interleukins, among others, have been discovered. SCD mice have also demonstrated evidence of large and small blood vessel endothelial activation, with increased VCAM, ICAM, and PECAM-1 and nuclear factor-κB levels similar to those observed in persons with SCD.

The most common clinical manifestation of SCD is acute episodic pain; however, treatment options are limited and primarily involve symptomatic treatment and the use of opioids. Humanized SCD transgenic mice show features of pain similar to humans, offering a model for investigating the mechanisms of pain in SCD and development of novel nonopioid targeted analgesic therapies. The SCD mouse models are invaluable for the evaluation of experimental drugs in vivo and for the preclinical studies that are discussed here.

In 1948, Watson observed that HbF ameliorates the clinical severity of SCD, ushering in one of the most intense areas of research in the globin field. The mechanism of HbF benefit involves the formation of hybrid ($\alpha_2\gamma\beta$) hemoglobin molecules that do not participate in the polymerization process (Figure I-1F). Early diagnosis of SCD allows initiation of therapy to induce HbF with hydroxyurea starting in infancy and before hemoglobin switching is complete. Prophylactic treatment with hydroxyurea and other standard-of-care measures including education, immunizations, and penicillin prophylaxis ameliorate clinical severity and disease complications and prolong survival to adulthood.

In general, reversing hemoglobin switching to increase HbF expression is desirable in persons with SCD. For the past 40 years, mechanisms involved in hemoglobin switching have been the subject of intense investigation because understanding the normal process facilitates new therapeutic approaches for hemoglobinopathies. Insights have been gained from the finding that genetic modifiers of SCD that increase HbF result from rare deletions within the *HBB* locus or point mutations in the γ-globin gene promoters producing HPFH.

To date, hydroxyurea is the only FDA-approved agent that induces HbF in persons with SCD; this agent works as a ribonucleotide reductase inhibitor. Hydroxyurea also mediates other beneficial effects in SCD, being an NO donor and anti-inflammatory drug. In the Multicenter Study of Hydroxyurea (MSH) reported in 1995, two-thirds of adults had a favorable response with clinically significant decreases in pain crises. These findings led to the FDA approval of hydroxyurea for SCD in 1998. A subsequent study publishing 9 years of follow-up of the original MSH cohort demonstrated a reduction in death rate of approximately 40%, and HbF levels were inversely related to mortality.

Subsequent clinical trials confirmed the efficacy and safety of hydroxyurea in children. The HUG-KIDS study group demonstrated changes in hematologic variables similar to those observed in adults, with no apparent adverse effect on growth. The subsequent BABY HUG randomized trial of hydroxyurea in children with sickle cell anemia aged 9 to 18 months showed decreased pain crises and dactylitis and increased HbF, thus demonstrating the efficacy and safety of hydroxyurea. These results provide the basis for the current recommendation to offer hydroxyurea therapy to infants with sickle cell anemia at 9 months of age regardless of clinical symptoms.

Reactivation of HbF expression by pharmacologic agents is an important therapeutic approach for treating SCD and continues to be an intense area of investigation. Over the past 4 decades, >70 pharmacologic agents displayed the ability to induce HbF synthesis mainly in tissue culture systems, and a few were tested in preclinical mouse models and human clinical trials. Agents such as 5-azacytidine, decitabine, butyrate, and short-chain fatty acid derivatives, among others, show clinical potential. These agents induce HbF by diverse mechanisms including DNA methyl transferase and histone deacetylase inhibition, enhanced chromatin interaction of DNA binding proteins, and cell signaling activation. Efforts to develop additional safe and effective agents for the treatment of SCD are underway.

The comprehensive discussion of SCD pathophysiology in the next 8 chapters highlights both the tremendous accomplishments in our basic understanding of disease mechanisms and the significant challenges that we still face in translating our deeper understanding into a better comprehension of the variability in SCD manifestations and complications at the individual patient level. Only by linking our current knowledge in these 2 separate areas, we will be able to achieve fundamental changes in tailoring the multiple available treatment modalities to the individual pediatric and adult patients affected by SCD.

Hemoglobin S Polymerization and Sickle Cell Disease: An Overview

Author: William A. Eaton

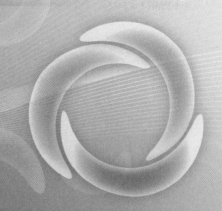

Polymerization of hemoglobin S is the root cause of the pathology of sickle cell disease. It has been 70 years since the legendary 20th-century genius of chemistry, Linus Pauling, discovered that aggregation of an abnormal hemoglobin into "rigid rods" is responsible for sickle cell disease.[1,2] Pauling left several important questions unanswered that have motivated an enormous amount of basic research since then. These include the following: What is the structure of his "rigid rods?"[3] What are the thermodynamics, kinetics, and mechanisms of polymerization? How can the disease be treated? This overview will briefly describe research that has played a major role in answering these questions. A more extensive account of polymerization and its role in disease pathogenesis and therapy can be found in 4 previous reviews[4-7] and in Chapter 2 of this book.

Fiber Structure

The low-resolution structure of the sickle fiber was determined using transmission electron microscopy and sophisticated image reconstruction methods by Stuart Edelstein.[8,9] A few years earlier, Warner Love had solved the x-ray structure of deoxyhemoglobin S, but it was not clear at the time whether his structure, which showed the details of the β-globin 6 intermoleocular contact, had any relationship to the fibers that form in sickle cells.[10] Edelstein recognized that he could construct a 14-stranded fiber structure that is consistent with both the fiber-diffraction data of Magdoff-Fairchild et al[11] and the orientation of the hemoglobin S molecules in the fiber determined by polarized optical absorption data on single sickled cells[12] by helically twisting 7 double strands of the x-ray structure.[8,9] Subsequent polymerization studies by Ronald Nagel, Ruth Benesch, Rheinhold Benesch, and their colleagues on mixtures of hemoglobin S with non-S hemoglobin variants were critically important for building the detailed molecular model, which is the current operative model today.[13,14]

Thermodynamics

A gel of hemoglobin S is very much like a crystal solution equilibrium, that is, a mixture of 2 phases, 1 solid and 1 liquid, as theoretically predicted by Allen Minton[15] and confirmed in experiments.[16-18] The thermodynamics become considerably more complex when considering the control of polymerization by oxygen and mixtures of hemoglobin S with non-S hemoglobins such as hemoglobins A and F. Understanding how oxygen controls polymerization is the result of careful solubility studies, the direct measurement of binding of oxygen to the fibers, and the application of the Monod, Wyman, and Changeux (MWC) model. Hofrichter[19] performed the first solubility measurement using carbon monoxide as a surrogate for oxygen, and later this was done using oxygen by Sunshine et al.[20] Application of linear dichroism in these studies allowed the measurement of the polymer binding curve of a gel because molecules in the liquid phase are randomly oriented and therefore make no contribution to the spectral changes of the fiber as oxygen binds. The linear dichroism experiments of Sunshine and colleagues showed that polymer binding is noncooperative; their solubility results were beautifully explained using the elegant polyphasic thermodynamic linkage relation of Gill and Wyman, which relates the solubility to the binding curves of hemoglobin in the polymer and liquid phases and includes activity coefficients.[20-22] The activity coefficients multiply the measured concentration to give the thermodynamically effective concentration and are large due to excluded volume effects in the concentrated protein solutions. At 35 g/dL, for example, the activity coefficient is about 100, so the solution behaves as if the concentration were 3500 g/dL. The work of Allen Minton and Philip Ross was primarily responsible for first recognizing the importance of activity coefficients[18,23,24] (Figure I-2).

The solubility results, as well as the solid-state nuclear magnetic resonance determination of the average polymer fraction in sickled red cells,[25] are also almost quantitatively explained by postulating that only the T quaternary structure can enter the fiber,[19,20,26] which is consistent with structural modeling by Eduardo Padlan.[27] The MWC model does quite an impressive job, because there are no adjustable parameters in the calculation. Extending the MWC model to include tertiary conformational changes[28,29] results in a quantitative explanation of the solubility data, albeit with one adjustable parameter.[30]

Polymerization in mixtures of hemoglobin S with non-S hemoglobins is much more theoretically complex. Allen Minton

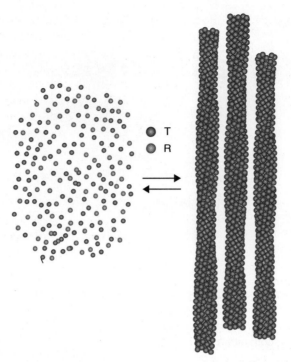

T
R

FIGURE I-2 **Schematic structure of gel with hemoglobin S (HbS) partially saturated with oxygen showing that only the T quaternary structure enters the fiber.** The total concentration of free HbS tetramers (left) is the solubility, which is an accurate measure of the thermodynamic stability of the fiber (right).

is responsible for the original theory on the copolymerization of non-S hemoglobins.[26] However, his equations only applied to the unachievable situation in which the total hemoglobin concentration of the solution is equal to the solubility (under these conditions, polymerization takes an infinite amount of time). When the total concentration is larger than the solubility (ie, the solution is supersaturated), the theoretical description becomes much more mathematically complicated.[21] Experimental results from many different laboratories[21] show that there is little or no copolymerization of the homotetramers $\alpha_2\beta_2{}^A$, a copolymerization probability for the hybrid $\alpha_2\beta^A\beta^S$ of about 0.4, and a copolymerization probability of 0 to 0.1 for the hybrid $\alpha_2\gamma\beta^S$. Tetramers that do not polymerize increase the measured solubility and add to the excluded volume in the liquid phase, further increasing the complexity of the theory.

There remain quite significant differences in measurements of copolymerization of hemoglobin F from different laboratories,[21] which, given the importance of the role of hemoglobin F today, should be repeated. Moreover, there is only a single study on the solubility of S/F, S/A, and S/A$_2$ mixtures as a function of ligand saturation, albeit with carbon monoxide as a surrogate for oxygen and using red cell lysates instead of purified hemoglobins.[31]

Kinetics and Mechanism

In slow temperature-jump experiments, a delay prior to the appearance of polymers was almost simultaneously reported from 3 different laboratories in 1974, by Hofrichter et al[32] using

birefringence and calorimetry, by Malfa and Steinhardt[33] using viscosity, and by Moffat and Gibson[34] using turbidity. It was not until the work of Ferrone et al[35,36] that a mechanism was proposed that could explain both the existence of a delay and a high concentration dependence (~30th power in Hofrichter et al[32]). Ferrone's experiments used photodissociation of the carbon monoxide complex of hemoglobin S to create deoxyhemoglobin S at any temperature in milliseconds instead of the tens of seconds to a minute in the earlier slow temperature-jump experiments. This method also made it possible to observe subsecond polymer formation on cells from patients with homozygous SS disease, which showed that there was little or no difference between polymerization of deoxyhemoglobin S in purified solutions and in red cells from patients with the disease.[37] Ferrone's double nucleation mechanism, in which secondary nucleation occurs on the surface of preexisting fibers, also accounts for the observation of large fluctuations in delay times in small volumes as a result of the stochastic appearance of the first fiber,[35,36,38,39] as well as the remarkable finding that the rate of formation of the first fiber exhibits approximately twice the concentration dependence of the delay time (up to 80th power of the concentration).[39,40] The mechanism has stood the test of time.[41] The double nucleation mechanism is now being used to explain the aggregation kinetics of the Alzheimer peptide.[42]

It has recently been discovered that the delay time can be obtained to reasonable accuracy if the supersaturation is known (ie, the ratio of total hemoglobin concentration to solubility, each multiplied by an activity coefficient), no matter what the composition of the solution—partial ligand saturation, mixtures of any kind, pH, and so on.[43] There are much more solubility data than delay time data, so this universal relation between delay time and supersaturation has become a valuable tool for theoretical calculations of sickling on any time scale.[30,44]

Disease Pathogenesis and Therapy

Given the recent large number of studies on processes that are sequelae of polymerization,[45-47] it has become a nontrivial statement to say that the root cause of pathology in sickle cell disease is polymerization of hemoglobin.[48] The discovery of the kinetics led to the hypothesis that a major determinant of severity in sickle cell disease is the delay time relative to the transit time through the microcirculation.[4,49] This concept created a coherent synthesis of a large amount of information on disease pathogenesis with a single postulate: Factors that decrease the delay time or increase the transit time through the microcirculation, for example, by increased adherence,[50] increase clinical severity, whereas factors that increase the delay time, such as the presence of hemoglobin A or fetal hemoglobin, and shorten the transit time are associated with decreased clinical severity. Schechter and coworkers proposed an alternative theory for pathogenesis,[5,25,48] discussed in Chapter 2, in which the amount of polymer formed at equilibrium is the key quantity. The dynamical scenario received strong support from the experiments of Mozzarelli et al,[51] which showed that almost all cells would be sickled were polymerization at equilibrium under in vivo conditions, suggesting that once fetal hemoglobin disappears, patients survive because the majority of cells escape the microcirculation before fibers form. A flaw in the Mozzarelli experiments is that sickling was determined on a nonphysiologic time scale. Their conclusion, however, is strongly supported by recent kinetic experiments at partial saturation with carbon monoxide and calculations of in vivo sickling in which oxygen is dissociated from red cells on the in vivo seconds timescale.[30,52] It should be noted that because both the delay time and the fraction polymerized depend on the supersaturation of the solution,[53] correlations of polymerization with disease severity that ignore the kinetics are, nevertheless, perfectly valid.[54]

There have been dramatic advances in curing sickle cell disease using hematopoietic stem cell transplantation, with gene therapy cures on the horizon.[47,55] However, these treatments are not available to the vast majority of patients in the world suffering from sickle cell disease and may not be for many decades because they require advanced medical facilities. Consequently, what is urgently needed now for patients in low-income countries is an inexpensive antisickling pill. Therapy will not require a drug that completely inhibits sickling, but one that allows more cells to escape the microcirculation before fibers form by increasing the delay time. Because there are several mechanisms for increasing delay times other than

by increasing fetal hemoglobin synthesis, there is cause for optimism.[7] Fortunately, there are now high-throughput, sensitive kinetic methods for making measurements on intact cells (Eaton and colleagues, unpublished results) and large libraries available for drug screening.. There is a growing confidence among sickle cell researchers that effective antisickling drugs for sickle cell disease, in addition to hydroxyurea, are about to be discovered.

Acknowledgment

The author thanks Dr. Frank Ferrone for his valuable comments on the manuscript. This work was supported by the intramural research program of the National Institute of Diabetes and Digestive and Kidney Diseases.

References

1. Pauling L, Itano HA, Singer SJ, Wells IC. Sickle cell anemia, a molecular disease. *Science.* 1949;110:543-548.
2. Eaton WA. Linus Pauling and sickle cell disease. *Biophys Chem.* 2003;100:109-116.
3. Pauling L. Abnormality of hemoglobin molecules in hereditary hemolytic anemias. *Harvey Lect.* 1954;49:216-241.
4. Eaton WA, Hofrichter J. Hemoglobin-S gelation and sickle-cell disease. *Blood.* 1987;70(5):1245-1266.
5. Noguchi CT, Schechter AN, Rodgers GP. Sickle cell disease pathophysiology. *Baillieres Clin Haematol.* 1993;6(1):57-91.
6. Bunn HF. Mechanisms of disease: pathogenesis and treatment of sickle cell disease. *N Engl J Med.* 1997;337(11):762-769.
7. Eaton WA, Bunn HF. Treatment of sickle cell disease by targeting Hb S polymerization. *Blood.* 2017;129(20):2719-2726.
8. Dykes GW, Crepeau RH, Edelstein SJ. Three-dimensional reconstruction of the fibres of sickle cell haemoglobin. *Nature.* 1978;272:506-510.
9. Dykes GW, Crepeau RH, Edelstein SJ. 3-Dimensional reconstruction of the 14-filament fibers of hemoglobin S. *J Mol Biol.* 1979;130(4):451-472.
10. Wishner BC, Ward KB, Lattman EE, Love WE. Crystal structure of sickle cell deoxyhemoglobin S at 5 A resolution. *J Mol Biol.* 1975;98(1):179-194.
11. Magdoff-Fairchild B, Swerdlow PH, Bertles JF. Intermolecular organization of deoxygenated sickle hemoglobin determined by X-ray diffraction. *Nature.* 1972;239(5369):217-219.
12. Hofrichter J, Hendricker DG, Eaton WA. Structure of hemoglobin S fibers. Optical determination of molecular orientation in sickled erythrocytes. *Proc Natl Acad Sci USA.* 1973;70(12):3604-3608.
13. Carragher B, Bluemke DA, Gabriel B, Potel MJ, Josephs R. Structural analysis of polymers of sickle cell hemoglobin 1. Sickle hemoglobin fibers. *J Mol Biol.* 1988;199(2):315-331.
14. Cretegny I, Edelstein SJ. Double strand packing in hemoglobin-S fibers. *J Mol Biol.* 1993;230:733-738.
15. Minton AP. Thermodynamic model for gelation of sickle cell hemoglobin. *J Mol Biol.* 1974;82(4):483-498.
16. Williams RC. Concerted formation of a gel of hemoglobin S. *Proc Natl Acad Sci USA.* 1973;70(5):1506-1508.
17. Ross PD, Hofrichter J, Eaton WA. Calorimetric and optical characterization of sickle cell hemoglobin gelation. *J Mol Biol.* 1975;96(2):239-253.

18. Ross PD, Hofrichter J, Eaton WA. Thermodynamics of gelation of sickle cell hemoglobin. *J Mol Biol.* 1977;115(2):111-134.

19. Hofrichter J. Ligand binding and the gelation of sickle cell hemoglobin. *J. Mol. Biol.* 1979;128(3):335-369.

20. Sunshine HR, Hofrichter J, Ferrone FA, Eaton WA. Oxygen binding by sickle-cell hemoglobin polymers. *J Mol Biol.* 1982;158(2):251-273.

21. Eaton WA, Hofrichter J. Sickle cell hemoglobin polymerization. *Adv Prot Chem.* 1990;40:63-279.

22. Gill SJ, Spokane R, Benedict RC, Fall K, Wyman J. Ligand-linked phase equilibria of sickle cell hemoglobin. *J Mol Biol.* 1980;140: 299-312.

23. Ross PD, Minton AP. Analysis of non-ideal behavior in concentrated hemoglobin solutions. *J Mol Biol.* 1977;112(3):437-452.

24. Minton AP. Non-ideality and thermodynamics of sickle cell hemoglobin gelation. *J Mol Biol.* 1977;110(1):89-103.

25. Noguchi CT, Torchia DA, Schechter AN. Determination of deoxyhemoglobin S polymer in sickle erythrocytes upon deoxygenation. *Proc Natl Acad Sci USA.* 1980;77(9):5487-5491.

26. Minton AP. Relations between oxygen saturation and aggregation of sickle cell hemoglobin. *J Mol Biol.* 1976;100(4):519-542.

27. Padlan EA, Love WE. Refined crystal structure of deoxyhemoglobin S, 2. Molecular interactions in the crystal. *J Biol Chem.* 1985;260(14):8280-8291.

28. Henry ER, Bettati S, Hofrichter J, Eaton WA. A tertiary two-state allosteric model for hemoglobin. *Biophys Chem.* 2002;98(1-2): 149-164.

29. Henry ER, Mozzarelli A, Viappiani C, et al. Experiments on hemoglobin in single crystals and silica gels distinguish among allosteric models. *Biophys J.* 2015;109(6):1264-1272.

30. Henry ER, Cellmer T, Dunkelberger EB, et al. Allosteric control of hemoglobin S fiber formation by oxygen and its relation to the pathophysiology of sickle cell disease. *Proc Natl Acad Sci USA.* Submitted for publication.

31. Poillon WN, Kim BC, Rodgers GP, Noguchi CT, Schechter AN. Sparing effect of hemoglobin F and hemoglobin A2 on the polymerization of hemoglobin S at physiological ligand saturations. *Proc Natl Acad Sci USA.* 1993;90(11):5039-5043.

32. Hofrichter J, Ross PD, Eaton WA. Kinetics and mechanism of deoxyhemoglobin-S gelation: new approach to understanding sickle-cell disease. *Proc Natl Acad Sci USA.* 1974;71(12):4864-4868.

33. Malfa R, Steinhardt J. Temperature-dependent latent period in the aggregation of sickle cell hemoglobin. *Biochem Biophys Res Comm.* 1974;59(3):887-893.

34. Moffat K, Gibson QH. Rates of polymerization and depolymerization of sickle cell hemoglobin. *Biochem Biophys Re. Comm.* 1974;61(1):237-242.

35. Ferrone FA, Hofrichter J, Sunshine HR, Eaton WA. Kinetic studies on photolysis induced gelation of sickle cell hemoglobin suggest a new mechanism. *Biophys J.* 1980;32:361-377.

36. Ferrone FA, Hofrichter J, Eaton WA. Kinetics of sickle hemoglobin polymerization 2. A double nucleation mechanism. *J Mol Biol.* 1985;183(4):611-631.

37. Coletta M, Hofrichter J, Ferrone FA, Eaton WA. Kinetics of sickle hemoglobin polymerization in single red-cells. *Nature.* 1982;300(5888):194-197.

38. Hofrichter J. Kinetics of sickle hemoglobin polymerization 3. Nucleation rates determined from stochastic fluctuations in polymerization progress curves. *J Mol Biol.* 1986;189:553-571.

39. Cao ZQ, Ferrone FA. A 50th order reaction predicted and observed for sickle hemoglobin nucleation. *J Mol Biol.* 1996; 256(2):219-222.

40. Christoph GW, Hofrichter J, Eaton WA. Understanding the shape of sickled red cells. *Biophys J.* 2005;88(2):1371-1376.

41. Ferrone FA. The delay time in sickle cell disease after 40 years: a paradigm assessed. *Am J Hematol.* 2015;90(5):438-445.

42. Cohen SIA, Linse S, Luheshi LM, et al. Proliferation of amyloid-beta 42 aggregates occurs through a secondary nucleation mechanism. *Proc Natl Acad Sci USA.* 2013;110(24):9758-9763.

43. Cellmer T, Ferrone FA, Eaton WA. Universality of supersaturation ratio in protein fiber formation. *Nat Struct Mol Biol.* 2016;23:459-471.

44. Dunkelberger EB, Metaferia B, Cellmer T, Henry ER. Theoretical simulation of red cell sickling upon deoxygenation based on the physical chemistry of sickle hemoglobin fiber formation. *J Phys Chem B.* 2018;122(49):11579-11590.

45. Kato GJ, Steinberg MH, Gladwin MT. Intravascular hemolysis and the pathophysiology of sickle cell disease. *J Clin Invest.* 2017;127(3):750-760.

46. Sundd P, Gladwin MT, Novelli EM. Pathophysiology of sickle cell disease. *Ann Rev Pathol.* 2019;14:263-292.

47. Telen MJ, Malik P, Vercellotti GM. Therapeutic strategies for sickle cell disease: towards a multi-agent approach. *Nat Rev Drug Discov.* 2019;18(2):139-158.

48. Noguchi CT, Schechter AN. The intracellular polymerization of sickle hemoglobin and its relevance to sickle-cell disease. *Blood.* 1981;58(6):1057-1068.

49. Eaton WA, Hofrichter J, Ross PD. Delay time of gelation: possible determinant of clinical severity in sickle-cell disease. *Blood.* 1976;47(4):621-627.

50. Hebbel RP, Boogaerts MAB, Eaton JW, Steinberg MH. Erythrocyte adherence to endothelium in sickle cell anemia: a possible determinant of clinical severity. *N Engl J Med.* 1980;302(18):992-995.

51. Mozzarelli A, Hofrichter J, Eaton WA. Delay time of hemoglobin-S polymerization prevents most cells from sickling in vivo. *Science.* 1987;237(4814):500-506.

52. Yosmanovich D, Rotter M, Aprelev A, Ferrone FA. Calibrating sickle cell disease. *J Mol Biol.* 2016;428(8):1506-1514.

53. Hofrichter J, Ross PD, Eaton WA. Supersaturation in sickle cell hemoglobin solutions. *Proc Natl Acad Sci USA.* 1976;73:3034-3039.

54. Brittenham GM, Schechter AN, Noguchi CT. Hemoglobin S polymerization - primary determinant of the hemolytic and clinical severity of the sickling syndromes. *Blood.* 1985;65(1):183-189.

55. Orkin SH, Bauer DE. Emerging genetic therapy for sickle cell disease. *Ann Rev Med.* 2019;70:257-271.

Genetic Basis of Sickle Cell Disease

Authors: *Martin H. Steinberg, Swee Lay Thein*

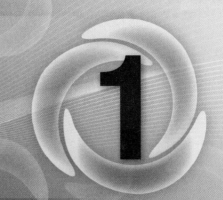

Chapter Outline

Overview

Subsequent to its ancient origin in Africa, the sickle hemoglobin (HbS) gene spread to the Western Hemisphere, Europe, the Middle East, and the Indian subcontinent by slave trading, war, and migration (Figure 1-1). The phenotype of sickle cell disease is caused by several common and many rare genotypes. All have in common at least 50% HbS in the blood. Among these genotypes, the most frequent and severe clinically is homozygosity for the HbS gene (HbSS or sickle cell anemia), followed by compound heterozygosity for the HbS and the hemoglobin C (HbC) gene (HbSC disease) and compound heterozygosity for HbS and various β thalassemia genes (HbS-β thalassemia). The HbS gene is associated with 5 common β-globin gene haplotypes, named after regions of high gene frequency in Africa, the Middle East, and India. These haplotypes have a loose association with the severity of disease that is explained by the characteristic fetal hemoglobin (HbF) level of each haplotype. HbF is the major modulator of the phenotype of sickle cell disease; it inhibits the polymerization of HbS that initiates the pathophysiology of disease, and it also dilutes the intraerythrocytic HbS concentration, a key factor in the sickling kinetics. Because HbS polymerization is the key mechanism that triggers all

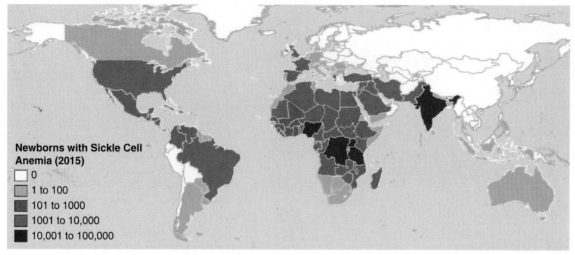

FIGURE 1-1 **World distribution of sickle cell anemia with expected numbers of newborns.** Adapted from Piel FB, Steinberg MH, Rees DC. Sickle cell disease. *N Engl J Med*. 2017;376:1561-1573. doi:10.1056/NEJMra1510865.

other pathophysiologic events, preventing poly-merization has been of prime therapeutic interest. Decades have been devoted to understanding how the HbF genes are almost totally turned off after birth and whether and how this switch from fetal to adult hemoglobin gene expression can be reversed by drugs or cellular therapeutics. In this chapter, we prepare the reader for understanding the pathophysiologic basis of the complications of sickle cell disease and the future therapeutic landscape by discussing the origin and genetic background of the HbS mutation, the most com-mon genotypes of this disease, the regulation of gene expression within the globin gene clusters, and genetic variants that might explain disease heterogeneity.

Evolution and Structure of Human Hemoglobin

Billions of years of evolution have morphed ancient protein motifs that functioned in bacteria and protists as electron trans-porters and nitric oxide (NO) dioxygenases to human hemoglo-bin that transports oxygen and metabolizes NO.[1] The aboriginal, primitive monomeric protein has become a heterotetrameric protein encoded in 2 nonallelic gene clusters and provides an essential function of vertebrate life (Figure 1-2). Homozygosity or compound heterozygosity for a single mutation in the gene encoding one of the hemoglobin subunits, the β-hemoglobin gene (*HBB*; *rs334*, GAG-GTG; $β^7$ glu-val; E7V; MIM 603903), is found in all individuals with sickle cell disease. Via complex pathophysiologic paths, beginning with its polymerization, HbS leads to the many complications of this disorder.

Hemoglobin is a tetramer of 2 α-like and 2 β-like globin chains, with each chain containing an oxygen-carrying heme group.[2] Its pivotal role in the transport of oxygen, carbon diox-ide, and NO has been well studied and is discussed in Chapter 4

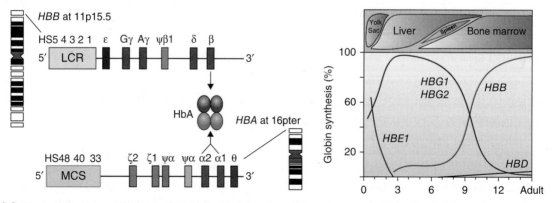

FIGURE 1-2 **The globin gene clusters with their associated coding genes and noncoding pseudogenes.** α-Globin and non–α-globin chains form dimers that then associate to form the tetrameric hemoglobin molecule. HS 48, 40, and 33 correspond respectively to R1, R2, and R3 in the multispecies conserved sequences (MCS) regulatory region.

in this volume.[3] Different hemoglobins are synthesized at different stages of human development in a process referred to as hemoglobin switching (embryonic → fetal → adult). The 3 embryonic hemoglobins are Gower I ($\zeta_2\varepsilon_2$), Gower II ($\alpha_2\varepsilon_2$), and Portland ($\zeta_2\gamma_2$). The switch from embryonic hemoglobin to HbF ($\alpha_2\gamma_2$) production occurs at 6 to 8 weeks' gestation, followed by the second "globin switch" from fetal to adult hemoglobin ($\alpha_2\beta_2$, HbA) that occurs slowly and is completed several months into the postnatal period. Each of the non–α-globin polypeptides is encoded by a structural gene found on the short arm of chromosome 11 (11p15.4) in the *HBB* cluster—a closely linked group of β-like genes that include, in addition to *HBB*, the embryonic ε-globin gene (*HBE*), fetal γ-globin genes (*HBG2* and *HBG1* [or *HBG2/1*]), and the other minor adult hemoglobin δ-globin gene (*HBD*) (Figure 1-2). *HBG2* and *HBG1* code for nearly identical γ-globin polypeptides, except at codon 136, where *HBG2* codes for glycine, whereas *HBG1* codes for alanine. *HBG1* and *HBG2* are identical in their function and in their capacity to inhibit HbS polymerization. In newborns, approximately two-thirds of γ-globin chains have glycine at position 136 ($^G\gamma$), whereas the remaining third have alanine ($^A\gamma$). This ratio falls during the switch from γ- to β-chain production and is nearly reversed in adults. In individuals who have the C-T variant (rs7482144) at −158 bp 5′ to the *HBG2* initiation site, also referred to as the *Xmn*1 $^G\gamma$ site, this "switch" does not occur,[4] perhaps because of derepression of *HBG2* expression.[5] Similarly, the α-like globin genes are closely linked in another cluster near the telomere of the short arm of chromosome 16 (16p13.3) (Figure 1-2). The α-globin gene cluster includes the ζ-globin gene (*HBZ*), whose protein is found in hemoglobins of the embryo and early fetus, and the duplicated α-globin genes (*HBA2* and *HBA1* [or *HBA2/1*]). *HBA2* and *HBA1* code for identical α-globin polypeptides but are expressed at different levels. The φ-globin gene (*HBQ1*) is expressed in early fetal life, but its function is unclear. Also of unknown function is the μ-globin gene (*HBM*), which has an open reading frame and might be expressed. In both α- and β-globin clusters, the genes are arranged 5′ to 3′ along the chromosome in the order of their developmental expression. Both globin gene clusters contain pseudogenes that are not protein coding (Figure 1-2).

Origin and Spread of the HbS Gene

The story of the first report of sickle cell anemia, the presence of a variant hemoglobin in the erythrocytes of patients and carriers, its inheritance, the structure of HbS, and how these singular discoveries revolutionized our understanding of genetic disease have often been recounted.[6-8] Pauling et al[9] first noticed that the hemoglobin of individuals with sickle cell disease migrated differently from normal hemoglobin in an electrical field and ascribed this to the presence of HbS. Validation for Pauling's suggestion was provided 8 years later in 1957 by Ingram,[10] who demonstrated that HbS was caused by a glutamic acid to valine substitution at position 6 of the β-globin chain of hemoglobin, followed by Goldstein et al,[11] who showed that this amino acid substitution arose from a single base change (A>T) at codon 6 (rs334). The convention for numbering amino acid residues in the human β-hemoglobin chain includes the cleaved initiator methionyl residue as amino acid residue 1, the N-terminal valine as 2, and so forth. Therefore, the HbS mutation becomes E7V rather than E6V, and the current numbering puts the HbS mutation in codon 7 rather than 6. In previous publications, the number assigned to the HbS mutation does not count the initiator methionyl. Until recently, it was hypothesized that the β^S mutation arose at least 4 times in Africa between 2000 and 4000 years ago and once in the Middle East or India (Figure 1-3). *Plasmodium falciparum* malaria was most likely the selective force involved in the increase of gene frequency that coincided with the expansion of agriculture. Recent studies that further elucidated the ancestry of the HbS mutation have suggested a more ancient unicentric origin.[12] Based on haplotypes derived from 27 phased SNPs (in LD with rs334) ascertained by whole-genome sequencing in 156 carriers rather than the much smaller number of SNPs detected by restriction fragment length polymorphisms, a common haplotype (HAP1) with a single genetic origin was proposed. This haplotype was related to the previously denominated Bantu, Cameroon, and Arab-Indian haplotypes from which were derived the Senegal and Benin haplotypes. A mutation age of 259 generations or about 7300 years (range, 3400-11,100 years) was calculated. This time corresponded to the Holocene Wet Phase and preceded the Bantu expansion. The origin was hypothesized to have occurred in West-Central Africa or in the Sahara when its climate was wet and rainy. Only a single Arab-Indian haplotype chromosome was included in these data, so the conclusions regarding the origins of this haplotype would be bolstered by additional studies.[12] Another analysis based on *HBB* sequencing in populations derived from African agriculturist and rainforest-dwelling populations supported a single origin of the HbS gene about 22,000 years ago in an agriculturist population that then was introduced into rainforest dwellers within the past 6000 years. Its prior presence in agriculturists might have been a consequence of their slash-and-burn farming lifestyle that permitted accumulation of standing water, allowing earlier exposure to malaria.[13]

Regulation Within the β-Globin Gene Complex

Expression of the β-globin gene is dependent on local promoter sequences and the upstream β-globin locus control region (β-LCR), which consists of 5 DNase I hypersensitive (HS) sites (designated HS1 to HS5) distributed between 6 and 20 kb 5′ of *HBE*. One HS site is approximately 20 kb downstream of *HBB*. All regulatory regions bind a number of key erythroid-specific

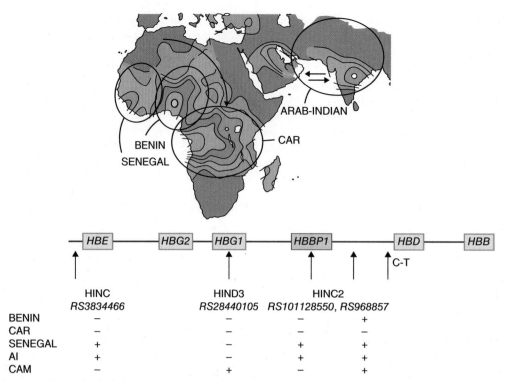

	HINC RS3834466	HIND3 RS28440105	HINC2 RS101128550, RS968857	
BENIN	−	−	−	+
CAR	−	−	−	−
SENEGAL	+	−	+	+
AI	+	−	+	+
CAM	−	+	−	+

FIGURE 1-3 Old world distribution of HbS gene haplotypes. The top panel shows the canonical haplotypes associated with the HbS gene. These haplotypes were derived from a small number of polymorphisms in the *HBB* gene cluster detected by restriction fragment length polymorphisms and were believed to reflect distinct origins of this gene (see text for additional discussion). In the lower panel, by using paternal and maternal phased polymorphism haplotypes, the pattern of 4 polymorphisms, *rs3834466*, *rs28440105*, *rs10128556*, and *rs968857*, obtainable from genome-wide association studies or sequencing can unequivocally and inexpensively ascertain the 5 common HbS-associated haplotypes.[156] A C-T polymorphisms 5′ to *HBD* is present only in the AI haplotype. CAR, Central African Republic.

transcription factors, notably GATA-1, GATA-2, NF-E2, KLF1 (also known as EKLF), and SCL; various cofactors (eg, FOG, p300); and factors that are more ubiquitous in their tissue distribution, such as Sp1.[14]

The *HBB* locus is a paradigm for tissue- and developmental stage–specific regulation; expression of each of the individual globin genes relies on a timely and direct physical interaction between the powerful β-LCR enhancer and gene promoter sequences. The interaction between the LCR and globin promoter is mediated through binding of erythroid-specific and ubiquitous transcription factors.[15,16] A dual mechanism has been proposed for the developmental expression: (1) gene competition for the upstream β-LCR, conferring advantage for the gene closest to the LCR; and (2) autonomous silencing (transcriptional repression) of the preceding gene.[17] The ability to compete for the β-LCR and autonomous silencing depends on the change in the abundance and repertoire of various transcription factors that favor promoter-LCR interaction. Although the ε- and γ-globin genes are autonomously silenced at the appropriate developmental stage, expression of the adult β-globin gene depends on lack of competition from the upstream γ-globin genes for the LCR sequences. Concordant with this mechanism, when the γ-globin genes are upregulated by point mutations in their promoters causing a nondeletion hereditary persistence of fetal hemoglobin (HPFH),

expression of the β-globin gene in *cis* is downregulated.[18] Further, mutations that affect the β-globin promoter, which removes competition for the β-LCR, are associated with higher than expected increases in γ- and δ-globin (HbA$_2$, α$_2$δ$_2$) expression.[19,20] Although the proposal of dual mechanism of gene competition for developmental expression of the globin genes was attractive, identification of the transcription factor genes *BCL11A* and *LRF* or *ZBTB7A*,[21-23] which autonomously silence the γ-globin genes in the switch to adult β-globin, proved elusive until the advent of genomics in the past 10 years.

The α-globin gene cluster also has an upstream regulatory locus consisting of 4 elements termed R1 to R4, 3 of which are in introns of the gene *NPRL3* (Figure 1-2). There is a developmental switch from embryonic ζ- to adult α-globin gene expression at about 6 weeks' gestation.[24] *BCL11A* and *LRF*, critical silencers of *HBG2/1*, are also likely to have roles in ξ-globin gene silencing.[25] All fetal and adult hemoglobins contain the same α-globin chain, so that switching in the α-globin cluster has little relevance in sickle cell disease.

Understanding the γ- to β-Globin Switch and HPFH

All adults continue to produce residual amounts of HbF that constitutes about 1% of the total hemoglobin. The level varies and is under strong genetic control.[26] In some individuals, however, synthesis of HbF persists into adult life in the absence of any hematological disorder; such individuals are considered to have HPFH. Historically, HPFH is classified as either pancellular or heterocellular, with the classification being based on a phenotypic description of the HbF distribution among the erythrocytes. Unraveling the genetic basis of the different entities of HPFH has provided much insight and further understanding of the switch from fetal to adult hemoglobin expression and has also led to the identification of the transcriptional repressors, validating the gene competition and autonomous silencing hypothesis proposed 20 years earlier.

Pancellular HPFH is rare and caused by either substantial deletions within the *HBB* cluster, including *HBB* itself, or single base substitutions or smaller deletions in either of the duplicated γ-globin gene promoters. These Mendelian forms of HPFH are characterized by elevations of HbF ranging from 10% to 40% in heterozygotes, and the HbF is present in all red blood cells, hence the term *pancellular*. Although the increases in HbF mirror the molecular diversity of HPFH mutations, within each molecular class, a range of HbF levels has been noted that can be explained by the underlying background of common HbF variation, as observed in healthy adults. In the Mendelian forms of nondeletion HPFH, the rare variants occur in 3 groups: in a cluster around −200, a single base substitution at −175, and a cluster at approximately −115 relative to the transcriptional start sites of *HBG2/1*. Although the mutations in these clusters have been shown to alter in vitro binding patterns of a variety of transcription factors (GATA-1, GATA-2, NF-E2, KLF1) with roles in globin gene regulation, identification of the transcription repressors binding to these sites was elusive.[14] *BCL11A* was identified as a major quantitative trait locus (QTL) for HbF by 2 independent genome-wide association studies (GWASs) in 2007 and 2008[21,22] and subsequently confirmed as a major repressor of γ-globin expression.[27,28] In a proof-of-principle experiment, reducing *bcl11a* in humanized sickle cell mice resulted in derepression of γ-globin (up to 30% HbF) with reversal of organ damage.[29] However, it had not been possible to demonstrate direct binding of BCL11A to γ-globin promoters, leading to the hypothesis that BCL11A activated the γ-globin gene indirectly via long-range interactions in the *HBB* complex through interaction with GATA-1 and SOX-6.[30,31] In 2018, evidence for direct binding of transcriptional repressors—BCL11A to the −115 region and ZBTB7A to the −200 region—finally provided a molecular explanation for the γ-globin activation in nondeletion HPFH.[32,33] It is now established that the regulatory circuit facilitating the switch from fetal to adult globin gene expression involves the proteins MYB, KLF1, BCL11A, and ZBTB7A. MYB activates *KLF1*,[34] which is a positive regulator of *BCL11A*[35,36] and *ZBTB7A*,[37] the 2 direct repressors of γ-globin genes (Figure 1-4). Thus, KLF1 has a dual effect on the switch: it preferentially activates adult globin genes,[38,39] and it silences fetal globin genes via activation of *BCL11A* and *ZBTB7A*.

Evolution of the QTLs That Modulate HbF Expression

The common variable persistence of HbF in adults constitutes the historical entity of heterocellular HPFH, where multiple genes, together with an environmental component, determine the HbF value measured in any individual. *Xmn1-HBG2* (*rs7482144*) on chromosome 11p, *HBS1L-MYB* intergenic region (HMIP) on chromosome 6q23, and *BCL11A* on chromosome 2p16 are QTLs for HbF, contributing to the complex inheritance of HbF levels in an individual.[40,41] Identification of these HbF QTLs mirrors the developing technology in genetic studies. Observations of variable HbF with different HbS globin gene haplotypes first suggested that the *HBB* cluster is a prime location for an HbF regulatory determinant. This element is represented by *rs7482144* 5′ of the Gγ-gene promoter. The first indication that chromosome 6q23 could be the location of an HbF QTL came from linkage association studies of an extended Asian-Indian family with β thalassemia and HPFH in which segregation analysis showed that the genetic determinant for HPFH was inherited independently from the *HBB* cluster.[42] However, it was the application of GWASs that led to association of HbF to the locus in intron 2 of the *BCL11A* gene on chromosome 2p16.[21,22] Hitherto, *BCL11A* was known as an oncogene involved in lymphoid development and leukemogenesis,[43-45] but its relevance to HbF and erythropoiesis was unsuspected. GWAS also reconfirmed the other 2 HbF QTLs: *Xmn1-HBG2* and HMIP. The association of these 3 QTLs with HbF has been replicated and validated throughout the world in healthy subjects as well as patients with β thalassemia and sickle cell disease (although at varying frequencies of the 3 variants).[46-51]

Functional studies in primary human erythroid progenitor cells and transgenic mice demonstrated that SNPs in intron 2 of *BCL11A* were responsible for the activity of this gene as a repressor of γ-globin gene expression.[52] Fine-mapping demonstrated that the most highly HbF-associated *BCL11A* variants are localized to a region marked by 3 erythroid-specific DNase I HS sites,[52] and near-saturating CRISPR-Cas 9 mutagenesis of the enhancer region in HUDEP-2 cells revealed that a critical HbF-regulating site resides within a 42-bp region at the (+58) enhancer element.[53] The comparatively large impact of this locus on HbF levels in sickle cell anemia is due to a combination of 2 separate factors; first, the effect size (β coefficient) of the variant is relatively large, and second, the haplotype carrying the HbF-boosting alleles of these markers is relatively frequent in African populations (generally 20% or larger, 1000 Genomes Project, phase 3), compared with the *Xmn1-HBG2* A allele and variants at *HBS1L-MYB* (generally <5% each). BCL11A, a zinc finger protein, binds TGACCA motifs present at 35 sites within the *HBB* gene cluster. Two of these sites are in the γ-globin gene promoters, and the distal of these 2 sites at positions −118 to −113 is the site of 2 point mutations and a 13-bp deletion associated with the phenotype of HPFH.[18] BCL11A binds preferentially to this site in adult erythroid progenitors. Preferential binding and occupancy of BCL11A in the −118 to −113 motif represses this promoter,[32,33] thus favoring

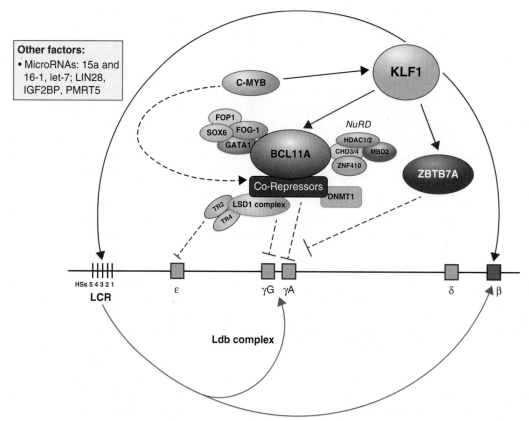

FIGURE 1-4 Current synthesis of HbF regulation in adults. Silencing of *HBG1/HBG2* in adult life is achieved by a network of transcription factors that enables binding of the 2 essential repressors, ZBTB7A and BCL11A, to the −200 and −115 regions of the γ-globin promoter, respectively. Both of these factors interact with the NuRD chromatin complex. Chromatin writers and erasers, such as DNMT, enable access of transcription factors to the *HBG1/2* promoters. Changes in the level of factors, such as the let-7 family of microRNAs, LIN28, and IGF2BP, in the fetal-to-adult transition have been observed, but how these influence globin gene expression remains incompletely understood. The network of HbF regulation also includes the chromatin-modeling factor FOP, the orphan nuclear receptors TR2/TR4 (part of the DRED complex),[71,72,91,92] and the protein arginine methyltransferase PRMT5. The roles of *KLF1* and *c-MYB* are likely to be indirect through coordinating expression of the direct repressor, *BCL11A*. ZNF410, a newly described HbF repressor, activates CHD4, silencing HBG expression.[92a,92b] Regulators of the key transcription factors, such as microRNAs 15a and 16-1 in controlling *MYB*, could also have a potential role in regulating HbF levels.

interaction of the upstream LCR with the β-globin gene promoters (Figure 1-4). The high-resolution studies of BCL11A binding sites *cis* to the *HBB* gene cluster suggest that promoter repression is the major mechanism of action of this protein that controls most of hemoglobin switching and that regions more distant to *HBG2/1* promoters, although potentially functional, are less likely to have major roles in switching from *HBG2/1* to *HBB* expression. Mutations changing the structure of BCL11A have not been reported, although deleterious variants have been modeled in silico and the effects of BCL11A on *HBG2/1* expression that have been described are a result of haploinsufficiency.[54,55] Naturally occurring microdeletions or point mutations encompassing *BCL11A* on chromosome 2p leading to haploinsufficiency of BCL11A have been reported in individuals with an autism-like neurologic syndrome; the mean HbF levels in these individuals are approximately 15%, equivalent to the levels encountered in individuals heterozygous for HPFH.[56-59]

With regard to HMIP, subsequent studies established that *MYB* is the relevant gene in the *HBS1L-MYB* region.[60,61] *MYB* encodes the MYB transcription factor that is essential for hematopoiesis and erythroid differentiation. The causal variants reside in 2 clusters within HMIP, at −84 and −71 kb, upstream of *MYB*.[61,62] The SNPs at these 2 regions disrupt binding of key erythroid enhancers, affecting long-range interactions with *MYB* and *MYB* expression and providing a functional explanation for the genetic association of the 6q *HBS1L-MYB* intergenic region with HbF and F cell levels.[61,63,64] A 3-bp deletion is one functional element in the *MYB* enhancers accounting for increased HbF expression in individuals who have the sentinel SNP *rs9399137* that was found to be common in Europeans and Asians but less common in African-derived populations.[47,65] A short fragment encompassing the 3-bp deletion polymorphism appears to have enhancer-like activity.[62,64] A 1283-bp long noncoding RNA (lncRNA) is transcribed from this enhancer, and γ-globin gene messenger RNA (mRNA) is increased 200-fold when this lncRNA was downregulated.[66] The *HBS1L-MYB* intergenic enhancers do not appear to affect expression of *HBS1L*, the other flanking gene.[61] A case report also excluded *HBS1L* as having a role in the regulation of HbF and erythropoiesis. In whole-exome sequencing of rare uncharacterized disorders, mutations in the *HBS1L* gene leading to a loss of function in the gene were identified in a female child.[67] The child had normal blood counts and normal HbF levels. Compelling evidence has also been provided that increased HbF effect can be mediated via downmodulation of *MYB*, at least in part, via targeting of its 3′ untranslated region by microRNAs 15a and 16-1. A delayed HbF to HbA switch, along with persistently elevated HbF levels, is one of the unique features in infants with trisomy 13[68]; these infants share in common increased dosage of a segment of chromosome 13q14 that encompasses the gene encoding microRNAs 15a and 16-1. *MYB* is a direct target of these microRNAs; increased expression of these microRNAs in primary human erythroid progenitor cells resulted in elevated fetal and embryonic hemoglobin gene expression.[27-29] Although *rs66650371* is associated with HbF in African sickle cell anemia patients, the low frequency of the minor allele in Africans and the very low minor allele frequency in Saudi sickle cell anemia with the Arab-Indian haplotype account for less of an effect of HMIP on HbF in these populations compared with its effects on HbF in normal Europeans or Chinese with β thalassemia. *MYB* was also causally implicated by fine-mapping, which identified rare missense *MYB* variants associated with HbF production.[69] It is proposed that MYB modulates HbF expression via 2 mechanisms: (1) indirectly through alteration of the kinetics of erythroid differentiation (low MYB levels accelerate erythroid differentiation, leading to release of early erythroid progenitor cells that are still synthesizing predominantly HbF)[70,71] and (2) directly via activation of *KLF1* and other repressors (eg, nuclear receptors TR2/TR4) of *HBG2/1*.[34,64,72] Modulation of *MYB* expression also provides a functional explanation for the association of the HMIP-2 SNPs with other erythroid traits, such as red cell count, mean corpuscular volume (MCV), mean corpuscular hemoglobin (MCH), and HbA$_2$ levels, and also with platelet and monocyte counts.[73-77]

Although the 3 HbF QTLs explain 25% to 50% of the genetic contribution to HbF levels, subsequent efforts in other cohorts have not identified new validated HbF QTLs, suggesting that the genetic variance that remains unaccounted for may be due to many common and/or rare alleles with small effects on the trait. One such example are rare variants in Kruppel-like factor 1 (*KLF1*). *KLF1* was discovered in 1993[78] and reemerged as a key transcription factor controlling HbF through genetic studies in a Maltese family with β thalassemia and HPFH that segregated independently of the *HBB* locus.[35] Numerous reports of different mutations in *KLF1* associated with increases in HbF soon followed; the HbF increases occurred either as a primary phenotype or in association with red blood cell disorders such as congenital dyserythropoietic anemia,[79] congenital nonspherocytic hemolytic anemia due to pyruvate kinase deficiency,[80] and sickle cell anemia. However, several GWASs of HbF, including ones in sickle cell anemia patients of African descent, failed to identify common *KLF1* variants.[81,82] On the contrary, targeted resequencing of *KLF1* identified variants that were overrepresented in southern China, where β thalassemia is more prevalent compared to North China. *KLF1* variants were also overrepresented in

patients with milder β thalassemia when compared to patients with thalassemia major.[83] KLF1 is a direct activator of *BCL11A* and is also essential for the activation of *HBB* expression.[36,84] Collectively, studies suggest that KLF1 is key in the regulatory circuit that controls the switch from *HBG2/1* to *HBB* expression; it not only preferentially activates *HBB*, providing a competitive edge, but also silences the γ-globin genes indirectly via activation of *BCL11A* and *ZBTB7A*. KLF1 may also contribute to the silencing of embryonic globin gene expression.[25,80,85] KLF1 has now emerged as a major erythroid transcription factor with pleiotropic roles underlying many of the previously uncharacterized anemias.[86]

ZBTB7A or *LRF* (leukemia/lymphoma-related factor), a C2H2 zinc finger protein, was identified through studies of its role in erythroid differentiation by Masuda et al.[23] Inactivation of either *BCL11A* or *LRF* in HUDEP-2 immortalized cells led to approximately 50% HbF, whereas in double knockout cells where *BCL11A* was also inactivated, HbF composed >90% of total hemoglobin. This suggested that the silencing pathway of *LRF* is independent of *BCL11A* and that the 2 factors account for the majority of HbF silencing.[23] To date, neither GWASs nor targeted searches for rare variants in individuals with elevated HbF have associated *LRF* genetic variation with HbF expression.[23,87] Disruption of ZBTB7A binding sites −195 to −197 and −201 to −202 bp 5′ to *HBG2/1* is associated with the phenotype of HPFH (Figure 1-4).[33,88]

A Current Synthesis of the Switch From Fetal to Adult Hemoglobin and Its Therapeutic Implications

In light of recent findings, the molecular machinery involved in hemoglobin switching centers on silencing of *HBG2/1*, which is achieved by a network of factors, with the major factors depicted in Figure 1-4. The emerging network of HbF regulation implicates numerous transcription factors in the fetal to adult globin switch, but recent findings focus on the transcriptional repressor proteins BCL11A and ZBTB7A, which provide the explanation for the nondeletion HPFH variants in the 2 dense clusters around the sites −200 and −115 bp 5′ to *HBG2/1*. Using genetically engineered cells that carry HPFH promoter variants, Martyn et al[33] showed that ZBTB7A and BCL11A bind to the −200 and −115 regions of the γ-globin promoter, respectively. Mutations in these regions disrupt binding of the respective transcription factors derepressing *HBG2/1* expression.[33] Independently, application of a technique named CUT&RUN also demonstrated clear occupancy of BCL11A at the −115 region.[32] The essential roles of BCL11A and ZBTB7A in *HBG2/1* silencing require the synchronization and coordination of several factors (Figure 1-4). DNA methylation at the γ-globin locus is recognized by the methylcytosine-binding domain (MBD) protein MBD2 that helps recruit the NuRD complex to the locus. Both BCL11A and ZBTB7A interact with the NuRD chromatin complex,[23,89] which includes 2 catalytic activities—the adenosine triphosphate (ATP)–dependent chromatin remodelers CHD3 and CHD4, as well as the histone deacetylases HDAC1 and HDAC2.[90] Interaction of BCL11A and ZBTB7A in erythroid cells occurred in distinct NuRD subcomplexes with no direct interaction with each other, suggesting that the silencing pathways of ZBTB7A and BCL11A are independent of each other.[23] Chromatin modifications that include both DNA methylation and methylation and acetylation of the histone tails are essential for access of transcription factors to promoters of *HBG2/1*. These modifications are recognized by a class of proteins referred to as chromatin "readers," which could be "writers" or "erasers." Targeting these readers and erasers is another pharmacotherapeutic approach for HbF induction. The observation that the CpG nucleotides in the promoters of *HBG2/1* are methylated in the adult stage led to the development of using 5-azacytidine and its analog, decitabine, as competitive inhibitors of DNA methyltransferase (DNMT1) for HbF induction. Changes in the levels of factors, such as the let-7 family of microRNAs, LIN28, and IGF2BP, in the fetal-to-adult transition created interest as potential therapeutic targets, but how these influence globin gene expression remains incompletely understood. The network of HbF regulation also includes the chromatin-modeling factor FOP, the orphan nuclear receptors TR2/TR4 (part of the DRED complex),[91,92] and the protein arginine methyltransferase PRMT5. The roles of KLF1 and MYB are likely to be indirect through coordinating expression of the direct repressors, such as BCL11A. Regulators of the key transcription factors, such as microRNA 15a and 16-1 in controlling MYB, could also have a potential role in controlling HbF levels.[91] A high HbF phenotype is also conditional on the presence of hemolysis, erythroid marrow expansion, and red blood cell turnover or stress erythropoiesis.

Acquisition of HbS Gene Haplotypes

More than 40 years ago, Kan and Dozy[93] published the first description of a SNP in humans and showed that this variant was frequently associated with inheritance of the HbS gene. This observation fueled the characterization of additional polymorphisms in the *HBB* gene cluster, which led to the definition of haplotypes associated with the HbS gene (reviewed in Nagel and Steinberg[8]). The HbS gene is found on 5 common haplotypes (Senegal, Benin, Bantu [Central African Republic or CAR], Cameroon, and Arab-Indian) (Figure 1-3).

The first studies of haplotypes of the HbS gene suggested that patients within different haplotype groups had different disease phenotypes and that the haplotype accounted for some of the remarkable heterogeneity of this Mendelian disease.[94-96] Patients with the Arab-Indian and Senegal haplotype had the mildest disease, patients with the CAR haplotype had the most severe disease, and patients with Benin and Cameroon haplotypes had intermediate disease. Although this generalization is likely to be true when the phenotypes of cohorts are compared, within each haplotype group, there is sufficient clinical heterogeneity to make ascertainment of haplotype valueless

for individual prognosis. Importantly, discrepant conclusions from haplotype-phenotype association studies might be a result of small cohorts of different ages, inclusion of haplotype compound heterozygotes, difficulty in haplotype assignment using unphased SNPs, imprecise phenotyping, and failure to control for the genotype of the α-globin gene cluster.

Each of the 5 typical HbS gene haplotypes is associated with a characteristic level of HbF. After controlling for α thalassemia, the clinical and hematologic variability among patient groups with different haplotypes is likely to be mediated by HbF levels. The mechanism accounting for variable HbF among haplotype groups remains unclear. In untreated adults, average HbF levels are about 10% in the Senegal haplotype and 17% in the Arab-Indian haplotype compared with 4% to 7% in the other 3 haplotypes. The aforementioned *rs7482144* 5′ to *HBG2* is present only in the Arab-Indian and the Senegal haplotypes. This SNP is associated with increased expression of only *HBG2* with a corresponding increase only in ^Gγ-globin. In contrast, the 2 transacting QTLs that modulate HbF gene expression affect *HBG2/1*.[97,98] *Rs7482144* is associated with reduced methylation in 6 CpG sites flanking the transcription start site of *HBG2*. Recent studies of BCL11A binding in the *HBG2/1* promoters, as discussed earlier, did not find evidence of binding in the region of *rs7482144*. However, CRISPR/Cas disruption of this motif was accompanied by increased *HBG2* expression, suggesting that this region is a binding site for an uncharacterized repressive factor.[5] BCL11A does bind within the promoter of *HBBP1*; *rs10128556* in this gene is in high LD with *rs7482144* in African ancestry sickle cell disease patients. It was suggested that this could be the functional SNP of the Senegal haplotype, but there are no mechanistic studies to support this and the bulk of *HBG2/1* silencing appears to occur by promoter repression.[32,69] Other *cis*-acting elements were located within the *HBD-HBG1* intergenic region, in the *HBB* LCR HS-2 core and approximately 530 bp 5′ to *HBB*. An additional candidate region was a 3.5-kb element near the 5′ portion of *HBD*, but this site is devoid of BCL11A binding sites.

Children with the Arab-Indian haplotype have HbF of about 30% and mild disease.[99,100] Uncovering the genetic elements in Arab-Indian haplotype sickle cell anemia that might either promote *HBG2/1* expression or decrease *HBG2/1* silencing favoring very high HbF might point to new targets for therapeutic HbF modulation. Progress toward achieving this goal has been slow. Variants *cis* to *HBG2/1* and in *ANTXR1* on chromosome 2 were exclusive to this haplotype and were associated with high HbF; however, a mechanistic basis for either of these associations has not been defined so causality cannot be assigned.[101-103] The association of the *ANTXR1* variant with HbF was first found during whole-genome sequencing of only 14 carefully selected Arab-Indian haplotype patients, 7 with high HbF and 7 with low HbF. However, this association was confirmed in independent cohorts of 120, 139, and 630 patients with this haplotype and was not present in 970 African American and Saudi patients with other haplotypes. Moreover, *ANTXR1* was expressed in erythroid progenitors, and its expression correlated inversely with HbF gene expression and protein levels. This locus explained about 10% of the HbF variance and was additive but independent of the effect of *BCL11A*. Like *BCL11A* and *MYB*, *ANTXR1* appeared to be a suppressor of HbF gene expression.[101] A 3-SNP subhaplotype of the *HBB* gene complex exclusive to patients with the Arab-Indian haplotype, T/A/T (*rs16912997*, *rs7482144*, and *rs101128556*), was hypothesized to mark a functional domain or a more extended haplotype of SNPs that might be required for optimal functional looping of the LCR to the *HBG2* promoter.[102]

In addition to the common haplotypes, 5% to 20% of HbS chromosomes have atypical haplotypes whose frequency is related to the degree of genetic admixture in the population examined. Most atypical haplotypes are a result of crossing-over events at a recombinational hotspot of about 9 kb 5′ to *HBB*. The hematologic and clinical phenotypes associated with atypical haplotypes appear to differ little from those of the common haplotypes.[104,105]

The original hope that defining different haplotypes associated with sickle cell anemia would provide a prognostic tool or lead to new ways of inducing HbF has not been realized. HbS gene- associated haplotypes have been very informative for epidemiologic and anthropologic studies. How a haplotype is mechanistically related to HbF level is largely unknown; the prognostic relevance of haplotype in individuals is minimal.

Genotypes of Sickle Cell Disease

Sickle cell disease is a clinical phenotype that results from 3 common genotypes—sickle cell anemia, HbSC disease, and the many varieties of HbS-β thalassemia—and many rare genotypes, some described only once.[106] Each genotype category has its own phenotypic characteristics, yet within each genotype, especially the common ones for which sufficient data are available, there is variability of phenotypic expression. For examples, HbSC disease is usually associated with about half the rate of complications as sickle cell anemia, but some patients have a clinical course similar to the most severe instances of sickle cell anemia, whereas other patients might not come to clinical attention until very late in life. The genetic basis of this intragenotype heterogeneity is rarely apparent for genotypes other than sickle cell anemia, where HbF and α thalassemia account for some of the heterogeneity. Table 1-1 lists the common genotypes, some rare genotypes, and selected associated clinical and laboratory features. Many other rare and "private" genotypes have been described, and some are discussed in Steinberg.[107]

Genetic Basis of Clinical Heterogeneity

The advent of high-throughput genomics raised the hope that its application to sickle cell anemia would illuminate the genetic basis for clinical heterogeneity and lead to an era of accurate prognosis and precision medicine. After 20 years of study, these hopes have been partially fulfilled, with the major breakthroughs being the discovery of most of the genetic variability modulating *HBG2/1* expression. We focus in this section on HbF, α thalassemia, and genes outside of the globin gene clusters as genetic modulators of disease severity. Based on the pathophysiology of disease, loci where genetic modulation could affect phenotype are shown in Figure 1-5.

Complications of sickle cell anemia can be divided into those associated with sickle vaso-occlusion and those that are a consequence of the intravascular destruction of varying numbers of sickle erythrocytes.[108,109] HbF appears to be most protective against complications that have been associated with vaso-occlusion and blood viscosity, such as acute painful episode, acute chest syndrome, and osteonecrosis. With the exception of leg ulceration, there is limited protection by HbF from complications closely associated with the severity of intravascular hemolysis, including cerebral, pulmonary, and systemic vasculopathy and nephropathy. This observation might be a result of the lysis of those sickle erythrocyte cells that contain insufficient HbF to protect them from HbS polymer-provoked injury. Liberation into the circulation of enough hemoglobin from these cells to deplete bioavailable NO is one trigger of the vasculopathic response associated with intravascular hemolysis.[110] Given the differential effects of HbF and α thalassemia on the subphenotypes associated with vaso-occlusion and hemolysis, the interaction of these disease-modifying factors might have clinical consequences. In a study of hydroxyurea-naive Senegalese children, patients with 3 to 6 minor alleles of the 3 HbF QTLs and homozygous for the $^{-3.7}$α-globin gene deletion had an increased frequency of vaso-occlusive episodes. The disease-ameliorating effects of higher HbF were present only in children without α thalassemia.[111]

HbF

HbS polymerization drives sickle cell disease pathophysiology. The rate and extent of polymerization are highly dependent on intracellular concentration of HbF and presence of non-S hemoglobin.[112] In addition to the diluting effect of intracellular HbF and HbA on intracellular HbS concentration, mixed hybrid tetramers of $\alpha_2\gamma\beta^S$ are largely excluded from the HbS polymer phase; hence, HbF is the most important modulator of the clinical and hematologic features of the disease. HbA_2 has a similar effect on polymerization but its low concentrations preclude clinical relevance. In adults, HbF expression is restricted to a subset of erythrocytes called F cells. These cells contain sufficient HbF (~6 pg) to allow their detection by flow cytometry (fluorescence-activated cell sorting). Otherwise, they differ little from non-F cells. The number of F cells present in an individual is genetically determined.[26,113] The total HbF level in any individual with sickle cell disease is determined by the absolute number of F cells, the amount of HbF per F cell, and the differential survival of F cells versus non-F cells.[114] The most compelling example of the primacy of HbF as an inhibitor of HbS polymerization is found in rare compound heterozygotes for HbS and gene deletion HPFH who have

TABLE 1-1 Genotypes of sickle hemoglobinopathies

Genotype	Percent HbS[a]	Percent HbF/A$_2$[b]	Phenotype[c]	Notes
Sickle cell anemia	100	1-20/3.5	See text	A$_2$ elevation often an artifact of HPLC
HbSC disease	50	1-10/2.5	About half the rate of HbSS complications	Proliferative retinopathy more common
HbS-β^0 thalassemia	100	1-20/4-6	Clinical: like HbSS Hematologic: microcytosis	Often difficult to distinguish from HbSS without genetic or family studies but indicator is the elevated hbA2 with hypochromic microcytic red cells in the absence of transfusion
HbS-β$^+$ thalassemia[d]	95-60	1-10/4-6	Variable but similar to HbSC; microcytosis	Phenotype depends in part on HbA levels that vary by thalassemia mutation
HbSD^{Punjab} (HBB 121 gln)	25-60	3-25/2.5	Variable but can be similar to HbSS	HbD separable by HPLC; not by electrophoresis
HbSE	~70	1-3/2.5	Milder than HbSC disease	HbE difficult to separate from HbA$_2$ on HPLC; DNA diagnosis best
HbSO^{Arab} (HBB 121 lys)	~60	3-8/2.5	More like HbSS than HbSC	Substitutions at HBB 121 can increase polymerization potential of HbS
HbS-HPFH	70	30/2	Microcytosis, near-normal PCV, no vaso-occlusive disease	Pancellular HPFH caused by deletion of HBB and HBD with continued expression of HBG2/1; HPFH can also be caused by nondeletion mutations in promoters of HBG2/1
HbS-Hope$^{(HBB\ 136\ asp)}$	42	Probably normal	Mild anemia, no vaso-occlusive disease	Hb Hope has high P$_{50}$ and mild instability
HbSS-G$^{(HBA\ 68\ lys)}$	33	The non-S hemoglobin consists of HbG and various hybrid tetramers	Like HbSS	HbG-Philadelphia is a common HBA variant

[a]Percent HbS ignores the presence of HbF and HbA$_2$.

[b]Percent HbF/A$_2$ values are dependent on age and usually reach stable adult levels by age 5 years. Normal HbA$_2$ is <3%; normal HbF is <1%.

[c]Estimation of phenotype or severity is relative to that of the HbS homozygote or HbSC disease, if more appropriate.

[d]In HbS-β$^+$ thalassemia, the balance of the remaining hemoglobin is HbA. Because of the many different β$^+$ thalassemia mutations, the percent HbA can vary widely and the phenotype varies accordingly. The most common mutations have about 20% HbS. In other compound heterozygote, the remaining hemoglobin is encoded by the β-globin variant in *trans* to the HbS gene. Most HBB variants with HbS do not have a clinical or hematologic phenotype. HbSS can also occur with HBA2/1 variants and have a phenotype of sickle cell disease. Any HbS genotype can be accompanied by α thalassemia, which, as discussed in the text, can alter clinical and hematologic phenotypes.

Note. At birth, the incidence of sickle cell anemia in African Americans has been estimated as 1 in 600, HbSC disease as 1 in 800, and HbS-β thalassemia as 1 in 1700.[157] Current worldwide population estimates have been provided by Piel et al.[158] Sickle cell anemia refers to homozygosity for the HbS gene, sometimes designated HbSS. Values in the table are averages in adults in the absence of transfusion or hydroxyurea.

Abbreviations: HPFH, hereditary persistence of fetal hemoglobin; HPLC, high-performance liquid chromatography; PCV, packed cell volume.

nearly 30% HbF distributed pancellularly so that each sickle erythrocyte contains about 10 pg. Compound heterozygotes of HbS-gene deletion HPFH are mostly asymptomatic with minor and clinically insignificant hematologic findings.[115] The clinical features of HbS-HPFH and polymerization modeling experiments suggest that >25% HbF in a pancellular expression pattern could "cure" sickle cell disease, and recent encouraging results achieving this goal are discussed later in this chapter.[116]

Table 1-2 summarizes the relationship between HbF concentration and the common complications of disease. High HbF is associated with a reduced rate of vaso-occlusive events and less so with hemolysis-related complications.[108,109] Studies at variance with these observations and disparities among study results might be a consequence of differing means of subphenotype assessment, nonhomogeneity of patient populations, small patient numbers, and different analytical approaches.

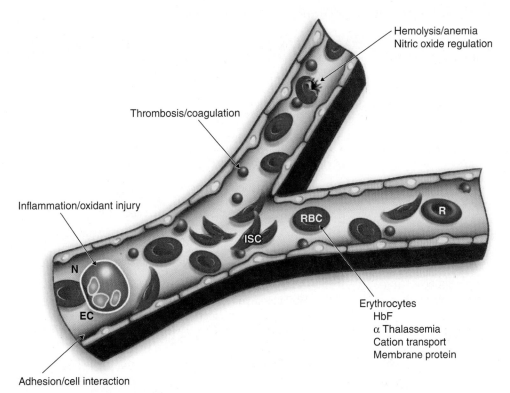

FIGURE 1-5 Potential loci of genetic variants impacting the phenotype of sickle cell disease. Based on an understanding of disease pathophysiology, it was possible to propose candidate genes whose variability might affect one of more disease subphenotypes. Genome-wide association studies and sequencing of exons or the entire genome have made it possible to detect associations that could not have been suspected from prior knowledge. The trade-off for increased sensitivity is reduced specificity, and to achieve statistical significance from these unbiased types of variant detection, large samples are needed if the effect of a variant on a phenotype is small. As a result, in sickle cell anemia, a rare disease, the results of most genotype-phenotype association studies have not been replicated. EC, endothelial cell; ISC, irreversibly sickled cell; N, neutrophil; R, reticulocyte; RBC, red blood cell.

The failure of HbF to modulate uniformly all complications of sickle cell disease might be related to the heterocellular distribution of HbF among sickle erythrocytes at both the baseline state and in response to hydroxyurea treatment. For absolute protection of the sickle erythrocyte from polymer-induced damage, it is proposed that 9 to 10 pg of HbF/F cell are required. Lesser amounts, although perhaps helpful, can leave the cell exposed to injury. Heterogeneity of HbF concentrations among F cells might explain why individuals with sickle cell anemia and similar total HbF levels—even 20% to 30% HbF—can have very different clinical and hematologic findings.[117]

α Thalassemia

α Thalassemia (MIM141850/141800) due to deletion of 1 or 2 α-globin genes is found in about 30% of most sickle cell disease populations of African descent and in 50% of sickle cell disease populations in the Middle East and India. In people of African descent, the most common α thalassemia variant is the $^{-3.7}$α-globin gene deletion. About 2% to 3% of patients are homozygous for this deletion. Various point mutations, the $^{-4.2}$α-globin gene deletion, and deletions removing both α-globin genes from a chromosome are uncommon causes of α thalassemia in sickle cell disease populations.

Genotype-phenotype associations in sickle cell anemia are limited to those involving the $^{-3.7}$α-globin gene deletion. α Thalassemia modulates sickle cell anemia by reducing the intracellular concentration of HbS, which in turn decreases HbS polymer-induced cellular damage, which attenuates hemolysis.[118] The hematologic and laboratory changes in sickle cell anemia–α thalassemia include higher hemoglobin concentration, lower MCV, higher HbA_2 level, lower reticulocyte count, lower bilirubin level, lower lactate dehydrogenase level, fewer dense and irreversibly sickled cells, and increased erythrocyte life span. The magnitude of these changes is related to the number of deleted α-globin genes. In addition to α thalassemia caused by gene deletion, *rs7203560* in *NPRL3* was associated with hemolysis after adjusting for the presence of gene deletion α thalassemia.[119] It was speculated that rs7203560 tagged enhancer variants that downregulated α-globin gene expression. Two other variants in the α-globin gene regulatory elements, rs11865131 and *rs11248850*, appeared to upregulate gene expression and were not associated with hemolysis.[120] In sickle cell anemia–α thalassemia, *rs11248850* and rs11865131 nullified the hemolysis-reducing effect of α thalassemia.[121] Regulatory elements of the α-globin gene cluster can up- or downregulate gene expression, and variants of these elements might account for some of the phenotypic heterogeneity of sickle cell anemia.

TABLE 1-2 **Association of HbF with subphenotypes of sickle cell anemia**

Subphenotype	Effects of HbF
Survival	High HbF prolongs survival in most untreated and hydroxyurea-treated cases
Painful episodes/dactylitis	High HbF reduces incidence
Acute chest syndrome	High HbF reduces rate
Leg ulcers	High HbF is protective
Osteonecrosis	Equivocal evidence for a protective effect
Priapism	Little or no evidence of a protective effect
Renal function/albuminuria	Little or no evidence of a protective effect
Cerebrovascular disease	Some evidence of a protective effect in infants; little evidence of protection in adults
Splenic sequestration/splenic function	Low HbF increases risk of sequestration and is associated with earlier loss of function; high HbF protective
Bacteremia	Little or no evidence of a protective effect
Cholelithiasis	High HbF protective
Retinopathy	Low HbF possibly increases capillary occlusion
Sickle vasculopathy/tricuspid regurgitant jet velocity	Little or no evidence of a protective effect
Pregnancy/perinatal death	Decreased risk
Erythrocyte survival	High intracellular HbF concentration increases red blood cell life span
Hemoglobin level	High HbF associated with increased level

Note. For most subphenotypes, both children and adults are included. The studies cited contain the largest sample size and the most rigorous experimental design, but no attempt was made to be exhaustive.[159]

Table 1-3 summarizes the effects of α thalassemia on the common subphenotypes of sickle cell anemia. Heterogeneity among patient populations that occasionally included individuals with HbSC disease and HbS-β+ thalassemia in addition to those with sickle cell anemia and small samples of different ages have resulted in some diversity of reported results. Because α thalassemia is an important determinant of hemolysis, its presence is usually associated with fewer complications that have been linked to intravascular hemolysis.[122] Paradoxically, patients with sickle cell anemia–α thalassemia do not have a reduction and might have an increase in vaso-occlusive complications, and this has been ascribed to increased blood viscosity that results from the higher hemoglobin level in sickle cell anemia patients with α thalassemia. In contrast to the results in patients with African-origin sickle cell anemia, a study of 2 groups of Indian patients with the Arab-Indian haplotype with similarly high HbF and F cell numbers found that fewer painful events and hospitalizations occurred in patients with coincident α thalassemia.[123]

Genetic Modulation by Nonglobin Genes

Both focused candidate gene–based association studies and agnostic GWASs studying the relationship between genetic variants and subphenotypes of sickle cell anemia have returned results far less conclusive than studies of HbF and α thalassemia. Most of the studies have not been replicated and suffer from small sample sizes, difficulty in precise phenotyping, small effects of the genetic variant on a phenotype, and problems of interpretation including adjustments for multiplicity. Apart from these factors, HbF and

TABLE 1-3 Associations of α thalassemia with subphenotypes of sickle cell anemia

Subphenotype	Effects of α thalassemia
Overall severity	Probably little effect
Stroke, silent infarction, transcranial Doppler velocity	Reduces risk
Painful episodes	Increases risk
Acute chest syndrome	Increases risk
Bacteremia	No effect
Osteonecrosis	Increases risk
Priapism	Reduces risk
Leg ulcers	Reduces risk
Sickle vasculopathy/tricuspid regurgitant jet velocity	Equivocal
Splenic sequestration/function	Reduces risk
Cholelithiasis	Reduces risk
Renal function/albuminuria/ glomerular hyperfiltration	Reduces risk
Retinopathy	Possibly reduces capillary occlusion

Note. Heterogeneity among populations of patients with sickle cell anemia, the study of small patient samples, inhomogeneity of the cohorts that sometimes include individuals with HbSC disease and HbS-β⁺ thalassemia, and age differences among subjects in different studies have resulted in some reports that diverge from the majority conclusions that are cited in this table. Data from references are in Steinberg and Sebastiani.[159]

α thalassemia have greater impact because they modify the process of HbS polymerization itself, HbF directly, and α thalassemia indirectly. In addition, high HbF is very common, and α thalassemia has a high gene frequency.

Regulation of Erythrocyte Volume

A heterogeneous red cell population is typical of sickle cell disease. Low-density cells include reticulocytes, and high-density cells can have an MCH concentration (MCHC) of 50 g/dL. Because the hematology and pathophysiology of sickle cell disease are driven by HbS polymerization, which in turn is affected by the cellular HbS concentration or cell density, it might be expected that mutations that increase cell density or reduce hydration will have phenotypic repercussions.[124] Common (or even rare) variants of the well-characterized Gardos channel (KCNN4) and K-Cl cotransport channels (KCC1, KCC3, KCC4) have not been associated with hematologic or clinical heterogeneity in sickle cell anemia.[125] In a secondary exploratory analysis, dense sickle cells were associated with an intronic variant of the calcium transporter ATPase, ATP2B4.

A mechanosensitive and deoxygenation-activated cation transport channel, or P^{sickle}, might be the product of the gene PIEZO1. A gain-of-function variant of this gene, E756del (rs572934641), is present in one-third of people of African descent and protects against malaria.[126] In 788 patients with sickle cell disease (sickle cell anemia or HbSC), there was no correlation between E756del and cation leak measured by P^{sickle} and hemoglobin, reticulocyte count and MCHC, or hospital admissions.[127] Based on whole-exome sequencing in 226 sickle cell disease patients, the E756del allele was associated with increased cell density, a result replicated in 375 additional patient samples based on imputation of the E756del genotype. There was no association with several markers of hemolysis, renal function, priapism, or leg ulcers. A polygenic score including genetic variants of PIEZO1, ATP2B4, and the rare variants of KCNN4 explained 6.3% of erythrocyte density variance.[128]

Despite the critical relationship between erythrocyte density and HbS polymerization, genetic variants affecting cell hydration have not yet been linked to hematologic or clinical heterogeneity of sickle cell disease, other than perhaps small differences in cell density.

Pain

Based on concordant genotype-phenotype studies in 3 independent cohorts, supported by in vivo physiologic studies in sickle cell anemia patients and bolstered by a firm scientific rationale provided by animal studies, the most robust genetic association with sickle cell pain is with variants of GCH1. This gene encodes a guanosine triphosphate cyclohydrolase and is rate limiting for tetrahydrobiopterin (BH4) synthesis. BH4 is a cofactor for NO synthases. In a discovery cohort of 228 patients and a replication cohort of 513 patients, rs8007267 in the promoter of GCH1 was a risk factor for pain crises. Cells from sickle cell anemia patients homozygous for the risk allele produced higher BH4. In vivo physiologic studies of traits likely to be modulated by GCH1 showed rs8007267 was associated with altered endothelial-dependent blood flow in females with sickle cell anemia. The GCH1 pain association was limited to females and attributable to a distinct African haplotype.[129] Independent studies of 131 patients with different genotypes of sickle cell disease confirmed the association of rs8007267 in GCH1 with acute care utilization rate and with chronic pain.[130]

In other studies, 16 SNPs in ADRB2, the β$_2$-adrenergic receptor that mediates neurotransmitter response in the sympathetic nervous system, were evaluated for their association with a chronic pain score in 136 patients, and 7 SNPs showed an association with either increased or decreased scores accounting for 2% to 15% of variance.[131] NR3C1, a glucocorticoid receptor gene, was associated with acute pain.[130] Rs3115229 in KIAA1109 located 63.7 kb upstream of this gene at 4q27 within an LD block of 4 genes, 3 of which were associated with inflammatory disease, was associated with acute painful events.[132] Forty variants in 17 pain-related genes were genotyped in 436 young Cameroonian patients, and 3 SNPs correlated with vaso-occlusive episodes and 5 SNPs correlated with hospitalization or consultation.[48] Haptoglobin HP-2 genotype was associated with pain in 199 children with sickle cell disease, an observation replicated in an additional 458 children.[133]

Pain, acute and chronic, is complex and likely to have multifactorial causes and is the most prominent clinical feature of sickle cell disease. Acute and chronic pain often coexist and can be difficult to separate. The imprecise nature of pain phenotypes and the huge impact of social and environmental elements make it hard to study pain in genetic association studies, and this is reflected in the underwhelming results of both candidate gene studies and GWASs of pain.

Hemolysis

Intravascular hemolysis is closely associated with many complications of sickle cell disease (Chapter 4). A hemolytic component that included reticulocyte count, lactate dehydrogenase, aspartate aminotransferase, and bilirubin levels was used in a genetic association study of 4 independent cohorts totaling >2000 patients. *Rs7203560* in *NPRL3* was associated with hemolysis independently of gene deletion α thalassemia or HbF level, leading to the hypothesis that regulatory loci tagged by *rs7203560* downregulated expression of these genes.

Bilirubin and Cholelithiasis

Unsurprisingly, considering the results of many previous studies, serum bilirubin levels and cholelithiasis were strongly associated with SNPs in *UGT1A1*. These studies included more than 4000 sickle cell disease patients, making them some of the largest of this type in this disease.[134]

Cerebrovascular Disease

Of the clinical subphenotypes of sickle cell disease, the clearest association markers have been found for stroke. In 130 stroke patients and 103 controls with sickle cell anemia, in addition to the known association of α thalassemia with reduced stroke risk, SNPs in *ANXA2*, *TEK*, *ADCY9*, and *TGFBR3* were associated with the risk of stroke. For 114 subjects not included in the original analysis, this model predicted the correct outcome for all 7 individuals with stroke and for 105 of 107 subjects without stroke, for an overall predictive accuracy of 98%.[135] Importantly, partial replication of this association was confirmed in an independent cohort in which 38 candidate SNPs in 22 genes were typed in 130 pediatric patients with thrombotic stroke and 103 patients without stroke. SNPs in the *ANXA2*, *TGFBR3*, and *TEK* genes were associated with increased stroke risk. α Thalassemia and an SNP in *ADCY9* were associated with a decreased stroke risk.[136] Other studies have associated different SNPs in *VCAM1* with increased and decreased risk of stroke.[137,138]

Other Subphenotypes

Multiple subphenotypes have been associated with several genes of the very large transforming growth factor-β (TGF-β)/Smad/bone morphogenetic protein (BMP) pathway that regulates diverse cellular processes important in the pathophysiology of sickle cell disease, including inflammation, fibrosis, cell proliferation and hematopoiesis, osteogenesis, angiogenesis, wound healing, and the immune response. GWASs, which provide an unbiased assessment of the genetic association with a phenotype, have not replicated candidate gene–based results, perhaps because the contribution of these variants to the phenotype is small.

Other genes outside of the globin gene clusters that have been associated with subphenotypes of sickle cell disease or with hematologic changes are shown in Table 1-4.

In genetic association studies, the phenotype must be sharply defined and consistently measured to differentiate cases from controls. This is often difficult because many complications are subjective without the precision needed for genetic association studies and some have a continuum of manifestations. For example, as discussed earlier for the pain phenotype, candidate gene studies and GWASs have often not returned replicable results. In contrast, laboratory phenotypes that can be reliably measured and analyzed as a continuous variable are more likely to be successful. Traits that are highly heritable with genetic regulation limited to a reasonably small set of genes with large effects on the phenotype have the highest chance of success, with prime examples being HbF and serum bilirubin.

Reversing the Hemoglobin Switch: Therapeutic Possibilities

The sole "cure" for sickle cell disease is hematopoietic stem cell transplantation from matched sibling donors, which has a success rate >95%. Unfortunately, this option is available to <15% of patients in the United States.[139] An alternative donor source that is being improved upon is haploidentical family members.[140] Genetic therapy uses the patient's own bone marrow stem cells (autologous stem cells) and is currently centered on mitigating HbS polymerization through synthesis of "antisickling" β-globin or induction of HbF.[141] Figure 1-6 displays current and potential genome-editing targets that include the β-globin gene itself, *BCL11A*, and the γ-globin gene promoters. The most promising of the gene addition approaches transfers lentiviral vectors containing an antisickling β-globin vector containing the HbA[T87Q] mutation and has been studied for >2 decades, with progress in β thalassemia exceeding that in sickle cell anemia.[142,143] Nevertheless, recent trials in sickle cell anemia resulted in nearly 50% HbA[T87Q], hemoglobin concentrations between 10 and 15 g/dL, and resolution of symptoms.[144]

A variety of genome editing approaches to induce HbF could be exploited based on delineation of the mechanisms involved in hemoglobin switching, coupled with recent progress in genome editing techniques.[145] Two phase I/II trials in sickle cell anemia aim to disrupt the *BCL11A* erythroid-specific enhancer[53] in patient CD34+ cells using CRISPR/Cas and zinc finger nucleases, thereby derepressing *HBG2/1* (ClinicalTrials. gov identifiers: NCT03745287 and NCT03653247). Another

TABLE 1-4 Genes outside of the globin gene clusters associated with subphenotypes of sickle cell anemia

Subphenotypes	Genes and effects
Survival	Multiple genes, including *TGFBR3*
Stroke, silent infarction	Multiple genes increase or decrease likelihood, including *VCAM1, ILR4, ADBR2, HLA, LDLR, ENPP1, GOLGB1* (see text)
Acute and chronic pain	*GCH1, KIAA1109, ADRB2, NR3C1, MBL2, CACNA2D3, DRD2, KCNS1, COMT, FAAH, OPRM1, ADRB2, UGT2B7, FAM193A, PLA2G4A, IL1A, LGALS3, HP* (see text) Single nucleotide polymorphisms could be associated with increased or decreased pain, and some associations were limited to children
Acute chest syndrome	Genes have been identified, eg, *COMMD7, HMOX1, NOS1, VEGFA,* but few studies have been validated
Bacteremia/infection	*MBL2;* contradictory evidence in different populations that it is low level protective Other genes include *CCL5,* various HLA alleles, *IGF1R,* TGF-β/SMAD/BMP pathway
Osteonecrosis	*MTHFR* (weak evidence) *BMP6;* results validated in 2 different populations
Priapism	*KL, TEK, TGFBR3, AQP1*
Leg ulcers	TGF-β/SMAD/BMP pathway, *KL,* possibly HLA alleles
Sickle vasculopathy/tricuspid regurgitant jet velocity	*BMP6, TGFBR3, ACVR1, BMP2, THBS1, DRD2*
Cholelithiasis	Promoter repeats in *UGT1A1* associated with serum bilirubin and gallstones
Renal function/albuminuria/glomerular hyperfiltration	*DARC* FY (associated with proteinuria), TGF-β/Smad/BMP pathway, *MYH9, APOL1, HMOX1, AGGF1, CYP4B1, TOR2A, PKD1L2, CD163*
Multiple subphenotypes	Duffy antigen receptor (*DARC*); no relationship to leg ulcers, nephropathy, priapism, osteonecrosis, response to opioids
Erythrocyte density	*ATP2B4, PIEZO1* increase cell density (see text)
Alloimmunization	HLA locus, chr5 rs75853687, *FCGR2C, CTLA4*
Hemolysis	*HBA2/1* deletions, *NPRL3, ADCY6* improve red cell survival

Note. These reports include primarily HbS homozygotes. Most studies are small, and their results should be considered exploratory because they often do not correct for coexistent α thalassemia, HbF level, age, sex, and multiplicity of testing. Mechanistic and functional studies to follow up these correlation analyses are nearly always lacking. Data from Steinberg and Sebastiani,[159] Piel et al,[160] Rodrigues et al,[161] Oliveira et al,[162] Williams and Thein,[163] and UpToDate (https://www.uptodate.com/contents/clinical-variability-in-sickle-cell-anemia).

approach to reducing expression of *BCL11A* involves a lentiviral vector containing lineage-specific short hairpin RNA suppressing *BCL11A* in erythroid cells (ClinicalTrials.gov identifier: NCT03282656).[146] An additional HbF-inducing lentiviral-based approach uses artificial transcription factors to "force" interaction between the γ-globin promoter and the LCR to engage high-level γ-globin gene expression.[147] An added advantage of the "forced looping" approach is the concomitant reduction in synthesis of β^S from the *cis* chromosome. An alternative gene editing approach for HbF elevation would be to mimic naturally occurring alleles associated with HPFH.[148-150] Disruption of the sites in the −200 and −115 regions upstream of *HBG1/2*, which are binding sites for the

transcription repressors ZBTB7A and BCL11A, are attractive targets for mimicking HPFH.

Early results of 2 trials targeting the *BCL11A* enhancer have been reported. One trial used autologous CD34+ cells that were edited with CRISPR-Cas9 using a guide RNA specific for the enhancer and demonstrated an increase of HbF from a baseline of 9.1% to 48% after 9 months, >99% F cells, a hemoglobin of 11 g/dL, and cessation of sickle vaso-occlusion.[151] In the other study, 3 patients treated with lentiviral-mediated shRNA knockdown of *BCL11A* were followed for 15 months; HbF ranged from 23.7% to 40.7%, F cells ranged from 67.7% to 76.4%, total hemoglobin was >11 g/dL, and acute vaso-occlusive events stopped.[152]

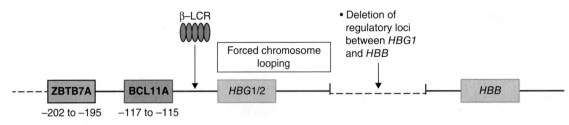

HbF induction –
1. Reducing *BCL11A* expression
   - BCL11A RNAi
   - Disruption of erythroid-specific BCL11A
2. Mimic HPFH variants
   - Recreate HPFH disruption of binding motifs for ZBTB7A or BCL11A
3. Forced chromosome looping using artificial transcription factors
   to engage high-level *HBG* expression

FIGURE 1-6 Genomic editing to reverse the hemoglobin switch. The *HBB* cluster showing regions affecting the fetal-to-adult hemo-globin switch that are being studied as possible loci for genomic manipulation to reverse this switch. HPFH, hereditary persistence of fetal hemoglobin; RNAi, RNA interference.

Delineation of the regulatory circuit in hemoglobin switching has also presented several therapeutic pharmacologic targets for HbF induction. Inhibition of lysine-specific histone demethylase 1 (LSD1) using RNA interference or by application of the monoamine oxidase inhibitor tranylcypromine in CD34+ cells resulted in increased HbF. Small-molecule inhibitors of LSD1 induced HbF in CD34+ cells, reduced sickling in transgenic sickle mice, and increased HbF in erythroid progeny of induced pluripotent stem cells from a patient with sickle cell disease.[153] Targeting DNA modification enzymes and chromatin remodelers is another promising pharmacotherapeutic approach for HbF induction. Inhibition of the histone lysine methyltransferases EHMT1 and EHMT2 prevents demethylation of H3K9, derepressing *HBG2/1* and inducing HbF. An orally available agent is highly selective and increases Pol II occupancy at the *HBG2/1* promoter in CD34+ cells while activating H3K9Ac. In a phase I trial (ClinicalTrials.gov identifier: NCT01685515), inhibition of DNA methyl transferase (DNMT1), a repressor of *HBG2/1* expression, using decitabine and tetrahydrouridine increased HbF 4% to 9%, with a larger increase in F cells, while markers of hemolysis improved and total hemoglobin increased 1 to 2 g/dL.[154] Histone deacetylase inhibitors targeting HDAC1 and HDAC2 are being evaluated as potential pharmacotherapeutic targets for reactivating HbF.[155]

Conclusion

The clinical and hematologic features of sickle cell disease are exceptionally diverse for a single-gene Mendelian disorder. Although obvious clinical differences exist among the most common genotypes of disease, within a single hemoglobin genotype such as sickle cell anemia, there is also clinical heterogeneity. The amount of HbF and its distribution among erythrocytes are the major modulators of disease severity because HbF inhibits the primary pathophysiologic process of HbS polymerization. α Thalassemia is the other major modulator of severity because of its effect on HbS concentration. Although it is highly likely that nonglobin genes play roles in the heterogeneity of phenotypic expression, conclusive evidence of these roles has been scant.

An increasingly complete understanding of switching in the *HBB* gene cluster has led to novel approaches to reversing the hemoglobin isotype switch in the *HBB* gene cluster, which has great therapeutic potential in β hemoglobinopathies.

Case Studies

Case 1. A 35-year-old woman was referred because of abnormal findings on a blood count obtained during preoperative screening. Her medical history was negative, and her physical examination was normal. Her children, ages 4 and 8 years, were normal. Hemoglobin concentration was 12.2 g/dL, MCV was 71 fL, and reticulocyte count was 1%. High-performance liquid chromatography (HPLC) examination of her hemoglobin showed 68% HbS, 30% HbF, and 2% HbA₂. HPLC of the children showed one with 59% HbA, 37% HbS, <1% HbF, and 3% HbA₂ and the other with 58% HbA, 30% HbF, and 2% HbA₂. The proband has sickle cell–HPFH, with a large deletion in her β-globin gene cluster that removed *HBB* and *HBD* but preserved *HBG2/1*. HbF was distributed pancellularly, endowing each erythrocyte with sufficient HbF to prevent HbS polymerization. Thus, despite an HbS concentration of nearly 70%, she had no signs or symptoms of sickle cell disease, and

Case Studies: Continued

except for microcytosis due to the failure of *HBG2/1* expression to equal that of *HBB* expression, she was normal hematologically. Because her husband was normal, each child had a 50% chance of having either sickle cell trait or the HPFH gene. In contrast to this case, compound heterozygotes for HbS and δβ thalassemia can have nearly identical findings on HPLC but have hemolytic anemia and symptoms of sickle cell disease because their erythrocyte HbF distribution is heterocellular.

Case 2. Dizygotic twin brothers with sickle cell anemia had distinctly different disease phenotypes. Their clinical and hematologic findings are shown next:

	Patient 1	Patient 2
Acute painful episodes	Uncommon	Frequent
Stroke	Yes	No
Leg ulcers	Yes	No
Tricuspid regurgitant velocity (m/s)	3.0	2.3
Hemoglobin (g/dL)	7.0	9.5
Reticulocytes (%)	18	7
MCV (fL)	100	80
Creatinine (g/dL)	1.6	0.7
Lactate dehydrogenase (IU)	550	220
HbF; HbA$_2$ (%)	5.0; 3.5	5.0; 4.5

Both patients were homozygous for the HbS gene; patient 2 was also homozygous for the $^{-3.7}$α-globin gene deletion, which is inherited independently of the HbS gene. As a result of coincident α thalassemia, there was a reduction in mean cell HbS concentration and improved circulatory competence of his erythrocytes. This reduction in hemolysis likely contributes to protection from cerebrovascular disease, pulmonary vasculopathy, and nephropathy. In contrast, increased hemoglobin level is often associated with more acute painful episodes because of increased blood viscosity. In sickle cell anemia–α thalassemia, HbA$_2$ is elevated because δ-globin chains compete more effectively than sickle β-globin chains for α-globin chains that are present in limiting amounts.

Case 3. During a visit to an obstetrician to discuss planning her first pregnancy, a 23-year-old woman with sickle cell trait was reassured that because her partner did not have sickle cell trait, she could not have an affected infant. After delivery, cord blood screening showed that her infant had an HbSF pattern, and follow-up HPLC studies at age 1 year showed 76% HbS, 20% HbF, and 4% HbA$_2$. Retesting her partner showed a hemoglobin of 13 g/dL, MCV of 62 fL, HbA of 94%, HbF of 1%, and HbA$_2$ of 5%, consistent with β thalassemia trait and suggesting that the infant had HbS-β^0 thalassemia. If one prospective partner has sickle cell trait, it is mandatory to have blood counts and HPLC done on the other prospective partner so that the odds of having an affected infant and the available reproductive options can be discussed and further testing done if indicated.

Case 4. A 38-year-old man presented with a 6-month history of worsening pruritis, jaundice, and ascites. He was previously well, rarely drank alcohol, and was not on regular medications or herbal remedies. Extensive workup for causes of liver disease was negative. Hematology showed the following: hemoglobin 10.5 g/dL, MCV 76.3 fL, and MCH 27.9 pg. Hemoglobin HPLC showed HbS of 49.6%, HbA of 41.3%, HbA$_2$ of 2.8%, and HbF of 0.5%. The patient had not received any blood transfusion. Although these results could easily be misinterpreted as the patient having HbS trait, the increase of HbS over HbA suggests compound heterozygosity for HbS and β thalassemia. DNA and family studies were pursued. The proband was a compound heterozygote for β^S and a novel very mild β thalassemia mutation (β IVS2-844 C-A), which was transmitted to both of his sons, and the liver pathology was ascribed as being related to sickle cell disease. His wife had completely normal hemoglobin profile and blood counts. One son had hemoglobin of 12.1 g/dL, MCV of 72.2 fL, MCH of 23.9 pg, HbA$_2$ of 3.5%, HbF of 0.4%, HbA of 96%, and heterozygosity for β IVS2-844 C-A. The other son had hemoglobin of 12.9 g/dL, MCV of 74.4 fL, MCH of 25.4 pg, HbA$_2$ of 3.9%, HbF of 0.7%, HbA of 95%, and heterozygosity for β IVS2-844 C-A. Rare compound heterozygotes with β^S and very mild β thalassemia mutations (β^S/β^{++} thalassemia) can mimic HbS carriers but with a reversed HbA/HbS ratio.

High-Yield Facts

◆ Coincident α thalassemia reduces the intensity of hemolysis in sickle cell anemia and the incidence of disease complications closely associated with hemolytic anemia, such as pulmonary and systemic vasculopathy, nephropathy, and leg ulcers.

◆ Patients with sickle cell anemia and similar HbF levels can have divergent clinical courses due to uneven and different distributions of HbF among their erythrocytes.

◆ Clinical features of HbS-HPFH and polymerization modeling experiments suggest that >25% HbF in a pancellular expression pattern could "cure" sickle cell disease.

◆ Variations in 3 QTLs, *BCL11A*, *MYB*, and a locus linked to the *HBB* cluster, account for a major portion of HbF variation among normal individuals and patients with sickle cell anemia.

◆ Delineation of the fetal-to-adult hemoglobin switching regulatory circuit has provided rational targets for directed genome editing and development of drugs for therapeutic induction of HbF.

References

1. Hardison R. Organization, evolution, and regulation of the globin genes. In: Steinberg MH, Forget BG, Higgs DR, Nagel RL, eds. *Disorders of Hemoglobin: Genetics, Pathophysiology, and Clinical Management.* Cambridge University Press; 2001:95-116.

2. Perutz MF, Rossmann MG, Cullis AF, Muirhead H, Will G, North ACT. Structure of haemoglobin: a three-dimensional fourier synthesis at 5.5-Å. resolution, obtained by x-ray analysis. *Nature.* 1960;185(4711):416-422.

3. Kim-Shapiro DB. Structure and function of hemoglobin and its dysfunction in sickle cell disease. In: Steinberg MH, Forget BG, Higgs DR, Weatherall DJ, eds. *Disorders of Hemoglobin: Genetics, Pathophysiology, and Clinical Management.* 2nd ed. Cambridge University Press; 2009:101-118.

4. Gilman JG, Huisman THJ. DNA sequence variation associated with elevated fetal ^{G}g globin production. *Blood.* 1985;66:783-787.

5. Weber L, Frati G, Felix T, et al. Editing a γ-globin repressor binding site restores fetal hemoglobin synthesis and corrects the sickle cell disease phenotype. *Sci Adv.* 2020;6:eaay9392.

6. Pauling L. Foreward. In: Embury SH, Hebbel RP, Mohandas N, Steinberg MH, eds. *Sickle Cell Disease: Basic Principles and Clinical Practice.* Lippincott-Raven; 1994:xvii-xix.

7. Ranney HM. Historical milestones In: Embury SH, Hebbel RP, Mohandas N, Steinberg MH, eds. *Sickle Cell Disease: Basic Principles and Clinical Practice.* Lippincott-Raven; 1994:1-5.

8. Nagel RL, Steinberg MH. Genetics of the β^S gene: origins, genetic epidemiology, and epistasis in sickle cell anemia. In: Steinberg MH, Forget BG, Higgs DR, Nagel RL, eds. *Disorders of Hemoglobin: Genetics, Pathophysiology, and Clinical Management.* Cambridge University Press; 2001:711-755.

9. Pauling L, Itano HA, Singer SJ, Wells IC. Sickle cell anemia: a molecular disease. *Science.* 1949;110(2685):543-548.

10. Ingram VM. Gene mutations in human haemoglobin: the chemical difference between normal and sickle cell haemoglobin. *Nature.* 1957;180(4581):326-328.

11. Goldstein J, Konigsberg W, Hill RJ. The structure of human hemoglobin: VI. The sequence of amino acids in the tryptic peptides of the β chain. *J Biol Chem.* 1963;238(6):2016-2027.

12. Shriner D, Rotimi CN. Whole-genome-sequence-based haplotypes reveal single origin of the sickle allele during the Holocene Wet Phase. *Am J Hum Genet.* 2018;102(4):547-556.

13. Laval G, Peyregne S, Zidane N, et al. Recent adaptive acquisition by African rainforest hunter-gatherers of the late Pleistocene sickle-cell mutation suggests past differences in malaria exposure. *Am J Hum Genet.* 2019;104(3):553-561.

14. Philipsen S, Hardison RC. Evolution of hemoglobin loci and their regulatory elements. *Blood Cells Mol Dis.* 2018;70:2-12. doi:10.1016/j.bcmd.2017.08.001

15. Bank A. Regulation of human fetal hemoglobin: new players, new complexities. *Blood.* 2006;107(2):435-443.

16. Kiefer CM, Hou C, Little JA, Dean A. Epigenetics of beta-globin gene regulation. *Mutat Res.* 2008;647(1-2):68-76.

17. Raich N, Enver T, Nakamoto B, Josephson B, Papayannopoulou T, Stamatoyannopoulos G. Autonomous developmental control of human embryonic globin gene switching in transgenic mice. *Science.* 1990;250:1147-1149.

18. Thein SL, Wood WG. The molecular basis of β thalassemia, δβ thalassemia, and hereditary persistence of fetal hemoglobin. In: Steinberg MH, Forget BG, Higgs DR, Weatherall DJ, eds. *Disorders of Hemoglobin: Genetics, Pathophysiology, and Clinical Management.* 2nd ed. Cambridge University Press; 2009:323-356.

19. Giardine B, Borg J, Higgs DR, et al. Systematic documentation and analysis of human genetic variation in hemoglobinopathies using the microattribution approach. *Nat Genet.* 2011;43(4):295-301.

20. Moi P, Faa V, Marini MG, et al. A novel silent beta-thalassemia mutation in the distal CACCC box affects the binding and responsiveness to EKLF. *Br J Haematol.* 2004;126(6):881-884.

21. Menzel S, Garner C, Gut I, et al. A QTL influencing F cell production maps to a gene encoding a zinc-finger protein on chromosome 2p15. *Nat Genet.* 2007;39(10):1197-1199.

22. Uda M, Galanello R, Sanna S, et al. Genome-wide association study shows BCL11A associated with persistent fetal hemoglobin and amelioration of the phenotype of beta-thalassemia. *Proc Natl Acad Sci USA.* 2008;105(5):1620-1625.

23. Masuda T, Wang X, Maeda M, et al. Transcription factors LRF and BCL11A independently repress expression of fetal hemoglobin. *Science.* 2016;351(6270):285-289.

24. Higgs DR. The molecular basis of alpha-thalassemia. *Cold Spring Harb Perspect Med.* 2013;3(1):a011718.

25. King AJ, Higgs DR. Potential new approaches to the management of the Hb Bart's hydrops fetalis syndrome: the most severe form of alpha-thalassemia. *Hematology Am Soc Hematol Educ Program.* 2018;2018(1):353-360.

26. Garner C, Tatu T, Reittie JE, et al. Genetic influences on F cells and other hematologic variables: a twin heritability study. *Blood.* 2000;95(1):342-346.

27. Sankaran VG, Menne TF, Xu J, et al. Human fetal hemoglobin expression is regulated by the developmental stage-specific repressor BCL11A. *Science.* 2008;322(5909):1839-1842.

28. Sankaran VG, Xu J, Ragoczy T, et al. Developmental and species-divergent globin switching are driven by BCL11A. *Nature.* 2009; 460(7259):1093-1097.

29. Xu J, Peng C, Sankaran VG, et al. Correction of sickle cell disease in adult mice by interference with fetal hemoglobin silencing. *Science.* 2011;334(6058):993-996.

30. Jawaid K, Wahlberg K, Thein SL, Best S. Binding patterns of BCL11A in the globin and GATA1 loci and characterization of the BCL11A fetal hemoglobin locus. *Blood Cells Mol Dis.* 2010;45(2):140-146.

31. Xu J, Sankaran VG, Ni M, et al. Transcriptional silencing of {gamma}-globin by BCL11A involves long-range interactions and cooperation with SOX6. *Genes Dev.* 2010;24(8):783-798.

32. Liu N, Hargreaves VV, Zhu Q, et al. Direct promoter repression by BCL11A controls the fetal to adult hemoglobin switch. *Cell.* 2018;173(2):430-442.e17.

33. Martyn GE, Wienert B, Yang L, et al. Natural regulatory mutations elevate the fetal globin gene via disruption of BCL11A or ZBTB7A binding. *Nat Genet.* 2018;50(4):498-503.

34. Bianchi E, Zini R, Salati S, et al. c-Myb supports erythropoiesis through the transactivation of KLF1 and LMO2 expression. *Blood.* 2010;116(22):e99-110.

35. Borg J, Papadopoulos P, Georgitsi M, et al. Haploinsufficiency for the erythroid transcription factor KLF1 causes hereditary persistence of fetal hemoglobin. *Nat Genet.* 2010;42(9):801-805.

36. Zhou D, Liu K, Sun CW, Pawlik KM, Townes TM. KLF1 regulates BCL11A expression and gamma- to beta-globin gene switching. *Nat Genet.* 2010;42(9):742-744.

37. Norton LJ, Funnell APW, Burdach J, et al. KLF1 directly activates expression of the novel fetal globin repressor ZBTB7A/LRF in erythroid cells. *Blood Adv.* 2017;1(11):685-692.

38. Nuez B, Michalovich D, Bygrave A, Ploemacher R, Grosveld F. Defective haematopoiesis in fetal liver resulting from inactivation of the EKLF gene. *Nature.* 1995;375(6529):316-318.

39. Perkins AC, Sharpe AH, Orkin SH. Lethal b-thalassaemia in mice lacking the erythroid CACCC-transcription factor EKLF. *Nature.* 1995;375(6529):318-322.

40. Menzel S, Thein SL. Genetic modifiers of fetal haemoglobin in sickle cell disease. *Mol Diagn Ther.* 2019;23(2):235-244.

41. Thein SL, Menzel S, Lathrop M, Garner C. Control of fetal hemoglobin: new insights emerging from genomics and clinical implications. *Hum Mol Genet.* 2009;18(R2):R216-R223.

42. Thein SL, Weatherall DJ. A non-deletion hereditary persistence of fetal hemoglobin (HPFH) determinant not linked to the beta-globin gene complex. In: Stamatoyannopoulos G, Nienhuis AW, eds. *Hemoglobin Switching, Part B: Cellular and Molecular Mechanisms.* Alan R Liss, Inc.; 1989:97-111.

43. Yu Y, Wang J, Khaled W, et al. Bcl11a is essential for lymphoid development and negatively regulates p53. *J Exp Med.* 2012;209(13):2467-2483.

44. Liu P, Keller JR, Ortiz M, et al. Bcl11a is essential for normal lymphoid development. *Nat Immunol.* 2003;4(6):525-532.

45. Yin B, Delwel R, Valk PJ, et al. A retroviral mutagenesis screen reveals strong cooperation between Bcl11a overexpression and loss of the Nf1 tumor suppressor gene. *Blood.* 2009;113(5):1075-1085.

46. Bhanushali AA, Patra PK, Nair D, Verma H, Das BR. Genetic variant in the BCL11A (rs1427407), but not HBS1-MYB (rs6934903) loci associate with fetal hemoglobin levels in Indian sickle cell disease patients. *Blood Cells Mol Dis.* 2015;54(1):4-8.

47. Menzel S, Rooks H, Zelenika D, et al. Global genetic architecture of an erythroid quantitative trait locus, HMIP-2. *Ann Hum Genet.* 2014;78(6):434-451.

48. Wonkam A, Mnika K, Ngo Bitoungui VJ, et al. Clinical and genetic factors are associated with pain and hospitalisation rates in sickle cell anaemia in Cameroon. *Br J Haematol.* 2018;180(1):134-146.

49. Wonkam A, Ngo Bitoungui VJ, Vorster AA, et al. Association of variants at BCL11A and HBS1L-MYB with hemoglobin F and hospitalization rates among sickle cell patients in Cameroon. *PLoS One.* 2014;9(3):e92506.

50. Mtatiro SN, Mgaya J, Singh T, et al. Genetic association of fetal-hemoglobin levels in individuals with sickle cell disease in Tanzania maps to conserved regulatory elements within the MYB core enhancer. *BMC Med Genet.* 2015;16(1):4.

51. Gardner K, Fulford T, Silver N, et al. g(HbF): a genetic model of fetal hemoglobin in sickle cell disease. *Blood Adv.* 2018;2(3):235-239.

52. Bauer DE, Kamran SC, Lessard S, et al. An erythroid enhancer of BCL11A subject to genetic variation determines fetal hemoglobin level. *Science.* 2013;342(6155):253-257.

53. Canver MC, Smith EC, Sher F, et al. BCL11A enhancer dissection by Cas9-mediated in situ saturating mutagenesis. *Nature.* 2015;527(7577):192-197.

54. Das SS, Mitra A, Chakravorty N. Diseases and their clinical heterogeneity: are we ignoring the SNiPers and micRomaNAgers? An illustration using beta-thalassemia clinical spectrum and fetal hemoglobin levels. *Genomics.* 2019;111(1):67-75.

55. Das SS, Chakravorty N. Identification of deleterious SNPs and their effects on BCL11A, the master regulator of fetal hemoglobin expression. *Genomics.* 2020;112(1):397-403.

56. Basak A, Hancarova M, Ulirsch JC, et al. BCL11A deletions result in fetal hemoglobin persistence and neurodevelopmental alterations. *J Clin Invest.* 2015;125(6):2363-2368.

57. Funnell AP, Prontera P, Ottaviani V, et al. 2p15-p16.1 microdeletions encompassing and proximal to BCL11A are associated with elevated HbF in addition to neurologic impairment. *Blood.* 2015;126(1):89-93.

58. Dias C, Estruch SB, Graham SA, et al. BCL11A haploinsufficiency causes an intellectual disability syndrome and dysregulates transcription. *Am J Hum Genet.* 2016;99(2):253-274.

59. Yoshida M, Nakashima M, Okanishi T, et al. Identification of novel BCL11A variants in patients with epileptic encephalopathy: expanding the phenotypic spectrum. *Clin Genet.* 2018;93(2):368-373.

60. Thein SL, Menzel S, Peng X, et al. Intergenic variants of HBS1L-MYB are responsible for a major quantitative trait locus on chromosome 6q23 influencing fetal hemoglobin levels in adults. *Proc Natl Acad Sci USA.* 2007;104(27):11346-11351.

61. Stadhouders R, Aktuna S, Thongjuea S, et al. HBS1L-MYB intergenic variants modulate fetal hemoglobin via long-range MYB enhancers. *J Clin Invest.* 2014;124(4):1699-1710.

62. Canver MC, Lessard S, Pinello L, et al. Variant-aware saturating mutagenesis using multiple Cas9 nucleases identifies regulatory elements at trait-associated loci. *Nat Genet.* 2017;49(4):625-634.

63. Stadhouders R, Thongjuea S, Andrieu-Soler C, et al. Dynamic long-range chromatin interactions control Myb proto-oncogene transcription during erythroid development. *Embo J.* 2012;31(4): 986-999.

64. Suzuki M, Yamazaki H, Mukai HY, et al. Disruption of the Hbs1l-Myb locus causes hereditary persistence of fetal hemoglobin in a mouse model. *Mol Cell Biol.* 2013;33(8):1687-1695.

65. Farrell JJ, Sherva RM, Chen ZY, et al. A 3-bp deletion in the HBS1L-MYB intergenic region on chromosome 6q23 is associated with HbF expression. *Blood.* 2011;117(18):4935-4945.

66. Morrison TA, Wilcox I, Luo HY, et al. A long noncoding RNA from the HBS1L-MYB intergenic region on chr6q23 regulates human fetal hemoglobin expression. *Blood Cells Mol Dis.* 2017;69:1-9.

67. Sankaran VG, Joshi M, Agrawal A, et al. Rare complete loss of function provides insight into a pleiotropic genome-wide association study locus. *Blood.* 2013;122(23):3845-3847.

68. Huehns ER, Hecht F, Keil JV, Motulsky AG. Developmental hemoglobin anomalies in a chromosomal triplication: D₁ trisomy syndrome. *Proc Natl Acad Sci USA.* 1964;51:89-97.

69. Galarneau G, Palmer CD, Sankaran VG, Orkin SH, Hirschhorn JN, Lettre G. Fine-mapping at three loci known to affect fetal hemoglobin levels explains additional genetic variation. *Nat Genet.* 2010;40(12):1049-1051.

70. Stamatoyannopoulos G. Control of globin gene expression during development and erythroid differentiation. *Exp Hematol.* 2005;33(3):259-271.

71. Jiang J, Best S, Menzel S, et al. cMYB is involved in the regulation of fetal hemoglobin production in adults. *Blood.* 2006;108(3):1077-1083.

72. Tallack MR, Perkins AC. Three fingers on the switch: Kruppel-like factor 1 regulation of gamma-globin to beta-globin gene switching. *Curr Opin Hematol.* 2013;20(3):193-200.

73. Tumburu L, Thein SL. Genetic control of erythropoiesis. *Curr Opin Hematol.* 2017;24(3):173-182.

74. Menzel S, Jiang J, Silver N, et al. The HBS1L-MYB intergenic region on chromosome 6q23.3 influences erythrocyte, platelet, and monocyte counts in humans. *Blood.* 2007;110(10):3624-3626.

75. Menzel S, Garner C, Rooks H, Spector TD, Thein SL. HbA2 levels in normal adults are influenced by two distinct genetic mechanisms. *Br J Haematol.* 2013;160(1):101-105.

76. Soranzo N, Spector TD, Mangino M, et al. A genome-wide meta-analysis identifies 22 loci associated with eight hematological parameters in the HaemGen consortium. *Nat Genet.* 2009;41(11):1182-1190.

77. van der Harst P, Zhang W, Mateo Leach I, et al. Seventy-five genetic loci influencing the human red blood cell. *Nature.* 2012;492(7429):369-375.

78. Miller IJ, Bieker JJ. A novel, erythroid cell-specific murine transcription factor that binds to the CACCC element and is related to the *Krüppel* family of nuclear proteins. *Mol Cell Biol.* 1993;13(5):2776-2786.

79. Arnaud L, Saison C, Helias V, et al. A dominant mutation in the gene encoding the erythroid transcription factor KLF1 causes a congenital dyserythropoietic anemia. *Am J Hum Genet.* 2010;87(5):721-727.

80. Viprakasit V, Ekwattanakit S, Riolueang S, et al. Mutations in Kruppel-like factor 1 cause transfusion-dependent hemolytic anemia and persistence of embryonic globin gene expression. *Blood.* 2014;123(10):1586-1595.

81. Bhatnagar P, Purvis S, Barron-Casella E, et al. Genome-wide association study identifies genetic variants influencing F-cell levels in sickle-cell patients. *J Hum Genet.* 2011;56(4):316-323.

82. Mtatiro SN, Singh T, Rooks H, et al. Genome wide association study of fetal hemoglobin in sickle cell anemia in Tanzania. *PLoS One.* 2014;9(11):e111464.

83. Liu D, Zhang X, Yu L, et al. KLF1 mutations are relatively more common in a thalassemia endemic region and ameliorate the severity of beta-thalassemia. *Blood.* 2014;124(5):803-811.

84. Esteghamat F, Gillemans N, Bilic I, et al. Erythropoiesis and globin switching in compound Klf1::Bcl11a mutant mice. *Blood.* 2013;121(13):2553-2562.

85. Magor GW, Tallack MR, Gillinder KR, et al. KLF1-null neonates display hydrops fetalis and a deranged erythroid transcriptome. *Blood.* 2015;125(15):2405-2417.

86. Perkins A, Xu X, Higgs DR, et al. Kruppeling erythropoiesis: an unexpected broad spectrum of human red blood cell disorders due to KLF1 variants. *Blood.* 2016;127(15):1856-1862.

87. Shaikho EM, Habara AH, Alsultan A, et al. Variants of ZBTB7A (LRF) and its β-globin gene cluster binding motifs in sickle cell anemia. *Blood Cells Mol Dis.* 2016;59:49-51.

88. Wienert B, Martyn GE, Funnell APW, Quinlan KGR, Crossley M. Wake-up sleepy gene: reactivating fetal globin for beta-hemoglobinopathies. *Trends Genet.* 2018;34(12):927-940.

89. Xu J, Bauer DE, Kerenyi MA, et al. Corepressor-dependent silencing of fetal hemoglobin expression by BCL11A. *Proc Natl Acad Sci USA.* 2013;110(16):6518-6523.

90. Bradner JE, Mak R, Tanguturi SK, et al. Chemical genetic strategy identifies histone deacetylase 1 (HDAC1) and HDAC2 as therapeutic targets in sickle cell disease. *Proc Natl Acad Sci USA.* 2010;107(28):12617-12622.

91. Suzuki M, Yamamoto M, Engel JD. Fetal globin gene repressors as drug targets for molecular therapies to treat the beta-globinopathies. *Mol Cell Biol.* 2014;34(19):3560-3569.

92. Shi L, Cui S, Engel JD, Tanabe O. Lysine-specific demethylase 1 is a therapeutic target for fetal hemoglobin induction. *Nat Med.* 2013;19(3):291-294.

92a. Vinjamur DS, Yao Q, Cole MA, McGuckin C, Ren C, Zeng J, Hossain M, Luk K, Wolfe SA, Pinello L, Bauer DE. (2020). ZNF410 represses fetal globin by devoted control of CHD4/NuRD [preprint]. University of Massachusetts Medical School Faculty Publications. Retrieved from https://escholarship.umassmed.edu/faculty_pubs/1820.

92b. Lan X, Ren R, Feng R, et al. ZNF410 uniquely activates the NuRD component CHD4 to silence fetal hemoglobin expression. *Blood.* 2020;136(1).

93. Kan YW, Dozy AM. Polymorphism of DNA sequence adjacent to human beta-globin structural gene: relationship to sickle mutation. *Proc Natl Acad Sci USA.* 1978;75(11):5631-5635.

94. Powars DR. Beta s-gene-cluster haplotypes in sickle cell anemia. Clinical and hematologic features. *Hematol Oncol Clin North Am.* 1991;5(3):475-493.

95. Powars DR. Sickle cell anemia: beta s-gene-cluster haplotypes as prognostic indicators of vital organ failure. *Semin Hematol.* 1991;28(3):202-208.

96. Powars D, Hiti A. Sickle cell anemia. Beta s gene cluster haplotypes as genetic markers for severe disease expression. *Am J Dis Child.* 1993;147(11):1197-1202.

97. Nagel, 1985 #143; Nagel, RL. et al. Hematologically and genetically distinct forms of sickle cell anemia in Africa. The Senegal type and the Benin type. *New Engl J Med.* 1985;312:880-884.

98. Shaikho EM, Farrell JJ, Chui DHK, Sebastiani P, Steinberg MH. Cis- and trans-acting expression QTL differentially regulate gamma-globin gene expression. *bioRxiv.* 2018.

99. Perrine SP, Brown MJ, Clegg JB, Weatherall DJ, May A. Benign sickle-cell anaemia. *Lancet.* 1972;2:1163.

100. Perrine RP, Pembrey ME, John P, Perrine S, Shoup F. Natural history of sickle cell anemia in Saudi Arabs. *Ann Intern Med.* 1978;88:1-6.

101. Vathipadiekal V, Farrell JJ, Wang S, et al. A candidate trans-acting modulator of fetal hemoglobin gene expression in the Arab-Indian haplotype of sickle cell anemia. *Am J Hematol.* 2016;91(11):1118-1122.

102. Vathipadiekal V, Alsultan A, Baltrusaitis K, et al. Homozygosity for a haplotype in the HBG2-OR51B4 region is exclusive to Arab-Indian haplotype sickle cell anemia. *Am J Hematol.* 2016;91(6):E308-E311.

103. Al-Ali ZA, Fallatah RK, Aljaffer EA, et al. ANTXR1 intronic variants are associated with fetal hemoglobin in the Arab-Indian haplotype of sickle cell disease. *Acta Haematol.* 2018;140(1):55-59.

104. Steinberg MH, Lu ZH, Nagel RL, et al. Hematological effects of atypical and Cameroon beta-globin gene haplotypes in adult sickle cell anemia. *Am J Hematol.* 1998;59(2):121-126.

105. Okumura JV, Silva DGH, Torres LS, et al. Atypical beta-S haplotypes: classification and genetic modulation in patients with sickle cell anemia. *J Hum Genet.* 2019;64(3):239-248.

106. Rees DC, Williams TN, Gladwin MT. Sickle-cell disease. *Lancet.* 2010;376(9757):2018-2031.

107. Steinberg MH. Other sickle hemoglobinopathies. In: Steinberg MH, Forget BG, Higgs DR, Weatherall DJ, eds. *Disorders of Hemoglobin: Genetics, Pathophysiology, and Clinical Management.* 2nd ed. Cambridge University Press; 2009:564-586.

108. Kato GJ, Gladwin MT, Steinberg MH. Deconstructing sickle cell disease: reappraisal of the role of hemolysis in the development of clinical subphenotypes. *Blood Rev.* 2007;21(1):37-47.

109. Kato GJ, Steinberg MH, Gladwin MT. Intravascular hemolysis and the pathophysiology of sickle cell disease. *J Clin Invest.* 2017;127(3):750-760.

110. Reiter CD, Wang X, Tanus-Santos JE, et al. Cell-free hemoglobin limits nitric oxide bioavailability in sickle cell disease. *Nat Med.* 2002;8(12):1383-1389.

111. Gueye Tall F, Martin C, Ndour EHM, et al. Combined and differential effects of alpha-thalassemia and HbF-quantitative trait loci in Senegalese hydroxyurea-free children with sickle cell anemia. *Pediatr Blood Cancer.* 2019;66:e27934.

112. Eaton WA, Bunn HF. Treating sickle cell disease by targeting HbS polymerization. *Blood.* 2017;129(20):2719-2726.

113. Khandros E, Huang P, Peslak SA, et al. Understanding heterogeneity of fetal hemoglobin induction through comparative analysis of F and A-erythroblasts. *Blood.* 2020;135(22):1957-1968.

114. Dover GJ, Boyer SH, Charache S, Heintzelman K. Individual variation in the production and survival of F cells in sickle-cell disease. *N Engl J Med.* 1978;299(26):1428-1435.

115. Ngo DA, Aygun B, Akinsheye I, et al. Fetal haemoglobin levels and haematological characteristics of compound heterozygotes for haemoglobin S and deletional hereditary persistence of fetal haemoglobin. *Br J Haematol.* 2012;156(2):259-264.

116. Henry ER, Cellmer T, Dunkelberger EB, et al. Allosteric control of hemoglobin S fiber formation by oxygen and its relation to the pathophysiology of sickle cell disease. *Proc Natl Acad Sci U S A.* 2020;11:201922004.

117. Steinberg MH, Chui DH, Dover GJ, Sebastiani P, Alsultan A. Fetal hemoglobin in sickle cell anemia: a glass half full? *Blood.* 2014;123(4):481-485.

118. Steinberg MH, Embury SH. Alpha-thalassemia in blacks: genetic and clinical aspects and interactions with the sickle hemoglobin gene. *Blood.* 1986;68(5):985-990.

119. Milton JN, Rooks H, Drasar E, et al. Genetic determinants of haemolysis in sickle cell anaemia. *Br J Haematol.* 2013;161(2):270-278.

120. Raffield LM, Ulirsch JC, Naik RP, et al. Common alpha-globin variants modify hematologic and other clinical phenotypes in sickle cell trait and disease. *PLoS Genet.* 2018;14(3):e1007293.

121. Milton JN, Shaikho EM, Steinberg MH. Haemolysis in sickle cell anaemia: effects of polymorphisms in alpha-globin gene regulatory elements. *Br J Haematol.* 2019;186(2):363-364.

122. Taylor JG, Nolan VG, Mendelsohn L, Kato GJ, Gladwin MT, Steinberg MH. Chronic hyper-hemolysis in sickle cell anemia: association of vascular complications and mortality with less frequent vasoocclusive pain. *PLoS One.* 2008;3(5):e2095.

123. Mukherjee MB, Lu CY, Ducrocq R, et al. Effect of alpha-thalassemia on sickle-cell anemia linked to the Arab-Indian haplotype in India. *Am J Hematol.* 1997;55(2):104-109.

124. Hofrichter J, Ross PD, Eaton WA. Kinetics and mechanism of deoxyhemoglobin S gelation: a new approach to understanding sickle cell disease. *Proc Natl Acad Sci USA.* 1974;71(12):4864-4868.

125. Ilboudo Y, Bartolucci P, Rivera A, et al. Genome-wide association study of erythrocyte density in sickle cell disease patients. *Blood Cells Mol Dis.* 2017;65:60-65.

126. Ma S, Cahalan S, LaMonte G, et al. Common PIEZO1 allele in African populations causes RBC dehydration and attenuates *Plasmodium* infection. *Cell.* 2018;173(2):443-455.e12.

127. Rooks H, Brewin J, Gardner K, et al. A gain of function variant in PIEZO1 (E756del) and sickle cell disease. *Haematologica.* 2019;104(3):e91-e93.

128. Ilboudo Y, Bartolucci P, Garrett ME, et al. A common functional PIEZO1 deletion allele associates with red blood cell density in sickle cell disease patients. *Am J Hematol.* 2018;93(11):E362-E365.

129. Belfer I, Youngblood V, Darbari DS, et al. A GCH1 haplotype confers sex-specific susceptibility to pain crises and altered endothelial function in adults with sickle cell anemia. *Am J Hematol.* 2014;89(2):187-193.

130. Jhun EH, Sadhu N, Yao Y, et al. Glucocorticoid receptor single nucleotide polymorphisms are associated with acute crisis pain in sickle cell disease. *Pharmacogenomics.* 2018;19(13):1003-1011.

131. Jhun EH, Sadhu N, Hu X, et al. Beta2-adrenergic receptor polymorphisms and haplotypes associate with chronic pain in sickle cell disease. *Front Pharmacol.* 2019;10:84.

132. Chaturvedi S, Bhatnagar P, Bean CJ, et al. Genome-wide association study to identify variants associated with acute severe vaso-occlusive pain in sickle cell anemia. *Blood.* 2017;130(5):686-688.

133. Willen SM, McNeil JB, Rodeghier M, et al. Haptoglobin genotype predicts severe acute vaso-occlusive pain episodes in children with sickle cell anemia. *Am J Hematol.* 2020;doi: 10.1002/ajh.25728.

134. Milton JN, Sebastiani P, Solovieff N, et al. A genome-wide association study of total bilirubin and cholelithiasis risk in sickle cell anemia. *PLoS One.* 2012;7(4):e34741.

135. Sebastiani P, Ramoni MF, Nolan V, Baldwin CT, Steinberg MH. Genetic dissection and prognostic modeling of overt stroke in sickle cell anemia. *Nat Genet.* 2005;37(4):435-440.

136. Flanagan JM, Frohlich DM, Howard TA, et al. Genetic predictors for stroke in children with sickle cell anemia. *Blood.* 2011;117(24):6681-6684.

137. Taylor JG, Tang DC, Savage SA, et al. Variants in the VCAM1 gene and risk for symptomatic stroke in sickle cell disease. *Blood.* 2002;100(13):4303-4309.

138. Hoppe C, Klitz W, Cheng S, et al. Gene interactions and stroke risk in children with sickle cell anemia. *Blood.* 2004;103(6):2391-2396.

139. Hsieh MM, Kang EM, Fitzhugh CD, et al. Allogeneic hematopoietic stem-cell transplantation for sickle cell disease. *N Engl J Med.* 2009;361(24):2309-2317.

140. Joseph JJ, Abraham AA, Fitzhugh CD. When there is no match, the game is not over: alternative donor options for hematopoietic stem cell transplantation in sickle cell disease. *Semin Hematol.* 2018;55(2):94-101.

141. Margin E, Miccio A, Cavazzana M. Lentiviral and genome-editing strategies for the treatment of β-hemoglobinopathies. *Blood.* 2019;134(15):1203-1213.

142. Ribeil JA, Hacein-Bey-Abina S, Payen E, et al. Gene therapy in a patient with sickle cell disease. *N Engl J Med.* 2017;376(9):848-855.

143. Thompson AA, Walters MC, Kwiatkowski J, et al. Gene therapy in patients with transfusion-dependent beta-thalassemia. *N Engl J Med.* 2018;378(16):1479-1493.

144. Kanter J, Tisdale JF, Mapare M, et al. Resolution of sickle cell disease manifestations in patients treated with lentiglobin gene therapy: updates results from the phase 1/2 HBG-206 group C study. *Blood.* 2019;134:990.

145. Orkin SH, Bauer DE. Emerging genetic therapy for sickle cell disease. *Annu Rev Med.* 2019;70:257-271. doi:10.1146/annurev-med-041817-125507

146. Brendel C, Guda S, Renella R, et al. Lineage-specific BCL11A knockdown circumvents toxicities and reverses sickle phenotype. *J Clin Invest.* 2016;126(10):3868-3878.

147. Breda L, Motta I, Lourenco S, et al. Forced chromatin looping raises fetal hemoglobin in adult sickle cells to higher levels than pharmacologic inducers. *Blood.* 2016;128(8):1139-1143.

148. Wienert B, Funnell AP, Norton LJ, et al. Editing the genome to introduce a beneficial naturally occurring mutation associated with increased fetal globin. *Nat Commun.* 2015;6:7085.

149. Traxler EA, Yao Y, Wang YD, et al. A genome-editing strategy to treat beta-hemoglobinopathies that recapitulates a mutation associated with a benign genetic condition. *Nat Med.* 2016;22(9):987-990.

150. Wienert B, Martyn GE, Kurita R, Nakamura Y, Quinlan KGR, Crossley M. KLF1 drives the expression of fetal hemoglobin in British HPFH. *Blood.* 2017;130(6):803-807.

151. Corbacioglu S, Cappellini MD, Chapin J, et al. Initial safety and efficacy results with a single dose of autologous crispr-cas9 modified CD34+ hematopoietic stem and progenitor cells in transfusion-dependent β-thalassemia and sickle cell disease. *Eur Soc Haematol.* 2020;EHA25:Abstr S280.

152. Esrick EB, Achebe M, Armant M. Validation of BCL11A as therapeutic target in sickle cell disease: results from the adult cohort of a pilot/feasibility gene therapy trial inducing sustained expression of fetal hemoglobin using post-transcriptional gene silencing. *Blood.* 2019;134:LBA-5.

153. Le CQ, Myers G, Habara A, et al. Inhibition of LSD1 by small molecule inhibitors stimulates fetal hemoglobin synthesis. *Blood.* 2019;133(22):2455-2459.

154. Molokie R, Lavelle D, Gowhari M, et al. Oral tetrahydrouridine and decitabine for non-cytotoxic epigenetic gene regulation in sickle cell disease: a randomized phase 1 study. *PLoS Med.* 2017;14(9):e1002382.

155. Shearstone JR, Golonzhka O, Chonkar A, et al. Chemical inhibition of histone deacetylases 1 and 2 induces fetal hemoglobin through activation of GATA2. *PLoS One.* 2016;11(4):e0153767.

156. Shaikho EM, Farrell JJ, Alsultan A, et al. A phased SNP-based classification of sickle cell anemia HBB haplotypes. *BMC Genomics.* 2017;18(1):608.

157. Motulsky AG. Frequency of sickling disorders in U.S. blacks. *N Engl J Med.* 1973;288(1):31-33.

158. Piel FB, Patil AP, Howes RE, et al. Global distribution of the sickle cell gene and geographical confirmation of the malaria hypothesis. *Nat Commun.* 2010;1:104. doi:10.1038/ncomms1104

159. Steinberg MH, Sebastiani P. Genetic modifiers of sickle cell disease. *Am J Hematol.* 2012;87(8):795-803.

160. Piel FB, Steinberg MH, Rees DC. Sickle cell disease. *N Engl J Med.* 2017;376(16):1561-1573.

161. Rodrigues C, Sell AM, Guelsin GAS, et al. HLA polymorphisms and risk of red blood cell alloimmunisation in polytransfused patients with sickle cell anaemia. *Transfus Med.* 2017;27(6):437-443.

162. Oliveira VB, Dezan MR, Gomes FCA, et al. -318C/T polymorphism of the CTLA-4 gene is an independent risk factor for RBC alloimmunization among sickle cell disease patients. *Int J Immunogenet.* 2017;44(5):219-224.

163. Williams TN, Thein SL. Sickle cell anemia and its phenotypes. *Annu Rev Genomics Hum Genet.* 2018;19:113-147.

Sickle Hemoglobin Polymerization

Authors: Daniel B. Kim-Shapiro,
Constance Tom Noguchi, Alan N. Schechter

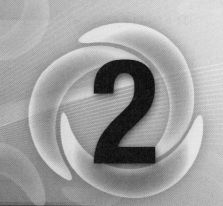

Chapter Outline

Overview

Sickle cell anemia is the most common form of sickle cell disease and is due to homozygosity of the substitution of valine for glutamate at the $\beta 6$ position, giving rise to mutant β^S-globin forming sickle hemoglobin (HbS, $\alpha_2\beta^S_2$). Other forms of sickle cell disease include hemoglobin SC disease where both HbS and HbC (caused by a glutamate to lysine substitution at the $\beta 6$ position giving rise to mutant β^C-globin) coexist and HbS-β thalassemia (combination of 1 mutant β^S-globin gene and mutation in the other β-globin gene resulting in reduced or no normal β-globin production). In all these cases, the dysfunction of HbS is the primary cause of the disease. Almost all of the major physiologic properties of HbS in dilute solution (eg, oxygen, carbon dioxide, 2,3-diphosphoglyceric acid [DPG], and hydrogen ion binding, as well as the cooperativity of oxygen binding) are normal. However, the low solubility upon deoxygenation of HbS, as compared to the very high solubility of the deoxy form of HbA ($\alpha_2\beta_2$), at the high concentrations inside the red cell, causes aggregation of the hemoglobin molecules, which is the major direct effect of the sickle mutations (β^SGlu6→Val). We assume that abnormal red cell flow properties in the circulation and the accompanying increase in hemolysis and thus all clinical manifestations can be traced back to this phenomenon. The major factors affecting the effective solubility inside the red cell are the intracellular hemoglobin composition and concentration and the oxygen saturation, whereas other cellular variables have smaller effects (see Figure 2-1 for overview of this paradigm).

This reduction of solubility upon deoxygenation in the erythrocyte from individuals with sickle cell disease (the sickle erythrocyte) leads to the intracellular formation of aggregates or polymers of HbS, which change many of the properties of the red cell. The most important change is the decrease in the intrinsic flexibility of the cell (necessary for passage through small arterioles) due to the presence of these intracellular arrays of polymer. Many other changes in the properties of the polymer-containing erythrocytes within the vascular bed beyond increased rigidity have been suggested as contributing to disease manifestations. These range from membrane abnormalities, including adhesion to other cells; intra- and extravascular fragility; and a large number of other "downstream" abnormalities, some of which can be directly correlated with the primary pathophysiologic event of intracellular deoxygenated HbS (deoxyHbS) polymerization. In this chapter, we review the polymerization process and how it may explain some of the protean biochemical and physiologic abnormalities that have been detected in the blood and tissues of sickle cell patients and animal models of this disease and are the basis of the systemic and organ-specific manifestations of the disease.

We also describe the factors—genetic, cellular, and physiologic—that modify the polymerization process and that are also the factors known to modify disease severity. Further, the many current approaches to treat this disease, a few of which have already shown some efficacy and have been approved by the US Food and Drug Administration (FDA) and other regulatory agencies, can also be largely conceptualized in the context of effects on intracellular deoxyHbS polymerization.

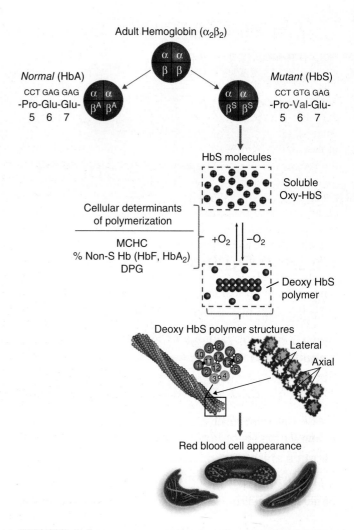

FIGURE 2-1 Overview of chapter. The mutant HbS molecules, with a valine residue at position 6 of the beta chains due to the GTG substitution for GAG in the sixth codon of the DNA, are soluble (however, in very concentrated solution) within the sickle erythrocyte in the oxygenated form (small red circles). Upon partial deoxygenation of the red cells, as in the normal transit through the human circulation, the deoxygenated (deoxy) HbS molecules in the cells (now shown as small blue circles in the middle of the diagram) begin to aggregate into strands that then grow and self-associate to form higher-order fibers. For illustrative purposes only, the deoxy molecules, as at total deoxygenation, are shown in this diagram.

These polymer fibers, as they accumulate and align further, decrease the flexibility of the sickle erythrocytes needed to transit the microcirculation but eventually will distort the shapes of these cells (shown as partially deoxygenated red cells at the bottom of the diagram), increase fragility-promoting hemolysis, and cause membrane damage. Although many factors determine the amount and detailed structure of the HbS polymer in the cells, at any oxygen saturation, the intracellular hemoglobin concentration and composition and 2,3-diphosphoglyceric acid (DPG) levels are probably the most important variables. This chapter is designed to summarize knowledge of the formation of intracellular HbS polymer, the primary pathophysiologic event in the sickle cell syndromes, and the expected effects of this process on the circulatory dynamics of these patients. Hb, hemoglobin; MCHC, mean corpuscular hemoglobin concentration; Oxy, oxygenated.

Classical Studies in Sickle Cell Disease

The 1910 report by James B. Herrick[1] of Chicago concerning a dental student from Grenada entitled "Peculiar Elongated and Sickle-Shaped Red Blood Corpuscles in a Case of Severe Anemia" is considered as the first report of a patient with this disease and is the basis of its descriptive designation. Among the studies of this disease relevant to this chapter up through the 1940s should be mentioned the findings of Hahn and Gillespie[2] in 1927 that sickling occurs upon deoxygenation of blood and those of Sherman[3] in 1940, who, using a polarizing microscope, found that sickled red cells become birefringent, suggesting some aligned intracellular material.

In 1949, Pauling et al[4] reported on the electrophoretic mobility of the hemoglobin from patients (the homozygous SS genotype) and normal individuals, as well as individuals with sickle trait who were "carriers" for sickle cell disease (the AS genotype). They suggested that the changed movement in the electrical field of the red cell proteins from the patients (and in some of the molecules from individuals with the sickle cell trait) was due to a change in the charge of the hemoglobin molecules (soon called sickle hemoglobin or HbS), indicating that it was abnormalities in this protein that were the basis of the disease. They also proposed that sickle cell disease could thus be considered a "molecular" disease, the first such designation. Eight years later, Vernon Ingram, using proteolytic digestion methods, identified an abnormal peptide in the hemoglobin protein and then the specific amino acid substitution (valine for glutamic acid) in HbS—work that was equally important for confirming the previously proposed linear relationship between DNA mutations and amino acid substitutions in proteins.[5]

In the 1950s and over subsequent decades, Max Perutz and his colleagues used x-ray crystallography to demonstrate the normal globular shape of HbA, that the globular shape of HbS and HbA were similar, and that the mutant amino acid residues were on the surface of the hemoglobin tetramer, suggesting intermolecular interactions.[6] By the early 1970s, these methods, and those of electron microscopy (Figure 2-2), were applied to the HbS intracellular polymer, as well as that formed from concentrated hemoglobin solutions in vitro to explore the geometry of the polymer phase, especially with regard to intermolecular interactions that would explain the reduction in solubility of HbS upon deoxygenation.[7]

Primary Pathophysiology of Sickle Cell Diseases and Disease Modifiers

As was discussed in more detail in the preceding chapter, HbS is formed due to a mutation in the gene coding for the β-globin chain of the normal, predominant adult human hemoglobin (HbA). Human hemoglobins are composed of 2 α-globin and 2 β-globin protein chains ($\alpha_2\beta_2$) each linked to

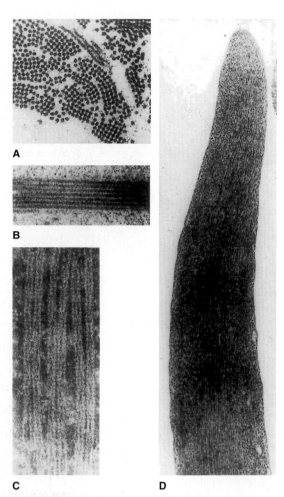

FIGURE 2-2 Electron micrographs of HbS polymer. A-B. Deoxygenated (deoxy) HbS fibers were prepared from centrifuge pellets of cell-free lysates. **C-D.** DeoxyHbS fibers from sickled cells. From Dean J, Schechter AN. Sickle-cell anemia: molecular and cellular bases of therapeutic approaches. *N Engl J Med*. 1978;299:752-763.

an iron-containing heme group. Hemoglobin, which is produced and transported in the erythrocytes of all mammals, has as its predominant function the transport of oxygen from the lungs to the tissues, but also transports carbon dioxide and is involved in nitric oxide metabolism. Hemoglobin has evolved to be an ideal physiological transporter of oxygen due to the cooperative binding of this gas that can be understood in terms of the Monod-Wyman-Changeaux/Perutz 2-state model involving a high oxygen affinity R-quaternary state and a low oxygen affinity T-quaternary state.[8] As oxygen binds to T-state molecules, the quaternary state (the arrangements of the 4 subunits with respect to each other) of the hemoglobin switches from the T-state to the R-state so that binding subsequent oxygen molecules is easier (Figure 2-3). In this way, hemoglobin is fully saturated at the lungs (where it is predominantly R-state) and delivers oxygen efficiently in the tissues where it switches partially to T-state.

HbS ($\alpha_2\beta_2^S$) with the glutamic acid at position 6 of each β-globin chain replaced with valine residues (β^SGlu6→Val) is due to the substitution of an adenine (A) in the coding triplet (GAG) for glutamic acid to a thymine (T), resulting in the

Oxy

Deoxy

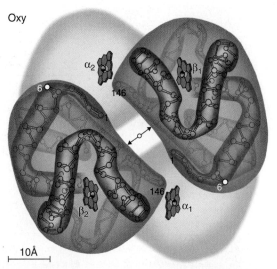
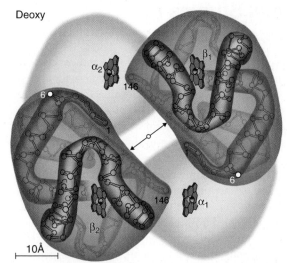

FIGURE 2-3 Conformation change between oxygenated (oxy) hemoglobin (oxyHb) and deoxygenated (deoxy) hemoglobin (deoxyHb). OxyHb (left) and deoxyHb (right) are drawn looking down the crystallographic dyad axis. The backbones of the β-globin chains are illustrated with residues 1 (amino-terminal end), 6 (site of sickle mutation), and 146 (carboxy-terminal end) numbered. Upon deoxygenation, the $α_1β_1$ and $α_2β_2$ dimers shift with the 2 β chains moving further apart as indicated by the arrow (allowing for 2,3-diphosphoglyceric acid binding), whereas the 2 α chains move slightly closer together with small changes in the position of the planar heme groups, the iron atoms, and the polypeptide chain tertiary structure. Illustration, Irving Geis. Image from the Irving Geis Collection. HHMI. Not to be used without permission.

coding triplet (GTG) for the valine amino acid residue. In the several types of sickle cell disease syndromes, the varying but large amounts of HbS in the patient's red cells aggregate upon deoxygenation, causing the formation of tactoids or liquid crystals of deoxyHbS in the sickle erythrocyte upon deoxygenation.[9] This intracellular formation of aggregates, or polymerization—the term used in the sickle cell field for the noncovalent interactions of the hemoglobin molecules—is the primary pathophysiologic event in this disease and what we believe underlies all other manifestations. The evidence for this fundamental relationship will be covered in this chapter. It should also be noted that understanding the polymerization process allows a comprehensive organization of the many factors that have been recognized as modifiers of the disease process as well as the potential therapies for this disease.[10]

Table 2-1 lists many of these disease modifiers, divided for convenience into those that might be considered primarily genetic, cellular, or physiologic in character as usually studied, although these distinctions are clearly arbitrary. Some of these factors, such as HbF ($α_2γ_2$) levels, mean corpuscular hemoglobin concentration (MCHC), and endothelial adhesion, have been extensively studied, whereas others, such as changes in the microvasculature or in tissue oxygen levels, have received much less attention. How these factors may be changed by the polymerization process or how they will be influenced by the process of polymerization will be noted in the following summary of both the structure and biophysics of the deoxyHbS polymer and the obvious consequences of the abnormal internal milieu of the red cell caused by its presence. It should also be noted that the deoxyHbS polymerization alters oxygen binding to the hemoglobin molecules and lowers the oxygen affinity of the intact HbS-containing erythrocyte.[11]

To understand the polymerization process, it is necessary to understand the contents of the HbS-containing erythrocyte.[12] In the cytoplasm of normal red blood cells, the hemoglobin molecules constitute about 95% of all proteins, and these

TABLE 2-1 Major modifiers of sickle cell disease

Genetic
HbF: Hereditary persistence of fetal hemoglobin, Hb F levels, F Cells
α Thalassemia: Coexistence of $(-α/-α)$ genotype
β Thalassemia: Heterozygous for $β°$, $β^-$ thalassemia
Heterozygosity for hemoglobin A, C, D, etc.
Cellular
Intracellular hemoglobin concentration: MCHC, density distribution
Other intracellular components: 2,3-DPG, pH, Ca^{2+}
Erythrocyte membrane abnormalities: Membrane changes, ISCs, vesicles
Cellular adhesion: Endothelial, leukocyte, platelet
Physiologic
Blood clotting factors: Thrombotic cofactors, platelets
Microvasculature: Arteriovenous shunts, arteriolar sphincters, vessel tone, NO, metabolism
Tissue oxygen levels: Po_2 levels, oxygen extraction

Abbreviations: 2,3-DPG, 2,3-diphosphoglyceric acid; ISC, irreversibly sickled cells; MCHC, mean corpuscular hemoglobin concentration; NO, nitric oxide; Po_2, partial pressure of oxygen.

hemoglobin molecules are usually distributed at about 97% HbA, 2% HbA$_2$, and about 0.5% HbF. In the red blood cells of individuals of the SS genotype (called sickle erythrocytes or sickle cells), HbA$_2$ remains at the same level, but HbF is frequently in the 5% to 8% range, with the remainder HbS. In sickle trait, HbS ranges from about 35% to 45% (in part due to variations in the number of α-globin genes), and the rest is HbA and small amounts of HbA$_2$ and HbF. It is these concentrations of the various hemoglobin species that determine the potential or tendency for polymerization to occur at any level of deoxygenation in the various sickle syndromes.

DeoxyHbS Polymer Structure

It was gradually realized by the 1960s that the abnormally shaped cells seen in deoxygenated preparations of blood from sickle cell patients contained aligned arrays of HbS.[7,13] These results from molecular imaging were also matched to the very-high-resolution x-ray structures determined for crystals of normal and sickle hemoglobin to allow gradual improvement in the resolution of the polymer structure. The present generally accepted structure of the deoxyHbS polymer, under usual or physiologic conditions, was finally elucidated with

data from both electron microscopy and x-ray crystallography for both cells and concentrated HbS solutions. The polymer is made of 7 twisted double strands so that the cross-section has 14 hemoglobin tetramers (Figure 2-4). One double strand is at the center of the fiber, and 6 double strands are twisted around those. The fiber is 21 nm in diameter, has a mean helical pitch of 270 nm, and has a variable length depending on the rate and time for its formation. Knowledge of the structure of the fiber is based largely on the assumption that the double strands in the fiber are very similar to double strands consisting of the 2-tetramer asymmetrical unit that forms when deoxyHbS crystallizes.[14]

These double strands contain axial contacts involving the β^{S}6 valine residue (Figure 2-4). Other contacts in the crystal have then been used to predict those in the HbS polymer.[15,16] Indeed, confirmed predictions of the effects of mutations in contact residues (obtained from the crystals) on measurements of deoxyHbS polymer solubility strongly support the notion that the crystal double strand is the basic unit of the 14-strand (7 double strands) HbS polymer. Other data supporting this important result include linear dichroism studies showing that HbS polymers and crystal double stands have the same hemoglobin orientations relative to the fiber axis. In

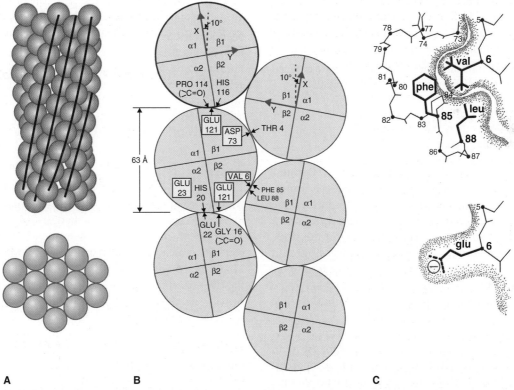

A **B** **C**

FIGURE 2-4 Deoxygenated (deoxy) HbS polymer structure based on electron microscopy and crystal structure. A. Model based on 14 HbS tetramers stacked to form a fiber structure and on-end view in the lower portion. **B.** Arrangement of double strand of deoxyHbS tetramers with arrows indicating intermolecular contact and boxes indicating side-by-side residues and suggested as contact points from studies of hemoglobin mutants and deoxyHbS gelation. **C.** Artistic interpretation of β^{S}6 valine intermolecular contact with an adjacent β-globin hydrophobic pocket involving β85 phenylalanine and β88 leucine; charge and size of normal β6 glutamic acid cannot be accommodated in the same geometry. From Dean J, Schechter AN. Sickle-cell anemia: molecular and cellular bases of therapeutic approaches. *N Engl J Med*. 1978;299:752-763; and Schechter AN, Noguchi CT, Rodgers GP. Sickle cell disease. In: Stamatoyannopoulos G, Nienhuis AW, Leder P, Majerus PW, eds. *The Molecular Basis of Blood Diseases*. Saunders; 1984.

addition to solubility measurements, measures of the kinetics of polymerization also have provided information on the contact residues between hemoglobin molecules.

The double-strand structure obtained in x-ray crystallography for deoxyHbS, and models building on these for the polymer, involve only 1 of the 2 β^S6 valine residues in each tetramer being involved in intermolecular contacts (Figure 2-2). However, some data suggest that more than one of these residues per tetramer are present in contact sites.[17] Future work is required to build models that fully account for all contacts and also to elucidate how the double strands and the deoxyHbS 14-strand fibers themselves are arranged with regard to each other. These contacts, especially those involving the β^S6 valine residue, are of great potential importance because the design of small molecules that inhibit one or more of them might be therapeutically useful.

The formation of such polymers will also tend to distort the shape of the cells from the normal biconcave form, and with extensive deoxygenation, comma-like or "sickled" cells will appear, sometimes with polymer protruding into the red cell membrane,[7] as is especially evident with the use of dithionite or similar chemicals to cause deoxygenation or after prolonged storage under hypoxic conditions. (Note the distinction between "sickled" or sickle-shaped cells and "sickle" cells, ie, red cells from individuals with the various sickle syndromes.) It should be noted that polymer may be formed inside cells without overt sickling (ie, that polymerization is a continuous process, not a 2-stage all-or-none process). Indeed, HbS-containing red cells of normal biconcave morphology but with significant amounts of intracellular polymer have reduced flexibility and presumably cause disease manifestations.

Thermodynamics of HbS Polymerization

The thermodynamics of HbS polymerization can be most simply defined in terms of a polymer phase with relatively immobile hemoglobin molecules and the solution phase with more rapidly moving hemoglobin molecules. The main determinant of HbS polymerization is the oxygenation state of the sickle red cell, which varies over a wide range as the red cells transit the circulation. The HbS concentration is also a very important variable, as is the hemoglobin composition when there are other hemoglobin species in the red cells, as in the sickle syndromes.

Solution-phase HbS behaves (especially in relatively dilute solutions) similarly to normal adult hemoglobin, HbA, in terms of cooperative oxygen binding[10] and other important functions, including the effects of allosteric modulators such as DPG and protons. In this context, the extent of deoxyHbS polymerization at equilibrium is primarily defined by 2 factors: the solubility of the hemoglobin (c_s) and the total concentration of hemoglobin (c_o) when c_o exceeds c_s.[18] The solubility is the maximum concentration that can exist in solution, analogous to a saturated salt solution with excess undissolved salt remaining in the solid phase. The concentration of deoxyHbS in the solution phase is equal to the solubility (about 16 g/dL at 37°C); when c_o exceeds c_s, the amount of HbS that exceeds c_s is in the polymer phase. However, c_s is very dependent on conditions, especially temperature and nonideality due to intracellular molecular crowding[18] (described later). Decreasing c_o or increasing c_s is the underlying goal of essentially all therapeutic strategies aimed directly at decreasing polymerization.

Only the quaternary T-state (approximately equivalent to the deoxyHbS tertiary conformation of the hemoglobin molecule; see Figure 2-3) of HbS enters the polymer phase.[19,20] Effectors that stabilize the R-state (or the oxygenated HbS conformation) will decrease the amount of polymer. Conversely, effectors that stabilize the T-state increase the polymer fraction. Thus, thermodynamically, oxygen is the greatest physiologically relevant effector, with deoxygenation promoting T-state hemoglobin and hence polymerization and oxygenation promoting R-state hemoglobin and hence depolymerization. However, the quaternary state (the T or R form) of hemoglobin also depends on the number of ligands bound, so this factor must be considered in detailed calculations.[19,20] One of the factors that affects this is the type of ligand; for example, carbon monoxide (CO) affects the solubility similarly to oxygen except that CO binds hemoglobin with much greater affinity. The effects of nitric oxide (NO) on polymerization are more complicated due to preferential binding to the α-globin subunits, so that for partial saturations, NO has a smaller effect on solubility than does oxygen or CO.[21] Recently, CO has again been studied as a potential therapy for sickle cell disease, as have agents that change the oxygen affinity itself (by covalent modification) and thus the ratio of T to R forms in the red cell.[22] NO effects on hemoglobin itself are not sufficient to be of therapeutic interest. Therapeutic strategies surrounding stabilization of the R-state (eg, increasing oxygen affinity) are discussed further later in this chapter.

Molecular Crowding

Another major factor that affects the degree of polymerization is molecular crowding due to the physical size of the hemoglobin molecule, which reduces the volume accessible to other hemoglobin or protein macromolecules in the solution (Figure 2-5).[18] More concentrated HbS leads to more polymerization. When the HbS concentration is very high, as it is within all erythrocytes (usually about 34 g/dL) but which can be exaggerated in dense red cells, the effects of crowding make the effective concentrations for the rates and extent of chemical reactions even higher. Two major consequences of such crowding are that one can have polymerization even at very high oxygen saturation values and the therapeutic goal of decreasing intracellular hemoglobin concentration becomes even more important.

Intracellular hemoglobin at the usual concentrations of about 34 g/dL inside the erythrocyte is highly "nonideal," because the molecules are closely packed, resulting in the relative lack of free water (which contains many dissolved ions). The effective hemoglobin concentration or activity is about 50 times greater than the calculated solute concentration in an

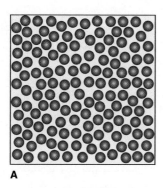
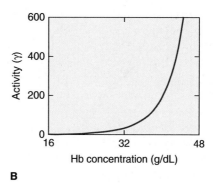

FIGURE 2-5 Schematic of molecular crowding and nonideality of hemoglobin (Hb) solutions at physiologic concentrations. A. Representation of the physical crowding of hemoglobin molecules at a concentration of 33 g/dL. **B.** The nonideal behavior of hemoglobin as indicated by the activity coefficient (γ) as a function of hemoglobin concentration (g/dL). From Noguchi CT. Polymerization in erythrocytes containing S and non-S hemoglobins. *Biophys J*. 1984;45(6):1153-1158. Reprinted with permission from Elsevier.

ideal solution when this so-called excluded volume* is not taken into account and is very sensitive to the intracellular concentrations of all proteins and ions. All hemoglobin molecules in the cells (eg, oxygenated HbS or non-S hemoglobins), even if they do not copolymerize, and other red cell proteins and molecules also exclude volume and thus tend to increase polymerization under any set of conditions. Therefore, both thermodynamic and kinetic studies suggest that changing hemoglobin S concentration (c_o), that is, MCHC, for example by swelling the sickle red cells, could have an important therapeutic benefit.[23,24]

This molecular crowding effect drastically changes the thermodynamics of deoxyHbS polymerization in the erythrocyte. The effects learned from solution measurements of deoxyHbS polymerization—the apparent 2-phase behavior, the differing solubility of the T and R structures, and the effects of non-S hemoglobins and of DPG and protons—all appear to hold for intracellular polymerization. However, the effects of non-ideality due to the very high intracellular concentrations of all macromolecules, especially hemoglobin, in the red cells greatly affect the relationship between polymer fraction and oxygen saturation.

Solid-state nuclear magnetic resonance methods have been used to measure intracellular deoxyHbS polymer, and the results are in agreement with predictions using non-ideality theory.[19,25,26] It was found that polymerization was detected at very high oxygen saturation values; in dense cells (with MCHC values of ≥40 g/dL), polymer was detected between 95% and 99% oxygen saturation (ie, there was almost no solubility of deoxyHbS under these conditions) (Figure 2-6).[25] In less dense cells, polymer was still detected at very high oxygen saturation levels. These results are due to the fact that although R-state HbS molecules may not enter the polymer phase themselves, by excluding volume, they do contribute to polymerization of T-state HbS molecules that are present. The possible implications of these results for models of pathophysiology will be described later.

*The excluded volume is the volume occupied by the hemoglobin molecules in the solution phase in the red cell interior, which is thus not available for other molecules to occupy, leading to "crowding," including of the hemoglobin molecules themselves. The term *non-ideality* refers to the deviation from the ideal gas law and the need for corrections for high effective concentrations of reagents and other factors.

Other Modifiers of Polymerization

DPG is a physiologically relevant effector. This major allosteric effector in the red cell stabilizes the deoxygenated T-state conformation by binding the central cavity of hemoglobin and noncovalently crosslinking the 4 subunits, thus promoting polymerization.[27] DPG decreases the nominal solubility about 15%. Inositol hexaphosphate (a nonphysiologic phosphate-containing molecule) stabilizes the T-state through a similar mechanism as DPG but is a stronger effector and decreases the solubility about 2-fold.[28] As noted later, biochemically decreasing intraerythrocytic DPG has become a proposed therapeutic goal.[29,30]

Temperature has a large effect on deoxyHbS solubility. Unlike most solutes that increase in solubility with temperature, deoxyHbS solubility decreases from 0°C to 35°C. Its value is at a minimum at about normal body temperature, where it is nominally about 0.16 g/mL, and increases at both higher and lower temperatures; at 0°C, the solubility is about 0.32 g/mL, approximately the value of the MCHC.[31] Thus, one can prepare cell-free deoxyHbS at concentrations between 0.16 and 0.32 g/mL on ice and have no polymerization and then observe polymerization when bringing the solution to body temperature.[32] pH also affects deoxyHbS solubility; however, it does not change very much in the physiologic range between about pH 6.5 and 7.5, but increases as the pH is increased or decreased above this range ex vivo. Thus, it is notable that the solubility is lowest near body temperature and at physiologic pH; this is why the effect of the mutation, the polymerization of deoxyHbS, so strongly affects red cell flow properties (called rheology) in the human circulation.

Lastly, the presence of other hemoglobin types in the red cell in addition to HbS has a profound effect on deoxyHbS solubility.[33-36] The extent of these effects depends on whether or not the other hemoglobin molecules copolymerize with deoxyHbS. Tetramers of normal adult hemoglobin (HbA) ($\alpha_2\beta_2$), fetal hemoglobin (HbF; $\alpha_2\gamma_2$), and HbA$_2$ ($\alpha_2\delta_2$) do not enter the deoxyHbS polymer phase in the oxygenated or deoxygenated states. However, these different hemoglobin molecules form tetramer hybrids composed of mixed dimers inside

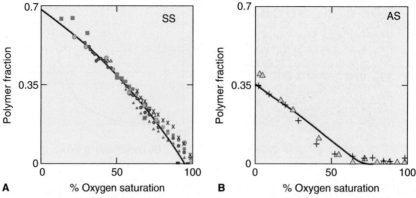

A

B

FIGURE 2-6 **Polymer fraction within intact sickle and sickle trait erythrocytes measured by ¹³C-nuclear magnetic resonance as a function of oxygen saturation from several patients (different symbols). A.** In sickle erythrocytes, polymer is detected at very high oxygen saturation values and increases as oxygen saturation decreases, reaching an average maximum of 70% of total hemoglobin at complete deoxygenation. The curve represents the calculated polymer fraction based on mean corpuscular hemoglobin concentration and hemoglobin composition. Dense cells cause the appearance of detectable polymer measured near 100% saturation. From Noguchi CT, Torchia DA, Schechter AN. Determination of deoxyhemoglobin-S polymer in sickle erythrocytes upon deoxygenation. *Proc Natl Acad Sci U S A.* 1980;77(9):5487-5491. **B.** In sickle trait erythrocytes, polymer fraction is detected at about 60% oxygen saturation and increases as oxygen saturation decreases to an average maximum of 35% to 40% at deoxygenation. From Noguchi CT, Torchia DA, Schechter AN. Polymerization of hemoglobin in sickle trait erythrocytes and lysates. *J Biol Chem.* 1981;256(9):4168-4171.

the red cell as well as in ex vivo solutions. For example, mixing HbS ($\alpha_2\beta_2^S$) with HbF ($\alpha_2\gamma_2$) results in a fraction of ($\alpha\beta^S$)($\alpha\gamma$) tetramer hybrids, roughly following the proportions expected from the binomial distribution. DeoxyHbS/HbF ($\alpha\beta^S$)($\alpha\gamma$) and deoxyHbS/HbA$_2$ ($\alpha\beta^S$)($\alpha\delta$) tetramer hybrids do not enter the deoxyHbS polymer phase, so these hemoglobins have a similar sparing effect on deoxyHbS solubility, which is greater than an equivalent amount of HbA, as deoxyHbS/HbA ($\alpha\beta^S$)($\alpha\beta$) hybrids copolymerize with deoxyHbS with a probability of about half that of deoxyHbS tetramers themselves (Figure 2-7). The greater sparing effect of both HbF and HbA$_2$ on deoxyHbS polymerization near physiologic ligand saturation and concentration values is also apparent from solubility measurements for hemolysates from patients with hemoglobin (HbF and/or HbA$_2$) up to 25%, as compared with solubility measured from sickle trait hemolysate or mixtures with HbC.[34,37,38]

Kinetics of HbS Polymerization

The kinetics of polymerization have been largely studied by temperature jump experiments (rapidly increasing the temperature from say 0°C to 37°C) and modeling oxygenated HbS by CO binding and using laser photolysis to dissociate CO from HbS solutions or cells, producing 100% T-state HbS from 100% R-state HbS within microseconds.[9,39,40] Polymerization was measured by changes in birefringence, turbidity, or light scattering.[39-41] Light scattering increases as particles get bigger, so that it increases during polymerization, which can easily be observed by measuring turbidity. These experiments, which begin with no polymer in the sample, thus follow both the initiation of the polymer (the nucleation event) and the growth and alignment of the polymerized deoxyHbS molecules.

The kinetics of deoxyHbS polymerization, as observed in these types of experiments, demonstrate an unusual

phenomenon: a long period of time when no polymerizations is observed, called the delay time, followed by exponential growth in detected polymer. In addition, the delay time itself is observed to follow a simple empirical law,

$$\frac{1}{t_d} = \lambda \left(\frac{c_0}{c_s} \right)^n ,$$

where t_d is the delay time, λ is a proportionality constant, and the exponent n is on the order of 15 to 30.[40] The ratio c_0/c_s is

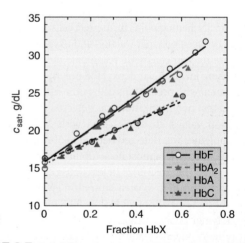

FIGURE 2-7 **Solubility of mixtures of deoxygenated HbS with HbF, HbA$_2$, HbA, and HbC.** Solubility (c_{sat}) values for mixtures of HbS with HbF or HbA$_2$ show the larger sparing effect with increasing fraction of HbX (F or A$_2$) compared with lower c_{sat} values for comparable mixtures of HbS with HbA or HbC. Solubility (c_{sat}) was determined at 30°C in physiologic buffer using total hemoglobin concentrations (c_0) of 27 to 30 g/dL. From Poillon WN, Kim BC, Rodgers GP, Noguchi CT, Schechter AN. Sparing effect of hemoglobin-F and hemoglobin-A2 on the polymerization of hemoglobin-S at physiological ligand saturations. *Proc Natl Acad Sci U S A.* 1993;90(11):5039-5043. Copyright 1993 National Academy of Sciences.

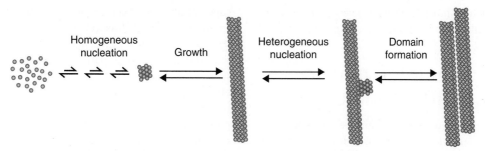

FIGURE 2-8 Model for polymerization kinetics of deoxygenated (deoxy) HbS solutions. During homogeneous nucleation, deoxyHbS tetramers (circles) aggregate to form a critical nucleus, a rate-limiting step that gives rise to a characteristic delay time and is greatly dependent on total deoxyHbS concentration. Addition of more deoxyHbS tetramers and polymer growth proceed rapidly, and additional nuclei may form on preexisting polymer fibers, giving rise to heterogeneous nucleation. Polymer growth and formation of multiple strands of polymer lead to domain formation. From Noguchi CT, Schechter AN. Sickle hemoglobin polymerization in solution and in cells. *Ann Rev Biophys Biophys Chem.* 1985;14:239-263, based on Ferrone FA, Hofrichter J, Eaton WA. Kinetics of sickle hemoglobin polymerization. 1. Studies using temperature-jump and laser photolysis techniques. *J Mol Biol.* 1985;183(4):591-610.

referred to as the supersaturation ratio, and because n is so high, small changes in this ratio can lead to large changes in the delay time. For example, with a deoxyHbS solubility of 0.16 g/mL, taking the intraerythrocytic HbS concentration from 0.34 g/mL to 0.30 g/mL (eg, by hydrating the cell) would increase the delay time by 1 to 2 orders of magnitude. Delay times associated with deoxyHbS polymerization in sickle erythrocytes appear widely distributed, from 1 millisecond to >100 seconds, and depend on intracellular hemoglobin composition and concentration.[42]

The kinetics of deoxyHbS polymerization from polymer-free solutions have been explained by a double nucleation mechanism (Figure 2-8).[43] The process begins with homogeneous nucleation where addition of deoxyHbS tetramers to the growing aggregate is thermodynamically unfavorable until a critical nucleus is made. Once a critical nucleus of deoxyHbS molecules is formed, adding additional deoxyHbS molecules is more favorable thermodynamically than their dissociation, and the polymer grows. Heterogeneous nucleation involves the formation of another deoxyHbS fiber on the surface of existing fibers. Thus, the more polymer there is, the more surface area for heterogeneous nucleation there is, and thereby the more polymerization. The delay time is the period of time required to form a critical nucleus combined with the time required to form enough polymer to be detected because small amounts of polymer are not detectable by usual means.[44] Following the delay time in these model systems, polymerization grows exponentially due to heterogeneous nucleation. These kinetic results seem similar for processes occurring in the cell, although most studies have been with hemoglobin solutions.[32,45]

However, physiologically, the growth of polymer in the cells in the body is expected to be a more complex process with the gradual desaturation of red cells as they transit from large arteries to the small arterioles and then to the capillaries of the microcirculation. The relevant physicochemical processes depend on the starting conditions of the erythrocytes (whether they have residual polymers) as they leave the lung and the rate of deoxygenation as the cells release oxygen for metabolic processes in the tissues, starting in the arterial system.[44]

HbS Polymer Depolymerization (Melting)

Just as polymers grow when the total deoxyHbS concentration exceeds the solubility, depolymerization (or polymer "melting") occurs when the solubility (c_s) is greater than solution-phase concentration of deoxyHbS (c_0).[39,46] Physiologically, polymer melting would occur to some extent upon oxygenation during the venous return from tissues, due to arterial to venous shunting and countercurrent oxygen exchange, but probably occurs to a much greater extent at the lungs and is generally believed to be very rapid.

Polymer melting can be separated into that which occurs at the ends of the polymers (end melting) and that which occurs at the sides of the polymers (side melting).[47] There is a dynamic equilibrium between HbS tetramers in solution and those at the ends of the polymer. In other words, HbS molecules are constantly coming on and off the ends, with the total concentrations in the polymer and monomer phases each being constant at equilibrium. Thus, oxygen-induced polymer melting can occur in 2 ways at the polymer ends: deoxyHbS molecules can come off the polymer and then bind oxygen (so that now they would stay in the solution phase), or the deoxyHbS molecules at the ends of the polymers can bind oxygen converting to R-state and then dissociate from the polymer. Side melting occurs by oxygen binding to deoxyHbS molecules away from the ends, which breaks the polymers and makes more ends, thereby facilitating end melting.

Recent kinetic analyses using high-resolution spatiotemporal optics have been used to modify the detailed previous models of growth and melting and suggest that the mechanism of fiber growth is based on very inefficient adding of tetramers, with constant addition and removal at the ends of the growing fiber.[48]

Few models, however, have attempted to model the alignment and disalignment (upon melting) of the 14 stranded fibers with each other to form macroscopic bundles, which are important because they can distort the shape of the cell, and even that of the cell membrane, and likely have a great effect on the important overall flexibility of the cell itself.

Kinetic and Thermodynamic Models of Pathophysiology

In Figure 2-9, we show our model of an overall view of the pathophysiology of sickle cell disease with reference to intracellular polymer formation. The kinetics of deoxyHbS polymerization have been proposed to play a major role in determining the severity of sickle cell disease. Assuming there is very little or no polymer when the sickle blood cells leave the lungs, if the delay time is long enough, the red cells can make it through hypoxic tissue without sickling. Indeed, it was proposed that the length of the delay time prevents most red blood cells from sickling in vivo, even though they would sickle at equilibrium.[45] As mentioned earlier, according to this "kinetic hypothesis," a small change in the supersaturation ratio changes the delay time greatly so that small changes in the deoxyHbS solubility or MCHC could be therapeutically very efficacious.

Another view is that pathology is dependent on the steady-state (quasi-equilibrium) concentration of polymer in the red blood cell and not the kinetics of its formation. This view is based on the finding from the measurements of intracellular polymerization, noted earlier, that sickle red blood cells contain polymers at very high hemoglobin oxygen saturation values.[19] Measurement of mean arterial oxygen saturation in patients differs in detail depending on the method used, but all show significant arterial desaturation from a very young age, which worsens through adolescence and suggests that relevant values of blood leaving the lungs of patients are perhaps in the 85% to 90% saturation range.[49,50] In this case, it is unlikely that all polymer melts during the transit through the lungs, and thus, nucleation (or delay time) kinetics would not be relevant in the patient's body.[44,46] Rather, the relevant factors are the relationship of polymer growth and alignment in decreasing sickle red

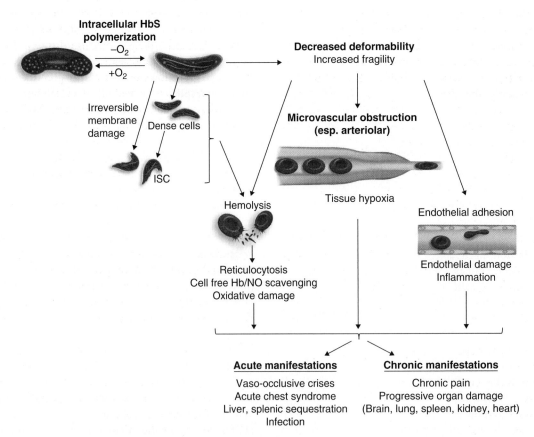

FIGURE 2-9 Schematic outline for the possible cellular pathophysiology of sickle cell anemia. Repeated cycles of intracellular polymerization-depolymerization in sickle erythrocytes can lead to dehydration, giving rise to dense cells, resulting in more polymer at any oxygen saturation. Reversible intracellular polymerization also leads to membrane damage and the formation of irreversibly sickled cells (ISCs), which are also largely in the dense cell fraction. Dense cells have reduced flexibility due to high mean corpuscular hemoglobin concentration and membrane rigidity but primarily because of the increased tendency of polymer formation at any oxygen saturation. In parallel to reduced flexibility or as a result of it, hemolysis and endothelial adhesion may also impair rheologic behavior. These processes lead to the acute and chronic manifestations of the disease. Hb, hemoglobin; NO, nitric oxide. Adapted from Noguchi CT, Schechter AN, Rodgers GP. Sickle cell disease pathophysiology. *Baillieres Clin Haematol.* 1993;6(1):57-91. Adapted with permission from Elsevier.

cell flexibility and the increasing resistance to blood flow in the terminal arterioles as oxygen levels continue to decrease before the capillary beds are reached.[51] Increasing growth and alignment of the polymer occur as deoxygenation proceeds, which results in further rigidity of the cells and decreases of flow of these sickle cells through the microcirculation.

This "thermodynamic" model also emphasizes the notion that morphologic sickling is not itself much of a determinant of poor sickle red cell rheology, as is the intracellular polymer content, which increases before overt sickling occurs. Whether or not there will be red cell–containing polymers on the arterial side of the circulation depends not only on the deoxyHbS solubility at these relativity high oxygen saturation values, but also on the kinetics of polymer melting. The issue is how fast polymers that are present in sickle cells melt upon reoxygenation as cells return to the lungs. If polymers persist after traversing the pulmonary circulation and into low-oxygen tissues, there would not be an effect due to the delay time. As noted earlier, early studies have suggested that polymer melting upon oxygenation is quite fast; however, some studies suggest that polymer melting might be too slow for full polymer melting to occur in all cells before entering the arterial tree.[46,52]

Although the kinetic and steady-state theories may seem incongruent, that is not necessarily so. First, it should be pointed out that both theories support the notion that a major therapeutic goal is to decrease the total intraerythrocytic hemoglobin concentration, c_o, and/or increase the solubility, c_s. Second, whether kinetics (particularly the delay time) or quasi-equilibrium thermodynamics has most relevance to pathology may lie somewhere in between the 2 models. Perhaps for dense cells (discussed later), significant amounts of deoxyHbS are always in the polymer phase, even in the arterial circulation. For these cells, there is no delay time. However, for less dense cells, there may be little to no deoxyHbS in the polymer phase in the arterial circulation and the delay time would be important in minimizing the pathologic effects of this subset of cells.

Of note, both the kinetics and thermodynamics of deoxyHbS polymerization, particularly with mixtures of HbA and HbS found in sickle trait or as a result of increasing HbF in red cells (pharmacologically or genetically), provide a strong explanation for the lack of clinical manifestations associated with sickle trait and the sparing effect of HbF.[53] Thermodynamically, the distribution of hemoglobins in sickle trait cells results in little polymer appearing at oxygen saturation values >60% (Figure 2-6); the only organ in which polymer effects are usually seen is the renal medulla, in which low oxygen saturation values are associated with cellular dehydration. The kinetic analyses also show that mixtures of 60% HbA and 40% HbS, to be expected in sickle trait (AS genotype), have much slower polymerization kinetics. HbF effects are similar but manifest at lower levels than for HbA. It should be noted that increasing HbF is only of value if the total intracellular hemoglobin concentration does not change (ie, MCHC remains almost constant); if HbF were just added to the cell and significantly increased MCHC, there would be no advantage from

the thermodynamic or kinetic viewpoint, but fortunately in most studies up to now (for unclear reasons), MCHC does not change with therapeutic increases in HbF.

Cellular Heterogeneity

The red cells of normal individuals have a narrow range of intracellular hemoglobin concentrations, based on the packing of about 250 million hemoglobin tetramers inside each biconcave disk-shaped cell of about 7 μM diameter and 2 μM thickness, with a normal volume of about 90 fL. This range, classically characterized by the value of the MCHC, closely varies around 34 g/dL, with reticulocytes being somewhat less dense. In the blood of sickle cell disease patients, the MCHC value is quite similar, but there tends to be a much wider distribution, going from values of about 25 g/dL to 40 g/dL or greater due to increased numbers of reticulocytes as well as the appearance of "dense" cells.[54]

These dense cells are thought to form in the circulation from repeated cycles of oxygenation and deoxygenation and resulting ion fluxes, as described later. The dense cells, for the reasons described earlier, would be expected to have faster kinetics of polymerization upon deoxygenation (even if polymer is already present and delay time does not occur) or a higher polymer fraction at any oxygen saturation value. Thus, these cells would likely contribute disproportionately to the manifestations of the disease; this phenomenon, related very closely to the basic polymerization process, surprisingly has not been clearly confirmed in clinical studies.[55]

In addition to the usual dense or high MCHC cells, another cellular phenomenon, the presence of so-called irreversibly sickled cells (ISCs), has been noted in the blood of sickle cell disease patients for many decades. These cells are now understood to be those with very high MCHC values, so the intracellular deoxyHbS polymer does not easily melt, for example, on exposure to room air, and it is necessary to use 100% oxygen or CO to fully restore these cells to normal morphology, except for some evidence of extensive membrane damage.[56] However, only a small percentage (usually about 5%-10%[57,58]) of the red cells in the peripheral circulation of most sickle cell patients seem to have these membrane changes, but ISC numbers appear to correlate with more severe illness. Numbers of dense sickle red blood cells (which include a fraction of ISCs) have been shown to correlate with hemolysis, as well as skin ulcers, priapism, and renal dysfunction.[59] However, attempts to directly correlate them with specific clinical manifestations, such as vaso-occlusive crises, have not been successful.

With respect to therapy, for the reasons described earlier for both the kinetic and thermodynamic models of pathophysiology, decreasing the numbers of dense cells or, better, lowering the densities of all cells would be expected to have a large benefit related to reduced polymerization. Clinical trials of several agents with such effects have shown some lowering of MCHC and even decreases in hemolysis, but end points based on vaso-occlusive crises were not improved. Recent screening studies have identified other agents that lower MCHC, but these have themselves led to hemolysis due to excess swelling of the red cells so are unlikely to be clinically useful.

Another manifestation of cellular heterogeneity is that HbF is usually not distributed uniformly among red cells, as it is in most forms of hereditary persistence of fetal hemoglobin (HPFH).[60] In certain of the syndromes with elevated HbF, the elevations are primarily in a subset of cells designated as F-cells, whereas other cells may have the usual very low percentages of HbF. Various strategies to increase HbF may also result in such heterogeneity, but one would optimally like all cells to have enhanced HbF levels. Otherwise, the cells not changed would have the same potential for intracellular polymerization.

The fact that intracellular polymerization (and/or sickling) results in red cell membrane abnormalities has been known for many decades.[61] Early on, it was noted that the membrane lipid profile seems to change with time with respect to which lipids are on the outer and which are on the inner surface of the cell. This phenomenon has been associated with evidence that sickle cells promote thrombotic processes.[62] Another phenomenon related to cellular effects of polymerization, and possibly also related to thrombosis as well as other clinical phenomena, is the release of membrane vesicles and shrinkage of the membranes of sickle cells in circulation.[62] These changes seem to be correlated with the appearance of the dense cells.

Genetic Heterogeneity Effects on Intracellular Polymerization

In addition to classical sickle cell disease (the SS genotype), there are several diverse sickle syndromes with highly variable severity, and much of this heterogeneity is due to genetic effects on polymerization.[63,64] Figure 2-10 presents a list of the major sickle cell syndromes in rough increasing order of their clinical severity and approximate calculations of polymerization tendency matched against projected changes in this parameter due to increasing HbF levels.[65] This variability in polymerization tendency (at about 70% oxygen saturation) is largely explained by differences in intracellular hemoglobin composition and concentration. Indeed, the heterogeneity of sickle cell disease, as compared to other Mendelian diseases even in patients homozygous for the sickle mutation (ie, of the SS genotype), has been one of the paradoxes of these conditions. Intracellular polymerization may be variable in each syndrome due to changes in levels of non-S hemoglobins, HbF in particular, and in MCHC values and red cell density distributions. There may also be contributions within each syndrome due to little-studied variability in oxygen availability in the lungs (eg, effects of shunting, fibrosis), oxygen extraction in the tissues for metabolic processes, and anatomic and functional details of the microcirculation.[66]

As was noted earlier, the most common sickle syndrome but, fortunately, the one with almost no manifestations of disease is the basic heterozygous condition of sickle trait (AS genotype) in which the percent HbA tends to be significantly greater than that of HbS.[67] Besides known effects on the kidneys of the AS individuals,[68] whether there are other effects such as susceptibility to stress-induced sudden death remains very controversial.[69] Figure 2-11 diagrams the effect of the presence of either HbA or HbF on the expected fraction of HbS molecules in the polymer phase at complete deoxygenation, but as previously shown (Figure 2-6), decreases in polymer tendency due to these other hemoglobin species are manifest at any oxygen saturation.[38,70] Indeed, in sickle trait cells, there would be no polymer detected until about 60% saturation.[71]

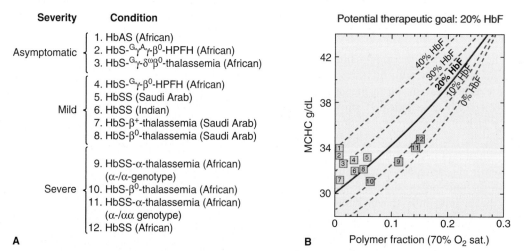

FIGURE 2-10 **Variation in polymerization potential among the sickle syndromes. A.** Approximate classification of the sickling hemoglobinopathies by reported clinical severity. **B.** The dashed curves show the relationship between calculated polymer fraction at 70% oxygen saturation and mean corpuscular hemoglobin concentration (MCHC) (g/dL). The red line indicates the calculated polymer fraction for 20% HbF at varying MCHC. The numbered squares represent mean values for polymer formation calculated based on red cell hemoglobin composition (S, F, A$_2$, A) and MCHC at 70% oxygen saturation for the sickle syndromes indicated in part A. From Noguchi CT, Rodgers GP, Serjeant G, Schechter AN. Levels of Fetal Hemoglobin Necessary for Treatment of Sickle-Cell Disease. New England Journal of Medicine. 1988;318(2):96-99 and Brittenham GM, Schechter AN, Noguchi CT. Hemoglobin-S Polymerization—Primary Determinant of the Hemolytic and Clinical Severity of the Sickling Syndromes. Blood. 1985;65(1):183-189. This research was originally published in Blood. (c) the American Society of Hematology. Used with permission.

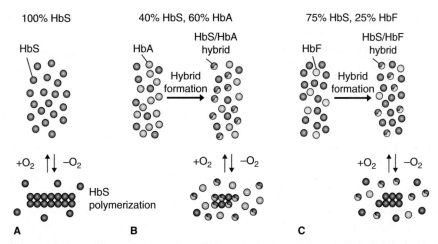

FIGURE 2-11 Diagrammatic representation of the sparing effect of HbA and HbF on oxygen-dependent polymerization of HbS.
A. Polymerization of fully deoxygenated (deoxy) HbS near physiologic concentration at equilibrium is illustrated for 100% HbS solution, whereas no polymer is formed with fully oxygenated HbS. **B.** In a mixture of 40% HbS and 60% HbA (comparable to sickle trait), deoxyHbA does not enter into the polymer phase, whereas the deoxyHbS/HbA hybrids polymerizes at 0.4 times the probability of deoxyHbS. **C.** The sparing effect of HbF is shown for a mixture of 75% HbS and 25% HbF where deoxyHbF and deoxyHbS/HbF hybrid do not enter into the polymer phase, resulting in a polymer fraction comparable with 40% HbS and 60% HbA. At physiologic oxygen saturation values, the differential effects are similar. Adapted from Noguchi CT. Polymerization in erythrocytes containing S and non-S hemoglobins. *Biophys J.* 1984;45(6):1153-1158.

For the usual SS genotype, the amount of fetal hemoglobin is perhaps the major determinant of sickle cell disease manifestations and severity.[72] The effects on polymerization of levels of 25% HbF, sometimes achieved with hydroxyurea therapy, is shown schematically in Figure 2-11.[34,36] In the 1940s, it was noted that morphologic sickling of cells and disease manifestations were markedly reduced until about 6 months of life, and this was ascribed to the alternate form of hemoglobin, now called HbF, that predominates at birth and for months afterward.[73,74] Subsequently, it was noted that individuals with HPFH, in whom fetal hemoglobin is about 15% to 30%, are essentially asymptomatic.[75] Later population studies, both in areas of the Middle East with prevalence of the Arab-India haplotype with relatively high HbF levels and in other groups with smaller elevations of HbF levels, showed that those with high values tend to present with milder disease or phenotype.[76]

Genome-wide association studies have helped identify polymorphisms in genes that are involved in fetal hemoglobin expression both *cis* and *trans* to the β-globin locus, and these studies support the predominant role of polymerization in determining the disease pathophysiology while paving the way for potential new treatments, based on increasing HbF levels pharmacologically or via gene therapy.[60,77] One variant that has been associated with elevated HbF is the MYB transcription factor, which regulates HbF directly and by altering the kinetics of erythropoiesis itself.[78] The transcriptional repressor BCL11A (B-cell lymphoma/leukemia 11A) has been identified as an important regulator of HbF levels that interacts with the locus control region of the β-globin locus. Inhibition of this regulatory protein could lead to elevated HbF levels, but doing so would affect other genes.[78] However, extensive work on BCL11A continues.

The other major genetic polymorphism that affects polymerization is α thalassemia due to deletion of one of the duplicated α-globin genes ($\alpha\alpha/\alpha\alpha$) in the heterozygous ($\alpha-/\alpha\alpha$) or homozygous ($\alpha-/\alpha-$) form, which reduces MCHC, with a greater reduction in the homozygous ($\alpha-/\alpha-$) form.[79,80] In addition, the total intraerythrocytic percentage of HbA_2 is higher due to reduction in α-globin production and the greater affinity of δ-globin than β^S-globin to α-globin in dimer formation of ($\alpha\delta$) compared with ($\alpha\beta^S$).[81] Thus, c_o of HbS is lower in sickle cell patients with homozygous α thalassemia, and one would expect less polymerization and the disease to be less severe with respect to the level of anemia. However, other aspects of pathology are not clearly improved. There is increased risk for acute chest syndrome and osteonecrosis but lower risk of leg ulcers and priapism, in stark contrast to what has been designated as the hyperhemolysis subphenotype.[82] It is thought that the increased levels of total hemoglobin, due to reduced hemolysis, causes the blood to become slightly more viscous, which may counteract the beneficial effects of the α thalassemia on polymerization.[83] These results must be factored into evaluation of any therapeutic strategy that increases overall hemoglobin levels, such as increases in oxygen affinity, because these effects may result in the therapy not ameliorating all manifestations of the disease.

The coexistence of one gene for HbC (β^CGlu6→Lys) and one gene for HbS (β^SGlu6→Val) causes hemoglobin SC disease ($\alpha_2\beta^S\beta^C$), which is relatively frequent in the African American population.[84] This disease is in general slightly less severe with respect to most manifestations than SS disease, except that retinopathy is more common. Despite the heterozygous state of the β^S6 mutation in SC disease and that HbC itself does not polymerize (although it can crystallize in the homozygous state), the deoxyHbS/HbC hybrid ($\alpha\beta^S$)($\alpha\beta^C$), like the deoxyHbS/HbA hybrid ($\alpha\beta^S$)($\alpha\beta$), copolymerizes with deoxyHbS tetramers with a probability of about half that of deoxyHbS.[37] The higher percentage of HbS (50%) compared with HbS (40%) in sickle trait and the higher MCHC in SC disease increases the polymerization tendency in SC erythrocytes compared to AS erythrocytes and likely contributes to disease pathology.[25] It should also be noted that individuals with SC disease have higher total hemoglobin values (about 11.5 g/dL) than SS individuals (perhaps closer to a mean of 9 g/dL),[85] and this itself may also contribute to some of the pathology, as noted later.

It has been possible to correlate the apparent disease severity in the entire spectrum of sickle syndromes, which include coexisting β thalassemia of several types (both β° and β⁺, and the ones described earlier [HPFH, α thalassemia]), and their effects on polymerization tendency (eg, polymer fraction calculated at equilibrium at about 70% oxygen saturation) with their known clinical severity (Figure 2-10).[70,86] Such correlations have led to the conclusion that whereas 60% HbA, as in sickle trait, will ameliorate almost all manifestations of the disease, 30% HbF (or HbA$_2$) will have about the same beneficial effect.[34,86] On this basis, it can be estimated that drugs that increase HbF, such as hydroxyurea, need to reach levels of 20% to 30% HbF to obtain very strong benefit and amelioration of most or all symptoms of the disease. It is likely that lower levels (15%-20%) will have some benefit, as indicated by population studies, but not be completely efficacious. Further increases in HbF must occur without any increase in the mean intracellular hemoglobin levels and most effectively be distributed in similar amounts in virtually all red cells so that they may be considered as F-cells (which basically indicates that various methods of quantitation detect the presence of HbF in these cells).[87]

Calculations of polymer tendency or potential at any specified oxygen saturation may be used to compare likely benefits, based on effects on polymerization of different therapeutic strategies.[10] Thus, one can estimate that a reduction of MCHC by 5% or 10%, as seen with α thalassemia and some of the pharmacologic methods of swelling red cells by interfering with ion channels, would have about the same beneficial effects as increasing levels of HbF by about 10%.[65]

Pathophysiologic Consequences of Intracellular DeoxyHbS Polymerization

As noted earlier, intracellular deoxyHbS polymerization is the primary functional cause of sickle cell disease (ie, all pathology of the disease is ultimately derived from this process). DeoxyHbS polymerization initially affects many properties of the red blood cell, particularly decreasing cell deformability and increasing fragility.[88,89] The rigidity of these intracellular gels, as measured, for example, by Young's modulus, increases greatly with polymer mass.[90] Thus, the phase transition of polymerization dramatically increases the internal viscosity of the red blood cell, which causes a huge decrease in the deformability and increase in fragility of red blood cells, without necessitating any independent effects on the red cell membrane. These rigid cells are expected to block small blood

vessels, beginning in the terminal arterial tree where resistance due to smooth muscle tissue around the vessel is high and cell deformability is necessary for passage.[91]

Once there is such an occlusion, blood flow is likely impaired and further deoxygenation can occur, resulting in further polymerization and thus leading to tissue hypoxia and the complex panoply of tissue and organ damage.[89] Some have likened this to a "vicious cycle," but there must be compensatory mechanisms that correct these deviations; otherwise, all the red cells in the body would be expected to participate in a lethal situation. The vaso-occlusive processes in these small blood vessels and the processes that follow their dissolution (possibly by vessel relaxation or availability of oxygen) have been likened to the phenomenon of ischemia-reperfusion injury where the major pathology appears to occur from the return of oxygen and the formation of reactive oxygen species rather than from the initial hypoxia.[89] Whether this construct has been heuristically valuable in understanding the pathology of this disease or in devising therapies is not clear yet.

Episodic pain in diverse parts of the body, including limbs and abdomen, is generally one of the most common manifestations of sickle cell disease and is a common reason for pain therapy and, at times, hospitalization.[92] These pain episodes are usually referred to as *vaso-occlusive crises* due to early understanding of the pathology of this disease.[93,94] However, investigators have not actually been able to show that occlusive events occur in any particular tissues of patients to correlate with these pain episodes; in fact, the pathophysiologic basis of their origin is not understood to any extent, nor has any detailed correlation with changes in the rheologic properties of the sickle cells been accomplished. It could be that these pain crises reflect changes in the microcirculation and not the red cells per se.

In addition to microvascular occlusion caused by intracellular deoxyHbS polymerization in sickle red blood cells, another consequence of decreased deformability of both oxygenated and deoxygenated blood cells is increased viscosity.[56,89] Blood is a non-Newtonian fluid so that the viscosity decreases as the shear rate increases, for example, when the blood flows faster in a given vessel.[95] The viscosity of oxygenated blood containing sickle red cells is greater than that containing normal cells at all shear rates for the same hematocrit.[56] However, the viscosity of oxygenated blood from patients with sickle cell anemia is generally lower than that of healthy normal individuals due to the lower hematocrit of the patients, but the viscosity of partially deoxygenated blood from patients with sickle cell disease is higher.[96] This effect may contribute to pathology in large vessels where occlusion per se is less likely. Thus, increased viscosity, as in the higher blood hemoglobin values in hemoglobin SC disease or coexisting α thalassemia, may itself have a deleterious effect.[97]

The deformability of sickle red blood cells, even in the oxygenated form, is also decreased due to dehydration and increases in MCHC, which result in increased internal viscosity; red cell membrane stiffness itself also contributes a small amount to these parameters but is not a primary effect.[98] However, cycles of deoxyHbS polymerization and depolymerization (as would be expected normally in the body) lead to increased ion permeability for several ions, including calcium.[99] Calcium influx activates the Gardos channel (a calcium-dependent K channel), which leads to potassium ion efflux and dehydration of the cells.[100] Dehydration not only decreases the deformability of the red cells, but also increases the intraerythrocytic hemoglobin concentration, c_o, which increases polymerization, which, in turn, may further increase calcium leak, potassium efflux, and dehydration.[101] This might be expected to cause another vicious cycle, but again, there must be compensatory mechanisms. Agents targeting the Gardos channel and related ion channels to prevent cellular dehydration are being studied as potential therapies for the sickle disease syndromes.[23]

DeoxyHbS polymer–containing cells are highly fragile in various ex vivo assays and are likely to undergo accelerated destruction or hemolysis in small arterioles, arterial sphincters, and probably extravascular spaces.[82] This is even true of cells that have not gone through multiple cycles of polymerization and depolymerization causing membrane abnormalities, which may have effects on properties such as blood clotting and adhesive interactions with other cells. However, membrane stiffness or rigidity itself is not likely to be a major contributor to such hemolysis. Intravascular hemolysis leads to anemia, which although usually well compensated may, under certain circumstances, require transfusion therapy, but also causes other pathophysiologic processes related to the released contents of the red cell, including hemoglobin and various enzymes and other compounds.[82] Further membrane fragments and vesicles have been detected and associated with disease processes.[102] In particular, enhanced tendency for thrombotic effects has been associated with these phenomena, as noted earlier.

The released HbS would be expected to scavenge NO much more readily than when it is encapsulated inside the red blood cell and may cause many pathologic effects associated with decreased NO availability, including enhanced interactions and adhesion with circulating and endothelial cells, platelet activation, and other inflammatory processes (see later).[82] The released hemoglobin (initially as tetramers [$\alpha_2\beta_2$]) is primarily in the ferrous form, due to plasma-reducing conditions, but can be oxidized to the ferric (methemoglobin) form, which more readily dissociates to hemoglobin ($\alpha\beta$) dimers, and this species can more easily lose the heme group, which may in turn release free iron.[82] In recent years, much attention has also focused on the potential toxic effects of the released heme moieties and of iron itself. Various ways of decreasing the concentrations of these in the circulation, such as infusions of haptoglobin or hemopexin, are being studied for their potential therapeutic value.[103]

Another major effect of polymerization is the decrease in the oxygen affinity of sickle cells as compared to normal erythrocytes. Although the cooperativity of oxygen binding—the allosteric effect noted in the sigmoidal nature of the curve of saturation versus partial pressure of oxygen (Po_2) and its sensitivity to pH and DPG—is little changed, the P50 is increased from the usual value of 27 mm Hg to about 33 mm Hg.[11]

This effect is due primarily to the fact that the energetics of polymerization compete with the energetics of oxygen binding, so that higher oxygen levels are needed to achieve the same levels of saturation, and to changes in the cooperativity of oxygen binding to the polymer phase. In addition, intracellular DPG levels in sickle red cells are increased as compared to cells from normal individuals, which would also decrease the expected P50 for oxygen.[27,104] This phenomenon would be expected to increase the amount of oxygen delivered to tissues at any Po_2 and may be a compensatory mechanism. In addition, the change in oxygen affinity due to polymerization would only occur under conditions in which polymer is already formed in the cells of the body, not in cells with no polymer as assumed in the kinetic model.

As noted earlier, there are other well-studied pathophysiologic mechanisms that appear to be more distantly related to polymerization. For example, in recent years, much attention has focused on endothelial injury itself in the blood vessels of sickle cell disease patients.[105] Early studies on sickle red cell adhesion to endothelial cells raised the question regarding whether these interactions were deleterious to the endothelium.[106,107] This potential has led to extensive studies of receptors that might be involved in the red cell/endothelial adhesion processes and of molecules—both of low molecular weight and monoclonal antibodies that affect one or more of the receptors—as potential therapeutic agents.[108,109] However, deoxygenated sickle cells appear to bind to endothelium less well than oxygenated cells, and the reticulocytes themselves, which are increased due to hemolysis in the sickle cell syndromes, have increased endothelial binding. Thus, the pathophysiologic role of this phenomenon is still not well understood. However, studies in sickle cell disease on hemolysis and increased circulating heme groups and iron atoms, NO depletion, and increased reactive oxygen species have also pointed to expected effects on endothelial cells.[110] These cells have been implicated in many other diseases and pathologic processes, although in general, the integrity of these cells is not easily ascertained.

Evidence for interactions of the sickle cells with platelets and white blood cells has also been noted, and the latter has been used to explain the apparent role of white blood cells in worsening some aspects of sickle cell severity, but this hypothesis is very controversial because white blood cell counts are influenced by many factors.[105,110] Even more distantly related to polymerization is a recent focus on inflammation (sometimes denoted as sterile inflammation) in the pathogenesis of sickle cell disease. Many parameters related to inflammation have been studied, especially in mouse models of this disease, but it is not yet clear how these effects may relate back to the events resulting from the mutation in the gene for the β-chain of hemoglobin or if their minimization will affect patient disease manifestations.[110,111] One recent pathophysiologic proposal involves a scenario in which polymerization leads to red blood cell fragility and thus hemolysis, which promotes inflammation and adhesion of circulating blood cells due to the release of many red cell components as well as oxidative changes.[110]

Pathophysiologic Basis of Sickle Cell Therapeutic Approaches

Table 2-2 shows a conceptual framework for the rapidly increasing numbers of clinical trials of potential therapies for sickle cell disease with respect to what aspects of intracellular deoxyHbS polymerization or its effects might be improved by each of these agents. Therapies that are now part of standard of care and those approved by the FDA are italicized; others undergoing particularly active development are denoted with a question mark.

This outline, like that in Table 2-1, is divided into groups that may be considered as primarily changing genetic, cellular, or physiologic properties, but these distinctions are arbitrary. However, in view of the fact that almost 1000 clinical trials in sickle cell disease are now registered at ClinicalTrials.gov at the time of preparation of this chapter and others may also be underway, it is important to have some framework to think about these many approaches. Many of these approaches, especially those that are based on new genetic technologies, have been underway for years and are discussed in other chapters in this book. Thus, we will confine ourselves to briefly noting some approaches that are related directly to intracellular polymerization or its effects.

Cellular Approaches

Blood transfusion, either as addition or exchange of units of normal (including AS genotype) whole blood or red cells, is perhaps the oldest approach of all of these approaches[112] and is described in another chapter in this book. It has been used for treatment of chronic anemia, especially with regard to symptomatic manifestations (but these are usually less severe than, for example, in many of the thalassemia syndromes), and for acute manifestations such as with the splenic syndromes.[112] Exchange transfusions have also been shown to be efficacious in prevention of stroke and other cerebral manifestations in patients at high risk for these complications and in improving outcomes in pregnancy.[113] There is some uncertainty regarding the levels of replacement of the sickle red cells that should be accomplished as well as the frequency of the procedures. Lowering the fraction of SS cells below 30% is a common goal and is supported by in vitro studies of the flow properties mixtures of normal and sickle red cells.

Reducing polymerization by administration of compounds that bind to HbS at polymer contact sites is a logical approach but also one that encounters several hurdles.[10] Primary among these problems is the fact that sickle erythrocytes contain several millimolar hemoglobin tetramers (mostly HbS), so that one would need to achieve very high intracellular concentrations of any drug, especially because these contact sites are on the surface of the hemoglobin molecules and are likely to have weak affinities for any noncovalent interactions. In addition, red cells are not easily permeable to molecules like peptides that have been developed by computer structural modeling for such inhibition of contact sites. Equally important, although not often recognized, is that non-ideality effects will result as the very large intracellular concentrations of such compounds will also tend to lower solubilities ("salting out") even as they also inhibit aggregation.

As noted earlier, cycles of deoxyHbS polymerization and depolymerization lead to calcium influx, activation of the Gardos channel with associated potassium efflux, and dehydration.[23] Mechanically activated increased cation permeability is likely due primarily to the PIEZO1 channel. In addition, activity of the K-Cl cotransport channel leads to dehydration through water efflux, and inhibition of these channels has also been a therapeutic target along with targeting the Gardos channel and other ion flux controls.[114]

Dehydration increases the MCHC and the intraerythrocytic concentration of HbS and thus polymerization at any oxygen saturation, as well as its rate. One promising way to decrease MCHC is to increase red blood cell volume.[24] Magnesium has been shown to inhibit K-Cl cotransport, and dietary Mg^{2+} has been studied in clinical trials, while several Gardos channel inhibitors have been studied in phase III clinical trials.[23] However, although some of these agents have

TABLE 2-2 Pathophysiologic bases of sickle cell therapeutic approaches

Genetic
Replace sickle cell precursors (allogeneic *stem cell transplants*)
Increase HbF to inhibit HbS polymerization (*HU*, ?gene therapy)
Replace β^S gene (?gene therapy, ?CRISPR/cas)
Cellular
Replace sickle red cells (*blood transfusion*)
Chemical inhibition of HbS polymerization (?CO)
Decrease intracellular HbS concentration
Increase HbS oxygen affinity (*GBT440*)
Decrease DPG concentration
Physiologic
Increase microvascular blood flow (?NO, ?nitrite)
Counter effects of cell-free hemoglobin (?haptoglobin, ?hemopexin)
Decrease red cell oxidative stress (*L-glutamine*)
Inhibit sickle red cell adhesion (*crizanlizumab*)
Inhibit secondary inflammation

Note. Therapies that are now part of standard of care, and those approved by the US Food and Drug Administration are italicized; others undergoing particularly active development are denoted by a question mark (?).

Abbreviations: CO, carbon monoxide; DGP, 2,3-diphosphoglyceric acid; HU, hydroxyurea; NO, nitric oxide.

increased hemoglobin levels, none has reduced the frequency and severity of painful crises, and the clinical studies of these agents have largely been abandoned.

Decreasing the concentration of DPG in the sickle red cells might have several therapeutic advantages, and attempts to affect the enzymatic systems responsible for its formation and metabolism are being employed to this end.[30] Lowering DPG levels will tend to shift the T/R equilibrium from the T to the R form, as with the agents that covalently stabilize the R form. However, although individually the effects are small, DPG both stabilizes the polymer fiber and lowers intracellular pH; thus, lowering its levels might have these benefits in decreasing intracellular deoxyHbS polymer.

Increasing oxygen affinity has recently become a major therapeutic thrust. Because only T-state HbS polymerizes and oxygen promotes the formation of R-state hemoglobin, increasing oxygen affinity will increase HbS solubility at any defined oxygen pressure.[10] Several methods to increase oxygen affinity of HbS that have been considered include using agents that stabilize the R-state by binding to the N-terminus of α chains, binding to the cysteine residue at the β 93 position, heme-ligand binding, or destabilizing the T-state by decreasing DPG.[30,115-117]

Early efforts at R-state stabilization with CO, and even methemoglobin formation, were successful at least in increasing red blood cell survival.[118] However, because the CO liganded hemoglobin molecules do not participate in oxygen delivery and CO binds hemoglobin molecules with an affinity 200 times that of oxygen, it is not clear that the overall effect will be beneficial. Tissues need continuous high levels of oxygen delivery, and the CO-liganded molecules are essentially inert to these processes. More recently, a CO-bound pegylated hemoglobin product was administered to patients in a phase IB trial with the rationale that, in addition to minimizing polymerization, the slowly released CO itself would be beneficial in inhibiting inflammation.[119]

Ligation of the β 93 cysteine with, for example, glutathione and other thiol compounds, also tends to stabilize the R-state and decreases polymerization. One agent binds to β cysteine 112 and stabilizes the R-state in multiple ways, doing so better than other thiol compounds that bind β 93, and has been suggested as a lead molecule for treatment of sickle cell disease as these reagents do not totally inhibit the function of the hemoglobin molecules that have been reacted, as with CO.[119] Derivatives of vanillin stabilize the R-state by binding the N-terminus of the α chains and also tend to destabilize the polymer and have been under development for some time.[117,120]

Perhaps the most currently discussed compound that acts through this R-state stabilization method is GBT440 (voxelotor).[121] GBT440 partitions about 150:1 in the red blood cells versus plasma. With 500 μM GBT440, the P50 of HbS in whole blood decreases from about 29 mm Hg to 18 mm Hg. Recently, this agent has been shown to increase hemoglobin levels in a small group of patients, but as noted earlier, it is still not clear in principle if such an agent will be beneficial because the nonmodified hemoglobin molecules must then give up

their oxygen to the tissues and will presumably enter into the polymer phase and impair the behavior of the red cells.

It can be argued that the increase in hemoglobin levels will itself result in extra molecules to deliver oxygen so that the fraction in the polymer phase (and perhaps the kinetics) will be improved; however, as noted earlier, there is reason to believe that increasing total hemoglobin (as in coexisting α thalassemia) may worsen some aspects of disease pathophysiology due to increases in effective blood viscosity.[122,123]

Recently, there has been much study on the increase in oxygen affinity with the drug GBT440, based on the hypothesis that it will result in a significant increase in blood hemoglobin (and hematocrit) levels and the extra hemoglobin molecules in circulation will result in less need for oxygen removal from each cell.[124] Thus, if the increase in hemoglobin molecules is greater than the reduction in optimally functioning hemoglobin molecules due to the chemical reactions, there will be a net decrease in polymer in each cell for the same level of oxygen delivery. Using the methods we have described earlier, we calculate that these changes in hemoglobin levels, which have been reported as about 0.5 to 1.0 g/dL with standard dosing, would amount to about a 5% to 10% increase in oxygen delivery molecules and would have about the same effects as increasing HbF by almost 10%.

In addition, erythropoietin, by increasing the number of oxygen-carrying hemoglobin molecules, should have a similar therapeutic effect, without any need for changes in other parameters such as HbF levels, which were the goals of therapeutic studies with this agent several decades ago.[125] However, as noted for coexisting α thalassemia, the increase in red cell numbers may itself contribute to increased viscosity and other deleterious effects, which might negate the therapeutic benefits. Indeed, in early studies of hydroxyurea to increase HbF and of other agents, phlebotomy was part of the protocol if hematocrit or hemoglobin levels rose beyond a prefixed level. Although increases in hemoglobin levels may reflect decreased hemolysis and improvement in polymerization-related fragility, it may also reflect compensatory mechanisms that are not entirely beneficial to the patient.

Physiologic Approaches

We have emphasized that disease pathology is a result of the decrease in sickle red cell flexibility with respect to that which is needed due to the resistance of the small blood vessels, or microcirculation. Because the properties of the microcirculation vary from tissue to tissue and because the propulsive force of the heart varies in time and in different parts of the body, it is not surprising that different organs may reflect the effects of the basic pathophysiologic mechanisms in this disease in very different ways. Thus, the factors that affect vascular resistance are clearly of great importance in understanding the manifestations of sickle cell disease.[110] The basic neural and humoral control of blood flow has been studied for a century and a half, and there is much information about these mechanisms and agents that are known to affect them, some of which may be of use in developing therapies for the sickle cell syndromes.

In recent years, perhaps the greatest interest has been in the role of NO as a vasodilator and its ability to be transported in the body, similar to a hormone.[126] This endocrine function of NO was originally attributed to the reversible formation of S-nitrosohemoglobin, but most work now points to circulating nitrite ions and their reduction by deoxyheme proteins (including deoxyHbS) to NO. Delivery of NO may be effected via dietary nitrate (reduced in the oral cavity to nitrite) or by inhalation or infusions of nitrite ions themselves, as well as by NO inhalation itself. Although all of these methods have difficulties, especially related to the ratio of toxicity to benefit and the evidence that circulating cell-free hemoglobin in sickle cell patients may itself tend to destroy NO bioactivity, much research continues in this area.[127]

Related to these processes is the recent concern about the toxic effects of red cell contents released by intravascular hemolysis, especially hemoglobin itself, which generates free heme and iron. Some of these globin molecules may enter tissues and cause pathology, but some effects may occur in the vasculature itself. Recent studies have focused on the potential use of haptoglobin to remove globin chains and of hemopexin to remove heme groups from the circulation.[128]

Among the metabolic abnormalities that occur in sickle cells, especially as a result of polymerization cycles, are changes in the redox properties, including increases in various reactive oxygen species (ROS).[129] Much pathology has been attributed to ROS, including destruction of NO, but this area of research remains controversial. However, work over the past 2 decades has provided evidence that exogenous L-glutamine can correct some of the abnormalities in the redox properties of sickle cells.[130] One clinical trial has shown that ingestion of this agent lowers crisis frequency, and its use to treat sickle cell disease patients has been approved by the FDA.[131]

Conclusion

Biophysical studies in the past half-century have given us much information about the structure of the deoxyHbS polymer that forms inside the red cells of patients with sickle syndromes, as well as the kinetics and thermodynamics of its formation, both in solutions and in cells. How red cells with polymer behave in the human vasculature—in blood vessels of all types and sizes—under the range of physiologic and pathologic changes that occur in patients is much less understood. In particular, the conditions under which the red cells themselves or their interactions with other cells in the circulation impede blood flow and undergo hemolysis require the use of new imaging techniques as well as in vitro flow systems that simulate the human circulation. Such studies need to focus on the vasculature—including its rheologic characteristics and changes in oxygen levels in particular, as well as the formation of various effectors of flow such as NO, endothelin, and other hormones and clotting factors—as well as the properties of the red cell itself.

The role of these rheologic abnormalities in contributing to disease manifestations is also little understood. In particular, disease effects in each of the major organs (eg, the brain, lungs, heart, kidneys, eye) seem to differ greatly, and these differences may reflect individuality of oxygen metabolism and vascular properties for each organ. In addition to these, pain crises, which are often treated as the primary end point for evaluation of therapies, may reflect as yet undiscovered processes; for example, crises may relate to changes in blood vessels rather than in the red cells or their interactions. Related to these differences is the likelihood that various therapies may improve pathology in some organs and not others. Improvement in crisis frequency or severity may not reflect benefit in all organs or mortality. These possibilities were anticipated in the work a decade ago that suggested that occlusion and hemolysis contributed very differently to the complex of symptoms and disease manifestations from individual to individual.[132]

Last, the disease-related processes that have increasingly occupied sickle cell research, such as cellular adhesion effects, inflammation, and thrombosis, are difficult to relate back directly to intracellular deoxyHbS polymerization or to quantitate with respect to their importance to potential sickle cell disease therapy. If these approaches are to prove valuable in the study of these syndromes, we believe such relationships must be explored and characterized in detail.

High-Yield Facts

- Intracellular HbS polymerization is the primary cause of the clinical manifestations of sickle cell disease.
- Whereas the oxygenated forms of both HbA and HbS are highly soluble, the HbS mutation (β^SGlu6→Val) results in the very low intracellular solubility of deoxyHbS compared to highly soluble deoxyHbA ($\alpha_2\beta_2$), resulting in the intracellular aggregation of the deoxyHbS molecules. This causes sickle red cells to have abnormal flow properties in the circulation, leading to impaired oxygen delivery to the tissues and increases in hemolysis, the effects of which are assumed to be the primary bases of the many pathophysiologic disease processes.
- Major factors affecting the effective HbS solubility inside the red cell are the oxygen saturation and the intracellular hemoglobin composition and concentration; the latter is very sensitive because of the nonideal behavior of intracellular hemoglobin.

High-Yield Facts (Cont.)

◆ Secondary changes in HbS polymer–containing erythrocytes within the vascular bed contributing to disease manifestations have been suggested as including membrane abnormalities, adhesion to other cells, intra- and extravascular fragility, endothelial abnormalities, and resulting inflammation.

◆ Disease severity correlates with determnations of HbS polymer fraction as a function of oxygen saturation for the different genetic sickle syndromes, but other genetic, cellular, and physiologic factors that modify the polymerization process may also affect disease severity.

◆ The benefits of therapeutic agents, such as hydroxurea, to increase HbF levels are primarily due to inhibition of intracellular HbS polymerization, but the complex downstream effects of this process may explain the organ-specific manifestations of sickle cell disease.

◆ Other current therapeutic approaches include replacing HbS with HbA or other hemoglobins with a lower propensity to polymerize, increasing the oxygen affinity of HbS, decreasing cellular interactions or inflammation, and decreasing levels of cell-free hemoglobin due to hemolysis. Some approaches have shown partial clinical efficacy and have received approval from the US Food and Drug Administration.

References

1. Herrick JB. Peculiar elongated and sickle shaped red blood corpuscles in a case of severe anemia. *Arch Intern Med.* 1910;6: 517-521.

2. Hahn EV, Gillespie E.B. Report of a case greatly improved by splenectomy and further observation on mechanism of sickle formation. *Arch Intern Med.* 1927;39:233-254.

3. Sherman IJ. The sickling phenomenon with special reference to the differentiation of sickle cell anemia. *Bull Johns Hopkins Hosp.* 1940;67:309-324.

4. Pauling L, Itano H, Singer SJ, Wells IC. Sickle cell anemia, a molecular disease. *Science.* 1949;110:543-548.

5. Ingram VM. A specific chemical difference between the globins of normal human and sickle cell anemia hemoglobin. *Nature.* 1956;178:792-794.

6. Perutz MF, Mitchison JM. State of haemoglobin in sickle-cell anaemia. *Nature.* 1950;166(4225):677-679.

7. Bertles JF, Dobler J. Reversible and irreversible sickling: a distinction by electron microscopy. *Blood.* 1969;33(6):884-898.

8. Eaton WA, Henry ER, Hofrichter J, Mozzarelli A. Is cooperative oxygen binding by hemoglobin really understood? *Nat Struct Biol.* 1999;6(4):351-358.

9. Eaton WA, Hofrichter J. Sickle cell hemoglobin polymerization. *Adv Protein Chem.* 1990;40:63-279.

10. Eaton WA, Bunn HF. Treating sickle cell disease by targeting HbS polymerization. *Blood.* 2017;129(20):2719-2726.

11. May A, Huehns ER. The concentration dependence of the oxygen affinity of haemoglobin S. *Br J Haematol.* 1975;30(3):317-335.

12. Forget BG, Bunn HF. Classification of the disorders of hemoglobin. *Cold Spring Harb Perspect Med.* 2013;3(2):a011684.

13. Dobler J, Bertles JF. The physical state of hemoglobin in sickle-cell anemia erythrocytes in vivo. *J Exp Med.* 1968;127(4):711-714.

14. Cretegny I, Edelstein SJ. Double strand packing in hemoglobin-S fibers. *J Mol Biol.* 1993;230(3):733-738.

15. Nagel RL, Johnson J, Bookchin RM, et al. Beta-chain contact sites in the haemoglobin S polymer. *Nature.* 1980;283(5750): 832-834.

16. Edelstein SJ. Molecular topology in crystals and fibers of hemoglobin S. *J Mol Biol.* 1981;150(4):557-575.

17. Rotter MA, Kwong S, Briehl RW, Ferrone FA. Heterogeneous nucleation in sickle hemoglobin: experimental validation of a structural mechanism. *Biophys J.* 2005;89(4):2677-2684.

18. Minton AP. Non-ideality and the thermodynamics of sickle-cell hemoglobin gelation. *J Mol Biol.* 1977;110(1):89-103.

19. Noguchi CT, Torchia DA, Schechter AN. Determination of deoxyhemoglobin-S polymer in sickle erythrocytes upon deoxygenation. *Proc Natl Acad Sci U S A.* 1980;77(9):5487-5491.

20. Sunshine HR, Hofrichter J, Ferrone FA, Eaton WA. Oxygen binding by sickle-cell hemoglobin polymers. *J Mol Biol.* 1982;158(2):251-273.

21. Xu XL, Lockamy VL, Chen KJ, et al. Effects of iron nitrosylation on sickle cell hemoglobin solubility. *J Biol Chem.* 2002;277(39):36787-36792.

22. Belcher JD, Gomperts E, Nguyen J, et al. Oral carbon monoxide therapy in murine sickle cell disease: beneficial effects on vaso-occlusion, inflammation and anemia. *PLoS One.* 2018; 13(10):e0205194.

23. Brugnara C. Sickle cell dehydration: pathophysiology and therapeutic applications. *Clin Hemorheol Microcirc.* 2018;68(2-3): 187-204.

24. Li Q, Henry ER, Hofrichter J, et al. Kinetic assay shows that increasing red cell volume could be a treatment for sickle cell disease. *Proc Natl Acad Sci U S A.* 2017;114(5):E689-E696.

25. Noguchi CT, Torchia DA, Schechter AN. Intracellular polymerization of sickle hemoglobin: effects of cell heterogeneity. *J Clin Invest.* 1983;72(3):846-852.

26. Schechter AN, Torchia DA, Noguchi CT. Erythrocyte nonuniformity and the intracellular polymerization of sickle hemoglobin. *Biophys J.* 1983;41(2):A226-A226.

27. Poillon WN, Kim BC. 2,3-Diphosphoglycerate and intracellular pH as interdependent determinants of the physiologic solubility of deoxyhemoglobin S. *Blood.* 1990;76(5):1028-1036.

28. Briehl RW. Gelation of sickle-cell hemoglobin .4. phase-transitions in hemoglobin S gels: separate measures of aggregation and solution-gel equilibrium. *J Mol Biol.* 1978;123(4):521-538.

29. Garel MC, Arous N, Calvin MC, Craescu CT, Rosa J, Rosa R. A recombinant bisphosphoglycerate mutase variant with acid phosphatase homology degrades 2,3-diphosphoglycerate. *Proc Natl Acad Sci U S A*. 1994;91(9):3593-3597.

30. Poillon WN, Kim BC, Labotka RJ, Hicks CU, Kark JA. Antisickling effects of 2,3-diphosphoglycerate depletion. *Blood*. 1995;85(11):3289-3296.

31. Ross PD, Hofrichter J, Eaton WA. Thermodynamics of gelation of sickle cell deoxyhemoglobin. *J Mol Biol*. 1977;115(2):111-134.

32. Ferrone FA, Hofrichter J, Eaton WA. Kinetics of sickle hemoglobin polymerization. 1. Studies using temperature-jump and laser photolysis techniques. *J Mol Biol*. 1985;183(4):591-610.

33. Moffat K. Gelation of sickle cell hemoglobin: effects of hybrid tetramer formation in hemoglobin mixtures. *Science*. 1974;185(4147):274-277.

34. Poillon WN, Kim BC, Rodgers GP, Noguchi CT, Schechter AN. Sparing effect of hemoglobin-F and hemoglobin-A2 on the polymerization of hemoglobin-S at physiological ligand saturations. *Proc Natl Acad Sci U S A*. 1993;90(11):5039-5043.

35. Noguchi CT, Torchia DA, Schechter AN. Polymerization of hemoglobin in sickle trait erythrocytes and lysates. *J Biol Chem*. 1981;256(9):4168-4171.

36. Sunshine HR, Hofrichter J, Eaton WA. Gelation of sickle-cell hemoglobin in mixtures with normal adult and fetal hemoglobins. *J Mol Biol*. 1979;133(4):435-467.

37. Bunn HF, Noguchi CT, Hofrichter J, Schechter GP, Schechter AN, Eaton WA. Molecular and cellular pathogenesis of hemoglobin-Sc disease. *Proc Natl Acad Sci U S A*. 1982;79(23):7527-7531.

38. Noguchi CT. Polymerization in erythrocytes containing S and non-S hemoglobins. *Biophys J*. 1984;45(6):1153-1158.

39. Moffat K, Gibson QH. The rates of polymerization and depolymerization of sickle cell hemoglobin. *Biochem Biophys Res Commun*. 1974;61:237-242.

40. Hofrichter J, Ross PD, Eaton WA. Kinetics and mechanism of deoxyhemoglobin-S gelation: A new approach to understanding sickle-cell disease. *Proc Natl Acad Sci U S A*. 1974;71:4864-4848.

41. Ferrone FA, Hofrichter J, Eaton WA. Laser-induced photolysis as a probe of sickle-cell hemoglobin gelation. *Biophys J*. 1978;21(3):A50-A50.

42. Coletta M, Hofrichter J, Ferrone FA, Eaton WA. Kinetics of sickle hemoglobin polymerization in single red-cells. *Nature*. 1982;300(5888):194-197.

43. Ferrone FA, Hofrichter J, Eaton WA. Kinetics of sickle hemoglobin polymerization. 2. A double nucleation mechanism. *J Mol Biol*. 1985;183(4):611-631.

44. Ferrone FA. The delay time in sickle cell disease after 40 years: a paradigm assessed. *Am J Hematol*. 2015;90(5):438-445.

45. Mozzarelli A, Hofrichter J, Eaton WA. Delay time of hemoglobin-S polymerization prevents most cells from sickling in vivo. *Science*. 1987;237(4814):500-506.

46. Huang Z, Hearne L, Irby CE, King SB, Ballas SK, Kim-Shapiro DB. Kinetics of increased deformability of deoxygenated sickle cells upon oxygenation. *Biophys J*. 2003;85(4):2374-2383.

47. Turner MS, Briehl RW, Ferrone FA, Josephs R. Twisted protein aggregates and disease: the stability of sickle hemoglobin fibers. *Phys Rev Lett*. 2003;90:12.

48. Wang JC, Kwong S, Ferrone FA, Turner MS, Briehl RW. Fiber depolymerization: fracture, fragments, vanishing times, and stochastics in sickle hemoglobin. *Biophys J*. 2009;96(2):655-670.

49. Needleman JP, Franco ME, Varlotta L, et al. Mechanisms of nocturnal oxyhemoglobin desaturation in children and adolescents with sickle cell disease. *Pediatr Pulmonol*. 1999;28(6):418-422.

50. Ahmed S, Siddiqui AK, Sison CP, Shahid RK, Mattana J. Hemoglobin oxygen saturation discrepancy using various methods in patients with sickle cell vaso-occlusive painful crisis. *Eur J Haematol*. 2005;74(4):309-314.

51. Higgins JM, Eddington DT, Bhatia SN, Mahadevan L. Review of an in vitro microfluidic model of sickle cell vaso-occlusion. *Transfus Clin Biol*. 2008;15(1-2):12-13.

52. Agarwal G, Wang JC, Kwong S, et al. Sickle hemoglobin fibers: mechanisms of depolymerization. *J Mol Biol*. 2002;322(2):395-412.

53. Klings ES, Christman BW, McClung J, et al. Increased F-2 isoprostanes in the acute chest syndrome of sickle cell disease as a marker of oxidative stress. *Am J Respir Crit Care Med*. 2001;164(7):1248-1252.

54. Seakins M, Gibbs WN, Milner PF, Bertles JF. Erythrocyte Hb-S concentration. An important factor in the low oxygen affinity of blood in sickle cell anemia. *J Clin Invest*. 1973;52(2):422-432.

55. Brousse V, El Hoss S, Bouazza N, et al. Prognostic factors of disease severity in infants with sickle cell anemia: a comprehensive longitudinal cohort study. *Am J Hematol*. 2018;93(11):1411-1419.

56. Chien S, Usami S, Bertles JF. Abnormal rheology of oxygenated blood in sickle cell anemia. *J Clin Invest*. 1970;49(4):623-634.

57. Asakura T, Hirota T, Nelson AT, Reilly MP, OheneFrempong K. Percentage of reversibly and irreversibly sickled cells are altered by the method of blood drawing and storage conditions. *Blood Cells Mol Dis*. 1996;22(24):297-306.

58. Rodgers GP, Noguchi CT, Schechter AN. Irreversibly sickled erythrocytes in sickle-cell anemia: a quantitative reappraisal. *Am J Hematol*. 1985;20(1):17-23.

59. Bartolucci P, Brugnara C, Teixeira-Pinto A, et al. Erythrocyte density in sickle cell syndromes is associated with specific clinical manifestations and hemolysis. *Blood*. 2012;120(15):3136-3141.

60. Steinberg MH, Sebastiani P. Genetic modifiers of sickle cell disease. *Am J Hematol*. 2012;87(8):795-803.

61. Kuypers FA. Hemoglobin S polymerization and red cell membrane changes. *Hematol Oncol Clin North Am*. 2014;28(2):155-179.

62. Lim MY, Ataga KI, Key NS. Hemostatic abnormalities in sickle cell disease. *Curr Opin Hematol*. 2013;20(5):472-477.

63. Brittenham GM, Schechter AN, Noguchi CT. Hemoglobin S polymerization: primary determinant of the hemolytic and clinical severity of the sickling syndromes. *Blood*. 1985;65(1):183-189.

64. Ware RE, de Montalembert M, Tshilolo L, Abboud MR. Sickle cell disease. *Lancet*. 2017;390(10091):311-323.

65. Noguchi CT, Rodgers GP, Serjeant G, Schechter AN. Levels of fetal hemoglobin necessary for treatment of sickle-cell disease. *N Engl J Med*. 1988;318(2):96-99.

66. Rees DC, Williams TN, Gladwin MT. Sickle-cell disease. *Lancet*. 2010;376(9757):2018-2031.

67. Bunn HF, Forget BG, Ranney HM. Hemoglobinopathies. *Major Probl Intern Med*. 1977;12:1-291.

68. Gupta AK, Kirchner KA, Nicholson R, et al. Effects of alpha-thalassemia and sickle polymerization tendency on the urine-concentrating defect of individuals with sickle-cell trait. *J Clin Invest*. 1991;88(6):1963-1968.

69. Liem RI, Chan C, Vu TT, et al. Association among sickle cell trait, fitness, and cardiovascular risk factors in CARDIA. *Blood*. 2017;129(6):723-728.

70. Brittenham GM, Schechter AN, Noguchi CT. Hemoglobin-S polymerization: primary determinant of the hemolytic and clinical severity of the sickling syndromes. *Blood*. 1985;65(1):183-189.

71. Noguchi CT, Torchia DA, Schechter AN. Determination of sickle hemoglobin polymer in SS and AS erythrocytes. *Blood Cells*. 1982;8(2):225-235.

72. Jackson JF, Odom JL, Bell WN. Amelioration of sickle cell disease by persistent fetal hemoglobin. *JAMA*. 1961;177:867-869.

73. Watson J. The significance of the paucity of sickle cells in newborn Negro infants. *Am J Med Sci*. 1948;215(4):419-423.

74. Watson J. A study of sickling of young erythrocytes in sickle cell anemia. *Blood*. 1948;3(4):465-469.

75. Natta CL, Niazi GA, Ford S, Bank A. Balanced globin chain synthesis in hereditary persistence of fetal hemoglobin. *J Clin Invest*. 1974;54(2):433-438.

76. Kato GJ, Piel FB, Reid CD, et al. Sickle cell disease. *Nat Rev Dis Primers*. 2018;4:18010.

77. Habara A, Steinberg MH. Genetic basis of heterogeneity and severity in sickle cell disease. *Exp Biol Med*. 2016;241(7):689-696.

78. Paikari A, Sheehan VA. Fetal haemoglobin induction in sickle cell disease. *Br J Haematol*. 2018;180(2):189-200.

79. Noguchi CT, Dover GJ, Rodgers GP, et al. Alpha-thalassemia changes erythrocyte heterogeneity in sickle-cell disease. *J Clin Invest*. 1985;75(5):1632-1637.

80. Steinberg MH, Embury SH. Alpha-thalassemia in blacks: genetic and clinical aspects and interactions with the sickle hemoglobin gene. *Blood*. 1986;68(5):985-990.

81. Noguchi CT, Eaton WA, Schechter AN, Torchia DA, Bunn HF. Gelation of mixtures of hemoglobins-S and hemoglobins-C and intracellular polymerization in SC-erythrocytes. *Fed Proc*. 1982;41(3):653-653.

82. Kato GJ, Steinberg MH, Gladwin MT. Intravascular hemolysis and the pathophysiology of sickle cell disease. *J Clin Invest*. 2017;127(3):750-760.

83. Serjeant GR, Vichinsky E. Variability of homozygous sickle cell disease: the role of alpha and beta globin chain variation and other factors. *Blood Cells Mol Dis*. 2018;70:66-77.

84. Nagel RL, Fabry ME, Steinberg MH. The paradox of hemoglobin SC disease. *Blood Rev*. 2003;17(3):167-178.

85. Bannerman RM, Serjeant B, Seakins M, England JM, Serjeant GR. Determinants of haemoglobin level in sickle cell-haemoglobin C disease. *Br J Haematol*. 1979;43(1):49-56.

86. Noguchi CT, Rodgers GP, Schechter AN. Intracellular polymerization of sickle hemoglobin: disease severity and therapeutic goals. *Prog Clin Biol Res*. 1987;240:381-391.

87. Steinberg MH, Chui DH, Dover GJ, Sebastiani P, Alsultan A. Fetal hemoglobin in sickle cell anemia: a glass half full? *Blood*. 2014;123(4):481-485.

88. Bessis M, Feo C, Jones E. Quantitation of red cell deformability during progressive deoxygenation and oxygenation in sickling disorders (the use of an automated Ektacytometer). *Blood Cells*. 1982;8(1):17-28.

89. Ballas SK, Mohandas N. Sickle red cell microrheology and sickle blood rheology. *Microcirculation*. 2004;11(2):209-225.

90. Zakharov MN, Aprelev A, Turner MS, Ferrone FA. The microrheology of sickle hemoglobin gels. *Biophys J*. 2010;99(4):1149-1156.

91. Torres Filho IP, Kerger H, Intaglietta M. pO2 measurements in arteriolar networks. *Microvasc Res*. 1996;51(2):202-212.

92. Tran H, Gupta M, Gupta K. Targeting novel mechanisms of pain in sickle cell disease. *Blood*. 2017;130(22):2377-2385.

93. Novelli EM, Gladwin MT. Crises in sickle cell disease. *Chest*. 2016;149(4):1082-1093.

94. Uwaezuoke SN, Ayuk AC, Ndu IK, Eneh CI, Mbanefo NR, Ezenwosu OU. Vaso-occlusive crisis in sickle cell disease: current paradigm on pain management. *J Pain Res*. 2018;11:3141-3150.

95. Carden MA, Fay ME, Lu X, et al. Extracellular fluid tonicity impacts sickle red blood cell deformability and adhesion. *Blood*. 2017;130(24):2654-2663.

96. Lu XR, Chaudhury A, Higgins JM, Wood DK. Oxygen-dependent flow of sickle trait blood as an in vitro therapeutic benchmark for sickle cell disease treatments. *Am J Hematol*. 2018;93(10):1227-1235.

97. Renoux C, Romana M, Joly P, et al. Effect of age on blood rheology in sickle cell anaemia and sickle cell haemoglobin C disease: a cross-sectional study. *PLoS One*. 2016;11(6):e0158182.

98. Mohandas N, Hebbel RP. Erythrocyte deformability, fragility, and rheology. In: Embury SH, Hebbel RP, Mohandas N, Steinberg MH, eds. *Sickle Cell Disease*. Raven Press; 1994:205-216.

99. Lew VL, Ortiz OE, Bookchin RM. Stochastic nature and red cell population distribution of the sickling-induced Ca2+ permeability. *J Clin Invest*. 1997;99(11):2727-2735.

100. Weiner DL, Brugnara C. Hydroxyurea and sickle cell disease: a chance for every patient. *JAMA*. 2003;289(13):1692-1694.

101. Nash GB, Johnson CS, Meiselman HJ. Rheologic impairment of sickle RBCs induced by repetitive cycles of deoxygenation-reoxygenation. *Blood*. 1988;72(2):539-545.

102. Hierso R, Lemonne N, Villaescusa R, et al. Exacerbation of oxidative stress during sickle vaso-occlusive crisis is associated with decreased anti-band 3 autoantibodies rate and increased red blood cell-derived microparticle level: a prospective study. *Br J Haematol*. 2017;176(5):805-813.

103. Belcher JD, Chen CS, Nguyen J, et al. Heme triggers TLR4 signaling leading to endothelial cell activation and vaso-occlusion in murine sickle cell disease. *Blood*. 2014;123(3):377-390.

104. Charache S, Grisolia S, Fiedler AJ, Hellegers AE. Effect of 2,3-diphosphoglycerate on oxygen affinity of blood in sickle cell anemia. *J Clin Invest*. 1970;49(4):806-812.

105. Kato GJ, Hebbel RP, Steinberg MH, Gladwin MT. Vasculopathy in sickle cell disease: biology, pathophysiology, genetics, translational medicine, and new research directions. *Am J Hematol*. 2009;84(9):618-625.

106. Hebbel RP. Beyond hemoglobin polymerization: the red-blood cell membrane and sickle disease pathophysiology. *Blood*. 1991;77(2):214-237.

107. Hebbel RP, Osarogiagbon R, Kaul D. The endothelial biology of sickle cell disease: inflammation and a chronic vasculopathy. *Microcirculation*. 2004;11(2):129-151.

108. Telen MJ. Beyond hydroxyurea: new and old drugs in the pipeline for sickle cell disease. *Blood*. 2016;127(7):810-819.

109. Telen MJ, Malik P, Vercellotti GM. Therapeutic strategies for sickle cell disease: towards a multi-agent approach. *Nat Rev Drug Discov*. 2019;18(2):139-158.

110. Sundd P, Gladwin MT, Novelli EM. Pathophysiology of sickle cell disease. *Annu Rev Pathol*. 2019;14:263-292.

111. Keleku-Lukwete N, Suzuki M, Panda H, et al. Nrf2 activation in myeloid cells and endothelial cells differentially mitigates sickle cell disease pathology in mice. *Blood Adv*. 2019;3(8):1285-1297.

112. Marouf R. Blood transfusion in sickle cell disease. *Hemoglobin*. 2011;35(5-6):495-502.

113. Biller E, Zhao Y, Berg M, et al. Red blood cell exchange in patients with sickle cell disease-indications and management: a review and consensus report by the therapeutic apheresis subsection of the AABB. *Transfusion*. 2018;58(8):1965-1972.

114. Brown FC, Conway AJ, Cerruti L, et al. Activation of the erythroid K-Cl cotransporter Kcc1 enhances sickle cell disease

pathology in a humanized mouse model. *Blood.* 2015;126(26): 2863-2870.

115. Kassa T, Strader MB, Nakagawa A, Zapol WM, Alayash AI. Targeting beta Cys93 in hemoglobin S with an antisickling agent possessing dual allosteric and antioxidant effects. *Metallomics.* 2017;9(9):1260-1270.

116. Nakagawa A, Ferrari M, Schleifer G, et al. A triazole disulfide compound increases the affinity of hemoglobin for oxygen and reduces the sickling of human sickle cells. *Mol Pharm.* 2018;15(5):1954-1963.

117. Pagare PP, Ghatge MS, Musayev FN, et al. Rational design of pyridyl derivatives of vanillin for the treatment of sickle cell disease. *Bioorg Med Chem.* 2018;26(9):2530-2538.

118. Beutler E. Effect of carbon-monoxide on red-cell life-span in sickle-cell disease. *Blood.* 1975;46(2):253-259.

119. Misra H, Bainbridge J, Berryman J, et al. A phase Ib open label, randomized, safety study of SANGUINATE™ in patients with sickle cell anemia. *Rev Brasil Hematol Hemoter.* 2017;39(1):20-27.

120. Abraham DJ, Mehanna AS, Wireko FC, Whitney J, Thomas RP, Orringer EP. Vanillin, a potential agent for the treatment of sickle cell anemia. *Blood.* 1991;77(6):1334-1341.

121. Metcalf B, Chuang CH, Dufu K, et al. Discovery of GBT440, an orally bioavailable R-state stabilizer of sickle cell hemoglobin. *ACS Med Chem Lett.* 2017;8(3):321-326.

122. Higgs DR, Aldridge BE, Lamb J, et al. The interaction of alpha-thalassemia and homozygous sickle-cell disease. *N Engl J Med.* 1982;306(24):1441-1446.

123. Hebbel RP, Hedlund BE. Sickle hemoglobin oxygen affinity-shifting strategies have unequal cerebrovascular risks. *Am J Hematol.* 2018;93(3):321-325.

124. Estepp JH. Voxelotor (GBT440), a first-in-class hemoglobin oxygen-affinity modulator, has promising and reassuring pre-clinical and clinical data. *Am J Hematol.* 2018;93(3):326-329.

125. Ferreira FA, Benites BD, Costa FF, Gilli S, Olalla-Saad ST. Recombinant erythropoietin as alternative to red cell transfusion in sickle cell disease. *Vox Sang.* 2019;114(2):178-181.

126. Schechter AN, Gladwin MT. Hemoglobin and the paracrine and endocrine functions of nitric oxide. *N Engl J Med.* 2003;348(15):1483-1485.

127. DeMartino AW, Kim-Shapiro DB, Patel RP, Gladwin MT. Nitrite and nitrate chemical biology and signalling. *Br J Pharmacol.* 2019;176(2):228-245.

128. Belcher JD, Chen CS, Nguyen J, et al. Haptoglobin and hemopexin inhibit vaso-occlusion and inflammation in murine sickle cell disease: Role of heme oxygenase-1 induction. *PLoS One.* 2018;13:4.

129. Meng FT, Kassa T, Strader MB, Soman J, Olson JS, Alayash AI. Substitutions in the subunits of sickle-cell hemoglobin improve oxidative stability and increase the delay time of sickle-cell fiber formation. *J Biol Chem.* 2019;294(11):4145-4159.

130. Quinn CT. L-Glutamine for sickle cell anemia: more questions than answers. *Blood.* 2018;132(7):689-693.

131. Niihara Y, Miller ST, Kanter J, et al. A phase 3 trial of L-glutamine in sickle cell disease. *N Engl J Med.* 2018;379(3):226-235.

132. Taylor JG, Nolan VG, Mendelsohn L, Kato GJ, Gladwin MT, Steinberg MH. Chronic hyper-hemolysis in sickle cell anemia: association of vascular complications and mortality with less frequent vasoocclusive pain. *PLoS One.* 2008;3:5.

Vaso-Occlusion in Sickle Cell Disease

Authors: *Huihui Li, Paul S. Frenette*

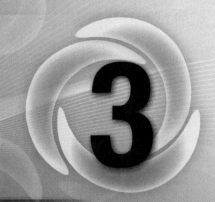

Chapter Outline

Overview

Repetitive vaso-occlusive episodes (VOEs) are the most common clinical manifestation of sickle cell disease (SCD). A VOE occurs when the microcirculation is temporarily or permanently obstructed by cellular aggregates, causing ischemic injury to the supplied organs and inducing pain. Acute pain and chronic organ damage provoked by the vascular occlusion may require emergency department visits or hospitalization for affected patients. Clinical presentations induced by VOE are variable and summarized in Table 3-1.[1,2] Although acute pain is a major reason for hospital admission and permanent organ damage is a frequent cause of mortality in SCD patients,[3,4] whether these 2 manifestations are linked remains unclear. VOE-associated ischemia in local tissue can indeed lead to organ dysfunction, but the etiology of these injuries is very complicated and not yet fully understood. For instance, the primary cause of acute chest syndrome is still debated, although it is thought to be a combination of infection, fat embolism, hypoventilation, and occlusion of the pulmonary vasculature.[5] VOE can be triggered by multiple circumstances such as dehydration, infection and/or fever, cold, stress, acidosis, hypoxia, and pain itself.[4] In addition, environmental factors, such as geographic altitude, weather, and air pollution, are likely to play an important role in triggering VOE.[2,6] Changes in these factors may promote red blood cell (RBC) sickling and initiate an inflammatory response with a cascade of cellular interactions among endothelial cells, leukocytes, and platelets and lead to vaso-occlusion in SCD patients. In this chapter, we will review the pathophysiology of

TABLE 3-1 Organ manifestations of vaso-occlusive events

Location	Complication	Presentation
Pulmonary	Acute chest syndrome	Pulmonary infection, fever, pleuritic chest pain
Kidney	Acute renal dysfunction	Hyposthenuria, hematuria, proteinuria
Spleen	Splenic sequestration, splenic infarction	Splenomegaly, drop in hemoglobin, abdominal pain and distension, sepsis from encapsulated organisms
Hepatobiliary	Acute intrahepatic cholestasis, hypoxic liver injury	Abdominal pain, hepatomegaly, hepatic necrosis and fibrosis
Skeletal/skin	Dactylitis, avascular necrosis	Swollen hands and feet, pain
Penis	Priapism	Painful sustained erection

VOE and discuss the implications for the development of suitable biomarkers of disease activity and therapeutic targets to prevent, treat, or cure the disease.

Fundamental Science Background

Endothelial Cells in Hemostasis

Endothelial cells form the lining of blood and lymphatic vessels and create a single-layered interface between circulating blood cells and the vessel wall. In addition to acting as conduit for blood transportation, endothelial cells regulate vessel permeability for fluid filtration and immune cell recruitment at the site of inflammation, while maintaining the vessel tone.[7,8] At steady state, endothelial cells repel platelet binding by the presence of negatively charged heparin sulphate proteoglycans on their surface[9,10] and can restrict platelet activation by secreting prostaglandin I_2 (PGI$_2$; also known as prostacyclin).[9-11] The effect of PGI$_2$ can be strengthened by nitric oxide (NO), which is produced by endothelial NO synthases (eNOS).[12,13] NO released by the endothelium functions as vasodilator to maintain vessel tone[14,15] and also plays an important role in

inhibiting platelet adhesion.[13] Mice lacking a functional eNOS gene (*NOS3*) displayed remarkably reduced bleeding time compared to wild-type mice, suggesting that presence of NO can significantly delay platelet recruitment and activation and hence play an important role in hemostasis.[16] Additionally, resting endothelial cells limit their interaction with leukocytes and platelets by sequestering the leukocyte interactive proteins, such as P-selectin and activating chemokines, and platelet-activating proteins, such as von Willebrand factor (vWF), within specialized secretory vesicles known as Weibel-Palade bodies (WPBs).[17,18] Another important function of NO is to inhibit WPBs surfacing up to the endothelial membrane, thereby preventing leukocyte and platelets activation.[19] Thus, endothelial cells at resting conditions synthesize different inhibitors to prevent formation of cell aggregates and maintain hemostasis.

Inflammation-Induced Cellular Interactions

Endothelial cells can rapidly respond to changes of the microenvironment (Figure 3-1A). A rapid response can occur within seconds in response to vasoactive stimuli independently of new gene expression.[20] A typical rapid response occurs after activation by ligands that bind to the extracellular domains of heterotrimeric G-protein–coupled receptors (GPCRs).[20] GPCRs represent a set of large and diverse protein receptors encoded by different genes that transduce intracellular signals for various extracellular ligands, including hormones, neurotransmitters, and sensory stimuli.[21,22] Intracellular signals transduced through endothelial heterotrimeric GPCRs result in influx of calcium ion and induction of cell signaling.[20] In this acute response, WPBs undergo exocytosis and bring P-selectin to the cell surface.[23] At the same time, phosphatidylcholine, a major phospholipid component of cell membrane, gets cleaved and acetylated into forms of platelet-activating factor (PAF).[24] Expression of P-selectin and PAF on endothelial membrane is important for leukocyte recruitment and extravasation.[25] Signaling through heterotrimeric GPCRs can last for 10 to 20 minutes and is followed by a more sustained inflammatory response that is triggered by endotoxin and inflammatory cytokines such as tumor necrosis factor-α (TNFα) and interleukin (IL)-1.[20] These mediators initiate a serial kinase cascade that activates the transcription factors nuclear factor-κB (NF-κB) and activator protein 1 (AP1).[26] These transcription factors induce a range of new genes for synthesis of proinflammatory proteins. Among these proteins are the adhesion molecules E-selectin, intercellular adhesion molecule 1 (ICAM1), and vascular cell adhesion molecule 1 (VCAM1), which are essential for leukocyte adhesion on endothelial cells.[10,20] PGI$_2$ synthesis is also enhanced to continuously increase plasma protein leakage into the tissue. Endothelial cells can also capture chemokines synthesized by other cells and present them on the heparin sulphate proteoglycans on the cell surface. All together, these changes facilitate leukocytes' firm attachment and induce leukocyte extravasation into tissue.[20] Because these responses involve transcription and translation of new proteins, this type of endothelial cell activation requires more time to be initiated.

Leukocytes are recruited to the inflammatory site and interact with endothelial cells by a tightly regulated cascade of adhesive and signaling events to facilitate their migration. Neutrophils, as the most abundant immune cells in the circulation, are activated to fight invading pathogens and keep the infection from spreading.[27] Neutrophil adhesion cascade includes slow rolling, polarization, arrest and intraluminal crawling, and migration.[28,29] The initial step to capture (or tether) neutrophils to the vessel wall is mediated by the P-selectin glycoprotein ligand 1 (PSGL1), E-selectin ligand 1 (ESL1), or L-selectin expressed on neutrophil membrane.[30,31] Neutrophil PSGL1 interacts with all 3 selectins, whereas ESL1 binds to E-selectin exclusively. L-selectin can bind a variety of endothelial molecules and, most importantly, interacts with PSGL1 from other neutrophils.[32,33] The interactions of selectins with their ligands enable neutrophils to adhere to inflamed endothelial cells and roll.[29,34] Studies have shown that ESL1 cooperates with PSGL1 to initiate tethering and networks with CD44 to slow down neutrophil rolling velocities.[35] Chemokines are secreted by activated endothelial cells or other cells, such as mast cells and platelets, and can bind with heparin sulphate proteoglycans on cell surface to recruit neutrophils to the site of inflammation.[20] Chemokines interact with specific neutrophil GPCRs including CXCR2, which binds to multiple chemokine receptors such as CXCL1, CXCL2, CXCL5, CXCL6, and CXCL7 on mouse neutrophils to regulate neutrophil mobilization; in human neutrophils, CXCR1 is also involved in CXCL8 detection.[29] Neutrophils also express other GPCRs, such as CCR2, CCR3, CCR5, CXCR3, and CXCR4, that expand their abilities to respond to more chemokines.[29] Binding of chemokines and their receptors activates integrin adhesion receptor of β2 and β1 families, and this leads to a change in integrin structure known as inside-out signaling, which increases ligand binding affinity and facilitates leukocyte attachment.[28] Conformational transformation at the same time allows integrins to receive signal and forms nano- and microclusters that further increase ligand interactions and avidity, in a phenomenon referred to as outside-in signaling.[28] The β2 integrins LFA1 (αLβ2) and MAC1 (also known as macrophage receptor 1, CD11b-CD18, and αMβ2) are functionally most important for controlling neutrophil rolling, arrest, and migration.[29] When LFA1 is partially activated through intracellular signaling pathways induced by PSGL1, it exhibits intermediate affinity to endothelial ICAM1 to decrease leukocyte rolling velocity.[36,37]

During transition from rolling to adhesion, neutrophils rapidly polarize; redistribute chemokine receptors, activated β2 integrins, and actin-remodeling GTPase clusters at their leading edge; and concentrate heavily glycosylated proteins such as PSGL1, L-selectin, and CD44, and other components involved in membrane retraction at its trailing edge (uropod).[35,38,39] Rearrangement of these microdomains is important for chemokine-driven movement of leukocytes

on and across the endothelium and initiate leukocyte-leukocyte interactions that facilitate secondary tethering to capture more leukocytes to the site of inflammation.[32,33]

The close interactions of rolling neutrophils with endothelial cells and exposure to chemokines enable binding of leukocyte integrins with endothelial immunoglobulin superfamily members, such as ICAM1 and VCAM1, and achieve firm arrest on the endothelium.[29] LFA1, at full activation, interacts with ICAM1 to firmly arrest leukocytes, which is immediately followed by MAC1/ICAM1-dependent crawling to probe for suitable sites for subsequent transmigration.[28,40] Experimental evidence suggests that MAC1/ICAM1-mediated neutrophil crawling relies on LFA1-induced outside-in signaling through the guanine nucleotide exchange factor VAV1, a major regulator for actin cytoskeleton remodeling during polarization and migration.[40] Other E-selectin–mediated signals transduced by ESL1 can also locally activate MAC1 at the leading edge of crawling neutrophils.[39] Following appropriate chemoattractant stimulation, leukocytes may choose to transmigrate into inflamed tissue, most commonly at the endothelial cell junction (paracellular) or sometimes directly through the endothelial cell body (transcellular). Paracellular transmigration involves engagement of several adhesion molecules and activation of junctional molecules, including ICAM1/2, VCAM1, JAM-A/C, PECAM1, CD99, and ESAM, which permit neutrophils to "squeeze" through endothelial junctions.[41] Transcellular route is initiated by forming actin-rich and ICAM1 clusters containing "transmigration cup" on the endothelial surface to wrap leukocytes.[41] During transcellular migration, activation of molecules, such as ICAM1, PECAM1, CD99, and JAM-A, facilitates leukocytes to pass through the transcellular channel formed between the apical and basal membrane of endothelial cells, leaving the endothelial junctions intact.[41]

Neutrophils' rapid and precise response to inflammatory stimuli is based on molecules stored in a variety of intracellular granules. These granule proteins control adhesion, transmigration, phagocytosis, and formation of neutrophil extracellular traps (NETs). Neutrophil secretory organelles contain azurophilic (primary), specific (secondary), and gelatinase (tertiary) granules, the multivesicular bodies (MVBs), and secretory vesicles.[29] With mild stimulation, these vesicles rapidly mobilize to the surface to initiate neutrophils' response by upregulating adhesion molecules and chemotactic receptors. With strong or repetitive stimulations, the neutrophil toxic granular cargoes are delivered either into the phagosome to eradicate microbes intracellularly or by exocytosis to kill extracellular bacteria.[29] Hence, neutrophil degranulation can be beneficial by removing infectious microbes, but may also be harmful by inducing endothelial dysfunction and systemic inflammation.[29] In addition to degranulation and phagocytosis, neutrophils can modify their chromatin and expel it into the extracellular space to trap and kill microbes, a phenomenon called NET formation.[42]

Recruitment of neutrophils at inflammatory sites may also be facilitated by platelets. Platelets are discoid-shaped fragments derived from bone marrow megakaryocytes and have

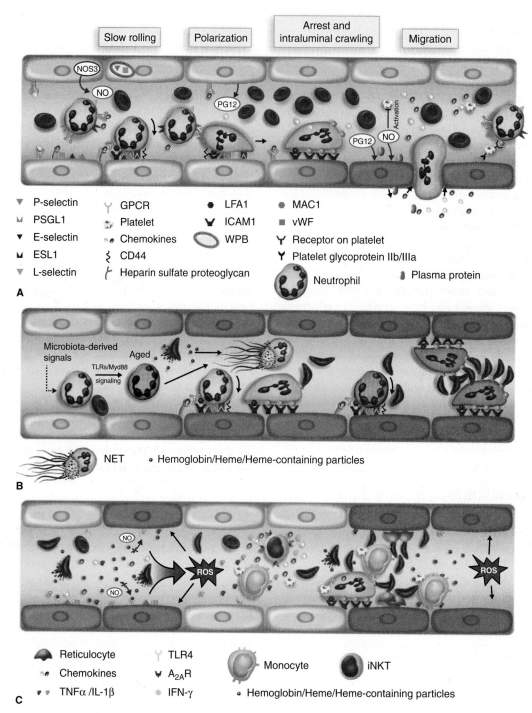

FIGURE 3-1 A. Cellular interactions induced by inflammation. Presence of stimuli triggers inflammatory responses, which release chemokines and cytokines at inflammatory sites to activate endothelial cells and platelets and quickly recruit immune cells such as neutrophils acting as front-line defense to clear harmful substances. When endothelial cells are activated, P-selectin rapidly surfaces to bind with neutrophils and initiate neutrophil rolling, followed by E-selectin and vascular cell adhesion molecule 1 (VCAM1), which mediate slow rolling, leading to adhesion. During transition from rolling to adhesion, neutrophils rapidly undergo polarization to rearrange microdomains that enable secondary tethering. Neutrophils firmly arrest on the endothelial cells via integrin interactions with their counterreceptors on endothelial cells and begin intraluminal crawling to survey the vasculature and probe for a suitable site for transmigration. Finally, neutrophils transmigrate through endothelial cells and arrive at the inflammatory site to remove harmful substances and cease the inflammation response. Additionally, activated platelets not only can "bridge" the endothelial and neutrophil interactions, but also facilitate the inflammatory response by secreting chemokines to activate endothelial cells and recruit more neutrophils. Inflammation is also negatively controlled by nitric oxide (NO). Presence of NO can prevent Weibel-Palade bodies (WPBs), which contain adhesion molecules, such as P-selectin and von Willebrand factor (vWF), from translocating to the surface of endothelial cells and releasing their content. NO, together with prostaglandin I_2 (PGI2), produces vasodilation, enhancing vascular permeability and increasing plasma protein leakage from blood into tissue. The extravasated plasma proteins can support the attachment, survival, and migration of invading neutrophils at inflammatory sites. ESL1, E-selectin ligand 1; GPCR, G-protein–coupled receptor; ICAM1, intercellular adhesion molecule 1; LFA1, β2 integrin αLβ21; MAC1, macrophage receptor 1/CD11b-CD18/αMβ2; PSGL1, P-selectin glycoprotein ligand 1.

a major role in maintaining vascular integrity and hemostasis. Platelets have 3 major types of storage granules: dense granules, lysosomes, and α-granules, of which α-granules are the most abundant.[43] Although the exact content of these granules remains incompletely known, they contain a diverse range of chemokines including CXCL1, CXCL4 (also known PF4), CXCL5, CXCL7, CXCL8 (IL-8), CXCL12, serotonin, and others.[43] Upon activation, platelets release these cytokines to regulate leukocyte movement, migration from the vasculature into the tissue, and other proinflammatory functions such as phagocytosis and generation of reactive oxygen species (ROS).[43] Furthermore, α-granules also contain P-selectin, which may initiate platelet-leukocyte binding through P-selectin/PSGL1 interaction, followed by firm adhesion mediated by leukocyte MAC1 and platelet glycoprotein (GP) Ib or platelet-bound fibrinogen or by leukocyte MAC1 to platelet ICAM2 binding.[39,44] Activated endothelial cells can rapidly trap platelets on their surface via platelet GPIIb/IIIa and endothelial-bound vWF.[45] In addition to directly promoting leukocyte adhesion to endothelial cells, endothelium-bound immobilized platelets can interact with leukocyte via P-selectin, acting as a bridge and further promoting leukocyte adhesion.[45] Although inflammation is generally thought to be beneficial to the host (eg, by providing protection against bacterial infection), it can be harmful when dysregulated as it is the case in SCD.

Alterations in Sickle Cell Disease

Mutated hemoglobin S (HbS) is prone to polymerize and cause SCD RBC membrane distortion. The repeated HbS polymerization and depolymerization process leads to membrane rigidity and susceptibility to undergo hemolysis or removal by the reticuloendothelial system.[1] Clinical data suggest that the total percentage of sickled cells (including reversibly and irreversibly sickled cells) increases 1 to 3 days prior to the onset of VOE and gradually decreases as patients recover.[46] In addition, a prospective study on 36 SCD patients over the course of 5 years reported that the RBC deformability (ability of erythrocytes to change shape under high shear force without hemolysis) was reduced prior to or at the time of VOE, and as the episode resolved, the RBC deformability reverted to values even higher than steady state, together with a reduced percentage of rigid cells.[47] Increased RBC deformability after recovery from VOE is likely due to lysis or removal of the most fragile SCD RBCs and to a lesser extent due to blockade of sickle RBCs (sRBCs) in the microcirculation.

Seminal in vitro adhesion experiments conducted nearly 40 years ago have revealed that sRBCs are more adherent to endothelial cells.[48,49] Subsequent studies proposed several possible adhesion mechanisms involving all major classes of cell adhesion molecules.[50,51] The finding that low-density (immature) RBCs were more adherent compared to high-density RBCs led to a working model in which the immature reticulocytes were initially recruited, followed by trapping of dense and rigid (irreversible) sickle cells.[50,52,53] Even though reticulocyte counts are occasionally used as a biomarker of disease severity,[54] there is no clinical evidence that direct suppression of reticulocyte counts or their adhesion has any impact on VOE. On the other hand, when blood cell trafficking was directly monitored by intravital microscopy of cremaster muscle, SCD RBCs were found to interact primarily with leukocytes that are firmly adherent to endothelial cells, causing temporary or permanent vessel obstruction.[55] These observations have suggested a pivotal role of leukocytes in initiating VOE.

Role of Neutrophils

Neutrophils are activated by inflammatory stimuli and signals from damaged endothelial cells and play an essential role in promoting vaso-occlusion. Neutrophils were first implicated in the SCD pathogenesis by observations that neutrophils could bind dense sRBCs in vitro.[56] As mentioned earlier, in

---

B. Role of neutrophils in vaso-occlusion. Neutrophil slow rolling on endothelial selectins initiates their activation, leading to firm adhesion mediated by integrins. Adherent neutrophils, after receiving a secondary wave of activation signals transduced by E-selectin, express activated MAC1 integrin, which captures circulating sickle red blood cells (RBCs) to induce a temporary or prolonged obstruction of venular blood flow. Recent studies show that an "aged" subset of neutrophils is the most active in capturing RBCs. Aging of neutrophils in the circulation is accelerated by the encounter of microbiota-derived signals through toll-like receptor (TLR)/Myd88 signaling pathways. Aged neutrophils exhibit enhanced MAC1 activation and neutrophil extracellular trap (NET) formation. Additionally, aged neutrophils exhibit increased neutrophil adhesion and elevated neutrophil-RBC interactions and play an important role in promoting vaso-occlusion in sickle cell disease (SCD). NET formation can also be boosted by heme and promotes acute pulmonary injury in SCD.

C. Multicellular contributions to vaso-occlusion. RBC sickling leads to changes in the surface membrane that increase RBC adhesion irritating the endothelium. Chronic hemolysis also causes the release of heme, which amplifies the inflammatory response in part through the toll-like receptor 4 (TLR4) signaling pathway. Free hemoglobin can also react with NO, depleting its bioavailability and generating reactive oxygen species (ROS) that damages endothelial cells. Additionally, endothelial cell activation can be further enhanced by proinflammatory cytokines such as tumor necrosis factor-α (TNFα) and interleukin (IL)-1β secreted from activated monocytes. Endothelial cell activation consequently upregulates adhesion molecules and recruits more neutrophils. When firmly adhered on the endothelial cells, neutrophils capture circulating sickle RBCs and initiate vaso-occlusion. Platelets may also contribute by secreting cytokines to activate neutrophils and endothelial cells, and by forming aggregates with monocytes and neutrophils. Invariant natural killer T (iNKT) cells are activated through its adenosine 2A receptor ($A_{2A}R$) and may also participate in pulmonary dysfunction and vaso-occlusion via interferon-γ (IFN-γ) and the secretion of other cytokines.

vivo analysis of the microcirculation in sickle Berkeley mice has revealed that the recruitment of a dense population of adherent leukocytes and the interactions of sRBCs with these leukocytes in postcapillary venules initiated VOE, whereas SCD mice deficient in P- and E-selectin exhibited defective recruitment of leukocytes to the vessel wall and were protected from vaso-occlusion.[55] Follow-up experiments demonstrated that Gr1+ neutrophils are the major leukocyte subpopulation that adhere on activated endothelial cells and capture circulating RBCs in TNFα-stimulated SCD mice.[34] The mechanism by which adherent neutrophils capture circulating RBC is via the MAC1 integrin. The interactions between neutrophils and RBCs are propagated and enhanced by surgical trauma and TNFα stimulation, leading to acute, lethal vaso-occlusion[39] (Figure 3-1B). Activation of MAC1 on adherent neutrophils requires a secondary wave of activation signals promoted by E-selectin binding. Inactivation of either MAC1 or E-selectin leads to reduced vaso-occlusion and prolonged survival of SCD mice.[39,57] Inhibition of selectin through a carbohydrate mimetic of the tetrasaccharide sialyl Lewis^x (sLe^x), a component of selectin ligands found on leukocytes and monocytes, significantly reduces leukocyte–endothelial cell adhesion and improves survival of SCD mice.[58] Recent studies using micro-fluidic flow chambers demonstrate that human SCD-derived neutrophil rolling on endothelial E-selectin may be preferentially mediated by sLe^x presented by neutrophil L-selectin.[59] In addition to selectin-dependent interactions, blocking of endothelin receptor on leukocytes[60] or targeting endothelin-1 molecules by omega-3 fatty acid[61] may reduce neutrophil-endothelium interactions and lower inflammation in SCD mice, suggesting that endothelin-1 may also participate in neutrophil activation and recruitment during VOE.

Excessive heme accumulation from RBC hemolysis triggers NET formation in the pulmonary vasculature of SCD mice[62] (Figure 3-1B). The fundamental function of NETs is the formation of extracellular fibers from granule proteins and chromatin to trap bacteria and prevent them from spreading.[42] In SCD mice, after TNFα challenge, NETs in the pulmonary vasculature appear to contribute to acute lung injury, and the lung damage is significantly prevented or delayed by the NET-dismantling reagent DNAse I or the heme scavenger molecule hemopexin.[62] Independent studies have also found that heme infusion dramatically induces acute lung injury in SCD mice.[63]

Circulating neutrophils have long been considered as a homogenous population. However, recent data suggest that neutrophils, as they age in the circulation, gradually upregulate CXCR4 and downregulate L-selectin expression.[64] Aged neutrophils represent an overly active proinflammatory subset that exhibits enhanced MAC1 integrin activation. Neutrophils are regulated by the gut microbiota from their products and metabolites that can diffuse into circulation and induce neutrophil aging through TLR/Myd88-dependent pathways (Figure 3-1B). In addition, the microbiota can also diffuse into the bone marrow and be sensed by mesenchymal stem cells, which synthesize cytokines that support lineage differentiation from hematopoietic stem cells (HSCs).[65] In SCD mice, aged

neutrophils are significantly expanded compared to wild-type mice, and upregulation of aged neutrophils strongly correlates with increased neutrophil adhesion, MAC1 activation, neutrophil-RBC interactions, and NETs formation[64] (Figure 3-1B). Microbiota depletion using broad-spectrum antibiotics normalizes aged neutrophil numbers, reduces vaso-occlusion, and prolongs survival.[64] Consistent with murine data, SCD patients exhibit high numbers of circulating aged neutrophils, and these numbers are reduced in patients on penicillin prophylaxis.[64] SCD patients start to take penicillin at a young age to prevent morbidity and mortality from *Streptococcus pneumoniae* infection[66]; however, the function of antibiotics in VOE remains unknown. This study implies that antibiotic treatment may be a potential therapy for VOE in SCD patients, and this should be evaluated further in clinical trials.

Hemolysis and NO Pathways

When RBCs undergo hemolysis, free hemoglobin is released into the plasma. At steady state, free hemoglobin can quickly bind with scavenger proteins such as haptoglobin and form complexes that are cleared from plasma. In SCD patients, HbS polymerization induces excessive RBC lysis, which overwhelms the clearance and detoxifying system, allowing free hemoglobin to react with NO in circulation to produce methemoglobin and nitrate. This ultimately depletes NO bioavailability and generates ROS that promote inflammation.[67] Additionally, free hemoglobin can form hemoglobin/heme-loaded microparticles, which may lead to vascular dysfunction and activate endothelial cells to express adhesion molecules promoting vaso-occlusion (Figure 3-1C).[68-70] Heme can also activate neutrophil and platelets, whose roles are discussed in the relevant sections.

Endothelial-derived NO, produced by NOS3, suppresses platelet activation,[13] restrains adhesion molecules in WPBs,[19] and diffuses to adjacent smooth muscle cells to promote vasodilation and regulate vessel tone. NO consumption and subsequent hemoglobin oxidation occur via 2 reactions: (1) NO deoxygenation of oxygenized hemoglobin, which generates nitrate (NO_2^-) and ferric hemoglobin (Hb-Fe^{3+}), and (2) iron nitrosylation of deoxygenized hemoglobin, which occurs by direct iron binding of NO to ferrous hemoglobin (Hb-Fe^{2+}).[71] In SCD patients, levels of NO metabolites (eg, L-arginine and NOx) are significantly reduced at time of crisis and return to normal during hospitalization, suggesting NO depletion is associated with vaso-occlusion.[5] In SCD mice, when NO bioavailability is increased by either hydroxyurea or phosphodiesterase 9 (PDE9) inhibitors, leukocyte adhesion and leukocyte-RBC interactions are reduced, together with extended life span survival, implying that upregulation of the NO pathway can help resolve VOE.[72]

Hemoglobin undergoes peroxidation by H_2O_2 to generate superoxide $O_2^{\bullet-}$, and increased ROS can damage endothelial cells and induce vaso-occlusion.[71] In addition to directly binding to hemoglobin, NO bioavailability can be further reduced by its reaction with superoxide $O_2^{\bullet-}$ to form NO_3^-. In vitro experiments demonstrate that oxidant stress increases monocytes and reticulocyte adhesion, indicating that injury or activation of endothelium can contribute to VOE in SCD.[73]

Free heme is released from free hemoglobin upon oxidation and is a mediator of inflammation and vascular injury. In SCD mice, heme-induced inflammation, vaso-occlusion, and coagulation can be effectively relieved by treatment with the heme scavenger hemopexin.[74] Hemolysis-induced oxidative stress provokes disruption of RBC membrane phospholipid asymmetry followed by membrane vesiculation resulting in the release of heme-contained microparticles.[74,75] RBC microparticles deliver toxic heme to damage endothelial cells and trigger vaso-occlusion.[70] Heme rapidly (approximately 5 minutes) activates NF-κB and mobilizes WPBs to upregulate P-selectin and vWF expression on endothelial cells, a process regulated by endothelial TLR4 signaling.[76] Damage-associated molecular patterns (DAMPs) generated from erythrocyte hemolysis products propagate inflammation and oxidative stress, further impairing the redox balance.[74] Thus, free hemoglobin released from intravascular hemolysis reduces NO bioavailability and generates free heme and DAMPs that disrupt vessel tone and lead to endothelial dysfunction.

Platelets and Other Blood Cells Contributing to SCD Inflammation

Platelets are activated in SCD patients under steady-state conditions, and the activation is further enhanced during VOE.[77,78] Cytokines released from activated platelets promote vaso-occlusion and generate ROS in SCD mice[43] (Figure 3-1C). In an in vitro microfluidic system, human SCD-derived platelets accumulated around arrested neutrophils, leading to increased number and extended duration of neutrophil-platelet interactions compared to control normal human blood samples.[78] In addition to leukocyte MAC1 binding with platelet GPIb or ICAM2,[39,44] the serine/threonine kinase isoform AKT2, which regulates the translocation and activation of MAC1 on neutrophils, is reported to play an essential role in neutrophil crawling and neutrophil-platelet interactions on activated endothelial cells during inflammation[79] (Figure 3-1C). AKT2 inhibition reduces neutrophil-platelet aggregates isolated from SCD patients and suppresses neutrophil adhesion and neutrophil-platelet aggregation in SCD mice, hence improving blood flow.[79] Activated platelets express CD40L, which has similar structure and similar effect as TNFα. Platelet-expressed CD40L binds to endothelial CD40 to promote secretion of chemokines, such as IL-8 and CCL2, and upregulation of adhesion molecules.[80] Despite these exciting data collected from in vivo experiments, clinical trials that target platelet activation have yielded disappointing results thus far. In a phase III clinical trial, prasugrel, a P2Y12 antagonist that decreases platelet activation, did not significantly prevent VOE.[81]

Other leukocytes, such as monocytes and invariant natural killer T (iNKT) cells, are also activated as a part of the inflammatory response and participate in the initiation or prevention of VOE in SCD (Figure 3-1C). Monocytes secrete proinflammatory cytokines, such as TNFα or IL-1β, that activate the NF-κB pathway in endothelial cells to upregulate the expression of surface adhesion molecules such as E-selectin, ICAM1, and VCAM1, and consequently promote leukocyte-endothelial binding.[82] Although the mechanisms that contribute to monocyte activation in SCD are still inconclusive, studies show that platelet binding to monocytes leads to monocyte activation. SCD patients show a 2- to 3-fold increase in platelet-monocyte aggregates, and levels of TNFα or IL-1β are elevated by 20- to 30-fold compared to controls, suggesting activation of monocytes in SCD patients.[83] Interestingly, a population of CD14low CD16+ monocytes (also known as patrolling monocytes), which normally scavenge damaged cells and debris from the vasculature, was found to have a beneficial effect in VOE in SCD mice.[84] This set of monocytes expresses high levels of anti-inflammatory heme oxygenase (HO-1), a heme-degrading enzyme, and is significantly increased in SCD patients compared to controls.[84] Heme-mediated VOE induced by sRBC infusion is exacerbated in patrolling monocyte–deficient mice, and this phenomenon is reversed with patrolling monocyte transfer.[84] The role of monocytes in VOE is controversial, and additional studies are required to categorize monocytes into specific subpopulations with their precise functionalities.

iNKT cells are a subset of T cells that produce significant amounts of proinflammatory cytokines[85] and play an important role in promoting pulmonary inflammation and dysfunction in SCD. For example, there are increased numbers of total and activated CD69+ interferon-γ (IFN-γ)-positive iNKT cells in lung, liver, and spleen of NY1DD SCD mice, and these cells are hyperresponsive to hypoxia/reoxygenation.[85] iNKT cells are activated and induce pulmonary dysfunction by a pathway involving overexpression of IFN-γ and production of chemokines (eg, CXCL9, CXCL10) for chemokine receptor CXCR3, which can be prevented by genetic deficiency or antibody inhibition, resulting in inactivation of iNKT cells.[85] Additional studies suggest that iNKT cells overexpress their adenosine 2A receptor ($A_{2A}R$) during painful VOE in SCD patients, and elevated $A_{2A}R$ may function through a counterregulatory mechanism intended to inhibit activation of iNKT cells[86] (Figure 3-1C). During VOE, iNKT cells from SCD patients are activated to express high levels of $A_{2A}R$ in an NF-κB–dependent manner.[86,87] Treatment of SCD mice with $A_{2A}R$ agonist resulted in dose-dependent reversal of pulmonary dysfunction, and when SCD mice are genetically depleted of lymphocytes by crossing with Rag1−/− mice, animals show reduced pulmonary injury. The protection from lung injury can be abrogated by transfer of 10^6 purified iNKT cells.[88] A phase II trial failed to demonstrate any significant difference in pain score or length of hospital stay between treatment and placebo groups relative to the percentage of iNKT cell reduction (cutoff of depletion >30%).[89] Another phase I compound, NNKTT120, specifically induced rapid iNKT cell depletion without serious adverse effects in SCD patients, and its function in VOE is being investigated in follow-up clinical trials.[90]

The onset of VOE is triggered by multiple interrelated pathways that may act in a vicious cycle. SCD RBCs may directly interact with endothelial cells or undergo hemolysis and consume NO, liberate heme together with other inflammatory cytokines that induce ROS, activate endothelial cells, and recruit neutrophils to the inflammatory site. Neutrophils attach on the activated endothelial cells and trap circulating SCD RBCs to form a complex that temporarily or permanently reduces flow to initiate VOE. The inflammatory microenvironment in SCD also triggers activation of other cells, such as platelets, monocytes, and iNKT cells, that either secrete chemokines or inflammatory cytokines to recruit more neutrophils to the site or directly interact with other cells to form aggregates. Clogged vessels have further delays in oxygen delivery, thereby inducing more severe hypoxia, which amplifies the subsequent signals that worsen VOE. Understanding the details of dysfunctional signaling pathways that initiate vaso-occlusion in SCD has led to the development of new agents for disease treatment.

Clinical Biomarkers of Vaso-occlusion

Understanding the natural history and disease progression of SCD patients to select those who are at high risk of complications could lead to personalized treatment and better prognosis. Monitoring changes in blood cellular parameters or circulating biomarkers may allow early detection or even prevent acute complications and guide therapeutic decisions.

Disease Severity and Changes in Blood Cell Parameters

The fundamental element that determines disease severity is the type of mutated hemoglobin gene inherited from the parents and the levels of fetal hemoglobin (HbF) present in steady state. The most severe form of SCD is due to inheritance of homozygous hemoglobin S mutation (HbSS), a subtype with a 50% to 60% prevalence in SCD patient cohorts from the United States, Caribbean, United Kingdom, and Europe.[1] In the compound heterozygous condition, namely HbSC (HbS with HbC, 25%-30% prevalence in SCD patients), HbS/β+ (HbS with mild β thalassemia and presence of 10%-25% hemoglobin A, 5%-10% prevalence in SCD patients), and HbS/β0 (HbS with severe β thalassemia, 1%-3% prevalence in SCD patients), the severity of clinical manifestations is variable.[1] There is also a 1% to 2% prevalence of compound heterozygous conditions of HbS with other β-globin variants, and the outcome severity depends on the β-globin gene mutation.[1] The inheritance of both HbA and HbS is commonly referred to as sickle cell trait, which carries a largely benign phenotype.[1] Another important regulator of disease severity is the level of HbF. In general, expression of HbF is gradually replaced by adult β-globin after birth, and SCD patients who express relatively high levels of HbF have reduced VOE, acute chest syndrome, and a lower rate of early mortality.[91]

Reticulocytes in SCD are known to bind to activated endothelial cells and may play a role in endothelial cells' inflammatory phenotype and VOE.[92] The percentage of reticulocytes in the circulation is also inversely related to RBC life span.[93] It has been suggested that reticulocyte counts in SCD children may function as a predictor of SCD severity.[54] Five out of 6 studies that have assessed reticulocyte counts have reported that more brisk reticulocytosis correlates with higher transcranial Doppler velocities (indicating increased blood flow velocity) and increased risk of stroke and early hospitalization for VOE and splenic sequestration, but is not associated with acute chest syndrome or death.[54] It is not clear whether higher reticulocyte counts directly contribute to disease severity or whether they merely represent a biomarker of disease severity.

The function of neutrophils in promoting VOE is documented in many reports. As the clinical manifestations have become more severe, leukocytosis and neutrophilia are well documented.[94] A recent study also demonstrates that microvascular oxygen consumption and neutrophil counts are further elevated in SCD patients during VOE.[95] Increased oxygen consumption more likely reflects the local density and activity of intravascular blood cells rather than the metabolic demands of erythropoiesis at distant sites.[95] Multiple case reports show that when myeloid growth factors such as granulocyte-macrophage colony-stimulating factor (GM-CSF) or granulocyte colony-stimulating factor (G-CSF) are given to SCD patients to mobilize HSCs, patients develop severe or fatal VOE together with dramatic leukocytosis.[96-98] However, suppression of overstimulated leukocytes by a chemotherapy drug—hydroxyurea—quickly resolved acute complications in a patient,[96] suggesting a direct role of leukocytes in acute disease manifestations. Leukocytosis also positively correlates with early death, silent brain infracts, hemorrhagic strokes, and acute chest syndrome in SCD patients,[82] suggesting the critical role of leukocytes, and neutrophils in particular, in SCD morbidity and mortality.

Together with increased neutrophils, many reports show strong correlations among monocyte counts, iNKT cell counts, and platelet numbers with the onset of VOE in SCD patients,[83,86,99,100] suggesting these cells may also participate. Different from neutrophils, which further increase prior to the onset of VOE, platelet count is high at steady state and declines during acute VOE.[101] It is recommended that SCD patients receive a low dose of hydroxyurea as standard treatment (maintenance dose) with neutrophil counts between 2000 and 25,000/μL, reticulocyte counts between 80,000 and 95,000/μL, and platelets counts between 80,000 and 95,000/μL; in addition, increasing the dose to a maximum of 35 mg/kg body weight when blood cell counts exceed these values should be considered.[102] Acute complications of SCD involve the activation of multiple cells, and emerging therapies have been designed to target these different cell populations. Monitoring changes in cellular numbers in SCD patients can guide practitioners to gauge disease severity and may also confirm the effectiveness of treatments in these patients.

Biomarkers of Vaso-occlusion

Molecular biomarkers include by-products of activated cells in the blood circulation that can be objectively measured to predict, diagnose, and monitor a pathogenic process. Even though

TABLE 3-2 Biomarkers of vaso-occlusion

Biomarker	Source	Effect	References
ICAM1	Endothelial cells	Released from endothelial cells, bind to leukocyte LFA1 and MAC1	104-106
VCAM1	Endothelial cells	Released from endothelial cells, bind to α4β1	104-106
P-selectin	Endothelial cells/platelets	Released from endothelial cells and platelets, bind to leukocyte PSGL1	104, 105
E-selectin	Endothelial cells	Released from endothelial cells, bind to leukocyte ESL1	104, 105
Prostaglandins	Endothelial cells	Vasodilators and suppress platelets-endothelium adhesion	9, 10, 109
IL-1β	Monocytes	Inflammatory mediator	83, 108, 114
IL-6	Monocytes	Inflammatory mediator	107, 108, 116, 171
IL-10	Monocytes	Anti-inflammatory	108, 171
TNFα	Monocytes	Inflammatory mediator	83, 107, 171
PlGF	Immature erythrocytes	Promotes monocyte activation	110, 111
CRP	Liver	Inflammatory mediator	107, 113, 115

Abbreviations: CRP, C-reactive protein; ICAM1, intercellular adhesion molecule 1; IL, interleukin; PlGF, placenta growth factor; TNFα, tumor necrosis factor-α; VCAM1, vascular cell adhesion molecule 1.

overexpressed adhesion molecules on activated cell surfaces play an important role in promoting cellular interactions and inducing vaso-occlusion, measuring adhesion either ex vivo or in vivo remains difficult. Studies of adhesion molecule expression, as discussed in prior sections, are often performed to understand disease mechanisms or response to new drugs, but these have not been extensively explored as markers of disease activity.[103] Vaso-occlusion can be triggered and worsened by dysfunctional endothelial cells and inflammation, and the biomarkers from these activities have been measured and correlated with disease activity (Table 3-2). Activation of endothelial cells leads to increased secretion of soluble ICAM1, VCAM1, P-selectin, E-selectin, and prostaglandins, with the first 3 biomarkers being independently associated with the risk of mortality in SCD cohort studies.[104-106] Inflammatory cytokines, such as IL-1β, IL-6, IL-10, and TNFα, and other markers such as placenta growth factor (PlGF) and C-reactive protein (CRP) are elevated at steady state and in VOE,[83,107-116] suggesting a potential role in monitoring and identifying disease progression.

Microparticles derived from multiple cell sources, including RBCs, platelets, monocytes, and endothelial cells, are increased in SCD patients at steady state and further increased in acute VOE.[117] Microparticles were first observed and implicated in the SCD pathogenesis when experimental data demonstrated that the plasma membrane undergoes outward budding in the process of RBC sickling.[118] The biological function of microparticles may include intercellular communication or the dissemination of inflammatory signals.[119,120] However, the role of microparticles as biomarkers remains controversial. Some studies show that microparticles are increased after hydroxyurea treatment,[121,122] while others claim a reduction of microparticles after treatment.[117,123,124]

Because vaso-occlusion can be triggered by an array of events (eg, infections, hypoxia, physical stress), it is challenging to identify a single biomarker of VOE. However, biomarkers may help risk stratify SCD patients for research and therapy and predict and monitor response to pharmacologic treatments.

Current and Emerging Therapies

The present cure for SCD is through stem cell transplantation from matched bone marrow or cord blood stem cells.[1] Despite the fact that event-free survival can be close to 90% with human leukocyte antigen–matched donor cells, stem cell transplantation has limitations: only 10% to 20% of patients have unaffected matched sibling donors, and the results using matched unrelated donors or unrelated cord blood units are suboptimal.[1] Current data revealed that the main problem for failure of unrelated donor marrow transplantation is due to graft-versus-host disease (GVHD).[125] In combination with a T-cell depletion strategy, bone marrow transplantation from haploidentical donors of a first-degree relative show reduced severity of GVHD.[126] Details of transplantation and transfusion therapies are reviewed in other chapters. In the following sections, we will briefly review currently approved and promising therapies.

Hydroxyurea

Hydroxyurea (HU) has beneficial effects in SCD patients and has been used since the late 1980s.[127] Based on the seminal Multicenter Study of Hydroxyurea (MSH) phase III trial data, where HU led to a 40% reduction in the incidence of VOE, acute chest syndrome, and hospitalization,[128] HU was approved by the US Food and Drug Administration (FDA) for symptomatic SCD adult patients in 1998. Trials of HU in pediatric populations followed in Europe and the United States. A phase I/II trial (HUG-KIDS) including patients aged 5 to 15 years demonstrated that HU significantly reduced diseased-related complications with no evidence of long-term toxicities.[91,129] In a subsequent trial (BABY HUG), HU treatment in infants aged 9 to 18 months did not prevent organ damage.[130,131] However, HU significantly reduced pain, dactylitis, transfusion, and hospital admissions. HU also led to significantly improved splenic and renal function as well as decreased transcranial Doppler velocity, suggesting a reduced stroke risk.[130,131] In 2017, HU was approved by the FDA to use in children aged 2 to 18 years.

Specific mechanisms have been extensively studied to understand how HU reduces VOE. As shown in Figure 3-2A, HU reduces vaso-occlusion by upregulating HbF production, interfering with HbS polymerization, and inhibiting cellular interactions and adhesion events that promote VOE. Studies have demonstrated that HU generally induces an additional 8% to 18% HbF level over baseline, and SCD children exhibit higher baseline HbF levels compared to adults.[132,133] A possible mechanism of HbF induction by HU implicates a bone marrow shift to a stressed state from the repetitive pharmacologic injury of daily drug use, which favors the output of RBCs containing higher HbF content.[102,134] RBCs containing high HbF concentrations are referred to as F cells and have reduced RBC membrane damage and hemolysis.[134] A major mechanism of HU may also be related to its effect on suppressing WBC counts, as well as decreasing adhesion molecule expression on endothelial cells and RBCs[102,135] (Figure 3-2A). Additionally, HU serves as an NO donor to enhance NO-induced vasodilation and improve blood flow[134] (Figure 3-2A). HU-induced NO availability also participates in boosting HbF synthesis through stimulation of soluble guanylyl cyclase–related signaling pathways.[136,137] In murine SCD models, long-term HU treatment consistently demonstrated its inhibitory effect on leukocytes without any impact on organ damage, but showed no effect on HbF concentration[138] due to the fact that HbF is not operative in this transgenic mouse model.[139] In sum, HU has pleiotropic benefits in SCD, but because of its limitations, including its failure to prevent organ damage in young children, side effect profile, and lack of response in some patients, there has been an effort to explore other approaches to the treatment of SCD.

L-Glutamine

L-Glutamine was approved by the FDA to treat SCD in 2017, but studies on the function of L-glutamine in SCD remain limited. Based on earlier work showing that glutamine bioavailability is associated with decreased nicotinamide adenine dinucleotide (NAD) redox potential and increased oxidative stress in RBC[140-142] (Figure 3-2B), Niihara et al[143] conducted a clinical trial of L-glutamine at 30 g/d for 4 weeks in 7 individuals with SCD. They showed that L-glutamine led to a significant increase in NAD redox potential, suggesting its potential function in reducing oxidative stress in erythrocytes.[143] In a follow-up in vitro experiment, L-glutamine treatment reduced patient-derived sickle erythrocyte adhesion to endothelial cells, suggesting that it may play a beneficial role in VOE.[144] In a recent phase III clinical trial conducted by Niihara et al,[145] L-glutamine administered at the dose of 0.3 g/kg body weight twice daily for a total of 48 weeks significantly lowered the rate of VOE and hospitalization in SCD patients. Two-thirds of patients were taking HU concurrently. The current recommended dose of L-glutamine in SCD appears to be well tolerated with only gastrointestinal side effects and headache,[145] but long-term safety data are lacking. There are also concerns about the safety of L-glutamine in critically ill patients because of evidence of higher mortality rates compared to placebo in this population.[146,147] Moreover, the function of L-glutamine alone in SCD patients who do not tolerate HU remains unclear.

Potential Therapeutic Targets

The activation of a cascade of events, including hemolysis, inflammation, and expression of adhesion molecules, can initiate and propagate VOE. Agents inhibiting these steps currently under investigation and showing promising beneficial effects are summarized in Table 3-3. In general, we classify these treatments into 4 major categories.

HbF Inducers

HbF has long been known to decrease the polymerization of HbS and ameliorate VOE manifestations. In a phase I clinical trial, decitabine showed a 4% to 9% increase in HbF in SCD patients by suppressing DNA methyltransferase 1 (DNMT1), which, together with BCL11A, functions as an HbF corepressor.[148] Histone deacetylase inhibitors also promote HbF production by increasing acetylation of the Hb promoter to increase transcription.[149] For example, sodium 2,2-dimethylbutyrate (HQK-1001) showed a 2% increase in HbF by treatment alone.[150] On the contrary, in another phase II clinical trial, HQK-1001 failed to demonstrate an increase in HbF production.[151] Other HbF inducers, such as pomalidomide, metformin, and panobinostat, are still undergoing clinical trials with no conclusive results currently available.

Antipolymerization Agents

HbS polymerization and subsequent cell "sickling" are promoted by HbS deoxygenation and higher hemoglobin concentration. The antisickling agent voxelotor (also known as GBT-440) increases the hemoglobin oxygen affinity and

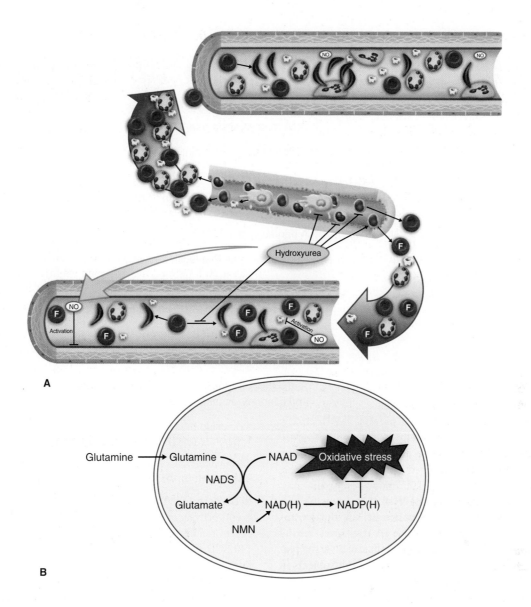

FIGURE 3-2 A. Hydroxyurea treatment in sickle cell disease (SCD). Hydroxyurea can reduce vaso-occlusion via multiple pathways. It promotes the production of erythrocytes containing high levels of HbF (F cells). Red blood cells (RBCs) containing increased HbF are less likely to adopt a sickle shape from hemoglobin polymerization and undergo hemolysis. Hydroxyurea also reduces leukocyte (neutrophil) and platelet counts and lowers expression of adhesion molecules and adhesion on endothelial cells. Hydroxyurea functions as a nitric oxide (NO) donor to enhance vasodilation, improve blood flow, and alleviate vaso-occlusive episodes.

B. Glutamine reduces RBC oxidative stress in SCD. Glutamine is transported across the membrane, and reacts with nicotinic acid adenine dinucleotide (NAAD) to generate reduced nicotinamide adenine dinucleotide [NAD(H)], which is converted to reduced nicotinamide adenine dinucleotide phosphate [NADP(H)] to reduce oxidative injury. NADS, nicotinamide adenine dinucleotide synthase; NMN, nicotinamide mononucleotide.

subsequently reduces sickling of RBC. In a phase I/II clinical trial, voxelotor (dose of 500-1000 mg/d) increased hemoglobin levels in all SCD patients and also reduced hemolysis and the percentage of sickled RBC.[152] In a phase III clinical trial of voxelotor (dose of 1500 or 900 mg/d) in 274 patients, a significant increase in the percentage of hemoglobin and a decline in hemolysis markers were observed.[153] However, the rate of VOE was not statistically different compared to the control groups.[153]

Antiadhesion Agents

Cellular adhesion interactions are important for VOE initiation. Rivipansel (also known as GMI-1070) is a small-molecule pan-selectin inhibitor that has the strongest activity against E-selectin.[58] In a phase II clinical trial, administration of rivipansel led to a marked (83%) reduction in cumulative intravenous opioid analgesic requirements,[154] and a phase III clinical trial is currently ongoing. In a phase II trial, crizanlizumab (also known as SEG101), a humanized anti–P-selectin

TABLE 3-3 Ongoing trials of new drugs to prevent or treat vaso-occlusive episodes

Category	Compound name	Mechanism of action[a]	Clinical phase (ClinicalTrials.gov identifier)
HbF inducer	Decitabine	DNA methyltransferase 1 inhibitor	I (NCT01685515)
	HQK-1001	Histone deacetylase inhibitor	II (NCT01322269)
			II (NCT01601340)
Antisickling	GBT-440 (voxelotor)	Stabilizes HbS by increasing oxygen and hemoglobin affinity	III (NCT03036813)
Antiadhesion	Rivipansel (GMI-1017)	A pan-selectin inhibitor	III (NCT02187003)
	Crizanlizumab (SEG101)	Humanized anti–P-selectin antibody	III (NCT03814746)
	Intravenous immunoglobin	Inhibits neutrophil activation and neutrophil–sickle red blood cell interactions	II (NCT01757418)
	Sevuparin	L-selectin inhibitor	II (NCT02515838)
Anti-inflammation	NKTT120	Humanized monoclonal antibody against invariant natural killer T cells	I (NCT01783691)
	Omega-3 fatty acid	Suppresses endothelin-1 on endothelial cells and alters membrane fatty acids	NCT02973360
	Arginine	Increases nitric oxide bioavailability	II (NCT02447874)

[a]Some drugs have multiple mechanisms of action.

antibody, led to a 45% lower rate of VOE at the expense of a higher rate of adverse effects (eg, arthralgia, diarrhea) compared to the placebo group.[155] A phase III trial investigating the efficacy and safety of 2 doses of crizanlizumab versus placebo, with or without HU, in adolescent and adult subjects in VOE (STAND) is nearing completion, and results are expected in the near future; approval by the FDA has been announced. In addition, intravenous immunoglobulin (IVIG) has led to decreased neutrophil adhesion and RBC-neutrophil interactions and reduced neutrophil MAC1 activation in VOE in a phase I clinical trial; analysis of a phase II trial is underway. Finally, sevuparin, which antagonizes L-selectin in a dose-dependent manner, is currently in a phase II clinical trial to study its role for acute treatment of vaso-occlusion in SCD.[156]

Anti-inflammatory Agents

Inflammation is a key factor in propagating VOE. iNKT cells have been suggested to contribute to inflammation.[82] In a phase II clinical trial, regadenoson, an $A_{2A}R$ agonist that functions as anti-iNKT cell monoclonal antibody, failed to sufficiently reduce iNKT cells and showed no effect on VOE in SCD patients.[90] Another humanized monoclonal antibody that specifically depletes iNKT cells (NKTT120) was shown to decrease iNKT cell activity by 50% during VOE in a phase I study.[90] Data on NKTT120 influencing VOE severity are still unavailable.

Omega-3 fatty acids, normally found in fish oil, have an anti-inflammatory effect in SCD mice[61] and reduced the frequency of pain episodes from 7.8 pain events per year to 3.8 events per year in SCD patients.[157] Subsequently, in a large, single-center, randomized, double-blind, placebo-controlled trial with 140 SCD patients, omega-3 fatty acid treatment decreased the rate of VOE and transfusion frequency.[158] A phase II, multicenter, randomized, double-blind, placebo-controlled, parallel-group, dose-finding trial (SCOT) is currently ongoing.

Hemolysis is tightly associated with inflammation by generating an excess of free hemoglobin to deplete NO bioavailability and elevate free heme levels in circulation, which consequently contribute to initiation of VOE. NO inhalation in SCD patients did not improve the course of VOE.[159] L-Arginine, an amino acid that can be oxidized into NO, significantly reduced painful VOE in SCD children[160] and adults,[161] and a phase II study on the function of arginine in increasing plasma bioavailable NO in SCD children is ongoing. Haptoglobin and hemopexin bound to free hemoglobin and heme, respectively, to reduce their toxicities.[74] Administration of haptoglobin or hemopexin inhibits VOE in unchallenged SCD mice, demonstrating their beneficial effect in hemolysis-driven manifestations.[162,163] Although there are no therapeutically purified proteins available, therapeutic administration of these proteins is an interesting new area of drug development in SCD.

Genetic Therapy and Editing

Gene therapy to correct autologous HSCs may obviate the limitations of HSC transplantation in SCD, such as availability of matched donors and risks of GVHD and graft rejection. Gene therapy approaches using lentiviral vectors to insert a functional β-globin or γ-globin gene in autologous HSCs have been tested in clinical trials. In a phase I/II clinical trial (NCT02151526), LentiGlobin BB305, a vector containing an antisickling β-globin gene (β^{T87Q}), demonstrated robust levels of antisickling β-globin in a patient with SCD, preventing recurrence of crisis and improvement of biomarkers for 15 months after treatment.[164] Other lentiviral vectors that contain β-globin gene (βAS3) or utilize a γ-globin coding sequence embedded in a β-globin gene are also being studied, and results from these clinical trials are awaited (NCT02247843 and NCT02186418, respectively).[165] The downside of lentiviral-based gene therapy is that the elements delivered via the vector may integrate into the genome in a semi-random manner and increase the potential of genotoxicity due to unintentional dysregulation of functional genes.[165] However, it is worth noting that no genotoxicity has been reported in the decade-long clinical trial experience with lentiviral vectors thus far.[165]

Emerging gene editing technologies aim at achieving precise genetic modifications in the patients' own HSCs. The key disadvantage of some gene editing strategies has been the need to create a targeted DNA double-strand break (DSB) and to rely on cells to repair in a nonhomologous end joining method, which frequently results in gene disruption or knockout. Currently, in the presence of a homologous donor template, genetic correction uses zinc-finger nuclease[166] or CRISPR/Cas9 approaches[167] to repair the DSB via homologous recombination to precisely correct β^s at the sixth codon. With sufficient correction of β^s, SCD would indeed be cured. In addition, other approaches, such as overexpressing HbF by genetic knockout of its repressor gene *BCL11A* by CRISPER/Case9,[168] are also evaluated in preclinical studies.

Gene correction remains at the preclinical stage for the treatment of SCD because there are persisting hurdles. First, it is difficult to mobilize and obtain HSCs from SCD patients by conventional G-CSF–mediated methods because G-CSF stimulates neutrophil production and induces complications in SCD patients.[96-98] Trials using other HSC mobilization agents such as plerixafor in SCD patients are underway.[169,170] Second, HSCs are difficult to maintain ex vivo and invariably lose long-term repopulating potential after

genetic manipulation.[165,167] Finally, pretransplant conditioning has induced toxicity/morbidity in SCD patients and needs to be optimized for gene editing therapies. Reduced-intensity pretransplant conditioning (NCT02186418) and antibody-mediated nonchemotherapy conditioning (NCT02963064) are currently being clinically tested.

Conclusion

We are entering an exciting era characterized by an advanced knowledge of the pathophysiology and factors contributing to the severity of SCD. Novel treatments hold further promise to interrupt or reverse VOE and reduce or prevent the occurrence of organ damage, which impacts patients' life quality and expectancy. In addition, there are exciting new curative gene therapy strategies. However, the high cost of the new drugs and the technical challenges of gene therapy will limit availability in resource-poor countries where most people affected by SCD reside. It is also likely that single drugs will not cover all manifestations or complications of this disease, and multiagent approaches may be required.[165] Thus far, L-glutamine and many other potential drug candidates have shown additive effects with HU.[145,152,155] It is conceivable to combine an HbF inducer and an anti-inflammatory agent, or an antisickling agent with an antiadhesion drug, together or sequentially, to deliver broader and stronger therapeutic effects. Other strategies, such as manipulating microbiota, should also be considered and studied further to limit inflammation and disease manifestations.[64] Clinical trials and rigorous planning will be required to ensure the safety and efficiency of these approaches to deliver the best outcome considering the complexity and multiplicity of SCD manifestations.

Acknowledgment

We thank Dr. Chunliang Xu for advice and lively discussions. This work was supported by the F32 grant from the National Heart, Lung, and Blood Institute (1F32HL142243-01A1, to H.L.) and R01 grants from from the National Institutes of Health (HL069438, DK056638, DK116312, and DK112976 to P.S.F.).

High-Yield Facts

- VOEs occur when the microcirculation is temporarily or permanently obstructed by heterotypic cellular aggregates, causing ischemic injury to the supplied organs and inducing pain.

- VOEs can be triggered by multiple circumstances such as dehydration, infection, fever, cold, stress, acidosis, hypoxia, and pain itself.[4] In addition, environmental factors, such as geographic altitude, weather, and air pollution, are likely to play an important role in triggering VOE.[2,6]

- In addition to sRBCs, cells such as endothelial cells, leukocytes, and platelets are reported to participate interactively to initiate VOE. When blood cell trafficking was directly monitored by intravital microscopy of cremaster muscle, sRBCs were found to interact primarily with neutrophils that are firmly adherent to endothelial cells, causing temporary or permanent vessel obstruction.[34,55]

High-Yield Facts (Cont.)

◆ The activation of a cascade of events, including hemolysis, inflammation, and expression of adhesion molecules, can initiate and propagate VOE.

◆ VOE severity is closely correlated with neutrophil counts. Additionally, biomarkers that reflect activation of endothelial cells or levels of inflammatory cytokines are elevated at steady state and in VOE.

◆ Hydroxyurea, L-glutamine, and crizanlizumab are drugs approved by the FDA to treat VOE in SCD patients. Other potential therapies such as hemoglobin F inducers, antipolymerization agents, antiadhesion agents, and anti-inflammatory agents are currently under investigation.

◆ Gene therapy approaches using lentiviral vectors to insert a functional β-globin or γ-globin gene in autologous HSCs have been tested in clinical trials. Nevertheless, gene correction approaches using zinc-figure nuclease[166] or CRISPR/Cas9 approaches[167] remain under investigation.

References

1. Ware RE, de Montalembert M, Tshilolo L, Abboud MR. Sickle cell disease. *Lancet*. 2017;390(10091):311-323.

2. Houwing ME, de Pagter PJ, van Beers EJ, et al. Sickle cell disease: Clinical presentation and management of a global health challenge. *Blood Rev*. 2019;37:100580.

3. Powars DR, Chan LS, Hiti A, Ramicone E, Johnson C. Outcome of sickle cell anemia: a 4-decade observational study of 1056 patients. *Medicine (Baltimore)*. 2005;84(6):363-376.

4. Ballas SK, Lusardi M. Hospital readmission for adult acute sickle cell painful episodes: frequency, etiology, and prognostic significance. *Am J Hematol*. 2005;79(1):17-25.

5. Morris CR, Kuypers FA, Larkin S, Vichinsky EP, Styles LA. Patterns of arginine and nitric oxide in patients with sickle cell disease with vaso-occlusive crisis and acute chest syndrome. *J Pediatr Hematol Oncol*. 2000;22(6):515-520.

6. Xu C, Frenette PS. Seasonal manifestations of sickle cell disease activity. *Nat Med*. 2019;25(4):536-537.

7. Jourde-Chiche N, Fakhouri F, Dou L, et al. Endothelium structure and function in kidney health and disease. *Nat Rev Nephrol*. 2019;15(2):87-108.

8. Balda MS, Matter K. Tight junctions. *J Cell Sci*. 1998;111 (Pt 5):541-547.

9. Pearson JD. Endothelial cell function and thrombosis. *Baillieres Best Pract Res Clin Haematol*. 1999;12(3):329-341.

10. van Hinsbergh VW. Endothelium: role in regulation of coagulation and inflammation. *Semin Immunopathol*. 2012;34(1): 93-106.

11. Moncada S. Eighth Gaddum Memorial Lecture. University of London Institute of Education, December 1980. Biological importance of prostacyclin. *Br J Pharmacol*. 1982;76(1):3-31.

12. Radomski MW, Palmer RM, Moncada S. Comparative pharmacology of endothelium-derived relaxing factor, nitric oxide and prostacyclin in platelets. *Br J Pharmacol*. 1987;92(1):181-187.

13. Radomski MW, Palmer RM, Moncada S. The role of nitric oxide and cGMP in platelet adhesion to vascular endothelium. *Biochem Biophys Res Commun*. 1987;148(3):1482-1489.

14. Rees DD, Palmer RM, Moncada S. Role of endothelium-derived nitric oxide in the regulation of blood pressure. *Proc Natl Acad Sci U S A*. 1989;86(9):3375-3378.

15. Shesely EG, Maeda N, Kim HS, et al. Elevated blood pressures in mice lacking endothelial nitric oxide synthase. *Proc Natl Acad Sci U S A*. 1996;93(23):13176-13181.

16. Freedman JE, Sauter R, Battinelli EM, et al. Deficient platelet-derived nitric oxide and enhanced hemostasis in mice lacking the NOSIII gene. *Circ Res*. 1999;84(12):1416-1421.

17. Knipe L, Meli A, Hewlett L, et al. A revised model for the secretion of tPA and cytokines from cultured endothelial cells. *Blood*. 2010;116(12):2183-2191.

18. Middleton J, Neil S, Wintle J, et al. Transcytosis and surface presentation of IL-8 by venular endothelial cells. *Cell*. 1997;91(3):385-395.

19. Matsushita K, Morrell CN, Cambien B, et al. Nitric oxide regulates exocytosis by S-nitrosylation of N-ethylmaleimide-sensitive factor. *Cell*. 2003;115(2):139-150.

20. Pober JS, Sessa WC. Evolving functions of endothelial cells in inflammation. *Nat Rev Immunol*. 2007;7(10):803-815.

21. Bjarnadottir TK, Gloriam DE, Hellstrand SH, Kristiansson H, Fredriksson R, Schiöth HB. Comprehensive repertoire and phylogenetic analysis of the G protein-coupled receptors in human and mouse. *Genomics*. 2006;88(3):263-273.

22. Oldham WM, Hamm HE. Heterotrimeric G protein activation by G-protein-coupled receptors. *Nat Rev Mol Cell Biol*. 2008;9(1):60-71.

23. Birch KA, Ewenstein BM, Golan DE, Pober JS. Prolonged peak elevations in cytoplasmic free calcium ions, derived from intracellular stores, correlate with the extent of thrombin-stimulated exocytosis in single human umbilical vein endothelial cells. *J Cell Physiol*. 1994;160(3):545-554.

24. Prescott SM, Zimmerman GA, McIntyre TM. Human endothelial cells in culture produce platelet-activating factor (1-alkyl-2-acetyl-sn-glycero-3-phosphocholine) when stimulated with thrombin. *Proc Natl Acad Sci U S A*. 1984;81(11):3534-3538.

25. Lorant DE, Patel KD, McIntyre TM, et al. Coexpression of GMP-140 and PAF by endothelium stimulated by histamine or thrombin: a juxtacrine system for adhesion and activation of neutrophils. *J Cell Biol*. 1991;115(1):223-234.

26. Martin MU, Wesche H. Summary and comparison of the signaling mechanisms of the Toll/interleukin-1 receptor family. *Biochim Biophys Acta*. 2002;1592(3):265-280.

27. Nauseef WM, Borregaard N. Neutrophils at work. *Nat Immunol*. 2014;15(7):602-611.

28. Scheiermann C, Kunisaki Y, Jang JE, Frenette PS. Neutrophil microdomains: linking heterocellular interactions with vascular injury. *Curr Opin Hematol.* 2010;17(1):25-30.

29. Ley K, Hoffman HM, Kubes P, et al. Neutrophils: New insights and open questions. *Sci Immunol.* 2018;3(30):eaat4579.

30. Kansas GS. Selectins and their ligands: current concepts and controversies. *Blood.* 1996;88(9):3259-3287.

31. Vestweber D, Blanks JE. Mechanisms that regulate the function of the selectins and their ligands. *Physiol Rev.* 1999;79(1): 181-213.

32. Eriksson EE, Xie X, Werr J, Thoren P, Lindbom L. Importance of primary capture and L-selectin-dependent secondary capture in leukocyte accumulation in inflammation and atherosclerosis in vivo. *J Exp Med.* 2001;194(2):205-218.

33. Sperandio M, Smith ML, Forlow SB, et al. P-selectin glycoprotein ligand-1 mediates L-selectin-dependent leukocyte rolling in venules. *J Exp Med.* 2003;197(10):1355-1363.

34. Chiang EY, Hidalgo A, Chang J, Frenette PS. Imaging receptor microdomains on leukocyte subsets in live mice. *Nat Methods.* 2007;4(3):219-222.

35. Hidalgo A, Peired AJ, Wild M, Vestweber D, Frenette PS. Complete identification of E-selectin ligands on neutrophils reveals distinct functions of PSGL-1, ESL-1, and CD44. *Immunity.* 2007;26(4):477-489.

36. Zarbock A, Abram CL, Hundt M, Altman A, Lowell CA, Ley K. PSGL-1 engagement by E-selectin signals through Src kinase Fgr and ITAM adapters DAP12 and FcR gamma to induce slow leukocyte rolling. *J Exp Med.* 2008;205(10):2339-2347.

37. Zarbock A, Lowell CA, Ley K. Spleen tyrosine kinase Syk is necessary for E-selectin-induced alpha(L)beta(2) integrin-mediated rolling on intercellular adhesion molecule-1. *Immunity.* 2007;26(6):773-783.

38. Ridley AJ, Schwartz MA, Burridge K, et al. Cell migration: integrating signals from front to back. *Science.* 2003;302(5651): 1704-1709.

39. Hidalgo A, Chang J, Jang JE, Peired AJ, Chiang EY, Frenette PS. Heterotypic interactions enabled by polarized neutrophil microdomains mediate thromboinflammatory injury. *Nat Med.* 2009;15(4):384-391.

40. Phillipson M, Heit B, Parsons SA, et al. Vav1 is essential for mechanotactic crawling and migration of neutrophils out of the inflamed microvasculature. *J Immunol.* 2009;182(11): 6870-6878.

41. Filippi MD. Neutrophil transendothelial migration: updates and new perspectives. *Blood.* 2019;133(20):2149-2158.

42. Brinkmann V, Reichard U, Goosmann C, et al. Neutrophil extracellular traps kill bacteria. *Science.* 2004;303(5663):1532-1535.

43. Thomas MR, Storey RF. The role of platelets in inflammation. *Thromb Haemost.* 2015;114(3):449-458.

44. Evangelista V, Manarini S, Sideri R, et al. Platelet/polymorphonuclear leukocyte interaction: P-selectin triggers protein-tyrosine phosphorylation-dependent CD11b/CD18 adhesion: role of PSGL-1 as a signaling molecule. *Blood.* 1999;93(3):876-885.

45. Mine S, Fujisaki T, Suematsu M, Tanaka Y. Activated platelets and endothelial cell interaction with neutrophils under flow conditions. *Intern Med.* 2001;40(11):1085-1092.

46. Kenny MW, Meakin M, Worthington DJ, Stuart J. Erythrocyte deformability in sickle-cell crisis. *Br J Haematol.* 1981;49(1): 103-109.

47. Ballas SK, Smith ED. Red blood cell changes during the evolution of the sickle cell painful crisis. *Blood.* 1992;79(8):2154-2163.

48. Hoover R, Rubin R, Wise G, Warren R. Adhesion of normal and sickle erythrocytes to endothelial monolayer cultures. *Blood.* 1979;54(4):872-876.

49. Hebbel RP, Yamada O, Moldow CF, Jacob HS, White JG, Eaton JW. Abnormal adherence of sickle erythrocytes to cultured vascular endothelium: possible mechanism for microvascular occlusion in sickle cell disease. *J Clin Invest.* 1980;65(1):154-160.

50. Kaul DK, Finnegan E, Barabino GA. Sickle red cell-endothelium interactions. *Microcirculation.* 2009;16(1):97-111.

51. Telen MJ. Role of adhesion molecules and vascular endothelium in the pathogenesis of sickle cell disease. *Hematology Am Soc Hematol Educ Program.* 2007:84-90.

52. Mohandas N, Evans E. Sickle erythrocyte adherence to vascular endothelium. Morphologic correlates and the requirement for divalent cations and collagen-binding plasma proteins. *J Clin Invest.* 1985;76(4):1605-1612.

53. Barabino GA, McIntire LV, Eskin SG, Sears DA, Udden M. Rheological studies of erythrocyte-endothelial cell interactions in sickle cell disease. *Prog Clin Biol Res.* 1987;240:113-127.

54. Meier ER, Fasano RM, Levett PR. A systematic review of the literature for severity predictors in children with sickle cell anemia. *Blood Cells Mol Dis.* 2017;65:86-94.

55. Turhan A, Weiss LA, Mohandas N, Coller BS, Frenette PS. Primary role for adherent leukocytes in sickle cell vascular occlusion: a new paradigm. *Proc Natl Acad Sci U S A.* 2002;99(5):3047-3051.

56. Hofstra TC, Kalra VK, Meiselman HJ, Coates TD. Sickle erythrocytes adhere to polymorphonuclear neutrophils and activate the neutrophil respiratory burst. *Blood.* 1996;87(10):4440-4447.

57. Chen G, Chang J, Zhang D, Pinho S, Jang JE, Frenette PS. Targeting Mac-1-mediated leukocyte-RBC interactions uncouples the benefits for acute vaso-occlusion and chronic organ damage. *Exp Hematol.* 2016;44(10):940-946.

58. Chang J, Patton JT, Sarkar A, Ernst B, Magnani JL, Frenette PS. GMI-1070, a novel pan-selectin antagonist, reverses acute vascular occlusions in sickle cell mice. *Blood.* 2010;116(10): 1779-1786.

59. Morikis VA, Chase S, Wun T, Chaikof EL, Magnani JL, Simon SI. Selectin catch-bonds mechanotransduce integrin activation and neutrophil arrest on inflamed endothelium under shear flow. *Blood.* 2017;130(19):2101-2110.

60. Koehl B, Nivoit P, El Nemer W, et al. The endothelin B receptor plays a crucial role in the adhesion of neutrophils to the endothelium in sickle cell disease. *Haematologica.* 2017;102(7):1161-1172.

61. Kalish BT, Matte A, Andolfo I, et al. Dietary omega-3 fatty acids protect against vasculopathy in a transgenic mouse model of sickle cell disease. *Haematologica.* 2015;100(7):870-880.

62. Chen G, Zhang D, Fuchs TA, Manwani D, Wagner DD, Frenette PS. Heme-induced neutrophil extracellular traps contribute to the pathogenesis of sickle cell disease. *Blood.* 2014;123(24):3818-3827.

63. Ghosh S, Adisa OA, Chappa P, et al. Extracellular hemin crisis triggers acute chest syndrome in sickle mice. *J Clin Invest.* 2013;123(11):4809-4820.

64. Zhang D, Chen G, Manwani D, et al. Neutrophil ageing is regulated by the microbiome. *Nature.* 2015;525(7570):528-532.

65. Zhang D, Frenette PS. Crosstalk between neutrophils and the microbiota. *Blood.* 2019;133(20):2168-2177.

66. Gaston MH, Verter JI, Woods G, et al. Prophylaxis with oral penicillin in children with sickle cell anemia. A randomized trial. *N Engl J Med.* 1986;314(25):1593-1599.

67. Reiter CD, Wang X, Tanus-Santos JE, et al. Cell-free hemoglobin limits nitric oxide bioavailability in sickle-cell disease. *Nat Med.* 2002;8(12):1383-1389.

68. Donadee C, Raat NJ, Kanias T, et al. Nitric oxide scavenging by red blood cell microparticles and cell-free hemoglobin as a mechanism for the red cell storage lesion. *Circulation.* 2011;124(4):465-476.

69. Jana S, Strader MB, Meng F, et al. Hemoglobin oxidation-dependent reactions promote interactions with band 3 and oxidative changes in sickle cell-derived microparticles. *JCI Insight.* 2018;3(21):e120451.

70. Camus SM, De Moraes JA, Bonnin P, et al. Circulating cell membrane microparticles transfer heme to endothelial cells and trigger vasoocclusions in sickle cell disease. *Blood.* 2015;125(24):3805-3814.

71. Schaer DJ, Buehler PW, Alayash AI, Belcher JD, Vercellotti GM. Hemolysis and free hemoglobin revisited: exploring hemoglobin and hemin scavengers as a novel class of therapeutic proteins. *Blood.* 2013;121(8):1276-1284.

72. Almeida CB, Scheiermann C, Jang JE, et al. Hydroxyurea and a cGMP-amplifying agent have immediate benefits on acute vaso-occlusive events in sickle cell disease mice. *Blood.* 2012;120(14):2879-2888.

73. Sultana C, Shen Y, Rattan V, Johnson C, Kalra VK. Interaction of sickle erythrocytes with endothelial cells in the presence of endothelial cell conditioned medium induces oxidant stress leading to transendothelial migration of monocytes. *Blood.* 1998;92(10):3924-3935.

74. Kato GJ, Steinberg MH, Gladwin MT. Intravascular hemolysis and the pathophysiology of sickle cell disease. *J Clin Invest.* 2017;127(3):750-760.

75. Connes P, Alexy T, Detterich J, Romana M, Hardy-Dessources MD, Ballas SK. The role of blood rheology in sickle cell disease. *Blood Rev.* 2016;30(2):111-118.

76. Belcher JD, Chen C, Nguyen J, et al. Heme triggers TLR4 signaling leading to endothelial cell activation and vaso-occlusion in murine sickle cell disease. *Blood.* 2014;123(3):377-390.

77. Villagra J, Shiva S, Hunter LA, Machado RF, Gladwin MT, Kato GJ. Platelet activation in patients with sickle disease, hemolysis-associated pulmonary hypertension, and nitric oxide scavenging by cell-free hemoglobin. *Blood.* 2007;110(6):2166-2172.

78. Bennewitz MF, Jimenez MA, Vats R, et al. Lung vaso-occlusion in sickle cell disease mediated by arteriolar neutrophil-platelet microemboli. *JCI Insight.* 2017;2(1):e89761.

79. Li J, Kim K, Hahm E, et al. Neutrophil AKT2 regulates heterotypic cell-cell interactions during vascular inflammation. *J Clin Invest.* 2014;124(4):1483-1496.

80. Henn V, Slupsky JR, Gräfe M, et al. CD40 ligand on activated platelets triggers an inflammatory reaction of endothelial cells. *Nature.* 1998;391(6667):591-594.

81. Heeney MM, Hoppe CC, Abboud MR, et al. A Multinational Trial of Prasugrel for Sickle Cell Vaso-Occlusive Events. *N Engl J Med.* 2016;374(7):625-635.

82. Zhang D, Xu C, Manwani D, Frenette PS. Neutrophils, platelets, and inflammatory pathways at the nexus of sickle cell disease pathophysiology. *Blood.* 2016;127(7):801-809.

83. Wun T, Cordoba M, Rangaswami A, Cheung AW, Paglieroni T. Activated monocytes and platelet-monocyte aggregates in patients with sickle cell disease. *Clin Lab Haematol.* 2002;24(2):81-88.

84. Liu Y, Jing F, Yi W, et al. HO-1hi patrolling monocytes protect against vaso-occlusion in sickle cell disease. *Blood.* 2018;131(14):1600-1610.

85. Van Kaer L, Parekh VV, Wu L. Invariant natural killer T cells: bridging innate and adaptive immunity. *Cell Tissue Res.* 2011;343(1):43-55.

86. Field JJ, Lin G, Okam MM, et al. Sickle cell vaso-occlusion causes activation of iNKT cells that is decreased by the adenosine A2A receptor agonist regadenoson. *Blood.* 2013;121(17):3329-3334.

87. Lin G, Field JJ, Yu JC, et al. NF-κB is activated in CD4+ iNKT cells by sickle cell disease and mediates rapid induction of adenosine A2A receptors [published correction appears in *PLoS One.* 2015;10(2):e0117760]. *PLoS One.* 2013;8(10):e74664.

88. Wallace KL, Linden J. Adenosine A2A receptors induced on iNKT and NK cells reduce pulmonary inflammation and injury in mice with sickle cell disease. *Blood.* 2010;116(23):5010-5020.

89. Field JJ, Majerus E, Gordeuk VR, et al. Randomized phase 2 trial of regadenoson for treatment of acute vaso-occlusive crises in sickle cell disease [published correction appears in *Blood Adv.* 2017 Oct 19;1(23):2058]. *Blood Adv.* 2017;1(20):1645-1649.

90. Field JJ, Majerus E, Ataga KI, et al. NNKTT120, an anti-iNKT cell monoclonal antibody, produces rapid and sustained iNKT cell depletion in adults with sickle cell disease. *PLoS One.* 2017;12(2):e0171067.

91. Wang WC, Helms RW, Lynn HS, et al. Effect of hydroxyurea on growth in children with sickle cell anemia: results of the HUG-KIDS Study. *J Pediatr.* 2002;140(2):225-229.

92. Papageorgiou DP, Abidi SZ, Chang HY, et al. Simultaneous polymerization and adhesion under hypoxia in sickle cell disease. *Proc Natl Acad Sci U S A.* 2018;115(38):9473-9478.

93. Hebbel RP. Reconstructing sickle cell disease: a data-based analysis of the "hyperhemolysis paradigm" for pulmonary hypertension from the perspective of evidence-based medicine. *Am J Hematol.* 2011;86(2):123-154.

94. Anyaegbu CC, Okpala IE, Akren'Ova YA, Salimonu LS. Peripheral blood neutrophil count and candidacidal activity correlate with the clinical severity of sickle cell anaemia (SCA). *Eur J Haematol.* 1998;60(4):267-268.

95. Rowley CA, Ikeda AK, Seidel M, et al. Microvascular oxygen consumption during sickle cell pain crisis. *Blood.* 2014;123(20):3101-3104.

96. Abboud M, Laver J, Blau CA. Granulocytosis causing sickle-cell crisis. *Lancet.* 1998;351(9107):959.

97. Adler BK, Salzman DE, Carabasi MH, Vaughan WP, Reddy VV, Prchal JT. Fatal sickle cell crisis after granulocyte colony-stimulating factor administration. *Blood.* 2001;97(10):3313-3314.

98. Pieters RC, Rojer RA, Saleh AW, Saleh AE, Duits AJ. Molgramostim to treat SS-sickle cell leg ulcers. *Lancet.* 1995;345(8948):528.

99. Wongtong N, Jones S, Deng Y, Cai J, Ataga KI. Monocytosis is associated with hemolysis in sickle cell disease. *Hematology.* 2015;20(10):593-597.

100. Shome DK, Jaradat A, Mahozi AI, et al. The platelet count and its implications in sickle cell disease patients admitted for intensive care. *Indian J Crit Care Med.* 2018;22(8):585-590.

101. Alhandalous CH, Han J, Hsu L, et al. Platelets decline during vaso-occlusive crisis as a predictor of acute chest syndrome in sickle cell disease. *Am J Hematol.* 2015;90(12):E228-E229.

102. Platt OS. Hydroxyurea for the treatment of sickle cell anemia. *N Engl J Med.* 2008;358(13):1362-1369.

103. Telen MJ. Biomarkers and recent advances in the management and therapy of sickle cell disease. *F1000Res.* 2015;4:F1000.

104. Kato GJ, Martyr S, Blackwelder WC, et al. Levels of soluble endo-thelium-derived adhesion molecules in patients with sickle cell disease are associated with pulmonary hypertension, organ dys-function, and mortality. *Br J Haematol.* 2005;130(6):943-953.

105. Zorca S, Freeman L, Hildesheim M, et al. Lipid levels in sickle-cell disease associated with haemolytic severity, vascular dysfunction and pulmonary hypertension. *Br J Haematol.* 2010;149(3):436-445.

106. Conran N, Fattori A, Saad ST, Costa FF. Increased levels of solu-ble ICAM-1 in the plasma of sickle cell patients are reversed by hydroxyurea. *Am J Hematol.* 2004;76(4):343-347.

107. Hibbert JM, Hsu LL, Bhathena SJ, et al. Proinflammatory cytok-ines and the hypermetabolism of children with sickle cell dis-ease. *Exp Biol Med (Maywood).* 2005;230(1):68-74.

108. Qari MH, Dier U, Mousa SA. Biomarkers of inflammation, growth factor, and coagulation activation in patients with sickle cell disease. *Clin Appl Thromb Hemost.* 2012;18(2):195-200.

109. Graido-Gonzalez E, Doherty JC, Bergreen EW, Organ G, Telfer M, McMillen MA. Plasma endothelin-1, cytokine, and pros-taglandin E2 levels in sickle cell disease and acute vaso-occlusive sickle crisis. *Blood.* 1998;92(7):2551-2555.

110. Brittain JE, Hulkower B, Jones SK, et al. Placenta growth factor in sickle cell disease: association with hemolysis and inflamma-tion. *Blood.* 2010;115(10):2014-2020.

111. Perelman N, Selvaraj SK, Batra S, et al. Placenta growth factor activates monocytes and correlates with sickle cell disease sever-ity. *Blood.* 2003;102(4):1506-1514.

112. Garrido VT, Sonzogni L, Mtatiro SN, Costa FF, Conran N, Thein SL. Association of plasma CD40L with acute chest syn-drome in sickle cell anemia. *Cytokine.* 2017;97:104-107.

113. Okocha C, Manafa P, Ozomba J, Ulasi T, Chukwuma G, Aneke J. C-reactive protein and disease outcome in nigerian sickle cell disease patients. *Ann Med Health Sci Res.* 2014;4(5):701-705.

114. Pitanga TN, Oliveira RR, Zanette DL, et al. Sickle red cells as danger signals on proinflammatory gene expression, leukotriene B4 and interleukin-1 beta production in peripheral blood mono-nuclear cell. *Cytokine.* 2016;83:75-84.

115. Mohammed FA, Mahdi N, Sater MA, Al-Ola K, Almawi WY. The relation of C-reactive protein to vasoocclusive crisis in chil-dren with sickle cell disease. *Blood Cells Mol Dis.* 2010;45(4):293-296.

116. Pathare A, Al Kindi S, Alnaqdy AA, Daar S, Knox-Macaulay H, Dennison D. Cytokine profile of sickle cell disease in Oman. *Am J Hematol.* 2004;77(4):323-328.

117. Hebbel RP, Key NS. Microparticles in sickle cell anaemia: prom-ise and pitfalls. *Br J Haematol.* 2016;174(1):16-29.

118. Allan D, Limbrick AR, Thomas P, Westerman MP. Release of spectrin-free spicules on reoxygenation of sickled erythrocytes. *Nature.* 1982;295(5850):612-613.

119. Suades R, Padro T, Badimon L. The role of blood-borne microparticles in inflammation and hemostasis. *Semin Thromb Hemost.* 2015;41(6):590-606.

120. Hargett LA, Bauer NN. On the origin of microparticles: from "platelet dust" to mediators of intercellular communication. *Pulm Circ.* 2013;3(2):329-340.

121. Brunetta DM, De Santis GC, Silva-Pinto AC, Oliveira de Oliveira LC, Covas DT. Hydroxyurea increases plasma concen-trations of microparticles and reduces coagulation activation and fibrinolysis in patients with sickle cell anemia. *Acta Haema-tol.* 2015;133(3):287-294.

122. Piccin A, Murphy C, Eakins E, et al. Circulating micropar-ticles, protein C, free protein S and endothelial vascular

123. Westerman M, Pizzey A, Hirschman J, et al. Microvesicles in haemoglobinopathies offer insights into mechanisms of hyper-coagulability, haemolysis and the effects of therapy. *Br J Haema-tol.* 2008;142(1):126-135.

124. Nebor D, Romana M, Santiago R, et al. Fetal hemoglobin and hydroxycarbamide moduate both plasma concentration and cellular origin of circulating microparticles in sickle cell anemia children. *Haematologica.* 2013;98(6):862-867.

125. Shenoy S, Eapen M, Panepinto JA, et al. A trial of unrelated donor marrow transplantation for children with severe sickle cell disease. *Blood.* 2016;128(21):2561-2567.

126. Abraham A, Jacobsohn DA, Bollard CM. Cellular therapy for sickle cell disease. *Cytotherapy.* 2016;18(11):1360-1369.

127. Gardner RV. Sickle cell disease: advances in treatment. *Ochsner J.* 2018;18(4):377-389.

128. Charache S, Terrin ML, Moore RD, et al. Effect of hydroxyurea on the frequency of painful crises in sickle cell anemia. Inves-tigators of the Multicenter Study of Hydroxyurea in Sickle Cell Anemia. *N Engl J Med.* 1995;332(20):1317-1322.

129. Kinney TR, Helms RW, O'Branski EE, et al. Safety of hydroxyurea in children with sickle cell anemia: results of the HUG-KIDS study, a phase I/II trial. Pediatric Hydroxyurea Group. *Blood.* 1999;94(5):1550-1554.

130. Wang WC, Ware RE, Miller ST, et al. Hydroxycarbamide in very young children with sickle-cell anaemia: a multi-centre, randomised, controlled trial (BABY HUG). *Lancet.* 2011;377(9778):1663-1672.

131. Bernaudin F, Verlhac S, Arnaud C, et al. Impact of early tran-scranial Doppler screening and intensive therapy on cerebral vasculopathy outcome in a newborn sickle cell anemia cohort. *Blood.* 2011;117(4):1130-1436.

132. Ware RE, Eggleston B, Redding-Lallinger R, et al. Predictors of fetal hemoglobin response in children with sickle cell anemia receiving hydroxyurea therapy. *Blood.* 2002;99(1):10-14.

133. Meier ER, Byrnes C, Weissman M, Noel P, Luban NL, Miller JL. Expression patterns of fetal hemoglobin in sickle cell erythro-cytes are both patient- and treatment-specific during childhood. *Pediatr Blood Cancer.* 2011;56(1):103-109.

134. Green NS, Barral S. Emerging science of hydroxyurea therapy for pediatric sickle cell disease. *Pediatr Res.* 2014;75(1-2):196-204.

135. Gambero S, Canalli AA, Traina F, et al. Therapy with hydroxyurea is associated with reduced adhesion molecule gene and protein expression in sickle red cells with a concomitant reduction in adhesive properties. *Eur J Haematol.* 2007;78(2):144-151.

136. Lou TF, Singh M, Mackie A, Li W, Pace BS. Hydroxyurea gen-erates nitric oxide in human erythroid cells: mechanisms for gamma-globin gene activation. *Exp Biol Med (Maywood).* 2009;234(11):1374-1382.

137. Cokic VP, Smith RD, Beleslin-Cokic BB, et al. Hydroxyurea induces fetal hemoglobin by the nitric oxide-dependent acti-vation of soluble guanylyl cyclase. *J Clin Invest.* 2003;111(2):231-239.

138. Lebensburger JD, Pestina TI, Ware RE, Boyd KL, Persons DA. Hydroxyurea therapy requires HbF induction for clin-ical benefit in a sickle cell mouse model. *Haematologica.* 2010;95(9):1599-1603.

139. Paszty C, Brion CM, Manci E, et al. Transgenic knockout mice with exclusively human sickle hemoglobin and sickle cell dis-ease. *Science.* 1997;278(5339):876-878.

markers in children with sickle cell anaemia. *J Extracell Vesicles.* 2015;4:28414.

140. Zerez CR, Lachant NA, Lee SJ, Tanaka KR. Decreased erythrocyte nicotinamide adenine dinucleotide redox potential and abnormal pyridine nucleotide content in sickle cell disease. *Blood.* 1988;71(2):512-515.

141. Niihara Y, Zerez CR, Akiyama DS, Tanaka KR. Increased red cell glutamine availability in sickle cell anemia: demonstration of increased active transport, affinity, and increased glutamate level in intact red cells. *J Lab Clin Med.* 1997;130(1):83-90.

142. Quinn CT. l-Glutamine for sickle cell anemia: more questions than answers. *Blood.* 2018;132(7):689-693.

143. Niihara Y, Zerez CR, Akiyama DS, Tanaka KR. Oral L-glutamine therapy for sickle cell anemia: I. Subjective clinical improvement and favorable change in red cell NAD redox potential. *Am J Hematol.* 1998;58(2):117-121.

144. Niihara Y, Matsui NM, Shen YM, et al. L-glutamine therapy reduces endothelial adhesion of sickle red blood cells to human umbilical vein endothelial cells. *BMC Blood Disord.* 2005;5:4.

145. Niihara Y, Miller ST, Kanter J, et al. A phase 3 trial of l-glutamine in sickle cell disease. *N Engl J Med.* 2018;379(3):226-235.

146. Heyland D, Muscedere J, Wischmeyer PE, et al. A randomized trial of glutamine and antioxidants in critically ill patients [published correction appears in *N Engl J Med.* 2013 May 9;368(19):1853. Dosage error in article text.]. *N Engl J Med.* 2013;368(16):1489-1497.

147. Heyland DK, Elke G, Cook D, et al. Glutamine and antioxidants in the critically ill patient: a post hoc analysis of a large-scale randomized trial. *JPEN J Parenter Enteral Nutr.* 2015;39(4):401-409.

148. Molokie R, Lavelle D, Gowhari M, et al. Oral tetrahydrouridine and decitabine for non-cytotoxic epigenetic gene regulation in sickle cell disease: a randomized phase 1 study. *PLoS Med.* 2017;14(9):e1002382.

149. Paikari A, Sheehan VA. Fetal haemoglobin induction in sickle cell disease. *Br J Haematol.* 2018;180(2):189-200.

150. Kutlar A, Reid ME, Inati A, et al. A dose-escalation phase IIa study of 2,2-dimethylbutyrate (HQK-1001), an oral fetal globin inducer, in sickle cell disease. *Am J Hematol.* 2013;88(11):E255-E260.

151. Reid ME, El Beshlawy A, Inati A, et al. A double-blind, placebo-controlled phase II study of the efficacy and safety of 2,2-dimethylbutyrate (HQK-1001), an oral fetal globin inducer, in sickle cell disease. *Am J Hematol.* 2014;89(7):709-713.

152. Howard J, Hemmaway CJ, Telfer P, et al. A phase 1/2 ascending dose study and open-label extension study of voxelotor in patients with sickle cell disease. *Blood.* 2019;133(17):1865-1875.

153. Vichinsky E, Hoppe CC, Ataga KI, et al. A phase 3 randomized trial of voxelotor in sickle cell disease. *N Engl J Med.* 2019;381(6):509-519.

154. Telen MJ, Wun T, McCavit TL, et al. Randomized phase 2 study of GMI-1070 in SCD: reduction in time to resolution of vaso-occlusive events and decreased opioid use. *Blood.* 2015;125(17):2656-2664.

155. Ataga KI, Kutlar A, Kanter J, et al. Crizanlizumab for the prevention of pain crises in sickle cell disease. *N Engl J Med.* 2017;376(5):429-439.

156. White J, Lindgren M, Liu K, Gao X, Jendeberg L, Hines P. Sevuparin blocks sickle blood cell adhesion and sickle-leucocyte rolling on immobilized L-selectin in a dose dependent manner. *Br J Haematol.* 2019;184(5):873-876.

157. Tomer A, Kasey S, Connor WE, Clark S, Harker LA, Eckman JR. Reduction of pain episodes and prothrombotic activity in sickle cell disease by dietary n-3 fatty acids. *Thromb Haemost.* 2001;85(6):966-974.

158. Daak AA, Ghebremeskel K, Hassan Z, et al. Effect of omega-3 (n-3) fatty acid supplementation in patients with sickle cell anemia: randomized, double-blind, placebo-controlled trial. *Am J Clin Nutr.* 2013;97(1):37-44.

159. Gladwin MT, Kato GJ, Weiner D, et al. Nitric oxide for inhalation in the acute treatment of sickle cell pain crisis: a randomized controlled trial. *JAMA.* 2011;305(9):893-902.

160. Morris CR, Kuypers FA, Lavrisha L, et al. A randomized, placebo-controlled trial of arginine therapy for the treatment of children with sickle cell disease hospitalized with vaso-occlusive pain episodes. *Haematologica.* 2013;98(9):1375-1382.

161. Eleutério RMN, Nascimento FO, Araújo TG, et al. Double-blind clinical trial of arginine supplementation in the treatment of adult patients with sickle cell anaemia. *Adv Hematol.* 2019;2019:4397150.

162. Vercellotti GM, Zhang P, Nguyen J, et al. Hepatic Overexpression of hemopexin inhibits inflammation and vascular stasis in murine models of sickle cell disease. *Mol Med.* 2016;22:437-451.

163. Belcher JD, Chen C, Nguyen J, et al. Haptoglobin and hemopexin inhibit vaso-occlusion and inflammation in murine sickle cell disease: Role of heme oxygenase-1 induction. *PLoS One.* 2018;13(4):e0196455.

164. Ribeil JA, Hacein-Bey-Abina S, Payen E, et al. Gene Therapy in a patient with sickle cell disease. *N Engl J Med.* 2017;376(9):848-855.

165. Telen MJ, Malik P, Vercellotti GM. Therapeutic strategies for sickle cell disease: towards a multi-agent approach. *Nat Rev Drug Discov.* 2019;18(2):139-158.

166. Hoban MD, Cost GJ, Mendel MC, et al. Correction of the sickle cell disease mutation in human hematopoietic stem/progenitor cells. *Blood.* 2015;125(17):2597-2604.

167. Dever DP, Bak RO, Reinisch A, et al. CRISPR/Cas9 β-globin gene targeting in human haematopoietic stem cells. *Nature.* 2016;539(7629):384-389.

168. Traxler EA, Yao Y, Wang YD, et al. A genome-editing strategy to treat β-hemoglobinopathies that recapitulates a mutation associated with a benign genetic condition. *Nat Med.* 2016;22(9):987-990.

169. Lagresle-Peyrou C, Lefrère F, Magrin E, et al. Plerixafor enables safe, rapid, efficient mobilization of hematopoietic stem cells in sickle cell disease patients after exchange transfusion. *Haematologica.* 2018;103(5):778-786.

170. Boulad F, Shore T, van Besien K, et al. Safety and efficacy of plerixafor dose escalation for the mobilization of CD34(+) hematopoietic progenitor cells in patients with sickle cell disease: interim results. *Haematologica.* 2018;103(5):770-777.

171. Sarray S, Saleh LR, Lisa Saldanha F, Al-Habboubi HH, Mahdi N, Almawi WY. Serum IL-6, IL-10, and TNFalpha levels in pediatric sickle cell disease patients during vasoocclusive crisis and steady state condition. *Cytokine.* 2015;72(1):43-47.

Hemolysis and Endothelial Dysfunction

Authors: Gregory J. Kato, Mark T. Gladwin

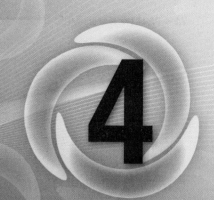

Chapter Outline

Overview

Sickle cell anemia (SCA) is characterized by severe chronic hemolysis that gives rise to anemia. There are many pathophysiologic responses to the hemolysis and to its resulting anemia. Most of these responses are adaptive in the short term, but some of these can have maladaptive consequences in the long term. The most harmful form of hemolysis is intravascular hemolysis, which releases the contents of red blood cells directly into plasma. Cell-free hemoglobin, free heme, arginase, and methylated arginines reduce nitric oxide (NO) bioavailability and promote oxidative stress and inflammation. Cell-free hemoglobin scavenges NO in a rapid, nearly diffusion-limited dioxygenase reaction. Both cell-free hemoglobin and free heme promote intense oxidative stress and serve as damage-associated molecular patterns (DAMPs). This activates the innate immune system to produce inflammatory cytokines, promoting adhesion molecule expression on blood cells and endothelial cells. Multilayered adaptive mechanisms have evolved to clear hemoglobin and heme, including haptoglobin and hemopexin. However, the severe chronic hemolysis in SCD saturates the haptoglobin system and depletes both haptoglobin and hemopexin. Arginase and methylarginine limit the activity of NO synthase to increase NO production to compensate for the destruction of NO. The physiologic consequences of decreased NO bioavailability include chronic vasoconstriction, proliferative arteriopathy, and increased platelet aggregation and clotting, especially in the pulmonary vasculature. Severe anemia results in high erythropoietin secretion, with increased circulating placenta growth factor (PlGF) and endothelin-1, a potent vasoconstrictor. Severe anemia also induces red cell content of 2,3-diphosphoglycerate (2,3-DPG), which lowers oxygen affinity and basal oxygen saturation and promotes HbS polymerization. Severe hemolytic anemia increases the risk of gallstones, systemic and pulmonary hypertension, leg ulceration, priapism, nephropathy, and stroke.

Historical Aspects of Hemolysis in Sickle Cell Disease

In the first case report of SCA in the English language, Herrick[1] reported anemia as a feature but did not elaborate on its possible mechanism. In 1923, Sydenstricker et al[2] reported 2 children with SCA, including the first reported necropsy. They observed that "yellow sclerae," "bile in the urine," and "brown granules in the Kuppfer cells of the liver and in the epithelium of the kidney tubules … suggest most strongly that there is a hemolytic factor in the production of the anemia." We would recognize this description today as (1) scleral icterus from indirect hyperbilirubinemia, the result of increased heme turnover; (2) increased urinary excretion of bilirubin; (3) possibly hemoglobinuria due to intravascular hemolysis exceeding the renal threshold for hemoglobin reabsorption; and (4) accumulation of iron as hemosiderin in the macrophages of the liver and the epithelium of the renal tubules. These are all well-established indicators of the extensive chronic extravascular and intravascular hemolysis that will be the focus of this chapter. By 1924, several authors alluded to the deduced role of hemolysis in SCA.

William Crosby was an influential figure in hematology in the 1950s and 1960s. He served as director of the Division of Medicine at Walter Reed Army Hospital, moving to Boston to serve as the chief of hematology at the New England Medical Center Hospitals and professor of medicine at Tufts University School of Medicine. Among his many publications on iron trafficking and hemolysis, a 1955 treatise in the *American Journal of Medicine* entitled, "The Metabolism of Hemoglobin and Bile Pigments in Hemolytic Diseases," stands as a landmark summary of the understanding of the pathophysiology of hemoglobin turnover in hemolysis, especially in SCA.[3] He performed calculations that estimated that two-thirds of hemolysis at steady state in SCA is extravascular and one-third is intravascular. No subsequent calculations or assays have improved upon that estimate or disproven it.

Crosby was senior author on a publication by David Sears and colleagues in *Blood* in 1966.[4] They observed prominent excretion of hemoglobin and hemosiderin in urine from patients with sickle cell disease (SCD) and observed similarity with paroxysmal nocturnal hemoglobinuria, a condition known to feature intravascular hemolysis.

In 1966, in an article published in the *British Journal of Haematology*, Graham and Beryl Serjeant and Paul Milner linked hemolysis in SCA to the number of circulating irreversibly sickled cells.[5] Graham and Beryl Serjeant conducted the Jamaican Cohort Study of Sickle Cell Disease, contributing natural history data in SCD over decades. Milner founded the

Comprehensive Sickle Cell Center at the Medical College of Georgia, where he served for >20 years.

In 1966, Neely et al[6] reported serum lactate dehydrogenase (LDH) and plasma hemoglobin as useful markers of intravascular hemolysis in patients with SCD. Graphs and analyses in that day included no statistical analysis, and they noted no particular relationship between the 2 markers. However, digitization of their data points and formal correlation testing decades later showed a statistically significant correlation that would be satisfying to current-day journal reviewers and editors.[7] In 1971, Naumann et al[8] showed that plasma hemoglobin levels acutely rise during a vaso-occlusive pain crisis. These latter 2 publication authorships both included Lemuel Diggs, a highly underappreciated, acutely intuitive clinician-researcher from the University of Tennessee at Memphis, who founded the sickle cell program at the inception of St. Jude's Children's Research Hospital. In *Blood* in 1968, Muller-Eberhard et al[9] showed that haptoglobin and hemopexin are depleted in the plasma of patients with SCA. A *JAMA* review article by Thomas Bensinger and Peter Gillette[10] summarized the 1974 state of knowledge of hemolysis in SCD, which dramatically expanded over the next 30 years.

Fundamental Science of Hemolysis in SCD

Breakdown of red blood cells prior to their expected 120-day senescence is considered hemolysis. The life span of sickle erythrocytes can be even shorter than 20 days, indicating very rapid hemolysis among the most severe of red cell diseases in humans. SCD accelerates the aging of red cells through multiple pathways. Excessive potassium ion loss promotes water loss, which concentrates sickle hemoglobin in dense, fragile red cells. This increases polymerization of sickle hemoglobin, leading to rigid red cells. Anemia-induced low oxygen affinity kinetically favors polymerization even further. Prominent oxidative stress depletes red cell antioxidants and damages red cell membranes. Membrane damage triggers microparticle shedding and hemolysis. These pathways are presented in more detail later in this chapter.

Normal Red Cell Turnover

In healthy humans, the red cell life span is approximately 120 days, after which time red cells become senescent.[11] During erythropoiesis, nuclear DNA is transcribed to mRNA and translated into the full complement of red cell proteins, including hemoglobin, cytoskeletal and membrane proteins, and a set of metabolic enzymes, especially involved in generation of adenosine triphosphate (ATP), reduced nicotinamide adenine dinucleotide (NADH), and reduced nicotinamide adenine dinucleotide phosphate (NADPH). After extrusion of the nucleus during normoblast differentiation and the attrition of existing mRNA, the red cell becomes completely dependent upon its existing proteins for cellular function. As these enzymes gradually lose function over months, the red cell

loses its catalytic antioxidant function and accumulates oxidant injury, leading to external membrane exposure of phosphatidylserine. This signals its removal by cognate receptors on macrophages. Oxidant injury can also damage cell surface proteins, marked by malondialdehyde production, and cause hemoglobin to denature and generate a hemichrome that crosslinks band 3, the major membrane-spanning protein in the red cell. This results in a conformational change in band 3 that exposes cryptic antigens that bind to preformed circulating immunoglobulin (Ig) G antibodies. The antibody binding results in phagocytosis by macrophages through Fc receptors. Erythrophagocytosis by macrophages leads to breakdown of the red cells in endosomes, releasing heme into the cytoplasm where it is broken down by heme oxygenase-1 (HO-1) and converted by several enzymatic steps to bilirubin. These mechanisms result in clearance of normal red cells at the limit of their life span. Red cell heme is catabolized and its iron recycled. In SCD, many pathways are affected, promoting accelerated extravascular hemolysis and the development of intravascular hemolysis (Figure 4-1).

Defective Ion Transport

HbS polymerization promotes loss of intracellular sodium and potassium, due to dysfunction of the K-Cl cotransporter (KCC), Gardos calcium-dependent potassium transport (KCCN4), and P_{sickle}, the polymerization-induced membrane permeability, most likely mediated by the mechanosensitive ion channel PIEZO1.[12] The cation imbalance leads to water loss, increasing the intracellular concentration of HbS, which accelerates HbS polymerization exponentially.[13]

Dense Red Cells and Irreversibly Sickled Cells

Normal red cells become denser as they age, reflecting ion loss that results in loss of intracellular water. The markedly increased ion loss and water loss in sickle erythrocytes results in red cell dehydration.[12,14] These dehydrated red cells are denser, increasing the mean corpuscular hemoglobin concentration (MCHC). The more highly concentrated HbS promotes polymerization far more readily, with exponentially more polymerization with small rises in MCHC. This effect also stabilizes the polymers of HbS, leading to irreversibly sickled cells (ISCs). These ISCs are more stable to osmotic pressure but more sensitive to mechanical stress and prone to entrapment and clearance in the spleen and peripheral microcirculation. Patients with SCD with greater percentages of circulating dense red cells have markers of more intense hemolytic anemia, including higher serum bilirubin and LDH and lower hemoglobin and hematocrit.[15] These correlations imply that dense red cells themselves are cleared through hemolysis at a greater rate.

T-State Stabilization

Deoxygenation of HbS induces the hemoglobin conformation (called tight or T-state) that exposes the nonpolar amino acid

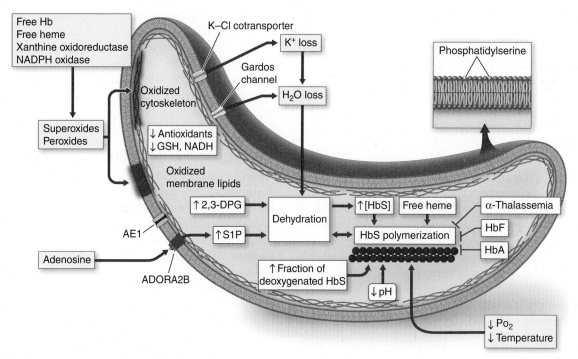

FIGURE 4-1 Erythrocyte changes in sickle cell disease. Polymerization of sickle hemoglobin (Hb) is the central driving factor in these changes, leading to a diverse, multifactorial erythrocyte pathophysiology. Recurrent cycles of polymerization-depolymerization give rise to oxidized and denatured hemoglobin, its binding to the band 3–anion exchanger membrane protein (AE1), oxidized cytoskeletal proteins and lipids, dysregulation of the K-Cl cotransporter and the Gardos channel, and externalization of phosphatidylserine. These changes potentiate erythrocyte rigidity and fragility. Extracellular oxidative stress from products of hemolysis and oxidase activities amplifies the oxidative membrane damage. Compensatory pathways increase intracellular 2,3-diphosphoglycerate (2,3-DPG) and sphingosine-1-phosphate (S1P), which decrease the affinity of hemoglobin for oxygen and favor the polymerizing conformation of HbS. α Thalassemia trait or coexpression of HbF or HbA, decreases the degree of HbS polymerization. Adapted from Kato GJ, Piel FB, Reid CD, et al. Sickle cell disease. *Nat Rev Dis Primers*. 2018;4:18010. Adapted by permission from Springer Nature.

residues that interact with adjacent HbS molecules to polymerize (see Chapter 2). Cycles of HbS polymerization and depolymerization occur as red cells are oxygenated and deoxygenated, generating hemichromes and denatured, deoxygenated HbS molecules that associate with band 3. Deoxygenated (deoxy) HbS displaces key glycolytic enzymes from band 3 inhibition, accelerating the glycolytic pathway and its by-product 2,3-DPG, already increased as a well-characterized physiologic response to anemia.[16,17] Very high levels of intraerythrocytic 2,3-DPG promote low oxygen affinity and increase deoxyHbS and the T-state HbS conformation that favors its polymerization, accelerating the processes described later.[18] There is one unconfirmed report that sickle red cells produce high levels of sphingosine-1-phosphate that binds to hemoglobin, further contributing to T-state stabilization.[19]

Oxidative Stress in the Red Cell

The second major pathway in sickle erythrocytes that accelerates hemolysis involves oxidant stress. Band 3 dysfunction also inhibits the activity of the hexose monophosphate shunt pathway, resulting in impaired production of NADPH and reduced glutathione, crucial defense molecules against antioxidant stress.[16,17] Cyclic HbS polymerization promotes the release of intracellular free heme, which associates with the red cell membrane and appears to drive production of peroxides and hydroxyl radicals.[20] Excessive oxidase activities

of extracellular and intracellular enzymes such as xanthine oxidase,[21] NADPH oxidase,[22,23] and uncoupled NO synthase[24] generate superoxides. Sickle hemoglobin has an accentuated pseudoperoxidase activity involving prominence of the ferryl state of heme iron, resulting in oxidation of important residues of βCys93 and promoting detachment of heme from hemoglobin.[25] Ischemia-reperfusion pathophysiology due to transient vaso-occlusion contributes more superoxides (discussed more extensively in Chapter 6). These superoxides can react with NO, producing highly oxidative peroxynitrites. These multiple oxidant pathways are marked by oxidation of sulfhydryls in red cell proteins. Oxidation of membrane components includes membrane lipid peroxidation, oxidation of protein 4.2, β-actin, and impaired ubiquitination of α-spectrin. The oxidative membrane damage renders erythrocytes more rigid and more susceptible to mechanical damage. In murine sickle red cells, oxidation of the active site of the flippase enzyme inhibits normal shuttling of phosphatidylserine (PS) to the inner leaflet of the plasma membrane, leading to accumulation of externally exposed PS, a signal of senescence that induces phagocytosis by macrophages.[26] Reticulocytes have intracellular hybrid endocytic-autophagic vacuoles that fuse inside out with the plasma membrane, exposing the vacuole's PS. This pathway is amplified in SCD.[27] PS-positive red cells accumulate to higher levels in patients with decreased splenic function due to splenectomy or splenic atrophy.[27] PS-positive sickle erythrocytes can also become sequestered by adherence to endothelial cells.[28]

Extracellular Vesicle Production

Repetitive cycles of HbS polymerization lead to disruption of the vertical connections of the red cell plasma lipid membrane to the underlying protein cytoskeleton.[29] This disruption may be caused in part by the oxidation of cytoskeletal proteins and lipid peroxidation described earlier, with increased vesiculation triggered by oxidizing agents and thermal stress.[30] The segments of detached lipid membrane bud off and are prone to detach as extracellular vesicles, formerly called microparticles or microvesicles. Red cell–derived extracellular vesicles join other complex particles derived from platelets and monocytes, now known to include exosomes.[31] These are currently being extensively investigated.[32]

Extravascular Versus Intravascular Hemolysis

As sickle erythrocytes accumulate cellular damage, such as protein and lipid oxidation and PS externalization, they become recognized by macrophages that clear the damaged or senescent red cells via erythrophagocytosis. This occurs mainly in the spleen, until the development of age-related splenic dysfunction and atrophy in early childhood. After that, erythrophagocytosis by macrophages in the liver and marrow is dominant. Red cells in erythrophagocytic vacuoles are broken down, and hemoglobin is proteolyzed, yielding heme, which then exits the vacuole through heme transporter Hrg1 into the cytoplasm.[33] Heme traffics to the endoplasmic reticulum, where the first step of heme breakdown by HO-1 initiates its conversion eventually to bilirubin. This reaction generates carbon monoxide as a by-product. Excess heme induces oxidation of Keap-1, which releases transcription factor Nrf2 to the nucleus, where it activates production of more HO-1 and a program of antioxidant enzymes. This pathway allows adaptive responses to the oxidant stress of the iron released from heme by the HO-1 reaction. The iron is stored in the macrophage in ferritin complexes or exported into plasma via ferroportin for transport to developing erythroid cells and other iron-utilizing cells. Sickle cell turnover through macrophages in this extravascular pathway accounts for roughly two-thirds of total hemolysis.[3] This seems to be a highly adaptive pathway for disposal of abnormal red cells.

Roughly one-third of damaged sickle erythrocytes rupture in the circulation, called intravascular hemolysis. This is a far more threatening form of hemolysis that can cause acute and chronic injury to the vasculature, which is detailed in the following section. The first line of defense against intravascular hemolysis is haptoglobin, which scavenges cell-free hemoglobin and shields its oxidant potential.[34] Haptoglobin binding also keeps hemoglobin from extravasating into the endothelial-vascular smooth muscle junction and into the renal tubules. Haptoglobin-hemoglobin complexes bind to CD163 receptors on macrophages, where they are taken up by receptor-mediated endocytosis and broken down largely by the same mechanisms as erythrophagocytosis.

Biochemical Pathways Affected by Intravascular Hemolysis in SCD

Depletion of Haptoglobin and Hemopexin

Haptoglobin is consumed in the process of escorting hemoglobin to the macrophages, and haptoglobin becomes completely depleted chronically in most SCD patients, leading to increased oxidant stress (Figure 4-2).[35] Cell-free hemoglobin without haptoglobin binds to CD163 for clearance, albeit inefficiently.[36] Some free hemoglobin can be scavenged by apo-L1 high-density lipoprotein (HDL) particles,[37] although this appears to make the HDL proinflammatory.[38] Cell-free hemoglobin that becomes oxidized to methemoglobin or denatured is prone to release free heme. The heme can bind transiently to albumin, but when it binds to hemopexin, the resulting high-affinity complexes are cleared through CD91 receptors mainly on hepatocytes and to a lesser extent on macrophages. Plasma hemopexin is depleted by this process in patients with SCD by about 85% to 90%.[35,39,40] The hepatocytes and macrophages catabolize heme through HO-1, eventually to bilirubin.

Impaired NO Bioavailability

Intravascular hemolysis produces several products that compromise NO bioavailability: hemoglobin, arginase-1, and proteins that bear methylated arginines (Figure 4-3).[41] This is compounded by increased activity of enzymes that produce reactive oxygen species that react with NO. NO synthase activity may also be compromised by deficiency of tetrahydrobiopterin and by thrombospondin dysregulation. Each of these pathways will be reviewed in detail later in this chapter.

Cell-free hemoglobin potently and rapidly scavenges NO in a nearly diffusion-limited reaction (Figures 4-3 and 4-4). This reaction of oxyhemoglobin with NO was used by biochemistry researchers to scavenge NO during in vitro experiments.[42] In 2002, the Gladwin group showed strong evidence that this fast and irreversible deoxygenation reaction occurs in vivo in patients with SCD.[43] The reaction produces a defect in vasodilation characterized by NO resistance, which is proportional to the plasma concentration of free hemoglobin. The reaction is also detectable when NO donors are incubated with plasma samples from patients compared to healthy controls. Independent investigations have demonstrated biochemical and physiologic evidence that increased cell-free plasma hemoglobin and depletion of haptoglobin are associated with a defect in systemic vasodilatory function[44-47] and with echocardiographic or pulmonary artery catheterization markers of increased pulmonary artery pressure.[47-52] In wild-type animals, induction of hypotonic hemolysis releases cell-free hemoglobin and induces hypertension, endothelial adhesiveness, and leukocyte recruitment to endothelial surfaces, all mitigated

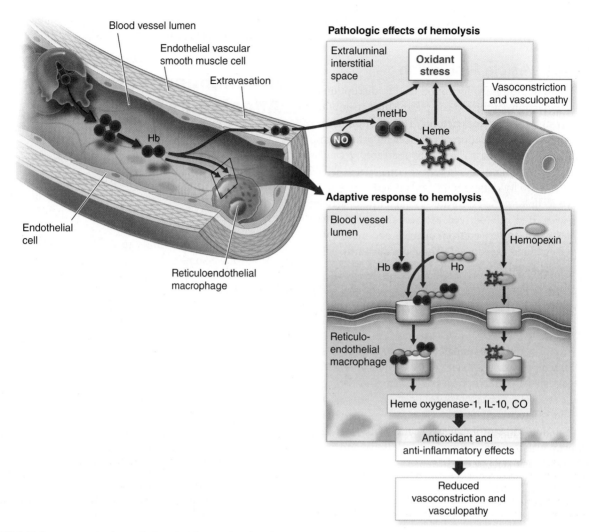

FIGURE 4-2 Intravascular hemolysis adaptive and pathophysiologic pathways. Erythrocytes that lyse in the circulation release hemoglobin (Hb) into blood plasma. Adaptive responses include the capture of free plasma hemoglobin by haptoglobin, which chaperones free hemoglobin to its receptor CD163 on macrophages, mainly in the spleen, liver, and bone marrow. Haptoglobin becomes depleted in this process. When haptoglobin supply is inadequate to capture all the free hemoglobin, the free hemoglobin tends to leak into the perivascular space, where it scavenges nitric oxide (NO) and induces oxidative stress. Oxidized hemoglobin releases free heme, which mediates potent oxidative stress and inflammatory pathway activation. Hemopexin captures the free heme and carries it to CD91 on hepatocytes and macrophages. RBC, red blood cell; IL-10, interleukin-10.

by NO donors.[53,54] Chronic or repeated infusion of cell-free hemoglobin potentiates the effect of hypoxia to induce pulmonary arterial hypertension in wild-type rats.[55,56] The hemoglobin-scavenging protein haptoglobin mitigates vascular dysfunction in mouse models of SCD[57,58] and in other models of hemolysis.[59]

Arginase-1 is present in red cells and released into plasma during intravascular hemolysis (see Figures 4-3 and 4-4). This ectopic arginase-1 converts plasma L-arginine into ornithine, reducing plasma levels of L-arginine, the obligate substrate for NO synthase to produce NO. A reduced ratio of L-arginine to ornithine predicts risk of elevated tricuspid regurgitant velocity (TRV) and mortality in SCD.[60] An arginase inhibitor mitigates sickle cell vasculopathy in mice.[61] Several studies indicate that arginine supplementation has therapeutic potential in SCD.[62-64]

Asymmetric dimethylarginine (ADMA) is derived from proteolysis of proteins containing methylated arginines. It is a naturally occurring competitive inhibitor of NO synthase found at high levels in plasma of patients with SCD. Its level closely correlates with the degree of intravascular hemolysis in SCD,[65-69] suggesting that it is derived from methylated red cell proteins.[70] It is associated with elevated TRV and early mortality in SCD.[65,67,71] ADMA is strongly associated with vasculopathy and chronic kidney disease in other human diseases.[72]

There is some evidence of **uncoupled NO synthase** in SCD.[24] In this complex situation, the normal coupling between the oxidase activity and the reductase activity of the 2 NO subunits is lost. This can be caused by deficiency of L-arginine, by ADMA, or by deficiency or oxidation of tetrahydrobiopterin, a required cofactor for NO synthase and some other important

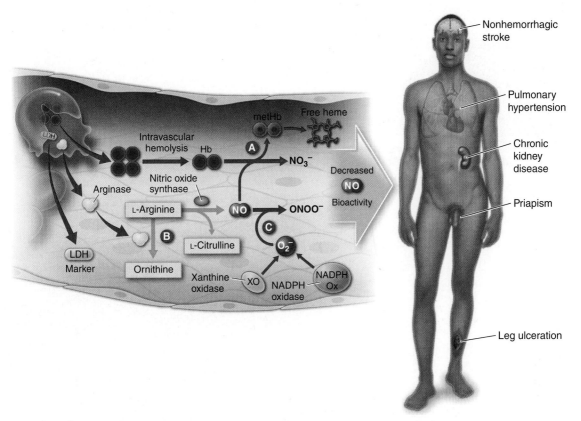

FIGURE 4-3 Intravascular hemolysis impairs nitric oxide (NO) bioavailability. Intravascular hemolysis decompartmentalizes hemoglobin, arginase-1, and lactate dehydrogenase (LDH) into blood plasma. **A.** Free plasma hemoglobin reacts with NO, resulting in methemoglobin (metHb) and inert nitrate (NO_3^-). Free heme may also be released from metHb. **B.** Arginase-1 depletes plasma L-arginine by converting it to ornithine. This depletes substrate from NO synthase. **C.** High activity of xanthine oxidase and reduced nicotinamide adenine dinucleotide phosphate (NADPH) oxidase produce superoxides, which can also deplete NO by converting it to peroxynitrite, a potent oxidizing species. The resulting decrease in NO bioactivity contributes to a vasculopathy endophenotype in sickle cell disease associated with stroke, pulmonary hypertension, chronic kidney disease, priapism, and leg ulceration.

enzymes. Uncoupling of NO synthase has 2 consequences: (1) the production of NO is compromised; and (2) the oxidase activity produces reactive oxygen species, which can directly interfere with vasodilation and vascular health and also neutralize NO.

Circulating **heme** can be released from oxidized or denatured hemoglobin (Figure 4-4). Composed of a porphyrin ring plus an atom of iron, it is normally in the oxidized +3 state when it is not a prosthetic group on hemoglobin or another hemoprotein. Heme is very hydrophobic, and in blood plasma, most of the heme is carried on albumin, which provides a low-affinity, high-abundance binding activity. Heme can become bound to the high-affinity, lower-abundance binding sites on hemopexin, which traffics heme to the CD91 receptor for heme-hemopexin complexes, concentrated on hepatocytes and on macrophages. Heme becomes internalized, and its breakdown is initiated by HO-1, an adaptive enzyme for vascular health, including in SCD.

There is now extensive evidence in sickle cell mouse models that free heme promotes a wide range of acute complications. Acute intravenous injection of heme triggers acute pulmonary vaso-occlusion, a mouse model of the acute chest syndrome.[73,74]

Heme induces neutrophils to become activated and to release neutrophil extracellular traps (NETs), networks of DNA that promote lung inflammation.[75] Heme also induces rapid release of PlGF, an angiogenic peptide with inflammatory cytokine properties implicated in sickle cell pulmonary hypertension[76,77] and also in vaso-occlusion.[78] Heme induces acute hepatopathy, and it triggers an HO-1 protective response and a potentially pathologic PlGF response in a variety of organs, including heart.[79] Heme qualifies as a DAMP by virtue of activating multiple inflammatory response pathways (Figure 4-4).[80,81]

Systemic Oxidative Stress

It is difficult to imagine another disease with more oxidative stress than in SCD. Cell-free hemoglobin and free heme promote extensive oxidative stress through a variety of chemical pathways, including the Fenton reaction and ferryl ion formation (Figure 4-4).[25,82] Several mechanisms produce abundant reactive oxygen species: (1) uncoupling of NO synthase; (2) ischemia-reperfusion biology; (3) increased activity of xanthine oxidoreductase and NADPH oxidase; and (4) depletion of catalytic and noncatalytic antioxidants in cells, especially red cells. These pathways are discussed in more detail in Chapter 6.

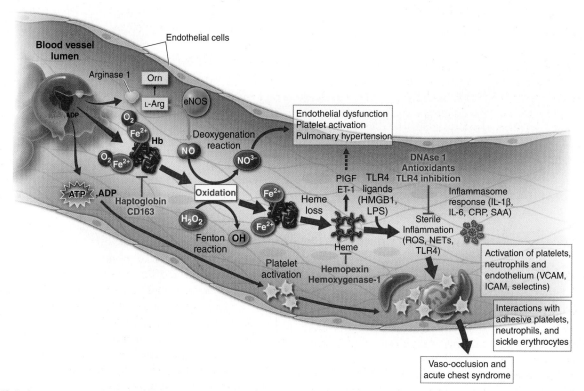

FIGURE 4-4 **Contribution of intravascular hemolysis to vasculopathy.** Erythrocytes release several products of hemolysis into plasma that alter vasomotor tone and cell adhesiveness. Free hemoglobin (Hb) consumes nitric oxide (NO) and triggers oxidative stress. Oxidized hemoglobin can release free heme, which activates many inflammatory pathways, especially amplification of toll-like receptor 4 (TLR4) pathways. Hemolysis also releases arginase-1 into plasma, which depletes the substrate for NO synthase, L-arginine. Adenine nucleotides released from red cells activate platelet adhesiveness and secretion of high-mobility group-1 (HMGB-1), a ligand for TLR4. Under the influence of inflammatory cytokines, oxidative stress, and decreased NO bioavailability, adhesion receptors are activated on neutrophils, platelets, endothelial cells, and erythrocytes. Intravascular hemolysis modifies the pathophysiology of sickle cell disease through diminished NO bioavailability, oxidative stress, and inflammatory activation of cell adhesiveness. ADP, adenosine diphosphate; ATP, adenosine triphosphate; CRP, C-reactive protein; ET-1, endothelin-1; ICAM, intercellular adhesion molecule; IL, interleukin; LPS, lipopolysaccharide; NETs, neutrophil extracellular traps; PlGF, placenta growth factor; RBC, red blood cell; ROS, reactive oxygen species; SAA, serum amyloid A; VCAM, vascular cell adhesion molecule.

Platelet Activation

Products of hemolysis promote platelet activation (Figure 4-4). Free hemoglobin carries bound adenosine diphosphate, which is a potent platelet activator.[83] Free hemoglobin induces dysfunction in platelet mitochondria, which also appears to contribute to platelet activation.[84] Free hemoglobin also scavenges NO, which normally serves to suppress platelet activation.[85] HMGB1, a nuclear protein that is released during cellular injury, also activates platelets.[86] The percentage of activated platelets in adults with SCD correlates with the pulmonary artery pressure estimated by echocardiography.[85] It is unclear whether the activated platelets contribute directly to pulmonary vasculopathy or whether platelet activation serves as a marker of additional mechanisms. These findings parallel the results of platelet activation investigations in the general population related to cerebrovascular or coronary arteriosclerosis. One of the prominent indicators of platelet activation is cell surface exposure of P-selectin, a molecule with increasing importance in SCD vascular biology. Recent evidence of inflammasome activation in platelets from sickle cell mice connects platelet biology to sterile inflammation in the innate immune system (Chapter 5).[32]

Endothelial Activation and Dysfunction

NO is known to suppress activation of endothelial cells, and its decreased bioavailability in SCD is associated with endothelial activation (Figure 4-4). A biomarker of endothelial cell activation, soluble vascular cell adhesion molecule 1 (sVCAM1), is highly elevated in SCD and correlated with markers of hemolysis.[87,88] Plasma levels of sVCAM1 are also associated with markers of pulmonary hypertension and renal and hepatic dysfunction and with death.[87] NO-mediated vasodilation is impaired in SCD, both in terms of NO production upon endothelial stimulus with acetylcholine and shear stress, and deficient response to NO donors such as sodium nitroprusside constitutes NO resistance.[47,89-95] This failure of endothelial NO production to produce adequate NO-mediated vasodilation is a form of endothelial dysfunction. Despite this defect in NO production and response, the endothelium can stimulate robust vasodilation in response to acetylcholine, presumably mediated by a compensatory increase in vasodilatory prostaglandin signaling.[89,90,92] Thrombospondin-1 in the plasma binds to its receptor CD47 to repress NO synthase activity, and high levels of thrombospondin-1 contribute to endothelial dysfunction, especially in the pulmonary circulation.[96]

DAMPs and Sterile Inflammation

Products of hemolysis activate sterile inflammation via the innate immune system, as mentioned earlier.[80,81] Free hemoglobin and especially free heme are potent DAMPs, affecting neutrophils, monocytes, and platelets, and potentiating vaso-occlusion in SCD, apparently by stimulating cell adhesion (Figure 4-4).[41,57,80,97,98] Free hemoglobin reduces the effects of NO, which normally suppresses these cells.[41] Heme augments interleukin-6 (IL-6) expression in circulating monocytes in response to lipopolysaccharide, an activator of the toll-like receptor 4 (TLR4) pathway.[99] Free heme activates P-selectin expression on endothelial cells and activates the complement pathway via the TLR4 pathway in vivo in sickle cell mice.[100-102] It appears that the most potent activation of the innate immune system is due to products of intravascular hemolysis.

Secondary Effects of More Severe Anemia

In patients with SCD, the intensity of hemolysis is the primary determinant of the severity of anemia. More severe anemia induces a higher level of compensatory erythropoietin and erythroblast hyperplasia. This in turn is associated with a higher level of PlGF,[103] an angiogenic and inflammatory factor that stimulates production of endothelin-1, a potent vaso-constrictor associated with pulmonary hypertension in SCD.[77,104] Heme can further activate PlGF secretion, as noted in the previous sections.[76] From a hemodynamic perspective, severe anemia induces a marked increase in cardiac output, resulting in a doubling of blood flow in all organs. This hemodynamic effect is believed to contribute to hyperfiltration in the kidney, a precursor to albuminuria and eventual chronic kidney disease in SCD.[105] The potential effects of highly increased blood flow in the cerebral and pulmonary circulations has not been formally investigated in SCD. It is well known outside of SCD that large congenital ventricular septal defects in the heart that double pulmonary blood flow are sufficient to induce pulmonary hypertension over 20 years, even without anemia.

Adaptive Potential of Hemolysis

The direct and indirect responses to hemolysis and its by-products are largely pathologic, with maladaptive activation of the innate immune system and excessive cell adhesion. However, there are some adaptive responses to hemolysis. Chief among them is the heme-induced expression of HO-1. Its primary activity is to initiate the breakdown of heme, but its products, biliverdin and bilirubin, have protective effects. Furthermore, HO-1 activity produces carbon monoxide, which regulates a whole protective program of responses. HO-1 also has additional nonenzymatic effects that are poorly understood, but also vasculoprotective.[106] The protective effects of high-level HO-1 activity are emphasized by the finding that enforced gene expression of HO-1 reduces disease severity in the sickle cell mouse.[107] Enforced HO-1 expression is antiatherogenic in the mouse,[108] and abundant expression of HO-1 may account for the paucity of atherosclerosis in adults and mice with SCD.[109] Inhaled carbon monoxide also has shown beneficial effects in the sickle cell mouse.[110] Heme also induces NAD(P)H quinone dehydrogenase 1 (*NQO1*) and other antioxidant program genes that presumably provide an adaptive response to the oxidative stress of SCD.

The Hemolysis Endophenotype

There is considerable variation in the severity of hemolysis among patients with SCD, with steady-state hemoglobin ranging from 5 to 12 g/dL. Much of this variation arises from individual patient differences in the intensity of hemolysis, as evidenced by clinical biomarkers of hemolytic intensity, such as serum bilirubin, LDH, and aspartate aminotransferase levels and reticulocyte count (Figure 4-5). Degree of haptoglobin and

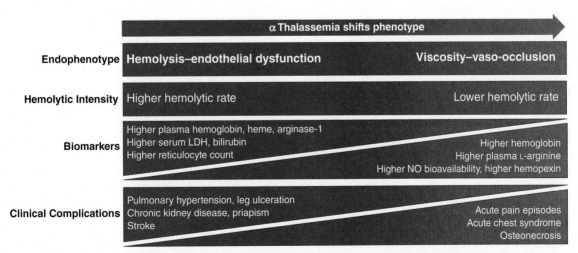

FIGURE 4-5 Intravascular hemolysis drives a clinical endophenotype. The hemolysis–endothelial dysfunction endophenotype exists in a spectrum with a viscosity–vaso-occlusion endophenotype, depending on the intensity of intravascular hemolysis. Clinical markers of intravascular hemolysis identify a subgroup of patients with sickle cell disease prone to pulmonary hypertension, leg ulceration, chronic kidney disease, priapism, and stroke. Higher total hemoglobin level and associated indicators of lower intensity of hemolysis are associated with higher total blood viscosity and higher incidence of acute pain episodes, acute chest syndrome, and osteonecrosis Co-inheritance of alpha-thalassemia trait shifts the phenotype from hemolysis to viscosity. LDH, lactate dehydrogenase; NO, nitric oxide.

TABLE 4-1 Subphenotypes of sickle cell disease and their association with hyperhemolysis, α thalassemia, and high expression of fetal hemoglobin.

Clinical features	Effect of hyperhemolytic subphenotype	Effects of α thalassemia	Protection by HbF
Painful episodes/dactylitis	Reduces risk	Increases risk	Protective
Acute chest syndrome	Neutral	Increases risk	Protective
Leg ulcers	Increases risk	Reduces risk	Equivocal
Osteonecrosis	Reduces risk	Increases risk	Equivocal
Priapism	Increases risk	Reduces risk	Not protective
Renal function/albuminuria/hemoglobinuria	Increases risk	Reduces risk	Not protective
Stroke, increased TCD velocity	Increases risk	Reduces risk	Not protective in infants; possibly protective in adults
Bilirubinemia/cholelithiasis	Increases risk	Reduces risk	Protective
Retinopathy	Neutral	Equivocal	Possibly protective
Sickle vasculopathy/high TRV/systemic hypertension	Increases risk	Equivocal	Not protective[112,214-217]
Mortality	Increases risk	Protective	Protective

Note. Hyperhemolysis is inferred from a combination of increased serum concentration of indirect bilirubin and lactate dehydrogenase. α Thalassemia was ascertained by gene analysis. For nearly every subphenotype, it is possible to find some contradictory evidence because of differences in cohort age distributions, sample size, phenotype definitions, and analytical approaches. Because of space limitations, many studies are not included. For most subphenotypes, both children and adults are included.
Abbreviations: HbF, fetal hemoglobin; TCD, transcranial Doppler; TRV, tricuspid regurgitant velocity.

hemopexin depletion can also serve as an indicator of hemolytic intensity. There is a long list of clinical complications of SCD, but there is a clinical constellation that epidemiologically occurs disproportionately in SCD patients with more severe hemolytic anemia (Table 4-1).

Gallstones

Contrary to gallstones in the general population, in patients with any form of chronic hemolytic anemia, gallstones are formed from the products of hemolysis. Classic symptoms of cholelithiasis can develop as early as adolescence with SCD, leading to early cholecystectomy. Up to half of all HbSS patients may undergo cholecystectomy, often in the second decade of life.[111] The gallstones are composed of calcium bilirubinate, a product of heme breakdown and excretion of large amounts of conjugated bilirubin into the gallbladder. These stones are visible in abdominal x-rays and computed tomography scans, in contrast to usual gallstones, which are radiolucent.

Pulmonary Hypertension

Elevated mean pulmonary artery pressure (mPAP) >25 mm Hg is found by pulmonary artery catheterization in approximately 10% of adults with SCD, meeting the traditional World Health Organization (WHO) definition for pulmonary hypertension. These patients have clearly higher mortality rates.

Recent revision to the WHO definition has lowered the diagnosis threshold to mPAP >20 mm Hg with pulmonary vascular resistance >3 Wood units, due to the high risk of death in all pulmonary arterial hypertension groups studied. The prevalence has not yet been reassessed in SCD by these new criteria. Another 25% of patients have higher than normal pulmonary artery systolic pressure estimated by echocardiography, and these patients have an intermediate mortality rate. These patients have lower hemoglobin levels than the rest of the SCD population.[112,113] About half of these patients have precapillary pulmonary hypertension caused by chronically increased vascular tone and intima-media proliferative remodeling and in situ thrombosis in the pulmonary arteries.[113-115] Extensive clinical correlation and mechanistic studies in animal models document that intravascular hemolysis promotes reduced NO bioavailability, as described in earlier sections. About half of SCD patients with pulmonary hypertension have a restrictive cardiomyopathy that promotes heart failure with preserved ejection fraction.[116] This complication also occurs mainly in the most anemic patients, apparently due to left ventricular hypertrophy as a consequence of chronically increased cardiac output to compensate for decreased oxygen-carrying capacity due to severe anemia. Fibrosis from inflammatory pathway activation also appears to play a role.[117] These topics are covered in greater detail in the chapters on pulmonary and cardiac complications of SCD (Chapters 14 and 15).

Leg Ulcers

Leg ulcers afflict approximately 15% of patients with SCD at some point in their life. These develop most frequently in patients with the most severe hemolytic anemia, marked by lowest hemoglobin level and highest serum LDH level.[118-120] They are epidemiologically linked to the prevalence of pulmonary hypertension.[114,119]

Nephropathy

Sickle cell nephropathy begins in childhood with hyperfiltration, a response induced by high cardiac output and renal blood flow due to severe anemia. Products of hemolysis appear to also play a role, because the nephropathy is also associated with HO-1 induction and inflammation, responses induced by heme deposition in the renal tubules.[121] Hemoglobinuria due to high-grade intravascular hemolysis is a marker of risk of progression of chronic kidney disease in SCD.[122] As nephropathy progresses, secretion of erythropoietin becomes deficient, compounding the hemolytic anemia with erythroid hypoplasia.[123] Sickle cell kidney disease is discussed further in Chapter 16.

Priapism

Persistent, often painful penile erection is common in males with SCD. It occurs most frequently in males with the most intense steady-state hemolytic anemia.[124] Priapism occurs more frequently in patients with a history of leg ulcers or nephropathy.[124] It is discussed in detail in Chapter 19.

Ischemic Stroke

Cerebrovascular disease and stroke have an unusually early onset in children with SCD, with median age at onset of 7 years. Both clinical stroke and its well-accepted predictor, elevated transcranial Doppler velocity, are detected in the SCD patients with the most intense hemolytic anemia.[125,126] Stroke pathophysiology and management are discussed in Chapter 9.

Genetic Modifiers

Most of the variation in steady-state hemolysis in SCD clearly comes from genetic modifiers. These are gene variants inherited independent of the HbS mutation. Some of these gene variants are known, but many still await identification. The main genetic variants affecting hemolytic rate in SCD are hereditary persistence of fetal hemoglobin (HPFH), α thalassemia trait, glucose-6-phosphate dehydrogenase (G6PD) deficiency, and male sex, discussed further in the following sections.

HPFH

Fetal hemoglobin levels vary considerably among patients with SCD. Hereditary persistence of fetal hemoglobin (HPFH) is associated with significantly lower frequency of acute painful episodes, acute chest syndrome, and osteonecrosis.[127] Higher fetal hemoglobin levels also reduce hemolysis, but there is no documented mitigation of hemolysis-associated complications, including pulmonary hypertension, stroke, or priapism.

This seemingly paradoxical situation might arise because of the heterocellular distribution of fetal hemoglobin expression. Although sickle red cells expressing high levels of fetal hemoglobin have a prolonged life span, the sickle red cells in the same patient that lack fetal hemoglobin actually have accelerated hemolysis. This dichotomous red cell life span is observed in the blood of SCD patients with higher fetal hemoglobin induced by hydroxyurea.[128]

α Thalassemia Trait

In patients with SCD in whom α thalassemia trait is coinherited, the red cells are more deformable,[129-131] intensity of hemolytic anemia is less severe, and the hemoglobin level is higher.[132-137] In what might be considered a Mendelian randomization experiment, SCD patients with α thalassemia trait have a lower prevalence of hemolysis-associated complications, such as stroke risk,[125,138-147] priapism,[124] leg ulcers,[134,148-150] nephropathy,[135,151-154] and gallstones.[155,156] They conversely have a higher rate of complications also linked to higher hemoglobin level in SCD, including vaso-occlusive crisis,[130,134,140,157-161] osteonecrosis,[148,162-164] and acute chest syndrome.[148] These issues are summarized in Table 4-1. In general, the antihemolytic effects of α thalassemia trait are protective against stroke, priapism, leg ulcers, nephropathy, and gallstones. Its role in pulmonary hypertension has not been well investigated.

G6PD Deficiency

In patients with SCD, deficiency of G6PD has been associated with more intense hemolysis in SCD.[165] It has also been associated with increased risk of the hemolysis-associated complications of cerebrovascular disease and stroke,[125,142,166,167] but this finding has been inconsistent.[146,168,169]

Male Sex

There is evidence that males have more intense hemolysis, especially in SCD.[90,170-172]

Potential Therapeutic Targets

The hemolysis–endothelial dysfunction axis presents a candidate pathway for therapeutic intervention. Several therapeutic efforts have been mounted to mitigate the effects of hemolysis on NO pathways through administration of NO, chemical donors of NO, inhibitors of cyclic guanosine monophosphate (cGMP) hydrolysis, reduction of hemolysis, or mitigation of the effects of the products of hemolysis. We will review these targets with an emphasis on clinical trial data.

Inhaled NO

Efforts to correct the NO deficiency in patients with SCD with inhaled NO (iNO) gas have been ineffective. A pilot study of iNO in children with SCD in the emergency department showed reduction of acute pain.[173] This positive result was somewhat surprising, because iNO has a half-life in blood of <1 second, which is not nearly enough for NO to be carried from the lungs to the systemic circulation where vaso-occlusion and pain occur. Indeed, a large phase II trial of children and adults with SCD hospitalized with acute pain showed no benefit.[174] Case reports have suggested possible benefit of iNO in acute chest syndrome, but no randomized controlled trials have been conducted to pursue this potential indication.

NO Donor: L-Arginine

This is the normal physiologic substrate for NO production by NO synthase. The plasma level of L-arginine is reduced by red cell arginase-1 released into plasma during intravascular hemolysis, as discussed earlier. Several pilot studies have evaluated the feasibility and preliminary efficacy of L-arginine administration in patients with SCD.[62,64,175] More recently, phase II clinical trials have suggested improvements in vascular function with oral L-arginine supplementation in patients with SCD.[63,176] The therapeutic potential of L-arginine treatment to reduce severity of acute pain episodes is currently being evaluated in a phase II randomized controlled trial (NCT02536170).

Alternative NO Donors: Nitrite

The nitrite anion can be converted to NO by xanthine oxidoreductase, hemoglobin, and a variety of other globins.[177] In adults with SCD, sodium nitrite infusion into the forearm circulation induced regional vasodilation.[91] The effect was blunted compared to normal controls, similar to other NO donors such as sodium nitroprusside and consistent with NO resistance in SCD. A topical formulation of sodium nitrite has been tested in adults with SCD and nonhealing leg ulcers.[178] It induced dose-dependent effects, including increased regional blood flow and decreases in ulcer pain and size over 4 weeks. It is currently in a phase II clinical trial (NCT02863068).

Increasing cGMP Production via Soluble Guanylyl Cyclase Agonists

Soluble guanylyl cyclase (sGC) is the principal effector of NO on intracellular content of cGMP. Pharmacologic stimulators of sGC such as riociguat may hypothetically bypass the NO deficiency in SCD, augmenting sGC activity in the presence or absence of NO. The current STERIO-SCD trial is a randomized controlled trial of an sGC stimulator, riociguat, in adults with hypertension, elevated TRV, or proteinuria (NCT02633397). Riociguat is already approved by the US Food and Drug Administration for the treatment of pulmonary arterial hypertension or chronic thromboembolic pulmonary hypertension, and some patients with SCD have already been prescribed it for those indications with apparent benefit.[179] Another sGC stimulator, olinciguat, is also in an early-phase clinical trial (NCT03285178). There is also evidence that sGC activity is further compromised in SCD due to oxidation of its heme prosthetic group.[180] A second class of sGC agonists called sGC activators specifically activate oxidized or heme-deficient sGC proteins. This class of agents offers even more interesting potential as an alternative mechanism to increase intracellular cGMP.[181]

Increasing cGMP by Inhibiting Its Hydrolysis via Phosphodiesterase 5

NO exerts its activity primarily by increasing cGMP in vascular smooth muscle, endothelial cells, and blood cells. This cGMP pathway promotes vasorelaxation and decreased cell adhesiveness. Sildenafil boosts cGMP levels by inhibiting hydrolysis of cGMP by phosphodiesterase 5 (PDE5). Single-arm studies suggested benefit of sildenafil in relieving exercise impairment associated with high TRV in adults with SCD.[182,183] Sildenafil was approved in the general population for pulmonary arterial hypertension in 2005. A large randomized controlled trial of sildenafil in adolescents and adults with SCD, elevated TRV, and impaired exercise capacity was halted due to safety reasons. Patients in the sildenafil group required 2.5-fold more hospitalizations for acute pain than patients in the placebo group.[184] Because of the early termination of the trial, only a fraction of the planned efficacy data were collected and no clinical benefit could be discerned. Although the mechanism of this increased pain remains unproven, cGMP in the spinal cord has been shown to play an important role in pain sensitivity.[185,186] Sildenafil subsequently has been shown to amplify pain in a rodent model.[187] Future investigational attempts to increase cGMP in SCD will need to focus on agents that do not increase pain sensitivity.

Increasing cGMP by Inhibiting Its Hydrolysis via Phosphodiesterase 9

Hematopoietic cells, including neutrophils, hydrolyze cGMP through phosphodiesterase 9 (PDE9). In a sickle cell mouse model activated with tumor necrosis factor-α, a PDE9 inhibitor decreased leukocyte rolling in the microvasculature.[188] The PDE9 inhibitor PF-04447943 is reported to be well tolerated in adults with SCD. It reduced the number and size of circulating platelet-monocyte and platelet-neutrophil aggregates, mainly when PF-04447943 was administered in combination with hydroxyurea.[189] There was also a nonsignificant trend toward reduced levels of circulating soluble E-selectin.

Decreasing Hemolysis With Exchange Transfusion

This intervention reduces hemolysis significantly when applied on a regular monthly basis. It also keeps the fraction of circulating sickle red cells low. Preliminary data indicate a favorable effect on pulmonary hypertension in patients with SCD, specifically with improvement in functional class and pulmonary vascular resistance.[190] A large-scale randomized trial of chronic blood exchange transfusions in adults with chronic cardiopulmonary or renal dysfunction (SCD-CARRE) is underway (NCT04084080).

Decreasing Hemolysis With Senicapoc

Basal overactivity of the Gardos potassium channel (KCNN4) in sickle red cells causes loss of potassium ions and water, concentrating intracellular HbS and promoting its polymerization.[13]

The Gardos channel inhibitor senicapoc decreases hemolysis in adults with SCD.[191] The resulting higher hemoglobin was not associated with reduction in acute pain episodes, with post hoc analysis conversely showing increased pain episode frequency in patients with SCA.[192] This response is reminiscent of the effect of α thalassemia trait, which in patients with SCA promotes higher hemoglobin with markers of decreased hemolysis combined with higher frequency of acute pain episodes (see earlier section on α thalassemia trait). In senicapoc-treated patients who had an increase in hemoglobin of at least 0.5 g/dL, the reduction in hemolysis was associated with a fall in serum N-terminal prohormone of brain natriuretic peptide (NT-proBNP),[193] a marker of ventricular stress and pulmonary artery pressure.[194] The NT-proBNP response to hemolytic reduction by senicapoc supports the model of hemolysis-linked pathophysiology in SCD.[41,195] Senicapoc has not been studied further in patients with SCD. It might hypothetically be expected to reduce severity of the hemolytic–endothelial dysfunction endophenotype in general.

Decreasing Hemolysis With Voxelotor

This agent is an aldehyde that forms a Schiff base with the amino terminus of α-globin, stabilizing the nonpolymerizing relaxed (R-state) conformation. Like senicapoc, voxelotor significantly reduces hemolysis in patients with SCD.[196] There is not yet any evidence that voxelotor reduces or augments acute pain episode frequency in SCD, but a study is ongoing (NCT03036813). This agent may have potential to reduce the severity of the hemolysis–endothelial dysfunction endophenotype, and it is being evaluated in an expanded-access program (NCT03943615).

Decreasing Hemolysis by Increasing Fetal Hemoglobin

The inconsistent and paradoxical protective effects of genetically determined fetal hemoglobin have been discussed earlier. The effects of hydroxyurea on hemolysis and associated complications are also inconsistent and unclear. Some case series have suggested that hydroxyurea may reverse early cases of pulmonary hypertension.[197,198] However, this has not been well investigated. Among the multiple effects of hydroxyurea, it has NO donor effects that could affect vascular function independent of fetal hemoglobin effects.[199,200] The relationship of hydroxyurea with leg ulcers remains highly controversial, possibly due to the presumed antiproliferative effects on hydroxyurea on wound healing. The complex effects of fetal hemoglobin and hydroxyurea yield some paradoxical relationships that remain incompletely understood.

Decreasing Hemolysis Through Induced Iron Deficiency

When hemoglobin production in SCD is limited by decreased synthesis of α-globin due to α-thalassemia trait, hemolysis decreases significantly. This seems to occur due to the reduction of intracellular hemoglobin concentration, a critical factor in HbS polymerization. Iron deficiency also limits hemoglobin production, and case reports suggest that iron deficiency reduces hemolytic intensity in patients with SCD.[201,202] Sickle cell mouse experiments provide supportive results. A mutation that interferes with iron absorption results in reduced hemolysis and higher hemoglobin level in a sickle cell mouse.[203] A clinical trial of repeated serial phlebotomy to reduce iron in patients with SCD could be feasible.[204]

Mitigating the Effects of Hemolysis With Haptoglobin and Hemopexin

These vasculoprotective plasma proteins become depleted in SCD because they are consumed as they chaperone hemoglobin and heme from plasma during intravascular hemolysis.[205] When injected into sickle cell mice, they each have activity in reducing vaso-occlusion, oxidative stress, organ injury, and inflammatory macrophage response induced by free heme or hemoglobin.[35,57,73,74,97,206] Hemopexin is entering clinical trials in SCD [NCT04285827].

Mitigating the Effects of Hemolysis by Enhancing the Compensatory Response

Heme and hemoglobin released from lysed red cells induce an adaptive response, as previously described. This response is mediated in large part by the oxidant stress sensor transcription factor, Nrf2, which activates transcription of HO-1, antioxidant enzymes, and many other adaptive genes. Non-oxidative pharmacologic activators of Nrf2 have been highly investigated, starting with sulforaphane, which is found in various foods, especially broccoli sprouts. Preclinical experiments in sickle cell mice suggest a potential benefit from activating the Nrf2 pathway.[207-211] A pilot trial of broccoli sprout extract suggests that it is well tolerated in patients with SCD.[212] Merely enhancing HO-1 expression genetically has produced beneficial effects in the sickle cell mouse.[213]

Conclusion

There have never been more agents in development for SCD and there have never been as many active clinical trials as there are now. The near future seems to hold even more activity in this area. These efforts include modulation of hemolysis or its resulting deficiency of NO. Recent and ongoing randomized clinical trials in patients with SCD help to determine validity of the hypothetical therapeutic targets in the hemolysis-NO pathophysiologic pathway. The quite large number of negative clinical trials in the cardiovascular field present a sober reality that therapeutic intervention in patients is far more complex than in laboratory animals. Trials can yield negative results when the original causal inferences are flawed. However, they can provide negative results due to nuances of outcome selection and protocol execution, even when the scientific premises are sound. Successes and failures will help to hone the clinical trial designs in this clinically heterogeneous patient population.

Over the next few years, randomized controlled trials will be completed addressing the many targets identified in the preceding section. In addition, many new approaches will complete early-phase clinical trials to assess feasibility and early indications of a signal of potential activity. These results will help to guide prioritization of reduction of hemolysis, blocking its vasculotoxic products, and augmentation of NO or cGMP signaling. It is of immense importance to complete these active and pending trials as soon as possible.

The physiologic defense mechanisms to prevent and react to hemolysis are biologically redundant and overlapping. For example, haptoglobin, hemopexin, and transferrin each serves to sequester and chaperone the circulating forms of biologically active, potentially toxic iron in plasma.[205] Optimal therapeutic defense against hemolysis may require each of these components working in synchrony. Prevention of hemolysis may be the best medicine, although the lessons from hemolysis reduction by senicapoc or α thalassemia trait show that hemolysis reduction can shift to a vaso-occlusion–hyperviscosity endophenotype.

These principles suggest that combination therapy to reduce vaso-occlusion and hemolysis in parallel may be required. The balancing of these factors will require improved biomarkers to personalize this approach to the wide phenotypic variation among patients with SCD. Curative-intent treatments such as hematopoietic cell transplantations and gene therapy approaches will not be widely available or applicable in the foreseeable future, with drug therapy more nearly on the horizon. Patients with SCD may lead the way in developing proof of principle for the amelioration of hemolysis-associated morbidities.

High-Yield Facts

- HbS induces ion and osmotic dysfunction and oxidant stress that cause loss of membrane integrity.
- Although a smaller fraction of hemolysis occurs in the intravascular compartment than in macrophages, this intravascular hemolysis is more toxic to vascular health.
- Cell-free hemoglobin scavenges NO, promoting vascular dysfunction.
- The hemolysis–endothelial dysfunction endophenotype is marked by lower hemoglobin and higher serum bilirubin and LDH.
- Patients with this endophenotype also have higher plasma arginase activity and depleted plasma arginine.
- The endophenotype includes increased risk of stroke, pulmonary hypertension, leg ulcers, priapism, chronic kidney disease, and gallstones.
- A wide variety of approaches are in clinical trial to reduce hemolysis and treat its consequences, including deficient NO-cGMP signaling.

References

1. Herrick JB. Peculiar elongated and sickle-shaped red blood corpuscles in a case of severe anemia. *Arch Intern Med.* 1910; 6(5):517-521.
2. Sydenstricked VP, Mulherin WA, Houseal RW. Sickle cell anemia: report of two cases in children, with necropsy in one case. *Am J Dis Child.* 1923;26(2):132-154.
3. Crosby WH. The metabolism of hemoglobin and bile pigment in hemolytic disease. *Am J Med.* 1955;18(1):112-122.
4. Sears DA, Anderson PR, Foy AL, Williams HL, Crosby WH. Urinary iron excretion and renal metabolism of hemoglobin in hemolytic diseases. *Blood.* 1966;28(5):708-725.
5. Serjeant GR, Serjeant BE, Milner PF. The irreversibly sickled cell; a determinant of haemolysis in sickle cell anaemia. *Br J Haematol.* 1969;17(6):527-533.
6. Neely CL, Wajima T, Kraus AP, Diggs LW, Barreras L. Lactic acid dehydrogenase activity and plasma hemoglobin elevations in sickle cell disease. *Am J Clin Pathol.* 1969;52(2):167-169.
7. Kato GJ, Nouraie SM, Gladwin MT. Lactate dehydrogenase and hemolysis in sickle cell disease. *Blood.* 2013;122(6):1091-1092.
8. Naumann HN, Diggs LW, Barreras L, Williams BJ. Plasma hemoglobin and hemoglobin fractions in sickle cell crisis. *Am J Clin Pathol.* 1971;56(2):137-147.
9. Muller-Eberhard U, Javid J, Liem HH, Hanstein A, Hanna M. Plasma concentrations of hemopexin, haptoglobin and heme in patients with various hemolytic diseases. *Blood.* 1968;32(5): 811-815.
10. Bensinger TA, Gillette PN. Hemolysis in sickle cell disease. *Arch Intern Med.* 1974;133(4):624-631.
11. Mohandas N, Gallagher PG. Red cell membrane: past, present, and future. *Blood.* 2008;112(10):3939-3948.
12. Joiner CH, Franco RS. The activation of KCL cotransport by deoxygenation and its role in sickle cell dehydration. *Blood Cells Mol Dis.* 2001;27(1):158-164.
13. Brugnara C. Sickle cell dehydration: pathophysiology and therapeutic applications. *Clin Hemorheol Microcirc.* 2018;68(2-3): 187-204.
14. Brugnara C. Sickle cell disease: from membrane pathophysiology to novel therapies for prevention of erythrocyte dehydration. *J Pediatr Hematol Oncol.* 2003;25(12):927-933.
15. Bartolucci P, Brugnara C, Teixeira-Pinto A, et al. Erythrocyte density in sickle cell syndromes is associated with specific clinical manifestations and hemolysis. *Blood.* 2012;120(15): 3136-3141.
16. Rogers SC, Ross JG, d'Avignon A, et al. Sickle hemoglobin disturbs normal coupling among erythrocyte O2 content, glycolysis, and antioxidant capacity. *Blood.* 2013;121(9):1651-1662.

17. Chu H, McKenna MM, Krump NA, et al. Reversible binding of hemoglobin to band 3 constitutes the molecular switch that mediates O2 regulation of erythrocyte properties. *Blood.* 2016;128(23):2708-2716.

18. Oder E, Safo MK, Abdulmalik O, Kato GJ. New developments in anti-sickling agents: can drugs directly prevent the polymerization of sickle haemoglobin in vivo? *Br J Haematol.* 2016;175(1):24-30.

19. Zhang Y, Berka V, Song A, et al. Elevated sphingosine-1-phosphate promotes sickling and sickle cell disease progression. *J Clin Invest.* 2014;124(6):2750-2761.

20. Hebbel RP. Beyond hemoglobin polymerization: the red blood cell membrane and sickle disease pathophysiology. *Blood.* 1991;77(2):214-237.

21. Aslan M, Freeman BA. Oxidant-mediated impairment of nitric oxide signaling in sickle cell disease: mechanisms and consequences. *Cell Mol Biol (Noisy-le-grand).* 2004;50(1):95-105.

22. Wood KC, Hebbel RP, Granger DN. Endothelial cell NADPH oxidase mediates the cerebral microvascular dysfunction in sickle cell transgenic mice. *FASEB J.* 2005;19(8):989-991.

23. George A, Pushkaran S, Konstantinidis DG, et al. Erythrocyte NADPH oxidase activity modulated by Rac GTPases, PKC, and plasma cytokines contributes to oxidative stress in sickle cell disease. *Blood.* 2013;121(11):2099-2107.

24. Wood KC, Hebbel RP, Lefer DJ, Granger DN. Critical role of endothelial cell-derived nitric oxide synthase in sickle cell disease-induced microvascular dysfunction. *Free Rad Biol Med.* 2006;40(8):1443-1453.

25. Alayash AI. Oxidative pathways in the sickle cell and beyond. *Blood Cells Mol Dis.* 2018;70:78-86.

26. de JK, Kuypers FA. Sulphydryl modifications alter scramblase activity in murine sickle cell disease. *BrJ Haematol.* 2006;133(4):427-432.

27. Mankelow TJ, Griffiths RE, Trompeter S, et al. Autophagic vesicles on mature human reticulocytes explain phosphatidylserine-positive red cells in sickle cell disease. *Blood.* 2015;126(15):1831-1834.

28. Setty BN, Kulkarni S, Stuart MJ. Role of erythrocyte phosphatidylserine in sickle red cell-endothelial adhesion. *Blood.* 2002;99(5):1564-1571.

29. Liu SC, Derick LH, Zhai S, Palek J. Uncoupling of the spectrin-based skeleton from the lipid bilayer in sickled red cells. *Science.* 1991;252(5005):574-576.

30. Rank BH, Moyer NL, Hebbel RP. Vesiculation of sickle erythrocytes during thermal stress. *Blood.* 1988;72(3):1060-1063.

31. Romana M, Connes P, Key NS. Microparticles in sickle cell disease. *Clin Hemorheol Microcirc.* 2018;68(2-3):319-329.

32. Vats R, Brzoska T, Bennewitz MF, et al. Platelet extracellular vesicles drive inflammasome-IL1beta-dependent lung injury in sickle cell disease. *Am J Respir Crit Care Med.* 2020;201(1):33-46.

33. White C, Yuan X, Schmidt PJ, et al. HRG1 is essential for heme transport from the phagolysosome of macrophages during erythrophagocytosis. *Cell Metab.* 2013;17(2):261-270.

34. Andersen CBF, Stodkilde K, Saederup KL, et al. Haptoglobin. *Antioxid Redox Signal.* 2017;26(14):814-831.

35. Yalamanoglu A, Deuel JW, Hunt RC, et al. Depletion of haptoglobin and hemopexin promote hemoglobin-mediated lipoprotein oxidation in sickle cell disease. *Am J Physiol Lung Cell Mol Physiol.* 2018;315(5):L765-L774.

36. Schaer DJ, Schaer CA, Buehler PW, et al. CD163 is the macrophage scavenger receptor for native and chemically modified hemoglobins in the absence of haptoglobin. *Blood.* 2006;107(1):373-380.

37. Nielsen MJ, Petersen SV, Jacobsen C, et al. Haptoglobin-related protein is a high-affinity hemoglobin-binding plasma protein. *Blood.* 2006;108(8):2846-2849.

38. Ji X, Feng Y, Tian H, et al. The mechanism of proinflammatory HDL generation in sickle cell disease is linked to cell-free hemoglobin via haptoglobin. *PLoS One.* 2016;11(10):e0164264.

39. Vendrame F, Olops L, Saad STO, Costa FF, Fertrin KY. Differences in heme and hemopexin content in lipoproteins from patients with sickle cell disease. *J Clin Lipidol.* 2018;12(6):1532-1538.

40. Santiago RP, Guarda CC, Figueiredo CVB, et al. Serum haptoglobin and hemopexin levels are depleted in pediatric sickle cell disease patients. *Blood Cells Mol Dis.* 2018;72:34-36.

41. Kato GJ, Steinberg MH, Gladwin MT. Intravascular hemolysis and the pathophysiology of sickle cell disease. *J Clin Invest.* 2017;127(3):750-760.

42. Doyle MP, Hoekstra JW. Oxidation of nitrogen oxides by bound dioxygen in hemoproteins. *J Inorg Biochem.* 1981;14(4):351-358.

43. Reiter CD, Wang X, Tanus-Santos JE, et al. Cell-free hemoglobin limits nitric oxide bioavailability in sickle-cell disease. *Nat Med.* 2002;8(12):1383-1389.

44. Kaul DK, Liu XD, Chang HY, Nagel RL, Fabry ME. Effect of fetal hemoglobin on microvascular regulation in sickle transgenic-knockout mice. *J Clin Invest.* 2004;114(8):1136-1145.

45. Kaul DK, Liu XD, Fabry ME, Nagel RL. Impaired nitric oxide-mediated vasodilation in transgenic sickle mouse. *Am J Physiol Heart Circ Physiol.* 2000;278(6):H1799-H1806.

46. Hanson MS, Xu H, Flewelen TC, et al. A novel hemoglobin-binding peptide reduces cell-free hemoglobin in murine hemolytic anemia. *Am J Physiol Heart Circ Physiol.* 2013;304(2):H328-H336.

47. Detterich JA, Kato RM, Rabai M, Meiselman HJ, Coates TD, Wood JC. Chronic transfusion therapy improves but does not normalize systemic and pulmonary vasculopathy in sickle cell disease. *Blood.* 2015;126(6):703-710.

48. Janka JJ, Koita OA, Traore B, et al. Increased pulmonary pressures and myocardial wall stress in children with severe malaria. *J Infect Dis.* 2010;202(5):791-800.

49. Atichartakarn V, Chuncharunee S, Archararit N, et al. Prevalence and risk factors for pulmonary hypertension in patients with hemoglobin E/beta-thalassemia disease. *Eur J Haematol.* 2014;92(4):346-353.

50. Rafikova O, Williams ER, McBride ML, et al. Hemolysis-induced lung vascular leakage contributes to the development of pulmonary hypertension. *Am J Respir Cell Mol Biol.* 2018;59(3):334-345.

51. Brittain EL, Janz DR, Austin ED, et al. Elevation of plasma cell-free hemoglobin in pulmonary arterial hypertension. *Chest.* 2014;146(6):1478-1485.

52. Nakamura H, Kato M, Nakaya T, et al. Decreased haptoglobin levels inversely correlated with pulmonary artery pressure in patients with pulmonary arterial hypertension: a cross-sectional study. *Medicine (Baltimore).* 2017;96(43):e8349.

53. Almeida CB, Souza LE, Leonardo FC, et al. Acute hemolytic vascular inflammatory processes are prevented by nitric oxide replacement or a single dose of hydroxyurea. *Blood.* 2015;126(6):711-720.

54. Minneci PC, Deans KJ, Zhi H, et al. Hemolysis-associated endothelial dysfunction mediated by accelerated NO inactivation by decompartmentalized oxyhemoglobin. *J Clin Invest.* 2005;115(12):3409-3417.

55. Buehler PW, Baek JH, Lisk C, et al. Free hemoglobin induction of pulmonary vascular disease: evidence for an inflammatory mechanism. *Am J Physiol Lung Cell Mol Physiol*. 2012;303(4):L312-L326.

56. Bilan VP, Schneider F, Novelli EM, et al. Experimental intravascular hemolysis induces hemodynamic and pathological pulmonary hypertension: association with accelerated purine metabolism. *Pulm Circ*. 2018;8(3):2045894018791557.

57. Belcher JD, Chen C, Nguyen J, et al. Haptoglobin and hemopexin inhibit vaso-occlusion and inflammation in murine sickle cell disease: role of heme oxygenase-1 induction. *PLoS One*. 2018;13(4):e0196455.

58. Chintagari NR, Nguyen J, Belcher JD, Vercellotti GM, Alayash AI. Haptoglobin attenuates hemoglobin-induced heme oxygenase-1 in renal proximal tubule cells and kidneys of a mouse model of sickle cell disease. *Blood Cells Mol Dis*. 2015;54(3):302-306.

59. Boretti FS, Buehler PW, D'Agnillo F, et al. Sequestration of extracellular hemoglobin within a haptoglobin complex decreases its hypertensive and oxidative effects in dogs and guinea pigs. *J Clin Invest*. 2009;119(8):2271-2280.

60. Morris CR, Kato GJ, Poljakovic M, et al. Dysregulated arginine metabolism, hemolysis-associated pulmonary hypertension, and mortality in sickle cell disease. *JAMA*. 2005;294(1):81-90.

61. Steppan J, Tran HT, Bead VR, et al. Arginase inhibition reverses endothelial dysfunction, pulmonary hypertension, and vascular stiffness in transgenic sickle cell mice. *Anesth Analg*. 2016;123(3):652-658.

62. Benites BD, Olalla-Saad ST. An update on arginine in sickle cell disease. *Expert Rev Hematol*. 2019;12(4):235-244.

63. Eleuterio RMN, Nascimento FO, Araujo TG, et al. Double-blind clinical trial of arginine supplementation in the treatment of adult patients with sickle cell anaemia. *Adv Hematol*. 2019;2019:4397150.

64. Morris CR. Arginine therapy shows promise for treatment of sickle cell disease clinical subphenotypes of hemolysis and arginine deficiency. *Anesth Analg*. 2017;124(4):1369-1370.

65. El-Shanshory M, Badraia I, Donia A, Abd El-Hameed F, Mabrouk M. Asymmetric dimethylarginine levels in children with sickle cell disease and its correlation to tricuspid regurgitant jet velocity. *Eur J Haematol*. 2013;91(1):55-61.

66. Landburg PP, Teerlink T, Biemond BJ, et al. Plasma asymmetric dimethylarginine concentrations in sickle cell disease are related to the hemolytic phenotype. *Blood Cells Mol Dis*. 2010;44(4):229-232.

67. Kato GJ, Wang Z, Machado RF, Blackwelder WC, Taylor JG, Hazen SL. Endogenous nitric oxide synthase inhibitors in sickle cell disease: abnormal levels and correlations with pulmonary hypertension, desaturation, haemolysis, organ dysfunction and death. *Br J Haematol*. 2009;145(4):506-513.

68. Landburg PP, Teerlink T, Muskiet FA, et al. Plasma concentrations of asymmetric dimethylarginine, an endogenous nitric oxide synthase inhibitor, are elevated in sickle cell patients but do not increase further during painful crisis. *Am J Hematol*. 2008;83(7):577-579.

69. Schnog JB, Teerlink T, van der Dijs FP, Duits AJ, Muskiet FA. Plasma levels of asymmetric dimethylarginine (ADMA), an endogenous nitric oxide synthase inhibitor, are elevated in sickle cell disease. *Ann Hematol*. 2005;84(5):282-286.

70. D'Alecy LG, Billecke SS. Massive quantities of asymmetric dimethylarginine (ADMA) are incorporated in red blood cell proteins and may be released by proteolysis following hemolytic stress. *Blood Cells Mol Dis*. 2010;45(1):40.

71. Haymann JP, Hammoudi N, Stankovic Stojanovic K, et al. Renin-angiotensin system blockade promotes a cardio-renal protection in albuminuric homozygous sickle cell patients. *Br J Haematol*. 2017;179(5):820-828.

72. Fulton MD, Brown T, Zheng YG. The biological axis of protein arginine methylation and asymmetric dimethylarginine. *Int J Mol Sci*. 2019;20(13):3322.

73. Belcher JD, Chen C, Nguyen J, et al. Heme triggers TLR4 signaling leading to endothelial cell activation and vaso-occlusion in murine sickle cell disease. *Blood*. 2014;123(3):377-390.

74. Ghosh S, Adisa OA, Chappa P, et al. Extracellular hemin crisis triggers acute chest syndrome in sickle mice. *J Clin Invest*. 2013;123(11):4809-4820.

75. Chen G, Zhang D, Fuchs TA, Manwani D, Wagner DD, Frenette PS. Heme-induced neutrophil extracellular traps contribute to the pathogenesis of sickle cell disease. *Blood*. 2014;123(24):3818-3827.

76. Wang X, Mendelsohn L, Rogers H, et al. Heme-bound iron activates placenta growth factor in erythroid cells via erythroid Kruppel-like factor. *Blood*. 2014;124(6):946-954.

77. Sundaram N, Tailor A, Mendelsohn L, et al. High levels of placenta growth factor in sickle cell disease promote pulmonary hypertension. *Blood*. 2010;116(1):109-112.

78. Gu JM, Yuan S, Sim D, et al. Blockade of placental growth factor reduces vaso-occlusive complications in murine models of sickle cell disease. *Exp Hematol*. 2018;60:73-82.e3.

79. Gbotosho OT, Ghosh S, Kapetanaki MG, et al. Cardiac expression of HMOX1 and PGF in sickle cell mice and haem-treated wild type mice dominates organ expression profiles via Nrf2 (Nfe2l2). *Br J Haematol*. 2019;187(5):666-675.

80. Mendonca R, Silveira AA, Conran N. Red cell DAMPs and inflammation. *Inflamm Res*. 2016;65(9):665-678.

81. Gladwin MT, Ofori-Acquah SF. Erythroid DAMPs drive inflammation in SCD. *Blood*. 2014;123(24):3689-3690.

82. Repka T, Hebbel RP. Hydroxyl radical formation by sickle erythrocyte membranes: role of pathologic iron deposits and cytoplasmic reducing agents. *Blood*. 1991;78(10):2753-2758.

83. Helms CC, Marvel M, Zhao W, et al. Mechanisms of hemolysis-associated platelet activation. *J Thromb Haemost*. 2013;11(12):2148-2154.

84. Cardenes N, Corey C, Geary L, et al. Platelet bioenergetic screen in sickle cell patients reveals mitochondrial complex V inhibition, which contributes to platelet activation. *Blood*. 2014;123(18):2864-2872.

85. Villagra J, Shiva S, Hunter LA, Machado RF, Gladwin MT, Kato GJ. Platelet activation in patients with sickle disease, hemolysis-associated pulmonary hypertension, and nitric oxide scavenging by cell-free hemoglobin. *Blood*. 2007;110(6):2166-2172.

86. Vogel S, Arora T, Wang X, et al. The platelet NLRP3 inflammasome is upregulated in sickle cell disease via HMGB1/TLR4 and Bruton tyrosine kinase. *Blood Adv*. 2018;2(20):2672-2680.

87. Kato GJ, Martyr S, Blackwelder WC, et al. Levels of soluble endothelium-derived adhesion molecules in patients with sickle cell disease are associated with pulmonary hypertension, organ dysfunction, and mortality. *Br J Haematol*. 2005;130(6):943-953.

88. Vilas-Boas W, Cerqueira BA, Zanette AM, Reis MG, Barral-Netto M, Goncalves MS. Arginase levels and their association with Th17-related cytokines, soluble adhesion molecules (sICAM-1 and sVCAM-1) and hemolysis markers among steady-state sickle cell anemia patients. *Ann Hematol*. 2010;89(9):877-882.

89. Scoffone HM, Krajewski M, Zorca S, et al. Effect of extended-release niacin on serum lipids and on endothelial function in adults with sickle cell anemia and low high-density lipoprotein cholesterol levels. *Am J Cardiol.* 2013;112(9):1499-1504.

90. Gladwin MT, Schechter AN, Ognibene FP, et al. Divergent nitric oxide bioavailability in men and women with sickle cell disease. *Circulation.* 2003;107(2):271-278.

91. Mack AK, McGowan VR II, Tremonti CK, et al. Sodium nitrite promotes regional blood flow in patients with sickle cell disease: a phase I/II study. *Br J Haematol.* 2008;142(6):971-978.

92. Belhassen L, Pelle G, Sediame S, et al. Endothelial dysfunction in patients with sickle cell disease is related to selective impairment of shear stress-mediated vasodilation. *Blood.* 2001;97(6):1584-1589.

93. de Montalembert M, Aggoun Y, Niakate ASI. Endothelial-dependent vasodilation is impaired in children with sickle cell disease. *Blood.* 2006;108(11):1709-1710.

94. Zawar SD, Vyawahare MA, Nerkar M, Jawahirani AR. Non-invasive detection of endothelial dysfunction in sickle cell disease by Doppler ultrasonography. *J AssocPhysicians India.* 2005;53:677-680.

95. Blum A, Yeganeh S, Peleg A, et al. Endothelial function in patients with sickle cell anemia during and after sickle cell crises. *J ThrombThrombolysis.* 2005;19(2):83-86.

96. Novelli EM, Little-Ihrig L, Knupp HE, et al. Vascular TSP1-CD47 signaling promotes sickle cell-associated arterial vasculopathy and pulmonary hypertension in mice. *Am J Physiol Lung Cell Mol Physiol.* 2019;316(6):L1150-L1164.

97. Vinchi F, Costa da Silva M, Ingoglia G, et al. Hemopexin therapy reverts heme-induced proinflammatory phenotypic switching of macrophages in a mouse model of sickle cell disease. *Blood.* 2016;127(4):473-486.

98. Guarda CCD, Santiago RP, Fiuza LM, et al. Heme-mediated cell activation: the inflammatory puzzle of sickle cell anemia. *Expert Rev Hematol.* 2017;10(6):533-541.

99. Dagur PK, McCoy JP, Nichols J, et al. Haem augments and iron chelation decreases toll-like receptor 4 mediated inflammation in monocytes from sickle cell patients. *Br J Haematol.* 2018;181(4):552-554.

100. Merle NS, Boudhabhay I, Leon J, Fremeaux-Bacchi V, Roumenina LT. Complement activation during intravascular hemolysis: implication for sickle cell disease and hemolytic transfusion reactions. *Transfus Clin Biol.* 2019;26(2):116-124.

101. Vercellotti GM, Dalmasso AP, Schaid TR Jr, et al. Critical role of C5a in sickle cell disease. *Am J Hematol.* 2019;94(3):327-337.

102. Merle NS, Paule R, Leon J, et al. P-selectin drives complement attack on endothelium during intravascular hemolysis in TLR-4/heme-dependent manner. *Proc Natl Acad Sci U S A.* 2019;116(13):6280-6285.

103. Gonsalves CS, Li C, Mpollo MS, et al. Erythropoietin-mediated expression of placenta growth factor is regulated via activation of hypoxia-inducible factor-1alpha and post-transcriptionally by miR-214 in sickle cell disease. *Biochem J.* 2015;468(3):409-423.

104. Patel N, Gonsalves CS, Malik P, Kalra VK. Placenta growth factor augments endothelin-1 and endothelin-B receptor expression via hypoxia-inducible factor-1 alpha. *Blood.* 2008;112(3):856-865.

105. Belisario AR, da Silva AA, Silva CV, et al. Sickle cell disease nephropathy: an update on risk factors and potential biomarkers in pediatric patients. *Biomark Med.* 2019;13(11):967-987.

106. Gall T, Balla G, Balla J. Heme, heme oxygenase, and endoplasmic reticulum stress: a new insight into the pathophysiology of vascular diseases. *Int J Mol Sci.* 2019;20(15):3675.

107. Belcher JD, Mahaseth H, Welch TE, Otterbein LE, Hebbel RP, Vercellotti GM. Heme oxygenase-1 is a modulator of inflammation and vaso-occlusion in transgenic sickle mice. *J Clin Invest.* 2006;116(3):808-816.

108. Ishikawa K, Sugawara D, Wang X, et al. Heme oxygenase-1 inhibits atherosclerotic lesion formation in ldl-receptor knock-out mice. *Circ Res.* 2001;88(5):506-512.

109. Wang H, Luo W, Wang J, et al. Paradoxical protection from atherosclerosis and thrombosis in a mouse model of sickle cell disease. *Br J Haematol.* 2013;162(1):120-129.

110. Belcher JD, Gomperts E, Nguyen J, et al. Oral carbon monoxide therapy in murine sickle cell disease: beneficial effects on vaso-occlusion, inflammation and anemia. *PLoS One.* 2018;13(10):e0205194.

111. Shah R, Taborda C, Chawla S. Acute and chronic hepatobiliary manifestations of sickle cell disease: a review. *World J Gastrointest Pathophysiol.* 2017;8(3):108-116.

112. Gladwin MT, Sachdev V, Jison ML, et al. Pulmonary hypertension as a risk factor for death in patients with sickle cell disease. *N Engl J Med.* 2004;350(9):886-895.

113. Parent F, Bachir D, Inamo J, et al. A hemodynamic study of pulmonary hypertension in sickle cell disease. *N Engl J Med.* 2011;365(1):44-53.

114. Mehari A, Alam S, Tian X, et al. Hemodynamic predictors of mortality in adults with sickle cell disease. *Am J Respir Crit Care Med.* 2013;187(8):840-847.

115. Anthi A, Machado RF, Jison ML, et al. Hemodynamic and functional assessment of patients with sickle cell disease and pulmonary hypertension. *Am J Respir Crit Care Med.* 2007;175(12):1272-1279.

116. Sachdev V, Machado RF, Shizukuda Y, et al. Diastolic dysfunction is an independent risk factor for death in patients with sickle cell disease. *J Am Coll Cardiol.* 2007;49(4):472-479.

117. Niss O, Quinn CT, Lane A, et al. Cardiomyopathy with restrictive physiology in sickle cell disease. *JACC Cardiovasc Imaging.* 2016;9(3):243-252.

118. Kato GJ, McGowan V, Machado RF, et al. Lactate dehydrogenase as a biomarker of hemolysis-associated nitric oxide resistance, priapism, leg ulceration, pulmonary hypertension, and death in patients with sickle cell disease. *Blood.* 2006;107(6):2279-2285.

119. Nolan VG, Adewoye A, Baldwin C, et al. Sickle cell leg ulcers: associations with haemolysis and SNPs in Klotho, TEK and genes of the TGF-beta/BMP pathway. *Br J Haematol.* 2006;133(5):570-578.

120. Minniti CP, Kato GJ. Critical reviews: how we treat sickle cell patients with leg ulcers. *Am J Hematol.* 2016;91(1):22-30.

121. Nath KA, Belcher JD, Nath MC, et al. Role of TLR4 signaling in the nephrotoxicity of heme and heme proteins. *Am J Physiol Renal Physiol.* 2018;314(5):F906-F914.

122. Saraf SL, Zhang X, Kanias T, et al. Haemoglobinuria is associated with chronic kidney disease and its progression in patients with sickle cell anaemia. *Br J Haematol.* 2014;164(5):729-739.

123. Ataga KI, Orringer EP. Renal abnormalities in sickle cell disease. *Am J Hematol.* 2000;63(4):205-211.

124. Nolan VG, Wyszynski DF, Farrer LA, Steinberg MH. Hemolysis-associated priapism in sickle cell disease. *Blood.* 2005;106(9):3264-3267.

125. Bernaudin F, Verlhac S, Chevret S, et al. G6PD deficiency, absence of alpha-thalassemia, and hemolytic rate at baseline are significant independent risk factors for abnormally high cerebral velocities in patients with sickle cell anemia. *Blood.* 2008;112(10):4314-4317.

126. Ohene-Frempong K. Stroke in sickle cell disease: demographic, clinical, and therapeutic considerations. *Semin Hematol.* 1991; 28(3):213-219.

127. Lettre G, Bauer DE. Fetal haemoglobin in sickle-cell disease: from genetic epidemiology to new therapeutic strategies. *Lancet.* 2016;387(10037):2554-2564.

128. Franco RS, Yasin Z, Palascak MB, Ciraolo P, Joiner CH, Rucknagel DL. The effect of fetal hemoglobin on the survival characteristics of sickle cells. *Blood.* 2006;108(3):1073-1076.

129. Ballas SK, Connes P, Investigators of the Multicenter Study of Hydroxyurea in Sickle Cell A. Rheological properties of sickle erythrocytes in patients with sickle-cell anemia: the effect of hydroxyurea, fetal hemoglobin, and alpha-thalassemia. *Eur J Haematol.* 2018;101(6):798-803.

130. Renoux C, Connes P, Nader E, et al. Alpha-thalassaemia promotes frequent vaso-occlusive crises in children with sickle cell anaemia through haemorheological changes. *Pediatr Blood Cancer.* 2017;64:8.

131. Serjeant BE, Mason KP, Kenny MW, et al. Effect of alpha thalassaemia on the rheology of homozygous sickle cell disease. *BrJ Haematol.* 1983;55(3):479-486.

132. De Ceulaer K, Higgs DR, Weatherall DJ, Hayes RJ, Serjeant BE, Serjeant GR. Alpha-thalassemia reduces the hemolytic rate in homozygous sickle-cell disease. *N Engl J Med.* 1983;309(3): 189-190.

133. Embury SH, Dozy AM, Miller J, et al. Concurrent sickle-cell anemia and alpha-thalassemia: effect on severity of anemia. *N Engl J Med.* 1982;306(5):270-274.

134. Olatunya OS, Albuquerque DM, Adekile A, Costa FF. Influence of alpha thalassemia on clinical and laboratory parameters among nigerian children with sickle cell anemia. *J Clin Lab Anal.* 2019;33(2):e22656.

135. Raffield LM, Ulirsch JC, Naik RP, et al. Common alpha-globin variants modify hematologic and other clinical phenotypes in sickle cell trait and disease. *PLoS Genet.* 2018;14(3):e1007293.

136. Nouraie M, Lee JS, Zhang Y, et al. The relationship between the severity of hemolysis, clinical manifestations and risk of death in 415 patients with sickle cell anemia in the US and Europe. *Haematologica.* 2013;98(3):464-472.

137. Milton JN, Rooks H, Drasar E, et al. Genetic determinants of haemolysis in sickle cell anaemia. *Br J Haematol.* 2013;161(2):270-278.

138. Adams RJ, Kutlar A, McKie V, et al. Alpha thalassemia and stroke risk in sickle cell anemia. *Am J Hematol.* 1994;45(4): 279-282.

139. Hsu LL, Miller ST, Wright E, et al. Alpha thalassemia is associated with decreased risk of abnormal transcranial Doppler ultrasonography in children with sickle cell anemia. *J Pediatr Hematol Oncol.* 2003;25(8):622-628.

140. Neonato MG, Guilloud-Bataille M, Beauvais P, et al. Acute clinical events in 299 homozygous sickle cell patients living in France. French Study Group on Sickle Cell Disease. *EurJ Haematol.* 2000;65(3):155-164.

141. Saraf SL, Akingbola TS, Shah BN, et al. Associations of alpha-thalassemia and BCL11A with stroke in Nigerian, United States, and United Kingdom sickle cell anemia cohorts. *Blood Adv.* 2017;1(11):693-698.

142. Joly P, Garnier N, Kebaili K, et al. G6PD deficiency and absence of alpha-thalassemia increase the risk for cerebral vasculopathy in children with sickle cell anemia. *Eur J Haematol.* 2016;96(4):404-408.

143. Belisario AR, Nogueira FL, Rodrigues RS, et al. Association of alpha-thalassemia, TNF-alpha (-308G>A) and VCAM-1 (c.1238G>C) gene polymorphisms with cerebrovascular disease in a newborn cohort of 411 children with sickle cell anemia. *Blood Cells Mol Dis.* 2015;54(1):44-50.

144. Cox SE, Makani J, Soka D, et al. Haptoglobin, alpha-thalassaemia and glucose-6-phosphate dehydrogenase polymorphisms and risk of abnormal transcranial Doppler among patients with sickle cell anaemia in Tanzania. *Br J Haematol.* 2014;165(5):699-706.

145. Domingos IF, Falcao DA, Hatzlhofer BL, et al. Influence of the betas haplotype and alpha-thalassemia on stroke development in a Brazilian population with sickle cell anaemia. *Ann Hematol.* 2014;93(7):1123-1129.

146. Flanagan JM, Frohlich DM, Howard TA, et al. Genetic predictors for stroke in children with sickle cell anemia. *Blood.* 2011;117(24):6681-6684.

147. Belisario AR, Rodrigues CV, Martins ML, Silva CM, Viana MB. Coinheritance of alpha-thalassemia decreases the risk of cerebrovascular disease in a cohort of children with sickle cell anemia. *Hemoglobin.* 2010;34(6):516-529.

148. Steinberg MH, Rosenstock W, Coleman MB, et al. Effects of thalassemia and microcytosis on the hematologic and vasoocclusive severity of sickle cell anemia. *Blood.* 1984;63(6):1353-1360.

149. Koshy M, Entsuah R, Koranda A, et al. Leg ulcers in patients with sickle cell disease. *Blood.* 1989;74(4):1403-1408.

150. Higgs DR, Aldridge BE, Lamb J, et al. The interaction of alpha-thalassemia and homozygous sickle-cell disease. *N Engl J Med.* 1982;306(24):1441-1446.

151. Geard A, Pule GD, Chetcha Chemegni B, et al. Clinical and genetic predictors of renal dysfunctions in sickle cell anaemia in Cameroon. *Br J Haematol.* 2017;178(4):629-639.

152. Saraf SL, Shah BN, Zhang X, et al. APOL1, alpha-thalassemia, and BCL11A variants as a genetic risk profile for progression of chronic kidney disease in sickle cell anemia. *Haematologica.* 2017;102(1):e1-e6.

153. Guasch A, Zayas CF, Eckman JR, Muralidharan K, Zhang W, Elsas LJ. Evidence that microdeletions in the alpha globin gene protect against the development of sickle cell glomerulopathy in humans. *J Am Soc Nephrol.* 1999;10(5):1014-1019.

154. Lamarre Y, Romana M, Lemonne N, et al. Alpha thalassemia protects sickle cell anemia patients from macro-albuminuria through its effects on red blood cell rheological properties. *Clin Hemorheol Microcirc.* 2014;57(1):63-72.

155. Alsultan A, Aleem A, Ghabbour H, et al. Sickle cell disease subphenotypes in patients from Southwestern Province of Saudi Arabia. *J Pediatr Hematol Oncol.* 2012;34(2):79-84.

156. Haider MZ, Ashebu S, Aduh P, Adekile AD. Influence of alpha-thalassemia on cholelithiasis in SS patients with elevated Hb F. *Acta Haematologia.* 1998;100(3):147-150.

157. Gill FM, Sleeper LA, Weiner SJ, et al. Clinical events in the first decade in a cohort of infants with sickle cell disease. Cooperative Study of Sickle Cell Disease. *Blood.* 1995;86(2):776-783.

158. Billett HH, Kim K, Fabry ME, Nagel RL. The percentage of dense red cells does not predict incidence of sickle cell painful crisis. *Blood.* 1986;68(1):301-303.

159. Bailey S, Higgs DR, Morris J, Serjeant GR. Is the painful crisis of sickle-cell disease due to sickling? *Lancet.* 1991;337(8743):735.

160. Abuamer S, Shome DK, Jaradat A, et al. Frequencies and phenotypic consequences of association of alpha- and beta-thalassemia alleles with sickle-cell disease in Bahrain. *Int J Lab Hematol.* 2017;39(1):76-83.

161. Darbari DS, Onyekwere O, Nouraie M, et al. Markers of severe vaso-occlusive painful episode frequency in children and adolescents with sickle cell anemia. *J Pediatr.* 2012;160(2):286-290.

162. Milner PF, Kraus AP, Sebes JI, et al. Sickle cell disease as a cause of osteonecrosis of the femoral head. *N Engl J Med.* 1991;325(21):1476-1481.

163. Ballas SK, Talacki CA, Rao VM, Steiner RM. The prevalence of avascular necrosis in sickle cell anemia: correlation with alpha-thalassemia. *Hemoglobin.* 1989;13(7-8):649-655.

164. Milner PF, Kraus AP, Sebes JI, et al. Osteonecrosis of the humeral head in sickle cell disease. *Clin Orthop Relat Res.* 1993(289):136-143.

165. Benkerrou M, Alberti C, Couque N, et al. Impact of glucose-6-phosphate dehydrogenase deficiency on sickle cell anaemia expression in infancy and early childhood: a prospective study. *Br J Haematol.* 2013;163(5):646-654.

166. Thangarajh M, Yang G, Fuchs D, Ponisio MR, et al. Magnetic resonance angiography-defined intracranial vasculopathy is associated with silent cerebral infarcts and glucose-6-phosphate dehydrogenase mutation in children with sickle cell anaemia. *Br J Haematol.* 2012;159(3):352-359.

167. Hellani A, Al-Akoum S, Abu-Amero KK. G6PD Mediterranean S188F codon mutation is common among Saudi sickle cell patients and increases the risk of stroke. *Genet Test Mol Biomarkers.* 2009;13(4):449-452.

168. Miller ST, Milton J, Steinberg MH. G6PD deficiency and stroke in the CSSCD. *Am J Hematol.* 2011;86(3):331.

169. Belisario AR, Rodrigues Sales R, Evelin Toledo N, Velloso-Rodrigues C, Maria Silva C, Borato Viana M. Glucose-6-phosphate dehydrogenase deficiency in brazilian children with sickle cell anemia is not associated with clinical ischemic stroke or high-risk transcranial Doppler. *Pediatr Blood Cancer.* 2016;63(6):1046-1049.

170. Raslan R, Shah BN, Zhang X, et al. Hemolysis and hemolysis-related complications in females vs. males with sickle cell disease. *Am J Hematol.* 2018;93(11):E376-E380.

171. Kanias T, Lanteri MC, Page GP, et al. Ethnicity, sex, and age are determinants of red blood cell storage and stress hemolysis: results of the REDS-III RBC-Omics study. *Blood Adv.* 2017;1(15):1132-1141.

172. Kanias T, Sinchar D, Osei-Hwedieh D, et al. Testosterone-dependent sex differences in red blood cell hemolysis in storage, stress, and disease. *Transfusion.* 2016;56(10):2571-2583.

173. Weiner DL, Hibberd PL, Betit P, Cooper AB, Botelho CA, Brugnara C. Preliminary assessment of inhaled nitric oxide for acute vaso-occlusive crisis in pediatric patients with sickle cell disease. *JAMA.* 2003;289(9):1136-1142.

174. Gladwin MT, Kato GJ, Weiner D, et al. Nitric oxide for inhalation in the acute treatment of sickle cell pain crisis: a randomized controlled trial. *JAMA.* 2011;305(9):893-902.

175. Morris CR, Kuypers FA, Lavrisha L, et al. A randomized, placebo-controlled trial of arginine therapy for the treatment of children with sickle cell disease hospitalized with vaso-occlusive pain episodes. *Haematologica.* 2013;98(9):1375-1382.

176. Cox SE, Ellins EA, Marealle AI, et al. Ready-to-use food supplement, with or without arginine and citrulline, with daily chloroquine in Tanzanian children with sickle-cell disease: a double-blind, random order crossover trial. *Lancet Haematol.* 2018;5(4):e147-e160.

177. Kim-Shapiro DB, Gladwin MT. Nitric oxide pathology and therapeutics in sickle cell disease. *Clin Hemorheol Microcirc.* 2018;68(2-3):223-237.

178. Minniti CP, Gorbach AM, Xu D, et al. Topical sodium nitrite for chronic leg ulcers in patients with sickle cell anaemia: a phase 1 dose-finding safety and tolerability trial. *Lancet Haematol.* 2014;1(3):e95-e103.

179. Weir NA, Conrey A, Lewis D, Mehari A. Riociguat use in sickle cell related chronic thromboembolic pulmonary hypertension: a case series. *Pulm Circ.* 2018;8(4):2045894018791802.

180. Potoka KP, Wood KC, Baust JJ, et al. Nitric oxide-independent soluble guanylate cyclase activation improves vascular function and cardiac remodeling in sickle cell disease. *Am J Respir Cell Mol Biol.* 2018;58(5):636-647.

181. Makrynitsa GI, Zompra AA, Argyriou AI, Spyroulias GA, Topouzis S. Therapeutic targeting of the soluble guanylate cyclase. *Curr Med Chem.* 2019;26(15):2730-2747.

182. Machado RF, Martyr S, Kato GJ, et al. Sildenafil therapy in patients with sickle cell disease and pulmonary hypertension. *Br J Haematol.* 2005;130(3):445-453.

183. Derchi G, Forni GL, Formisano F, et al. Efficacy and safety of sildenafil in the treatment of severe pulmonary hypertension in patients with hemoglobinopathies. *Haematologica.* 2005;90(4):452-458.

184. Machado RF, Barst RJ, Yovetich NA, et al. Hospitalization for pain in patients with sickle cell disease treated with sildenafil for elevated TRV and low exercise capacity. *Blood.* 2011;118(4):855-864.

185. Schmidtko A, Tegeder I, Geisslinger G. No NO, no pain? The role of nitric oxide and cGMP in spinal pain processing. *Trends Neurosci.* 2009;32(6):339-346.

186. Hannig G, Tchernychev B, Kurtz CB, Bryant AP, Currie MG, Silos-Santiago I. Guanylate cyclase-C/cGMP: an emerging pathway in the regulation of visceral pain. *Front Mol Neurosci.* 2014;7:31.

187. Patil CS, Padi SV, Singh VP, Kulkarni SK. Sildenafil induces hyperalgesia via activation of the NO-cGMP pathway in the rat neuropathic pain model. *Inflammopharmacology.* 2006;14(1-2):22-27.

188. Almeida CB, Scheiermann C, Jang JE, et al. Hydroxyurea and a cGMP-amplifying agent have immediate benefits on acute vaso-occlusive events in sickle cell disease mice. *Blood.* 2012;120(14):2879-2888.

189. Charnigo RJ, Beidler D, Rybin D, et al. PF-04447943, a phosphodiesterase 9A inhibitor, in stable sickle cell disease patients: a phase ib randomized, placebo-controlled study. *Clin Transl Sci.* 2019;12(2):180-188.

190. Turpin M, Chantalat-Auger C, Parent F, et al. Chronic blood exchange transfusions in the management of pre-capillary pulmonary hypertension complicating sickle cell disease. *Eur Respir J.* 2018;52(4):1800272.

191. Ataga KI, Smith WR, De Castro LM, et al. Efficacy and safety of the Gardos channel blocker, senicapoc (ICA-17043), in patients with sickle cell anemia. *Blood.* 2008;111(8):3991-3997.

192. Ataga KI, Reid M, Ballas SK, et al. Improvements in haemolysis and indicators of erythrocyte survival do not correlate with acute vaso-occlusive crises in patients with sickle cell disease: a phase III randomized, placebo-controlled, double-blind study of the Gardos channel blocker senicapoc (ICA-17043). *Br J Haematol.* 2011;153(1):92-104.

193. Minniti CP, Wilson J, Mendelsohn L, et al. Anti-haemolytic effect of senicapoc and decrease in NT-proBNP in adults with sickle cell anaemia. *Br J Haematol.* 2011;155(5):634-636.

194. Machado RF, Hildesheim M, Mendelsohn L, Remaley AT, Kato GJ, Gladwin MT. NT-pro brain natriuretic peptide levels and the risk of death in the cooperative study of sickle cell disease. *Br J Haematol.* 2011;154(4):512-520.

195. Kato GJ, Gladwin MT, Steinberg MH. Deconstructing sickle cell disease: reappraisal of the role of hemolysis in the development of clinical subphenotypes. *Blood Rev.* 2007;21(1):37-47.

196. Vichinsky E, Hoppe CC, Ataga KI, et al. A phase 3 randomized trial of voxelotor in sickle cell disease. *N Engl J Med.* 2019;381(6):509-519.

197. Olnes M, Chi A, Haney C, et al. Improvement in hemolysis and pulmonary arterial systolic pressure in adult patients with sickle cell disease during treatment with hydroxyurea. *Am J Hematol.* 2009;84(8):530-532.

198. Pashankar FD, Carbonella J, Bazzy-Asaad A, Friedman A. Longitudinal follow up of elevated pulmonary artery pressures in children with sickle cell disease. *Br J Haematol.* 2009;144(5):736-741.

199. Cokic VP, Beleslin-Cokic BB, Tomic M, Stojilkovic SS, Noguchi CT, Schechter AN. Hydroxyurea induces the eNOS-cGMP pathway in endothelial cells. *Blood.* 2006;108(1):184-191.

200. King SB. N-hydroxyurea and acyl nitroso compounds as nitroxyl (HNO) and nitric oxide (NO) donors. *Curr Top Med Chem.* 2005;5(7):665-673.

201. Castro O, Poillon WN, Finke H, Massac E. Improvement of sickle cell anemia by iron-limited erythropoiesis. *Am J Hematol.* 1994;47(2):74-81.

202. Haddy TB, Castro O. Overt iron deficiency in sickle cell disease. *Arch Intern Med.* 1982;142(9):1621-1624.

203. Das N, Xie L, Ramakrishnan SK, Campbell A, Rivella S, Shah YM. Intestine-specific disruption of hypoxia-inducible factor (hif)-2alpha improves anemia in sickle cell disease. *J Biol Chem.* 2015;290(39):23523-23527.

204. Castro O, Kato GJ. Iron restriction in sickle cell anemia: time for controlled clinical studies. *Am J Hematol.* 2015;90(12):E217.

205. Schaer DJ, Vinchi F, Ingoglia G, Tolosano E, Buehler PW. Haptoglobin, hemopexin, and related defense pathways-basic science, clinical perspectives, and drug development. *Front Physiol.* 2014;5:415.

206. Vercellotti GM, Zhang P, Nguyen J, et al. Hepatic overexpression of hemopexin inhibits inflammation and vascular stasis in murine models of sickle cell disease. *Mol Med.* 2016;22:437-451.

207. Panda H, Keleku-Lukwete N, Kuga A, Fuke N, et al. Dietary supplementation with sulforaphane attenuates liver damage and heme overload in a sickle cell disease murine model. *Exp Hematol.* 2019;77:51-60.e1.

208. Keleku-Lukwete N, Suzuki M, Panda H, et al. Nrf2 activation in myeloid cells and endothelial cells differentially mitigates sickle cell disease pathology in mice. *Blood Adv.* 2019;3(8):1285-1297.

209. Ghosh S, Hazra R, Ihunnah CA, Weidert F, Flage B, Ofori-Acquah SF. Augmented NRF2 activation protects adult sickle mice from lethal acute chest syndrome. *Br J Haematol.* 2018;182(2):271-275.

210. Ghosh S, Ihunnah CA, Hazra R, et al. Nonhematopoietic Nrf2 dominantly impedes adult progression of sickle cell anemia in mice. *JCI Insight.* 2016;1:4.

211. Krishnamoorthy S, Pace B, Gupta D, et al. Dimethyl fumarate increases fetal hemoglobin, provides heme detoxification, and corrects anemia in sickle cell disease. *JCI Insight.* 2017;2:20.

212. Doss JF, Jonassaint JC, Garrett ME, Ashley-Koch AE, Telen MJ, Chi JT. Phase 1 study of a sulforaphane-containing broccoli sprout homogenate for sickle cell disease. *PLoS One.* 2016;11(4):e0152895.

213. Belcher JD, Vineyard JV, Bruzzone CM, et al. Heme oxygenase-1 gene delivery by Sleeping Beauty inhibits vascular stasis in a murine model of sickle cell disease. *J Mol Med (Berl).* 2010;88(7):665-675.

214. Ataga KI, Moore CG, Jones S, et al. Pulmonary hypertension in patients with sickle cell disease: a longitudinal study. *Br J Haematol.* 2006;134(1):109-115.

215. Gordeuk VR, Campbell A, Rana S, et al. Relationship of erythropoietin, fetal hemoglobin, and hydroxyurea treatment to tricuspid regurgitation velocity in children with sickle cell disease. *Blood.* 2009;114(21):4639-4644.

216. Voskaridou E, Tsetsos G, Tsoutsias A, Spyropoulou E, Christoulas D, Terpos E. Pulmonary hypertension in patients with sickle cell/beta thalassemia: incidence and correlation with serum N-terminal pro-brain natriuretic peptide concentrations. *Haematologica.* 2007;92(6):738-743.

217. Sachdev V, Kato GJ, Gibbs JS, et al. Echocardiographic markers of elevated pulmonary pressure and left ventricular diastolic dysfunction are associated with exercise intolerance in adults and adolescents with homozygous sickle cell anemia in the United States and United Kingdom. *Circulation.* 2011;124(13):1452-1460.

Sterile Inflammation in Sickle Cell Disease

Authors: *Prithu Sundd, Solomon F. Ofori-Acquah*

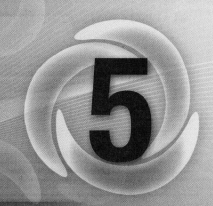

Chapter Outline

Overview

Studies over several decades have characterized 3 major events (hemoglobin S [HbS] polymerization described in Chapter 2, vaso-occlusion discussed in Chapter 3, and hemolysis-mediated endothelial dysfunction discussed in Chapter 4) that drive the pathobiology of sickle cell disease (SCD).[1-4] Recent findings have identified sterile inflammation as another underlying phenomenon that contributes to the pathophysiology of SCD. Sterile inflammation involves the activation of innate immune pathways, in the absence of infection, in diverse vascular cells in response to the release of a variety of damage-associated molecular pattern molecules (DAMPs) from dying or damaged cells or tissues.[1,5,6] Several DAMPs and innate immune pathways that contribute to inflammation and end-organ damage in SCD have been identified.[1,5] They trigger disturbances in the innate immune system that appear to promote infection, acute systemic painful vaso-occlusive episode (VOE), acute chest syndrome (ACS), and chronic organ damage in SCD patients.[1,2,4,7-16] The improved understanding of these molecular pathways has also led to identification of new therapeutic targets to attenuate both acute and chronic complications of SCD.[1,3,9,17-19] This chapter serves to inform readers of the current understanding of the role and mechanism of sterile inflammation in SCD. The next section of this chapter describes hematologic findings that inspired recent studies to explore the role of sterile inflammation in SCD. The following section describes pathways and phenomena that have been found to contribute to sterile inflammation in SCD. We then describe how our current understanding of sterile inflammation is inspiring new avenues of therapy for SCD. Next, we discuss how insights in sterile inflammation are guiding contemporary research in SCD. Finally, we end the chapter with concluding remarks.

Footprints of Sterile Inflammation in SCD

VOE, ACS, and Chronic Organ Injury

Studies conducted in SCD mice and patients over the past 2 decades have identified several immunologic and hematologic abnormalities (clockwise in Figure 5-1 and described in the following text) that suggest a role for sterile (noninfectious)

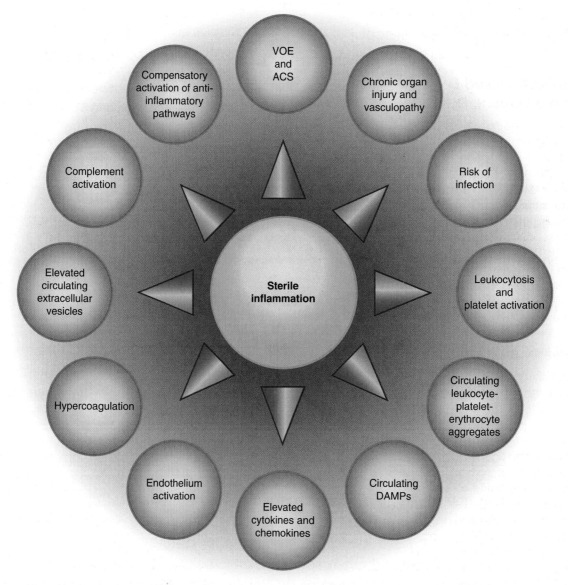

FIGURE 5-1 Footprints of sterile inflammation in sickle cell disease (SCD). Immunologic and hematologic abnormalities (clockwise) that suggest a role for sterile inflammation in acute and chronic pathobiology of SCD. ACS, acute chest syndrome; DAMPs, damage-associated molecular pattern molecules; VOE, acute systemic painful vaso-occlusive episode.

inflammation in acute and chronic pathobiology of SCD.[1] Occlusions in various vascular beds promote the development of acute systemic painful VOE, which is the primary reason for emergency medical care among SCD patients.[4] Clinical evidence suggests that VOE is frequently a leading prodrome to ACS, particularly among adult patients. ACS is a severe acute lung injury (ALI) in SCD; it is one of the leading causes of mortality among this patient population.[4,15,20] ACS is associated with 3 major findings at diagnosis: hypoxia, multilobular pulmonary infiltrates, and acute anemia (decrease in hemoglobin [Hb]).[11] Infectious bronchopneumonia and bacteremia are also major risk factors for ACS.[11,16,21-27] Other causes include pulmonary vaso-occlusion and infarction, pulmonary fat embolism, and/or sudden decrease in Hb (acute hemolysis) in the absence of clinically detectable infection, suggesting a potential contribution of sterile inflammatory response.[1,4,9,11,14,15,20,28-34] The importance of sterile inflammation in SCD is also supported by clinical evidence of chronic vasculopathy and progressive multiorgan damage with aging.[2,4,9,17,35,36]

Chronically Activated Blood Cells Prime Immune Response

SCD patients are highly sensitive to bacterial or viral infection. ACS can develop with exposure to relatively less severe infectious triggers that are harmless in healthy subjects.[11,14-16,22,24,27,29,37-42] This suggests there is an underlying sterile inflammatory state that lowers the threshold for infection in SCD.[1] SCD patients have elevated numbers of neutrophils, monocytes, and platelets at baseline and raised circulating neutrophil-platelet-erythrocyte as well as monocyte-platelet aggregates, which correlate with disease severity.[43-52] The leukocytes and platelets in the blood of SCD patients are activated.[34,49,50,53-57] Thrombocytopenia during VOE is associated with ACS, which suggests a role for platelet activation and sequestration at sites of lung vaso-occlusion.[20,31,32,34,58,59]

Inflammatory Mediators

The inflammatory milieu in SCD is evident by raised proinflammatory circulating erythroid and tissue-derived DAMPs.[5] DAMPs circulating in the blood of patients and transgenic mice with SCD include cell-free hemoglobin (Hb), heme, adenosine diphosphate (ADP), uric acid, high mobility group box 1 (HMGB1), and nucleosomes.[4,5,33,60-63] The concentrations of several inflammatory cytokines are also elevated in the blood of SCD patients. They include interleukin (IL)-1α, IL-1β, IL-6, IL-8, IL-12, tumor necrosis factor-α (TNF-α), prostaglandin E_2 (PGE_2), monocyte chemoattractant protein-1 (MCP-1), macrophage inflammatory protein-1α (MIP-1α), interferon-γ (IFN-γ), highly sensitive C-reactive protein (hs-CRP), and leukotriene B4 (LTB4).[30,64-70] In addition to circulating cytokines, both protein and mRNA levels are significantly elevated for IL-1β, sCD40L, and IL-6 in platelets[71]; TNF-α, IL-8, IL-1β, and the heme catabolizing

enzyme heme oxygenase-1 (HO-1) in mononuclear cells[65,72]; and IL-8, IFN-γ, and inducible nitric oxide synthase (iNOS) in neutrophils[65] of SCD patients compared to healthy control subjects. Studies in mice have revealed that the endothelium is activated in diverse vascular beds in SCD characterized by the upregulation of selectins (P- and E-selectin), vascular cell adhesion molecule 1 (VCAM1), intercellular adhesion molecule 1 (ICAM1), von Willebrand factor (vWF), and major leukocyte chemoattractants such as keratinocyte-derived chemokine (KC [CXCL1]) on endothelial cells.[2,3,5,62] Soluble VCAM1 (sVCAM1) and ultra-large vWF multimers probably released by activated endothelial cells are also elevated in the plasma of SCD patients.[73-77]

Hemostatic Activation

The inflammatory milieu in SCD may also contribute to the coagulopathy typical of the disease. Markers of thrombin generation and coagulation, such as prothrombin fragment F1+2, thrombin-antithrombin III complexes, and D-dimers, are significantly increased in the plasma of SCD patients at steady state and increase further during VOE.[68,78-82] Activation of both extrinsic and intrinsic coagulation pathways contributes to the hypercoagulable state in SCD. Levels of factor (F) VII and activated FVII are reduced in SCD patients compared to control subjects, and there is aberrant expression of tissue factor (TF) on circulating endothelial cells and monocytes and elevated whole blood TF procoagulant activity.[82-85] Similarly, plasma levels of intrinsic coagulation system proteins including FXII, prekallikrein, and high-molecular-weight kininogen are decreased in SCD patients at steady state and decreased further during VOE.[86-88] Low levels of natural anticoagulants protein C and protein S in patients provide additional evidence of hypercoagulation in SCD.[89-91]

Extracellular Vesicles, Complement Activation, and Anti-Inflammatory Pathways

Extracellular vesicles (EVs) derived from sickle erythrocytes, platelets, neutrophils, monocytes, and endothelial cells are significantly elevated in the plasma of patients and transgenic mice with SCD, and the levels correlate with disease severity.[79,92-94] As described later in this chapter, these EVs contribute to sterile inflammation in SCD by carrying cytokines such as IL-1β and IL-8, HO-1, HMGB1, and heme and also promote coagulation by presenting TF as well as negatively charged phospholipids such as phosphatidyl serine.[79,94-99] Complement is activated in both patients and mice with SCD. Deposition of complement C3 and C5b-9 has been observed in kidney biopsies of SCD nephropathy patients and tissues of SCD mice.[100] Erythrocytes isolated from hospitalized SCD patients have increased levels of bound C3, suggestive of activated alternative complement pathway.[101] Sterile inflammation in SCD is also supported by the compensatory activation of the nuclear factor erythroid-2–related factor-2

(Nrf2)-dependent anti-inflammatory and antioxidant pathway to provide cytoprotection.[65,102-106]

Pathways Leading to Sterile Inflammation in SCD

Basic and translational studies on SCD patient blood samples and transgenic SCD mice have led to our current understanding of the role and mechanism of sterile inflammation in SCD. As shown in Figure 5-2 and described in the following text, hemolysis and erythrocyte sickling secondary to Hb polymerization, nitric oxide depletion, endothelial dysfunction, ischemia-reperfusion injury secondary to vaso-occlusion, release of

DAMPs, and activation of innate immune pathways synergize to promote sterile inflammation in SCD.[1,2,5]

HbS Polymerization

Intraerythrocytic HbS deoxygenation in tissues with high oxygen demand promotes the exposure of hydrophobic motifs on individual deoxygenated (T-state) HbS tetramers.[4,107] As a result, β^s-globin chains on different deoxygenated HbS tetramers bind to each other to hide the hydrophobic motifs, thus initiating the nucleation of an HbS polymer. These HbS polymers grow rapidly to form long fibers that increase cellular rigidity and distort the erythrocyte membrane, leading to erythrocyte sickling, cellular energetic failure and stress, dehydration,

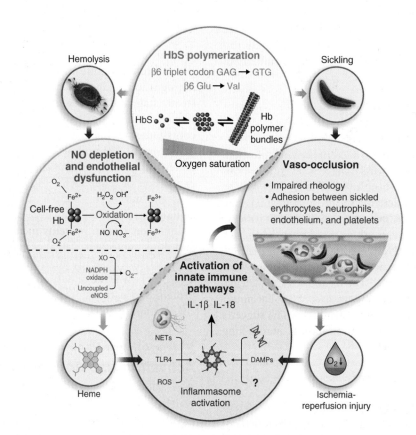

FIGURE 5-2 **Pathways promoting sterile inflammation in sickle cell disease (SCD).** Yellow circle: Single nucleotide polymorphism in β-globin gene leading to substitution of valine for glutamic acid at the sixth position in β-globin chain. Following deoxygenation, the mutated hemoglobin S (HbS) molecules polymerize to form bundles. The polymer bundles result in erythrocyte sickling (clockwise), which results in impaired rheology of the blood and aggregation of sickle erythrocytes with neutrophils, platelets, and endothelial cells to promote stasis of blood flow referred to as vaso-occlusion (blue circle). Vaso-occlusion promotes ischemia-reperfusion injury (clockwise). Hemoglobin (Hb) polymer bundles (yellow circle) also promote hemolysis or lysis of erythrocytes (counterclockwise) that releases cell-free Hb into the blood circulation. Oxygenated Hb (Fe^{2+}) promotes endothelial dysfunction (green circle) by depleting endothelial nitric oxide (NO) reserves to form nitrate (NO_3^-) and methemoglobin. Alternatively, Hb can also react with hydrogen peroxide (H_2O_2) through the Fenton reaction to form hydroxyl free radical (OH·) and methemoglobin (Fe^{3+}). Also, NADPH oxidase, xanthine oxidase (XO), and uncoupled endothelial NO synthase (eNOS) generate oxygen free radicals to promote endothelial dysfunction. Methemoglobin (Fe^{3+}) degrades to release cell-free heme (counterclockwise), which is a major erythrocyte damage-associated molecular pattern molecule (DAMP). Reactive oxygen species (ROS) generation, toll-like receptor 4 (TLR4) activation, neutrophil extracellular trap (NET) generation, release of tissue- or cell-derived DAMPs, DNA, and other unknown factors (?) triggered by cell-free heme or ischemia-reperfusion injury can promote innate immune signaling by activating the inflammasome pathway in vascular and inflammatory cells to release interleukin (IL)-1β (purple circle). Finally, activated innate immune pathways further promote vaso-occlusion through a feedback loop by promoting adhesiveness of neutrophils, platelets, and endothelial cells. Adapted from Sundd P, Gladwin MT, Novelli EM. Pathophysiology of sickle cell disease. *Annu Rev Pathol.* 2019;14:263-292.

impaired rheology, and premature hemolysis[4,107,108] (yellow circle in Figure 5-2). We refer readers to Chapter 2 (on HbS polymerization) to learn further about this topic.

Vaso-occlusion

Intravital imaging studies of transgenic humanized SCD mice and in vitro flow chamber studies over the past decade have contributed to our current understanding of vaso-occlusion (blue circle in Figure 5-2) as an interplay of impaired blood rheology, increased adhesiveness of erythrocytes with inflammatory cells and vascular endothelium, and hemostatic activation.[3] Blood rheology is driven by hematocrit, plasma viscosity, and erythrocyte deformability.[108] Increased blood viscosity as a result of reduced sickle erythrocyte deformability due to Hb polymerization and erythrocyte dehydration contributes to impaired flow of blood through capillaries and postcapillary venules of tissues with high oxygen demand.[108] Rigid sickle erythrocytes may become mechanically sequestered in the microcirculation to promote transient vaso-occlusion.[4,107] Sickling-dependent damage to erythrocyte membrane promotes exposure of adhesion molecules and binding motifs not expressed normally on erythrocytes such as phosphatidyl serine (PS), basal cell adhesion molecule-1/Lutheran (B-CAM-1/Lu), integrin-associated protein (IAP), and ICAM4.[107-109] Chronic anemia promotes premature release of so-called "stress" reticulocytes from the bone marrow,[4] which are decorated with adhesion molecules such as $\alpha 4\beta 1$ integrin (VLA-4) and CD36.[109] Besides impaired blood rheology, adhesion of erythrocytes and reticulocytes to leukocytes, platelets, and endothelial cells also promotes vaso-occlusion in SCD.[2,3,34,110] The endothelial dysfunction (discussed next) may contribute to upregulation of selectins (P- and E-selectin), VCAM1, ICAM1, and major leukocyte chemoattractants such as KC (mouse) or IL-8 (humans) on endothelial cells.[2,3,5] Activation of innate immune pathways in SCD (discussed later in this chapter) may also promote activation of neutrophils, monocytes, and platelets, leading to their increased adhesion to each other and the endothelium.[2,3,5] Activation of both extrinsic and intrinsic pathways of coagulation also contributes to vaso-occlusion, and activated leukocytes, platelets, and endothelial cells have been implicated in progression of SCD-related coagulopathy.[111] Readers are advised to read Chapter 3 (on vaso-occlusion in SCD) to learn more about cellular and molecular mechanisms of vaso-occlusion.

Nitric Oxide Depletion, Endothelial Dysfunction, and Oxidative Stress

Nitric oxide (NO) produced by endothelial cells serves to inhibit inflammation by increasing cyclic guanosine monophosphate (cGMP) levels in both platelets and endothelial cells, attenuating oxidative stress, and inhibiting inflammasome activation in leukocytes.[1,2,54,112-122] As shown in Figure 5-2 (green circle), NO generated by endothelial cells reacts with the oxygenated heme groups (Fe^{2+}) of cell-free Hb at nearly diffusion-limited rates (10^7 M^{-1} s^{-1}) to generate methemoglobin and nitrate (NO_3^-).[123-125] This dioxygenation reaction is irreversible and so fast that it results in the immediate depletion of intravascular NO.[126,127] Under normal physiologic conditions, the reaction of NO with Hb is restricted by the diffusional barriers imposed by the compartmentalization of Hb within the erythrocyte.[128-133] Due to intravascular hemolysis, the diffusional barriers are disrupted and the cell-free Hb depletes NO, promoting platelet activation (degranulation, P-selectin exposure, and $\alpha IIb\beta 3$ activation), endothelial activation and dysfunction (upregulation of P- and E-selectin, ICAM1, and VCAM1), and inflammation.[1,2,4,7,14,15,35,54,113,128,134-136] In addition to the dioxygenation reaction, cell-free Hb also undergoes Fenton and peroxidase reactions (green circle in Figure 5-2) to generate reactive oxygen species (ROS).[137,138] Superoxide (O_2^-), an abundant ROS in SCD, reacts with NO to form peroxynitrite ($ONOO^-$) and its conjugate peroxynitrous acid, contributing further to the reduced NO bioavailability and leading to enhanced platelet activation and inflammation in SCD.[6,35,136,139-141] Intravascular hemolysis in SCD also results in the release of arginase-1, which converts L-arginine to ornithine and urea, thus impairing NO synthesis and further promoting inflammation.[114,142,143] Abundant ROS may also promote inflammation and endothelial dysfunction by oxidizing soluble guanylate cyclase (sGC), which is the target for NO-mediated anti-inflammatory signaling.[144] Readers are advised to read Chapter 4 (on hemolysis and endothelial dysfunction) to learn more about hemolysis and NO depletion–mediated vascular injury in SCD. In addition to promoting NO depletion and oxidative stress, Hb is also oxidized and degrades to release cell-free heme and heme iron (Figure 5-2). Extracellular Hb and heme activate innate immune pathways through toll-like receptor 4 (TLR4) and inflammasome signaling, which is discussed in the following paragraphs.[1,5,33,62,94,145] These 2 primary hemolysis products are erythrocyte DAMPs (eDAMPs) that further promote and propagate sterile inflammation, oxidative stress, and vascular injury.[1,2,5] Release of Hb and erythrocyte ADP during hemolysis stimulates platelet activation and activates hypercoagulation pathways to promote vascular thrombosis, thus further contributing to vaso-occlusion.[53,54,146,147]

Heme-Induced Activation of Endothelial Cells and Leukocytes

Heme (ferrous protoporphyrin IX) or the oxidized form hemin (ferric protoporphyrin IX) released following oxidation of Hb is a potent TLR4 agonist that contributes to a proinflammatory, pro-oxidative, and procoagulant state in SCD, characterized by activated leukocytes, platelets, endothelial cells, TF, cytokine storm, NO depletion, and generation of ROS.[5,33,60,62,63,111,148] Intravenous administration of purified hemin promotes ALI and pulmonary vascular congestion in SCD mice, which was prevented following therapeutic inhibition or genetic deletion of endothelial TLR4.[33] In another study,[62] extracellular hemin was shown to promote endothelial activation, leading to increased neutrophil adhesion and vaso-occlusion in skin venules, NADPH oxidase (NOX)-mediated ROS generation, and death in SCD mice, which was also inhibited following inhibition or genetic deletion of endothelial TLR4. Heme-laden erythrocyte-derived microparticles have been shown to promote endothelial activation, ROS generation, and vaso-occlusion in the kidney of SCD mice by adhering and delivering heme to the endothelial cells.[149] Heme has also been shown to promote TLR4 activation in macrophages, which promotes release of TNF-α, KC, and LTB4.[148,150,151] Thus, extracellular heme seems to promote sterile inflammation in SCD by stimulating TLR4-dependent innate immune signaling in endothelial and mononuclear cells. Interestingly, heme appears to act through G-protein–coupled receptor (GPCR)-dependent signaling to promote neutrophil migration, oxidative burst, neutrophil extracellular trap (NET) generation, IL-8 production, and increased neutrophil survival.[152-155] However, the GPCR receptor for heme on neutrophils remains unknown.[148] Activated neutrophils release NETs, which are mesh-like structures composed of decondensed chromatin decorated with neutrophil proteases and citrullinated histones.[156] Diverse inflammatory agonists release neutrophil NETs to promote the activation of innate immune response leading to tissue injury.[156-159] Most recently,[63] extracellular heme was shown to promote oxidative burst, leading to release of NETs by neutrophils in the lung microcirculation of TNF-α–challenged SCD mice, which was inhibited following administration of hemopexin. Indeed, circulating markers of NETs such as nucleosomes and elastase–α$_1$-antitrypsin are significantly elevated in the plasma of SCD patients at steady state and increase further during VOE.[61] TLR4 inhibition reduces P-selectin-PSGL-1–dependent platelet-neutrophil aggregation in SCD human blood flowing through microfluidic flow channels in vitro.[34] Although it is unclear how extracellular heme promotes platelet activation in SCD, an early study showed that heme enhances ADP- and epinephrine-dependent platelet aggregation.[160] Heme activates the secretion of placenta growth factor (PlGF), a peptide hormone with both inflammatory cytokine and angiogenic properties that is related to vasculopathy in SCD, which preliminarily contributes to vaso-occlusion.[161-164] SCD patients have increased risk for contracting bacterial infections with detrimental outcomes compared to healthy control humans.[11,14] The molecular pathophysiology that contributes to this infection susceptibility remains incompletely understood. Heme promotes cytoskeletal disruption, leading to impaired bacterial clearance, phagocytosis, and migration by monocytes, macrophages, and neutrophils in a process involving guanine nucleotide exchange factor DOCK8-mediated activation of the guanosine triphosphate–binding Rho family protein Cdc42.[165] This suggests heme may be involved in the increased susceptibility of SCD patients to bacterial infections. Taken together, these studies suggest that extracellular heme promotes TLR4 activation in mononuclear leukocytes and endothelial cells, generation of ROS by vascular cells, and NET generation by neutrophils in SCD (purple circle in Figure 5-2).

Release of Cell- and Tissue-Derived DAMPs

Vaso-occlusion contributes to ischemia-reperfusion injury and release of cell- and tissue-derived DAMPs, which along with eDAMPs promote sterile inflammation in SCD (Figure 5-2).[1-3,5,94] Readers are advised to refer to Chapter 6 (on ischemia-reperfusion injury and oxidative stress) to learn more about this topic. Repeated episodes of vaso-occlusion and reperfusion contribute to ischemia-reperfusion injury by promoting transient hypoxia, ROS generation, microvascular dysfunction, activation of innate and adaptive immune responses, and cell death.[49,166-171] ROS-dependent oxidative damage of cellular proteins, lipids, DNA, and ribonucleic acids contributes to activation of cell death programs such as apoptosis, necrosis, autophagy, and NETosis (release of NETs by neutrophils), which contributes to release of tissue- and cell-derived DAMPs such as oxidized DNA and plasma membrane fragments, chromatin-binding protein such as HMGB1, adenosine triphosphate, mitochondrial proteins such as cardiolipin, loss of mitochondrial membrane potential, cytoplasmic proteins, proteases, lysosomal products, histones, and nucleosomes.[171-173] These DAMPs promote innate immune responses by priming TLR signaling in endothelial cells and leukocytes, leading to activation of nuclear factor-κB (NF-κB), mitogen-activated protein kinase (MAPK), and type I interferon pathways, resulting in proinflammatory cytokine and chemokine inductions.[174] HMGB1 is elevated in the plasma of SCD patients and mice, and the levels are increased further during VOE in patients and after hypoxia-reoxygenation challenge in mice.[175] HMGB1 was shown to promote TLR4 activity in plasma of both SCD patients and mice.[175]

Inflammasome Activation and EV Generation

Both hemolysis—through the release of eDAMPs—and ischemia-reperfusion injury secondary to vaso-occlusive events—through release of cell- and tissue-derived DAMPs—have the potential to activate the innate immune signaling pathways.[174,176] Studies conducted over the past decade have identified inflammasome pathways as key regulators of sterile inflammation.[174,177-179] Nucleotide-binding domain and leucine-rich repeat receptors (NLRs) or absent in melanoma 2 (AIM2)-like receptors (ALRs) are the major components of the inflammasome complex.

Inflammasomes are multimeric cytoplasmic pattern recognition receptor complexes that are activated to process and release the activated cytokines IL-1β and IL-18 into the extracellular space in response to cell- and tissue-derived DAMPs, ROS, TLR4 activation, double-stranded DNA, NETs, and other cell- or tissue-derived danger signals.[157,177,178] Once released into the extracellular space, IL-1β binds to leukocyte and vascular wall IL-1 receptor (IL-1R) to promote IL-1β–dependent downstream innate immune signaling leading to activation of neutrophils, platelets, E-selectin, P-selectin, VCAM1, ICAM1, and chemokines such as IL-8 on endothelial cells to further promote vaso-occlusion[2,3] (Figure 5-2). Readers are advised to refer to more detailed reviews on the role of inflammasomes in sterile inflammation.[177-179]

The NOD-like receptor family pyrin domain containing 3 (NLRP3) inflammasome is the most widely studied inflammasome complex. It is composed of NLRP3, apoptosis-associated speck-like protein containing a caspase recruitment domain (ASC), and caspase-1.[177] Recently, purified hemin was shown to promote NLRP3–ASC–caspase-1 inflammasome activation in lipopolysaccharide (LPS)-primed macrophages, leading to IL-1β release.[176] Deletion of NLRP3, ASC, caspase-1, or IL-1R attenuated hemolysis-induced lethality in mice, suggesting a role for NLRP3 inflammasome activation and systemic release of IL-1β in promoting hemolysis-dependent sterile inflammation.[176] The NLRP3–ASC–caspase-1 inflammasome activation in macrophages was dependent on heme-induced NOX2 activation, mitochondrial ROS production, and K^+ efflux.[176] NLRP3 and IL-1β are elevated in peripheral blood mononuclear cells (PBMCs) of SCD patients compared to those of control human subjects, and incubation of control human PBMCs with sickle erythrocytes increased expression of NLRP3, caspase-1, IL-1β, and IL-18.[72] Serum levels of IL-1β, IL-6, and IL-8 are elevated in SCD patients compared to healthy control subjects.[64,67-70] Although NLRP3 and other inflammasome complexes are expressed in monocytes, macrophages, neutrophils, platelets, and endothelial cells,[176,180-183] heme is a potent inflammasome activator,[176] and IL-1β is significantly elevated in the serum of SCD patients,[64,72] the contribution of inflammasome activation and IL-1β release by these different cell types in promoting sterile inflammation in SCD remains incompletely understood. The inflammatory milieu in SCD promotes TLR4-dependent activation of the NLRP3–ASC–caspase-1 inflammasome pathway in platelets, which is enhanced by the presence of nanogram levels of a TLR4 ligand (pathogen-associated molecular patterns [PAMPs]) such as LPS[94] (Figure 5-3). The NLRP3 inflammasome complex is activated in SCD human platelets at steady state (not in crisis), activation is enhanced following treatment with nanogram doses of LPS, and inhibition of the inflammasome pathway abolishes platelet-neutrophil aggregation in SCD human blood in vitro and prevents intravenous LPS-induced pulmonary vaso-occlusion in SCD mice in vivo.[94]

The combined guidelines of the International Society on Extracellular Vesicles (ISEV) and the International Society of Thrombosis and Hemostasis (ISTH) recommend the use of the umbrella term *extracellular vesicles (EVs)* to collectively define both platelet-derived exosomes (<150 nm) and microparticles (>150 nm).[184,185] Platelet-derived EVs account for >75% of all the EVs in SCD patient blood,[93] and the circulating levels are significantly elevated during ACS.[79,92] Vats and Brzoska et al[94] found that NLRP3-infammasome activation in SCD platelets led to generation of IL-1β, IL-8, and cleaved caspase-1 carrying platelet EVs (Figure 5-3). These platelet EVs contributed to lung vaso-occlusion by promoting caspase-1 and IL-1β–dependent activation of neutrophils and platelets to form large aggregates, which occluded pulmonary arterioles in SCD mice (Figure 5-3). These findings suggest that the inflammatory milieu in SCD is defined by a primed TLR4/inflammasome/IL-1β–dependent innate immune pathway creating an enhanced basal inflammatory state, which provokes a robust inflammatory response to innocuous levels of PAMPs. This enhanced sensitivity may explain the high risk of bacterial or viral infection and development of lung injury in SCD patients after exposure to relatively mild infectious triggers.[11,14-16,22-24,27,29,37-42] Platelet EVs may contribute to sterile inflammation in SCD by several other mechanisms that require further investigation. IL-1β carrying platelet EVs may also activate the IL-1 receptor on platelets by an autocrine loop[182,186] to further promote generation of platelet EVs (orange curved arrow in Figure 5-3). Activated platelets trapped within the platelet-neutrophil aggregates may undergo degranulation[187] to locally generate IL-1β carrying EVs (gray dotted arrow in Figure 5-3). IL-1β carrying platelet EVs may also promote the activation of vascular endothelium,[181] fibrin deposition leading to coagulation, and monocyte-platelet aggregation, which are all hallmarks of sterile inflammation (Figure 5-1). Inhibition of inflammasome and the IL-1β–dependent innate immune pathway thus offers an attractive therapeutic strategy to halt the progression of ACS in high-risk patients hospitalized with VOE.

Current and Future Therapies Targeting Sterile Inflammation in SCD

As shown in Figure 5-4, our current understanding of the molecular and cellular pathways of sterile inflammation in SCD has inspired several potential therapeutic strategies (blue circle in Figure 5-4).[1,9,17-19] This topic is addressed in detail in Part III of this book (Emerging Therapeutics). Although the outcome of the activation of innate immune pathways is sterile inflammation, the genesis of sterile inflammation in SCD is a direct or indirect consequence of several pathologic processes (described in Figure 5-2) including hemolysis and erythrocyte sickling secondary to HbS polymerization, NO depletion, ROS production, endothelial dysfunction, ischemia-reperfusion injury secondary to vaso-occlusion, and release of eDAMPs and cell- or tissue-derived DAMPs, which ultimately triggers the activation of innate immune pathways in SCD. Therefore, therapies targeting the aforementioned upstream events would also reduce sterile inflammation in SCD. Such therapies have been proposed or are currently being tested to attenuate disease severity (Figure 5-4). As shown in Figure 5-4 (yellow circle), some of the approved or potential therapies attenuate hemolysis and sickling by either inhibiting HbS polymerization or rescuing erythrocyte deformability by inducing fetal Hb (HbF) expression (hydroxyurea, metformin, and sodium butyrate), stabilizing the R-state conformation of HbS (GBT440/voxelotor), preventing erythrocyte dehydration (senicapoc), or serving as carbon monoxide (CO) donors (pegylated bovine carboxyhemoglobin).[18,188,189] Several antiadhesion therapies are also approved or being tested to attenuate vaso-occlusion–associated ischemia-reperfusion injury (blue circle

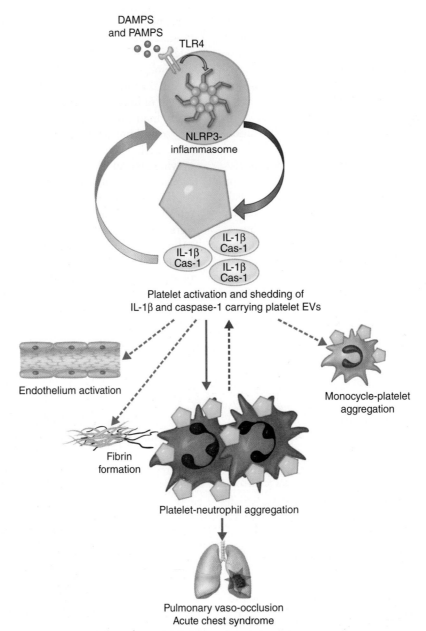

FIGURE 5-3 Platelet inflammasome activation and extracellular vesicle generation. The inflammatory milieu in sickle cell disease (SCD) (damage-associated molecular patterns [DAMPs]) primes toll-like receptor 4 (TLR4)–dependent activation of NLRP3–ASC–caspase-1 inflammasome in platelets (green), which is enhanced by the presence of TLR4 agonists (pathogen-associated molecular patterns [PAMPs]) at low concentrations that are innocuous under healthy conditions. Inflammasome-dependent Caspase-1 activation promotes platelet activation (blue curved arrow), leading to shedding of interleukin (IL)-1β and caspase-1 carrying extracellular vesicles (EVs; shown in yellow) by platelets. Platelet EVs promote IL-1β and caspase-1–dependent platelet-neutrophil aggregation in lung arterioles (red solid arrows), leading to pulmonary vaso-occlusion. IL-1β carrying platelet EVs may activate the IL-1 receptor on platelets by an autocrine loop to further promote generation of platelet EVs (orange curved arrow). In addition, activated platelets trapped within the platelet-neutrophil aggregates may undergo degranulation to locally generate EVs (gray dotted arrow). IL-1β carrying platelet EVs may also promote the activation of vascular endothelium, fibrin deposition leading to coagulation, and monocyte-platelet aggregation (brown dotted arrows). ASC, apoptosis-associated speck-like protein containing a caspase recruitment domain; Cas-1, caspase-1; NLRP3, NOD-like receptor family, pyrin domain containing 3.

in Figure 5-4). These therapies target P-selectin (crizanlizumab) and E-selectin (rivipansel), CD11b/CD18 (intravenous immunoglobulin), platelet glycoprotein Ibα inhibitor (CCP-224), or MAPK (MEK inhibitors) to prevent erythrocyte adhesion. These agents prevent endothelial dysfunction by scavenging cell-free Hb or heme (haptoglobin or hemopexin), promoting NO production (hydroxyurea, oral or intravenous nitrite, inhaled NO, and oral arginine), and reducing oxidative stress (L-glutamine and antioxidants). The emerging role of innate immune pathways (described in Figure 5-2) in SCD-associated morbidity suggests that anti-inflammatory approaches such as therapies to promote induction of heme degradation enzyme HO-1 (MP4CO), scavenging of ROS (antioxidants and L-glutamine), inhibition of TLR4 signaling, degradation of NETs

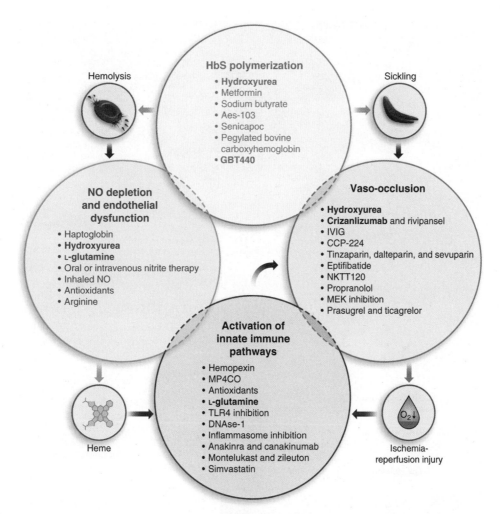

FIGURE 5-4 **Current and future therapies targeting sterile inflammation in sickle cell disease (SCD).** Yellow circle: Drugs capable of modulating hemoglobin (Hb) polymerization, erythrocyte dehydration, and Hb oxygen affinity. Blue circle: Drugs capable of preventing vaso-occlusion by inhibiting adhesive interactions between leukocytes/platelets/endothelial cells and erythrocytes. Green circle: Drugs capable of preventing nitric oxide (NO) depletion, reactive oxygen species (ROS) generation, endothelial dysfunction by scavenging Hb and ROS or promoting NO synthesis. Purple circle: Drugs capable of preventing the activation of innate immune pathways by scavenging heme and ROS, digesting neutrophil extracellular traps (NETs), inhibiting toll-like receptor 4 (TLR4) or inflammasome activation, and inhibiting IL-1β–dependent innate immune signaling. Drugs approved by the US Food and Drug Administration (hydroxyurea, GBT440, Crizanlizumab, and L-glutamine) are shown in bold. HbS, hemoglobin S; IVIG, intravenous immunoglobulin. Adapted from Sundd P, Gladwin MT, Novelli EM. Pathophysiology of sickle cell disease. *Annu Rev Pathol.* 2019;14:263-292.

(DNase-1), leukotriene inhibition, and inhibition of inflammasome or IL-1β–dependent signaling may also be beneficial in SCD.[1,2,5,17-19,190] IL-1R antagonist (anakinra) and IL-1β–blocking antibody (canakinumab) are already approved by US Food and Drug Administration as anti-inflammatory biologic drugs for the treatment of rheumatoid arthritis[191] and NLRP3-inflammasome–mediated cryopyrin-associated periodic syndrome (CAPS),[192] respectively. There is a strong evidence to investigate repurposing these anti-inflammatory drugs in SCD.

Future Scientific Investigations

Our current understanding of sterile inflammation opens up new avenues of basic and translational research in SCD. First, the NLRP3-inflammasome contributes to sterile inflammation in SCD[94]; however, other inflammasome complexes[178] or

inflammasome-independent pathways may also be involved. Second, generation of NETs has been implicated in promoting oxidative stress, sterile inflammation, and organ injury in SCD, but the molecular mechanisms that drive NET production in SCD are poorly defined. Recent evidence suggests that both protein arginine deiminase 4 (PAD4)-dependent and -independent pathways can contribute to NET generation under diverse inflammatory conditions. Therefore, it is critical to investigate which of these pathways is important in SCD.[193] Studies in mice have primarily explored the role of innate immunity in promoting sterile inflammation in SCD (representative findings shown in Figure 5-5); however, SCD is a chronic inflammatory condition, and a possible dysregulation in the adaptive immune system such as the role of cytotoxic and regulatory T cells or humoral response mediated by B cells warrants future investigation. Recent findings suggest

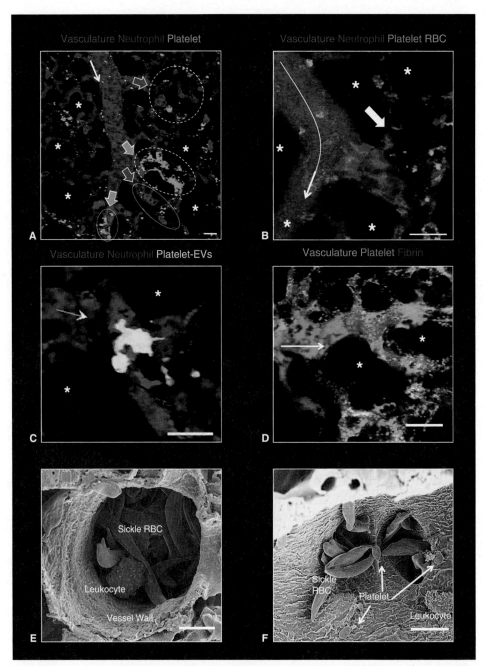

FIGURE 5-5 Vaso-occlusive pathophysiology in SCD mice. A-D. Representative quantitative fluorescence intravital lung microscopy (qFILM) images of lung microvasculature in live SCD mice following induction of vaso-occlusive crisis by intravenous (IV) challenge with a nanogram-dose (0.1 μg/kg) LPS which does not induce crisis in control mice. Pulmonary arteriole micro-embolism by neutrophil-platelet aggregates (**A**) and neutrophil-platelet-RBC aggregates (**B**) in lung of SCD mouse. (**C**) Platelet-derived extracellular vesicles (yellow) bound to neutrophils (red) in the pulmonary arteriole of SCD mouse. (**D**) Pulmonary arteriole thrombi in SCD mouse. **E-F.** Scanning electron micrographs showing vaso-occlusion in lung of SCD mice. White arrows in A-D-flow direction. Scale bars 20 μm. *denote alveoli. A, B adapted from Bennewitz et al JCI Insight 2017 Jan 12;2(1):e89761. C adapted from Vats et al AJRCCM, 2020;201(1):33-46. Adapted with permission of the American Thoracic Society. Copyright © 2020 American Thoracic Society. All rights reserved.

a contribution of platelet-derived EVs in promoting lung inflammation in SCD (Figures 5-3 and 5-5C). Although platelet-derived EVs are the most abundant species of circulating EVs in SCD,[79,92,93] the contribution of EVs derived from other cells types (eg, endothelial cells, erythrocytes, neutrophils, and monocytes) may also be important. EVs may carry several cytokines, DAMPs, and microRNAs and may serve as interorgan communication vehicles to promote multiorgan dysfunction (a hallmark of SCD) by contributing to sterile inflammation at both the protein and transcriptional levels. Finally, existing and future genome-wide association studies should be interrogated to identify single nucleotide polymorphisms in innate immune pathways that can predict the severity of sterile inflammation in SCD. Such studies may lead to identification of patient populations that may benefit from experimental anti-inflammatory therapy.

Conclusion

In the last century, SCD was primarily characterized as a simple monogenic red blood cell disorder. Based on this definition, the diverse acute and chronic morbidities of SCD were attributed to the underlying Hb polymerization and erythrocyte sickling leading to recurrent vaso-occlusive events. Over the past 3 decades, several new pathologic processes in SCD (described in Figures 5-2, 5-3, and 5-5) downstream to Hb polymerization and sickling have been identified. These processes activate innate immune pathways that were previously associated only with host defense from infection or progression of autoimmune disorders. Studies of noninfectious chronic inflammation, or *sterile inflammation*, allow us to modify the characterization of SCD as an autoinflammatory disease.

As described in this chapter, recognition of the importance of sterile inflammation in SCD has inspired several innovative anti-inflammatory therapies for this prototypical Hb polymerization disorder. Future findings in autoinflammatory research in SCD will be generalizable to many other diseases affecting the innate immune system.

Acknowledgment

P.S. was supported by grants (1R01HL128297-01 and 1R01HL141080-01A1) from the National Institutes of Health, National Heart, Lung, and Blood Institute and grant 18TPA34170588 from the American Heart Association. S.O.-A. was supported by grants R01HL106192 and U01HL117721.

High-Yield Facts

- Sickle cell disease (SCD) is an autoinflammatory disease.
- Erythrocyte- and tissue-derived damage-associated molecular pattern molecules (DAMPs) activate innate immune pathways to promote sterile inflammation in SCD.
- Sterile inflammation contributes to the acute and chronic pathophysiology of SCD.
- Inhibition of toll-like receptor 4, inflammasome, and interleukin-1β pathway can be a potential therapy in SCD.
- Future SCD research should explore the role of extracellular vesicles, adaptive immunity, and single nucleotide polymorphisms in immune pathways.

References

1. Sundd P, Gladwin MT, Novelli EM. Pathophysiology of sickle cell disease. *Annu Rev Pathol.* 2019;14:263-292.
2. Kato GJ, Steinberg MH, Gladwin MT. Intravascular hemolysis and the pathophysiology of sickle cell disease. *J Clin Invest.* 2017;127:750-760.
3. Zhang D, Xu C, Manwani D, Frenette PS. Neutrophils, platelets, and inflammatory pathways at the nexus of sickle cell disease pathophysiology. *Blood.* 2016;127:801-809.
4. Rees DC, Williams TN, Gladwin MT. Sickle-cell disease. *Lancet.* 2010;376:2018-2031.
5. Gladwin MT, Ofori-Acquah SF. Erythroid DAMPs drive inflammation in SCD. *Blood.* 2014;123:3689-3690.
6. Kato GJ, Gladwin MT, Steinberg MH. Deconstructing sickle cell disease: reappraisal of the role of hemolysis in the development of clinical subphenotypes. *Blood Rev.* 2007;21:37-47.
7. Gladwin MT. Cardiovascular complications and risk of death in sickle-cell disease. *Lancet.* 2016;387:2565-2574.
8. Gladwin MT, Barst RJ, Gibbs JS, et al. Risk factors for death in 632 patients with sickle cell disease in the United States and United Kingdom. *PLoS One.* 2014;9:e99489.
9. Novelli EM, Gladwin MT. Crises in sickle cell disease. *Chest.* 2016;149:1082-1093.
10. Platt OS, Brambilla DJ, Rosse WF, et al. Mortality in sickle cell disease. Life expectancy and risk factors for early death. *N Engl J Med.* 1994;330:1639-1644.
11. Vichinsky EP, Neumayr LD, Earles AN, et al. Causes and outcomes of the acute chest syndrome in sickle cell disease. National Acute Chest Syndrome Study Group. *N Engl J Med.* 2000;342:1855-1865.
12. Ballas SK, Lieff S, Benjamin LJ, et al. Definitions of the phenotypic manifestations of sickle cell disease. *Am J Hematol.* 2010;85:6-13.
13. Hamideh D, Alvarez O. Sickle cell disease related mortality in the United States (1999-2009). *Pediatr Blood Cancer.* 2013;60:1482-1486.
14. Gladwin MT, Vichinsky E. Pulmonary complications of sickle cell disease. *N Engl J Med.* 2008;359:2254-2265.
15. Miller AC, Gladwin MT. Pulmonary complications of sickle cell disease. *Am J Respir Crit Care Med.* 2012;185:1154-1165.
16. Strouse JJ, Reller ME, Bundy DG, et al. Severe pandemic H1N1 and seasonal influenza in children and young adults with sickle cell disease. *Blood.* 2010;116:3431-3434.
17. Kato GJ, Piel FB, Reid CD, et al. Sickle cell disease. *Nat Rev Dis Primers.* 2018;4:18010.
18. Telen MJ. Beyond hydroxyurea: new and old drugs in the pipeline for sickle cell disease. *Blood.* 2016;127:810-819.
19. Telen MJ, Malik P, Vercellotti GM. Therapeutic strategies for sickle cell disease: towards a multi-agent approach. *Nat Rev Drug Discov.* 2019;18:139-158.
20. Chaturvedi S, Ghafuri DL, Glassberg J, Kassim AA, Rodeghier M, DeBaun MR. Rapidly progressive acute chest syndrome in

individuals with sickle cell anemia: a distinct acute chest syndrome phenotype. *Am J Hematol.* 2016;91:1185-1190.

21. Vichinsky EP, Styles LA, Colangelo LH, Wright EC, Castro O, Nickerson B. Acute chest syndrome in sickle cell disease: clinical presentation and course. Cooperative Study of Sickle Cell Disease. *Blood.* 1997;89:1787-1792.

22. Thomas AN, Pattison C, Serjeant GR. Causes of death in sickle-cell disease in Jamaica. *Br Med J.* 1982;285:633-635.

23. Norris CF, Smith-Whitley K, McGowan KL. Positive blood cultures in sickle cell disease: time to positivity and clinical outcome. *J Pediatr Hematol Oncol.* 2003;25:390-395.

24. Chulamokha L, Scholand SJ, Riggio JM, Ballas SK, Horn D, DeSimone JA. Bloodstream infections in hospitalized adults with sickle cell disease: a retrospective analysis. *Am J Hematol.* 2006;81:723-728.

25. Vaishnavi C. Translocation of gut flora and its role in sepsis. *Indian J Med Microbiol.* 2013;31:334-342.

26. Munoz P, Cruz AF, Rodriguez-Creixems M, Bouza E. Gram-negative bloodstream infections. *Int J Antimicrob Agents.* 2008; 32(Suppl 1):S10-S14.

27. Neumayr L, Lennette E, Kelly D, et al. Mycoplasma disease and acute chest syndrome in sickle cell disease. *Pediatrics.* 2003;112:87-95.

28. Desai PC, Ataga KI. The acute chest syndrome of sickle cell disease. *Exp Opin Pharmacother.* 2013;14:991-999.

29. Manci EA, Culberson DE, Yang YM, et al. Causes of death in sickle cell disease: an autopsy study. *Br J Haematol.* 2003;123: 359-365.

30. Adegoke SA, Kuti BP, Omole KO, Smith OS, Oyelami OA, Adeodu OO. Acute chest syndrome in sickle cell anaemia: higher serum levels of interleukin-8 and highly sensitive C-reactive proteins are associated with impaired lung function. *Paediatr Int Child Health.* 2018;38:244-250.

31. Anea CB, Lyon M, Lee IA, et al. Pulmonary platelet thrombi and vascular pathology in acute chest syndrome in patients with sickle cell disease. *Am J Hematol.* 2016;91:173-178.

32. Mekontso Dessap A, Deux JF, Abidi N, et al. Pulmonary artery thrombosis during acute chest syndrome in sickle cell disease. *Am J Respir Crit Care Med.* 2011;184:1022-1029.

33. Ghosh S, Adisa OA, Chappa P, et al. Extracellular hemin crisis triggers acute chest syndrome in sickle mice. *J Clin Invest.* 2013;123:4809-4820.

34. Bennewitz MF, Jimenez MA, Vats R, et al. Lung vaso-occlusion in sickle cell disease mediated by arteriolar neutrophil-platelet microemboli. *JCI Insight.* 2017;2:e89761.

35. Gladwin MT, Sachdev V. Cardiovascular abnormalities in sickle cell disease. *J Am Coll Cardiol.* 2012;59:1123-1133.

36. Chaturvedi S, DeBaun MR. Evolution of sickle cell disease from a life-threatening disease of children to a chronic disease of adults: the last 40 years. *Am J Hematol.* 2016;91:5-14.

37. Barrett-Connor E. Bacterial infection and sickle cell anemia. An analysis of 250 infections in 166 patients and a review of the literature. *Medicine (Baltimore).* 1971;50:97-112.

38. Craddock PR. Bacterial infection in sickle-cell anemia. *N Engl J Med.* 1973;288:1301-1302.

39. Wong WY, Powars DR, Chan L, Hiti A, Johnson C, Overturf G. Polysaccharide encapsulated bacterial infection in sickle cell anemia: a thirty year epidemiologic experience. *Am J Hematol.* 1992;39:176-182.

40. Makani J, Mgaya J, Balandya E, et al. Bacteraemia in sickle cell anaemia is associated with low haemoglobin: a report of 890

41. admissions to a tertiary hospital in Tanzania. *Br J Haematol.* 2015;171:273-276.

41. Navalkele P, Ozgonenel B, McGrath E, Lephart P, Sarnaik S. Invasive pneumococcal disease in patients with sickle cell disease. *J Pediatr Hematol Oncol.* 2017;39:341-344.

42. Zarrouk V, Habibi A, Zahar JR, et al. Bloodstream infection in adults with sickle cell disease: association with venous catheters, *Staphylococcus aureus*, and bone-joint infections. *Medicine (Baltimore).* 2006;85:43-48.

43. Kenny MW, George AJ, Stuart J. Platelet hyperactivity in sickle-cell disease: a consequence of hyposplenism. *J Clin Pathol.* 1980;33:622-625.

44. Mohan JS, Lip GY, Bareford D, Blann AD. Platelet P-selectin and platelet mass, volume and component in sickle cell disease: relationship to genotype. *Thromb Res.* 2006;117:623-629.

45. Westwick J, Watson-Williams EJ, Krishnamurthi S, et al. Platelet activation during steady state sickle cell disease. *J Med.* 1983;14:17-36.

46. Curtis SA, Danda N, Etzion Z, Cohen HW, Billett HH. Elevated steady state WBC and platelet counts are associated with frequent emergency room use in adults with sickle cell anemia. *PLoS One.* 2015;10:e0133116.

47. Frelinger AL 3rd, Jakubowski JA, Brooks JK, et al. Platelet activation and inhibition in sickle cell disease (pains) study. *Platelets.* 2014;25:27-35.

48. Dominical VM, Samsel L, Nichols JS, et al. Prominent role of platelets in the formation of circulating neutrophil-red cell heterocellular aggregates in sickle cell anemia. *Haematologica.* 2014;99:e214-217.

49. Polanowska-Grabowska R, Wallace K, Field JJ, et al. P-selectin-mediated platelet-neutrophil aggregate formation activates neutrophils in mouse and human sickle cell disease. *Arterioscler Thromb Vasc Biol.* 2010;30:2392-2399.

50. Wun T, Cordoba M, Rangaswami A, Cheung AW, Paglieroni T. Activated monocytes and platelet-monocyte aggregates in patients with sickle cell disease. *Clin Lab Haematol.* 2002;24:81-88.

51. Miller ST, Sleeper LA, Pegelow CH, et al. Prediction of adverse outcomes in children with sickle cell disease. *N Engl J Med.* 2000;342:83-89.

52. Wongtong N, Jones S, Deng Y, Cai J, Ataga KI. Monocytosis is associated with hemolysis in sickle cell disease. *Hematology.* 2015;20:593-597.

53. Cardenes N, Corey C, Geary L, et al. Platelet bioenergetic screen in sickle cell patients reveals mitochondrial complex V inhibition, which contributes to platelet activation. *Blood.* 2014;123:2864-2872.

54. Villagra J, Shiva S, Hunter LA, Machado RF, Gladwin MT, Kato GJ. Platelet activation in patients with sickle disease, hemolysis-associated pulmonary hypertension, and nitric oxide scavenging by cell-free hemoglobin. *Blood.* 2007;110:2166-2172.

55. Wun T, Paglieroni T, Rangaswami A, et al. Platelet activation in patients with sickle cell disease. *Br J Haematol.* 1998;100: 741-749.

56. Inwald DP, Kirkham FJ, Peters MJ, et al. Platelet and leucocyte activation in childhood sickle cell disease: association with nocturnal hypoxaemia. *Br J Haematol.* 2000;111:474-481.

57. Zhang D, Chen G, Manwani D, et al. Neutrophil ageing is regulated by the microbiome. *Nature.* 2015;525:528-532.

58. Gardner K, Thein SL. Super-elevated LDH and thrombocytopenia are markers of a severe subtype of vaso-occlusive crisis in sickle cell disease. *Am J Hematol.* 2015;90:E206-E207.

59. Alhandalous CH, Han J, Hsu L, et al. Platelets decline during vaso-occlusive crisis as a predictor of acute chest syndrome in sickle cell disease. *Am J Hematol.* 2015;90:E228-E229.

60. Setty BN, Betal SG, Zhang J, Stuart MJ. Heme induces endothelial tissue factor expression: potential role in hemostatic activation in patients with hemolytic anemia. *J Thromb Haemost.* 2008;6:2202-2209.

61. Schimmel M, Nur E, Biemond BJ, et al. Nucleosomes and neutrophil activation in sickle cell disease painful crisis. *Haematologica.* 2013;98:1797-1803.

62. Belcher JD, Chen C, Nguyen J, et al. Heme triggers TLR4 signaling leading to endothelial cell activation and vaso-occlusion in murine sickle cell disease. *Blood.* 2014;123:377-390.

63. Chen G, Zhang D, Fuchs TA, Wagner DD, Frenette PS. Heme-induced neutrophil extracellular traps contribute to the pathogenesis of sickle cell disease. *Blood.* 2014;123:3818-3827.

64. Alagbe AE, Justo Junior AS, Ruas LP, et al. Interleukin-27 and interleukin-37 are elevated in sickle cell anemia patients and inhibit in vitro secretion of interleukin-8 in neutrophils and monocytes. *Cytokine.* 2018;107:85-92.

65. Lanaro C, Franco-Penteado CF, Albuqueque DM, Saad ST, Conran N, Costa FF. Altered levels of cytokines and inflammatory mediators in plasma and leukocytes of sickle cell anemia patients and effects of hydroxyurea therapy. *J Leukoc Biol.* 2009;85:235-242.

66. Francis RB Jr, Haywood LJ. Elevated immunoreactive tumor necrosis factor and interleukin-1 in sickle cell disease. *J Natl Med Assoc.* 1992;84:611-615.

67. Goncalves MS, Queiroz IL, Cardoso SA, et al. Interleukin 8 as a vaso-occlusive marker in Brazilian patients with sickle cell disease. *Braz J Med Biol Res.* 2001;34:1309-1313.

68. Qari MH, Dier U, Mousa SA. Biomarkers of inflammation, growth factor, and coagulation activation in patients with sickle cell disease. *Clin Appl Thromb Hemost.* 2012;18:195-200.

69. Duits AJ, Schnog JB, Lard LR, Saleh AW, Rojer RA. Elevated IL-8 levels during sickle cell crisis. *Eur J Haematol.* 1998;61: 302-305.

70. Carvalho MOS, Araujo-Santos T, Reis JHO, et al. Inflammatory mediators in sickle cell anaemia highlight the difference between steady state and crisis in paediatric patients. *Br J Haematol.* 2018;182:933-936.

71. Davila J, Manwani D, Vasovic L, et al. A novel inflammatory role for platelets in sickle cell disease. *Platelets.* 2015;26:726-729.

72. Pitanga TN, Oliveira RR, Zanette DL, et al. Sickle red cells as danger signals on proinflammatory gene expression, leukotriene B4 and interleukin-1 beta production in peripheral blood mononuclear cell. *Cytokine.* 2016;83:75-84.

73. Krishnan S, Siegel J, Pullen G Jr, Hevelow M, Dampier C, Stuart M. Increased von Willebrand factor antigen and high molecular weight multimers in sickle cell disease associated with nocturnal hypoxemia. *Thromb Res.* 2008;122:455-458.

74. Chen J, Hobbs WE, Le J, Lenting PJ, de Groot PG, Lopez JA. The rate of hemolysis in sickle cell disease correlates with the quantity of active von Willebrand factor in the plasma. *Blood.* 2011;117:3680-3683.

75. Sakhalkar VS, Rao SP, Weedon J, Miller ST. Elevated plasma sVCAM-1 levels in children with sickle cell disease: impact of chronic transfusion therapy. *Am J Hematol.* 2004;76:57-60.

76. Schnog JB, Rojer RA, MacGillavry MR, Ten Cate H, Brandjes DPM, Duits AJ. Steady-state sVCAM-1 serum levels in adults with sickle cell disease. *Ann Hematol.* 2003;82:109-113.

77. Duits AJ, Rojer RA, van Endt T, et al. Erythropoiesis and serum sVCAM-1 levels in adults with sickle cell disease. *Ann Hematol.* 2003;82:171-174.

78. Peters M, Plaat BE, ten Cate H, Wolters HJ, Weening RS, Brandjes DP. Enhanced thrombin generation in children with sickle cell disease. *Thromb Haemost.* 1994;71:169-172.

79. Tomer A, Harker LA, Kasey S, Eckman JR. Thrombogenesis in sickle cell disease. *J Lab Clin Med.* 2001;137:398-407.

80. Ataga KI, Moore CG, Hillery CA, et al. Coagulation activation and inflammation in sickle cell disease-associated pulmonary hypertension. *Haematologica.* 2008;93:20-26.

81. Francis RB Jr. Elevated fibrin D-dimer fragment in sickle cell anemia: evidence for activation of coagulation during the steady state as well as in painful crisis. *Haemostasis.* 1989;19: 105-111.

82. Kurantsin-Mills J, Ofosu FA, Safa TK, Siegel RS, Lessin LS. Plasma factor VII and thrombin-antithrombin III levels indicate increased tissue factor activity in sickle cell patients. *Br J Haematol.* 1992;81:539-544.

83. Solovey A, Gui L, Key NS, Hebbel RP. Tissue factor expression by endothelial cells in sickle cell anemia. *J Clin Invest.* 1998;101:1899-1904.

84. Key NS, Slungaard A, Dandelet L, et al. Whole blood tissue factor procoagulant activity is elevated in patients with sickle cell disease. *Blood.* 1998;91:4216-4223.

85. Shet AS, Aras O, Gupta K, et al. Sickle blood contains tissue factor-positive microparticles derived from endothelial cells and monocytes. *Blood.* 2003;102:2678-2683.

86. Gordon EM, Klein BL, Berman BW, Strandjord SE, Simon JE, Coccia PF. Reduction of contact factors in sickle cell disease. *J Pediatr.* 1985;106:427-430.

87. Verma PS, Adams RG, Miller RL. Reduced plasma kininogen concentration during sickle cell crisis. *Res Commun Chem Pathol Pharmacol.* 1983;41:313-322.

88. Miller RL, Verma PS, Adams RG. Studies of the kallikrein-kinin system in patients with sickle cell anemia. *J Natl Med Assoc.* 1983;75:551-556.

89. el-Hazmi MA, Warsy AS, Bahakim H. Blood proteins C and S in sickle cell disease. *Acta Haematol.* 1993;90:114-119.

90. Francis RB Jr. Protein S deficiency in sickle cell anemia. *J Lab Clin Med.* 1988;111:571-576.

91. Tam DA. Protein C and protein S activity in sickle cell disease and stroke. *J Child Neurol.* 1997;12:19-21.

92. Tantawy AA, Adly AA, Ismail EA, Habeeb NM, Farouk A. Circulating platelet and erythrocyte microparticles in young children and adolescents with sickle cell disease: relation to cardiovascular complications. *Platelets.* 2013;24:605-614.

93. Zahran AM, Elsayh KI, Saad K, et al. Circulating microparticles in children with sickle cell anemia in a tertiary center in upper Egypt. *Clin Appl Thromb Hemost.* 2019;25:1076029619828839.

94. Vats R, Brzoska T, Bennewitz MF, et al. Platelet extracellular vesicles drive inflammasome-IL1β-dependent lung injury in sickle cell disease. *Am J Respir Crit Care Med.* 2020;201: 33-46.

95. Wu Y. Contact pathway of coagulation and inflammation. *Thromb J.* 2015;13:17.

96. Tait JF, Gibson D. Measurement of membrane phospholipid asymmetry in normal and sickle-cell erythrocytes by means of annexin V binding. *J Lab Clin Med.* 1994;123:741-748.

97. Kuypers FA, Lewis RA, Hua M, et al. Detection of altered membrane phospholipid asymmetry in subpopulations of human

red blood cells using fluorescently labeled annexin V. *Blood*. 1996;87:1179-1187.

98. van Tits LJ, van Heerde WL, Landburg PP, et al. Plasma annexin A5 and microparticle phosphatidylserine levels are elevated in sickle cell disease and increase further during painful crisis. *Biochem Biophys Res Commun*. 2009;390:161-164.

99. Kannemeier C, Shibamiya A, Nakazawa F, et al. Extracellular RNA constitutes a natural procoagulant cofactor in blood coagulation. *Proc Natl Acad Sci U S A*. 2007;104:6388-6393.

100. Merle NS, Grunenwald A, Rajaratnam H, et al. Intravascular hemolysis activates complement via cell-free heme and heme-loaded microvesicles. *JCI Insight*. 2018;3(12):e96910.

101. Wang RH, Phillips G Jr, Medof ME, Mold C. Activation of the alternative complement pathway by exposure of phosphatidylethanolamine and phosphatidylserine on erythrocytes from sickle cell disease patients. *J Clin Invest*. 1993;92:1326-1335.

102. Liu Y, Jing F, Yi W, et al. HO-1(hi) patrolling monocytes protect against vaso-occlusion in sickle cell disease. *Blood*. 2018;131:1600-1610.

103. Ghosh S, Ihunnah CA, Hazra R, et al. Nonhematopoietic Nrf2 dominantly impedes adult progression of sickle cell anemia in mice. *JCI Insight*. 2016;1:e81090.

104. Nath KA, Grande JP, Haggard JJ, et al. Oxidative stress and induction of heme oxygenase-1 in the kidney in sickle cell disease. *Am J Pathol*. 2001;158:893-903.

105. Jison ML, Munson PJ, Barb JJ, et al. Blood mononuclear cell gene expression profiles characterize the oxidant, hemolytic, and inflammatory stress of sickle cell disease. *Blood*. 2004;104:270-280.

106. Belcher JD, Mahaseth H, Welch TE, Otterbein LE, Hebbel RP, Vercellotti GM. Heme oxygenase-1 is a modulator of inflammation and vaso-occlusion in transgenic sickle mice. *J Clin Invest*. 2006;116:808-816.

107. Bunn HF. Pathogenesis and treatment of sickle cell disease. *N Engl J Med*. 1997;337:762-769.

108. Barabino GA, Platt MO, Kaul DK. Sickle cell biomechanics. *Annu Rev Biomed Eng*. 2010;12:345-367.

109. Kaul DK, Finnegan E, Barabino GA. Sickle red cell-endothelium interactions. *Microcirculation*. 2009;16:97-111.

110. Manwani D, Frenette PS. Vaso-occlusion in sickle cell disease: pathophysiology and novel targeted therapies. *Blood*. 2013;122:3892-3898.

111. Sparkenbaugh E, Pawlinski R. Interplay between coagulation and vascular inflammation in sickle cell disease. *Br J Haematol*. 2013;162:3-14.

112. Reiter CD, Wang X, Tanus-Santos JE, et al. Cell-free hemoglobin limits nitric oxide bioavailability in sickle-cell disease. *Nat Med*. 2002;8:1383-1389.

113. Rother RP, Bell L, Hillmen P, Gladwin MT. The clinical sequelae of intravascular hemolysis and extracellular plasma hemoglobin: a novel mechanism of human disease. *JAMA*. 2005;293:1653-1662.

114. Morris CR, Kato GJ, Poljakovic M, et al. Dysregulated arginine metabolism, hemolysis-associated pulmonary hypertension, and mortality in sickle cell disease. *JAMA*. 2005;294:81-90.

115. Nouraie M, Lee JS, Zhang Y, et al. The relationship between the severity of hemolysis, clinical manifestations and risk of death in 415 patients with sickle cell anemia in the US and Europe. *Haematologica*. 2013;98:464-472.

116. Hsu LL, Champion HC, Campbell-Lee SA, et al. Hemolysis in sickle cell mice causes pulmonary hypertension due to global impairment in nitric oxide bioavailability. *Blood*. 2007; 109:3088-3098.

117. Radomski MW, Palmer RM, Moncada S. Comparative pharmacology of endothelium-derived relaxing factor, nitric oxide and prostacyclin in platelets. *Br J Pharmacol*. 1987;92:181-187.

118. de Graaf JC, Banga JD, Moncada S, Palmer RM, de Groot PG, Sixma JJ. Nitric oxide functions as an inhibitor of platelet adhesion under flow conditions. *Circulation*. 1992;85:2284-2290.

119. Mellion BT, Ignarro LJ, Ohlstein EH, Pontecorvo EG, Hyman AL, Kadowitz PJ. Evidence for the inhibitory role of guanosine 3', 5'-monophosphate in ADP-induced human platelet aggregation in the presence of nitric oxide and related vasodilators. *Blood*. 1981;57:946-955.

120. Azuma H, Ishikawa M, Sekizaki S. Endothelium-dependent inhibition of platelet aggregation. *Br J Pharmacol*. 1986;88:411-415.

121. Hernandez-Cuellar E, Tsuchiya K, Hara H, et al. Cutting edge: nitric oxide inhibits the NLRP3 inflammasome. *J Immunol*. 2012;189:5113-5117.

122. Lundberg JO, Gladwin MT, Weitzberg E. Strategies to increase nitric oxide signalling in cardiovascular disease. *Nat Rev Drug Discov*. 2015;14:623-641.

123. Eich RF, Li T, Lemon DD, et al. Mechanism of NO-induced oxidation of myoglobin and hemoglobin. *Biochemistry*. 1996; 35:6976-6983.

124. Exner M, Herold S. Kinetic and mechanistic studies of the peroxynitrite-mediated oxidation of oxymyoglobin and oxyhemoglobin. *Chem Res Toxicol*. 2000;13:287-293.

125. Olson JS, Foley EW, Rogge C, Tsai AL, Doyle MP, Lemon DD. No scavenging and the hypertensive effect of hemoglobin-based blood substitutes. *Free Radic Biol Med*. 2004;36:685-697.

126. Nakai K, Ohta T, Sakuma I, et al. Inhibition of endothelium-dependent relaxation by hemoglobin in rabbit aortic strips: comparison between acellular hemoglobin derivatives and cellular hemoglobins. *J Cardiovasc Pharmacol*. 1996;28:115-123.

127. Lancaster JR Jr. A tutorial on the diffusibility and reactivity of free nitric oxide. *Nitric Oxide*. 1997;1:18-30.

128. Schechter AN, Gladwin MT. Hemoglobin and the paracrine and endocrine functions of nitric oxide. *N Engl J Med*. 2003;348:1483-1485.

129. Nagel RL, Gibson QH. The binding of hemoglobin to haptoglobin and its relation to subunit dissociation of hemoglobin. *J Biol Chem*. 1971;246:69-73.

130. Kristiansen M, Graversen JH, Jacobsen C, et al. Identification of the haemoglobin scavenger receptor. *Nature*. 2001;409: 198-201.

131. Liao JC, Hein TW, Vaughn MW, Huang KT, Kuo L. Intravascular flow decreases erythrocyte consumption of nitric oxide. *Proc Natl Acad Sci U S A*. 1999;96:8757-8761.

132. Vaughn MW, Kuo L, Liao JC. Effective diffusion distance of nitric oxide in the microcirculation. *Am J Physiol*. 1998; 274:H1705-H1714.

133. Liu X, Miller MJ, Joshi MS, Sadowska-Krowicka H, Clark DA, Lancaster JR Jr. Diffusion-limited reaction of free nitric oxide with erythrocytes. *J Biol Chem*. 1998;273:18709-18713.

134. Reiter CD, Wang X, Tanus-Santos JE, et al. Cell-free hemoglobin limits nitric oxide bioavailability in sickle-cell disease. *Nat Med*. 2002;8:1383-1389.

135. Gladwin MT, Lancaster JR, Freeman BA, Schechter AN. Nitric oxide's reactions with hemoglobin: a view through the SNO-storm. *Nat Med*. 2003;9:496-500.

136. Gladwin MT, Kato GJ. Cardiopulmonary complications of sickle cell disease: role of nitric oxide and hemolytic anemia. *Hematology Am Soc Hematol Educ Program*. 2005:51-57.

137. Sadrzadeh SM, Graf E, Panter SS, Hallaway PE, Eaton JW. Hemoglobin. A biologic fenton reagent. *J Biol Chem.* 1984;259: 14354-14356.

138. Reeder BJ. The redox activity of hemoglobins: from physiologic functions to pathologic mechanisms. *Antioxid Redox Signal.* 2010;13:1087-1123.

139. Aslan M, Ryan TM, Adler B, et al. Oxygen radical inhibition of nitric oxide-dependent vascular function in sickle cell disease. *Proc Natl Acad Sci U S A.* 2001;98:15215-15220.

140. Beckman JS, Koppenol WH. Nitric oxide, superoxide, and peroxynitrite: the good, the bad, and ugly. *Am J Physiol.* 1996;271: C1424-C1437.

141. Nur E, Biemond BJ, Otten HM, Brandjes DP, Schnog JJ, Group CS. Oxidative stress in sickle cell disease; pathophysiology and potential implications for disease management. *Am J Hematol.* 2011;86:484-489.

142. Morris CR, Kuypers FA, Larkin S, Vichinsky EP, Styles LA. Patterns of arginine and nitric oxide in patients with sickle cell disease with vaso-occlusive crisis and acute chest syndrome. *J Pediatr Hematol Oncol.* 2000;22:515-520.

143. Schnog JJ, Jager EH, van der Dijs FP, et al. Evidence for a metabolic shift of arginine metabolism in sickle cell disease. *Ann Hematol.* 2004;83:371-375.

144. Gladwin MT. Deconstructing endothelial dysfunction: soluble guanylyl cyclase oxidation and the NO resistance syndrome. *J Clin Invest.* 2006;116:2330-2332.

145. Almeida CB, Souza LE, Leonardo FC, et al. Acute hemolytic vascular inflammatory processes are prevented by nitric oxide replacement or a single dose of hydroxyurea. *Blood.* 2015;126:711-720.

146. Helms CC, Marvel M, Zhao W, et al. Mechanisms of hemolysis-associated platelet activation. *J Thromb Haemost.* 2013;11: 2148-2154.

147. Ataga KI. Hypercoagulability and thrombotic complications in hemolytic anemias. *Haematologica.* 2009;94:1481-1484.

148. Dutra FF, Bozza MT. Heme on innate immunity and inflammation. *Front Pharmacol.* 2014;5:115.

149. Camus SM, De Moraes JA, Bonnin P, et al. Circulating cell membrane microparticles transfer heme to endothelial cells and trigger vasoocclusions in sickle cell disease. *Blood.* 2015;125: 3805-3814.

150. Monteiro AP, Pinheiro CS, Luna-Gomes T, et al. Leukotriene B4 mediates neutrophil migration induced by heme. *J Immunol.* 2011;186:6562-6567.

151. Figueiredo RT, Fernandez PL, Mourao-Sa DS, et al. Characterization of heme as activator of Toll-like receptor 4. *J Biol Chem.* 2007;282:20221-20229.

152. Arruda MA, Rossi AG, de Freitas MS, Barja-Fidalgo C, Graca-Souza AV. Heme inhibits human neutrophil apoptosis: involvement of phosphoinositide 3-kinase, MAPK, and NF-kappaB. *J Immunol.* 2004;173:2023-2030.

153. Kono M, Saigo K, Takagi Y, et al. Heme-related molecules induce rapid production of neutrophil extracellular traps. *Transfusion.* 2014;54:2811-2819.

154. Graca-Souza AV, Arruda MA, de Freitas MS, Barja-Fidalgo C, Oliveira PL. Neutrophil activation by heme: implications for inflammatory processes. *Blood.* 2002;99:4160-4165.

155. Porto BN, Alves LS, Fernandez PL, et al. Heme induces neutrophil migration and reactive oxygen species generation through signaling pathways characteristic of chemotactic receptors. *J Biol Chem.* 2007;282:24430-24436.

156. Jorch SK, Kubes P. An emerging role for neutrophil extracellular traps in noninfectious disease. *Nat Med.* 2017;23:279-287.

157. Warnatsch A, Ioannou M, Wang Q, Papayannopoulos V. Inflammation. Neutrophil extracellular traps license macrophages for cytokine production in atherosclerosis. *Science.* 2015;349: 316-320.

158. Hu Z, Murakami T, Tamura H, et al. Neutrophil extracellular traps induce IL-1beta production by macrophages in combination with lipopolysaccharide. *Int J Mol Med.* 2017;39:549-558.

159. Liu D, Yang P, Gao M, et al. NLRP3 activation induced by neutrophil extracellular traps sustains inflammatory response in the diabetic wound. *Clin Sci (Lond).* 2019;133:565-582.

160. Malik Z, Creter D, Cohen A, Djaldetti M. Haemin affects platelet aggregation and lymphocyte mitogenicity in whole blood incubations. *Cytobios.* 1983;38:33-38.

161. Kapetanaki MG, Gbotosho OT, Sharma D, Weidert F, Ofori-Acquah SF, Kato GJ. Free heme regulates placenta growth factor through NRF2-antioxidant response signaling. *Free Radic Biol Med.* 2019;143:300-308.

162. Wang X, Mendelsohn L, Rogers H, et al. Heme-bound iron activates placenta growth factor in erythroid cells via erythroid Kruppel-like factor. *Blood.* 2014;124:946-954.

163. Sundaram N, Tailor A, Mendelsohn L, et al. High levels of placenta growth factor in sickle cell disease promote pulmonary hypertension. *Blood.* 2010;116:109-112.

164. Gu JM, Yuan S, Sim D, et al. Blockade of placental growth factor reduces vaso-occlusive complications in murine models of sickle cell disease. *Exp Hematol.* 2018;60:73-82 e73.

165. Martins R, Maier J, Gorki AD, et al. Heme drives hemolysis-induced susceptibility to infection via disruption of phagocyte functions. *Nat Immunol.* 2016;17:1361-1372.

166. Wallace KL, Linden J. Adenosine A2A receptors induced on iNKT and NK cells reduce pulmonary inflammation and injury in mice with sickle cell disease. *Blood.* 2010;116:5010-5020.

167. Kaul DK, Hebbel RP. Hypoxia/reoxygenation causes inflammatory response in transgenic sickle mice but not in normal mice. *J Clin Invest.* 2000;106:411-420.

168. Belcher JD, Bryant CJ, Nguyen J, et al. Transgenic sickle mice have vascular inflammation. *Blood.* 2003;101:3953-3959.

169. Osarogiagbon UR, Choong S, Belcher JD, Vercellotti GM, Paller MS, Hebbel RP. Reperfusion injury pathophysiology in sickle transgenic mice. *Blood.* 2000;96:314-320.

170. Belcher JD, Mahaseth H, Welch TE, et al. Critical role of endothelial cell activation in hypoxia-induced vasoocclusion in transgenic sickle mice. *Am J Physiol Heart Circ Physiol.* 2005;288: H2715-2725.

171. Eltzschig HK, Eckle T. Ischemia and reperfusion: from mechanism to translation. *Nat Med.* 2011;17:1391-1401.

172. Hotchkiss RS, Strasser A, McDunn JE, Swanson PE. Cell death. *N Engl J Med.* 2009;361:1570-1583.

173. Krysko DV, Agostinis P, Krysko O, et al. Emerging role of damage-associated molecular patterns derived from mitochondria in inflammation. *Trends Immunol.* 2011;32:157-164.

174. Chen GY, Nunez G. Sterile inflammation: sensing and reacting to damage. *Nat Rev Immunol.* 2010;10:826-837.

175. Xu H, Wandersee NJ, Guo Y, et al. Sickle cell disease increases high mobility group box 1: a novel mechanism of inflammation. *Blood.* 2014;124:3978-3981.

176. Dutra FF, Alves LS, Rodrigues D, et al. Hemolysis-induced lethality involves inflammasome activation by heme. *Proc Natl Acad Sci U S A.* 2014;111:E4110-E4118.

177. Elliott EI, Sutterwala FS. Initiation and perpetuation of NLRP3 inflammasome activation and assembly. *Immunol Rev.* 2015; 265:35-52.

178. Man SM, Kanneganti TD. Regulation of inflammasome activation. *Immunol Rev.* 2015;265:6-21.

179. Broz P, Dixit VM. Inflammasomes: mechanism of assembly, regulation and signalling. *Nat Rev Immunol* 2016;16: 407-420.

180. Bakele M, Joos M, Burdi S, et al. Localization and functionality of the inflammasome in neutrophils. *J Biol Chem.* 2014;289: 5320-5329.

181. Hottz ED, Lopes JF, Freitas C, et al. Platelets mediate increased endothelium permeability in dengue through NLRP3-inflammasome activation. *Blood.* 2013;122:3405-3414.

182. Hottz ED, Monteiro AP, Bozza FA, Bozza PT. Inflammasome in platelets: allying coagulation and inflammation in infectious and sterile diseases? *Mediat Inflamm.* 2015;2015:435783.

183. Xia M, Boini KM, Abais JM, Xu M, Zhang Y, Li PL. Endothelial NLRP3 inflammasome activation and enhanced neointima formation in mice by adipokine visfatin. *Am J Pathol.* 2014;184:1617-1628.

184. Aatonen MT, Ohman T, Nyman TA, Laitinen S, Gronholm M, Siljander PR. Isolation and characterization of platelet-derived extracellular vesicles. *J Extracell Vesicles.* 2014;6:3.

185. van der Pol E, Boing AN, Gool EL, Nieuwland R. Recent developments in the nomenclature, presence, isolation, detection and clinical impact of extracellular vesicles. *J Thromb Haemost.* 2016;14:48-56.

186. Brown GT, Narayanan P, Li W, Silverstein RL, McIntyre TM. Lipopolysaccharide stimulates platelets through an IL-1beta autocrine loop. *J Immunol.* 2013;191:5196-5203.

187. Eckly A, Rinckel JY, Proamer F, et al. Respective contributions of single and compound granule fusion to secretion by activated platelets. *Blood.* 2016;128:2538-2549.

188. Howard J, Hemmaway CJ, Telfer P, et al. A phase 1/2 ascending dose study and open-label extension study of voxelotor in patients with sickle cell disease. *Blood.* 2019;133:1865-1875.

189. Vichinsky E, Hoppe CC, Ataga KI, et al. A phase 3 randomized trial of voxelotor in sickle cell disease. *N Engl J Med.* 2019;381:509-519.

190. Belcher JD, Young M, Chen C, et al. MP4CO, a pegylated hemoglobin saturated with carbon monoxide, is a modulator of HO-1, inflammation, and vaso-occlusion in transgenic sickle mice. *Blood.* 2013;122:2757-2764.

191. Fleischmann RM, Tesser J, Schiff MH, et al. Safety of extended treatment with anakinra in patients with rheumatoid arthritis. *Ann Rheum Dis.* 2006;65:1006-1012.

192. Lachmann HJ, Kone-Paut I, Kuemmerle-Deschner JB, et al. Use of canakinumab in the cryopyrin-associated periodic syndrome. *N Engl J Med.* 2009;360:2416-2425.

193. Boeltz S, Amini P, Anders HJ, et al. To NET or not to NET:current opinions and state of the science regarding the formation of neutrophil extracellular traps. *Cell Death Differ.* 2019;26:395-408.

Ischemia-Reperfusion Pathobiology in Sickle Cell Anemia

Authors: *Robert P. Hebbel, John D. Belcher, Gregory M. Vercellotti*

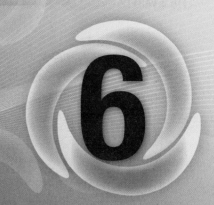

Chapter Outline

Overview

The polymerization of deoxygenated sickle hemoglobin provides the elemental basis for the pathophysiology of sickle cell anemia (SCA). Nonetheless, this disease still presents abundant uncertainties and mysteries, something particularly true for events involved in the occurrence, resolution, and consequences of sickle vaso-occlusion.[1] This chapter will describe the unique character of ischemia-reperfusion (I/R) pathophysiology occurring in SCA and why it likely plays a pivotal role in its pathophysiology. Indeed, some features of SCA are less easily explained, in particular the perpetuity, intensity, systematicity, complexity, and instability of its unique inflammatory state.[2-4]

Thus, we perceive I/R pathobiology to be the foundational engine that relentlessly drives inflammation because, in the specific sickle context, it establishes an inherent *cyclicity* (Figure 6-1). This would be the modern realization of the "vicious cycle" between erythrostasis and sickling/hemolysis posited by Ham and Castle in 1942. It is a context that reveals both the robust adaptability of human biology and its exquisite vulnerabilities.

Understanding I/R in SCA requires cognizance of the literature on experimental I/R and the human I/R-related diseases generally, the studies of sickle transgenic mice and humans with SCA, and the pathobiologies of the general medical analogs of SCA complications. Assembly of this puzzle illuminates the role that I/R likely plays in the vascular wall dysfunction and, therefore, clinical phenotype of SCA.

In focusing on I/R in the sickle context, we certainly do not argue that hemolysis is of no consequence. Indeed, sickle red cell hemolysis releases multiple agents that present danger to endothelium, including microparticles, cell-free hemoglobin and heme, procoagulant lipid, and arginase.[5] Such factors contribute to the sickle inflammatory state (Figure 6-1).

General Introduction to I/R

Fundamentally, I/R is the biology of *resolving* ischemia, the concept being that the reintroduction of oxygen to an ischemic area can, paradoxically, exacerbate local tissue injury. I/R thereby differs from the pathobiologies of simple hypoxia or infarction. Although I/R injury in general has been explored in great detail, many of the measurements used in experimental models cannot be applied to living humans. Nonetheless, sufficient human data have been collected to clearly demonstrate that I/R is an important participant in the pathobiology of human diseases affecting many organs. Prominent among these are myocardial infarction, stroke, organ transplantation,

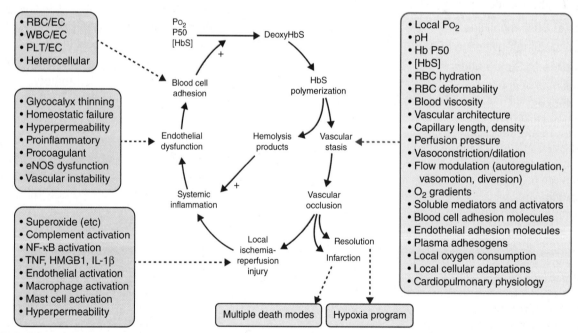

FIGURE 6-1 Ischemia-reperfusion pathobiology in sickle cell anemia. Ischemia-reperfusion cyclicity is the foundational engine that drives the inflammatory state, explaining its perpetuity, complexity, intensity, systematicity, and instability. The boxes indicate a few of the major actors. The result is a constant activating influence, causing blood cell adhesion to endothelium and thus slowing microvascular transit of red blood cells (RBCs) and enabling sickling and vaso-occlusion. DeoxyHbS, deoxygenated hemoglobin S; EC, endothelial cell; eNOS, endothelial nitric oxide synthase; Hb, hemoglobin; HbS, hemoglobin S; HMGB1, high mobility group box 1; IL-1β, interleukin-1β; NF-κB, nuclear factor-κB; O₂, oxygen; PLT, platelet; Po₂, partial pressure of oxygen; TNF, tumor necrosis factor; WBC, white blood cell. Modified, with permission, from Figure 1 of Hebbel RP, Elion J, Kutlar A. The missing middle of sickle therapeutics: multi-agent therapy, targeting risk, using biomarkers. *Am J Hematol.* 2018;93(12):1439-1443.

trauma, acute kidney injury, postpriapism erectile dysfunction, limb ischemia, and SCA.[6,7]

The pathobiology of I/R encompasses a vastly complex systems biology,[4,6-9] the details of which vary somewhat among experimental animals and organs. Therefore, we first present a generic, composite version of I/R injury as a general introduction. Then we focus on I/R in SCA, in which several disease features uniquely confer greater complexity and vulnerability. For conceptual clarity, we here (somewhat arbitrarily) parse "I/R pathobiology" into its triggering vascular event, the consequent development of *local* "I/R injury," followed by the systematization of inflammation that ultimately causes widespread, pathogenic vascular wall disturbances.

A Triggering Event

The disparate human diseases involving I/R injury have in common a loss of blood flow as the triggering event. However, this can be precipitated in different ways: thrombosis in myocardial infarction; crush injury in trauma; whole-organ ischemia in transplantation; and so on. The trigger in SCA is unique in multiple respects, as we shall see later.

Local I/R Injury

Note that I/R injury per se is a *local* event, affecting endothelium, vessel wall, and parenchymal cells. Its severity is governed mostly by duration and extent of the ischemia.[6]

The *ischemia phase* is probably similar in all I/R contexts. As oxygen depletion ensues, cell metabolism shifts to anaerobic glycolysis. Xanthine oxidoreductase (XOR) begins converting to its xanthine oxidase (XO) form, and adenosine triphosphate (ATP) is depleted and converted to hypoxanthine. ATP-dependent pumps run down, and intracellular hypercalcemia and acidification develop. Antioxidant levels fall. The cytoskeleton becomes disorganized, and intracellular membranes become compromised. Finally, there is irreversible opening of mitochondrial permeability transition pores and uncoupling of the electron transport chain. If ischemia is reversed quickly enough, this catastrophic cascade can be interrupted, and full recovery can occur. At the other end of the spectrum, all modes of cell death can occur. In between lies I/R injury.

The *reperfusion phase*, as defined by multiple experimental models, tends to begin with specific key processes. Upon reintroduction of oxygen, the newly formed XO uses accumulated hypoxanthine to robustly generate superoxide (O_2^-).[8,9] Soon, other O_2^- sources contribute, with uncoupled endothelial nitric oxide synthase (eNOS) tending to be a major source in the *local* I/R injury area.[9] Excess O_2^- reacts with and lowers NO concentrations, but where this occurs is governed by the compartmentalization of the O_2^- generation. Endothelial cells, for example, have both inwardly and outwardly oriented nicotinamide adenine dinucleotide phosphate (NADPH) oxidases. Combined with the presence of abundant iron, a variety of reactive oxygen species (ROS) and reactive nitrogen species are generated.

Nuclear factor-κB (NF-κB) is activated, and inflammatory mediators of many types can erupt volcanically or take days to be released. Prominent among them are interleukin (IL)-1β and the "sentinel cytokine" tumor necrosis factor (TNF) and the "alarmin" high mobility group box 1 (HMGB1). Complement activation generates anaphylatoxins, C3a and C5a, that activate leukocytes and endothelium. This leads to granulocyte recruitment to the vessel wall and fosters generation of the membrane attack complex (C5b-9) that can damage endothelial cells.

Endothelial cells are activated and injured, and their barrier function degrades. Within the local injury area, tissue macrophages, newly arriving blood cells, and endothelial cells assume inflammatory phenotypes. Resident mast cells degranulate and release large amounts of histamine and TNF, probably the earliest inducers of endothelial permeability barrier failure. Eventually many other permeabilizers also contribute. This barrier hyperpermeability renders subendothelial spaces accessible to soluble factors, and it fosters transmigration of blood leukocytes attracted especially by monocyte chemotactic protein 1 and HMGB1. Neutrophils infiltrate the local site early, followed on longer timescales by blood monocytes, and eventually, virtually every type of immune or inflammatory cell becomes involved.[7]

The *"no-reflow" phenomenon* refers to reperfusion-enabled plugging of nearby capillaries by locally activated white blood cells (WBCs), resulting in even further expansion of the local I/R injury area. Other contributors can include endothelial cell swelling, compressive tissue edema, vasoconstrictors, and dysregulated vasomotion/autoregulation. In general medicine, this is believed to occur fairly commonly (eg, after myocardial infarction and stroke), especially following revascularization maneuvers. Interestingly, no-reflow can contribute to a "perfusion paradox" wherein microvascular blood flow is sluggish despite macrovascular hyperemia (this is a peculiar but characteristic feature of SCA).[10]

Adaptive Responses to I/R

In response to these I/R injury phases, local tissues manifest programmed responses that should be adaptive and corrective. Examples include increased HIF-1α, Nrf2, heme oxygenase-1 (HO-1), eNOS, and KLF2; changes that protect barrier function; and even adaptive leukocyte changes. Nrf2 activation is particularly important because it induces antioxidant enzymes and HO-1.[11] However, innumerable biological mediators can be Janus-like, able to exert either benefit or harm. Specific context is everything.

Conditioning

Experimental and clinical research has shown that "conditioning" approaches can manipulate innate adaptive plasticity to induce ischemic tolerance.[6] For example, *preconditioning* can protect from future I/R events, and *postconditioning* can blunt severity of a (very) recent event. Accomplishing ischemic tolerance typically requires exposure to a "sweet spot" between too little and too much ischemia exposure.

Encouragingly, the brain has proven quite amenable to such protection, with endothelial cells, neurons, and glia all exhibiting successful development of ischemic tolerance.[12] Indeed, it is suspected that achieving cerebral ischemic tolerance requires converting a dysfunctional cerebrovascular endothelium to a fully functional one. Interestingly, induction of cerebral ischemia tolerance has been confirmed (in experimental models) after transient focal or global cerebral ischemia, hyper- or hypothermia, hypoxia, inhaled anesthetics, seizures, and lipopolysaccharide administration. Even transfer of preconditioned monocytes can induce a degree cerebral of ischemic tolerance in recipients.[13]

Even *remote conditioning* is possible; applying ischemia at one location can induce ischemia tolerance in a different organ. In addition, some research hints that remote-conditioning maneuvers can be periodically repeated to offer long-term preventative benefit.

Pharmacologic conditioning has been used to induce ischemic tolerance. In a rodent model, pretreatment of kidney donors with simvastatin induced conditioning changes durable enough to protect the organ from I/R injury after its transplantation into a new host.[14] Similarly, using a sickle mouse model, we found that lovastatin exerted protective benefit vis-à-vis I/R impact on vascular endothelium.[15] Alternatively, increasing activity of Nrf2[16,17] or its succedent partner HO-1[11] has proven to be protective in experimental I/R. It has been suggested that nitrite may offer conditioning benefits.[18]

I/R in SCA

With its triad of pathogenic vectors—vaso-occlusion, anemia, and hemolysis—SCA presents a unique context for I/R pathobiology. For SCA patients, extant data are consistent with an underlying I/R pathophysiology, and no data are incompatible with it. Nonetheless, matching human SCA to I/R pathophysiology is, to some extent, an exercise in pattern recognition. However, experimentation using sickle transgenic mice (mice in which the genes for human α- and β^S-globins have been added or swapped in) has clearly established the relevance and participation of I/R pathophysiology.

Experimental I/R and Sickle Transgenic Mice

Even at their unmanipulated baseline, sickle transgenic mice exhibit many aberrancies that are typical features of I/R injury pathobiology in general.[4] Many of these typical I/R footprints also are evident in SCA. However, finding an aberrancy in baseline sickle mice or humans does not prove it developed from I/R per se.

Far more powerful in elucidating presence and nature of sickle I/R, we expose the sickle mouse to transient hypoxia/reoxygenation (H/R). Thus, our regimen imposes moderate hypoxia (7%-11% oxygen) for 1 to 4 hours, followed by return to room air. This is intended simply to increase the likelihood that sickling occurs (somewhere) in a manageable experimental time window. Applied to the normal mouse, such H/R has no substantial effect because no occlusion develops. Applied to the sickle mouse, however, this H/R model does induce sickling and occlusion during hypoxia, followed by reperfusion-enabled brisk development of an unambiguous I/R response.[2,15,19-24]

The Unique I/R Trigger in SCA

Sickle vaso-occlusion is a consequence of deoxygenated hemoglobin S (HbS) polymerization resulting in increased red blood cell (RBC) rigidity and sickling. Yet, for most sickle RBCs to develop such changes, their microvascular transit must be slowed. The current understanding of SCA holds that abnormal adhesion of RBCs and/or leukocytes to endothelium causes such slowing, thus enabling and triggering vaso-occlusion. However, this description is deceptively simple.

It must be emphasized that *many* inherent features of human vascular biology inevitably participate in determining the rate of an RBC's transit across any given capillary (see the right-hand box in Figure 6-1). Some of these determinants can change over time, even on the timescale of microvascular transit (~1 second). Some exhibit heterogeneities even within a single arteriole-capillary-venule "unit." They can vary from patient to patient, organ to organ, or time to time. All of these nuances are probably important; none is yet understood. Therefore, our notional understanding of sickle vaso-occlusion is far from complete.

Nonetheless, it is predictable that I/R triggering and occurrence have multiple aspects unique to SCA (Table 6-1). It could be that I/R-triggering vaso-occlusions in SCA can vary in size, but it is probable that they are microvascular in nature. Notwithstanding the seeming stochasticity of acute pain episodes, we suspect that in SCA vaso-occlusions are occurring nearly constantly, hence the characteristic constant presence, yet instability, of inflammatory biomarkers (Figure 6-2). In this construct, it follows that a *clinically* evident vaso-occlusion derives from the stochastic coincidence

TABLE 6-1 Features of ischemia-reperfusion (I/R) occurring in the sickle context that are not considerations in other I/R diseases

- Instigation is determined by multiple factors, many of which are *not* stable in time.[a]
- Occlusive mechanism can vary among organs and persons and from time to time.
- Occlusion/ischemia is microvascular rather than large vessel.
- Tissue mass involved per individual occlusion may be small.
- Occlusions are multifocal.
- Occlusions occur frequently, possibly incessantly.
- Occlusive events recur lifelong.
- Resulting systemic inflammatory state is often perpetual, unresolving, and unstable.
- I/R events occur in context of preexisting vascular vulnerabilities.
- A new event occurs in a complex context already fashioned by prior events and their sequelae.

[a]Governors of oxygenated blood flow in sickle cell anemia include all the parameters listed in Figure 6-1 (right-hand box).

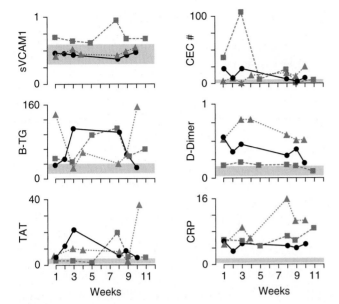

FIGURE 6-2 **The chaotic "steady state."** Values for 6 clinical biomarkers of inflammation were measured repeatedly over 11 weeks. The 3 subjects (red, blue, and black symbols) all had historically mild disease, and each was asymptomatic for at least 3 months before, during, and for at least 3 months after these measures were made. Gray bars indicate range for concurrently studied normals. B-TG, thromboglobulin; CEC, circulating endothelial cells; CRP, C-reactive protein; sVCAM1, soluble vascular cell adhesion molecule 1; TAT, thrombin-antithrombin complexes. Modified, with permission, from Figure 2 of Hebbel RP, Elion J, Kutlar A. The missing middle of sickle therapeutics: multi-agent therapy, targeting risk, using biomarkers. *Am J Hematol*, 2018;93(12):1439-1443. Experiment was performed by Dr. Colleen Morton.

of multiple microvascular occlusions disturbing a larger volume of tissue.

Differential Susceptibilities

It is known that I/R pathophysiology (and its impact) can be influenced by several types of preexisting features that confer differential susceptibilities. *Among organs,* the classical perception of general susceptibilities to *local* I/R injury has been brain > heart > kidney > intestine > liver > skeletal muscle > lung.[6] *Among individuals,* a number of factors establish differences in outcome of I/R. An individual's genetic background can influence vulnerability.[6] For example, Duffy-null status (highly prevalent in sub-Saharan Africa) increases severity should acute lung injury occur.[25] I/R impact also can be influenced by epigenetic factors.[6] For example, prenatal hypoxia induces epigenetic changes that augment consequences from postnatal myocardial I/R. The microbiome can impact I/R, which in turn can modify the microbiome.[6,26] Likewise, classical cardiologic comorbidities can accentuate the impact of an I/R event.[27] They must have the same effect in SCA as well.

Preexisting Vulnerabilities in SCA

In SCA, there are additional biosystem features that comprise unique preexisting vulnerabilities vis-à-vis the effects of I/R pathobiology. Most prominently, the *sickle mutation* itself

creates opportunity for recurrent I/R events by establishing cyclicity (Figure 6-1). Thus, laid bare, the grand pathophysiologic cycle consists of adhesion causing sickling/occlusion causing adhesion, and so on.

Chronic anemia elevates HIF-1α, which, in isolation, confers some tolerance to hypoxia and ischemia. However, this is far more complicated in inflammatory environments. For example, in experimental gut I/R, HIF-1α actually promoted pathogenic inflammatory responses, including remote acute lung injury.[28] Thus, our programmed adaptive responses can be maladaptive in a different context.

Systemic endothelial dysfunction (in the broad sense of the term) must pose the greatest danger in the sickle context. It comprises a template of vulnerability (ie, a "primed" state ready to respond briskly and robustly to I/R events). One example of functional priming is the damage associated molecular pattern (DAMP) toll-like receptor 4 (TLR4)–dependent activation of the NLRP3 inflammasome in endothelial cells[29] and monocytes/macrophages that accelerates IL-1β release by those cells. Another is the status of marginated leukocytes in the pulmonary microcirculation (discussed later in this chapter). These types of heightened readiness can only result in magnified adverse impact from potential vascular stressors. A specific example is that the pulmonary artery response to any given vasoconstrictor (eg, hypoxia, platelet-activating factor, plasma hemoglobin) is greatly augmented if eNOS is not contributing properly at the outset.[5]

Opaque simultaneity is perhaps the most confounding of all preexisting vulnerabilities. Any new I/R event in SCA would be superimposed upon a milieu already undergoing active fashioning by prior I/R event onset and/or evolution and/or resolution, in addition to preconditioning and/or postconditioning and/or remote-conditioning effects. All may be contributing simultaneously. This biologic complexity, additionally aggravated by multiple time dependencies, seems to be a strong candidate explanation for the perplexing randomness of vaso-occlusive crises in SCA.

I/R Footprints in Sickle Mice

Establishing reperfusion unleashes a dispersal of activating mediators from the *local* I/R injury throughout the vascular system. The result can be systemic inflammation that expands and recruits multiple biosystem involvements. Such systematization of robust inflammation is a characteristic and clinically impactful feature of clinical SCA (see Figure 6-1).

Studies of sickle transgenic mice have revealed and characterized I/R in the sickle context. In general, the more severe-phenotype sickle mouse models (eg, SS-BERK) exhibit greater abnormality at baseline than does the mild-phenotype sickle mouse (NY1DD). However, H/R provocation causes the NY1DD mild phenotype to shift toward that of the active/inflammatory phenotype exhibited by SS-BERK at baseline.[15] In aggregate, the I/R-like features of sickle mice at their unmanipulated baseline are delineated in Table 6-2, which also indicates features further amplified once the sickle mouse is undergoing H/R-provoked I/R.

TABLE 6-2 Footprints of ischemia-reperfusion pathobiology observed in sickle transgenic mice at baseline

Blood cells
  Leukocytosis[a]
  ↑ Activation of monocytes[a], neutrophils, platelets
  ↑ Platelet/leukocyte aggregates
  ↑ NF-κB activation (monocytes)[a]
Inflammatory markers and mediators in blood
  ↑ SAP, TNF[a], MCP-1, IL-6[a], IL-8, IL-1[a], TGF-β, INF-γ
  ↑ Cell-free hemoglobin/heme[a]
  ↑ HMGB1[a]
  ↑ Activated complement[a]
  ↑ Tissue complement deposition (liver, kidney, lung)
  ↑ PGE$_2$
  ↑ Histamine[a]
  ↑ Growth factors (PlGF, VEGF, EPO, PDGF, bFGF, angiopoietin-1, NGF)
  ↑ Blood microparticles
  ↑ PLA2 (red cells, blood)
  ↑ sVCAM1, sICAM1, soluble E-selectin
Coagulation activation
  ↑ Thrombin-antithrombin complexes[a]
  ↑ PAI-1
  ↑ Platelet activation
  ↑ Tissue factor on endothelial cells[a], leukocytes
Oxidative stress and footprints
  ↑ Endothelial generation of O$_2^-$ and H$_2$O$_2$[a]
  ↑ Hydroxyl radical generation
  ↑ NADPH oxidase activity (leukocytes, endothelial cells)
  ↑ XD to XO conversion (liver, lung)[a]
  ↑ Plasma XO
  ↑ XO on endothelium (thoracic aorta, pulmonary artery)[a]
  ↑ Myeloperoxidase (lung, liver)
  ↓ Antioxidants (NADH, GSH, SOD, catalase, GSH peroxidase)
  ↑ Lipid peroxidation[a]
  ↑ Tissue nitrotyrosine (liver, kidney, lung)[a]
  ↑ LDL oxidizability
  ↑ HO-1[a]
Vasoregulatory disruption
  Perfusion paradox (kidney, brain)
  ↑ O$_2^-$ consumption of NO
  ↓ NOx
  ↓ Response to vasoregulators
  ↑ Vascular instability
  ↓ Reduced arterial diameters
  ↑ ADMA[a]

  ↑ Arginase in plasma
  ↓ BH$_4$ availability
  ↑ eNOS uncoupling
  ↓ eNOS activity[a]
  ↓ NO bioavailability
  ↑ ET1[a]
  ↑ 8-Isoprostane
  ↑ Angiotensin II
  ↓ Microvascular flow (P-selectin dependent)[a]
Endothelial cells
  ↑ Endothelial barrier permeability (brain, lung)
  ↑ Adhesion molecule expression (P-selectin, VCAM1, ICAM1)[a]
  ↑ WBC adhesion to endothelium (P-selectin dependent)[a]
  ↑ RBC adhesion to endothelium (multiple mechanisms)
  ↑ WBC emigration to subendothelium[a]
  ↑ Tissue factor expression[a]
  ↑ Platelet adhesion
Organ and tissue effects
  Perfusion paradox (kidney, brain, heart)
  Intimal hyperplasia-arterial (heart, pulmonary, cerebrovascular)
  Fibrosis (liver, heart)
  ↑ NF-κB activation (liver, lung, kidney, blood monocytes, endothelial cells)[a]
  ↑ Activation of tissue macrophages and mast cells[a]
  ↓ Cerebral blood flow[a]
  ↓ Cerebral Po$_2$[a]
  ↓ Matching of oxygen supply/demand
  ↑ Cerebrovascular occlusions
  ↑ Multiorgan microvascular infarcts[a]
  ↑ Retinopathy
  ↑ iNOS activity (kidney, liver)[a]
  ↑ iNOS:eNOS ratio[a]
  ↑ MMP-9/12/13
  ↑ TIMP-2
  ↑ Inflammatory infiltrates[a]
  ↑ Vascular congestion[a]
  ↑ Thrombi in lung[a]
  ↑ Bronchoalveolar leukocytes, fluid, MMP, TNF, IL-6[a]
  ↑ Renal tubular apoptosis[a]
  ↑ Glomerular filtration
  ↑ Tissue mast cell activation[a]
  ↑ Neuroinflammatory mediators (histamine[a], tryptase, CGP, substance P)
  ↑ Pain behaviors[a]

[a]Feature documented to worsen further in sickle mice undergoing hypoxia/reoxygenation-provoked ischemia-reperfusion.

Abbreviations: ADMA, asymmetric dimethylarginine; BH$_4$, tetrahydrobiopterin; CGP, calcitonin gene-related peptide; eNOS, endothelial nitric oxide synthase; EPO, erythropoietin; ET1, endothelin 1; GSH, glutathione; H$_2$O$_2$, hydrogen peroxide; HMGB1, high mobility group box 1; HO-1, heme oxygenase-1; ICAM1, intercellular adhesion molecule 1; IL, interleukin; INF, interferon; iNOS, inducible nitic oxide synthase; MCP-1, monocyte chemoattractant protein 1; MMP, matrix metalloproteinase; NF-κB, nuclear factor-κB; NADH, reduced nicotinamide adenine dinucleotide; NADPH, reduced nicotinamide adenine dinucleotide phosphate; NGF, nerve growth factor; NO, nitric oxide; O$_2^-$, superoxide; PAI-1, plasminogen activator inhibitor-1; PDGF, platelet-derived growth factor; PGE$_2$, prostaglandin E$_2$; PLA2, phospholipase A2; PlGF, placental growth factor; Po$_2$, partial pressure of oxygen; RBC, red blood cell; s, soluble; SOD, superoxide dismutase; TGF, transforming growth factor; TIMP-2, tissue inhibitor of metalloproteinases 2; TNF, tumor necrosis factor; VCAM1, vascular cell adhesion molecule 1; VEGF, vascular endothelial growth factor; WBC, white blood cell; XD, xanthine dehydrogenase; XO, xanthine oxidase.

Oxidants

ROS (oxygen radicals) play diverse biologic roles, both adaptive and maladaptive, so many factors influence biologic outcome and clinical effects. Oxidants are generated to excess and play major roles in I/R states generally[9] and also in SCA. In sickle mice, excess oxygen radical generation occurs at baseline, with augmentation upon H/R provocation. Footprints of this process include increased (systemic) lipid peroxidation,[19] hydroxyl radical generation,[19] and tissue deposition of nitrotyrosine (the product of O_2^- reacting with NO).[30-32] Multiple O_2^- generators participate in this process.

XO is an early generator at the local I/R injury site. In sickle mice at baseline, tissues already reveal abnormal conversion of XOR to XO, and this is further increased upon H/R provocation,[19] accompanied by an increment in XO-dependent O_2^- generation.[19] In such mice, XO is found both in blood and layered onto endothelium (evidence of its prior release),[32] but its quantitative contribution to systemic extracellular O_2^- generation is unknown. Uncoupled eNOS develops in sickle mice and SCA,[33] but this tends to be a major O_2^- source only at *local* I/R injury sites.[9] *Mitochondria-derived* O_2^- is difficult to assess, but experimental models indicate it does contribute in I/R states.[9]

NADPH oxidase activation, however, seems likely to be the most prominent O_2^- generator (by both phagocytes and endothelial cells) during systematization of sickle I/R-triggered inflammation,[9] just as it generally is in I/R states and human arteriopathies.[34] In sickle mouse brain, microvascular leukocyte/endothelial adhesion (P-selectin–mediated) and occlusions are dependent upon endothelial NADPH oxidase.[35]

Myeloperoxidase from blood leukocytes has been found in excess in lungs of sickle mice.[36]

NO Synthases

NO synthases play complex roles. In I/R contexts, inducible NOS (iNOS) tends to be *upregulated* in vessel wall and parenchymal cells. In this respect, I/R mimics a peculiar feature of sepsis—a deficiency of NO production by eNOS coexists with a *surfeit* of NO production from iNOS.[37] Indeed, an abnormally high iNOS-to-eNOS expression ratio is seen in kidney and liver in sickle mouse I/R models.[10,20,38] Perhaps the most interesting implication of high iNOS activity is that in a high O_2^- endothelial environment, such as I/R and SCA, it would enhance formation of peroxynitrite, the major agent causing eNOS dysfunction in vascular diseases.[39] So, not surprisingly, increased presence of nitrotyrosine is seen in sickle mouse lung, increasing after H/R provocation.[31] Clearly, modeling and experimentation must take into account augmented iNOS activity.

NF-κB Activation

In sickle mice, H/R-provoked I/R increases NF-κB activation in tissues, monocytes, and endothelial cells, resulting in increased endothelial expression of vascular cell adhesion molecule 1 (VCAM1) and tissue factor.[15] There is a hint that VCAM1 expression is driven by p65/p65 homodimers. It is blunted by NF-κB inhibitors (curcumin, andrographolide, sulfasalazine),[40,41] lovastatin,[15] histone deacetylase inhibitors,[42] and TNF blockade.[24] Expression of endothelial tissue factor is inhibited by the same drugs, but its expression is dependent upon NF-κB in blood monocytes, not the NF-κB in endothelial cells themselves.[40]

Soluble Mediators

In I/R-triggered sterile inflammation, TNF, IL-1, and HMGB1 residing at the top of inflammatory networks are particularly prominent actors, each promoting expression and release of the others. Elevated in SCA and in sickle mice, each increases further upon H/R exposure, as do a host of other mediators (see Table 6-2).[4,43]

TNF is elaborated by blood monocytes in sickle mice with H/R-provoked I/R, causing endothelial activation and a host of pathobiologic features.[24] Supporting a prominent role, TNF blockade with etanercept ameliorates H/R-provoked vascular stasis, monocyte and endothelial activation, inflammatory biomarkers, cytopenias, and liver injury, and it also improves 3 surrogate indicators of pulmonary hypertension.

HMGB1, a classical DAMP, is elevated in blood of sickle mice and patients, and it increases further in response to H/R.[44] It can be released passively and actively, in particular from high-HMGB1 expressers such as endothelial cells and monocytes/macrophages. In I/R contexts, its release can even precede that of TNF. HMGB1 is a TLR4 signaling ligand and a dominant instigator of I/R-triggered sterile inflammatory responses, hence its description as the "nuclear weapon in the nuclear arsenal." It specifically engenders barrier hyperpermeability and development of intimal hyperplasia in human arterial diseases.[45]

IL-1β is found in excess in sickle mice and increases after H/R. Its processing and release are regulated by the NLRP3 inflammasome, which also plays a role in HMGB1 biology. Conversely, 2 TLR4 ligands (heme and HMGB1) are implicated in activation of the inflammasome, which appears to exist in a primed state in monocytes, endothelial cells, and platelets.[29,46-48]

Heme is readily liberated from cell-free methemoglobin S[49] and also signals via TLR4 to trigger Weibel-Palade disgorgement and P-selectin–mediated microvascular stasis.[50] In sickle mice, hypoxia-induced sickling increases hemolysis.

Cells

Multiple cell types are found systemically activated in I/R contexts. Activated monocytes travel and adhere to vascular endothelial cells, often followed by neutrophils, inducing endothelial inflammatory responses. Invariant natural killer T cells amplify inflammation. In sickle mice, activated neutrophil NETosis has been specifically implicated in cerebral thrombosis. Tissue resident macrophages and mast cells become activated. In sickle mice, H/R-provoked I/R induces tissue mast cell activation, resulting in neuroinflammatory responses and hyperalgesia.[51] In support, mast cell activation, inflammatory responses, and hyperalgesia are ameliorated with imatinib or cromolyn.

Complement

In sickle mice, H/R-provoked I/R induces complement activation fragments, with deposition of C5b-9 membrane attack complex in kidney, liver, and lung and on endothelium.[52] Experimental induction of C5a generation in sickle mice leads to expression of endothelial adhesion molecules, including P-selectin. In support, H/R-induced microvascular stasis (P-selectin dependent) was improved using antibodies blocking C5 cleavage or the C5a receptor.[52]

Coagulation

The well-known bidirectional activating communications between inflammation and coagulation are evident in sickle mice and patients at baseline.[53] In response to H/R provocation, sickle mice display increased thrombin-antithrombin complexes[53] and endothelial tissue factor expression.[15]

Growth Factors

Growth factors of many types are typically elevated in I/R, in both sickle mice and in SCA; in H/R-provoked sickle mice, they are increased further. These include placental growth factor (PlGF), fibroblast growth factor (FGF), hepatocyte growth factor (HGF), nerve growth factor (NGF), vascular endothelial growth factor (VEGF), erythropoietin, and others. These, too, are Janus-like, equally able to exert maladaptive effects or adaptive benefits. For example, the role of VEGF in causing blood-brain barrier hyperpermeability worsens acute stroke, yet VEGF exerts some neuroprotective and healing effects on brain cells.[54] Undoubtedly, the proliferative influence of excess growth factors contributes to arteriopathy in SCA.

Microparticles

Microparticles (MPs) are elevated in SCA patients, with a subpopulation being positive for functional tissue factor.[55] MPs also establish intercellular information transfer and thereby can impact biology. MP formation is a cell response to activation, so there are, no doubt, innumerable instances of MP formation in SCA, just as in inflammation and I/R generally. For example, MPs mobilized by hepatic I/R can injure healthy cells.[56] MPs released by inflammation-stressed brain endothelial cells can impair blood-brain barrier function and adversely impact astrocytes, depressing cerebral blood flow.[57] Heme-laden MPs from RBCs can induce endothelial ROS and vasodilatory dysfunction and trigger occlusion in sickle mice.[58]

Inflammation Resolution Mechanisms

Perpetuity and instability of the sickle inflammatory state indicate repeated, ongoing incitement and/or a failure of normal inflammation resolution mechanisms. The latter has been implicated in human diseases characterized by unresolving inflammation *absent* repeated incitement (eg, rheumatoid arthritis). Early evidence for such failure has been described in sickle mice.[59] It will be challenging to parse the proportionate contributions of repeated incitement versus resolution mechanistic failure.

Vascular Wall Consequences of I/R in SCA

The initial target and central effector of I/R-triggered pathobiology is the vascular endothelium: approximately 10^{13} endothelial cells covering >4000 m^2 that function as a distributed signaling network.[37] Not only does endothelium comprise the physical interface between blood and tissue, but also it establishes a functional linkage between the biologies of protective surveillance, inflammation, coagulation, vasoregulation, and the nervous system. To accomplish this, the endothelium must adeptly sense and adaptively integrate countless inputs to optimize vascular homeostasis and mitigate risk. Normally, individual endothelial cells within this vast network function with coordinate adaptivity. In SCA, normality is overwhelmed.

Indeed, endothelial dysfunction is a hallmark feature of I/R contexts,[6-9] as well as sickle mice and SCA. There are no discrete borderlines between endothelium that is normally "quiescent" versus physiologically "activated" versus pathobiologically "dysfunctional." Rather, these are conceptual states of an always active, vastly complicated, ever-readjusting continuum without singularities. Moreover, endothelial complexity is also fashioned by heterogeneities in location and time.[60] It is apparent that in SCA there is systemic "endothelial dysfunction" in all senses with which the term has been applied over the decades, including (in chronologic order) barrier hyperpermeability, prothrombotic phenotype, proinflammatory/proadhesive phenotype, and vasoregulatory dysfunction. In our view, the distinct pathobiological processes of I/R and hemolysis are codominant pathogenic vectors that biologically converge at the vessel wall (and at monocytes/macrophages)–in part via HMGB1 and free heme, respectively—to induce inflammation and endothelial dysfunction via TLR4 signaling (Figure 6-3).

Glycocalyx Thinning

The endothelial surface normally is covered by a glycocalyx layer, approximately 2 μm thick and having multiple components, with some membrane anchored and some not. Separating the cell surface and free-flowing plasma, the glycocalyx is a well-hydrated, porous gel with hydraulic permeability (a thick wet sponge). Its thickness and porosity are key determinants of endothelial function in all blood vessels.

Pathologic glycocalyx thinning is executed in response to O_2^-, TNF, oxidized low-density lipoprotein (oxLDL), activated complement, and abnormal shear stress. This is understood to be a feature of inflammatory states generally,[61-63] and it has been identified in I/R models. Thus, glycocalyx thinning is an expected pathogenic feature of SCA, although it has not been studied in this specific context.

Glycocalyx integrity is a commanding determinant of endothelial homeostasis, vulnerability, and dysfunction. Its thinning encumbers endothelial shear stress responsiveness (for which it is essential), thus promoting vasoregulatory dysfunction. Thinning impairs maintenance of receptor conformation and masking, thus allowing abnormal blood cell adhesion.

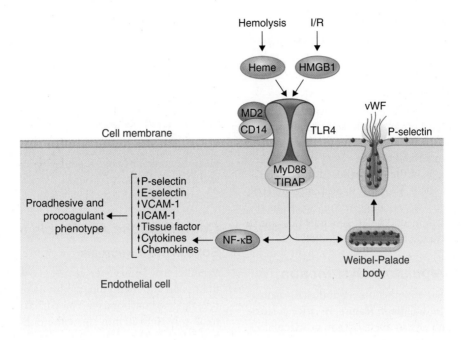

FIGURE 6-3 Pathobiological convergence of I/R and hemolysis. I/R and hemolysis both produce signaling ligands that converge at TLR4 (Toll-like receptor 4), a dominant driver of sterile inflammation. Prominent among these are HMGB1 (high mobility group box 1) and free heme, respectively. Thus, the two processes are co-dominant promoters of inflammation that biologically converge at the endothelial cell (and monocyte/macrophage) membrane. This figure is modified with permission from Figure 2 from Hebbel RP and Vercellotti GM, The multi-faceted role of ischemia/reperfusion in sickle cell anemia. *J Clin Invest* 2020; 130(3):1062-1072.

It disrupts the normal solute gradients, thus disturbing cation and channel homeostasis. It weakens surface fixation of important extracellular proteins (eg, thrombomodulin, extracellular superoxide dismutase, antithrombin).[61] It degrades endothelial permeability barrier function. In addition to all of this, glycocalyx degradation releases heparan sulfates that are TLR4 signaling ligands.[64]

Hyperpermeability

Endothelial permeability barrier function is normally actively regulated to control what reaches the subendothelium. Its breakdown is a universal and prominent feature of local I/R injury, beginning at onset of reperfusion and escalating with time.[65] Subsequently, hyperpermeability can become systemic upon spread of histamine, TNF, IL-1, thrombin, MCP-1, HMGB1, and VEGF. Eventually, platelet derivatives, proteases, oxidases, leukotrienes, and adenosines contribute as well. Such hyperpermeability is evident in sickle mice and in SCA patients,[66,67] in whom it would contribute to organ dysfunction. For example, hyperpermeability at the blood-brain barrier is exquisitely important in brain disease. Mast cells from sickle mice induce experimental barrier hyperpermeability.[68]

Adhesive Endothelium

Abnormally activated/adhesive endothelial surfaces in postcapillary venular endothelium are prominent in inflammation generally, I/R contexts,[6] and sickle mice.[15,41,69,70] In SCA, evidence includes elevated levels of soluble forms of adhesion receptors, plus their increased expression on circulating endothelial cells.[41,71]

Both oxygenated and deoxygenated sickle RBCs adhere abnormally to endothelial cells and thereby initiate occlusion.[72] Multiple underlying molecules and mechanisms have been implicated,[73] but only adhesion mediated by $\alpha_v\beta_3$, P-selectin, and intercellular adhesion molecule 4 (ICAM4; Landsteiner-Wiener) has been validated using an in vivo system. When this occurs in postcapillary venules, it can incite retrograde blockage of the microcirculation.[69,70] An underappreciated observation in sickle mice is that RBCs roll on endothelium, just as leukocytes do. Notably, exposure of endothelial cells to oxygenated or deoxygenated sickle RBCs induces an activating endothelial injury response.

Regarding leukocyte adhesion, multiple factors in sickle blood upregulate P-selectin (eg, C5a, heme, thrombin, HMGB1, TNF). Indeed, in sickle mice at baseline, there is elevated WBC/endothelial interaction and adhesion along with very sluggish microvascular flow.[70] H/R-provoked I/R worsens this dramatically and promotes leukocyte emigration into subendothelium. Importantly, these aberrancies are reversed by blocking P-selectin.[70]

Later experiments brought RBCs and WBCs together via a somewhat different role for E-selectin (although they did so only after administering sufficient TNF to artificially increase its already-elevated TNF level in the sickle mouse by many logs).[74] This revealed that, if an adherent WBC then engages E-selectin, the activated edge of that WBC can capture sickle RBCs. This highlights that heterocellular aggregates may be a third-mode of occlusion-initiation. In fact, heterocellular aggregates (eg, platelet/monocyte, WBC/RBC) can be found in the blood of sickle mice and patients. In general medicine, there is a notable association between presence of circulating platelet/monocyte aggregates and arterial disease.

Endothelial Heterogeneity

Locational heterogeneity of endothelial phenotype and function is a fundamental aspect of vascular biology.[60] Not surprisingly, in sickle mice, endothelial adhesion molecule expression patterns vary among organs and among vessel sizes within a given organ.[41] For example, in the H/R-exposed sickle mouse, we observed upregulation of VCAM1 in response to H/R, but only in postcapillary venules falling within a certain size range.[24] Such microenvironmental heterogeneities relevant to sickle vaso-occlusion have not been further studied.

Endothelial Vasoregulatory Dysfunction

Largely affecting arteriolar endothelium, endothelial vasoregulatory dysfunction is a hallmark feature in I/R,[6,75] sickle mice,[33] and SCA patients.[76] It can affect both microcirculatory (resistance) arteries[77] and large (conduit) arteries.[78] Tellingly, the vasoregulatory dysfunction caused by a *single* experimental I/R event was seen to persist for 3 months.[79] In this light, the perpetuity of vasoregulatory dysfunction in SCA is easily explained, although the agents causing it are debated.

It has been argued that consumption of NO by plasma hemoglobin is the cause of endothelial vasoregulatory dysfunction in SCA. Cell-free hemoglobin can lower the $NO:O_2^-$ ratio *outside* the endothelial cell, and hemoglobin access to subendothelial spaces[80] will be fostered by barrier hyperpermeability. However, in our view, this consumptive mechanism does not *cause* endothelial dysfunction per se; rather, it *mimics* (some) aspects of it.

eNOS uncoupling, however, is the mechanism of eNOS dysfunction in arterial diseases.[81] It is known to be caused by multiple factors within the endothelial cell, and at least 4 of these are clearly part of the sickle milieu. *Superoxide* generated by intracellular endothelial NADPH oxidizes (via peroxynitrite) both BH_4 (tetrahydrobiopterin) and the rate-limiting enzyme in its formation. When the BH_4:eNOS ratio falls to <1, eNOS becomes uncoupled[39] such that NO production is replaced by O_2^- production. Indeed, NADPH oxidase is believed to be the major cause of eNOS dysfunction in arterial wall diseases generally.[81]

TNF upregulates arginases within endothelial cells, resulting in lowered intracellular L-arginine availability, uncoupling eNOS.[82,83] This arginase effect is true for pulmonary artery endothelial cells in pulmonary hypertension.[84] Indeed, in sickle mice, chronic TNF blockade improved pulmonary hypertension.[24] *Asymmetric dimethylarginine*, an endogenous inhibitor, uncouples eNOS in a direct molar ratio. Its levels are elevated in I/R models, in sickle mice, and in virtually all SCA subjects.[85] *Chronic hypoxia* was observed to decrease endothelial cell L-arginine level,[86] possibly by exerting an adverse effect on the active L-arginine importer.

Vasoregulatory Instability

Vasoregulatory instability can result from I/R. For example, renal arteries from sickle mice were found to have marked and tonic upregulation of both vasodilators and vasoconstrictors.[10] We perceive this to be a state of enhanced risk for vascular instability.

Clinical Consequences of I/R in SCA

No organ pathologies in SCA are simply explained, but in our view, the complexity of I/R pathophysiology is *sufficient* for some and perhaps *necessary* for others. Here, we indicate which specific facet of I/R pathobiology likely underlies which clinical features.

Complications Ascribable to Local I/R Injury

Bone Marrow Necrosis

Whether I/R injury per se occurs within marrow space is unknown. Yet, high vulnerability is suggested by animal data revealing normal bone marrow partial pressure of oxygen (Po_2) to be only 10 to 20 mm Hg, with nonhomogeneous and erratic blood flow.[87] Thus, damage to marrow probably occurs often, certainly in conjunction with bone pain and fat embolization.

Brain Disease

Brain disease is common in SCA. The brain's exquisite susceptibility to I/R results from its aerobic dependence, low carbohydrate stores, high metabolic activity, high unsaturated fat content, low antioxidant levels, and rather high iron content. In some regions of brain, 5 minutes of ischemia are sufficient to cause neuronal death. In addition, massive amounts of toxic neurotransmitters are released by ischemic brain.[88] Much damage can result from small events.

I/R may specifically account for multiple brain pathologies in SCA, in particular because a fully functioning cerebrovascular endothelium is necessary for postischemic recovery.[12] For example, dysfunction of endothelium and endothelial/astrocyte interaction can directly depress cerebral perfusion. Brains in subjects with SCA exhibit hypoxia and microvascular hypoperfusion despite large-vessel hyperperfusion—again, the perfusion paradox.[89] This oxygen demand/supply mismatch includes impaired white matter blood flow despite increased cerebral blood flow.[90]

All of this creates risk for both large (clinical) and small (silent) strokes. Indeed, there are microinfarcts in sickle mouse cerebral cortex, just as in SCA.[91,92] A major factor is probably the I/R-initiated blood-brain barrier hyperpermeability, which in nonsickle studies has been specifically implicated in expanding stroke size, hemorrhagic transformation, occurrence of small and silent cerebral strokes, and induction of maladaptive neuro-rewiring that can degrade cognitive function.[93-95]

Pain

In sickle mice, nociceptive hypersensitivity is increased by H/R-provoked I/R, accounted for by inflammatory effects within the central nervous system and at the periphery. Mast cell activation and neuroinflammatory mediator release are believed to be causal, as specifically implicated in sickle mice.[51,68]

Heart

In SCA, the heart can reveal pathologic changes attributable to the effects of, and responses to, anemia, chronic inflammation, endothelial dysfunction, and microinfarctions. This is consistent with multifocal microvascular I/R events, although no experimental support for this has been sought in the sickle context specifically.

Liver

Liver in H/R-provoked sickle mice develops a hepatopathy resembling that seen in SCA: increases in inflammatory infiltrates and serum transaminases and a dramatic increase in the iNOS:eNOS activity ratio.[20] Such hepatic changes are classic features of whole-organ hepatic I/R models.

Kidney

Kidney in sickle mice exhibits great vulnerability to I/R injury, predictable from the organ's polymerization-favoring low Po_2, low pH, and high osmolality milieu.[10] At baseline, sickle mice already exhibit cortical hyperperfusion accompanying medullary hypoperfusion (again, the perfusion paradox), and in response to H/R exposure, they develop greatly exaggerated pathologic responses. This includes an abnormally elevated iNOS:eNOS activity ratio.[10,20] Glomerular hyperfiltration can follow glycocalyx thinning at the endothelial/glomerular basement membrane/podocyte barrier.

Lung

Lung is the organ least likely to develop direct *local* I/R injury in general medicine, probably due to its abundant oxygen and dual blood supply. Of note, however, if inspired oxygen tension is lowered enough, sickle mice do develop lung pathology, including bronchoalveolar fluid containing protein, leukocytes, and inflammatory mediators.[66] Whether or not this is due to primary, local I/R injury per se is unclear.

Other Organs

Other organs develop pathology that is consistent with I/R. I/R is believed to participate in retinopathy generally, with NADPH oxidase activation overwhelming the cytoprotective effect of Nrf2.[96] VEGF, induced by I/R, tends to be a primary driver of this by promoting both endothelial proliferation and barrier hyperpermeability, as seen in retinae of sickle mice.[97] I/R affecting the penis can cause postpriapism erectile tissue damage. Although the intestine has not been studied in the sickle context, it is plausible that abdominal pain (eg, during acute crisis) is caused by I/R, as it can be in general medicine.

Complications Ascribable to Remote Organ Injury

Acute Chest Syndrome

A classical complication of local I/R injury, remote organ injury is the (unpredictable) development of acute disease in an organ *distant* from an active local I/R injury site. In general medicine, the lung is by far the most frequent target, with injury typically occurring during severe systemic inflammatory response syndromes. The consequence is an acute lung injury syndrome for which 2 pathogenic factors are barrier hyperpermeability and selectin-mediated[98] pulmonary leukosequestration, sometimes involving microembolization. Such microvascular plugging can be severe enough to raise pulmonary artery pressure.[99]

In SCA itself, approximately 70% of acute chest syndrome cases develop during an acute inflammatory vaso-occlusive crisis. It perfectly matches the setting, timing, targeting, pathobiology, and acuity of classical I/R-driven remote organ injury of the lung.[4,6] Multiorgan failure in SCA is a particularly severe form of acute chest syndrome.[100]

The exquisite susceptibility of lung derives from multiple unique factors. In I/R, barrier permeabilizers are unleashed, and TNF is prominent because it permeabilizes both endothelial and epithelial barriers, and it inhibits epithelial reuptake of leaked fluid. In addition, the pulmonary circulation has multiple unique inherent features.[101] Lung capillaries are organized in series rather than in parallel. They make frequent, abrupt directional changes. Endothelial adhesion molecules are expressed capillaries. The capillary endothelium is constitutively activated such that, even under normal circumstances, the marginated WBC pool in the lung vastly exceeds that of other organs. In aggregate, these factors confer great susceptibility as a remote organ injury target during systemic inflammatory states.

Aseptic Necrosis

In general medicine, aseptic necrosis is suspected to be caused by remote organ injury complicating I/R. We hypothesize that in SCA this complication is caused by microembolization of fat and marrow, although there are no experimental data available.

Complications Ascribable to Inflammatory Systematization

The inherent cyclicity and instability that I/R can produce in SCA are the most compelling explanations for its unrelenting inflammatory state (see Figure 6-1). Indeed, the systematization of inflammation assembles the underlying maladaptive template of vulnerability that characterizes the vascular wall in SCA. We suggest that I/R is implicated in the "steady state," in sudden death, and in the arteriopathy of SCA.

Steady State

The *steady state*, in a sense, is propelled by I/R pathobiology. It represents a period of disease subsidence that is perceptional rather than biological, simply a label for periods when symptoms have not risen to the level of clinical recognition. In truth, there is nothing steady about the steady state, as is evident in the multitude of aberrancies exhibited by the sickle mouse (see Table 6-2) and in the chaotic fluctuations of inflammatory biomarkers in asymptomatic SCA subjects (see Figure 6-2).[102] The label "stochastic stasis" is an apt descriptor anticipating not only acute crises, but also the chaotic background of the pauses.

Sudden Death

Sudden death is a complication of SCA that tends to occur during acute vaso-occlusive crises. It may be that the inherently chaotic nature of ceaseless I/R pathobiology itself is a plausible explanation for this, with the agent of fatality being an abrupt rise in pulmonary artery pressure. Experimental data indicate that this could occur if a sudden increase in vasoconstricting influences is superimposed upon the *preexisting* endothelial dysfunction inherent in I/R and constantly present in SCA.[5]

Arteriopathy

Arteriopathy has been identified in cerebral, pulmonary, umbilical, renal, splenic, celiac, and penile arteries in SCA. Its etiology is undoubtedly multifactorial. We suggest that I/R-driven inflammation is a necessary etiologic factor, although unlikely to be sufficient.

In human biomedicine, the occurrence, location, timing, and severity of arteriopathic changes are determined by vascular microenvironments and their differential abilities to accommodate pathogenic forces.[60,103] Dramatically highlighting the maladaptive substructure that I/R can create, the endothelial dysfunction triggered by experimental I/R can continue for 3 months after the inciting I/R injury event.[79] This truly is a commanding chronicity of impact.

Histopathology of arterial wall lesions in SCA is *not* sickle specific.[2] Rather, it is the arterial wall's universal response to *endothelial injury*, intimal hyperplasia. In full-blown form, this includes intimal thickening, accompanying matrix increase, abnormalities of the internal elastic lamina, and proliferation of vascular smooth muscle cells. In general medicine, this can be caused by intravascular trauma, immune disease, abnormal shear stress, hypoxia, and inflammatory diseases, with the common denominator being induction of an endothelial inflammatory phenotype. In humans, it is the *chronicity* of endothelial insult that subserves arterial lesion development. From the endothelial cell's perspective, susceptibility to injury also derives from distinct microenvironmental risk states.

Inherent risk is unavoidable and created by normal vascular anatomy: vascular areas with curves and branching that create oscillatory, turbulent, nonlaminar flow.[104] In humans, these are well-known "atheroprone" locations because the endothelium there is always in a low-level inflammatory state, "primed" for exaggerated pathologic response to subsequent pathogenic stimuli. The possibility that the same locations perhaps exhibit subtle evidence of arteriopathy in SCA has not been adequately studied. It should be, though, because careful autopsy studies on normal children revealed that intimal thickening can be detected even during childhood, an initial step in the decades-long process of arteriopathy genesis.

Lesion location in SCA differs from that in atherosclerosis. This is not surprising because the anemic hyperemia of SCA puts far more arterial tree at risk, with abnormally high shear stress being harmful in itself.[104] A dramatic example of this is that the circle of Willis is at risk because the cerebral arteries diverge at rather acute angles, bestowing local shear stress disturbances when the flow rate is abnormally high.

Instructively, a rat model demonstrated that if brain perfusion became hyperemic it initiated middle cerebral artery intimal thickening.[105] Similarly, the anemic hyperemia is a strong candidate pathogenic factor for lesion development in SCA, including the pulmonary artery.

I/R-driven risk includes the aggregate vascular wall aberrancies that establish a chronically inflamed endothelium. Given this preexisting vulnerability, superimposition of additional insults increases likelihood of arterial disease. For example, extant classical atherosclerosis risk factors (eg, tobacco, diabetes, obesity) can amplify I/R impact,[103] and presumably would do so in SCA as well.

In fact, a *lipid-based hypothesis* is not irrational for SCA. It is well established in the atherosclerosis literature that oxLDL promotes intimal hyperplasia. It is plausible that it contributes to sickle arteriopathy as well. A possible scenario would be as follows.

In sickle blood, cell-free HbS rapidly auto-oxidizes and loses its heme,[49] which fosters formation of oxLDL.[106] So, regardless of steady-state levels, the *flux* of oxLDL from blood to endothelial cell can be elevated in SCA. If so, oxLDL presents itself to endothelium and subendothelium, enabled by hyperpermeability. Of note, even absent oxLDL in plasma, abnormal shear stress activates endothelial NADPH oxidase that can oxidize extant LDL in situ.[107]

At the endothelial receiving end, a receptor for oxLDL, LOX-1 (lectin-like oxidized low-density lipoprotein receptor), is described as overexpressed in sickle patients.[108] Experimentally, LOX-1 is induced by I/R,[109] and oxLDL/LOX-1 engagement strongly activates NADPH oxidase, causing eNOS dysfunction and intimal thickening.[110]

Therefore, we suggest that this scenario in SCA would contribute to vascular wall inflammation, dysfunction, and arteriopathy, even without visible lipid accumulations. In support, giving SCA mice an apolipoprotein A1 mimetic (which counters LDL oxidation) dramatically improves vasodilation capacity of sickle mouse arteries.[111]

Therapeutics for I/R

Therapeutics that target I/R in sickle pathophysiology must be *preventative* in intent and must confront a challenging systems biology problem.[3] Applying the parlance of that discipline, in sickle I/R, the "nodes" are the individual steps depicted in the grand cycle, whereas the pathobiologic trajectory is represented by the "edges," the arrows connecting the nodes (see Figure 6-1). Hidden within are the extraordinarily complex, overlapping, bidirectional signaling loops between and embedded within individual "nodes." These not only blur boundaries, but also can provide alternate activation routes should one be blocked. Thus, it seems unlikely that any single I/R-targeting drug could be sufficiently effective for I/R in SCA. Hence, we believe that multiagent combinations should be considered for targeting sickle I/R.[102]

The literature documents a great many drugs that exhibit efficacy in experimental I/R models of various types, there being a wealth of relevant potential targets.[3-9] The smaller universe of drugs tested to date in the sickle mouse with H/R-provoked I/R is provided in Table 6-3. Which of these (or other[112]) drugs should be used depends, of course, on the intended strategy.

Targeting I/R Initiation

After its initiation at the local I/R injury site, the pathobiology vastly arborizes, becoming more complex and developing into the labyrinthine inflammatory state described earlier. From this perspective, the single point of greatest vulnerability in I/R pathobiology is expected to be that specific initiation step.[102] For this targeting strategy, consideration should be given to the combination of daily oral allopurinol[19,113] (to inhibit early XO generation of O_2^-), daily oral sulfasalazine[40,41,113] (to inhibit NF-κB), and semiweekly subcutaneous etanercept[24] (to block TNF). Each of these drugs individually improves microvascular blood flow in the H/R-provoked sickle mouse. Rather than parenteral etanercept, one might substitute a daily oral statin to gain its endothelial-sparing and pharmacologic conditioning effects.[3,15] This would be a very low-cost approach.

Targeting Different Steps

Targeting different steps in the I/R cycle might be tried. Rationale for this strategy lies in the hope that a few key steps are *necessary* for pathobiology advancement (ie, its cyclicity). For this strategy, we would consider inhibiting leukocyte and RBC adhesion to endothelium by blocking P-selectin,[70] for which 2 agents are already identified—monthly intravenous crizanlizumab[114] and daily oral pentosan polysulfate sodium.[115] To this, we suggest adding an Nrf2 activator such as oral daily dimethyl fumarate (which helpfully also induces fetal hemoglobin)[16] plus monthly intravenous eculizumab (to block complement activation).[52] Each of these agents individually improves microvascular flow in sickle mice.

Efficacy Testing

As illustrated elsewhere, whether such drugs exert desired biologic impact in humans can be pilot tested using a tiny number of sickle subjects who are simply studied longitudinally.[102] This, for example, demonstrated oral sulfasalazine's efficacy in downregulating endothelial adhesion molecule expression, and it required only 3 SCA subjects. This approach could aid in establishing dosing and provide sufficient evidence to proceed to an actual pilot trial.

Conditioning Approaches

Conditioning approaches should be tested in the sickle context, as they potentially offer easier, less expensive, noninvasive, and more widely available preventative benefits. For example, could periodic mild limb ischemia be used to prevent stroke in SCA patients? Indeed, remote conditioning effects may be the reason that exercise training of sickle mice reduced their systemic inflammation.[116]

TABLE 6-3 Drugs inducing substantial vascular benefit in sickle mice undergoing hypoxia/reoxygenation-provoked ischemia-reperfusion

Antioxidant
Allopurinol[a]
SOD[a]
Catalase[a]
Dexamethasone[a]
Polynitroxyl albumin[a]
Haptoglobin[a]
Hemopexin[a]
HO-1 induction[a]
CO[a]
Biliverdin[a]
ϖ-3 fatty acid
Dimethyl fumarate
NF-κB inhibitor
Sulfasalazine[a]
Andrographolide
Curcumin
Didox[a]
Trimidox[a]
TLR4 blocker
TAK-242[a]
Immunomodulation
$A_{2A}R$ agonist
Endothelial sparing
Lovastatin
Anti-C5aR[a]
Anti-C5[a]
Antiadhesive
2-Fluorofucose[a]
Anti–P-selectin[a]
Anti-VCAM1[a]
Anti-ICAM1[a]
Histone deacetylase inhibitor
Trichostatin A[a]
Vorinostat
TNF blocker
Etanercept[a]
Infliximab
Vasomodulation
Inhaled NO
L-Arginine diet
eNOS gene therapy

[a]Efficacy also includes improving microvascular blood flow.

Abbreviations: CO, carbon monoxide; eNOS, endothelial nitric oxide synthase; HO-1, heme oxygenase-1; ICAM1, intercellular adhesion molecule 1; NF-κB, nuclear factor-κB; NO, nitric oxide; SOD, superoxide dismutase; TLR4, toll-like receptor 4; TNF, tumor necrosis factor; VCAM1, vascular cell adhesion molecule 1.

Conclusion

We view I/R pathobiology as the foundational driver of the unique inflammatory state characteristic of SCA (see Figure 6-1). Certainly, the effects of anemia and hemolysis contribute. However, the unique cyclicity created by I/R seems to be the most parsimonious explanation for sickle inflammation's perpetuity, intensity, systematicity, complexity, and instability. In addition, local I/R injury likely plays direct roles in clinical disease of multiple organs, in particular the brain. The subsequent systematization of inflammation creates a template of vulnerability that sets the stage for arteriopathy and possibly for sudden death and that defines the steady state itself. Remote organ injury can fully explain acute chest syndrome.

Laid bare, the grand pathobiologic I/R cycle in the sickle context (see Figure 6-1) is essentially as follows: occlusion causes adhesion causes occlusion. In reality, however, the cycle is a labyrinthine systems biology construct. Nonetheless, the notional "nodes" within the grand cycle identify rational I/R targets, and solid experimental data reveal beneficial effects when they are targeted in sickle mice.

High-Yield Facts

◆ The pathophysiology of sickle cell anemia (SCA) involves a singular form of ischemia-reperfusion (I/R), the pathobiology of resolving ischemia.

◆ In SCA, I/R is at least recurrent and is probably perpetual, with there being nothing steady about the "steady state."

◆ The systematization phase of I/R drives the uniquely complex systemic inflammatory state and systemic endothelial dysfunctional state of SCA.

◆ Effects of I/R and of hemolysis converge at toll-like receptor 4 (TLR4), as both high mobility group box 1 (HMGB1) from I/R and free heme from hemolysis are signaling ligands for this receptor that drives sterile inflammation.

◆ Local I/R undoubtedly underlies sickle stroke and its sequelae and disease in liver, kidney, heart, and marrow. I/R also likely contributes to pain.

◆ Acute chest syndrome is an example of remote organ injury caused at a site distant from an acute I/R injury event.

◆ The systematization of I/R inflammation underlies the arteriopathy of SCA, in that systemic endothelial dysfunction is the foundational source of arterial wall disease.

◆ I/R deserves consideration as a therapeutic target in SCA. In sickle transgenic mouse models of sickle I/R, 20 different drugs or manipulations have been shown to improve microvascular blood flow. Many of these agents are already in use in general medicine.

References

1. Embury SH. The not-so-simple process of sickle cell vasocclusion. *Microcirculation.* 2004;11(2):101-113.

2. Hebbel RP, Osarogiagbon R, Kaul D. The endothelial biology of sickle cell disease: inflammation and a chronic vasculopathy. *Microcirculation.* 2004;11(2):129-151.

3. Hebbel RP, Vercellotti GM, Nath KA. A systems biology consideration of the vasculopathy of sickle cell anemia: the need for multi-modality chemo-prophylaxis. *Cardiovasc Hematol Disord Drug Targets.* 2009;9(4):271–292.

4. Hebbel RP. Ischemia-reperfusion injury in sickle cell anemia: relationship to acute chest syndrome, endothelial dysfunction, arterial vasculopathy, and inflammatory pain. *Hematol Oncol Clin North Am.* 2014;28(2):181-198.

5. Hebbel RP. Reconstructing sickle cell disease: a data-based analysis of the "hyperhemolysis paradigm" for pulmonary hypertension from the perspective of evidence-based medicine. *Am J Hematol.* 2011;86(2):123-154.

6. Kalogeris T, Baines CP, Krenz M, Korthuis RJ. Ischemia/reperfusion. *Compr Physiol.* 2016;7(1):113-170.

7. Eltzschig HK, Eckle T. Ischemia and reperfusion--from mechanism to translation. *Nat Med.* 2011;17(11):1391-1401.

8. Carden DL, Granger DN. Pathophysiology of ischaemia-reperfusion injury. *J Pathol.* 2000;190(3):255-266.

9. Granger DN, Kvietys PR. Reperfusion injury and reactive oxygen species: the evolution of a concept. *Redox Biol.* 2015;6:524–551.

10. Nath KA, Hebbel RP. Sickle cell disease: renal manifestations and mechanisms. *Nat Rev Nephrol.* 2015;11(3):161-171.

11. Belcher JD, Chen C, Nguyen J, et al. Haptoglobin and hemopexin inhibit vaso-occlusion and inflammation in murine sickle cell disease: role of heme oxygenase-1 induction. *PLoS One.* 2018;13(4):e0196455.

12. Gidday JM. Cerebral preconditioning and ischaemic tolerance. *Nat Rev Neurosci.* 2006;7(6):437-448.

13. Garcia-Bonilla L, Brea D, Benakis C, et al. Endogenous protection from ischemic brain injury by preconditioned monocytes. *J Neurosci.* 2018;38(30):6722-6736.

14. Tuuminen R, Nykänen AI, Saharinen P, et al. Donor simvastatin treatment prevents ischemia-reperfusion and acute kidney injury by preserving microvascular barrier function. *Am J Transplant.* 2013;13(8):2019-2034.

15. Solovey A, Kollander R, Shet A, et al. Endothelial cell expression of tissue factor in sickle mice is augmented by hypoxia/reoxygenation and inhibited by lovastatin. *Blood.* 2004;104(3):840-846.

16. Belcher JD, Chen C, Nguyen J, et al. Control of oxidative stress and inflammation in sickle cell disease with the NRF2 activator dimethyl fumarate. *Antioxid Redox Signal.* 2017;26(14):748-762.

17. Zhu X, Oseghale AR, Nicole LH, Li B, Pace BS. Mechanisms of NRF2 activation to mediate fetal hemoglobin induction and protection against oxidative stress in sickle cell disease. *Exp Biol Med (Maywood)*. 2019;244(2):171-182.

18. Corti P, Gladwin MT. Is nitrite the circulating endocrine effector of remote ischemic preconditioning? *Circ Res.* 2014; 114(10):1554-1557.

19. Osarogiagbon UR, Choong S, Belcher JD, Vercellotti GM, Paller MS, Hebbel RP. Reperfusion injury pathophysiology in sickle transgenic mice. *Blood.* 2000;96(1):314-320.

20. Siciliano A, Malpeli G, Platt OS, et al. Abnormal modulation of cell protective systems in response to ischemic/reperfusion injury is important in the development of mouse sickle cell hepatopathy. *Haematologica.* 2011;96(1):24-32.

21. Aufradet E, DeSouza G, Bourgeaux V, et al. Hypoxia/reoxygenation stress increases markers of vaso-occlusive crisis in sickle SAD mice. *Clin Hemorheol Microcirc.* 2013;54(3):297-312.

22. Matte A, Recchiuti A, Federti E, et al. Resolution of sickle cell disease-associated inflammation and tissue damage with 17R-resolvin D1. *Blood.* 2019;133(3):252-265.

23. Belcher JD, Bryant CJ, Nguyen J, et al. Transgenic sickle mice have vascular inflammation. *Blood.* 2003;101(10):3953-3959.

24. Solovey A, Somani A, Belcher JD, et al. A monocyte-TNF-endothelial activation axis in sickle transgenic mice: therapeutic benefit from TNF blockade. *Am J Hematol.* 2017;92(11): 1119-1130.

25. Kangelaris KN, Sapru A, Calfee CS, et al. The association between a Darc gene polymorphism and clinical outcomes in African American patients with acute lung injury. *Chest.* 2012;141(5):1160-1169.

26. Zhang D, Frenette PS. Cross talk between neutrophils and the microbiota. *Blood.* 2019;133(20):2168-2177.

27. Ferdinandy P, Hausenloy DJ, Heusch G, Baxter GF, Schulz R. Interaction of risk factors, comorbidities, and comedications with ischemia/reperfusion injury and cardioprotection by preconditioning, postconditioning, and remote conditioning. *Pharmacol Rev.* 2014;66(4):1142-1174.

28. Feinman R, Deitch EA, Watkins AC, et al. HIF-1 mediates pathogenic inflammatory responses to intestinal ischemia-reperfusion injury. *Am J Physiol Gastrointest Liver Physiol.* 2010;299(4): G833-G843.

29. Erdei J, Tóth A, Balogh E, et al. induction of nlrp3 inflammasome activation by heme in human endothelial cells. *Oxid Med Cell Longev.* 2018;2018:4310816.

30. Aslan M, Ryan TM, Townes TM, et al. Nitric oxide-dependent generation of reactive species in sickle cell disease. Actin tyrosine induces defective cytoskeletal polymerization. *J Biol Chem.* 2003;278(6):4194-4204.

31. Pritchard KA Jr, Ou J, Ou Z, et al. Hypoxia-induced acute lung injury in murine models of sickle cell disease. *Am J Physiol Lung Cell Mol Physiol.* 2004;286(4):L705-L714.

32. Aslan M, Freeman BA. Redox-dependent impairment of vascular function in sickle cell disease. *Free Radic Biol Med.* 2007;43(11):1469-1483.

33. Hsu LL, Champion HC, Campbell-Lee SA, et al. Hemolysis in sickle cell mice causes pulmonary hypertension due to global impairment in nitric oxide bioavailability. *Blood.* 2007;109(7):3088-3098.

34. García-Redondo AB, Aguado A, Briones AM, Salaices M. NADPH oxidases and vascular remodeling in cardiovascular diseases. *Pharmacol Res.* 2016;114:110-120.

35. Wood KC, Hebbel RP, Granger DN. Endothelial cell NADPH oxidase mediates the cerebral microvascular dysfunction in sickle cell transgenic mice. *FASEB J.* 2005;19:989-991.

36. Zhang H, Xu H, Weihrauch D, et al. Inhibition of myeloperoxidase decreases vascular oxidative stress and increases vasodilatation in sickle cell disease mice. *J Lipid Res.* 2013;54(11): 3009-3015.

37. Aird WC. The role of the endothelium in severe sepsis and multiple organ dysfunction syndrome. *Blood.* 2003;101(10): 3765-3777.

38. Juncos JP, Grande JP, Croatt AJ, et al. Early and prominent alterations in hemodynamics, signaling, and gene expression following renal ischemia in sickle cell disease. *Am J Physiol Renal Physiol.* 2010;298(4):F892-F899.

39. Crabtree MJ, Tatham AL, Al-Wakeel Y, et al. Quantitative regulation of intracellular endothelial nitric-oxide synthase (eNOS) coupling by both tetrahydrobiopterin-eNOS stoichiometry and biopterin redox status: insights from cells with tet-regulated GTP cyclohydrolase I expression. *J Biol Chem.* 2009;284(2):1136-1144.

40. Kollander R, Solovey A, Milbauer LC, Abdulla F, Kelm RJ Jr, Hebbel RP. Nuclear factor-kappa B component p50 in blood mononucler cells regulates endothelial tissue factor expression in sickle transgenic mice: implications for the coagulopathy of sickle cell disease. *Transl Res.* 2010;155:170-177.

41. Solovey AA, Solovey AN, Harkness J, Hebbel RP. Modulation of endothelial cell activation in sickle cell disease: a pilot study. *Blood.* 2001;97(7):1937-1941.

42. Hebbel RP, Vercellotti GM, Pace BS, et al. The HDAC inhibitors trichostatin A and suberoylanilide hydroxamic acid exhibit multiple modalities of benefit for the vascular pathobiology of sickle transgenic mice. *Blood.* 2010;115(12):2483-2490.

43. Pathare A, Al Kindl S, Daar S, Dennison D. Cytokines in sickle cell disease. *Hematology.* 2003;8(5):329-337.

44. Xu H, Wandersee NJ, Guo Y, et al. Sickle cell disease increases high mobility group box 1: a novel mechanism of inflammation. *Blood.* 2014;124(26):3978-3981.

45. Cai J, Yuan H, Wang Q, et al. HMGB1-driven inflammation and intimal hyperplasia after arterial injury involves cell-specific actions mediated by TLR4. *Arterioscler Thromb Vasc Biol.* 2015;35(12):2579-2593.

46. Dutra FF, Alves LS, Rodrigues D, et al. Hemolysis-induced lethality involves inflammasome activation by heme. *Proc Natl Acad Sci U S A.* 2014;111(39):E4110-E4118.

47. Patanga TN, Oliveira RR, Zanette DL, et al. Sickle red cells as danger signals on proinflammatory gene expression, leukotriene B4 and interleukin-1 beta production in peripheral blood mononuclear cell. *Cytokine.* 2016;83:75-84.

48. Vogel S, Arora T, Wang X, et al. The platelet NLRP3 inflammasome is upregulated in sickle cell disease via HMGB1/TLR4 and Bruton tyrosine kinase. *Blood Adv.* 2018;2(20):2672-2680.

49. Hebbel RP, Morgan WT, Eaton JW, Hedlund BE. Accelerated autoxidation and heme loss due to instability of sickle hemoglobin. *Proc Natl Acad Sci U S A.* 1988;85(1):237-241.

50. Belcher JD, Chen C, Nguyen J, et al. Heme triggers TLR4 signaling leading to endothelial cell activation and vaso-occlusion in murine sickle cell disease. *Blood.* 2014;123(3):377-390.

51. Vincent L, Vang D, Nguyen J, et al. Mast cell activation contributes to sickle cell pathobiology and pain in mice. *Blood.* 2013;122(11):1853-1862.

52. Vercellotti GM, Dalmasso AP, Schaid TR Jr, et al. Critical role of C5a in sickle cell disease. *Am J Hematol.* 2019;94(3):327-337.

53. Sparkenbaugh E, Pawlinski R. Interplay between coagulation and vascular inflammation in sickle cell disease. *Br J Haem.* 2013;162:3-14.

54. Geiseler SJ, Morland C. The Janus face of VEGF in stroke. *Int J Mol Sci.* 2018;19:1362.

55. Hebbel RP, Key NS. Microparticles in sickle cell anaemia: promise and pitfalls. *Br J Haematol.* 2016;174(1):16-29.

56. Teoh NC, Ajamieh H, Wong HJ, et al. Microparticles mediate hepatic ischemia-reperfusion injury and are the targets of Diannexin (ASP8597). *PLoS One.* 2014;9(9):e104376.

57. Pan Q, He C, Liu H, et al. Microvascular endothelial cells-derived microvesicles imply in ischemic stroke by modulating astrocyte and blood brain barrier function and cerebral blood flow. *Mol Brain.* 2016;9(1):63.

58. Camus SM, De Moraes JA, Bonnin P, et al. Circulating cell membrane microparticles transfer heme to endothelial cells and trigger vascocclusions in sickle cell disease. *Blood.* 2015;125(24):3805-3814.

59. Matte A, Recchiuti A, Federti E, et al. Resolution of sickle cell disease-associated inflammation and tissue damage with 17R-resolvin D1. *Blood.* 2019;133(3):252-265.

60. Aird WC. Spatial and temporal dynamics of the endothelium. *J Thromb Haemost.* 2005;3(7):1392-1406.

61. Reitsma S, Slaaf DW, Vink H, van Zandvoort MA, oude Egbrink MG. The endothelial glycocalyx: composition, functions, and visualization. *Pflugers Arch.* 2007;454(3):345-359.

62. Becker BF, Jacob M, Leipert S, Salmon AHJ, Chappel D. Degradation of the endothelial glycocalyx in clinical settings: searching for the sheddases. *Br J Clin Pharmacol.* 2015;80(3):389-402.

63. Lipowsky HH. The endothelial glycocalyx as a barrier to leukocyte adhesion and its mediation by extracellular proteases. *Adv Exp Med Biol.* 2018;1097:51-68.

64. Schaefer L. Complexity of danger: the diverse nature of damage-associated molecular patterns. *J Biol Chem.* 2014;289(51): 35237-35245.

65. Rodrigues SF, Granger DN. Blood cells and endothelial barrier function. *Tissue Barriers.* 2015;3(1-2):e978720.

66. de Franceschi L, Baron A, Scarpa A, et al. Inhaled nitric oxide protects transgenic SAD mice from sickle cell disease-specific lung injury induced by hypoxia/reoxygenation. *Blood.* 2003;102(3):1087-1096.

67. Manci EA, Hillery CA, Bodian CA, Zhang ZG, Lutty GA, Coller BS. Pathology of Berkeley sickle cell mice: similarities and differences with human sickle cell disease. *Blood.* 2006;107(4):1651-1658.

68. Tran H, Mittal A, Sagi V, et al. Mast cells induce blood brain barrier damage in SCD by causing endoplasmic reticulum stress in the endothelium. *Front Cell Neurosci.* 2019;13:56.

69. Kaul DK, Fabry ME, Costantini F, Rubin EM, Nagel RL. In vivo demonstration of red cell-endothelial interaction, sickling and altered microvascular response to oxygen in the sickle transgenic mouse. *J Clin Invest.* 1995;96(6):2845-2853.

70. Kaul DK, Hebbel RP. Hypoxia/reoxygenation causes inflammatory response in transgenic sickle mice but not in normal mice. *J Clin Invest.* 2000;106(3):411-420.

71. Solovey A, Lin Y, Browne P, Choong S, Wayner E, Hebbel RP. Circulating activated endothelial cells in sickle cell anemia. *N Engl J Med.* 1977;337:1584-1590.

72. Hebbel RP, Yamada O, Moldow CF, Jacob HS, White JG, Eaton JW. Abnormal adherence of sickle erythrocytes to cultured vascular endothelium: possible mechanism for microvascular occlusion in sickle cell disease. *J Clin Invest.* 1980;65(1):154-160.

73. Hebbel RP. Perspectives series: cell adhesion in vascular biology. Adhesive interactions of sickle erythrocytes with endothelium. *J Clin Invest.* 1997;99(11):2561-2564.

74. Turhan A, Weiss LA, Mohandas N, Coller BS, Frenette PS. Primary role for adherent leukocytes in sickle cell vascular occlusion: a new paradigm. *Proc Natl Acad Sci U S A.* 2002;99(5):3047-3051.

75. Korthuis RJ. Mechanisms of I/R-induced endothelium-dependent vasodilator dysfunction. *Adv Pharmacol.* 2018;81:331-364.

76. Gladwin MT, Schechter AN, Ognibene FP, et al. Divergent nitric oxide bioavailability in men and women with sickle cell disease. *Circulation.* 2003;107(2):271-278.

77. Quillen JE, Sellke FW, Brooks LA, Harrison DG. Ischemia-reperfusion impairs endothelium-dependent relaxation of coronary microvessels but does not affect large arteries. *Circulation.* 1990;82(2):586-594.

78. Loukogeorgakis SP, van den Berg MJ, Sofat R, et al. Role of NADPH oxidase in endothelial ischemia/reperfusion injury in humans. *Circulation.* 2010;121(21):2310-2316.

79. Pearson PJ, Schaff HV, Vanhoutte PM. Long-term impairment of endothelium-dependent relaxations to aggregating platelets after reperfusion injury in canine coronary arteries. *Circulation.* 1990;81(6):1921-1927.

80. Schaer CA, Deuel JW, Schildknecht D, et al. Haptoglobin preserves vascular nitric oxide signaling during hemolysis. *Am J Respir Crit Care Med.* 2016;193(10):1111-1122.

81. Drummond GR, Selemidis S, Griendling KK, Sobey CG. Combating oxidative stress in vascular disease: NADPH oxidases as therapeutic targets. *Nat Rev Drug Discov.* 2011;10(6): 453-471.

82. Gao X, Xu X, Belmadani S, et al. TNF contributes to endothelial dysfunction by upregulating arginase in ischemia/reperfusion injury. *Arterioscler Thromb Vasc Biol.* 2007;27:1269-1275.

83. Zhang C, Wu J, Xu X, Potter BJ, Gao X. Direct relationship between levels of TNF-alpha expression and endothelial dysfunction in reperfusion injury. *Basic Res Cardiol.* 2010;105(4):453-464.

84. Xu W, Kaneko FT, Zheng S, et al. Increased arginase II and decreased NO synthesis in endothelial cells of patients with pulmonary arterial hypertension. *FASEB J.* 2004;18(14): 1746-1748.

85. Kato GJ, Wang Z, Machado RF, Blackwelder WC, Taylor JG, Hazen SL. Endogenous nitric oxide synthase inhibitors in sickle cell disease: abnormal levels and correlations with pulmonary hypertension, desaturation, hemolysis, organ dysfunction and death. *Br J Haematol.* 2009;145(4):506-513.

86. Block ER, Herrera H, Couch M. Hypoxia inhibits L-arginine uptake by pulmonary artery endothelial cells. *Am J Physiol.* 1995;269(5 Pt 1):L574-L580.

87. Spencer JA, Ferraro F, Roussakis E, et al. Direct measurement of local oxygen concentration in the bone marrow of live animals. *Nature.* 2014;508(7495):269-273.

88. Lee JM, Grabb MC, Zipfel GJ, Choi DW. Brain tissue responses to ischemia. *J Clin Invest.* 2000;106(6):723-731.

89. Detterich JA, Kato R, Bush A, et al. Sickle cell microvascular paradox-oxygen supply-demand mismatch. *Am J Hematol.* 2019;94(6):678-688.

90. Chai Y, Bush AM, Coloigner J, et al. White matter has impaired resting oxygen delivery in sickle cell patients. *Am J Hematol.* 2019;94(4):467-474.

91. Cahill LS, Gazdzinski LM, Tsui AK, et al. Functional and anatomical evidence of cerebral tissue hypoxia in young sickle cell anemia mice. *J Cereb Blood Flow Metab.* 2017;37(3): 994-1005.

92. Hyacinth HI, Sugihara CL, Spencer TL, Archer DR, Shih AY. Higher prevalence of spontaneous cerebral vasculopathy and cerebral infarcts in a mouse model of sickle cell disease. *J Cereb Blood Flow Metab.* 2019;39(2):342-351.

93. Wardlaw JM, Doubal F, Armitage P, et al. Lacunar stroke is associated with diffuse blood-brain barrier dysfunction. *Ann Neurol.* 2009;65(2):194-202.

94. Schoknecht K, David Y, Heinemann U. The blood-brain barrier-gatekeeper to neuronal homeostasis: clinical implications in the setting of stroke. *Semin Cell Dev Biol.* 2015;38:35-42.

95. Rajani RM, Quick S, Ruigrok SR, et al. Reversal of endothelial dysfunction reduces white matter vulnerability in cerebral small vessel disease in rats. *Sci Transl Med.* 2018;10:448.

96. Wei Y, Gong J, Yoshida T, et al. Nrf2 has a protective role against neuronal and capillary degeneration in retinal ischemia-reperfusion injury. *Free Radic Biol Med.* 2011;51(1):216-224.

97. Gupta K, Chen C, Lutty GA, Hebbel RP. Morphine promotes neovascularizing retinopathy in sickle transgenic mice. *Blood Adv.* 2019;3(7):1073-1083.

98. Seekamp A, Till GO, Mulligan MS, et al. Role of selectins in local and remote tissue injury following ischemia reperfusion. *Am J Pathol.* 1994;144(3):592-598.

99. Bengisun JS, Köksoy C, Bengisun JS, Bayraktaroğlu G, Camur A, Aras N. Ischemia and reperfusion injury: prevention of pulmonary hypertension and leukosequestration following lower limb ischemia. *Prostaglandins Leukot Essent Fatty Acids.* 1997;56(2):117-120.

100. Hassell KL, Eckman JR, Lane PA. Acute multiorgan failure syndrome: a potentially catastrophic complication of severe sickle cell pain episodes. *Am J Med.* 1994;96(2):155-162.

101. Reutershan J, Ley K. Bench-to-bedside review: acute respiratory distress syndrome: how neutrophils migrate into the lung. *Crit Care.* 2004;8(6):453-461.

102. Hebbel RP, Elion J, Kutlar A. The missing middle of sickle therapeutics: multi-agent therapy, targeting risk, using biomarkers. *Am J Hematol.* 2018;93(12):1439-1443.

103. Granger DN, Rodrigues SF, Yildirim A, Senchenkova EY. Microvascular responses to cardiovascular risk factors. *Microcirculation.* 2010;17(3):192–205.

104. Davies PF, Civelek M, Fang Y, Fleming I. The atherosusceptible endothelium: endothelial phenotypes in complex haemodynamic shear stress regions in vivo. *Cardiovasc Res.* 2013;99(2):315-327.

105. Onetti Y, Dantas AP, Pérez B, et al. Middle cerebral artery remodeling following transient brain ischemia is linked to early postischemic hyperemia: a target of uric acid treatment. *Am J Physiol Heart Circ Physiol.* 2015;308(8):H862-H874.

106. Belcher JD, Marker PH, Geiger P, et al. Low-density lipoprotein susceptibility to oxidation and cytotoxicity to endothelium in sickle cell anemia. *J Lab Clin Med.* 1999;133(6):605-612.

107. Hwang J, Ing MH, Salazar A, et al. Pulsatile versus oscillatory shear stress regulates NADPH oxidase subunit expression: implication for native LDL oxidation. *Circ Res.* 2003;93(12):1225-1232.

108. Chen M, Qiu H, Lin X, et al. Lectin-like oxidized low-density lipoprotein receptor (LOX-1) in sickle cell disease vasculopathy. *Blood Cells Mol Dis.* 2016;60:44-48.

109. Hu C, Chen J, Dandapat A, et al. LOX-1 abrogation reduces myocardial ischemia-reperfusion injury in mice. *J Mol Cell Cardiol.* 2008;44(1):76-83.

110. Ogura S, Kakino A, Sato Y, et al. Lox-1: the multifunctional receptor underlying cardiovascular dysfunction. *Circ J.* 2009;73(11):1993-1999.

111. Ou J, Ou Z, Jones DW, et al. L-4F, an apolipoprotein A-1 mimetic, dramatically improves vasodilation in hypercholesterolemia and sickle cell disease. *Circulation.* 2003;107(18):2337-2341.

112. Telen MJ, Malik P, Vercellotti GM. Therapeutic strategies for sickle cell disease: towards a multi-agent approach. *Nat Rev Drug Discov.* 2019;18(2):139-158.

113. Kaul DK, Liu XD, Choong S, Belcher JD, Vercellotti GM, Hebbel RP. Anti-inflammatory therapy ameliorates leukocyte adhesion and microvascular flow abnormalities in transgenic sickle mice. *Am J Physiol Heart Circ Physiol.* 2004;287(1):H293-H301.

114. Ataga KI, Kutlar A, Kanter J, et al. Crizanlizumab for the prevention of pain crises in sickle cell disease. *N Engl J Med.* 2017;376(5):429-439.

115. Kutlar A, Ataga KI, McMahon L, et al. A potent oral P-selectin blocking agent improves microcirculatory blood flow and a marker of endothelial cell injury in patients with sickle cell disease. *Am J Hematol.* 2012;87(5):536-539.

116. Charrin E, Dubé JJ, Connes P, et al. Moderate exercise training decreases inflammation in transgenic sickle cell mice. *Blood Cells Mol Dis.* 2018;69:45-52.

Mechanistic Insights on Sickle Cell Pathophysiology Learned From Transgenic Mouse Models

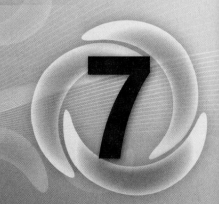

7

Authors: Kalpna Gupta, Lewis L. Hsu

Chapter Outline

Overview

This chapter will introduce how mouse models have provided insights on the pathobiology and comorbidities of sickle cell disease (SCD), including vaso-occlusion and pain, which are the clinical hallmarks of SCD. Types of transgenic sickle mouse models will be presented, highlighting the correlation between hemoglobin pattern, anemia, and acute microcirculatory obstruction. Translational research using sickle mice has provided insights into the mechanisms underlying acute and chronic pain (Figure 7-1). Sickle mice provide a platform for preclinical testing of pharmacologic agents for pain and other comorbidities of SCD. Insights gained from mouse models into vascular complications of SCD, including retinopathy, nephropathy, pulmonary hypertension, priapism, and leg ulcers, are discussed. Limitations of mouse models are described, and future directions are presented.

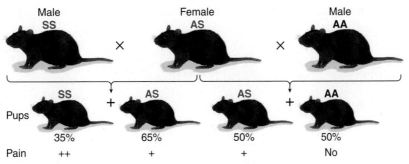

FIGURE 7-1 Matings of SS mice provide evidence of the survival disadvantage of sickle cell disease. The proportion of SS and AS is 35:65, instead of the 50:50 for litters of AS and AA, respectively. Data from the lab of Kalpna Gupta.

Why Mice?

No animals have spontaneously developed sickle hemoglobin (HbS) and sickle vaso-occlusive pain. Although several species of deer have crescent-shaped red blood cells, their deformation occurs with oxygenation rather than with deoxygenation, and the deer do not have hemolytic anemia or vaso-occlusion, so they cannot serve as models for human SCD.[1] Mice serve as an excellent model organism because of their relatively wide availability and ease of maintenance, cost-effectiveness, short life span, scope of genetic manipulations, and ability to model disease through diverse interventions including pharmacologic, cellular, surgical, and others. The inherent resilience of mice to manipulations provides flexibility in experimental design and consequent follow-up of disease processes. Mouse models have been developed to represent pathologic conditions by using genetic manipulations by gene insertions, deletions, or editing. Humanized mouse models are defined as "mice engrafted with functional human cells or tissues or expressing human transgenes."[2] These mice are a valuable asset because they afford an opportunity to intervene throughout the lifespan of the animal, which enables targeting the preventive strategies at the source before the sequelae of primary pathology leads to secondary complications. Mouse models of SCD have been developed using transgenic techniques. The goal was a mouse model for severe SCD that recapitulates extensive polymerization of HbS, hemolytic anemia, histologic and functional changes of vaso-occlusion, organ damage, and high mortality without treatment.

Types of Transgenic Sickle Mice

Overview and History

Milestones in the development of transgenic mouse models of SCD are summarized herein.[3-5] The overall premise is that the extent of HbS expression correlates with the severity of hematologic and pathophysiologic complications in the mice, just as in human SCD. Thus, the biophysical principles for polymerization of deoxygenated (deoxy) HbS that were described *in vitro* (Chapters 1 and 2) were recapitulated *in vivo* during the iterative development of transgenic sickle mice (Tables 7-1 and 7-2). The main feature for comparison between different strains of transgenic sickle mice is the level of HbS expression (right-hand column in Tables 7-1 and 7-2). For example, SAD mice express about 19% HbS and mild vaso-occlusive manifestations, whereas Townes and BERK mice express >90% HbS and severe manifestations of SCD including pain and organ pathology.[6-9] However, mouse models also differ in the level of mouse α-globins and mouse β-globins and the levels of transgenic human globins. Development of a series of transgenic mice strove for higher expression of human HbS and lower expression of mouse hemoglobin, as discussed later in this chapter. Inserting a transgene with the sickle β-globin gene and human β-globin locus control region (LCR) into mice resulted in expression of sickle β-globin in the mouse erythrocytes but very little SCD pathophysiology.[10] Subsequent studies *in vitro* demonstrated that both mouse β-globin and mouse α-globin inhibit sickle hemoglobin polymerization.[11]

β Thalassemia mice have low expression of mouse β-globins (Table 7-1, deletion of mouse β-major gene, continued expression of mouse β-minor gene). Using β thalassemic mice as a genetic background, transgenes expressing HbS were introduced, which generated several mouse models with a range of HbS, along with mouse α- and β-globins.

New York mice (NYDD1) express about 73% HbS and evince some features of mild SCD when exposed to 8% oxygen for 4 or more days. These features include glomerular and cerebral blood flow abnormalities, chronic oxidative stress, and a urine-concentrating defect.[12] Compound heterozygote mice were created with β thalassemia and sickle transgene, thus decreasing the amount of mouse β-globin, but they still displayed a mild phenotype of SCD.[13] NYDD1 is useful for renal and retinopathy studies.

SAD mice (Table 7-1) express "super" HbS that harbors 2 additional mutations known to enhance the polymerization process in sickle cell patients (Antilles β23-I and D-Punjab β121-N).[6] The SAD mouse is a hemizygote, expressing a low proportion (19%-26%) of human SAD hemoglobin. The SAD neonates are anemic (hematocrit, 32%), with a reduced weight and increased mortality. The SAD adults are not significantly anemic, but they have dehydrated red cells, related to the

TABLE 7-1 Transgenic mice expressing mouse and human sickle hemoglobins

Name	α	βmajor	βminor	α	βA	βS	βS-Antilles	βD-Punjab	Genetic strain C57BL/6
Normal	+	+	+/−						C57BL/6
Thal	+		+/−						C57BL/6
New York	+		+/−			+			C57BL/6
Hybrid	+		+/−			+	+		C57BL/6
Antilles	+		+/−				+		C57BL/6
SAD	+		+/−			+	+	+	C57BL/6 CBA/J

Note. Early mouse models of sickle cell disease still had mouse hemoglobin and added transgenes. The models began with a background of mouse β thalassemia: mildly anemic mice that lack expression of mouse β-major but still express mouse β-minor. Mouse α-globin is still expressed fully. The progressive development of these mouse models featured transgenic insertion of sickle β-globin (βS), then the double-mutant βS-Antilles, then the addition of βD-Punjab. However, the presence of mouse α and mouse β-minor reduces sickle polymerization, and these mice did not have severe manifestations of sickle cell disease.

Adapted from Sagi V, Song-Naba WL, Benson BA, Joshi SS, Gupta K. Mouse models of pain in sickle cell disease. *Curr Protoc Neurosci.* 2018;85:e54.

persistent activity of the KCl cotransport system and hypoxia-induced activation of the calcium-dependent potassium channel (Gardos channel). Older SAD mice develop sickle cell complications such as priapism, kidney defects, and a shorter survival.[8,14]

Knockout and transgenic techniques were developed and achieved greater success (Table 7-2). Mice with "knockout" of the mouse β-globin genes with transgenic insertion of human β sickle globin were generated in one laboratory, whereas mice with knockout of mouse α-globin genes were generated in another laboratory. Mice from the 2 laboratories were mated to create mice expressing exclusively human sickle hemoglobin.[8,15]

These mice are homozygous for the mouse α-globin null allele, are homozygous for the mouse β-globin null allele, and carry the sickle transgene [$Hba^{0/0} Hbb^{0/0} Tg(Hu\text{-}miniLCR\alpha1^G\gamma^A\gamma\delta\beta^S)$] called HbSS or SS, henceforth.

BERK mice were distributed widely to investigators from the Lawrence Berkeley laboratory at the University of California, and hence called *Berkeley model* (abbreviated as *BERK*) mice or *Paszty* sickle mice.[8] These mice display the major genetic, hematologic, and histopathologic features observed in severe human SCD, including severe anemia (hemoglobin, 5 g/dL).[3] BERK mice have been used in numerous laboratories as models

TABLE 7-2 Transgenic Townes and BERK mice express human α- and β-globins but no mouse α- and β-globins

Name	α	βmajor	βminor	α	βA	βS	βS-Antilles	Genetic strain
HbAA-control				+	+			Mixed
HbAS-hemi				+	+	+		Mixed
HbSS-homo				+		+		Mixed

Note. The transgenic Townes and BERK mouse models of severe sickle cell disease express human α- and human β-globins but do not express mouse α- and mouse β-globins. Some take the perspective that the erythrocyte membranes of these mice are still murine, but the contents of the erythrocyte are human. The HbSS-homozygote (HbSS-homo) has 2 transgenes for βS. The Townes HbAS-hemizygote (HbAS-hemi) has 1 transgene for βS and 2 transgene for βA. The Townes HbAA control has 2 transgenes for βA.

for severe SCD physiology, including vaso-occlusion, vascular biology, inflammation, and hemolysis.

Townes mice were developed by Townes and colleagues, who used 2 strategies to develop transgenic sickle mice.[15] The first strategy was gene knockout by generating a mouse that is homozygous for the same knockout of murine α- and β-globins as the BERK mouse but has 2 separate transgenes inserted, one for the human α-globin gene and one for the human βA-γ- or βS-globin genes.[15] However, due to limited availability, this 1997 knockout Townes sickle mouse has not been examined significantly. The second strategy was gene knock-in by replacing the mouse α-globin genes with a human globin gene (hα/hα) and the mouse β-globin genes with human βA-γ- or βS-γ-globin genes (-1400 γ-βS/-1400 γ-βS). The Townes knock-in model has baseline hemoglobin of 8.9 g/dL, similar to average patients with HbSS, and might be a more accurate genetic representation of SCD.[3] This model has severe hemolytic anemia due to erythrocyte sickling, reticulocytosis, splenic infarcts, kidney damage, and overall poor health.[7] This knock-in model published in 2006 is the Townes sickle mouse that has been widely distributed. The phenotype of the Townes knock-in mouse is less severe than that of BERK mice.[5]

Many insights on the fundamental science of SCD emerged from the comparisons of mice with different proportions of HbS, mouse hemoglobins, and human hemoglobin A (HbA). Elegant experiments on the impact of fetal hemoglobin (HbF) on SCD were made possible by creation of NY1KO mice with knockout of mouse hemoglobins and insertion of transgenes with 3 different levels of γ-globin expression.[16]

What Is a Suitable Control Mouse?

Mouse models for SCD have 2 homologous copies of the transgene allele for β-globin and can be regarded as homozygotes, but mice with 1 allele of transgene for β-globin are called hemizygotes (abbreviated hBERK or HbAS BERK) (Figure 7-1).[4] Studies showed that hemizygotes were not all equivalent to humans with sickle trait; other factors such as the type of other hemoglobins present (native mouse vs transgenic human HbA) and the balance of α- and β-globins could affect pathophysiologic manifestations such as the amount of reactive oxygen species (ROS). Additional features of the mouse such as polymorphisms in inflammatory response can also affect the phenotype of hemizygotes for HbS transgene.

HbAA-BERK mice (Figure 7-1) have the same mixed genetic background as BERK but exclusively express normal human HbA (human α- and βA-globins) without murine globins. These mice are the most appropriate control for the BERK mouse when the experiment is designed to compare the full effect of SCD versus normal. Similarly, the Townes sickle mouse has a well-matched control: HbAA-Townes mice have the same human α-globin gene (hα/hα), but the mouse β-globin gene was replaced with human Aγ- and βA-globin genes.

HbAS mice (or hBERK) express HbS at about 25% and have complex features that are not normal. Under normoxic conditions, hemizygotes have elevated ROS and prothrombotic markers, hyperalgesia, activated endothelium, and renal pathology.[17] Hemizygotes can be regarded as models of humans with sickle trait.[5, 9, 17-28] Under hypoxic conditions, hemizygotes show organ pathology, pain, and sensitivity to hypoxia.[9, 20, 26, 27] Experiments can be designed with conditions that cause sickle deformation only in homozygote sickle mice but not in hemizygotes, in order to focus on the impact of sickle vaso-occlusion.

Hemizygote mouse siblings have been used as controls in some studies, but it is important to recognize that they are not normal mice. The hemizygote (hBERK/HbAS BERK) can have a phenotype similar to that of SS BERK with increased cytokines and tissue factor and pain.[9, 29-32] hBERK mice also display endothelial activation, including elevated adhesion molecule expression under normoxia.[30] Trichostatin A, a histone deacetylase inhibitor, completely ameliorated vascular cell adhesion molecule 1 (VCAM1) and tissue factor expression in the pulmonary vein endothelium of these mice.[33] In our experience, these mice show improved survival compared to homozygous BERK mice. (unpublished observations, K.G.). Creation of ischemic open wounds led to morbidity in SS but not in HbAS/hBERK mice.[34] Therefore, due to constitutive sickle pathobiology, hBERK serves as an excellent model to define the mechanisms and functions that may be challenging to perform in fragile SS mice, such as those requiring survival surgery. Most importantly, hBERK/HbAS mice serve as excellent female breeding partners with male SS mice, which is important because female SS mice are challenging to breed (Figure 7-1).

Wild-type mice from a well-characterized inbred strain such as C57BL/6J can be used as the experimental control. The inbred strains of mice are easier to obtain than specific transgenic HbA control mice, and results can be compared to those of many other labs with the same strain. However, comparing wild-type mice with transgenic sickle mice can be confounded by genetic differences in many other traits unrelated to the sickle transgene, as described later in the section titled "Limitations of Using Sickle Mouse Models."

Studies of the hemolytic pathophysiology of SCD can be designed with control mice with lower levels of hemolysis due to lower levels of HbS or with human HbA. Positive controls for intense hemolysis can be mice with acute or chronic hemolysis that is not caused by HbS (eg, immune-mediated hemolysis, hereditary spherocytosis, or chemical damage by phenylhydrazine).[35, 36]

Adding genetic features to transgenic sickle mice can facilitate mechanistic studies of chronic factors in vaso-occlusion. Cross breeding the complex transgenic sickle mouse with another transgenic mouse can be laborious and susceptible to reproductive failure. However, elegant studies examined the role of endothelial factors in sickle vaso-occlusion by transplanting transgenic sickle mouse bone marrow into mice with knockout or overexpression of toll-like receptor 4 (TLR4).[37] Chimeric sickle cell mice with knockout of TLR4 did not have vaso-occlusion when challenged with infusion of heme. This result indicates that hemolysis triggers vaso-occlusion via TLR4. Similarly, the role of CD47 was examined by transplanting sickle mouse marrow into CD47 knockout mice.[38] However, these transplanted mice may not recapitulate the evolutionary spectrum of injury, which can start early in life. Several genetic knockouts/deletions have been made recently on Townes and BERK mice by cross-breeding, including deletion of mast cells on BERK,[39] calpain 1 knockout on Townes,[40] cannabinoid receptor 2 knockout on BERK,[41, 42] and TLR4 knockout on BERK.[43]

Transgenic Sickle Mice Provide a Good Model for SCD but Also Fall Short

Models of Acute Sickle Vaso-occlusion

The unique polymerization response of HbS to acute hypoxia-reoxygenation (H/R) creates the clearest pattern of sickle pathophysiology in transgenic sickle mice. Experimental exposure of mice to 8% to 10% oxygen (normobaric hypoxia) followed by reoxygenation causes different levels of vaso-occlusion and ischemic injury that correlate strongly with the proportion of HbS in the red blood cells. Mice expressing exclusively HbS will have severe ischemic tissue damage and die with prolonged exposure to hypoxia.[6, 44, 45] Experimental preparations showed dramatic images of microcirculatory venules becoming occluded with sickled red cells upon *in vivo* video microscopy. Mice with lower percentages of HbS and presence of native mouse hemoglobins have relatively less ischemia and vaso-occlusion and can tolerate longer periods of hypoxia.[3, 44, 46] The ability to design experiments with hypoxic challenge to isolate the impact of HbS polymerization in pathophysiology has been a major scientific contribution of transgenic sickle mice.

Under normoxic conditions, higher expression of HbS correlates with more severe hemolytic anemia and elevation of ROS, inflammatory markers, and thrombotic markers.[5, 47, 48] When normoxic sickle mice are administered inflammatory triggers such as tumor necrosis factor-α (TNF-α) or lipopolysaccharide, those with higher HbS have exaggerated inflammatory responses compared to controls.[29, 37, 49, 50] Increased hyperalgesia was observed following H/R in BERK and Townes mice, which serves as a model for vaso-occlusive crisis (VOC) pain.[51, 52] Experimental designs can feature control mice with lower levels of hemolysis due to lower levels of HbS or with human HbA. To focus on the effects of intense hemolysis, sickle mice can also be compared to mice with acute or chronic hemolysis that is not caused by HbS.[35, 36] Thus, some labs design comprehensive experiments incorporating wild-type mice, transgenic HbA mice, hemizygous mice, mildly affected transgenic sickle mice, and severely affected transgenic sickle mice.[33, 50, 53] Comparing these multiple groups of mice permits dissection of the effects of vaso-occlusion, sickle hemoglobin, and the transgenic background. Obviously, this rigorous study design requires substantial investment of resources for statistically significant sample size in each of these multiple types of mice.

Additional comprehensive reviews of sickle mice are available.[3, 4, 8, 14, 54-56]

Limitations of Using Sickle Mouse Models

Experience with transgenic sickle mice has revealed pitfalls and limitations of these animal models. Careful experimental design can focus on what is relevant to human SCD, elucidate pathophysiologic mechanisms, and test candidate therapies while avoiding these pitfalls and limitations.

Transgenic sickle mice are physiologically fragile. Laboratory conditions tolerated by wild-type mice can cause high mortality in transgenic sickle mice; these conditions include dehydration, cold temperatures, transportation, and anesthesia. Breeding efficiency is low: transgenic sickle mice suffer higher mortality during pregnancy and in the newborn period.[57] A standard practice in lab mouse colonies is to enrich the diet of pregnant mice to improve their viability, and many laboratories maintain their sickle transgenic mice on customized enriched diets such as "sickle chow" (Purina Mills, St. Louis, MO). Sickle chow is a super-enriched feed containing additional vitamins, antioxidants, and L-arginine, which produces free nitric oxide. A version without supplemental arginine is also available.[8, 58] Both chows have been examined for their therapeutic benefit as dietary supplements for sickle mice.[57, 59]

Genetic admixture in sickle mice poses several challenges. Transgenic mice were originally developed on a mixed genetic background because certain inbred strains were more efficient for insertion of the transgene.[8, 15] C57BL/6 mice are the most widely used mice for laboratory studies and were chosen for sequencing in the landmark mouse genomic sequencing project.[60] FVB/N mice have large pronuclei and large litter sizes, which made this strain a favorite for injecting transgenes.[61] Cell lines from the 129 strain tolerate the gene knockout process.[62] The BERK mouse had a genetic background that included C57BL/6, FVB/N, 129, DBA/2, and Black Swiss.[8] The heterogeneity of genetic background was obvious in simple features; often one litter of mice from transgenic sickle parents had pups with 2 or 3 different coat colors. Mice have polymorphisms in many other features relevant to sickle cell pathophysiology, such as the differences between inbred strains in cellular and chemokine inflammatory response and mitochondrial oxidant response.[63-65] With a mixed strain background, individual transgenic sickle mice or controls could show different properties caused by unsuspected polymorphisms that are separate from the effect of the sickle transgene. For example, early retinal degeneration occurred in some BERK mice but was linked to the homozygous mutation (rd1) independent of the sickle transgene.[20]

Genetic drift can cause an isolated gene pool to become enriched in some polymorphisms that are unrelated to the sickle transgene and introduce confounders. Data might not be reproducible in any other lab because of the uniqueness of a certain lab's mouse colony. Genetic drift is more likely in colonies of BERK mice, with their known background of mixed strains, than in colonies of transgenic sickle mice that have been backcrossed to homozygosity for nearly all genes of a single mouse strain (eg, congenic transgenic sickle mice such as BERK on C57BL/6, JAX catalog #031677). Accordingly, systematic backcrossing of transgenic sickle mice onto the C57BL/6 background strain is conducted by some labs to reduce genetic drift.[5] However, even mice that are considered fully backcrossed after 10 or more generations can still retain several genes from the mixed strains in the transgenic founder mouse embryonic stem cell: DNA flanking the inserted transgene ("congenic footprint") plus randomly distributed DNA elsewhere.[66] Thus, some investigators renew their transgenic sickle mouse colonies every few years with imported animals from Jackson Labs.

Explicit study of modifier genes is now possible with genetic modification by transgenic techniques, CRISPR, or bone marrow transplant (TLR4, E-selectin, or hemopexin).[37, 67-69]

HbF upregulation is the target of hydroxyurea, decitabine, and other candidate therapies for SCD. Unlike β-globin development in humans, mice do not have native mouse HbF. This limitation in mice was addressed by introducing transgenes with human γ-globin under the control of a miniLCR (Townes mice). Other studies took advantage of the absence of mouse HbF to study the effects of hydroxyurea separate from HbF induction.[69-71]

Some have pointed out that BERK mice have a mild α thalassemia phenotype because they are deficient in α-globin genes and thus not an exact hematologic model for most people with SCD who have all human α-globin genes. BERK mice "differed from humans with SCD in having splenomegaly, splenic hematopoiesis, more severe hepatic infarcts, less severe pulmonary manifestations, no significant vascular intimal hyperplasia, and only a trend toward vascular medial hypertrophy."[20]

Although humans and mice share the characteristics of mammals and an estimated 99% of their genes, species differences can limit the utility of mouse models for certain features of human SCD. For example, mice can differ in pharmacokinetics. Some solutions to species differences in pharmacokinetics are as easy as adjusting hydroxyurea dosing in order to obtain similar plasma levels.[72] However, for other agents such as 5-hydroxymethyl-2-furfural that show promising data in transgenic sickle mice,[73] species differences in metabolism could cause great complexity in predicting the level of risk for adverse effects in humans.[74, 75]

Another prominent difference between mice and humans is the brain development and cerebral vasculature. Concerns about growth impairment from hydroxyurea in mice, fortunately, have not been borne out by growth data in human children with SCD.[76-78] Ischemic stroke and hemorrhagic stroke are highly prevalent in human SCD but have not been found in transgenic sickle mice. However, recently, microscopic infarcts of the cerebral cortex in aged Townes mice were observed.[79] Stroke models have been created by disruption of carotid artery flow.

The small smooth (lissencephalic) mouse brain is suboptimal as an animal model for stroke compared to the gyrencephalic human-like brains in larger animals.[80] We can also speculate that the blood flow is less turbulent in the mouse carotid artery, which is straight, than in the human carotid artery with its well-known siphon curvature.

Bones are a prime target for SCD damage, and some studies have demonstrated microinfarcts and osteopenia,[81] but bones differ in certain respects between mice and humans. The quadrupedal gait of mice places very different weight-bearing loads on their hip joints compared to the bipedal gait of humans. Transgenic HbS mice do not develop avascular necrosis spontaneously. Like other rodents, mice have teeth that continue to grow in adulthood, unlike humans with primary teeth that are then replaced by the set of adult teeth. To conduct mechanistic studies of SCD-related dental pulp necrosis in animal models, species with a dental eruption pattern similar to humans (eg, dog or sheep) would be required.[82-84] The mouse immune system is not as complex as the human immune system,[85] so that hematopoietic stem cell transplants are less likely to be rejected by mice. The human chemokine interleukin-8 (IL-8) is one of the mediators of inflammatory response in SCD and is implicated in pain symptoms,[86-89] but mice do not have a homolog for IL-8 (reviewed by Guenet[90]).

The spleen in severe human SCD (homozygous HbSS) becomes scarred and involuted but can become enlarged and show hypersplenism pathophysiology in sickle β thalassemia or SCD with high HbF. Instead of involution, the spleens of transgenic sickle mice show massive enlargement with erythroid precursors and hypersplenism. Reducing splenomegaly is a marker for cure of the transgenic sickle mouse by transplant or gene therapy.[6, 91-100]

Additional differences are obvious between human and mouse physiology and include detoxification, smell, reproduction, communication, and socialization. However, creative experimental designs can be applied; for instance, Gupta compared sickle mice that were allowed to mate versus sickle mice kept isolated and without mating.

Chronic Vasculopathy of SCD

Several debilitating complications of SCD result from chronic vascular damage. Retinopathy, nephropathy, and pulmonary hypertension can require years to develop, and the interaction of genetic and environmental factors has emerged from epidemiologic studies. Priapism and leg ulcers are vascular complications with an intermittent pattern that make mechanisms difficult to study in humans. Studies in mouse models permit elegant experimental manipulation of risk factors to elucidate mechanisms of these vasculopathies, as described in the following sections and in Figure 7-2.

Retinopathy

Proliferative sickle retinopathy (PSR) is a devastating vascular complication of SCD with very little preventive therapy and, thus, a prime topic for mouse model experiments. The blood-retina barrier is considered a part of the blood-brain

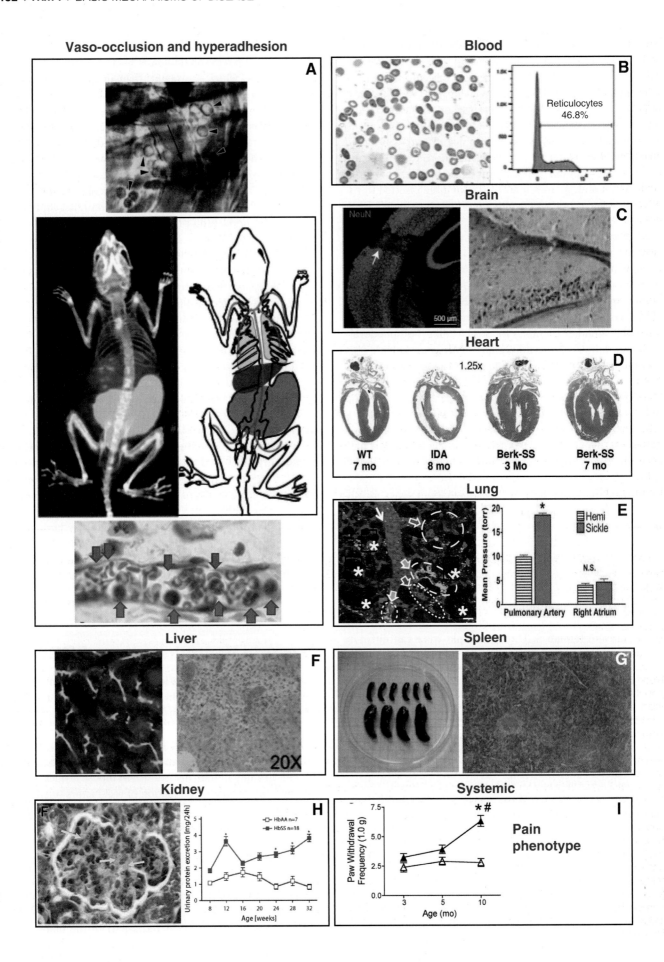

Vaso-occlusion and hyperadhesion

Blood

Brain

Heart

Lung

Liver

Spleen

Kidney

Systemic

Pain phenotype

barrier (BBB) but has not received the same attention as BBB and perhaps has unique features and heterogeneity compared with BBB and other barriers. Examining the retina is critical to fully appreciate the gateway function of retinal vasculature for targeted therapies. Using phage sub-libraries injected in mice, distinct signatures were found in different central nervous systems (CNS).[101] Neuroimaging of brain is also significantly advanced to obtain functional and phenotypic data on human brain vasculature. However, retinal vasculature remains a challenge to analyze using such technology. Needless to say, interventions and molecular analysis of human retina are not possible to the extent that they can be performed in mice. Most of the retinopathy models are induced models using vascular endothelial growth factor (VEGF) or oxygenation/laser, which cannot mimic the evolutionary spectrum and disease-driven pathology of the retina.[102] Limitations exist in human models based on diabetic retinopathy, with a high risk of bias and reduced applicability and most models focusing on low-risk patients.[103]

Of the various types of sickle mice listed in Tables 7-1 and 7-2, only 30% of NY1DD mice >15 months old developed bilateral choroidal retinopathy.[20, 104] BERK SS mice develop retinal detachment early in age due to a $Pde6b^{rd1}$ (rd1) mutation, independent of HbS, and are therefore not suited to examine retinopathy.[20] Townes SS mice do not have the rd1 or $Crb1^{rd8}$ mutations that are known to cause retinal pathology and have been shown to develop age-dependent pigmentary and retinal pathology indicative of retinopathy but show variability in severity and manifestation.[105] However, authors note that Townes SS

mice develop cataract or severe retinal hemorrhage, preventing retinal imaging, and some became too sick and/or died unexpectedly. Therefore, Townes mice do not appear to be suitable for examining retinopathy. However, NY1DD sickle mice have been well characterized using the highly sensitive technique of visualizing retinal vasculature phenotype with ADPase activity and show features of PSR.[106-108] ADPase is specific to retinal vasculature and is also observed in angioblasts.[109, 110] ADPase is expressed on the plasma membrane of the endothelial cells and plays a critical role in preventing platelet aggregation, which is stimulated by adenosine phosphatase (ADP), the substrate for ADPase.[111] Involvement of leukocytes was suggested in human diabetic choroid and in sickle retinopathy.[112, 113] The levels of adhesion molecules intercellular adhesion molecule 1 (ICAM1), VCAM1, and P-selectin were higher in humans with SCD compared to control subjects, and their levels were parallel to an increase in polymorphonucleate (PMN) leukocytes.[113] PMNs increased with disease progression in the retina. The role of adhesion molecule–mediated leukocyte adhesion in sickle vasculopathy is well established, and therefore, it would be important to know whether leukocyte-targeted anti–P- and/or anti–E-selectin therapies would ameliorate PSR. Sickle mouse models can provide translational insights for mechanism-based interventions to develop sickle cell retinopathy–targeted therapies.

Many features of retinopathy in NY1DD mice resemble human PSR including occluded nonperfused areas, hairpin loops, arteriovenous anastomoses, loss of arterial and venous architecture, pigmented lesions likely from the migration of

---

FIGURE 7-2 Representative pathology of sickle mice. Panel (**A**) shows the contribution of sickle mouse models to the elucidation of vaso-occlusion and hyperadhesion in SCD. Photomicrograph of cremaster venules after 3-hr hypoxia and 18 hr of reoxygenation showing a large number of emigrated leukocytes adjacent to a venule (arrowheads). Large arrows depict the flow direction (*top*, adapted from J Clin Invest. 2000;106(3):411-420). PET/CT scan of a mouse (alongside a schematic drawing) 24 hours after injection of a PET tracer that binds the adhesion molecule VLA-4 after challenge with LPS. The mouse had massive splenomegaly and increased tracer uptake in the humeri and femurs, indicating areas of hyperadhesion (*middle*, courtesy of Lydia Perkins, PhD and adapted from Blood Advances 2020, in press). Histology of a venule in the dorsal skin after 1 hr of hypoxia and 1 hr of reoxygenation. The venule has a suspected vascular obstruction. Blue arrowheads point to leukocytes that appear to be adherent to the vascular endothelium, and white arrows point to misshapen RBCs inside the venule (*bottom*, adapted from American Journal of Hematology 77:117–125 (2004). The **lateral panels** show representative pathology in key organs of sickle mice. Clockwise, the blood panel (**B**) shows evidence of sickling and hemolysis in sickle mice by peripheral smear evaluation, where anisopoikilocytosis, target cells, polychromasia and nucleated RBCs are observed (*left*, adapted from Science 31 Oct 1997:Vol. 278, Issue 5339, pp. 873-876), and by flow cytometry of thiazole orange-stained RBCs, revealing brisk reticulocytosis (*right*, courtesy of Enrico Novelli, MD). The brain panel (**C**) shows a spontaneous cortical microinfarct (arrow), as shown by the region devoid of NeuN staining, a marker of neuronal viability (*left*, adapted from J Cereb Blood Flow Metab. 2019 Feb;39(2):342-351), and pyknotic nuclei in the C3 field of the hippocampus (*right*, adapted from Neurobiol Dis. 2016 Jan;85:60-72). The heart panel (**D**) shows biventricular hypertrophy and left atrial dilation as early as 3 mo of age and worsening by 7 mo in sickle mice as compared to wild type mice and mice exposed to iron deficiency anemia for 3 mo (adapted from PNAS August 30, 2016 113 (35) E5182-E5191). The lung panel (**E**) shows a quantitative fluorescence intravital lung microscopy image of an arteriole microembolism with neutrophil (red)-platelet (green) aggregates after LPS challenge. The arrow denotes blood flow and the asterisks denote alveoli (*left*, adapted from Bennewitz et al JCI Insight. 2017 Jan 12; 2(1):e89761), and elevated mean pulmonary artery pressure in sickle mice as compared to hemizygous controls, denoting pulmonary hypertension (*right*, adapted from Blood. 2007 Apr 1;109(7):3088-98). The liver panel (**F**) shows quantitative liver intravital imaging using TXR-dextran (red) and carboxyfluorescein (green) for blood and bile duct staining, respectively, revealing loss of blood flow from vaso-occlusion in the liver (*left*), and hepatic fibrosis (*right*, courtesy of Tirthadipa Pradhan, PhD). The spleen panel (**G**) shows that sickle mice have splenomegaly (lower half of Petri dish) as compared to control mice (*left*) and marked histological disorganization of the spleen with reduction of clearly defined splenic white pulp, and expanded red pulp (*right*, adapted from Am J Pathol. 2012 Nov; 181(5): 1725–1734). The kidney panel (**H**) shows glomerular changes, including mesangial hyperplasia (arrows, *left*, adapted from Blood (2006) 107 (4): 1651–1658), and proteinuria exacerbating with age in sickle mice (*right*, adapted from Blood Adv (2019) 3 (9): 1460–1475). The systemic panel (**I**) shows increased nociception in sickle mice (solid triangles) as compared to non-sickling controls, as evidenced by higher paw withdrawal frequency in response to monofilament challenge (adapted from *Blood*. 2010 Jul 22; 116(3):456-65). PET/CT: positron emission tomography/computed tomography; LPS: lipopolysaccharide; NeuN: neuronal nuclei; TXR: Texas Red; mo: months.

retinal pigment epithelial cells, and corkscrew-like structures resembling microangiopathy in human sickle retinopathy.[104, 108] Differences also exist between mouse and human sickle retinopathy: (1) retinal occlusions occur in the mid retina predominantly in mice compared to the periphery in human PSR; (2) retinal neovascularization is more common in humans compared to choroidal neovascularization in mice; (3) sea fan neovascularization is typical in human PSR as compared to few large neovascular formations in sickle mice; and (4) prominence of retinal hemorrhage lesions in human PSR are rarely observed in mice. Some of these differences were overcome in mice after chronic treatment with morphine for >10 months.[108] Although morphine is used to treat pain via the CNS, it can promote angiogenesis via the mitogenic and survival-promoting signaling pathways of mitogen-activated protein kinase/extracellular signal-regulated kinases (MAPK/ERK) and protein kinase B (PKB/Akt), respectively, and by coactivation of VEGF receptor-2 (VEGFR2) signaling and by platelet-derived growth factor receptor β (PDGFRβ)-mediated pericyte recruitment and activation.[108, 114–116] Unfortunately, these proangiogenic effects of morphine contribute to retinal neovascularization in NY1DD mice with increased vessel branching in the periphery as well as mid retina and presence of hemorrhagic areas, which are reminiscent of human PSR.[108] This raises the possibility that opioid use for pain in patients with SCD may be contributing to some of the differences observed between NY1DD mice and human PSR. Morphine stimulates TNF-α release from mast cells, which leads to increased expression of ICAM1, VCAM1, and endothelial leukocyte adhesion molecule 1 (ELAM1) on microvascular endothelial cells from neonatal human foreskins, suggesting that morphine may promote endothelial-leukocyte interaction.[117, 118] Morphine also stimulates vascular permeability.[119] Together, these observations on NY1DD mice support the notion that opioids contribute to human PSR, which needs to be validated in clinical studies to develop targeted therapies and alternatives to opioids.

Nephropathy

The kidney is a key target organ in SCD. Sickle nephropathy differs from other types of nephropathies and is characterized by hyposthenuria, glomerular hyperfiltration, albuminuria, papillary necrosis and hematuria, chronic kidney disease, and end-stage renal disease[120] (see Chapter 16). Modeling sickle nephropathy in sickle mice has included several studies of the vasoactive peptide endothelin-1 (ET-1) using physiologic and other invasive surgical procedures in HbSS Townes mice, some of which may not be possible in human subjects.[121] Complementary to this observation, ET-1 receptor type A (ETA) blockade with the specific antagonist atrasentan is being investigated in a phase III trial (Study of Diabetic Nephropathy with Atrasentan). In this trial, nephroprotection was provided in a restrictive cohort of overt diabetic kidney disease patients.[122] Fluid retention was one of the major risk factors in diabetic kidney disease. Using B6;129$Hba^{tm1(HBA)Tow}Hbb^{tm2(HBG1,HBB*)Tow}$/ $Hbb^{tm3(HBG1,HBB)Tow}$/J mice (Townes knock-in HbSS mice),[7] the selective ETA receptor antagonist ambrisentan and the

nonselective ETA/ETB receptor antagonist A-182086 suggested nephroprotection in the tubules and glomerular vasculature and prevented immune cell infiltration.[121]

Hypoxia accentuates renal manifestations of SCD in SAD1 mice. Bosentan, an endothelin receptor antagonist, prevents hypoxia-induced pulmonary and renal microvascular congestion, immune cell infiltration, and death of sickle mice.[46] Several transgenic sickle mice studies thus demonstrate the potential of ETA blockade in preventing or ameliorating sickle nephropathy. In SCD with increased renal clearance, it remains to be seen whether ETA blockade would provide nephroprotection. ETA blockade has also been effective in reducing pain in Townes sickle mice (discussed later in this chapter). Therefore, ETA appears to be a treatable target for pain and organ damage.

Using BERK SS mice, fibrinogen was shown to contribute to renal disease by engaging neutrophils/macrophages through αMβ2 integrin receptors.[123] Fibg390-396A mutation in these mice had a renal protective effect; however, it did not affect any other organ.

Opioids also influence renal pathobiology. It is challenging to modulate opioids in patients suffering from pain. Therefore, transgenic sickle mice have provided insights on the effects of analgesic opioids on renal pathobiology.[124] Podocyte foot effacement, a key contributor of albuminuria, could be visualized by electron microscopy in HbSS-BERK sickle mice treated with chronic morphine.[125] Complementary to podocyte pathology, morphine exacerbated albuminuria accompanied by impaired renal function, including increased blood urea nitrogen (BUN) and decreased clearance of BUN in HbSS-BERK sickle mice. Morphine's adverse effects in the sickle kidney were mediated by activation of platelet-derived growth factor receptor β (PDGFRβ) signaling via mesangial cell proliferation and glomerulomegaly.[125] In addition to demonstrating the adverse effects of opioids on nephropathy, sickle mice provide insights into a mechanism-based treatable target, PDGFRβ. Treatment with sunitinib, an inhibitor of PDGFR tyrosine kinase, inhibited glomerular mesangial cell proliferation.[125, 126] In other studies in mice and patients with SCD, imatinib, an inhibitor of receptor tyrosine kinases including that of PDGFRβ, prevented acute and chronic pain (described in detail later in this chapter).[39, 127, 128] Thus, sickle mice have provided critical insights into treatable targets for nephropathy. Novel renal protective therapies are being examined in sickle mouse models.[121, 123, 129, 130] A role for complement deposition in glomerular pathophysiology has been demonstrated in sickle mice.[131] The impact of mixed chimeric bone marrow transplantation on renal dysfunction was also examined in sickle mice,[98] as well as similar levels of chimerism afforded by gene therapy.[94]

Pulmonary Hypertension

Sickle mice can develop severe pulmonary hypertension with aging, spontaneously in BERK mice and with hypoxia (9% oxygen) in SAD mice. Hemolysis is implicated as a major driver of pulmonary hypertension.[35] Pulmonary hypertension was associated with higher levels of heme oxygenase-1, endothelial nitric oxide synthase, and phosphodiesterase 5 (PDE5). Combined therapy with a PDE5 inhibitor and NCX1443 reduced severity of pulmonary hypertension.[132] Thrombospondin-1 and plasma CD47 promote pulmonary hypertension in sickle mice; sickle mice that were CD47 knockout had less pulmonary hypertension.[38] A series of studies in sickle mice demonstrate a role for the angiogenic growth factor placental growth factor (PlGF) in pulmonary hypertension, at the junction of inflammation, vasoconstriction, and airway hyperresponsiveness.[133]

Priapism

Priapism is another very painful manifestation of SCD. Clinical trials of priapism are difficult because the episodes are unpredictable and men with priapism might not seek care. Transgenic sickle mice have spontaneous priapism, but experimental triggering of priapism is also possible.[134, 135] This mouse model has provided insights on how multiple steps of nitric oxide vasoregulation are dysfunctional and examined possible therapies.[136]

Leg Ulcers

Chronic painful skin ulcers in the perimalleolar areas are a common complication of adult SCD, but knowledge about the pathophysiology is scant. Wound healing is slow, and the SCD leg ulcers can be worsened by trauma; therefore, it is unethical to perform sequential biopsies on patients.[137-139] Sickle mice do not develop spontaneous leg ulcers, but a model has been developed that studies healing from an excisional surgical wound in old SAD mice.[138]

Abnormal wound healing correlated with impaired blood and lymphatic angiogenesis in the wound beds and poor mobilization of endothelial progenitor cells from the bone marrow. The wounds of SAD mice had abnormally low secretion of C-X-C motif chemokine 12 (CXCL12) by keratinocytes and inflammatory cells. Local therapy with endothelial progenitor cells or recombinant CXCL12 injections restored wound angiogenesis and rescued the healing defect, together with mobilization of circulating endothelial progenitor cells. Deferoxamine injection of the wound accelerated healing in BERK sickle mice, and remodeling was associated with chelation of excess free iron.[140]

Transgenic Sickle Mice in Translational Science

Preclinical Testing of Pharmaceutical Agents

The development of voxelotor (GBT440) exemplifies the utility of sickle mice in drug discovery in SCD.[141] We will highlight other illustrative examples of transgenic sickle mice as drug development platforms, but a full review is beyond the scope of this chapter.

Transgenic sickle mice were used by Kean et al.[98] to develop costimulatory blockade (CTLA4-Ig and anti-CD40L) to facilitate hematopoietic stem cell transplantation with tolerance to mismatch of major histocompatibility complex. Transgenic sickle mice were used by Silva et al.[136] to examine possible therapy for priapism using nitric oxide pathways; efficient conduct of these studies was made possible by experimental methods to induce priapism in the mice, while studies in humans would be limited by the intermittent and unpredictable occurrence of priapism. Similarly, agents to treat SCD pain, such as cannabinoids, could efficiently be tested in transgenic sickle mice.[9, 41, 51] Vinjamur et al.[142] used transgenic sickle mice to examine small-molecule candidates to manipulate γ-globin gene repression by BCL11. Pulmonary hypertension therapy with endothelin receptor antagonists is being examined in sickle mice; these studies would be impractical in humans because of the length of follow-up required.[143] Prior to human clinical trials of agents to inhibit conformational change of sickle hemoglobin under deoxygenated conditions such as 5-hydroxymethyl-furfural (5-HMF) and voxelotor, preclinical testing was conducted to demonstrate that these agents would not have dangerous off-target binding to molecules other than hemoglobin.[144] Transgenic sickle mice were also used to screen for adverse effects of the hematopoietic stem cell mobilizer plerixafor as the foundation for a clinical trial of plerixafor in patients with SCD.[145]

Mechanistic insights on hydroxyurea have subsequently emerged from mouse experiments that adjusted the dosing of hydroxyurea for mice pharmacodynamics.[72] Transgenic sickle mouse studies showed that lack of HbF induction by hydroxyurea in sickle mice does not abrogate its acute vascular benefits.[70, 71] Hydroxyurea can modulate inflammation and actually improved survival of pneumococcal sepsis and pneumonia in transgenic sickle mice;[69] experimentally administering a bacterial infection obviously would not be possible in human clinical trials. Other mice provided data on the teratogenic potential of hydroxyurea and partial mechanistic explanation for variability in hydroxyurea dose-response.[146, 147] Additional mechanistic studies on hydroxyurea examine modulation of angiogenesis and hypoxia-inducible factor 1α and protection from renal tubular damage.[148, 149]

Neurobehavioral Modeling of Pain in Transgenic Sickle Mice

Mouse models are essential to examine mechanisms of pain in SCD, including the dissection of the specific nociceptive, inflammatory, and neuropathic components of pain; the discovery of novel treatable targets; and mechanisms of pain associated with psychosocial spinothalamic pathways. It is challenging to study pain in humans with SCD because the presentation of pain is heterogeneous, with significant overlap between chronic pain and the unpredictable, acute pain of VOC, so teasing out chronic and acute pain is almost impossible. Another limitation of studies of pain in humans is that the effect of chronic opioid use in many patients is difficult to ascertain, since opioids cannot always be withdrawn without adverse, short-term repercussions. Humanized transgenic mice have offered unique insights into discovery of peripheral and central mechanisms, treatable

TABLE 7-3 Features of hyperalgesia (pain) in sickle mice using sensory testing with and without stimuli

Pain characteristic	Device	Response	Sensory stimuli	Clinical interpretation
Thermal (heat)	Hargreaves' apparatus	Paw withdrawal latency	Heat targeted to the plantar surface of the hind paw	Sensitive to temperature extremes
Thermal (cold)	Cold plate	Paw withdrawal latency and frequency	Cold at 4°C	Develop acute pain upon cold exposure; often leads to ED visit
Mechanical	von Frey monofilaments	Paw withdrawal frequency	Application of filament to the plantar surface of the hind paw	Sensitive to touch and wind speed
Deep tissue/ musculoskeletal	Grip force meter	Grip force exerted	None	Pain in joints
Facial expression	Mouse grimace scale	Orbital tightening, ear position, nose bulge, cheek bulge	None	Facial expression in infants and children
Conditioned place preference	Chambers at different temperatures	Time spent in specific chamber	None	Aversive to cold
Vocalization after discharge	None	Vocalization	None	NA

Abbreviations: ED, emergency department; NA, not applicable.

targets, and integrative approaches with translational potential to understand and treat pain in SCD.

Characteristic Features of Pain in Sickle Mice and Similarities with Human Sickle Pain

The chronic pain phenotype in transgenic BERK sickle mice was first characterized using behavioral assays that include evaluation of (1) mechanical hyperalgesia by paw withdrawal frequency in response to application of von Frey filaments, (2) thermal hyperalgesia by paw withdrawal latency to a radiant heat source and paw withdrawal frequency and latency on a cold plate, and (3) deep tissue hyperalgesia measured by a computerized grip force measure instrument.[9, 51] Subsequently, hypersensitivity to mechanical and thermal stimuli was validated in sickle patients with the application of quantitative sensory testing (QST) (Tables 7-3 and 7-4).[150-156] Both BERK and Townes sickle mice demonstrated greater hypersensitivity to heat, cold, and mechanical stimuli with increasing age,[9, 52] similar to the findings of decreased pain threshold in response to the same stimuli with increasing age in patients with SCD.[150, 155] Higher sickle pain intensity in females is reported in human subjects with SCD,[157, 158] which was also observed in both homozygous BERK and Townes sickle mouse models.[9, 52] Similar to patients with SCD who require high opioid doses to alleviate pain as compared to other pain conditions,[159, 160] relatively higher dose of opioids are required to treat hyperalgesia in sickle mice compared to

other mouse models of pain.[9, 52] Biochemically, higher levels of substance P (SP), a known neurotransmitter mediating chronic pain, have been reported in patients with SCD at steady state, with further increases with pain.[161, 162] Similarly, higher SP has been observed in the plasma, dorsal root ganglia (DRG), and skin secretagogue of sickle mice.[9, 39, 163] Peripherally, cutaneous nociceptors of sickle mice *in vivo* and *ex vivo* from skin nerve preparation exhibited enhanced sensitization and increased response to heat, cold, and mechanical stimuli.[42, 164, 165] Importantly, nociceptors on the second-order neurons in the spinal dorsal horn in BERK sickle mice were shown to be hypersensitive in electrophysiologic recordings suggestive of central sensitization.[166] Such direct hyperexcitability and direct interrogation of neuronal physiology is not possible in human subjects. However, analysis of QST and neuroimaging data reveals sensitization of CNS and altered brain connectivity in patients with SCD.[167-169] Subjecting sickle mice to H/R evokes pathobiology similar to human acute VOC, characterized by significantly enhanced sickling of RBCs, ischemic injuries, and augmented inflammation.[45] H/R treatment leads to acute and significantly higher hyperalgesic response compared to the basal chronic hyperalgesia in sickle mice.[9, 52] H/R-evoked hyperalgesia in sickle mice and its resolution using investigational drugs targeting underlying sickle pathobiology and novel nonopioid pain receptors have been reported in multiple studies.[9, 39, 51, 163, 170-175] Altogether, BERK and Townes transgenic sickle mice recapitulate the features of both acute

TABLE 7-4 Similarities in sensory testing for pain/hyperalgesia between mice and human subjects with SCD

Pain characteristic	Device	Response	Sensory stimuli	Clinical interpretation
Thermal (heat)	Hargreaves' apparatus	Paw withdrawal latency	Heat targeted to the plantar surface of the hind paw	QST measures of lower heat detection threshold and heat pain threshold in sickle patients QST for thermal sensitivity is measured using Thermal Sensory Analyzer (Medoc, Ramat Yishai, Israel) that employs cold temperature to the skin via Peltier-based thermode
Thermal (cold)	Cold plate	Paw withdrawal latency and frequency	Cold at 4°C	Low temperature related to higher hospital admissions for VOC events, and association of high wind velocity with acute VOC events Patients experience VOCs after exposure to cold water Higher pain intensity in colder months QST measures of lower cold detection threshold and cold pain threshold in sickle patients, and worse cold sensitivity in sickle children and adolescents during VOC
Mechanical	von Frey monofilaments	Paw withdrawal frequency	Application of filament to the plantar surface of the hind paw	QST measures of sickle children demonstrating lower mechanical threshold using brush and pinprick at steady state and using von Frey elements during VOC
Deep tissue/ musculoskeletal	Grip force meter	Grip force exerted	None	Description of musculoskeletal pain in arms, chest, and lower back in sickle adult patients using the Nordic musculoskeletal symptoms questionnaire and the SF-36 Health Survey
Facial expression	Mouse grimace scale	Orbital tightening, ear position, nose bulge, cheek bulge	None	Not documented
Conditioned place preference	Chambers at different temperatures	Time spent in specific chamber	None	Not documented
Vocalization after discharge	Pressure-zone microphone	Vocalization	None	Not documented

Abbreviations: QST, quantitative sensory testing; SF-36, Short Form-36; VOC, vaso-occlusive crisis.

and chronic human sickle pain and serve as effective preclinical models to analyze the complex neurobiology of sickle pain, identify treatable targets, and test effectiveness of targeted therapeutics.

Mechanisms of Sickle Pain and Its Resolution

SCD causes oxidative stress, inflammation, and recurrent VOC-induced ischemia-reperfusion injury, which may underlie peripheral and central sensitization via activation of nociceptors and/or direct injury of the neurons.[176] Due to central sensitization, antidromic release of neuropeptides from the spinal cord to the periphery, in turn, evokes further inflammation and nociceptor activation, thus facilitating a perpetual cycle of heightened peripheral and central sensitization and resultant pain. These observations provide a possible explanation for challenges in treating pain in SCD. Modulation of top-down pain inhibitory mechanisms may also impact pain perception. Nearly a decade ago, Kohli et al.[9] found distorted neurovascular architecture in the dorsal skin of sickle mice. In addition to decreased expression of μ-opioid receptors and with increased expression of pain-related neurotransmitters calcitonin gene-related peptide (CGRP) and SP in sickle mice skin, increased phosphorylation of nociceptive signaling pathways of MAPK were observed. These findings complement the observation that sickle mice have hyperalgesia.[9] Since then, multiple preclinical mouse studies helped to identify molecular and cellular effectors of sickle pain.

Peripheral and Central Neuroimmune Axis Affects Sickle Pain

The discovery that mast cells mediate pain was the foremost demonstration of neuroimmune interactions affecting sickle pain.[39] Our results suggest that activated mast cells in the sickle microenvironment release tryptase, which may activate protease activated receptor 2 (PAR2) on nerve fibers, leading to the release of SP and CGRP from peripheral nerve endings. SP stimulates vascular permeability, thus causing neurogenic inflammation.[39] Persistent mast cell activation in a feedforward loop orchestrated by SP and other inflammatory mediators possibly contributes to the sustained sensitization of the peripheral nociceptors. Treating sickle mice with imatinib mesylate (a receptor tyrosine kinase inhibitor) alone and cromolyn sodium (a mast cell stabilizer) with morphine elicited significant analgesic response along with reduction of mast cell activation, expression of SP/CGRP, systemic inflammation, and neuroinflammation.[39, 138] Additionally, mast cells may cause neurovascular dysfunction via direct physical interactions through extracellular traps.[177] Mast cells also contribute to BBB dysfunction via the endoplasmic reticulum stress-mediated pathway in sickle mice.[178] Sickle patients have higher plasma levels of SP, tryptase, and glial fibrillary acidic protein (GFAP; a marker of neuroinflammation),[161, 162, 179, 180] and patients with SCD who received imatinib for chronic myeloid leukemia experienced an amelioration of their SCD phenotype.[127, 128, 181] Thus, mast cell–targeted therapeutics may alleviate SCD pain.

Serpins are genes encoding serine protease inhibitors (eg, α_1-antitrypsin [A1AT]) that regulate endogenous elastase activity, which is elevated in SCD.[171, 182-186] Clinically, patients with SCD exhibit a positive association of A1AT plasma levels with hemolytic and inflammation markers.[185, 186] We found downregulation of serpins[170] and increased elastase activity in sickle mice DRG, and treating sickle mice with human plasma–derived A1AT (US Food and Drug Administration [FDA] approved and also known as Prolastin-C) reduced pain in these mice, suggesting that repurposing of A1AT could prevent pain in SCD.[171] Thus, dysregulation of serpin-mediated elastase homeostasis constitutes another neuroimmune axis affecting mechanisms of SCD pain.

In sickle mouse spinal cord (compared to control mice), microglial and astrocyte activation was prominent, with concomitant elevation of ROS, SP, and GFAP, all of which were reduced with simultaneous reduction in hyperalgesia in sickle mice treated with coenzyme Q10 (Co-Q10) and curcumin.[187] Co-Q10 was found to reduce VOC frequency in patients with SCD.[188] Therefore, central mechanisms of SCD pain entail oxidative stress and neuroimmune interactions by glial activation in the SCD microenvironment. It is noteworthy that neurochemical alterations in sickle mice are replicative of their presentation in SCD subjects.

Druggable Targets for SCD Pain Treatment

Pain and Neuromodulatory Receptors

Opioids are the mainstay of SCD pain management despite their known adverse effects.[176] Potentiation of morphine analgesia when coadministered with cromolyn sodium in sickle mice suggests that targeting mast cell activation is necessary for more effective analgesia in SCD.[39, 138] The possibility that nonopioid therapies may be more effective in treating pain has been tested in sickle mice. Targeting nociceptin opioid receptors with the small-molecule, high-affinity agonist AT-200 in sickle mice reduced hyperalgesia, which was accompanied by attenuation of inflammation and mast cell activation and was devoid of tolerance.[163]

Treating sickle mice with nonselective and selective agonists of cannabinoid receptors (known to stimulate neuromodulatory effects) demonstrated amelioration of both chronic basal and H/R-evoked hyperalgesia via receptor-specific mechanisms to reduce neurogenic inflammation and mast cell activation.[39, 51] Many patients with SCD self-administer marijuana to relieve pain.[189] A human clinical trial testing the efficacy of vaporized cannabis in resolving SCD pain (ClinicalTrials.gov identifier: NCT01771731) showed a trend in reduction in pain with inhaled cannabis compared to placebo, but the difference was not statistically significant due to a relatively lower number of participants.[190]

Cellular Signaling Proteins

Recently, based on preclinical observations in sickle mice, targeting 2 novel proteins has shown efficacy in treating sickle pain clinically. Upregulation of Ca^{2+}/calmodulin protein kinase IIα (CaMKIIα, a cellular protein) was found in the DRG and spinal cord of sickle BERK mice, and inhibition of CaMKIIα with molecular antagonist or RNA silencing attenuated SCD pain descriptors in these mice.[172] In a recent clinical trial with a single dose of the CaMKIIα inhibitor trifluoperazine, 8 of 18 SCD patients reported a 50% reduction in chronic pain intensity.[173]

In the DRG of sickle mice, ET-1 and ETA expression was found to be elevated compared to control mice.[165] Genetic knockdown or pharmacologic inhibition of ETA effectively reduced chronic and H/R-evoked acute hyperalgesia in sickle mice, possibly through nuclear factor κ–light-chain enhancer of activated B cells (NF-κB)-mediated upregulation of the sodium ion channel Nav1.8.[174] Thus, targeting ET-1/ETA may provide alternate SCD pain therapeutics. As discussed earlier, ET-1-targeted therapies are in clinical trials for nephropathy, which may be supportive of clinical trials to relieve pain in SCD.

Targeting Nerve Regeneration

Expression of small proline-rich repeat protein 1A (SPRR1A), expressed primarily in DRG neurons and responsible for modulating nerve regeneration after peripheral injury, is suppressed in the DRG of sickle mice at a relatively young age, so much so that it is not further attenuated with either increasing age or H/R.[170, 191, 192] Based on the observations in sickle mice, subsequent examination of SPRR1A knockout C57BL/6 mice exhibited mechanical and thermal (both heat and cold) hyperalgesia compared to wild-type controls, indicating the contribution of SPRR1A in pain. SPRR1A-overexpressing BERK sickle mice exhibit reduced mechanical and cold hyperalgesia compared to BERK sickle mice.[175] Sickle pain can be neuropathic in nature,[193, 194] and utilization of neuropathic pain medications in children with SCD is associated with increasing age.[158] Therefore, downregulation of SPRR1A in sickle mice may reflect an inability to repair injured nerve fibers due to an ongoing noxious SCD environment. SPRR1A is also involved in the cornification of skin.[195] Earlier studies by the Gupta laboratory demonstrated a thinner epidermal layer and nerve fiber injury in the skin of sickle mice.[9] It is likely that increased sensitivity to noxious stimuli in sickle mice may be due to a thinner epidermis, including heightened sensitivity to cold. Moreover, thinner skin and reduced cornification may contribute to leg ulcers. Therefore, the transcriptomic analysis in sickle mice has provided insights into pain and associated comorbidities in SCD.

Nonpharmacologic Complementary and Integrative Approaches for SCD Pain Treatment

Complementary approaches can integrate traditional therapeutics to ease the burden of pain. Acupuncture is a well-recognized complementary approach, and a retrospective analysis found that patients with SCD reported significantly favorable outcomes of acupuncture in reducing pain.[196] Acupuncture therapy has been tested in a sickle mouse model. The novel method of electroacupuncture (EA) in freely moving, awake mice developed by the Gupta laboratory demonstrated responders with 3 different pain outcomes, namely high responders (>200% pain threshold increase), moderate responders (100%-200% pain threshold increase), and nonresponders (≤100% pain threshold increase).[197] A unique observation in these studies was that transgenic BERK mouse models of SCD as well as a transgenic mouse model of breast cancer showing the evolutionary spectrum of human breast cancer showed similar variability in response to EA. In contrast, chemically induced hyperalgesia with complete Freund's adjuvant (CFA) showed that >90% of wild-type mice had uniformly similar analgesic response to EA. These data clearly demonstrate that transgenic models of specific diseases recapitulate the variability observed in human subjects with specific disease conditions, whereas chemically induced, transient models such as CFA-induced pain may not elicit the response associated with specific clinical conditions. It is not surprising that most of the neuroscience data with sciatic nerve ligation or CFA-induced pain have been challenging to translate to clinical pain conditions.

All BERK mice used in the EA study were from the same colony, but differences existed in their neurochemistry, which may support the variability in analgesic response to EA. It was found that BERK mice showing moderate or low response to EA also had higher circulating and spinal SP. SP underlies the initiation and maintenance of pain via spinal p38 MAPK phosphorylation. Spinal inhibition of SP with the FDA-approved neurokinin-1 receptor antagonist netupitant potentiated the effectiveness of EA in nonresponders.[198] Therefore, it is likely that the variable response with EA/acupuncture that has been

reported clinically may be a consequence of the neurochemical makeup of the individual (mouse), which can be tested to predict response to therapy.

Transgenic sickle mice have also been used to explore the role of nutritional and behavioral interventions for pain, using experimental interventions that would be difficult to conduct in human clinical trials. An enriched diet (high-calorie protein diet supplemented with micronutrients) and companionship (male and female mice housed together) were compared to regular diet and single-gender confinement.[199] Surprisingly, the hyperalgesia was reduced in the male mice on the enriched diet and with female companionship, with a concurrent increase in the serotonin levels in the spinal dorsal horn and rostral ventromedial medulla region of the brain. These results indicate that a top-down inhibitory mechanism is in play via the spinothalamic inhibitory pathway.[199] The positive effect of companionship on pain reduction may be a result of activation of the sympathetic nervous system. Recent neurovascular studies in patients with SCD demonstrated inception of vasoconstriction at the anticipation of a painful event, although the event was absent.[200] This indicates that in the SCD pathobiology, the autonomic nervous system (ANS) may affect the perception of pain. Thus, modulation of the ANS via meditation, mindfulness, hypnosis, and other integrative approaches may moderate the perception of pain.[201] In summary, mouse models have plasticity to be modulated pharmacologically and genetically to simulate both acute and chronic pain in SCD, enabling the examination of molecular mechanisms that may not be possible to accomplish in human subjects.

Future Directions

The recent surge in clinical trials of pharmacologic agents and hematopoietic stem cell transplant strategies suggests that the field of SCD might have matured to a point where preclinical animal models may not be necessary. Cellular and molecular approaches to screening pharmacologic agents using microfluidics offer promise for potential drug discovery without an animal model. However, many scientific questions justify the use of mouse models. For example, the top-down mechanisms cited earlier require a complete neurovascular and neuroimmune central and peripheral orchestra, which cannot be replicated *ex vivo*. Certainly, behavioral analysis cannot be performed in *in vitro* systems. Pharmacologic screening for off-target toxicities in a whole mammalian system would still be needed as an intermediate safety testing stage before introducing a new candidate drug into human clinical trials. In addition, mice can still be used to test hypotheses that would be difficult to examine rigorously in human clinical trials. Control of environment, diet, or genetics can be far more rigorous in mouse experiments than in human studies. New imaging techniques such as high-resolution magnetic resonance imaging, multiphoton microscopy, and new contrast labels mean that serial noninvasive imaging can sometimes replace serial tissue samples.[79, 93, 202-207] Future studies could employ longitudinal cohort designs that do not require euthanizing many mice.

The advent of gene editing technology opens new possibilities for mouse models with multiple combinations of genes as a way to examine "precision medicine" in a mouse model. Introducing new genes with gene editing methods like CRISPR would avoid the problem of congenic footprint of DNA carried along with the transgene.[66] New gene editing methods also suggest that the HbS gene could be introduced into other species that overcome some of the limitations of mice. For example, human lung and brain anatomy is more similar to that of large mammals such as sheep or pigs than to that of mice.[80, 208] At this time, a porcine model of SCD has been created, but it remains to be seen if it would have a higher translational contribution in SCD compared to mouse models.

Acknowledgment

We thank Dr. Mark Gladwin and Dr. Enrico Novelli for creating Figure 7-2, and Dr. Anupam Aich and Dr. Donovan Argueta for help with some sections of this chapter. We are also thankful for the funding from National Institutes of Health grants U18 EB029354 and HL147562 to KG. *The content is solely the responsibility of the authors and does not necessarily represent the official views of the National Institutes of Health.*

Contributions

LH and KG defined the content, created figures, and cowrote the chapter. KG prepared the tables.

Conclusion

A variety of transgenic mouse models expressing human sickle hemoglobin have been created and have provided critical insights into the pathobiology and comorbidities of SCD, including vaso-occlusion and pain, the clinical hallmarks of SCD. Different mouse models have offered pathobiology-specific significance, such as the occurrence of retinopathy in NY1DD mice and constitutive chronic hyperalgesia in BERK and Townes mice. Critical insights into the mechanisms and translational significance have been gained from sickle mice into vascular pathobiology, inflammation, retinopathy, nephropathy, pulmonary hypertension, priapism, leg ulcers, and pain, both chronic and acute. Translational potential of sickle mouse models provides a platform for preclinical testing of pharmacologic agents for pain and other comorbidities of SCD. Like any other model system, sickle mouse models have limitations, which require attention during experimental design, data interpretation, and drawing conclusions.

High-Yield Facts

- Transgenic sickle mouse models have many similarities to severe sickle cell disease (SCD), including susceptibility to acute hypoxia, acute inflammation, pain, and chronic organ damage.

- Availability of transgenic mice expressing different levels of sickle hemoglobin (HbS) and/or mixed or exclusive mouse or human hemoglobins offers the plasticity of investigating specific comorbidities of SCD, but also imposes certain limitations. Consideration and caution in experimental design are warranted when using these mouse models. For example, New York mice are not appropriate for examining pain, but are the only known model of sickle retinopathy.

- Transgenic sickle mice have provided insights on the complex pathophysiology of HbS polymerization, hemolytic anemia, endothelial dysfunction, inflammation, thrombosis, and oxidant stress.

- Transgenic sickle mice offer new opportunities to examine pain, notably the interplay of chronic inflammation and neuropathic pain evoking peripheral and central sensitization. These mice offer SCD-specific development of mechanism-based novel pharmacologic and integrative interventions to treat pain and/or prevent pain from being evoked.

- Comparisons with the appropriate transgenic control mice with similar genetic background and genetic manipulations are critical for interpreting transgenic sickle mouse experimental data.

References

1. Esin A, Bergendahl LT, Savolainen V, Marsh JA, Warnecke T. The genetic basis and evolution of red blood cell sickling in deer. *Nat Ecol Evol.* Feb 2018;2(2):367-376. doi:10.1038/s41559-017-0420-3

2. Brehm MA, Shultz LD, Greiner DL. Humanized mouse models to study human diseases. *Curr Opin Endocrinol Diabetes Obes.* Apr 2010;17(2):120-5. doi:10.1097/MED.0b013e328337282f

3. Beuzard Y. Mouse models of sickle cell disease. *Transfus Clin Biol.* Feb-Mar 2008;15(1-2):7-11. doi:10.1016/j.tracli.2008.04.001

4. McColl B, Vadolas J. Animal models of beta-hemoglobinopathies: utility and limitations. *J Blood Med.* 2016;7:263-274. doi:10.2147/JBM.S87955

5. Sagi V, Song-Naba WL, Benson BA, Joshi SS, Gupta K. Mouse Models of Pain in Sickle Cell Disease. *Current Protocols in Neuroscience.* 2018/10/01 2018;85(1):e54. doi:10.1002/cpns.54

6. Trudel M, De Paepe ME, Chretien N, et al. Sickle cell disease of transgenic SAD mice. *Blood*. Nov 1 1994;84(9):3189-97.

7. Wu LC, Sun CW, Ryan TM, Pawlik KM, Ren J, Townes TM. Correction of sickle cell disease by homologous recombination in embryonic stem cells. *Blood*. Aug 15 2006;108(4):1183-8. doi:10.1182/blood-2006-02-004812

8. Pászty C, Brion CM, Manci E, et al. Transgenic knockout mice with exclusively human sickle hemoglobin and sickle cell disease. *Science*. Oct 1997;278(5339):876-8. doi:10.1126/science.278.5339.876

9. Kohli DR, Li Y, Khasabov SG, et al. Pain-related behaviors and neurochemical alterations in mice expressing sickle hemoglobin: modulation by cannabinoids. *Blood*. 2010/07/22 2010;116(3):456-465. doi:10.1182/blood-2010-01-260372.

10. Greaves DR, Fraser P, Vidal MA, et al. A transgenic mouse model of sickle cell disorder. *Nature*. Jan 11 1990;343(6254): 183-5. doi:10.1038/343183a0

11. Rhoda MD, Domenget C, Vidaud M, et al. Mouse alpha chains inhibit polymerization of hemoglobin induced by human beta S or beta S Antilles chains. *Biochim Biophys Acta*. Jan 29 1988;952(2):208-12.

12. Fabry ME, Costantini F, Pachnis A, et al. High expression of human beta S- and alpha-globins in transgenic mice: erythrocyte abnormalities, organ damage, and the effect of hypoxia. *Proc Natl Acad Sci U S A*. Dec 15 1992;89(24):12155-9.

13. Ryan TM, Townes TM, Reilly MP, et al. Human sickle hemoglobin in transgenic mice. *Science*. Feb 2 1990;247(4942):566-8.

14. Fabry ME. Transgenic animal models of sickle cell disease. *Experientia*. Jan 15 1993;49(1):28-36.

15. Ryan TM, Ciavatta DJ, Townes TM. Knockout-transgenic mouse model of sickle cell disease. *Science*. Oct 31 1997;278(5339):873-6.

16. Fabry ME, Suzuka SM, Weinberg RS, et al. Second generation knockout sickle mice: the effect of HbF. *Blood*. Jan 15 2001; 97(2):410-8. doi:10.1182/blood.v97.2.410

17. Diwan BA, Gladwin MT, Noguchi CT, Ward JM, Fitzhugh AL, Buzard GS. Renal pathology in hemizygous sickle cell mice. *Toxicol Pathol*. Mar-Apr 2002;30(2):254-62. doi:10.1080/01926230275355 9597

18. Sadler KE, Zappia KJ, O'Hara CL, et al. Chemokine (c-c motif) receptor 2 mediates mechanical and cold hypersensitivity in sickle cell disease mice. *Pain*. Aug 2018;159(8):1652-1663. doi:10.1097/j.pain.0000000000001253

19. Solovey A, Kollander R, Shet A, et al. Endothelial cell expression of tissue factor in sickle mice is augmented by hypoxia/reoxygenation and inhibited by lovastatin. *Blood*. Aug 1 2004;104(3): 840-6. doi:10.1182/blood-2003-10-3719

20. Manci EA, Hillery CA, Bodian CA, Zhang ZG, Lutty GA, Coller BS. Pathology of Berkeley sickle cell mice: similarities and differences with human sickle cell disease. *Blood*. 2006;107(4): 1651-1658. doi:10.1182/blood-2005-07-2839

21. Kaul DK, Zhang X, Dasgupta T, Fabry ME. Arginine therapy of transgenic-knockout sickle mice improves microvascular function by reducing non-nitric oxide vasodilators, hemolysis, and oxidative stress. *Am J Physiol Heart Circ Physiol*. Jul 2008; 295(1):H39-47. doi:10.1152/ajpheart.00162.2008

22. Nandedkar SD, Feroah TR, Hutchins W, et al. Histopathology of experimentally induced asthma in a murine model of sickle cell disease. *Blood*. Sep 15 2008;112(6):2529-38. doi:10.1182/ blood-2008-01-132506

23. Gladwin MT, Barst RJ, Castro OL, et al. Pulmonary hypertension and NO in sickle cell. *Blood*. Aug 5 2010;116(5):852-4. doi:10.1182/blood-2010-04-282095

24. Pritchard KA, Jr., Feroah TR, Nandedkar SD, et al. Effects of experimental asthma on inflammation and lung mechanics in sickle cell mice. *Am J Respir Cell Mol Biol*. Mar 2012;46(3): 389-96. doi:10.1165/rcmb.2011-0097OC

25. Zhang H, Xu H, Weihrauch D, et al. Inhibition of myeloperoxidase decreases vascular oxidative stress and increases vasodilatation in sickle cell disease mice. *J Lipid Res*. Nov 2013;54(11):3009-15. doi:10.1194/jlr.M038281

26. Zappia KJ, Guo Y, Retherford D, Wandersee NJ, Stucky CL, Hillery CA. Characterization of a mouse model of sickle cell trait: parallels to human trait and a novel finding of cutaneous sensitization. *Br J Haematol*. Nov 2017;179(4):657-666. doi:10.1111/bjh.14948

27. Noguchi CT, Gladwin M, Diwan B, et al. Pathophysiology of a sickle cell trait mouse model: human alpha(beta)(S) transgenes with one mouse beta-globin allele. *Blood Cells Mol Dis*. Nov-Dec 2001;27(6):971-7. doi:10.1006/bcmd.2001.0469

28. Szczepanek SM, McNamara JT, Secor ER, Jr., et al. Splenic morphological changes are accompanied by altered baseline immunity in a mouse model of sickle-cell disease. *Am J Pathol*. Nov 2012;181(5):1725-34. doi:10.1016/j.ajpath.2012.07.034

29. Holtzclaw JD, Jack D, Aguayo SM, Eckman JR, Roman J, Hsu LL. Enhanced pulmonary and systemic response to endotoxin in transgenic sickle mice. *Am J Respir Crit Care Med*. Mar 15 2004; 169(6):687-95. doi:10.1164/rccm.200302-224OC

30. Kaul DK, Liu XD, Choong S, Belcher JD, Vercellotti GM, Hebbel RP. Anti-inflammatory therapy ameliorates leukocyte adhesion and microvascular flow abnormalities in transgenic sickle mice. *Am J Physiol Heart Circ Physiol*. Jul 2004;287(1):H293-301. doi:10.1152/ajpheart.01150.2003

31. Lunzer MM, Yekkirala A, Hebbel RP, Portoghese PS. Naloxone acts as a potent analgesic in transgenic mouse models of sickle cell anemia. *Proc Natl Acad Sci U S A*. Apr 3 2007;104(14): 6061-5. doi:10.1073/pnas.0700295104

32. Beckman JD, Belcher JD, Vineyard JV, et al. Inhaled carbon monoxide reduces leukocytosis in a murine model of sickle cell disease. *Am J Physiol Heart Circ Physiol*. Oct 2009;297(4): H1243-53. doi:10.1152/ajpheart.00327.2009

33. Hebbel RP, Vercellotti GM, Pace BS, et al. The HDAC inhibitors trichostatin A and suberoylanilide hydroxamic acid exhibit multiple modalities of benefit for the vascular pathobiology of sickle transgenic mice. *Blood*. Mar 25 2010;115(12):2483-90. doi:10.1182/blood-2009-02-204990

34. Gupta K, Poonawala T, Levay-Young BK, Ericson ME, Ammbashankar NS, Hebbel RP. Abnormal Angiogenesis, Neurogenesis and Lymphangiogenesis in the Skin Underlies Delayed Wound Healing in the Sickle Mouse: Acceleration of Healing by Topical Opioids. Presented at American Society of Hematology Annual Meeting, Atlanta, Dec 2005. *Blood*. 2005;106(11):3177-3177.

35. Hsu LL, Champion HC, Campbell-Lee SA, et al. Hemolysis in sickle cell mice causes pulmonary hypertension due to global impairment in nitric oxide bioavailability. *Blood*. Apr 1 2007; 109(7):3088-98. doi:10.1182/blood-2006-08-039438

36. Hanson MS, Xu H, Flewelen TC, et al. A novel hemoglobin-binding peptide reduces cell-free hemoglobin in murine hemolytic anemia. *Am J Physiol Heart Circ Physiol*. Jan 15 2013; 304(2):H328-36. doi:10.1152/ajpheart.00500.2012

37. Belcher JD, Chen C, Nguyen J, et al. Heme triggers TLR4 signaling leading to endothelial cell activation and vaso-occlusion in murine sickle cell disease. *Blood*. Jan 16 2014;123(3):377-90. doi:10.1182/blood-2013-04-495887

38. Novelli EM, Little-Ihrig L, Knupp HE, et al. Vascular TSP1-CD47 signaling promotes sickle cell-associated arterial vasculopathy and pulmonary hypertension in mice. *Am J Physiol Lung Cell Mol Physiol.* Jun 1 2019;316(6):L1150-l1164. doi:10.1152/ajplung.00302.2018

39. Vincent L, Vang D, Nguyen J, et al. Mast cell activation contributes to sickle cell pathobiology and pain in mice. *Blood.* 2013/09/12 2013;122(11):1853-1862. doi:10.1182/blood-2013-04-498105

40. Nwankwo JO, Lei J, Xu J, Rivera A, Gupta K, Chishti AH. Genetic inactivation of calpain-1 attenuates pain sensitivity in a humanized mouse model of sickle cell disease. *Haematologica.* Oct 2016;101(10):e397-e400. doi:10.3324/haematol.2016.148106

41. Vincent L, Vang D, Nguyen J, Benson B, Lei J, Gupta K. Cannabinoid receptor-specific mechanisms to alleviate pain in sickle cell anemia via inhibition of mast cell activation and neurogenic inflammation. *Haematologica.* May 2016;101(5):566-77. doi:10.3324/haematol.2015.136523

42. Uhelski ML, Gupta K, Simone DA. Sensitization of C-fiber nociceptors in mice with sickle cell disease is decreased by local inhibition of anandamide hydrolysis. *Pain.* 2017/09 2017;158(9):1711-1722. doi:10.1097/j.pain.0000000000000966

43. Lei J, Paul J, Wang Y, Gupta M, Vang D, Thompson S, Jha R, Nguyen J, Peng F, Valverde Y, Lamarre Y, Gupta K. Heme causes pain in sickle mice via toll-like receptor 4-mediated ROS- and endoplasmic reticulum stress-induced glial activation. *Antioxid Redox Signal.* 2020 Aug 24. doi: 10.1089/ars.2019.7913. PMID: 32729340.

44. Kaul DK, Hebbel RP. Hypoxia/reoxygenation causes inflammatory response in transgenic sickle mice but not in normal mice. *J Clin Invest.* Aug 2000;106(3):411-20. doi:10.1172/jci9225

45. Osarogiagbon UR, Choong S, Belcher JD, Vercellotti GM, Paller MS, Hebbel RP. Reperfusion injury pathophysiology in sickle transgenic mice. *Blood.* Jul 1 2000;96(1):314-20.

46. Sabaa N, de Franceschi L, Bonnin P, et al. Endothelin receptor antagonism prevents hypoxia-induced mortality and morbidity in a mouse model of sickle-cell disease. *J Clin Invest.* May 2008; 118(5):1924-33. doi:10.1172/JCI33308

47. Hebbel RP, Osarogiagbon R, Kaul D. The endothelial biology of sickle cell disease: inflammation and a chronic vasculopathy. *Microcirculation.* Mar 2004;11(2):129-51.

48. Kollander R, Solovey A, Milbauer LC, Abdulla F, Kelm RJ, Hebbel RP. Nuclear factor-kappa B (NFkappaB) component p50 in blood mononuclear cells regulates endothelial tissue factor expression in sickle transgenic mice: implications for the coagulopathy of sickle cell disease. *Transl Res.* Apr 2010;155(4):170-7. doi:10.1016/j.trsl.2009.10.004

49. Turhan A, Jenab P, Bruhns P, Ravetch JV, Coller BS, Frenette PS. Intravenous immune globulin prevents venular vaso-occlusion in sickle cell mice by inhibiting leukocyte adhesion and the interactions between sickle erythrocytes and adherent leukocytes. *Blood.* Mar 15 2004;103(6):2397-400. doi:10.1182/blood-2003-07-2209

50. Solovey A, Somani A, Belcher JD, et al. A monocyte-TNF-endothelial activation axis in sickle transgenic mice: Therapeutic benefit from TNF blockade. *Am J Hematol.* Nov 2017;92(11):1119-1130. doi:10.1002/ajh.24856

51. Cain DM, Vang D, Simone DA, Hebbel RP, Gupta K. Mouse models for studying pain in sickle cell disease: effects of strain, age, and acuteness. *British journal of haematology.* 2012/02/15 2012;156(4):535-544. doi:10.1111/j.1365-2141.2011.08977.x

52. Lei J, Benson B, Tran H, Ofori-Acquah SF, Gupta K. Comparative Analysis of Pain Behaviours in Humanized Mouse Models of Sickle Cell Anemia. *PLOS ONE.* 2016/08/05 2016; 11(8):e0160608. doi:10.1371/journal.pone.0160608.

53. Belcher JD, Chen C, Nguyen J, et al. The fucosylation inhibitor, 2-fluorofucose, inhibits vaso-occlusion, leukocyte-endothelium interactions and NF-kB activation in transgenic sickle mice. *PLoS One.* 2015;10(2):e0117772. doi:10.1371/journal.pone.0117772

54. Nagel RL, Fabry ME. The panoply of animal models for sickle cell anaemia. *Br J Haematol.* Jan 2001;112(1):19-25. doi:10.1046/j.1365-2141.2001.02286.x

55. Beuzard Y. Transgenic mouse models of sickle cell disease. *Curr Opin Hematol.* Mar 1996;3(2):150-5.

56. Nagel RL. Lessons from transgenic mouse lines expressing sickle hemoglobin. *Proc Soc Exp Biol Med.* Apr 1994;205(4):274-81. doi:10.3181/00379727-205-43708

57. Jahagirdar OB, Mittal AM, Song-Naba WL, et al. Diet and gender influence survival of transgenic Berkley sickle cell mice. *Haematologica.* Feb 14 2019;104(8):e331-e334. doi:10.3324/haematol.2018.208322

58. Kaul DK, Fabry ME, Suzuka SM, Zhang X. Antisickling fetal hemoglobin reduces hypoxia-inducible factor-1alpha expression in normoxic sickle mice: microvascular implications. *Am J Physiol Heart Circ Physiol.* Jan 1 2013;304(1):H42-50. doi:10.1152/ajpheart.00296.2012

59. Tran H, Gupta M, Gupta K. Targeting novel mechanisms of pain in sickle cell disease. *Blood.* Nov 30 2017;130(22):2377-2385. doi:10.1182/blood-2017-05-782003

60. Mouse Genome Sequencing C, Waterston RH, Lindblad-Toh K, et al. Initial sequencing and comparative analysis of the mouse genome. *Nature.* Dec 5 2002;420(6915):520-62. doi:10.1038/nature01262

61. Taketo M, Schroeder AC, Mobraaten LE, et al. FVB/N: an inbred mouse strain preferable for transgenic analyses. *Proc Natl Acad Sci U S A.* Mar 15 1991;88(6):2065-9.

62. Eisener-Dorman AF, Lawrence DA, Bolivar VJ. Cautionary insights on knockout mouse studies: the gene or not the gene? *Brain Behav Immun.* Mar 2009;23(3):318-24. doi:10.1016/j.bbi.2008.09.001

63. Becker M, Reuter S, Friedrich P, et al. Genetic variation determines mast cell functions in experimental asthma. *J Immunol.* Jun 15 2011;186(12):7225-31. doi:10.4049/jimmunol.1100676

64. Amcheslavsky A, Zou W, Bar-Shavit Z. Toll-like receptor 9 regulates tumor necrosis factor-alpha expression by different mechanisms. Implications for osteoclastogenesis. *J Biol Chem.* Dec 24 2004;279(52):54039-45. doi:10.1074/jbc.M409138200

65. Scheffler K, Krohn M, Dunkelmann T, et al. Mitochondrial DNA polymorphisms specifically modify cerebral beta-amyloid proteostasis. *Acta Neuropathol.* Aug 2012;124(2):199-208. doi:10.1007/s00401-012-0980-x

66. Schalkwyk LC, Fernandes C, Nash MW, Kurrikoff K, Vasar E, Koks S. Interpretation of knockout experiments: the congenic footprint. *Genes Brain Behav.* Apr 2007;6(3):299-303. doi:10.1111/j.1601-183X.2007.00304.x

67. Wang H, Luo W, Wang J, et al. Paradoxical protection from atherosclerosis and thrombosis in a mouse model of sickle cell disease. *Br J Haematol.* Jul 2013;162(1):120-9. doi:10.1111/bjh.12342

68. Vercellotti GM, Zhang P, Nguyen J, et al. Hepatic Overexpression of Hemopexin Inhibits Inflammation and Vascular Stasis in Murine Models of Sickle Cell Disease. *Mol Med.* Sep 2016;22:437-451. doi:10.2119/molmed.2016.00063

69. Lebensburger JD, Howard T, Hu Y, et al. Hydroxyurea therapy of a murine model of sickle cell anemia inhibits the progression of

pneumococcal disease by down-modulating E-selectin. *Blood*. Feb 23 2012;119(8):1915-21. doi:10.1182/blood-2011-08-374447

70. Lebensburger JD, Pestina TI, Ware RE, Boyd KL, Persons DA. Hydroxyurea therapy requires HbF induction for clinical benefit in a sickle cell mouse model. *Haematologica*. Sep 2010;95(9):1599-603. doi:10.3324/haematol.2010.023325

71. Almeida CB, Scheiermann C, Jang JE, et al. Hydroxyurea and a cGMP-amplifying agent have immediate benefits on acute vaso-occlusive events in sickle cell disease mice. *Blood*. Oct 4 2012;120(14):2879-88. doi:10.1182/blood-2012-02-409524

72. Iyamu WE, Lian L, Asakura T. Pharmacokinetic profile of the anti-sickling hydroxyurea in wild-type and transgenic sickle cell mice. *Chemotherapy*. Jul-Aug 2001;47(4):270-8. doi:10.1159/000048534

73. Abdulmalik O, Safo MK, Chen Q, et al. 5-hydroxymethyl-2-furfural modifies intracellular sickle haemoglobin and inhibits sickling of red blood cells. *Br J Haematol*. Feb 2005;128(4):552-61. doi:10.1111/j.1365-2141.2004.05332.x

74. Sachse B, Meinl W, Sommer Y, Glatt H, Seidel A, Monien BH. Bioactivation of food genotoxicants 5-hydroxymethylfurfural and furfuryl alcohol by sulfotransferases from human, mouse and rat: a comparative study. *Arch Toxicol*. Jan 2016;90(1):137-48. doi:10.1007/s00204-014-1392-6

75. Pastoriza de la Cueva S, Alvarez J, Vegvari A, et al. Relationship between HMF intake and SMF formation in vivo: An animal and human study. *Mol Nutr Food Res*. Mar 2017;61(3)doi:10.1002/mnfr.201600773

76. Woo GH, Bak EJ, Nakayama H, Doi K. Molecular mechanisms of hydroxyurea(HU)-induced apoptosis in the mouse fetal brain. *Neurotoxicol Teratol*. Jan-Feb 2006;28(1):125-34. doi:10.1016/j.ntt.2005.08.002

77. Wang WC, Ware RE, Miller ST, et al. Hydroxycarbamide in very young children with sickle-cell anaemia: a multicentre, randomised, controlled trial (BABY HUG). *Lancet*. May 14 2011;377(9778):1663-72. doi:10.1016/S0140-6736(11)60355-3

78. Rana S, Houston PE, Wang WC, et al. Hydroxyurea and growth in young children with sickle cell disease. *Pediatrics*. Sep 2014;134(3):465-72. doi:10.1542/peds.2014-0917

79. Hyacinth HI, Sugihara CL, Spencer TL, Archer DR, Shih AY. Higher prevalence of spontaneous cerebral vasculopathy and cerebral infarcts in a mouse model of sickle cell disease. *J Cereb Blood Flow Metab*. Feb 2019;39(2):342-351. doi:10.1177/0271678X17732275

80. Sorby-Adams AJ, Vink R, Turner RJ. Large animal models of stroke and traumatic brain injury as translational tools. *Am J Physiol Regul Integr Comp Physiol*. Aug 1 2018;315(2):R165-R190. doi:10.1152/ajpregu.00163.2017

81. Xiao L, Andemariam B, Taxel P, et al. Loss of Bone in Sickle Cell Trait and Sickle Cell Disease Female Mice Is Associated With Reduced IGF-1 in Bone and Serum. *Endocrinology*. Aug 2016;157(8):3036-46. doi:10.1210/en.2015-2001

82. Costa CP, Thomaz EB, Souza Sde F. Association between Sickle Cell Anemia and Pulp Necrosis. *J Endod*. Feb 2013;39(2):177-81. doi:10.1016/j.joen.2012.10.024

83. Altaii M, Broberg M, Cathro P, Richards L. Standardisation of sheep model for endodontic regeneration/revitalisation research. *Arch Oral Biol*. May 2016;65:87-94. doi:10.1016/j.archoralbio.2016.01.008

84. Altaii M, Richards L, Rossi-Fedele G. Histological assessment of regenerative endodontic treatment in animal studies with different scaffolds: A systematic review. *Dent Traumatol*. Aug 2017;33(4):235-244. doi:10.1111/edt.12338

85. Sellers RS. Translating Mouse Models. *Toxicol Pathol*. Jan 2017;45(1):134-145. doi:10.1177/0192623316675767

86. Toledo SLO, Guedes JVM, Alpoim PN, Rios DRA, de BPM. Sickle cell disease: Hemostatic and inflammatory changes, and their interrelation. *Clin Chim Acta*. Feb 27 2019;doi:10.1016/j.cca.2019.02.026

87. Garrido VT, Proenca-Ferreira R, Dominical VM, et al. Elevated plasma levels and platelet-associated expression of the pro-thrombotic and pro-inflammatory protein, TNFSF14 (LIGHT), in sickle cell disease. *Br J Haematol*. Sep 2012;158(6):788-97. doi:10.1111/j.1365-2141.2012.09218.x

88. Laurance S, Pellay FX, Dossou-Yovo OP, et al. Hydroxycarbamide stimulates the production of proinflammatory cytokines by endothelial cells: relevance to sickle cell disease. *Pharmacogenet Genomics*. Apr 2010;20(4):257-68. doi:10.1097/FPC.0b013e32833854d6

89. McCall MK, Stanfill AG, Skrovanek E, Pforr JR, Wesmiller SW, Conley YP. Symptom Science: Omics Supports Common Biological Underpinnings Across Symptoms. *Biol Res Nurs*. Mar 2018;20(2):183-191. doi:10.1177/1099800417751069

90. Guenet JL. The mouse genome. *Genome Res*. Dec 2005;15(12):1729-40. doi:10.1101/gr.3728305

91. Poletti V, Urbinati F, Charrier S, et al. Pre-clinical Development of a Lentiviral Vector Expressing the Anti-sickling betaAS3 Globin for Gene Therapy for Sickle Cell Disease. *Mol Ther Methods Clin Dev*. Dec 14 2018;11:167-179. doi:10.1016/j.omtm.2018.10.014

92. Devadasan D, Sun CW, Westin ER, et al. Bone Marrow Transplantation after Nonmyeloablative Treosulfan Conditioning Is Curative in a Murine Model of Sickle Cell Disease. *Biol Blood Marrow Transplant*. Aug 2018;24(8):1554-1562. doi:10.1016/j.bbmt.2018.04.011

93. Vigil GD, Adami AJ, Ahmed T, et al. Label-free and depth resolved optical sectioning of iron-complex deposits in sickle cell disease splenic tissue by multiphoton microscopy. *J Biomed Opt*. Jun 2015;20(6):066001. doi:10.1117/1.JBO.20.6.066001

94. Pestina TI, Hargrove PW, Zhao H, et al. Amelioration of murine sickle cell disease by nonablative conditioning and gamma-globin gene-corrected bone marrow cells. *Mol Ther Methods Clin Dev*. 2015;2:15045. doi:10.1038/mtm.2015.45

95. Rogers FA, Lin SS, Hegan DC, Krause DS, Glazer PM. Targeted gene modification of hematopoietic progenitor cells in mice following systemic administration of a PNA-peptide conjugate. *Mol Ther*. Jan 2012;20(1):109-18. doi:10.1038/mt.2011.163

96. Pestina TI, Hargrove PW, Jay D, Gray JT, Boyd KM, Persons DA. Correction of murine sickle cell disease using gamma-globin lentiviral vectors to mediate high-level expression of fetal hemoglobin. *Mol Ther*. Feb 2009;17(2):245-52. doi:10.1038/mt.2008.259

97. Levasseur DN, Ryan TM, Pawlik KM, Townes TM. Correction of a mouse model of sickle cell disease: lentiviral/antisickling beta-globin gene transduction of unmobilized, purified hematopoietic stem cells. *Blood*. Dec 15 2003;102(13):4312-9. doi:10.1182/blood-2003-04-1251

98. Kean LS, Durham MM, Adams AB, et al. A cure for murine sickle cell disease through stable mixed chimerism and tolerance induction after nonmyeloablative conditioning and major histocompatibility complex-mismatched bone marrow transplantation. *Blood*. Mar 1 2002;99(5):1840-9. doi:10.1182/blood.v99.5.1840

99. Iannone R, Luznik L, Engstrom LW, et al. Effects of mixed hematopoietic chimerism in a mouse model of bone

marrow transplantation for sickle cell anemia. *Blood*. Jun 15 2001; 97(12):3960-5. doi:10.1182/blood.v97.12.3960.

100. Chen W, Wu X, Levasseur DN, et al. Lentiviral vector transduction of hematopoietic stem cells that mediate long-term reconstitution of lethally irradiated mice. *Stem Cells*. 2000;18(5):352-9. doi:10.1634/stemcells.18-5-352

101. Tang FHF, Staquicini FI, Teixeira AAR, et al. A ligand motif enables differential vascular targeting of endothelial junctions between brain and retina. *Proc Natl Acad Sci U S A*. Feb 5 2019; 116(6):2300-2305. doi:10.1073/pnas.1809483116

102. Shah M, Cabrera-Ghayouri S, Christie LA, Held KS, Viswanath V. Translational Preclinical Pharmacologic Disease Models for Ophthalmic Drug Development. *Pharm Res*. Feb 25 2019; 36(4):58. doi:10.1007/s11095-019-2588-5

103. Haider S, Sadiq SN, Moore D, Price MJ, Nirantharakumar K. Prognostic prediction models for diabetic retinopathy progression: a systematic review. *Eye (Lond)*. May 2019;33(5):702-713. doi:10.1038/s41433-018-0322-x

104. Lutty GA, McLeod DS, Pachnis A, Costantini F, Fabry ME, Nagel RL. Retinal and choroidal neovascularization in a transgenic mouse model of sickle cell disease. *Am J Pathol*. Aug 1994; 145(2):490-7.

105. Promsote W, Powell FL, Veean S, et al. Oral Monomethyl Fumarate Therapy Ameliorates Retinopathy in a Humanized Mouse Model of Sickle Cell Disease. *Antioxid Redox Signal*. Dec 10 2016;25(17):921-935. doi:10.1089/ars.2016.6638

106. McLeod DS, Goldberg MF, Lutty GA. Dual-perspective analysis of vascular formations in sickle cell retinopathy. *Arch Ophthalmol*. Sep 1993;111(9):1234-45. doi:10.1001/archopht.1993.01090090086026

107. Lutty GA, McLeod DS. Phosphatase enzyme histochemistry for studying vascular hierarchy, pathology, and endothelial cell dysfunction in retina and choroid. *Vision Res*. Dec 2005; 45(28):3504-11. doi:10.1016/j.visres.2005.08.022

108. Gupta K, Chen C, Lutty GA, Hebbel RP. Morphine promotes neovascularizing retinopathy in sickle transgeneic mice. *Blood Adv*. Apr 9 2019;3(7):1073-1083. doi:10.1182/bloodadvances.2018026898

109. Lessell S, Kuwabara T. Phosphatase Histochemistry of the Eye. *Arch Ophthalmol*. Jun 1964;71:851-60. doi:10.1001/archopht.1964.00970010867015

110. Lutty GA, McLeod DS. A new technique for visualization of the human retinal vasculature. *Arch Ophthalmol*. Feb 1992;110(2): 267-76. doi:10.1001/archopht.1992.01080140123039

111. Marcus AJ, Broekman MJ, Drosopoulos JH, et al. The endothelial cell ecto-ADPase responsible for inhibition of platelet function is CD39. *J Clin Invest*. Mar 15 1997;99(6):1351-60. doi:10.1172/JCI119294

112. Lutty GA, Cao J, McLeod DS. Relationship of polymorphonuclear leukocytes to capillary dropout in the human diabetic choroid. *Am J Pathol*. Sep 1997;151(3):707-14.

113. Kunz Mathews M, McLeod DS, Merges C, Cao J, Lutty GA. Neutrophils and leucocyte adhesion molecules in sickle cell retinopathy. *Br J Ophthalmol*. Jun 2002;86(6):684-90. doi:10.1136/bjo.86.6.684

114. Gupta K, Kshirsagar S, Chang L, et al. Morphine stimulates angiogenesis by activating proangiogenic and survival-promoting signaling and promotes breast tumor growth. *Cancer Res*. Aug 1 2002;62(15):4491-8.

115. Chen C, Farooqui M, Gupta K. Morphine stimulates vascular endothelial growth factor-like signaling in mouse retinal

116. Luk K, Boatman S, Johnson KN, et al. Influence of morphine on pericyte-endothelial interaction: implications for antiangiogenic therapy. *J Oncol*. 2012;2012:458385. doi:10.1155/2012/458385

117. Klein LM, Lavker RM, Matis WL, Murphy GF. Degranulation of human mast cells induces an endothelial antigen central to leukocyte adhesion. *Proc Natl Acad Sci U S A*. Nov 1989; 86(22):8972-6. doi:10.1073/pnas.86.22.8972

118. Walsh LJ, Trinchieri G, Waldorf HA, Whitaker D, Murphy GF. Human dermal mast cells contain and release tumor necrosis factor alpha, which induces endothelial leukocyte adhesion molecule 1. *Proc Natl Acad Sci U S A*. May 15 1991;88(10):4220-4. doi:10.1073/pnas.88.10.4220

119. Singleton PA, Moreno-Vinasco L, Sammani S, Wanderling SL, Moss J, Garcia JG. Attenuation of vascular permeability by methylnaltrexone: role of mOP-R and S1P3 transactivation. *Am J Respir Cell Mol Biol*. Aug 2007;37(2):222-31. doi:10.1165/rcmb.2006-0327OC

120. Naik RP, Derebail VK. The spectrum of sickle hemoglobin-related nephropathy: from sickle cell disease to sickle trait. *Expert Rev Hematol*. Dec 2017;10(12):1087-1094. doi:10.1080/17474086.2017.1395279

121. Kasztan M, Fox BM, Speed JS, et al. Long-Term Endothelin-A Receptor Antagonism Provides Robust Renal Protection in Humanized Sickle Cell Disease Mice. *J Am Soc Nephrol*. Aug 2017; 28(8):2443-2458. doi:10.1681/asn.2016070711

122. Heerspink HJL, Parving HH, Andress DL, et al. Atrasentan and renal events in patients with type 2 diabetes and chronic kidney disease (SONAR): a double-blind, randomised, placebo-controlled trial. *Lancet*. 05 2019;393(10184):1937-1947. doi:10.1016/S0140-6736(19)30772-X

123. Nasimuzzaman M, Arumugam PI, Mullins ES, et al. Elimination of the fibrinogen integrin alphaMbeta2-binding motif improves renal pathology in mice with sickle cell anemia. *Blood Adv*. May 14 2019;3(9):1519-1532. doi:10.1182/bloodadvances.2019032342

124. Gupta M, Msambichaka L, Ballas SK, Gupta K. Morphine for the treatment of pain in sickle cell disease. *ScientificWorldJournal*. 2015;2015:540154. doi:10.1155/2015/540154

125. Weber ML, Vang D, Velho PE, et al. Morphine promotes renal pathology in sickle mice. *International journal of nephrology and renovascular disease*. 2012 2012;5:109-118. doi:10.2147/IJNRD.S33813

126. Weber ML, Chen C, Li Y, et al. Morphine stimulates platelet-derived growth factor receptor-beta signalling in mesangial cells in vitro and transgenic sickle mouse kidney in vivo. *Br J Anaesth*. Dec 2013;111(6):1004-12. doi:10.1093/bja/aet221

127. Stankovic Stojanovic K, Thiolière B, Garandeau E, Lecomte I, Bachmeyer C, Lionnet F. Chronic myeloid leukaemia and sickle cell disease: could imatinib prevent vaso-occlusive crisis? *British Journal of Haematology*. 2011/10/01 2011;155(2):271-272. doi:10.1111/j.1365-2141.2011.08670.x

128. Murphy M, Close J, Lottenberg R, Rajasekhar A. Effectiveness of Imatinib Therapy for Sickle Cell Anemia and Chronic Myeloid Leukemia. *The American Journal of the Medical Sciences*. 2014/03/01 2014;347(3):254-255. doi:10.1097/MAJ.0000000000000228

129. Khaibullina A, Adjei EA, Afangbedji N, et al. RON kinase inhibition reduces renal endothelial injury in sickle cell disease mice. *Haematologica*. May 2018;103(5):787-798. doi:10.3324/haematol.2017.180992

130. Taylor C, Kasztan M, Tao B, Pollock JS, Pollock DM. Combined hydroxyurea and ETA receptor blockade reduces renal injury in the humanized sickle cell mouse. *Acta Physiol (Oxf)*. Feb 2019;225(2):e13178. doi:10.1111/apha.13178

131. Vercellotti GM, Dalmasso AP, Schaid TR, Jr., et al. Critical role of C5a in sickle cell disease. *Am J Hematol*. Mar 2019;94(3): 327-337. doi:10.1002/ajh.25384

132. Abid S, Kebe K, Houssaïni A, et al. New Nitric Oxide Donor NCX 1443: Therapeutic Effects on Pulmonary Hypertension in the SAD Mouse Model of Sickle Cell Disease. *J Cardiovasc Pharmacol*. 05 2018;71(5):283-292. doi:10.1097/FJC.0000000000000570

133. Kalra VK, Zhang S, Malik P, Tahara SM. Placenta growth factor mediated gene regulation in sickle cell disease. *Blood Rev*. Jan 2018;32(1):61-70. doi:10.1016/j.blre.2017.08.008

134. Bivalacqua TJ, Musicki B, Hsu LL, Gladwin MT, Burnett AL, Champion HC. Establishment of a transgenic sickle-cell mouse model to study the pathophysiology of priapism. *J Sex Med*. Sep 2009;6(9):2494-504. doi:10.1111/j.1743-6109.2009.01359.x

135. Sopko NA, Matsui H, Hannan JL, et al. Subacute Hemolysis in Sickle Cell Mice Causes Priapism Secondary to NO Imbalance and PDE5 Dysregulation. *J Sex Med*. Sep 2015;12(9):1878-85. doi:10.1111/jsm.12976

136. Silva FH, Karakus S, Musicki B, et al. Beneficial Effect of the Nitric Oxide Donor Compound 3-(1,3-Dioxoisoindolin-2-yl) Benzyl Nitrate on Dysregulated Phosphodiesterase 5, NADPH Oxidase, and Nitrosative Stress in the Sickle Cell Mouse Penis: Implication for Priapism Treatment. *J Pharmacol Exp Ther*. Nov 2016;359(2):230-237. doi:10.1124/jpet.116.235473

137. Halabi-Tawil M, Lionnet F, Girot R, Bachmeyer C, Lévy PP, Aractingi S. Sickle cell leg ulcers: a frequently disabling complication and a marker of severity. *Br J Dermatol*. Feb 2008; 158(2):339-44. doi:10.1111/j.1365-2133.2007.08323.x

138. Nguyen VT, Nassar D, Batteux F, Raymond K, Tharaux PL, Aractingi S. Delayed Healing of Sickle Cell Ulcers Is due to Impaired Angiogenesis and CXCL12 Secretion in Skin Wounds. *J Invest Dermatol*. Feb 2016;136(2):497-506. doi:10.1016/j.jid.2015.11.005

139. Delaney KM, Axelrod KC, Buscetta A, et al. Leg ulcers in sickle cell disease: current patterns and practices. *Hemoglobin*. 2013;37(4):325-32. doi:10.3109/03630269.2013.789968

140. Rodrigues M, Bonham CA, Minniti CP, Gupta K, Longaker MT, Gurtner GC. Iron Chelation with Transdermal Deferoxamine Accelerates Healing of Murine Sickle Cell Ulcers. *Adv Wound Care (New Rochelle)*. Oct 1 2018;7(10):323-332. doi:10.1089/wound.2018.0789

141. Oksenberg D, Dufu K, Patel MP, et al. GBT440 increases haemoglobin oxygen affinity, reduces sickling and prolongs RBC half-life in a murine model of sickle cell disease. *Br J Haematol*. Oct 2016;175(1):141-53. doi:10.1111/bjh.14214

142. Vinjamur DS, Bauer DE, Orkin SH. Recent progress in understanding and manipulating haemoglobin switching for the haemoglobinopathies. *Br J Haematol*. Mar 2018;180(5):630-643. doi:10.1111/bjh.15038

143. Fox BM, Kasztan M. Endothelin receptor antagonists in sickle cell disease: A promising new therapeutic approach. *Life Sci*. Aug 15 2016;159:15-19. doi:10.1016/j.lfs.2016.04.001

144. Oder E, Safo MK, Abdulmalik O, Kato GJ. New developments in anti-sickling agents: can drugs directly prevent the polymerization of sickle haemoglobin in vivo? *Br J Haematol*. Oct 2016; 175(1):24-30. doi:10.1111/bjh.14264

145. Choi E, Branch C, Cui MH, et al. No evidence for cell activation or brain vaso-occlusion with plerixafor mobilization in sickle cell mice. *Blood Cells Mol Dis*. Mar 2016;57:67-70. doi:10.1016/j.bcmd.2015.12.008

146. Sampson M, Archibong AE, Powell A, et al. Perturbation of the developmental potential of preimplantation mouse embryos by hydroxyurea. *Int J Environ Res Public Health*. May 2010;7(5):2033-44. doi:10.3390/ijerph7052033

147. Walker AL, Lancaster CS, Finkelstein D, Ware RE, Sparreboom A. Organic anion transporting polypeptide 1B transporters modulate hydroxyurea pharmacokinetics. *Am J Physiol Cell Physiol*. Dec 15 2013;305(12):C1223-9. doi:10.1152/ajpcell.00232.2013

148. Lopes FC, Ferreira R, Albuquerque DM, et al. In vitro and in vivo anti-angiogenic effects of hydroxyurea. *Microvasc Res*. Jul 2014; 94:106-13. doi:10.1016/j.mvr.2014.05.009

149. Park F, Soni H, Pressly JD, Adebiyi A. Acute hydroxyurea treatment reduces tubular damage following bilateral ischemia-reperfusion injury in a mouse model of sickle cell disease. *Biochem Biophys Res Commun*. Jul 12 2019;515(1):72-76. doi:10.1016/j.bbrc.2019.05.116

150. Brandow AM, Panepinto JA. Clinical Interpretation of Quantitative Sensory Testing as a Measure of Pain Sensitivity in Patients With Sickle Cell Disease. *Journal of pediatric hematology/oncology*. 2016/05 2016;38(4):288-293. doi:10.1097/MPH.0000000000000532

151. Campbell CM, Carroll CP, Kiley K, et al. Quantitative sensory testing and pain-evoked cytokine reactivity: comparison of patients with sickle cell disease to healthy matched controls. *Pain*. 2016/04 2016;157(4):949-956. doi:10.1097/j.pain.0000000000000473

152. Ezenwa MO, Molokie RE, Wang ZJ, et al. Safety and Utility of Quantitative Sensory Testing among Adults with Sickle Cell Disease: Indicators of Neuropathic Pain? *Pain practice : the official journal of World Institute of Pain*. 2016/03 2016;16(3):282-293. doi:10.1111/papr.12279

153. O'leary JD, Crawford MW, Odame I, Shorten GD, McGrath PA. Thermal pain and sensory processing in children with sickle cell disease. *The Clinical journal of pain*. 2014 2014;30(3):244-250. doi:10.1097/AJP.0b013e318292a38e.

154. Jacob E, Chan VW, Hodge C, Zeltzer L, Zurakowski D, Sethna NF. Sensory and thermal quantitative testing in children with sickle cell disease. *Journal of pediatric hematology/oncology*. 2015 2015;37(3):185-189. doi:10.1097/MPH.0000000000000214.

155. Brandow AM, Stucky CL, Hillery CA, Hoffmann RG, Panepinto JA. Patients with Sickle Cell Disease Have Increased Sensitivity to Cold and Heat. *American journal of hematology*. 2013/01/31 2013;88(1):37-43. doi:10.1002/ajh.23341

156. Bakshi N, Lukombo I, Shnol H, Belfer I, Krishnamurti L. Psychological Characteristics and Pain Frequency Are Associated With Experimental Pain Sensitivity in Pediatric Patients With Sickle Cell Disease. *The Journal of Pain*. 2017/10/01 2017;18(10): 1216-1228. doi:10.1016/j.jpain.2017.05.005

157. Franck LS, Treadwell M, Jacob E, Vichinsky E. Assessment of Sickle Cell Pain in Children and Young Adults Using the Adolescent Pediatric Pain Tool. *Journal of Pain and Symptom Management*. 2002/02/01 2002;23(2):114-120. doi:10.1016/S0885-3924(01)00407-9

158. Brandow AM, Farley RA, Dasgupta M, Hoffmann RG, Panepinto JA. The use of neuropathic pain drugs in children with sickle cell disease is associated with older age, female sex, and longer length of hospital stay. *Journal of pediatric*

hematology/oncology. 2015/01 2015;37(1):10-15. doi:10.1097/MPH.0000000000000265

159. Ruta NS, Ballas SK. The Opioid Drug Epidemic and Sickle Cell Disease: Guilt by Association. *Pain Medicine.* 2016/05/05 2016;17(10):1793-1798. doi:10.1093/pm/pnw074

160. Ballas SK. Comorbidities in aging patients with sickle cell disease. *Clin Hemorheol Microcirc.* 2018;68(2-3):129-145. doi:10.3233/CH-189003

161. Brandow AM, Wandersee NJ, Dasgupta M, et al. Substance P is increased in patients with sickle cell disease and associated with haemolysis and hydroxycarbamide use. *British journal of haematology.* 2016/10/19 2016;175(2):237-245. doi:10.1111/bjh.14300

162. Michaels LA, Ohene-Frempong K, Zhao H, Douglas SD. Serum Levels of Substance P Are Elevated in Patients With Sickle Cell Disease and Increase Further During Vaso-Occlusive Crisis. *Blood.* 1998/11/01 1998;92(9):3148 LP - 3151.

163. Vang D, Paul JA, Nguyen J, et al. Small-molecule nociceptin receptor agonist ameliorates mast cell activation and pain in sickle mice. *Haematologica.* 2015;100(12):1517-1525. doi:10.3324/haematol.2015.128736

164. Hillery CA, Kerstein PC, Vilceanu D, et al. Transient receptor potential vanilloid 1 mediates pain in mice with severe sickle cell disease. *Blood.* 2011/09/22 2011;118(12):3376-3383. doi:10.1182/blood-2010-12-327429

165. Zappia KJ, Garrison SR, Hillery CA, Stucky CL. Cold hypersensitivity increases with age in mice with sickle cell disease. *Pain.* 2014/12/03 2014;155(12):2476-2485. doi:10.1016/j.pain.2014.05.030

166. Cataldo G, Rajput S, Gupta K, Simone DA. Sensitization of nociceptive spinal neurons contributes to pain in a transgenic model of sickle cell disease. *Pain.* 2015/04 2015;156(4):722-730. doi:10.1097/j.pain.0000000000000104

167. Darbari DS, Hampson JP, Ichesco E, et al. Frequency of Hospitalizations for Pain and Association With Altered Brain Network Connectivity in Sickle Cell Disease. *J Pain.* Nov 2015;16(11):1077-86. doi:10.1016/j.jpain.2015.07.005

168. Darbari DS, Vaughan KJ, Roskom K, et al. Central sensitization associated with low fetal hemoglobin levels in adults with sickle cell anemia. *Scandinavian journal of pain.* 2017/10 2017;17:279-286. doi:10.1016/j.sjpain.2017.08.001

169. Case M, Zhang H, Mundahl J, et al. Characterization of functional brain activity and connectivity using EEG and fMRI in patients with sickle cell disease. *Neuroimage Clin.* 2017;14:1-17. doi:10.1016/j.nicl.2016.12.024

170. Paul JA, Aich A, Abrahante JE, et al. Transcriptomic analysis of gene signatures associated with sickle pain. *Scientific Data.* 2017/05/16 2017;4:170051. doi:10.1038/sdata.2017.51

171. Aich A, Paul J, Lei J, Wang Y, Bagchi A, Gupta K. Regulation of Elastase By SerpinA3N Contributes to Pain in Sickle Cell Disease. *Blood.* 2016;128(22):858-858. doi:10.1182/blood.V128.22.858.858

172. He Y, Chen Y, Tian X, et al. CaMKIIalpha underlies spontaneous and evoked pain behaviors in Berkeley sickle cell transgenic mice. *Pain.* Dec 2016;157(12):2798-2806. doi:10.1097/j.pain.0000000000000704

173. Molokie RE, Wilkie DJ, Wittert H, et al. Mechanism-Driven Phase I Translational Study of Trifluoperazine in Adults with Sickle Cell Disease. *European journal of pharmacology.* 2014/01/15 2014;723:419-424. doi:10.1016/j.ejphar.2013.10.062

174. Lutz BM, Wu S, Gu X, et al. Endothelin type A receptors mediate pain in a mouse model of sickle cell disease.

Haematologica. 2018/07 2018;103(7):1124-1135. doi:10.3324/haematol.2017.187013

175. Argueta DA, Aich A, Lei J, et al. Downregulation of Sprr1a Contributes to the Pathobiology of Sickle Cell Disease. *Blood.* 2019;134(Supplement_1):75-75. doi:10.1182/blood-2019-129004

176. Aich A, Jones MK, Gupta K. Pain and sickle cell disease. *Current Opinion in Hematology.* 2019 2019;26(3):131-138. doi:10.1097/MOH.0000000000000491.

177. Gupta K, Harvima IT. Mast cell-neural interactions contribute to pain and itch. *Immunol Rev.* Mar 2018;282(1):168-187. doi:10.1111/imr.12622

178. Tran H, Mittal A, Sagi V, et al. Mast Cells Induce Blood Brain Barrier Damage in SCD by Causing Endoplasmic Reticulum Stress in the Endothelium. *Frontiers in Cellular Neuroscience.* 2019 2019;13:56. doi:10.3389/fncel.2019.00056. eCollection 2019.

179. Kuei N, Patel N, Xu H, et al. Characteristics and Potential Biomarkers for Chronic Pain in Patients with Sickle Cell Disease. *Blood.* 2015;126(23):986-986. doi:10.1182/blood.V126.23.986.986

180. Savage WJ, Barron-Casella E, Fu Z, et al. Plasma glial fibrillary acidic protein levels in children with sickle cell disease. *American journal of hematology.* 2011/05 2011;86(5):427-429. doi:10.1002/ajh.21995

181. Close JL, Lottenberg R. Effectiveness of Imatinib Therapy for a Patient with Sickle Cell Anemia and Chronic Myelocytic Leukemia. *Blood.* 2009/11/20 2009;114(22):2559 LP - 2559.

182. Lard LR, Mul FPJ, Haas M, Roos D, Duits AJ. Neutrophil activation in sickle cell disease. *Journal of Leukocyte Biology.* 1999/09/01 1999;66(3):411-415. doi:10.1002/jlb.66.3.411

183. Afshar-Kharghan V, Thiagarajan P. Leukocyte adhesion and thrombosis. *Curr Opin Hematol.* Jan 2006;13(1):34-9. doi:10.1097/01.moh.0000190107.54790.de

184. Keegan PM, Surapaneni S, Platt MO. Sickle cell disease activates peripheral blood mononuclear cells to induce cathepsins k and v activity in endothelial cells. *Anemia.* 2012;2012:201781. doi:10.1155/2012/201781

185. Carvalho MOS, Souza ALCS, Carvalho MB, et al. Evaluation of Alpha-1 Antitrypsin Levels and SERPINA1 Gene Polymorphisms in Sickle Cell Disease. *Frontiers in Immunology.* 2017/11/06 2017;8:1491. doi:10.3389/fimmu.2017.01491

186. Schimmel M, Nur E, Biemond BJ, et al. Nucleosomes and neutrophil activation in sickle cell disease painful crisis. *Haematologica.* 2013/11/15 2013;98(11):1797-1803. doi:10.3324/haematol.2013.088021

187. Valverde Y, Benson B, Gupta M, Gupta K. Spinal glial activation and oxidative stress are alleviated by treatment with curcumin or coenzyme Q in sickle mice. *Haematologica.* 2016/02 2016;101(2):e44-e47. doi:10.3324/haematol.2015.137489

188. Thakur AS, Littaru GP, Moesgaard S, Dan Sindberg C, Khan Y, Singh CM. Hematological Parameters and RBC TBARS Level of Q 10 Supplemented Tribal Sickle Cell Patients: A Hospital Based Study. *Indian journal of clinical biochemistry : IJCB.* 2013/04 2013;28(2):185-188. doi:10.1007/s12291-012-0277-9

189. Ballas SK. Use of Marijuana in Patients with Sickle Cell Disease Increased the Frequency of Hospitalization for Acute Painful Vaso-Occlusive Crises. *Blood.* 2016;128(22):2498-2498. doi:10.1182/blood.V128.22.2498.2498

190. Abrams DI, Couey P, Dixit N, et al. Effect of Inhaled Cannabis for Pain in Adults With Sickle Cell Disease: A Randomized Clinical Trial. *JAMA Netw Open.* Jul 2020;3(7):e2010874. doi:10.1001/jamanetworkopen.2020.10874

191. Starkey ML, Davies M, Yip PK, et al. Expression of the regeneration-associated protein SPRR1A in primary sensory neurons and spinal cord of the adult mouse following peripheral and central injury. *The Journal of comparative neurology.* 2009/03/01 2009;513(1):51-68. doi:10.1002/cne.21944

192. Jing X, Wang T, Huang S, Glorioso JC, Albers KM. The transcription factor Sox11 promotes nerve regeneration through activation of the regeneration-associated gene Sprr1a. *Experimental neurology.* 2012/01 2012;233(1):221-232. doi:10.1016/j.expneurol.2011.10.005

193. Brandow AM, Farley RA, Panepinto JA. Neuropathic Pain in Patients with Sickle Cell Disease. *Pediatric blood & cancer.* 2014/03/26 2014;61(3):512-517. doi:10.1002/pbc.24838

194. Brandow AM, Zappia KJ, Stucky CL. Sickle cell disease: a natural model of acute and chronic pain. *Pain.* 2017/04 2017;158 Suppl(Suppl 1):S79-S84. doi:10.1097/j.pain.0000000000000824

195. Sark MW, Fischer DF, de Meijer E, van de Putte P, Backendorf C. AP-1 and ets transcription factors regulate the expression of the human SPRR1A keratinocyte terminal differentiation marker. *J Biol Chem.* Sep 18 1998;273(38):24683-92. doi:10.1074/jbc.273.38.24683

196. Lu K, Cheng M-CJ, Ge X, et al. A retrospective review of acupuncture use for the treatment of pain in sickle cell disease patients: descriptive analysis from a single institution. *The Clinical journal of pain.* 2014/09 2014;30(9):825-830. doi:10.1097/AJP.0000000000000036

197. Wang Y, Lei J, Gupta M, et al. Electroacupuncture in conscious free-moving mice reduces pain by ameliorating peripheral and central nociceptive mechanisms. *Scientific Reports.* 2016/09/30 2016;6:34493. doi:10.1038/srep34493.

198. Wang Y, Lei J, Jha RK, Kiven S, Gupta K. Substance P modulates electroacupuncture analgesia in humanized mice with sickle cell disease. *Journal of pain research.* 2019/08/01 2019;12:2419-2426. doi:10.2147/JPR.S210196

199. Tran H, Sagi V, Jarrett S, Badgaiyan R, Gupta K. Diet and companionship stimulate affective modulation of pain via serotonergic mechanisms. Under Review

200. Khaleel M, Puliyel M, Shah P, et al. Individuals with sickle cell disease have a significantly greater vasoconstriction response to thermal pain than controls and have significant vasoconstriction in response to anticipation of pain. *American journal of hematology.* 2017/11 2017;92(11):1137-1145. doi:10.1002/ajh.24858

201. Bhatt RR, Martin SR, Evans S, et al. The effect of hypnosis on pain and peripheral blood flow in sickle-cell disease: a pilot study. *Journal of pain research.* 2017/07/14 2017;10:1635-1644. doi:10.2147/JPR.S131859

202. Bennewitz MF, Watkins SC, Sundd P. Quantitative intravital two-photon excitation microscopy reveals absence of pulmonary vaso-occlusion in unchallenged Sickle Cell Disease mice. *Intravital.* Jul 7 2014;3(2):e29748. doi:10.4161/intv.29748

203. Bakeer N, James J, Roy S, et al. Sickle cell anemia mice develop a unique cardiomyopathy with restrictive physiology. *Proc Natl Acad Sci U S A.* Aug 30 2016;113(35):E5182-91. doi:10.1073/pnas.1600311113

204. Cahill LS, Gazdzinski LM, Tsui AK, et al. Functional and anatomical evidence of cerebral tissue hypoxia in young sickle cell anemia mice. *J Cereb Blood Flow Metab.* Mar 2017;37(3):994-1005. doi:10.1177/0271678X16649194

205. Chatel B, Messonnier LA, Bendahan D. Exacerbated in vivo metabolic changes suggestive of a spontaneous muscular vaso-occlusive crisis in exercising muscle of a sickle cell mouse. *Blood Cells Mol Dis.* Jun 2017;65:56-59. doi:10.1016/j.bcmd.2017.05.006

206. Cui MH, Suzuka SM, Branch NA, et al. Brain neurochemical and hemodynamic findings in the NY1DD mouse model of mild sickle cell disease. *NMR Biomed.* May 2017;30(5) doi:10.1002/nbm.3692

207. Wang Y, Wang X, Chen W, Gupta K, Zhu XH. Functional MRI BOLD response in sickle mice with hyperalgesia. *Blood Cells Mol Dis.* Jun 2017;65:81-85. doi:10.1016/j.bcmd.2017.03.005

208. Fard N, Saffari A, Emami G, Hofer S, Kauczor HU, Mehrabi A. Acute respiratory distress syndrome induction by pulmonary ischemia-reperfusion injury in large animal models. *J Surg Res.* Jun 15 2014;189(2):274-84. doi:10.1016/j.jss.2014.02.034

Pharmacologic Induction of Fetal Hemoglobin

Authors: *Abdullah Kutlar, Vivien A. Sheehan*

Chapter Outline

Overview

The presence of fetal hemoglobin (HbF, $\alpha_2\gamma_2$) is known to reduce the clinical complications of sickle cell disease (SCD). Pharmacologic agents able to induce HbF have been sought after for decades. Agnostic drug screens have been unsuccessful, and progress in identifying novel HbF-inducing agents was slowed by our limited understanding of γ-globin regulation. Our understanding of γ-globin induction was increased significantly by an unbiased genome-wide association study (GWAS) approach, which identified variants in the transcription factor B-cell lymphoma/leukemia 11A (BCL11A) and regulatory elements within the intergenic region HBS1L-MYB as associated with HbF levels. Functional studies subsequently established the roles of BCL11A, MYB, and KLF1 in γ-globin repression, and disruption of the BCL11A erythroid enhancer element is now a gene therapy target in >1 clinical trial. Gene therapy may provide a cure for SCD, either through HbF induction or correction of the causative mutation, but several technical and safety hurdles must be overcome before this therapy can be offered widely, particularly in low-resource countries, where 99% of individuals with SCD reside. Pharmacologic therapies to treat SCD are still needed, and hydroxyurea, developed for use in SCD almost 3 decades ago, remains the only widely used pharmacologic HbF inducer.

Hemoglobin Structure

Hemoglobin is composed of 2 α-like globin chains and 2 β-like globin chains, with a heme moiety in the middle. In humans, the β-globin gene locus is comprised of 5 different genes (*HBE1*, *HBG1*, *HBG2*, *HBD*, and *HBB*), all located on chromosome 11. The α-globin gene locus, located on chromosome 16, is composed of 3 genes (*HBZ*, *HBA1*, and *HBA2*). Early in fetal development, expression of embryonic globin gene (*HBE1*) declines and is replaced by expression of HbF (*HBG1*, *HBG2*). HbF has a higher oxygen affinity than the maternal hemoglobin A (HbA). After birth, in normal individuals, HbF is no longer needed and begins to be replaced by HbA, or adult hemoglobin ($\alpha_2\beta_2$).[1] HbF typically makes up <5% of the total hemoglobin at 6 months of age and becomes undetectable by 2 years of age.[2] Although all vertebrates studied have a switch from primitive to definitive erythropoiesis, only old world primates, humans, and some ruminants make HbF; this limits the availability of animal models in which to study hemoglobin switching and screen compounds to alter or reverse the switch from HbF to HbA.

Importance of HbF in Sickle Cell Anemia Pathophysiology

Sickle cell anemia (SCA) is caused by the autosomal recessive inheritance of a single base substitution (A-T) in the first exon of the β-globin gene (*HBB*). This substitution results in the replacement of a negatively charged, hydrophilic amino acid, glutamic acid, by a hydrophobic amino acid, valine, at position 6 [*HBB*; glu(E)6val(A); GAG-GTG; rs334]. This substitution is damaging, significantly altering the function of the protein. The hemoglobin tetramers that harbor the mutated β-globin chains polymerize and aggregate upon deoxygenation, changing the flexible, soft discoid red blood cells into stiff, sickle-shaped cells. This morphologic change in the red blood cell has given the disease and its causative mutation their name. The resulting hemoglobin is called hemoglobin S (HbS).

The presence of HbF in a cell containing HbS profoundly delays the polymerization of HbS that occurs under deoxygenated conditions. Mixtures of purified HbF and HbS have a much higher gelling concentration (41.0 g/dL) compared to mixtures of HbA and HbS (32.2 g/dL). HbA_2 has an equally potent antisickling effect, with mixtures of purified HbS and HbA_2 displaying a minimal gelling concentration of 41.0 g/dL. Addition of HbF to the growing HbS polymer prevents further extension, and shorter HbS polymers are less detrimental to red cell flexibility. The HbS polymer is stabilized when the hydrophobic β 6 Val of HbS on one strand binds to a hydrophobic patch at β 85-88 on the adjacent strand. Because γ-globin has a glutamine rather than a threonine at position 87, this weakens the hydrophobic interaction and truncates the growing HbS polymer.[3] This observation was used to design an "antisickling" recombinant globin molecule (β87T→ Q) used in one of the ongoing gene therapy trials for SCD.

To clarify the terminology used in this chapter, individuals homozygous for the sickle mutation have the HbSS genotype and have SCA. *Sickle cell disease (SCD)* is a broader clinical term that includes compound heterozygotes that also sickle under physiologic conditions, such as HbSC, HbS-β thalassemia, and other SCD variants. HbAS individuals are considered carriers of sickle cell trait and do not have SCD. Rare SCD genotypes, and the associated clinical phenotypes, are described in greater detail in Chapter 1.

The importance of HbF levels in SCD was first suggested by a pediatrician, Janet Watson, in 1948. She noted that SCD clinical complications were rare before the age of 1 year and connected this to the fact that HbF levels were still elevated at this early age.[4] The potential disease-modifying properties of HbF in SCD were further supported by the observation that patients with SCD who co-inherited a variant producing hereditary persistence of fetal hemoglobin (HPFH) were relatively asymptomatic. HPFH can be caused by deletions in *cis*-acting factors in the β-globin gene cluster, causing a decrease in β-globin production and leading to compensatory increases in γ-globin synthesis, mutations in the γ-globin gene (*HBG2*, *HBG1*) promoter regions that impair repression, or inheritance of an HbF-modulating quantitative trait locus, such as the *HBS1L-MYB* intergenic region (6q23) or *BCL11A* (2p16).[5,6]

There are 2 theories regarding the origin of SCD. The older theory posits that it arose spontaneously in 5 different geographic locations a few thousand years ago, whereas the newer theory contends it has a single, older origin. Five major sickle haplotypes have been described, named for the geographic locations the individuals with SCD originated from: Benin (BEN), Bantu or Central African Republic (CAR), Cameroon (CAM), Arab-Indian (ARAB), and Senegal (SEN). The SCD haplotypes were defined by restriction enzyme digest patterns. Several uncharacteristic or atypical haplotypes have also been described.[7-10] Each haplotype is associated with a characteristic average level of HbF (Arab-Indian > Senegal > Benin > Bantu); however, among patients homozygous for any haplotype, HbF levels vary. For example, in carriers of Senegal and Saudi-Indian haplotypes, the Xmn1 C-T restriction site polymorphism (158 bp upstream of *HBG2*) is associated with high HbF and γ-globin levels.[11-13] The reason for the significantly higher HbF levels in homozygotes for the Saudi-Indian haplotype compared to those with the homozygous Senegal haplotype is unclear.[14] Newer whole-genome sequencing approaches have led to a report that the sickle mutation did not arise multiple times, as the haplotype theory suggests, but instead originated in a single female individual during the Holocene Wet Phase.[15]

Although the pathophysiology of β thalassemia, characterized by insufficient or absent production of β-globin chains, is different from the pathophysiology of SCD, it can be ameliorated by induction of HbF. HbF can alleviate imbalanced non–α-globin to α-globin chain synthesis and its consequences, including ineffective erythropoiesis and hemolysis caused by precipitation of unpaired α-globin chains. More mechanistic details and studies related to HbF induction in α thalassemia can be found in Chapter 1.[16,17]

Hemoglobin Regulation

The β-like globin genes are linearly arranged in the same order they are expressed in during development: *HBE1*, *HBG1/HBG2*, and *HBD/HBB*. The 16-kb-long locus control region (LCR) located 40 to 60 kb upstream of the β-like gene cluster consists of 4 erythroid-specific DNase I hypersensitive sites made up of clusters of binding sites for transcription activators. The LCR regulates the expression of the β-like genes by direct interaction with the β-like globin promoters.[18] A complex combination of factors, including GATA1, TAL1, E2A, LMO2, and LDB1, mediates the formation of the DNA loop that brings the LCR into contact with the globin promoters.[19] β-Globin gene expression is tightly regulated by several mechanisms, including gene autonomous control, competition between the globin genes for the LCR,[20] and repressive elements that bind to the γ-δ intergenic region such as BCL11A.[21]

GWASs searching for variants associated with HbF levels in normal individuals identified BCL11A as a key negative regulator of γ-globin (*HBG1/HBG2*) expression.[22] The BCL11A protein is a C2H2-type zinc finger transcriptional repressor, with functions outside of HbF regulation in nonerythroid cells, including neuronal development. Although reduction in BCL11A expression would increase HbF, it is essential to regulate or alter only erythroid-specific aspects of *BCL11A* in order to avoid affecting neurocognitive development.[23] Fortunately, the precise binding site of BCL11A to the γ-globin promoter has been identified, and interruption of that site has been shown to induce HbF.[24]

Common variants within the intergenic region between guanosine triphosphate (GTP)-binding elongation factor *HBS1L* and myeloblastosis oncogene *MYB* on chromosome 6q are also associated with elevated HbF levels.[25] The MYB transcription factor is a key regulator of hematopoiesis, erythropoiesis, and HbF levels and modulates erythroid elements directly via activation of KLF1 and other γ-globin repressors, such as the nuclear receptors TR2/TR4, and indirectly through alterations in erythroid differentiation kinetics. Low MYB levels accelerate erythroid differentiation, leading to release of less mature erythroid progenitor cells that are larger and express more γ-globin; γ-globin is replaced by β-globin as the erythroid progenitor matures.[26]

Kruppel-like factor 1 (KLF1) is an erythroid-specific transcription factor that plays a key role in erythropoiesis. KLF1 increases β-globin production by directly activating β-globin expression through the β-globin promoter and decreases γ-globin production by directly activating its repressor, BCL11A. Some naturally occurring heterozygous *KLF1* mutations cause HPFH. Pharmacologic or genetic reduction of KLF1 levels may induce γ-globin and be a viable therapy for SCD.[27-29] Several other transcription factors have been implicated in embryonic/fetal β-like globin gene silencing. These include GATA1 in association with FOG1 and the NuRD complex, NF-E4,[30] LRF/ZBTB7A,[31] the TR2/TR4/DRED complex, and Ikaros in association with the PYR coregulatory complex.[32]

Developmental hemoglobin switching is also regulated epigenetically via several mechanisms, including alterations to higher-order chromatin structure, histone modifications, and DNA methylation. In erythroid cells from adults, the γ-globin gene exhibits increased cytosine methylation, loss of surrounding active histone modifications (eg, H3K36me3 and H3K27ac), and a decrease in chromatin accessibility compared with erythroid cells from fetuses or newborns.[33-35] γ-Globin expression is elevated by genetic or chemical inhibition of DNA methylation,[36] by the methyl-cytosine binding protein MBD2,[37] the histone arginine methyltransferase PRMT5,[38] the histone methyltransferases EHMT1 and EHMT2,[39] and histone deacetylases (HDACs). Chromatin regulators occupy the γ-globin promoter in the form of repressive complexes, including the DNA methylating enzyme DNMT3A, the lysine methyltransferase SUV4-20h1, the serine/threonine kinase CK2α, and components of NuRD[38,40] (Figure 8-1).

Lysine-specific demethylases (LSDs) also silence the γ-globin gene. LSD1 demethylates lysine 4 and lysine 9 in histone H3K4 and H3K9, respectively, decreasing DNA methylation of the γ-globin promoter.[41,42] In addition, LSD1, along with several other corepressors, is involved in TR2/TR4/DRED-mediated γ-globin gene silencing.[43] Inhibition of LSD1 results in increased γ-globin gene expression in transgenic mice, primate models, and cultured primary human erythroid cells. Small-molecule inhibitors of LSD1 can induce HbF in CD34+ cells, but because LSD1 is required for normal erythroid and myeloid maturation, its inhibition can cause adverse effects such as neutropenia.[42-44]

MicroRNAs (miRNAs) also play a role in hemoglobin switching. Lin28B proteins and their known target, the let-7 miRNA family, are involved in fetal to adult erythroid development. LIN28B has an inhibitory effect on BCL11A expression.[45] MiR-486-3p binds to the BCL11A mRNA and downregulates its expression, upregulating γ-globin gene expression in hematopoietic stem and progenitor cells (HSPCs).[46] miR-15a and miR-16-1 elevate HbF expression by acting on MYB.[47] Several other miRNAs, such as miR-221/222, miR-26b, miR-146a, and miR-96, are implicated in γ-globin regulation and hemoglobin switching, although their mechanism of action is not well characterized. Known molecular mechanisms of HbF regulation are summarized in Figure 8-1. Hemoglobin switching is described in greater detail in Chapter 1.

Pharmacologic Induction

Hydroxyurea

Hydroxyurea is the only widely used HbF inducer. It was approved for use in adult patients with SCD by the US Food and Drug Administration (FDA) in 1998 and the European Medicines Agency in 2007, and for patients with SCD aged 2 years or older in 2017. Hydroxyurea has a favorable side effect profile, daily oral dosing, and proven efficacy.[48,49] Several clinical trials have established that hydroxyurea prevents pain events and acute chest syndrome and reduces the need for

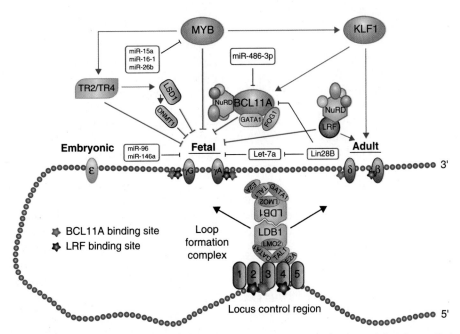

FIGURE 8-1 Regulation of fetal hemoglobin (HbF) production. *Cis* and *trans* regulators and the chromatin loop formation complex involved in hemoglobin switching. Reproduced, with permission, from Paikari A, Sheehan V. Fetal haemoglobin induction in sickle cell disease. *Br J Haematol.* 2018;180:189-200.

blood transfusions and hospitalizations.[50] A pediatric clinical trial found that hydroxyurea and phlebotomy were noninferior to chronic blood transfusions in children with SCD at higher risk for stroke, as determined by high transcranial Doppler ultrasound velocities (>200 cm/s).[51]

However, long-term observation of the Multicenter Study of Hydroxyurea in Patients With SCA (MSH) participants found that up to half of adult patients do not experience clinical improvement on hydroxyurea.[52] The clinical response of pediatric SCD patients to hydroxyurea is typically higher than that of adult patients. Although hydroxyurea has disease-modifying effects unrelated to the degree of HbF induction, including reduction in red cell adhesion and white blood cell count,[53] HbF is considered strongly associated with clinical response, with individuals who produce more HbF experiencing fewer disease-related complications.[54] HbF response to hydroxyurea may decline over time and leave adult patients with reduced disease-modifying effect as their chronic illness and related organ damage progress.[55] A better understanding of this decline in HbF response to hydroxyurea is needed. It is not clear if reduced response is related to patient age and bone marrow function or the duration of hydroxyurea use. Further investigation into the effects of prolonged hydroxyurea use and SCD on erythroid progenitors and the stem cell niche is needed to better understand the reduced clinical benefit of hydroxyurea in adult patients.

Despite being a mainstay of SCD therapy in high- to moderate-resource countries for >20 years, much is still unknown about how hydroxyurea induces HbF and why some patients produce several times more HbF in response to the drug than others. Many theories have been proposed to explain the mechanism by which hydroxyurea induces HbF.

One of the most widely accepted theories is that hydroxyurea causes a "stress erythropoiesis" response.[56,57] Stress erythropoiesis alters erythroid differentiation kinetics, resulting in a more immature erythroid progenitor, with HbF still highly expressed, to exit the bone marrow. This hypothesis is supported by the observation that other cytotoxic agents also induce HbF, such as busulfan[58] and methotrexate.[59] Another proposed mechanism for hydroxyurea-mediated HbF induction involves induction of the nitric oxide (NO)–cyclic guanosine monophosphate (cGMP) pathway.[60,61] Hydroxyurea acts as an NO donor; NO then stimulates intracellular soluble guanylate cyclase, which in turn increases cGMP and induces HbF via cGMP-dependent protein kinase (PKG).[62] Individuals with variants in *BCL11A* have a higher HbF response to hydroxyurea,[63] and hydroxyurea has been shown to decrease *BCL11A* expression in erythroid cells,[64] suggesting that hydroxyurea may induce HbF by decreasing expression of this γ-globin repressor.

DNA Methyltransferase Inhibitors

Direct modification of DNA by methylation of its cytidine residues is associated with transcriptional repression or silencing of genes.[65] Adult CpG nucleotides are methylated in the γ-globin promoters of adults, who also have low HbF, but not in the γ-globin promoters of infants with high HbF.[34] DNA methyltransferase (DNMT) inhibition, through knockdown of DNMT1 in human erythroid precursors, through DNMT1 knockout in transgenic mice, or via chemical inhibitors, results in reactivation of γ-globin expression.[44,66] These observations have led to investigations into the use of the competitive DNMT inhibitors and analogs of cytidine 5-azacytidine (5-Aza) and 2′deoxy-5-azacytidine (decitabine) for HbF induction.

5-Aza and decitabine are incorporated into the DNA, inactivating the DNMT enzymes that methylate DNA.[67] 5-Aza was one of the first HbF-inducing agents investigated; it was tested first in anemic baboons followed by patients with hemoglobinopathies. Concerns regarding the carcinogenic potential of 5-Aza and lack of an oral formulation at the time ended further clinical investigation. Hydroxyurea was pursued instead.

Decitabine is incorporated into DNA only, unlike 5-Aza, which is incorporated into both DNA and RNA.[68] It is a more potent inhibitor of DNMT, in addition to having a more favorable safety profile than 5-Aza. However, decitabine is limited by lack of intestinal absorption without suppression of cytidine deaminase. Oral administration of tetrahydrouridine (THU) 1 hour before decitabine overcomes this limitation. Combined decitabine-THU therapy is under investigation as an HbF-inducing agent for individuals with SCD in a phase I clinical trial (NCT01685515). Decitabine has a mutagenic effect in various cell lines, sparking concern that chronic decitabine use will increase cancer risk.[69] In addition, cytogenetic instability secondary to DNA hypomethylation produced by knocking out DNMT genes can cause chromosome instability and carcinogenesis in mouse models. However, in practice, decitabine has been noted to reactivate expression of a range of tumor-suppressor genes.[70,71]

HDAC Inhibitors

HDACs remove acetyl groups, primarily from histone lysine residues. Acetylated chromatin is more accessible to interacting proteins and is more likely to be transcribed.[72] Inhibition of HDAC activity results in more histone acetylation and, therefore, more gene expression.[33,73] In vitro studies in K562 cells, an erythroleukemia cell line, and in HSPCs have shown that HDAC inhibitors can induce HbF, likely through increased acetylation of the γ-globin promoter, leading to increased transcription (Figure 8-2).

Butyrate is an HDAC inhibitor that has been investigated as an HbF inducer. Butyrate increases the transcription and translation of γ-globin.[74] Intravenous infusions of arginine butyrate and oral administration of sodium phenylbutyrate increased HbF in patients with SCD and β thalassemia; however, oral butyrate compounds only produced a modest elevation of HbF, without a rise in total hemoglobin. Compliance was poor due to the unpleasant taste of the medication.[75] Intravenous administration required pulse treatments, and HbF response was variable. HbF increased the most in individuals with already high HbF levels. Panobinostat is a pan-HDAC inhibitor reported to have greater potency than sodium butyrate[76]; as of this writing, it is listed in ClinicalTrials.gov as being investigated in an active clinical trial (see Table 8-1).

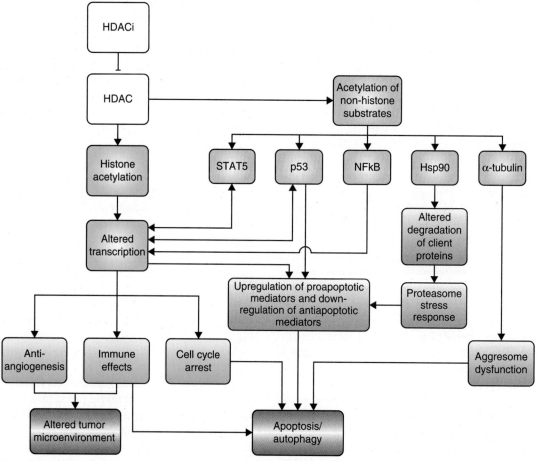

FIGURE 8-2 **Targets and downstream effects of histone deacetylase (HDAC) inhibition (HDACi).** Reprinted with permission of Springer Nature. Dickinson M, et al. Histone deacetylase inhibitors: potential targets responsible for their anti-cancer effect. Investigational New Drugs. 2010; 28(Suppl 1): 3–20.

Like butyrate and panobinostat, a variety of nonselective HDAC inhibitors have been shown to induce HbF in in vitro studies in HSPCs[77,78]; unfortunately, many are ineffective in vivo. In addition, the nonselective HDAC inhibitors may cause significant toxicity and adverse events, including thrombocytopenia and gastrointestinal side effects.[79,80] Development of potent, selective HDAC1/2 inhibitors that induce HbF with less toxicity remains a promising therapeutic approach for the treatment of SCD and β thalassemia.

Thalidomide Derivatives

Thalidomide has been used to treat patients with β thalassemia, producing significant increases in HbF and total hemoglobin.[81-83] The thalidomide derivatives pomalidomide and lenalidomide are antiangiogenic and immunomodulatory agents used in relapsed and refractory multiple myeloma; pomalidomide-treated multiple myeloma patients are known to experience elevation of HbF.[84] In a humanized mouse model of SCD, pomalidomide increased HbF production to a degree comparable to hydroxyurea but without myelosuppressive effects.[85] However, when pomalidomide was given in combination with hydroxyurea in a mouse model, the HbF-inducing activity of both drugs was lost. Pomalidomide can induce a fetal-like erythroid differentiation program, leading to reversal of γ-globin silencing in adult human erythroblasts by altering expression of BCL11A, SOX6, IKZF1, KLF1, and LSD1, which are known regulators of γ- and β-globin synthesis.[84]

Metformin

A commonly used diabetic drug, metformin, is under investigation as an HbF-inducing agent in an ongoing clinical trial (NCT02981329). Whole-exome sequencing and analysis of rare variants in patients with SCD found that individuals with variants predicted to be damaging in forkhead box O3 (FOXO3) had lower HbF levels. This suggested that FOXO3 was a positive regulator of HbF. Functional studies in human HSPCs confirmed the association[86] and led to the identification of metformin, a FOXO3 inducer, as a potential HbF-inducing agent. The mechanism by which metformin induces HbF remains to be elucidated but may be related to metabolic manipulation of erythroid progenitor cells (Figure 8-3). The possible role of metabolic manipulation in hemoglobin switching was suggested by the observation made by Perrine et al[87] >30 years ago that the infants of diabetic mothers showed a delay in the switch from fetal to adult hemoglobin.

Vitamin D

Vitamin D deficiency is common in individuals with SCD. A small study investigating the safety and efficacy of high-dose daily vitamin D in patients with SCD observed a modest increase in HbF with supplementation.[88] There are 8 clinical trials investigating vitamin D supplementation in individuals with SCD. Only one, NCT03417947, includes HbF levels as an end point.

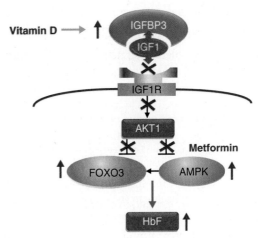

FIGURE 8-3 **Proposed metabolic regulation of hemoglobin switching.** HbF, hemoglobin F.

Of note, 1,25-dihydroxy vitamin D_3, the metabolically active form of vitamin D, induces FOXO3 via upregulation of insulin growth factor binding protein 3 (IGFBP3) and subsequent activation of the insulin signaling pathway (Figure 8-3).

Gene Therapy

The only curative therapy for SCD is hematopoietic stem cell transplant (HSCT). Best outcomes are obtained from a human leukocyte antigen (HLA)-matched related donor; unfortunately only 10% to 15% of patients have such a donor.[89] A prospective study of unrelated donor HSCT in SCD generated the conclusion that, without modifications to existing regimens, HSCT with unrelated donors is not safe for widespread adoption.[90] Gene therapy using autologous HSPCs would remove the limitation of matched related donor availability, the need for immunosuppressive drugs, and risk of graft-versus-host disease.

There are several possible gene-editing strategies that can be used to treat individuals with SCD: (1) correction of the causative A-T point mutation in *HBB*; (2) induction of HbF through introduction of an HPFH deletion,[91] downregulation of BCL11A, or double-strand breaks; and (3) gene addition of HBB, HBG1/2, or an antisickling γ-globin cassette.[92] Sufficient correction of the A-T mutation or HbF induction could be curative.[31,39] Different technologies can be used to achieve these goals. Lentiviral vectors have been used extensively in clinical trials, and the first patient with SCD reported to have been successfully treated with gene therapy received an ex vivo altered autologous transplant on the HGB-205 study.[93] Two other ongoing clinical trials are using lentiviral vectors, one to express γ-globin and the other to introduce a β-globin transgene that contains 3 antisickling mutations (NCT02186418 and NCT02151526). Other approaches include gene editing by zinc finger nucleases (ZFNs), transcription activator-like effector nucleases (TALENs), and clustered regularly interspaced short palindromic repeat (CRISPR)-associated nuclease 9 (Cas9).

Lentivirus-Based Gene Editing to Induce HbF in SCD

Two lentiviral gene therapy strategies for SCD under active investigation do not attempt to increase γ-globin, but instead seek to correct the *HBB* sickle mutation or produce a unique, "antisickling" β-globin. All current lentivirus-based clinical trials in individuals with hemoglobinopathies use a modified LCR to express genes in an erythroid-specific manner. The non-HbF approaches have the advantage of producing a gene product that can be easily distinguished from endogenous β-globin. Some of the HbF induction noted in trials employing that strategy may be due to stress erythropoiesis caused by the transplant procedure and therefore may not be sustained beyond the first year after transplant.

Most gene-based therapy trials in SCD use busulfan as a conditioning regimen; the Cincinnati Children's Medical Center has an open protocol to perform autologous stem cell transplants of ex vivo edited HSPCs following reduced-intensity conditioning with melphalan (NCT02186418). This protocol uses ex vivo lentiviral delivery of the γ-globin gene. To avoid excess unpaired β-globin-like chains, the trial investigators are preferentially enrolling HbSβ⁰ patients.

CRISPR/Cas9

CRISPR/Cas9 technology has been used to correct the sickle mutation in SCD patient–derived HSPCs[94-96] and to disrupt the BCL11A enhancer region, preventing BCL11A repression of γ-globin. A clinical trial of the latter approach is underway (NCT03745287). The advantage of HbF-inducing strategies is that they can be used in all SCD genotypes and in individuals with β-thalassemia. However, HbF induction must be sufficient to outcompete large amounts of HbS. A sickle mutation correction approach would be most effective in HbSS individuals alone, but has the advantage of decreasing HbS while generating HbA. CRISPR/Cas9 can also be used in a base-editing approach pared with a deaminase. CRISPR/Cas9 is used to locate the sickle mutation, and the deaminase changes the adenine to a guanine, producing HbG-Makassar, a naturally occurring hemoglobin variant that does not sickle. An A→ T change is not technically possible.[97]

Significant challenges (both common to all CRISPR/Cas9 applications and SCD specific) in bringing this technology to a clinical trial remain. First, off-target effects of editing are a major concern, and depending on the strategy, on-target insertions and deletions may also be problematic. Unbiased genome-wide off-target analysis of CRISPR/Cas9-edited HSPCs to rigorously identify all genomic changes is needed. Second, gene-editing efficiency needs to be very high to be curative because engraftment of gene-edited SCD HSPCs without selection is low.[95] Third, obtaining sufficient CD34+ cells for gene editing can be challenging because patients with SCD cannot be mobilized with granulocyte colony-stimulating factor (G-CSF), although plerixafor (typically used as an adjuvant stem cell mobilization agent with G-CSF in non-SCD patients) has been shown to be safe in individuals with SCD. The number of CD34+ cells needed is also greater than for an allogeneic transplant because ex vivo

gene editing is associated with cell death and edited cells show lower levels of engraftment. Multiple mobilization cycles with plerixafor may be needed for some patients.

CRISPR/Cas9 can be used to target known HbF repressors such as KLF1 and BCL11A.[98] However, these transcription factors also have essential roles in nonerythroid contexts. BCL11A plays a significant role in lymphoid and neuronal development, and *BCL11A* knockout is perinatal lethal in mice.[99,100] Because of this limitation, most strategies focus on the deletion of erythroid-specific BCL11A-binding sequences to prevent BCL11A-mediated repression of γ-globin expression. Another approach is repression of erythroid-specific BCL11A.[23] CRISPR/Cas9 was used to delete a 12-kb *BCL11A* enhancer located in the first intron of the *BCL11A* gene. The erythroid-specific transcription factor GATA1 interacts with this site and is essential for *BCL11A* expression, but only in erythroid cells. This editing resulted in a significant increase in γ-globin expression and production of HbF, suggesting that perturbation of defined critical sequences within the *BCL11A* enhancer may result in HbF levels meeting the yet undefined clinical threshold required to ameliorate the phenotype of SCD.[101]

TALENs

TALENs can be used to form a site-specific double-stranded DNA break. A TALEN monomer is made up of a DNA-binding domain (DBD) formed by tandem repeats of approximately 34 amino acids with each repeat recognizing 1 nucleotide. The DBD is fused to FokI nuclease; a TALEN pair is required to make the site-specific double-strand break within the spacer region. The therapeutic potential of TALEN in SCD has been investigated to target and correct the SCD mutation and to inactivate BCL11A with double-strand DNA break–induced mutagenesis in HSPCs. This approach, targeting exon 2 of *BCL11A*, had a 30% efficiency rate in human and nonhuman primate CD34+ cells in vitro. Colony-forming efficiency was slightly lower in *BCL11A*-edited CD34+ cells, but the lineage differentiation potential was unchanged. Increased γ- to β-globin ratio was obtained in both human and primate *BCl11A*-modified cells compared to control cells, and sustained HbF elevation was present at almost 1 year after transplant in a primate model.[102]

ZFNs

The first gene-editing technology used to correct single point mutations in the β-globin gene was ZFN, which was used to correct the sickle mutation in patient-derived induced pluripotent stem cells and CD34+ HSPCs. ZFNs have also been used to disrupt the *BCL11A* gene in human HSPCs, either within exon 2 or at the GATAA motif in the intronic erythroid-specific enhancer. Both targeting strategies upregulated γ-globin expression in erythroid cells to levels predicted to inhibit HbS polymerization (ie, ~20%). However, complete inactivation of *BCL11A* obtained by inducing biallelic frameshift mutations in *BCL11A* exon 2 prevented erythroid enucleation and significantly reduced engraftment in immunodeficient mice. Biallelic disruption of the GATAA motif in the erythroid enhancer of *BCL11A* did not negatively impact enucleation or impact engraftment.[103]

Ongoing Clinical Trials and Future Directions

The drawbacks of the available cell-based assays and animal model systems make identification of novel HbF-inducing agents challenging. Currently available in vitro systems used to screen compounds include K562 cells, an erythroleukemia cell line, human umbilical cord–derived erythroid progenitor (HUDEP) cells, and Bristol erythroid lineage adult (BEL-A) cells. K562 cells only produce γ-globin, which does not permit observation of the switch from γ- to β-globin. K562 cells may be too permissive; agents that increase γ-globin expression in K562 cells may fail to induce HbF when tested in vivo or in primary erythroid culture. HUDEP cells have been shown to be poorly drug inducible; more experience with BEL-A cells is needed. Formerly considered the gold standard for studying hemoglobin switching, erythroid cultures derived from human CD34+ cells subjected to a cocktail of growth factors to induce erythroid differentiation may also permit γ-globin induction using agents that fail to induce HbF in vivo.

The challenge in obtaining in vivo evidence of efficacy for an agent under investigation as an HbF inducer is that rodents do not naturally make HbF; sickle mouse models contain the entire human hemoglobin locus but may lack other components needed to interact with these human globin genes. Induction of HbF by agents such as decitabine and pomalidomide in a mouse model has been a major achievement; however, other agents that have demonstrated HbF induction in humans, such as hydroxyurea, do not induce HbF in sickle mice.

Clinical trials identified by a search of ClinicalTrials.gov using the keywords "sickle cell disease" and "fetal hemoglobin" are summarized in Table 8-1. Trials designed to optimize hydroxyurea use were omitted. The majority of the clinical trials investigate pharmacologic agents; 2 are gene therapy trials.

TABLE 8-1 Clinical trials involving fetal hemoglobin (HbF) induction in sickle cell disease (SCD) currently posted in ClinicalTrials.gov

Trial	Status at time of publication	Reported results
Study of decitabine and THU in patients with SCD; NCT01685515	Active, not recruiting	N/A
Gum arabic as an HbF agent in SCA; NCT02467257	Completed	None
Hydroxyurea and erythropoietin to treat SCA; NCT00270478	Completed	None
Study to determine the maximum-tolerated dose, safety, and effectiveness of pomalidomide for patients with SCD; NCT01522547	Completed	None
Effects of HQK-1001 in patients with SCD; NCT01601340	Terminated	None
Decitabine for high-risk SCD; NCT01375608	Completed	4.8% average HbF increase
Effectiveness of arginine as a treatment for SCA; NCT00513617	Completed	None for HbF induction
HbF induction treatment with metformin; NCT02981329	Recruiting	N/A
Gene transfer for patients with SCD; NCT02186418	Recruiting	N/A
Study of panobinostat in patients with SCD; NCT01245179	Recruiting	N/A
A study to evaluate the safety, pharmacokinetics, and biologic activity of INCB059872; NCT03132324	Terminated	None
Efficacy of vorinostat to induce HbF in SCD; NCT01000155	Terminated	None; closed due to slow accrual
A phase IIa-IIb trial to study the safety, tolerability, and efficacy of memantine as a long-term treatment of SCD; NCT03247218	Recruiting	N/A
A safety and efficacy study evaluating CTX001 in subjects with severe SCD; NCT03745287	Recruiting	N/A

Abbreviations: N/A, not applicable; None, closed or completed without reported results; SCA, sickle cell anemia; THU, tetrahydrouridine.

Other gene therapy are trials underway, but only the trials using an HbF induction strategy are included. The agents listed have made the leap to a clinical trial, a significant achievement. However, a large number of closed studies had no published or reported results, either because there was no significant effect or the study was unable to be completed. Until the recent FDA approval of L-glutamine (2016), crizanlizumab (2019), and voxelotor (2019) as agents for individuals with SCD, no other agents had achieved FDA approval for the treatment of SCD since hydroxyurea. These new agents do not increase HbF, but instead act on other aspects of SCD pathophysiology, as described in Chapter 32.

A frequently asked question pertaining to HbF induction in SCD is: What level of HbF is required for optimal modification of disease severity? Data from the pre-hydroxyurea era suggests that patients who have HbF levels >15% have less frequent vaso-occlusive crises and acute chest syndrome; those with >20% HbF are protected from stroke and pulmonary complications.[104] These levels are frequently achievable with hydroxyurea therapy. Some individuals with SCD may achieve HbF levels >40% on hydroxyurea, which is in the range of HbF seen in individuals with SCD and deletional HPFH (typical HbF levels of 35%-40%). Despite this, individuals with SCD who achieve HbF levels of 40% on hydroxyurea can experience complications of the disease, albeit much less frequently than individuals with more typical HbF levels. In contrast, most individuals with SCD and deletional HPFH are asymptomatic. This discrepancy can be readily explained by the difference in the distribution of HbF between the red blood cells (RBCs). Deletional HPFH produces a pancellular distribution of HbF; each RBC has the same percentage of HbF, and all cells are F-cells, meaning they contain enough HbF to prevent sickling. Hydroxyurea produces a heterocellular distribution of HbF; some RBCs contain more HbF than others, and there is a mixed population of F-cells and non–F-cells. Thus, to achieve a near-curative HbF response, it is of utmost importance that HbF induction is pancellular.

Now that there are 4 FDA-approved pharmacologic therapies for SCD, combinations of HbF induction by hydroxyurea and therapies targeting other aspects of SCD pathophysiology are possible. Clinical trials of the 3 recently FDA approved drugs (L-glutamine, crizanlizumab, and voxelotor) included patients on hydroxyurea. Crizanlizumab was shown to provide additional reduction in vaso-occlusive episodes in patients who were on a stable dose of hydroxyurea,[105] and individuals on hydroxyurea demonstrated an increase in total hemoglobin when treated with voxelotor.[106] Hydroxyurea should remain the backbone of SCD therapy, with additional agents added to address disease complications not prevented by hydroxyurea.

The power of unbiased genomic analyses to reveal biology that would not have been found through a candidate approach is demonstrated by the identification of the roles of BCL11A and HBS1L-MYB in γ-globin regulation. Large-scale whole-genome sequencing of thousands of patients with SCD is underway as part of the Transcriptomics in Precision Medicine (TOPMed) National Heart, Lung, and Blood Institute (NHLBI) initiative. It is possible that this work will identify other regulators of γ-globin that are more easily "druggable" than BCL11A or new targets for gene therapy. Gene therapy is a promising strategy and may lead to a cure for individuals in high-resource countries in the next 5 to 10 years, provided there are no unexpected setbacks.

However, despite our hope for autologous stem cell transplant of edited HSPCs as a cure for individuals with SCD, we must not neglect the search for inexpensive, well-tolerated pharmacologic agents that can be used in low-resource countries where SCD is endemic. It is essential that we have several therapeutics and strategies to offer our patients so that they can make choices that fit their health status, environment, pharmacogenomic status, and personal preferences. The 2010's saw exciting developments in sickle cell therapeutics, including the FDA approval of 3 new drugs in 4 years. This provides a unique opportunity to rationally design clinical trials of combination therapies for HbF induction, as well as combinations of HbF-inducing agents with drugs targeting downstream effects of sickling, provided that end points and biomarkers are chosen wisely.

Conclusion

The discovery of BCL11A as the key player in the perinatal γ- to β-globin switch as well as the major repressor of γ-globin expression has significantly improved our understanding of globin gene expression. Along with BCL11A, a number of transcriptional regulators form the "repressor complex" (Figure 8-1) and act in synergy with epigenetic mechanisms (histone deacetylation and methylation) in γ-globin silencing. Clinical trials have confirmed that reactivation of γ-globin expression can be achieved by (1) inhibition of the erythroid-specific expression of BCL11A, (2) targeting various members of the repressor complex such as the DRED complex with lysine specific demethylase 1 (LSD1), (3) targeting the NURD complex with HDAC inhibitors, and (3) DNMT1 inhibition. Despite this, the precise mechanism of action of certain drugs remains unclear; hydroxyurea, the most widely used antiswitching agent is an example, along with the FOXO3 enhancer metformin and thalidomide derivatives. Future research may further elucidate the mechanisms of action of these agents or identify new targets. Our current level of knowledge of the γ- to β-globin switch does support using antiswitching agents with different mechanisms of action in combination for optimal HbF induction in β-hemoglobinopathies.

High-Yield Facts

◆ The best-known modifier of sickle cell disease (SCD) is the level of fetal hemoglobin (HbF, $\alpha_2\gamma_2$), which exerts a strong anti-sickling effect when present in sufficient amounts in the red cell.

◆ Hydroxyurea, developed for use in SCD almost 3 decades ago, is the only widely used pharmacologic HbF inducer.

◆ It is still not known how hydroxyurea induces HbF and why up to half of adults with SCD do not exhibit clinical improvement.

◆ Identification of additional HbF-inducing agents has been slowed by our limited understanding of γ-globin regulation and lack of optimal in vitro and in vivo systems to screen compounds for HbF-inducing properties.

◆ Potential additional HbF-inducing agents under investigation include DNA methyltransferase inhibitors, histone deacetylase inhibitors, thalidomide derivatives, and agents that impact the insulin signaling pathway, such as metformin.

◆ Genome-wide association study approaches have identified that variants in B-cell lymphoma/leukemia 11A (BCL11A) and regulatory elements within the intergenic region HBS1L-MYB are associated with HbF levels.

◆ Disruption of the BCL11A erythroid enhancer element is now a gene therapy target in clinical trials.

◆ Pharmacologic HbF-inducing therapies are still needed because >99% of the world's SCD population lives in low-resource countries where implementation of gene-based therapies may not be possible.

References

1. Stamatoyannopoulos G. Control of globin gene expression during development and erythroid differentiation. *Exp Hematol.* 2005;33(3):259-271.

2. Thein SL, Menzel S. Discovering the genetics underlying foetal haemoglobin production in adults. *Br J Haematol.* 2009;145(4):455-467.

3. Nagel RL, Bookchin RM, Johnson J, et al. Structural bases of the inhibitory effects of hemoglobin F and hemoglobin A2 on the polymerization of hemoglobin S. *Proc Natl Acad Sci U S A.* 1979;76(2):670-672.

4. Watson J. The significance of the paucity of sickle cells in newborn negro infants. *Am J Med Sci.* 1948;215(4):419-423.

5. Galarneau G, Palmer CD, Sankaran VG, Orkin SH, Hirschhorn JN, Lettre G. Fine-mapping at three loci known to affect fetal hemoglobin levels explains additional genetic variation. *Nat Genet.* 2010;42(12):1049-1051.

6. Akinsheye I, Alsultan A, Solovieff N, et al. Fetal hemoglobin in sickle cell anemia. *Blood.* 2011;118(1):19-27.

7. Lapoumeroulie C, Dunda O, Ducrocq R, et al. A novel sickle cell mutation of yet another origin in Africa: the Cameroon type. *Hum Genet.* 1992;89(3):333-337.

8. Pagnier J, Mears JG, Dunda-Belkhodja O, et al. Evidence for the multicentric origin of the sickle cell hemoglobin gene in Africa. *Proc Natl Acad Sci U S A.* 1984;81(6):1771-1773.

9. Labie D, Pagnier J, Lapoumeroulie C, et al. Common haplotype dependency of high G gamma-globin gene expression and high Hb F levels in beta-thalassemia and sickle cell anemia patients. *Proc Natl Acad Sci U S A.* 1985;82(7):2111-2114.

10. Srinivas R, Dunda O, Krishnamoorthy R, et al. Atypical haplotypes linked to the beta S gene in Africa are likely to be the product of recombination. *Am J Hematol.* 1988;29(1):60-62.

11. Green NS, Fabry ME, Kaptue-Noche L, Nagel RL. Senegal haplotype is associated with higher HbF than Benin and Cameroon haplotypes in African children with sickle cell anemia. *Am J Hematol.* 1993;44(2):145-146.

12. Chang YC, Smith KD, Moore RD, Serjeant GR, Dover GJ. An analysis of fetal hemoglobin variation in sickle cell disease: the relative contributions of the X-linked factor, beta-globin haplotypes, alpha-globin gene number, gender, and age. *Blood.* 1995;85(4):1111-1117.

13. Pandey S, Pandey S, Mishra RM, Saxena R. Modulating effect of the -158 gamma (C->T) Xmn1 polymorphism in Indian sickle cell patients. *Mediterr J Hematol Infect Dis.* 2012;4(1):e2012001.

14. Habara AH, Shaikho EM, Steinberg MH. Fetal hemoglobin in sickle cell anemia: the Arab-Indian haplotype and new therapeutic agents. *Am J Hematol.* 2017;92(11):1233-1242.

15. Shriner D, Rotimi CN. Whole-genome-sequence-based haplotypes reveal single origin of the sickle allele during the holocene wet phase. *Am J Hum Genet.* 2018;102(4):547-556.

16. Thein SL. Molecular basis of beta thalassemia and potential therapeutic targets. *Blood Cells Mol Dis.* 2018;70:54-65.

17. Sripichai O, Fucharoen S. Fetal hemoglobin regulation in beta-thalassemia: heterogeneity, modifiers and therapeutic approaches. *Expert Rev Hematol.* 2016;9(12):1129-1137.

18. Kim A, Dean A. Chromatin loop formation in the beta-globin locus and its role in globin gene transcription. *Mol Cells.* 2012;34(1):1-5.

19. Breda L, Motta I, Lourenco S, et al. Forced chromatin looping raises fetal hemoglobin in adult sickle cells to higher levels than pharmacologic inducers. *Blood.* 2016;128(8):1139-1143.

20. Enver T, Raich N, Ebens AJ, Papayannopoulou T, Costantini F, Stamatoyannopoulos G. Developmental regulation of human fetal-to-adult globin gene switching in transgenic mice. *Nature.* 1990;344(6264):309-313.

21. Sankaran VG, Xu J, Byron R, et al. A functional element necessary for fetal hemoglobin silencing. *N Engl J Med.* 2011;365(9):807-814.

22. Uda M, Galanello R, Sanna S, et al. Genome-wide association study shows BCL11A associated with persistent fetal hemoglobin and amelioration of the phenotype of beta-thalassemia. *Proc Natl Acad Sci U S A.* 2008;105(5):1620-1625.

23. Bauer DE, Kamran SC, Lessard S, et al. An erythroid enhancer of BCL11A subject to genetic variation determines fetal hemoglobin level. *Science.* 2013;342(6155):253-257.

24. Liu N, Hargreaves VV, Zhu Q, et al. Direct promoter repression by BCL11A controls the fetal to adult hemoglobin switch. *Cell.* 2018;173(2):430-442 e417.

25. Thein SL, Menzel S, Peng X, et al. Intergenic variants of HBS1L-MYB are responsible for a major quantitative trait locus on chromosome 6q23 influencing fetal hemoglobin levels in adults. *Proc Natl Acad Sci U S A.* 2007;104(27):11346-11351.

26. Stadhouders R, Aktuna S, Thongjuea S, et al. HBS1L-MYB intergenic variants modulate fetal hemoglobin via long-range MYB enhancers. *J Clin Invest.* 2014;124(4):1699-1710.

27. Borg J, Papadopoulos P, Georgitsi M, et al. Haploinsufficiency for the erythroid transcription factor KLF1 causes hereditary persistence of fetal hemoglobin. *Nat Genet.* 2010;42(9):801-805.

28. Zhou D, Liu K, Sun CW, Pawlik KM, Townes TM. KLF1 regulates BCL11A expression and gamma- to beta-globin gene switching. *Nat Genet.* 2010;42(9):742-744.

29. Vinjamur DS, Alhashem YN, Mohamad SF, Amin P, Williams DC Jr, Lloyd JA. Kruppel-like transcription factor KLF1 is required for optimal gamma- and beta-globin expression in human fetal erythroblasts. *PLoS One.* 2016;11(2):e0146802.

30. Zhou W, Zhao Q, Sutton R, et al. The role of p22 NF-E4 in human globin gene switching. *J Biol Chem.* 2004;279(25):26227-26232.

31. Masuda T, Wang X, Maeda M, et al. Transcription factors LRF and BCL11A independently repress expression of fetal hemoglobin. *Science.* 2016;351(6270):285-289.

32. Bank A. Regulation of human fetal hemoglobin: new players, new complexities. *Blood.* 2006;107(2):435-443.

33. Forsberg EC, Downs KM, Christensen HM, Im H, Nuzzi PA, Bresnick EH. Developmentally dynamic histone acetylation pattern of a tissue-specific chromatin domain. *Proc Natl Acad Sci U S A.* 2000;97(26):14494-14499.

34. Mabaera R, Richardson CA, Johnson K, Hsu M, Fiering S, Lowrey CH. Developmental- and differentiation-specific patterns of human gamma- and beta-globin promoter DNA methylation. *Blood.* 2007;110(4):1343-1352.

35. Yin W, Barkess G, Fang X, et al. Histone acetylation at the human beta-globin locus changes with developmental age. *Blood.* 2007;110(12):4101-4107.

36. DeSimone J, Heller P, Hall L, Zwiers D. 5-Azacytidine stimulates fetal hemoglobin synthesis in anemic baboons. *Proc Natl Acad Sci U S A.* 1982;79(14):4428-4431.

37. Rupon JW, Wang SZ, Gaensler K, Lloyd J, Ginder GD. Methyl binding domain protein 2 mediates gamma-globin gene silencing in adult human betaYAC transgenic mice. *Proc Natl Acad Sci U S A.* 2006;103(17):6617-6622.

38. Zhao Q, Rank G, Tan YT, et al. PRMT5-mediated methylation of histone H4R3 recruits DNMT3A, coupling histone and DNA methylation in gene silencing. *Nat Struct Mol Biol.* 2009;16(3):304-311.

39. Renneville A, Van Galen P, Canver MC, et al. EHMT1 and EHMT2 inhibition induces fetal hemoglobin expression. *Blood.* 2015;126(16):1930-1939.

40. Rank G, Cerruti L, Simpson RJ, Moritz RL, Jane SM, Zhao Q. Identification of a PRMT5-dependent repressor complex linked to silencing of human fetal globin gene expression. *Blood.* 2010;116(9):1585-1592.

41. Rivers A, Vaitkus K, Ibanez V, et al. The LSD1 inhibitor RN-1 recapitulates the fetal pattern of hemoglobin synthesis in baboons (P. anubis). *Haematologica.* 2016;101(6):688-697.

42. Cui S, Lim KC, Shi L, et al. The LSD1 inhibitor RN-1 induces fetal hemoglobin synthesis and reduces disease pathology in sickle cell mice. *Blood.* 2015;126(3):386-396.

43. Cui S, Kolodziej KE, Obara N, et al. Nuclear receptors TR2 and TR4 recruit multiple epigenetic transcriptional corepressors that associate specifically with the embryonic beta-type globin promoters in differentiated adult erythroid cells. *Mol Cell Biol.* 2011;31(16):3298-3311.

44. Xu J, Bauer DE, Kerenyi MA, et al. Corepressor-dependent silencing of fetal hemoglobin expression by BCL11A. *Proc Natl Acad Sci U S A.* 2013;110(16):6518-6523.

45. Lee YT, de Vasconcellos JF, Yuan J, et al. LIN28B-mediated expression of fetal hemoglobin and production of fetal-like erythrocytes from adult human erythroblasts ex vivo. *Blood.* 2013;122(6):1034-1041.

46. Lulli V, Romania P, Morsilli O, et al. MicroRNA-486-3p regulates gamma-globin expression in human erythroid cells by directly modulating BCL11A. *PLoS One.* 2013;8(4):e60436.

47. Sankaran VG, Menne TF, Scepanovic D, et al. MicroRNA-15a and 16-1 act via MYB to elevate fetal hemoglobin expression in human trisomy 13. *Proc Natl Acad Sci U S A.* 2011;108(4):1519-1524.

48. Charache S, Barton FB, Moore RD, et al. Hydroxyurea and sickle cell anemia. Clinical utility of a myelosuppressive "switching" agent. The Multicenter Study of Hydroxyurea in Sickle Cell Anemia. *Medicine (Baltimore).* 1996;75(6):300-326.

49. Kinney TR, Helms RW, O'Branski EE, et al. Safety of hydroxyurea in children with sickle cell anemia: results of the HUG-KIDS study, a phase I/II trial. Pediatric Hydroxyurea Group. *Blood.* 1999;94(5):1550-1554.

50. Wykes C, Rees DC. The safety and efficacy of hydroxycarbamide in infants with sickle cell anemia. *Expert Rev Hematol.* 2011;4(4):407-409.

51. Ware RE, Davis BR, Schultz WH, et al. Hydroxycarbamide versus chronic transfusion for maintenance of transcranial doppler flow velocities in children with sickle cell anaemia-TCD With Transfusions Changing to Hydroxyurea (TWiTCH): a multicentre, open-label, phase 3, non-inferiority trial. *Lancet.* 2016;387(10019):661-670.

52. Steinberg MH, McCarthy WF, Castro O, et al. The risks and benefits of long-term use of hydroxyurea in sickle cell anemia: a 17.5 year follow-up. *Am J Hematol.* 2010;85(6):403-408.

53. Ferster A, Vermylen C, Cornu G, et al. Hydroxyurea for treatment of severe sickle cell anemia: a pediatric clinical trial. *Blood.* 1996;88(6):1960-1964.

54. Strouse JJ, Lanzkron S, Beach MC, et al. Hydroxyurea for sickle cell disease: a systematic review for efficacy and toxicity in children. *Pediatrics.* 2008;122(6):1332-1342.

55. Green NS, Manwani D, Qureshi M, Ireland K, Sinha A, Smaldone AM. Decreased fetal hemoglobin over time among youth with sickle cell disease on hydroxyurea is associated with higher urgent hospital use. *Pediatr Blood Cancer.* 2016;63(12):2146-2153.

56. Galanello R, Veith R, Papayannopoulou T, Stamatoyannopoulos G. Pharmacologic stimulation of Hb F in patients with sickle cell anemia. *Prog Clin Biol Res.* 1985;191:433-445.

57. Stamatoyannopoulos G, Veith R, Galanello R, Papayannopoulou T. Hb F production in stressed erythropoiesis: observations and kinetic models. *Ann N Y Acad Sci.* 1985;445:188-197.

58. Liang CC, Liu DP, Jia PC, Ao ZH, Chen SS, Yang KG. Augmentation of fetal hemoglobin in anemic monkeys by myleran. *Prog Clin Biol Res.* 1987;251:467-478.

59. Veith R, Dautenhahn AG, Roth RC. Methotrexate stimulates fetal hemoglobin production in anemic baboons. *Prog Clin Biol Res.* 1989;316B:363-370.

60. Cokic VP, Smith RD, Beleslin-Cokic BB, et al. Hydroxyurea induces fetal hemoglobin by the nitric oxide-dependent activation of soluble guanylyl cyclase. *J Clin Invest.* 2003;111(2):231-239.

61. Lou TF, Singh M, Mackie A, Li W, Pace BS. Hydroxyurea generates nitric oxide in human erythroid cells: mechanisms for gamma-globin gene activation. *Exp Biol Med (Maywood).* 2009;234(11):1374-1382.

62. Almeida CB, Scheiermann C, Jang JE, et al. Hydroxyurea and a cGMP-amplifying agent have immediate benefits on acute vaso-occlusive events in sickle cell disease mice. *Blood.* 2012;120(14):2879-2888.

63. Friedrisch JR, Sheehan V, Flanagan JM, et al. The role of BCL11A and HMIP-2 polymorphisms on endogenous and hydroxyurea induced levels of fetal hemoglobin in sickle cell anemia patients from southern Brazil. *Blood Cells Mol Dis.* 2016;62:32-37.

64. Grieco AJ, Billett HH, Green NS, Driscoll MC, Bouhassira EE. Variation in gamma-globin expression before and after induction with hydroxyurea associated with BCL11A, KLF1 and TAL1. *PLoS One.* 2015;10(6):e0129431.

65. van der Ploeg LH, Flavell RA. DNA methylation in the human gamma delta beta-globin locus in erythroid and nonerythroid tissues. *Cell.* 1980;19(4):947-958.

66. Charache S, Dover G, Smith K, Talbot CC Jr, Moyer M, Boyer S. Treatment of sickle cell anemia with 5-azacytidine results in increased fetal hemoglobin production and is associated with nonrandom hypomethylation of DNA around the gamma-delta-beta-globin gene complex. *Proc Natl Acad Sci U S A.* 1983;80(15):4842-4846.

67. Gnyszka A, Jastrzebski Z, Flis S. DNA methyltransferase inhibitors and their emerging role in epigenetic therapy of cancer. *Anticancer Res.* 2013;33(8):2989-2996.

68. Lavelle DE. The molecular mechanism of fetal hemoglobin reactivation. *Semin Hematol.* 2004;41(4 suppl 6):3-10.

69. Marquardt H, Marquardt H. Induction of malignant transformation and mutagenesis in cell cultures by cancer chemotherapeutic agents. *Cancer.* 1977;40(4 suppl):1930-1934.

70. Karpf AR, Lasek AW, Ririe TO, Hanks AN, Grossman D, Jones DA. Limited gene activation in tumor and normal epithelial cells treated with the DNA methyltransferase inhibitor 5-aza-2'-deoxycytidine. *Mol Pharmacol.* 2004;65(1):18-27.

71. Leone G, Voso MT, Teofili L, Lubbert M. Inhibitors of DNA methylation in the treatment of hematological malignancies and MDS. *Clin Immunol.* 2003;109(1):89-102.

72. Tse C, Sera T, Wolffe AP, Hansen JC. Disruption of higher-order folding by core histone acetylation dramatically enhances transcription of nucleosomal arrays by RNA polymerase III. *Mol Cell Biol.* 1998;18(8):4629-4638.

73. Cao H, Stamatoyannopoulos G, Jung M. Induction of human gamma globin gene expression by histone deacetylase inhibitors. *Blood.* 2004;103(2):701-709.

74. Weinberg RS, Ji X, Sutton M, et al. Butyrate increases the efficiency of translation of gamma-globin mRNA. *Blood.* 2005;105(4):1807-1809.

75. Sher GD, Ginder GD, Little J, Yang S, Dover GJ, Olivieri NF. Extended therapy with intravenous arginine butyrate in patients with beta-hemoglobinopathies. *N Engl J Med.* 1995;332(24):1606-1610.

76. Bradner JE, Mak R, Tanguturi SK, et al. Chemical genetic strategy identifies histone deacetylase 1 (HDAC1) and HDAC2 as therapeutic targets in sickle cell disease. *Proc Natl Acad Sci U S A.* 2010;107(28):12617-12622.

77. Cao H, Stamatoyannopoulos G. Histone deacetylase inhibitor FK228 is a potent inducer of human fetal hemoglobin. *Am J Hematol.* 2006;81(12):981-983.

78. Witt O, Monkemeyer S, Ronndahl G, et al. Induction of fetal hemoglobin expression by the histone deacetylase inhibitor apicidin. *Blood.* 2003;101(5):2001-2007.

79. Guha M. HDAC inhibitors still need a home run, despite recent approval. *Nat Rev Drug Discov.* 2015;14(4):225-226.

80. Subramanian S, Bates SE, Wright JJ, Espinoza-Delgado I, Piekarz RL. Clinical toxicities of histone deacetylase inhibitors. *Pharmaceuticals (Basel).* 2010;3(9):2751-2767.

81. Aguilar-Lopez LB, Delgado-Lamas JL, Rubio-Jurado B, Perea FJ, Ibarra B. Thalidomide therapy in a patient with thalassemia major. *Blood Cells Mol Dis.* 2008;41(1):136-137.

82. Fozza C, Pardini S, Giannico DB, et al. Dramatic erythroid response to low-dose thalidomide in two patients with transfusion independent thalassemia and severe post-transfusional alloimmune hemolysis. *Am J Hematol.* 2015;90(7):E141.

83. Li Y, Ren Q, Zhou Y, Li P, Lin W, Yin X. Thalidomide has a significant effect in patients with thalassemia intermedia. *Hematology.* 2018;23(1):50-54.

84. Dulmovits BM, Appiah-Kubi AO, Papoin J, et al. Pomalidomide reverses gamma-globin silencing through the transcriptional reprogramming of adult hematopoietic progenitors. *Blood.* 2016;127(11):1481-1492.

85. Meiler SE, Wade M, Kutlar F, et al. Pomalidomide augments fetal hemoglobin production without the myelosuppressive effects of hydroxyurea in transgenic sickle cell mice. *Blood.* 2011;118(4):1109-1112.

86. Zhang Y, Paikari A, Sumazin P, et al. Metformin induces FOXO3-dependent fetal hemoglobin production in human primary erythroid cells. *Blood.* 2018;132(3):321-333.

87. Perrine SP, Greene MF, Faller DV. Delay in the fetal globin switch in infants of diabetic mothers. *N Engl J Med.* 1985;312(6):334-338.

88. Dougherty KA, Bertolaso C, Schall JI, Smith-Whitley K, Stallings VA. Safety and efficacy of high-dose daily vitamin D3 supplementation in children and young adults with sickle cell disease. *J Pediatr Hematol Oncol.* 2015;37(5):e308-315.

89. Mentzer WC, Heller S, Pearle PR, Hackney E, Vichinsky E. Availability of related donors for bone marrow transplantation in sickle cell anemia. *Am J Pediatr Hematol Oncol.* 1994;16(1):27-29.

90. Shenoy S, Eapen M, Panepinto JA, et al. A trial of unrelated donor marrow transplantation for children with severe sickle cell disease. *Blood.* 2016;128(21):2561-2567.

91. Traxler EA, Yao Y, Wang YD, et al. A genome-editing strategy to treat beta-hemoglobinopathies that recapitulates a mutation associated with a benign genetic condition. *Nat Med.* 2016;22(9):987-990.

92. Urbinati F, Hargrove PW, Geiger S, et al. Potentially therapeutic levels of anti-sickling globin gene expression following lentivirus-mediated gene transfer in sickle cell disease bone marrow CD34+ cells. *Exp Hematol.* 2015;43(5):346-351.

93. Ribeil JA, Hacein-Bey-Abina S, Payen E, et al. Gene therapy in a patient with sickle cell disease. *N Engl J Med.* 2017;376(9):848-855.

94. Hsu PD, Scott DA, Weinstein JA, et al. DNA targeting specificity of RNA-guided Cas9 nucleases. *Nat Biotechnol.* 2013;31(9): 827-832.

95. DeWitt MA, Magis W, Bray NL, et al. Selection-free genome editing of the sickle mutation in human adult hematopoietic stem/progenitor cells. *Sci Transl Med.* 2016;8(360):360ra134.

96. Dever DP, Bak RO, Reinisch A, et al. CRISPR/Cas9 β-globin gene targeting in human haematopoietic stem cells. *Nature.* 2016;539:384-389.

97. Song CQ, Jiang T, Richter M, et al. Adenine base editing in an adult mouse model of tyrosinaemia. *Nat Biomed Eng.* 2020;4(1):125-130.

98. Shariati L, Khanahmad H, Salehi M, et al. Genetic disruption of the KLF1 gene to overexpress the gamma-globin gene using the CRISPR/Cas9 system. *J Gene Med.* 2016;18(10):294-301.

99. John A, Brylka H, Wiegreffe C, et al. Bcl11a is required for neuronal morphogenesis and sensory circuit formation in dorsal spinal cord development. *Development.* 2012;139(10): 1831-1841.

100. Liu P, Keller JR, Ortiz M, et al. Bcl11a is essential for normal lymphoid development. *Nat Immunol.* 2003;4(6):525-532.

101. Canver MC, Smith EC, Sher F, et al. BCL11A enhancer dissection by Cas9-mediated in situ saturating mutagenesis. *Nature.* 2015;527(7577):192-197.

102. Humbert O, Kiem H-P. Long-term increase in fetal hemoglobin expression in nonhuman primates following transplantation of autologous Bcl11a nuclease-edited HSCs. *Blood.* 2015;126(23):2035-2035.

103. Chang KH, Smith SE, Sullivan T, et al. Long-term engraftment and fetal globin induction upon BCL11A gene editing in bone-marrow-derived CD34+ hematopoietic stem and progenitor cells. *Mol Ther Methods Clin Dev.* 2017;4:137-148.

104. Powars DR, Weiss JN, Chan LS, Schroeder WA. Is there a threshold level of fetal hemoglobin that ameliorates morbidity in sickle cell anemia? *Blood.* 1984;63(4):921-926.

105. Kutlar A, Kanter J, Liles DK, et al. Effect of crizanlizumab on pain crises in subgroups of patients with sickle cell disease: a SUSTAIN study analysis. *Am J Hematol.* 2019;94(1):55-61.

106. Vichinsky E, Hoppe CC, Ataga KI, et al. A phase 3 randomized trial of voxelotor in sickle cell disease. *N Engl J Med.* 2019;381(6):509-519.

PART II
Clinical Complications of Sickle Cell Disease

Stroke and Cognitive Dysfunction

Authors: *Hanne Stotesbury, Robert J. Adams,*
Fenella J. Kirkham

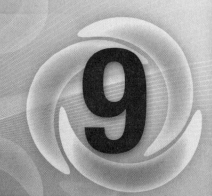

Chapter Outline

Overview

Among the most debilitating and poorly understood complications of sickle cell disease (SCD) are the conditions affecting the central nervous system (CNS), including cerebrovascular disease and diffuse structural abnormalities associated with clinical and silent stroke, seizures, headache, and cognitive impairment (Figure 9-1).[1] Neurologic complications affect at least 25% of SCD patients[2] and are often, but not always, associated with underlying large-vessel vasculopathy.[3] There is a broad spectrum of acute and chronic complications[1]; some of the risk factors are universal, but others appear to be specific and, in some cases, paradoxical.[4] Ischemic and hemorrhagic stroke may occur in the context of acute illness, including chest and vaso-occlusive crises, or "out of the blue."[5] In addition, seizures, headache, and coma are common in patients with SCD.[1,6-8] Advances in neuroimaging

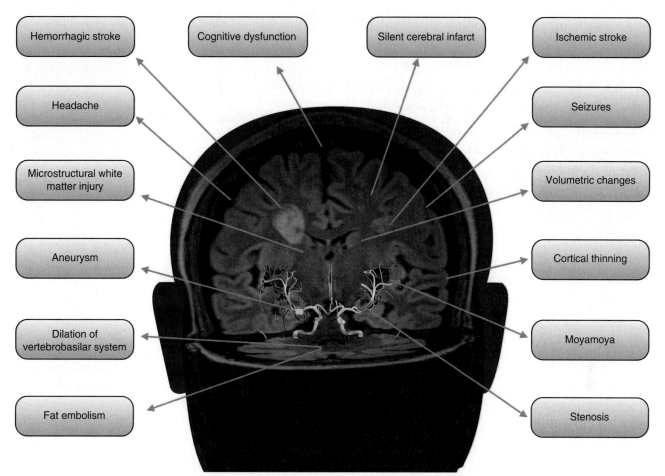

FIGURE 9-1 Neurologic complications in sickle cell disease (SCD). Time of flight angiography image overlaid on 3-dimensional rendered fluid-attenuated inversion recovery (FLAIR) image, edited to depict common neurologic complications in SCD. Adapted from Stotesbury H, Kawadler JM, Hales PW, Saunders DE, Clark CA, Kirkham FJ. Vascular instability and neurological morbidity in sickle cell disease: an integrative framework. *Front Neurol.* 2019;10:871.

have demonstrated evidence for large-vessel and, potentially, small-vessel involvement, along with hemodynamic stress, both in symptomatic clinical stroke and apparently asymptomatic patients with covert or silent cerebral infarction.[1] Screening for large-vessel vasculopathy with transcranial Doppler ultrasound (TCD; Cases 1 and 2) and magnetic resonance angiography (MRA; Cases 1, 2) and for parenchymal damage (ischemic and hemorrhagic; Cases 2-11) with magnetic resonance imaging (MRI) is now established.[1] Computed tomography (CT) may be essential for acute diagnosis and emergency management of ischemia (Case 3) or hemorrhage (Cases 9 and 11), and arterial or venous occlusion (Cases 3 and 4), although because the radiation dose is high, magnetic resonance,

including magnetic resonance venography (MRV; Case 7), should be organized, if possible. Management strategies currently focus on blood transfusion and hydroxyurea.[1] Follow-up from the Stroke Prevention in Sickle Cell Anemia (STOP) trials has demonstrated that if children aged 2 to 16 years with abnormal TCD cerebral blood flow velocities (time-averaged mean maximum velocity >200 cm/s; Case 1) are regularly transfused indefinitely, the majority of pediatric strokes are preventable.[9,10] The Transfusions Switching to Hydroxyurea (TWiTCH) trial showed noninferiority for continuing with hydroxyurea at maximum-tolerated dose in those with abnormal time-averaged mean maximum velocities, but normal MRA, transfused on the STOP protocol for 1 year.[11] Chronic transfusion for children aged

5 to 14 years with silent cerebral infarction was shown to prevent further infarction, particularly clinical stroke, in the Silent Infarct Transfusion (SIT) trial.[12] Bone marrow transplantation has been used for secondary stroke prevention in some, and revascularization is an option if there is intracranial vessel occlusion with collateral formation (moyamoya).[10]

As new treatments are developed, there is increasing interest in CNS end points.[13] Although there are evidence-based strategies for ischemic stroke prevention in children,[10] there are few data on which to base management of adults who remain at risk of hemorrhagic as well as ischemic stroke. Moreover, treatment is often burdensome, the specificity of screening is poor, and many children and adults continue to suffer progressive vasculopathy and/or recurrent cerebral injury, including silent cerebral infarction, as well as recurrent clinical stroke.[14] There are few evidence-based strategies to tackle cognitive difficulties in domains such as executive function and processing speed, which may be compromised in people with SCD with and without cerebral infarction[15-17] and may decline with age,[18] particularly if there is moyamoya on MRA.[19] This chapter defines and discusses what is known about the pathophysiology of the most well-described neurologic complications, before discussing clinical presentations, epidemiology, screening, management, and opportunities for future research.

Classification and Definitions

Vasculopathy

Vasculopathy is an umbrella term used to describe disease affecting blood vessels, irrespective of the underlying cause. To further classify the type and extent of cerebral vasculopathy, a wide-range of modality-specific radiologic grading scales exist.[20]

Clinical Stroke

Clinical stroke is defined by the World Health Organization as "a clinical syndrome consisting of rapidly developing clinical signs of focal (or global in case of coma) disturbance of cerebral function lasting more than 24 hours or leading to death with no apparent cause other than a vascular origin." Strokes occur when there is an interruption in the supply of blood to the brain, either due to an obstruction or failure of perfusion, referred to as an ischemic/infarctive stroke, or due to a bleed, referred to as a hemorrhagic stroke.

Silent Cerebral Infarction

More common than clinical stroke is evidence of infarction or ischemia on brain MRI in the absence of focal neurologic symptoms, typically referred to as *silent cerebral infarction*.[21] Although criteria vary, silent cerebral infarction is most commonly defined as a hyperintense region, consistent with infarction, visible in at least 2 imaging planes on T2-weighted or fluid-attenuated inversion recovery (FLAIR) MRI, measuring at least 3 mm in children and 5 mm in adults.[12,22]

Cognitive Impairment

Cognitive impairment is an umbrella term used to describe difficulties with learning, remembering, concentrating, or making decisions that significantly impact social and economic mobility, as well as quality of life. In the *Diagnostic and Statistical Manual of Mental Disorders*, Fourth Edition, a diagnosis of cognitive impairment additionally requires cognitive psychometric test results to fall >2 standard deviations below the norm for age.

Pathophysiology of Neurologic Morbidity

Autopsy Studies

The available autopsy studies indicate a role for vasculopathy in neurologic morbidity, with intimal thickening, smooth muscle layer hyalinization, fragmented elastic lamina, and microthrombi in segments of large vessels affected by occlusion[23-25] and aneurysm.[26] Microinfarcts in the deep white matter[24] occur not only in stroke patients, but also in patients with no history of neurologic complications, consistent with subtle structural injury. It has been postulated that this is similar to the "cerebral small-vessel disease" recognized in older adults without SCD,[27] but descriptions are vague, and there is no direct histologic evidence in support.[21] Acute demyelination[28] and venous sinus thrombosis[23,29,30] have also been documented.

Pathophysiology

Progressive large-vessel vasculopathy appears to be associated with distal ischemia, leading to focal ischemia with clinical or silent infaction.[31] Inflammation, hypercoagulation, and erythrocyte-leukocyte adhesion to the endothelium, particularly of the more adhesive reticulocytes, probably play a major role in progressive large-vessel vasculopathy and perhaps also in cerebral small-vessel disease and capillary pruning.[32,33] Clinical studies suggest that the risk of cerebral infarction is related to reticulocytosis,[34,35] platelet and leukocyte activation,[36] leukocyte count, P-selectin and L-selectin levels, and endothelial expression of vascular cell adhesion molecule 1 (VCAM1) variant, as well as degree of anemia and hypoxia and markers of hemolytic rate.[35]

To account for cases in which regional ischemic and hemorrhagic pathology develops concurrently, it has been postulated that endothelial dysfunction may lead either to a reparative response, involving intimal thickening and smooth muscle cell proliferation, or to fragmentation of the elastic lamina. The former would be expected to result in vessel narrowing and the development of stenosis, and the latter in vessel wall dilation and aneurysm formation. Local rheology, shear stress, and/or tissue characteristics may determine whether endothelial injury leads to focal narrowing or dilation.[31,32] However, although associated with an increased risk of ischemic events, observable large-vessel vasculopathy does not appear to account for all clinical or silent strokes or cognitive impairment in SCD.[31] Other mechanisms require further investigation, including thromboembolism from the venous circulation through pulmonary or cardiac right-to-left shunts[37] and direct hypoxic-ischemic exposure.[38]

Animal Models

There are mouse models of stroke in SCD that suggest that the mechanism of cerebrovascular disease involves inflammation, neutrophils, and thrombin generation,[39] with relative protection from atherosclerosis, at least in part related to upregulation of heme oxygenase.[40] Using quantitative MRI techniques, mice with the mild NY1DD sickle phenotype had abnormalities in white matter tissue consistent with edema and alterations in the cerebral hemodynamic response to oxygen related to oxidative stress.[41] There are also cerebrovascular abnormalities: compared with control mice, using 2-photon microscopy, the 13-month-old Townes humanized sickle mouse has wider and more tortuous capillaries with shorter branches and more occlusions; at autopsy, there are cortical infarcts.[42] Murine studies have also found volumetric differences in gray and white matter volumes, including in subcortical structures.[43,44] Moreover, older SCD mice show neuropathologic changes in the hippocampus and cerebellum that are not seen in control mice, including shrunken neurons, associated with memory impairment.[44] It may be possible to demonstrate responses to novel treatments using MRI in the sickle mouse and then in patients with SCD.

Imaging Studies

Structural Abnormalities on MRI

In patients with SCD, conventional qualitative radiologic techniques such as CT and MRI (T1-, T2-weighted FLAIR, diffusion-weighted imaging; Figure 9-2) are used to demonstrate hemorrhage, ischemia (clinical and silent),[5] and other compromise of the white and gray matter (eg, cerebral fat embolism[45] or posterior reversible encephalopathy syndrome; Table 9-1).[1,5] In those with overt ischemic stroke, patterns indicative of intracranial large-vessel vasculopathy (Table 9-1, Case 8) occur in over two-thirds, with over one-third showing

lesions consistent with major cerebral vessel occlusion, with or without moyamoya collaterals, and around one-third with distal insufficiency and cortical watershed border zone infarction; the remaining third have lesions consistent with subcortical or small cortical branch occlusion attributed to cerebral small-vessel disease and/or embolism (Case 2).[46] The distribution of silent cerebral infarction is not dissimilar, with up to 90% reportedly occurring in cortical watershed and deep watershed zones (Case 10).[47] Several authors have suggested that differences in lesion size and location, rather than underlying physiologic mechanism, may determine whether an ischemic insult is accompanied by overt symptoms (clinical stroke) or goes undetected (silent cerebral infarction).[38,48] Associated vascular abnormalities may be demonstrated on MRA of the intracranial (Table 9-1) and/or extracranial arteries (Table 9-1, Case 8) and MRV (Figure 9-2, Table 9-1); digital subtraction angiography is usually reserved for those in whom surgery is contemplated (eg, for aneurysm or moyamoya; Table 9-1, Case 9).[1] However, over the past 3 decades, quantitative neuroimaging studies have revealed that functionally significant macro- and microstructural abnormalities detectable by quantitative MRI techniques (Figure 9-2) may be far more prevalent.[49,50] There is evidence that the watershed border zones may be particularly vulnerable to structural injury also in patients without overt or silent stroke, with cortical thinning in the frontal cortex,[51] reduction in white matter density across periventricular regions,[48] and reduction in white matter integrity across the centrum semiovale.[52,53]

Vasculopathy

In addition to, and in the absence of, clinical and silent stroke, up to one-third of SCD patients may have vasculopathy on MRA (Figures 9-2 and 9-3).[54] Intra- and extracranial tortuosity[55] (Case 8) and steno-occlusive arteriopathy (Figure 9-3), often involving the distal internal carotid and the proximal anterior and middle cerebral arteries, are common, particularly in patients with clinical[56] and silent[57] infarction. MRA-defined vasculopathy in radiologically normal patients (Case 1) appears to be rarer, with one sample showing prevalence rates of 6.3%.[58] Incidence of progressive stenosis with compensatory collateral vessel formation, similar to that seen in moyamoya (Figure 9-3), is as high as 30% to 40% in SCD patients with large-vessel vasculopathy.[59]

Of note, findings vary widely due to inconsistent use of definitions and grading schemes for MRA-defined vasculopathy.[20,50] The studies that originally defined stenosis as >50% or >70% narrowing,[54] definitions used in the SWITCH[3] and SIT[58] trials, reported cohorts of patients who had had a clinical stroke. Severity of vasculopathy may more accurately be categorized as degree of signal loss (Figure 9-3),[60] rather than degree of stenosis, since MRA signal is based on velocity of flow and not structure of the vessel. In addition, stenosis, dissection, and occlusion also occur in the carotid and vertebral arteries in the neck (Figure 9-3, Case 8).[61] Despite the discrepancies in terminology and field of view, studies have consistently demonstrated associations between clinical and silent infarction and

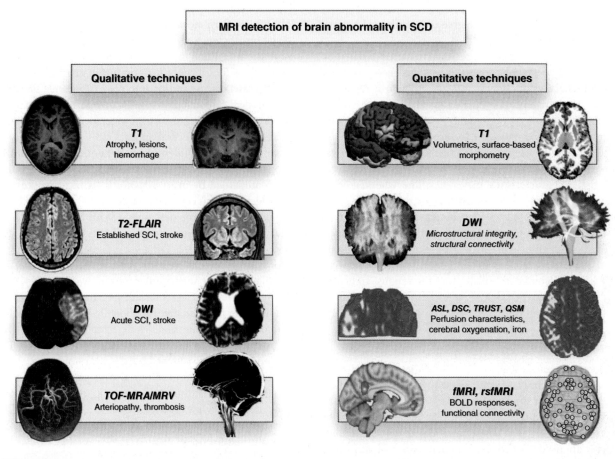

FIGURE 9-2 **Magnetic resonance imaging (MRI) detection of abnormality in sickle cell disease (SCD).** Showing common qualitative and quantitative MRI techniques that have yielded insight into neurologic complications in SCD patients. ASL, arterial spin labeling; BOLD, blood oxygenation level dependent; DSC, dynamic susceptibility contrast; DWI, diffusion-weighted imaging; FLAIR, fluid-attenuated inversion recovery; fMRI; functional MRI; QSM, quantitative susceptibility mapping; rsfMRI, resting-state functional MRI; SCI, silent cerebral infarction; TOF-MRA/MRV; time-of-flight magnetic resonance angiography/magnetic resonance venography; TRUST, T2-relaxation-under-spin-tagging. DWI qualitative images from Hussain Z, Hilal K, Ahmad M, et al. Clinicoradiological correlation of infarct patterns on diffusion-weighted magnetic resonance imaging in stroke. *Cureus*. 2018;10(3):e2260. doi:10.7759/cureus.2260. MRV qualitative image from https://medpix.nlm.nih.gov/case?id=4510eec0-5199-4e4b-b803-15723ae51c31. rsfMRI connectivity image from Dr. Jon Clayden (unpublished).

extra- and intracranial stenosis, with or without moyamoya collaterals (Figure 9-3).[57,58,62,63] Lesser degrees of vessel signal abnormalities (eg, turbulence on MRA) also appear to be associated with reduced white matter integrity[64] and lower gray and white matter volumes.[48]

Hemorrhagic Stroke

Although some authors have suggested independent pathways for the development of infarctive and hemorrhagic stroke, others have proposed a sequential moyamoya-like model of SCD vasculopathy,[65] in which early ischemic events are associated with stenosis and later hemorrhagic events with the development and eventual rupturing of friable and maximally dilated collateral vessels. This model is supported by case reports of collateral vessel hemorrhage in adult SCD cases with a history of ischemic stroke.[65] However, the majority of SCD-related intracerebral and subarachnoid hemorrhages are associated not with rupture of collateral vessels, but with intracerebral aneurysms (Table 9-1, Figure 9-3),[66] which are prevalent in SCD patients, particularly in the posterior circulation.[67,68] Although aneurysms

are not significantly associated with collateral vessel formation,[69] they do appear to form in the context of progressive vasculopathy, with a majority of aneurysm patients presenting with >1 aneurysm.[70] In a recent clinical case review of children with SCD, 5 of 7 patients with hemorrhagic stroke and/or aneurysm also had evidence of clinical or silent infarction (Case 10).[71] These findings may indicate concurrent development of ischemic and hemorrhagic pathology, with shared underlying mechanisms.[26] Further support for this notion comes from the identification of a number of common, albeit nonspecific, risk factors for both ischemic and hemorrhagic stroke, including low steady-state hemoglobin, recent acute chest syndrome, hypertension, and previous ischemic stroke.[4]

TCD

Time-averaged mean of the maximum velocity measured using TCD provides a noninvasive indication of cerebral blood flow velocity in intracranial vessels. Increased time-averaged mean of the maximum velocity may reflect stenotic vasculopathy or high cerebral blood flow.[38] In initial studies, abnormally high

TABLE 9-1 Acute clinicoradiologic syndromes in sickle cell disease

MR/CT	Vascular: MRA/V	Clinical and pathological findings	Treatment
	 (See Ref. 10 [Supp 5])	Sudden onset **stroke** with arterial territory infarct: stenosis, occlusion, dissection ICA, MCA, moyamoya. Exclude shunting	Transfuse–ideally exchange but top-up if not immediately available, O$_2$, ITU, consider thrombolysis in adults within 4.5 h, Stroke Unit
	 (See Ref. 21)	**Silent cerebral infarction:** no stroke but may have had seizures. ?Stenosis, occlusion, moyamoya ICA, MCA. ?Shunt at cardiac or pulmonary level	?Transfuse; ?hydroxyurea
	(See Ref. 45)	**Cerebral fat embolism:** no stroke but typically unconscious after painful crisis or ACS. May have cor pulmonale/shunt at cardiac or pulmonary level	Red cell exchange transfusion, ?plasma exchange, intensive care, inotropic support
	(See Case 5)	**PRES: Posterior reversible encephalopathy syndrome** after rapid transfusion, acute chest, hypertension	Treat seizures, hypertension, hypoxia
	 (See Cases 3 and 4)	**Venous sinus thrombosis:** presents with hemiplegia, seizures, coma. CT: empty delta, thrombus, CTV/MRV	?Transfuse; rehydrate, anticoagulate, if coma ?thrombolysis/thrombectomy, craniectomy for raised ICP
	(See Ref. 10 [Supp 5])	**Abscess:** seizures, headaches, coma, raised intracranial pressure, fever	Antibiotics Neurosurgeon Intensive care
	(See Case 9, Ref. 10 [Supp 5])	**Intracerebral haemorrhage:** sudden onset very severe headache, coma. Venous, hypertension, aneurysm	Neurosurgeon, interventional neuroradiologist Intensive care
	 (See Case 5, Ref. 10 [Supp 5])	**Subarachnoid haemorrhage:** sudden onset very severe headache, coma. Aneurysm, venous, hypertension	Neurosurgeon, interventional neuroradiologist Intensive care
	(See Case 11)	**Subdural haemorrhage:** headache, coma, raised intracranial pressure, skull infarction. Exclude trauma/NAI	Neurosurgeon Intensive care
	(See Case 10)	**Extradural haemorrhage:** headache, coma, raised intracranial pressure, skull infarction. Exclude NAI	Neurosurgeon Intensive care

Abbreviations: ACS, acute coronary syndrome; CT, computed tomography; CT, computed tomography angiography; ICA, internal carotid artery; ICP, intracranial pressure; ITU, intensive therapy unit; MCA, middle cerebral artery; MRA, magnetic resonance angiography; MRI, magnetic resonance imaging; MRV, magnetic resonance venography; NAI, nonaccidental injury; O$_2$, oxygen; SCI, silent cerebral infarction.

time-averaged mean of the maximum velocity showed 90% sensitivity and 100% specificity for the detection of intracranial arterial narrowing or occlusion defined by digital subtraction angiography.[72] However, in recent years, several studies have shown variable correlations between TCD, MRI, and MRA abnormalities.[3,73] Although abnormally high time-averaged mean of the maximum velocity was initially believed to reflect high-grade large-vessel stenosis in SCD patients, subsequent studies have revealed patients with high TCD and normal MRI and MRA.[74] Importantly, regardless of mechanism, nonimaging (Case 1) or imaging TCD (Case 2) is an effective screening tool to prevent stroke.[75] Children with abnormal time-averaged mean of the maximum velocity of ≥200 cm/s had a 3-year stroke risk of 40% compared to a risk of 7% in those with conditional time-averaged mean of the maximum velocity of 170 to 199 cm/s and low risk in those with time-averaged

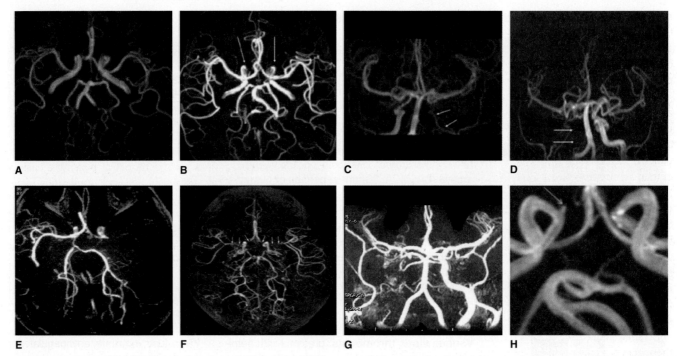

FIGURE 9-3 Vasculopathy on magnetic resonance angiography graded according to severity of signal loss. A. Grade 0: normal.
B. Grade 1: minor signal attenuation (turbulence) and normal-appearing vessel on magnetic resonance imaging. **C.** Grade 2: obvious signal attenuation but presence of distal flow (stenosis). **D.** Grade 3: signal loss and no distal flow (occlusion). **E.** Acute grade 3 occlusion, embolic.
F. Grade 4: occlusion with collaterals (moyamoya). **G.** Occlusion of the carotid in the neck in a patient with previous ataxia and an acute hemiplegia. **H.** Small unruptured aneurysm in an asymptomatic patient.

mean of the maximum velocity <170 cm/s.[76] However, low time-averaged mean of the maximum velocity or unobtainable TCD has also been observed in patients with history of stroke.[7]

Several studies have also established correlations between high time-averaged mean of the maximum velocity and cognitive impairment across a range of domains,[77,78] with results indicating that executive function may be particularly associated with TCD abnormalities. However, there have been no large, systematic studies on the relationship between TCD abnormalities and presence of silent cerebral infarction, and no studies investigating links with structural abnormalities. Nevertheless, in a retrospective review of 78 children (17 silent cerebral infarctions) who participated in the Cooperative Study of Sickle Cell Disease (CSSCD) and STOP trials, there was no relationship between TCD status and presence of silent cerebral infarction.[73]

Cerebral Venous Pathology

There is evidence for abnormalities of cerebral venous drainage in asymptomatic patients with SCD; for example, dural venous sinus diameter is greater in children with SCD with and without stroke than in controls.[79] A recent qualitative susceptibility-weighted imaging study found evidence of abnormal venular patterns in watershed zones of the periventricular white matter in adult SCD patients, with a lower density of long venules and a higher density of short venules.[80] Thrombosis may develop in the superficial or deep venous system, so CT or MRV (Case 7) should be included in acute neuroimaging protocols[81]; because recanalization often

occurs,[82] the opportunity for a diagnosis may be lost if neuroimaging is delayed.

Brain Volume

Quantitative T1-based morphometric studies (Figure 9-2) have reported volumetric changes in SCD patients. Studies in older children and adolescents (>9 years) have consistently reported lower white matter volume globally, and focally in frontal, parietal, and temporal lobes, as well as in the corpus callosum, brain stem, and cerebellum.[49,50,83] For gray matter volumes in late childhood and adolescence, findings are less consistent, with some studies finding few differences in gray matter volume globally or focally,[83,84] and others finding widespread differences in subcortical structures, including lower hippocampal, amygdala, thalamus, cerebellum, and basal ganglia volumes in SCD patients with no radiologic abnormality compared to controls.[85] Cortical morphometric findings in this age group have also been mixed, with 2 studies finding cortical thinning in regions with high metabolic activity in older children and adolescents with SCD[51,86] and a third study finding no differences.[83]

In the only cross-sectional study to examine volumetrics in a sample including younger patients and controls (>4 years), there was lower global gray matter volume in patients but no difference in white matter volume.[87] Differences were more pronounced in total subcortical gray matter volume than in cortical gray matter volume. Interestingly, there was a decrease in global gray matter volume with age in controls that was not observed in patients, which the authors attributed to abnormal brain maturation. A pattern consistent with abnormal maturation was also described in the only prospective longitudinal study of gray and white matter morphometry in SCD to date,[88,89] which included patients and controls between the ages of 3 and 16 years. In this study, change in global gray matter in patients was best captured by a model of linear decrease with age, whereas change in gray matter in controls was best described by a quadratic model in which there was an initial increase in global volume followed by a period of stabilization and slight decrease. Moreover, although change in global white matter in patients was best described by a model of linear increase, the rate of increase was approximately half of that observed in controls.

These results are consistent with a study tracking overall percent brain volume change over a 3-year period in children with SCD,[90] which showed rates of decline beyond those observed in healthy populations and similar to those seen in elderly populations with leukoaraiosis.[91] Although white matter volume has not been investigated in adults with SCD, linear decline in gray matter volume with age is consistent with the only morphometric study in adult sickle patients, where patients showed lower basal ganglia and thalamus volumes and thinner frontal lobe cortex compared to controls.[92] Taken together, these morphometric findings are indicative of abnormalities in brain size and growth that may begin early in development and persist into adulthood, irrespective of presence of clinical or silent cerebral infarction or large-vessel vasculopathy.

Brain Microstructure

Quantitative diffusion-weighted techniques, including diffusion tensor imaging (DTI; Figure 9-2), have been used to investigate microstructural white matter changes in SCD. Changes in white matter integrity, including widespread reductions in fractional anisotropy, have been found in all 4 of the DTI studies that have been conducted in SCD patients to date, one of which included adults up to the age of 45.[16,50,52,53,64,93,94] Affected regions have consistently included the corpus callosum and the centrum semiovale. In 3 of these studies, children without silent cerebral infarction were directly compared with age-matched controls.[53,93,94] All 3 studies found widespread reductions in fractional anisotropy in SCD patients, and 2 found increases in radial and mean diffusivity.[53,93] Because anisotropy and diffusivity are nonspecific indices of microstructural integrity,[95] findings could reflect axonal damage, disorganization of fibers, myelin loss, and/or a failure to adequately myelinate in SCD patients. Three studies have demonstrated relationships between indices of disease severity and structural injury; associations have been demonstrated between lower hemoglobin and reduced white matter volume[83] and fractional anisotropy,[93] and between lower peripheral oxygen saturation and increased radial diffusivity.[93] There have been no studies investigating the impact of socioenvironmental factors on brain structure in SCD.

Functional and Dynamic Pathologies

Hypercoagulability and Embolic Events

In the context of a hypercoagulable state[23,96] and intrapulmonary or intracardiac shunting,[37,97,98,99] with the additional risk of bone marrow necrosis and fat embolism syndrome (Table 9-1),[45,97,100-102] paradoxical embolic ischemic infarction may occur in SCD, particularly in regions affected less commonly.[48,103] One study found correlations between higher mean platelet volume levels and lower white matter volumes in SCD patients, suggesting an association between hypercoagulability, inflammation, and structural brain abnormalities.[83]

Cerebral Hemodynamics

Hemodynamic stress has been demonstrated using a variety of quantitative MRI techniques in SCD patients and is likely to contribute to the high density of infarction and structural abnormalities in the watershed border zone regions between adjacent arterial territories,[31,104] where vascular supply is inherently low[105] and an acute drop in the metabolic rate of oxygen utilization can lead to ischemia. The cerebral metabolic rate of oxygen utilization is defined as the product of arterial oxygen content, rate of blood delivery (ie, cerebral blood flow), and the percentage of oxygen extracted by the tissue (ie, oxygen extraction fraction). The following equations, derived from the Fick principle, show their relationship:

$$\text{Arterial oxygen content } (\text{Ca}_{\text{O}_2}) = (\text{Hb} \times 1.34 \times \text{Sa}_{\text{O}_2}) + (0.003 \times \text{Po}_2)$$

$$\text{Venous oxygen content } (\text{Cv}_{\text{O}_2}) = (\text{Hb} \times 1.34 \times \text{Sv}_{\text{O}_2}) + (0.003 \times \text{Po}_2)$$

where Sa_{O_2} and Sv_{O_2} are arterial and venous oxygen saturation, respectively; Po_2 is the partial pressure of oxygen; and Hb is hemoglobin.

$$\text{Oxygen delivery } (\text{DO}_2) = \text{Ca}_{\text{O}_2} \times \text{Cerebral blood flow (CBF)}$$

$$\text{Oxygen extraction fraction } (\text{OEF}) = (\text{Ca}_{\text{O}_2} - \text{Cv}_{\text{O}_2})/\text{Ca}_{\text{O}_2}$$

$$\text{Cerebral metabolic rate of oxygen utilization } (\text{CMRO}_2) = \text{Ca}_{\text{O}_2} \times \text{CBF} \times \text{OEF}$$

In patients with SCD, changes indicative of cerebral hemodynamic stress include altered arterial oxygen content, cerebral blood flow,[106] cerebrovascular reactivity,[107-109] and oxygen extraction fraction.[110,111] These changes, considered in turn in the following sections, may in part represent global compensatory responses to physiologic stressors associated with SCD pathophysiology,[104] including chronic and acute reductions in Ca_{O_2} secondary to anemic and hypoxic hypoxia.[60,112,113]

Arterial Oxygen Content

The terms *anemic hypoxia* and *hypoxemia* are often used to describe states in which arterial oxygen content is lower due to decreased or dysfunctional hemoglobin.[114] Arterial oxygen content may be further reduced in patients with SCD due to chronic daytime, nocturnal, and/or exercise-induced oxyhemoglobin desaturation,[115] which, when due to inadequate oxygenation in the lungs (eg, hypoventilation, ventilation-perfusion mismatch, shunting, altitude), is sometimes referred to as *hypoxic hypoxia*.[114] Altered sickle hemoglobin (HbS) oxygen affinity, elevated levels of dyshemoglobins, and pulse oximeter calibration for hemoglobin A (HbA) rather than HbS may also affect measured oxyhemoglobin saturation.

Patients with SCD are exposed to low oxygen saturation during acute and chronic hypoxic hypoxia secondary to airway obstruction and/or pulmonary complications, as well as during anemic hypoxia/hypoxemia secondary to low hemoglobin in the context of hemolysis.[116] Daytime desaturation, when defined from pulse oximetry as peripheral oxygen saturation (SpO_2) <96%, may affect up to 30% to 50% of patients with SCD.[117-122] In a study comparing steady-state patients with HbSS and HbSC patients, 44% of HbSS patients, but no HbSC patients, had daytime SpO_2 <96%, in association with previous acute chest syndrome and increasing age.[117] However, normal daytime saturation does not preclude nocturnal or postexercise desaturation,[115] although desaturation under one condition increases the likelihood of desaturation under another.[113,123] Some patients have chronically low oxygen saturation, which may be related to right-to-left shunting at the pulmonary or cardiac level, whereas obstructive sleep apnea is typically associated with chronic intermittent hypoxia, and acute chest syndrome may precipitate acute hypoxia,[124] particularly if there is large-scale polymerization of HbS.

There is increasing evidence for a role of hypoxic exposure in neurologic morbidity in SCD,[60,93,112,125-129] but the mechanisms have not been fully elucidated. There are compensatory physiologic responses to chronic sustained, chronic intermittent, and acute exposures,[124] which may prevent acute cellular hypoxia, defined as inadequate oxygenation at the tissue level,[130] but may increase the risk of intracranial vasculopathy.[60;131-133]

Cerebral Blood Flow, Cerebrovascular Reactivity, and Oxygen Extraction

In steady-state patients, there is evidence for an association between reduced arterial oxygen content and compensatory vessel dilation,[134] leading to increases in global cerebral blood flow and cerebral blood volume,[135] which appear to maintain cerebral oxygen delivery and metabolism when averaged globally.[110,136] However, the increase in cerebral blood flow observed in gray matter is not as high in white matter, and there is evidence that oxygen delivery in border zone white matter regions may be disproportionately reduced, going beyond the watershed effect alone.[137] Recent blood oxygenation level–dependent and arterial spin labeling MRI studies (Figure 9-2) have also demonstrated that increases in global cerebral blood flow are associated with reduced cerebrovascular reactivity to vasodilators, for example, carbon dioxide,[107,108,138,139] with the white matter particularly exhibiting disproportionate delays in cerebrovascular reactivity response times.[140] Studies suggest that a majority of SCD patients may approach the upper limit of dilatory capacity, with up to a quarter exhibiting negative reactivity or "steal,"[138] where blood is "stolen" from one cerebral region and given to another. Steal is thought to occur when there is a pressure gradient between regions (eg, when one

region is maximally dilated and unable to respond to a vasodilatory challenge).[141]

Baseline hemodynamic stress may be exacerbated with exposure to states in which metabolic demand is acutely increased (eg, if body temperature increases or arterial carbon dioxide tension increases during acute chest syndrome or if a seizure occurs)[142] or arterial oxygen content is acutely decreased (eg, with acute hypoxia during acute chest syndrome or an acute decrease in hemoglobin during a parvovirus aplastic crisis).[143] Autoregulatory vasodilation enables increases in cerebral blood flow within the autoregulatory range, which may maintain cerebral metabolic demand up to a point. However, when dilatory capacity is reached,[144,145] with or without steal, the watershed regions may be particularly vulnerable to hemodynamic ischemia associated with disproportionate reductions in oxygen delivery relative to metabolic demand.[146] Events that decrease CaO_2 are consistently associated with both clinical[2,112] and silent stroke in SCD.[21,57,147-149] Recent acute chest syndrome is also associated with ischemic stroke in the absence of large-vessel vasculopathy,[150,151] consistent with a role for reduced oxygen delivery.[152]

Other potential physiologic stressors in SCD patients include flow restriction related to focal vasculopathy, embolic vaso-occlusion, relative systemic hypotension, diastolic dysfunction, and/or altered cerebral autoregulation.[31] Cerebral blood flow may be decreased in arterial territories distal to vascular stenosis or occlusion,[153] as well as in border zone regions.[47,111] Positron emission tomography (PET),[135,154-158] xenon CT,[159] and gadolinium contrast, arterial-spin labeling, and dynamic susceptibility contrast MRI studies[103,111,153,160] have consistently reported focal hypometabolism and hypoperfusion in watershed regions vulnerable to silent cerebral infarction and microstructural damage. Even in "steady-state" patients with radiologically normal FLAIR and T2-weighted MRI, relatively reduced perfusion may be seen on MRI[153] and hypometabolism in watershed regions on PET.[154,156] In patients with higher hematocrit, either naturally or as a result of transfusion, the increased viscosity of blood containing HbS may further reduce perfusion in low-shear watershed regions.[32,161,162]

A state of hemodynamic compromise known as "misery perfusion" is often observed within the first 48 hours of an ischemic insult, involving reductions in focal cerebral blood flow that are accompanied by increases in focal oxygen extraction fraction, which may also serve to maintain cerebral metabolism up to a certain threshold.[163-166] Consistent with hemodynamic compromise, oxygen extraction fraction is abnormal globally[110,167] and in border zone regions[111] prone to silent cerebral infarction in SCD patients.[168] However, oxygen extraction fraction has been reported to be lower[167,169] or higher,[110,111,170] depending on the precise MRI method (ie, whether T2-relaxation-under-spin-tagging based or susceptibility based; Figure 9-2) as well as the calibration model used,[167,171] reflecting either compensation for or exacerbation of hemodynamic compromise. Reports of higher oxygen extraction fraction are broadly consistent with a previous PET study,[135] which is considered the gold standard for measurement of oxygen extraction. The finding of venous hyperintensities on arterial spin labeling MRI (Figure 9-2), indicative of arteriovenous shunting,[172] may explain these paradoxical results,[173] although there appears to be no relationship between venous hyperintensities and whole-brain oxygen extraction fraction,[171,172] underscoring the need for further validation of novel oxygen-sensitive MRI techniques in SCD populations.

Acute silent cerebral ischemic events (ASCIEs) are prevalent in SCD patients presenting with acute decreases in Cao_2,[174-178] as well as in "steady-state" patients undergoing MRI screening. Some ASCIEs appear to transition into later silent cerebral infarction, whereas others may be reversible. The incidence of ASCIE appears to be 10 times greater than that for silent cerebral infarction (47.3 vs 4.8 per 100 patient-years).[176] ASCIEs are likely to occur when the compensatory increases in dilatory capacity and oxygen extraction are exhausted; vascular instability may play a role.[31] Parallel measurement of cerebral blood flow, cerebrovascular reactivity, and oxygen extraction fraction might lead to better stratification of neurologic risk than TCD, particularly in adults, but further validation work, along with prospective studies with long-term follow-up, is required.

Clinical Presentations
Acute Cerebrovascular Complications
Ischemic Stroke

Ischemic insults are most common, accounting for up to 75% of SCD-related strokes,[179] and occur when there is an interruption in the supply of blood to the brain, either due to an obstruction or failure of perfusion (ie, ischemic/infarctive stroke). Hemiparesis is the typical presentation of isolated "out of the blue" ischemic stroke but may be preceded by anterior (hemiparesis) or posterior (ataxia, visual loss) transient ischemic attacks. Infarction is common in mid-childhood, between 2 and 10 years of age, but also occurs in adults as they age; risk factors may be different. Without secondary prophylaxis, recurrence of stroke occurs in as many as 67% of patients, with risk of recurrence greatest within 36 months of the initial event.[14] Treatment reduces, but does not abolish, the recurrence risk.[14,180]

Hemorrhagic Stroke

Patients with SCD are also at considerable risk of hemorrhagic stroke,[71] typically presenting with coma or severe headache. Intracerebral, intraventricular, subarachnoid, subgaleal, subdural, and extradural hemorrhage have all been described in SCD patients (Cases 5, 9, and 11).[1] Although intracranial hemorrhage has the highest incidence in young adults (age 20-30 years),[2] up to 3% of children are also affected.[71] Spontaneous intracranial hemorrhage "out of the blue" is commonly related to the rupture of small (2-9 mm) aneurysms at the bifurcations of major vessels; some may be seen on MRA in asymptomatic patients (Case 10). In addition to the vascular and hematologic risk factors for primary hemorrhagic "out of the blue" stroke, hemorrhagic stroke as a complication of another acute illness typically occurs after recent transfusion,[181] particularly if there is a rapid increase in hemoglobin and/or blood pressure. Other reasons for hypertension may also contribute

(eg, acute renal failure; treatment with cyclosporin, corticosteroids, or phenylephrine; and splenic sequestration).[181] Patients with prior infarction are at increased risk of hemorrhage as they age.[182]

Transient Ischemic Attacks

Patients with SCD also present with transient ischemic attacks. Although symptoms and signs usually resolve within 24 hours, many of these patients show evidence of recent cerebral infarction or atrophy on imaging, which may be indicative of more subtle structural tissue injury, and there is a long-term risk of stroke.[2]

Altered Mental Status

Altered mental status, including acute psychiatric manifestations as well as reduced conscious level, can occur in numerous contexts, including with acute chest syndrome or acute anemia (eg, aplastic secondary to parvovirus); after surgery, transfusion, or immunosuppression; and apparently spontaneously.[1] These patients may have had an ischemic or hemorrhagic cerebrovascular accident, although there is a wide differential of alternative focal and generalized vascular and nonvascular pathologies, including posterior reversible encephalopathy syndrome, cerebral fat embolism, and cerebral abscess (Table 9-1), as well as the effect of medication.

Seizures

Even in the context of a febrile or systemic illness, in patients with SCD, brain MRI should be undertaken for first seizure to exclude the possibility of a potentially treatable underlying cause, such as arterial ischemic stroke, venous sinus thrombosis, posterior reversible encephalopathy syndrome, fat embolism, or cerebral abscess (Table 9-1).[1] A history of seizures has been associated with silent cerebral infarction.[147] Recurrent seizures are 2 to 3 times more common than in the general population and are associated with earlier death.[183] The majority of patients with SCD and seizures have focal abnormality on neuroimaging or electroencephalography and cerebrovascular disease.[184]

Headaches

Headaches are one of the most common neurologic symptoms in SCD, both acutely and chronically.[1] In acute headache, hemorrhagic stroke must be considered (Cases 5, 9, and 11), particularly in older patients and those with a history of stroke, transient ischemic attack, seizure, neurologic symptoms, or focal neurologic findings.[185] Space-occupying lesion or idiopathic intracranial hypertension must be excluded in those with nocturnal or early morning headaches.[186] A neurologist should be consulted for all patients with SCD and new-onset acute headaches. Recurrent headaches and migraines are also common, but neither are associated with ischemia.[8] Referral to a neurologist is advised for assessment of recurrent headache and management with diet, psychological support, and prophylactic medication. Triptans for acute migrainous headaches are contraindicated because of the risk of cerebral ischemia.

Cognitive Impairment

Cognitive difficulties are common in SCD and may be particularly debilitating due to potential adverse effects on social and economic mobility,[187] disease self-management,[188,189] healthcare use,[190] mental health,[191,192] and quality of life.[188,193,194] Already in infancy, up to 50% of SCD patients show delay in early markers of cognition and expressive language.[195] There has been little research into risk factors, which may include hearing loss,[196-198] anemia, hypoxia,[127,199] vasculopathy, and brain injury.[200,201] Through childhood,[18,202,203] adolescence,[192,204,205] and adulthood,[206] patients continue to be at risk of impairment across a range of domains, including general intelligence, executive function, attention, visuospatial abilities, verbal abilities, processing speed, working memory, and visual and verbal short-term memory. Adaptive and behavioral difficulties increase with age.[207] Cognitive impairment may manifest as poorer school readiness during the preschool years,[208,209] academic difficulties during childhood through adolescence,[210-212] and employment difficulties during adulthood.[187] Patients presenting with such difficulties ought to be referred for neuropsychological assessment. Where resources allow, brief neuropsychological screening[213] ought to feature as part of routine care from early childhood.

Stroke was originally identified as the primary cause of cognitive impairment in SCD.[214] Subsequent work has indicated that, although clinical and silent stroke are typically associated with the greatest impairment, lower full-scale intelligence quotient (FSIQ) may be common even in patients with no radiologic MRI or MRA abnormality (Figure 9-4).[15] Findings have been mixed, however, with some studies reporting no differences in cognitive function between patients reported radiologically as normal and healthy controls.[93,203,215,216] Similar discrepancies have been observed between studies comparing cognitive function in patients with and without silent cerebral infarction. In studies finding no differences between patient MRI groups,[16,206] this appears not to be due to the absence of impairment in patients with silent stroke, but rather to a similar proportion of radiologically normal patients observed with impairment.[206] Inconsistent findings may be due to differences in study characteristics, definition of silent stroke

(ie, variability in scanner magnet strength and sequence), cognitive domains examined, neurodevelopmental trajectories, and social and economic factors.

In recent years, evidence has emerged indicating that quantitatively determined MRI abnormalities are associated with cognitive impairment in SCD patients with and without silent cerebral infarction. Lower gray matter volumes in SCD patients have been associated with decreased performance IQ in adults[92] and with decline in global cognitive function in children,[217] whereas decreases in white matter density in the corpus callosum independently predict performance on tests of processing speed, working memory, and distractibility, irrespective of presence of silent cerebral infarction.[218] Widespread reductions in the microstructural integrity of white matter have also been found to be associated with processing speed in patients with and without silent cerebral infarction (Figure 9-5).[16,219]

Vulnerable Domains

Although the majority of previous studies have focused on global functioning (eg, FSIQ), domain-specific tests appear to be more sensitive markers of cognitive impairment in SCD.[17] In patients with no radiologic abnormality, domain-specific tests of executive function and processing speed are at least twice as sensitive as global tests.[220] In patients with clinical or silent ischemic stroke, there are dose-dependent relationships between lesion size and the degree of visuospatial and verbal impairment, but not degree of executive dysfunction.[221,222] These findings may suggest that deficits in some domains (eg, verbal and visuospatial) are associated with lesion size and location,[215,218,223] whereas deficits in others (eg, executive function and processing speed) are associated with the severity of more subtle and diffuse effects of SCD on the brain (Figure 9-5).

Executive Function

Early studies of cognitive challenges in SCD relied almost entirely on measures of intelligence (IQ),[214] but concerns were later voiced about the ability of these to detect specific dysfunction.[221] Measures of executive function, superordinate processes that control and regulate lower level thought and behavior,[224] appear to be particularly sensitive to the cognitive

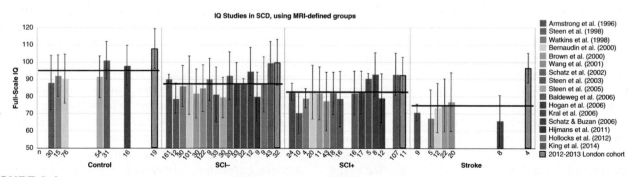

FIGURE 9-4 Full-scale intelligence quotient (FSIQ) in sickle cell disease (SCD). Overview of FSIQ literature in pediatric SCD using magnetic resonance imaging (MRI)-defined groups. Horizontal black lines represent mean FSIQ of the entire group, including previously unreported data from the 2012-2013 London cohort. Italicized numbers on x-axis indicate number of subjects in each group. SCI, silent cerebral infarction. Reproduced from Kawadler JM. Neuroimaging biomarkers in paediatric sickle cell disease. Doctoral thesis, University College London, 2015. https://discovery.ucl.ac.uk/id/eprint/1464063/. Accessed June 22, 2020.

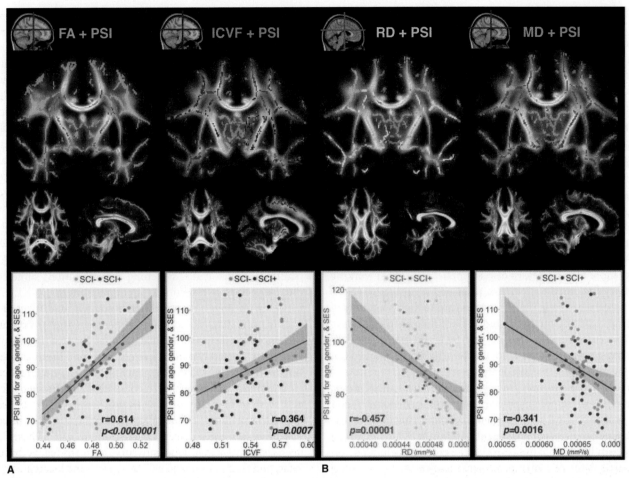

FIGURE 9-5 **White matter integrity and processing speed in sickle cell disease (SCD). A.** Blue voxels indicate areas in which fractional anisotropy (FA) correlated with processing speed index (PSI) (34,392 voxels, *P* <.05). Red voxels indicate areas in which intracellular volume fraction (ICVF) correlated with PSI (70,659 voxels, *P* <.05). **B.** Yellow voxels indicate areas in which radial diffusivity (RD) correlated with PSI (67,296 voxels, *P* <.05). Purple voxels indicate areas in which mean diffusivity (MD) correlated with PSI (82,663 voxels, *P* <.05). Results were age, sex, education decile (socioeconomic status [SES]), and threshold-free cluster enhancement corrected and overlaid on the group white matter skeleton (green) and the study-specific mean FA template. Adj, adjusted; SCI, silent cerebral infarction. Reproduced from Stotesbury H, Kirkham FJ, Kölbel M, et al. White matter integrity and processing speed in sickle cell anemia. *Neurology.* 2018;90(23):e2042-e2050. © 2019 The Authors.

difficulties associated with SCD.[220] Although disruptions to executive function can pose serious threats to development, deficits may be subtle and are often mistaken for immaturity in young children.

Although subtle executive function deficits are already observable at the group level during the preschool years,[225] slower processing speed does not appear to be.[226] It is possible that some core deficits only become apparent on particular tests once patients have reached a developmental stage at which significant gains are expected. Consistent with this notion, results from a recent meta-analysis reviewing cognitive function in SCD patients across the life span found that scores on tests of FSIQ, verbal reasoning, perceptual reasoning, and executive function decreased from preschool to school-aged samples.[17] According to one influential model,[227] the development of mature executive function, termed *executive control*, depends on 4 executive subdomains: attentional control, cognitive flexibility, goal setting, and information processing speed. Each executive domain matures at a different rate, with attentional control emerging early in infancy and maturing through early

childhood and cognitive flexibility, goal setting, and information processing speed emerging later and not maturing until early adolescence.[228] Deficits in executive function, according to this model, can occur as a result of underlying deficits in any of the executive subdomains.

Executive functions are thought to be subserved by a distributed set of frontally guided networks that mediate top-down control.[229] Regions implicated by lesion and neuroimaging studies include the "guiding" prefrontal cortex and the "guided" posterior cortex, subcortical structures, and thalamic pathway. The development of executive function has been shown to coincide with white matter development and the strengthening of synaptic connections between frontal and posterior areas. Strengthened frontal, parietal, and subcortical connectivity is also associated with age-related improvements in working memory, inhibition, and processing speed.

The development of executive networks may be particularly vulnerable to SCD pathology. Overt clinical and silent strokes appear to have primary influence on the integrity of executive function networks, occurring frequently in the frontal lobes[230,231] and in the deep white matter in the border zones between the anterior and middle cerebral artery distributions.[232] The pathways mediating executive function may also be compromised in SCD due to reductions in microstructural integrity in the absence of stroke; exposures including infection,[233] anemia, and hypoxia[125] may play a role.

Working Memory

Working memory, a process that is responsible for the short-term storage and manipulation of information, is often considered a key executive component and is typically further divided into separable subcomponents: the phonologic loop, central executive, and the visuospatial sketch pad.[234] Modality- and information-specific components have also been proposed.[235]

Although findings are mixed, children with SCD appear to make more errors on tasks of visuospatial and verbal working memory compared both to their peers and to normative values on standardized tests.[202,235,236] With regard to digit span tests of auditory working memory, studies have ranged from finding no differences between children with SCD and their peers,[219;202] to finding poorer performance on the digit span backward but not forward task,[235] to finding the opposite pattern of results.[237] Such discrepancies may be accounted for by methodologic differences or sample characteristics; both hematocrit[232] and hemoglobin[238] have been found to independently predict performance on digit span tasks in children with SCD.

A body of research indicates that the presence of lesions may be particularly detrimental to performance on tasks within this domain. There is evidence that compared to children with SCD without infarcts, children with SCD and frontal lesions make more errors on visual working memory tasks[239] and on digit span tasks.[240] Whereas White et al[241] did not observe a similar deficit in verbal working memory span, they did observe that children with SCD and frontal lesions failed to show the usual effect of word length on working memory span, an indication of phonologic loop dysfunction. Conversely, children with SCD and diffuse lesions were found to exhibit the usual effect of word length but showed a decline in verbal working memory span compared to peers with SCD without infarcts, an indication of difficulties with the central executive component of working memory. Schatz et al[231,242] provided evidence that both lesion and anterior corpus callosum volume independently predict performance across working memory tasks. Taken together, these results indicate that SCD-related working memory difficulties are moderated by lesion volume and location, as well as by the degree of tissue loss sustained, either secondary to or independently of infarction.

Studies have provided inconsistent results with respect to whether working memory deficits exist in the absence of stroke. None of the studies reporting significant deficits in working memory used MRI, the only current strategy to detect silent cerebral infarction; studies relying on clinical history may have included those with silent cerebral infarction in their samples. These findings are therefore inconclusive. However, there are reports that, after controlling for the effects of age

and hematocrit, abnormal TCD significantly predicts deficits in auditory working memory.[243-245]

Cognitive Flexibility, Inhibition, and Shifting

In models of executive function, cognitive flexibility is another major component, with inhibition and shifting typically featuring as the main subcomponents. Inhibition can broadly be defined as the ability to restrain the expression of an instinctive response.[246] Linked to inhibition, but with a more prolonged developmental trajectory, is the ability to adapt to changing conditions. This adaptive ability is thought to be measured by tasks in which participants are required to "shift" between task sets.[247]

Compared to their peers[237] and to normative values,[233] children with SCD have been shown to perform more poorly on the color-word interference (inhibition), trail-making (shifting), and sorting (switching and inhibition) subtests of the Delis-Kaplan Executive Function System (D-KEFS).[248] However, findings have not always been replicated.[93,125] As with working memory, methodologic differences and/or variations in sample characteristics could account for this discrepancy. Kral et al[249] found hematocrit to account for a significant portion of the variance in performance on the trail-making task.

Inhibition and switching, as measured by a range of tasks, also seem to be particularly vulnerable to stroke. The Test of Variable Attention (TOVA),[250] a test that among other cognitive processes relies on a substantial amount of shifting, has been shown to be highly sensitive to undetected silent cerebral infarction in children with SCD,[251] indicating that it may be a cost-effective screening tool for suspected cerebral injury. Craft et al[214] found deficits in switching and inhibition to be moderated by lesion type and location, but not volume; children with frontal lesions as a result of an overt stroke showed the greatest impairments. More recently, Hogan et al[239] provided evidence that compared to SCD and sibling controls, children with white matter lesions show a diminished event-related potential component difference between error and correct responses, an indication of weaker response monitoring systems. These results lend support to the distributed network model of executive function and provide a possible explanation for difficulties in children with lesions that do not involve the frontal cortex.

As with working memory, also in this domain, it is unclear whether deficits exist in the absence of stroke. The majority of studies that screened participants for the presence of silent cerebral infarction reported no differences in inhibition or in shifting between children with SCD without stroke and peer/sibling controls.[93,214,239] There have, however, been 2 exceptions to this. First, Andreotti et al[233] observed that children with SCD and without infarcts performed significantly below normative means on the trail-making and color-word interference test. Correlations were found between scores and plasma cytokine levels, a marker of inflammatory processes. However, because 16 of 25 participants had a comorbid diagnosis of asthma, a condition associated with elevated cytokines,[252] it is unclear whether the inflammation could be attributed to SCD pathology alone. Second, Hollocks et al[125] found that children with

SCD and no infarcts made more errors on the sorting test in comparison to normative means. A similar pattern of results was reported by Berg et al.[237] These findings indicate that the sorting test may be sensitive to executive dysfunction in SCD that is not associated with presence of silent cerebral infarction. However, because sorting tests engage multiple executive functions as well as more general cognitive processes that are not readily isolated, it is difficult to pinpoint which process or processes might be compromised. Given the lack of evidence for specific inhibition and shifting deficits in the absence of stroke, these findings may point to higher-level deficits in synchronizing the activity of several executive functions.

Processing Speed

Processing speed is often considered an executive subdomain and appears to be particularly sensitive to the effects of SCD on the brain; irrespective of the presence or absence of silent cerebral infarction, this is the domain showing the greatest disparity between adult SCD patients and controls.[206,253] Children with SCD are slower, but not less accurate, on tests of executive function and memory, potentially reflecting slower processing speed.[237,243,254,255] Patient performance is similar to that of controls across a range of cognitive tests, including tests of general intelligence and executive function, if processing speed is statistically controlled for.[256] These findings may suggest mediation of other deficits by slower processing in SCD and/or an overlap in the mechanisms underlying slower processing, lower FSIQ, and executive dysfunction. There is evidence that reduced processing speed is related to severity of anemia in SCD patients, including levels of hemoglobin and hematocrit. Socioeconomic factors, such as maternal education[16,257] and employment status, have also been implicated.

The behavioral significance of many of the structural and hemodynamic changes demonstrable using quantitative MRI remain elusive; relatively few studies have investigated potential correlates of cognitive difficulties. However, DTI abnormalities have been established as potential biomarkers of longitudinal hypoxic exposure in SCD,[93] and there is evidence for associations with reduced processing speed, irrespective of the presence of silent cerebral infarction (Figure 9-5).[219]

Neurodevelopment

Several authors have considered SCD in the framework of a neurodevelopmental disorder (Figure 9-6).[258] Although few of the clinical manifestations of SCD are apparent early in life, there are reports of mild neurologic abnormalities in infants with SCD aged 7 to 48 months[200] and of silent cerebral infarction occurring in the first year of life.[259] However, although children in the CSSCD were followed up and change in IQ was compared in those with and without silent cerebral infarction,[18] there have been no comprehensive longitudinal studies examining cognitive trajectories and their interaction with environmental and disease factors over time.

Cross-sectional studies have consistently reported negative associations between cognitive function and age in sickle patients, which may reflect cognitive decline.[18,77,244,260] Worsening of global cognitive ability has been demonstrated longitudinally in toddlers,[261] as well as in patients with severe vasculopathy[19] and in those with silent cerebral infarction and tissue loss.[217] In the CSSCD, processing speed was lower in older than younger patients, irrespective of silent cerebral infarction presence, which may indicate worsening of cognitive function even in children with no radiologic abnormality.[18] However, use of age-scaled rather than raw scores limits the conclusions that can be drawn regarding cognitive decline in

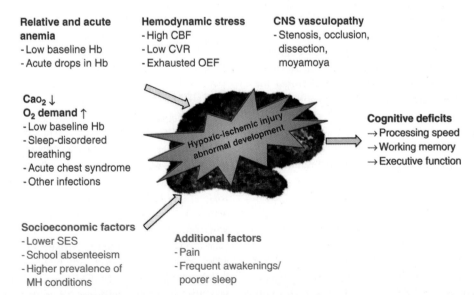

FIGURE 9-6 Sickle cell disease (SCD) as a neurodevelopmental disorder. An overview of key biologic, socioeconomic, and psychological factors in SCD. Cao_2, arterial oxygen content; CBF, cerebral blood flow; CNS, central nervous system; CVR, cerebrovascular reactivity; Hb, hemoglobin; MH, mental health; OEF, oxygen extraction fraction; SES, socioeconomic status. Adapted from DeBaun MR, Kirkham FJ. Central nervous system complications and management in sickle cell disease. *Blood.* 2016;127(7):829-838.

these studies, as a decrease in scaled scores could also reflect a failure to improve at the expected rate with no numerical change in raw score (ie, delay). In the absence of raw longitudinal data, the extent to which later cognitive impairment is causally related to earlier developmental delay and/or previous or ongoing pathophysiologic processes remains obscure. Early language delay is predictive of later academic performance, quality of life, and risk of stroke.[262] These findings highlight the clinical utility of cognitive screening but are potentially a reflection of more severe disease courses leading to worse outcomes. Whether sickle patients "grow into" some deficits with maturation and/or display catch-up in others is an open question, particularly because disease factors that may influence development may also change over time.

Disease and Socioeconomic Factors

There is cross-sectional evidence that early developmental delay and later cognitive impairment are associated with both environmental and disease-related variables (Figure 9-5).[78] In infants and preschoolers with SCD, studies consistently report relationships between early markers of cognitive development and socioenvironmental factors, including level of parental education, income, and stress.[207,261,263,264] However, socioenvironmental factors do not appear to sufficiently explain early developmental delay.[265] Although some studies of early cognitive development have also found associations with the severity of anemia[261,266,267] and peripheral oxygen desaturation (Spo$_2$),[127] others have not.[207,263–265]

During childhood, correlations between cognitive and disease-related variables[215,268,269] are more widely and consistently reported, and the effects of socioeconomic and environmental factors appear to persist.[204,268,270,271] In the baseline data of the SIT trial, presence of silent cerebral infarction was associated with a 5-point cross-sectional decrease in FSIQ, and absence of parental college education was associated with a 6-point decrease.[126] There was also a 1-point decrease for every 1% decrease in Spo$_2$.[126] In a French multicenter trial, silent cerebral infarction was only associated with cognitive dysfunction when accompanied by reduced hematocrit or thrombocytosis.[232] More recently, evidence was provided for a role of inflammation in cognitive dysfunction, with strong correlations found between elevated cytokine levels and executive dysfunction in SCD children with radiologically normal MRI.[233] Although there have been few studies in adult patients, there is evidence that associations with hematocrit remain and become stronger with age.[206]

Epidemiology

Clinical Stroke

In the absence of screening and prophylactic treatment, approximately 11% of SCD patients in the United States will suffer a stroke by their 20th birthday, and 24% by age 45.[2] In a systematic review of 10 cross-sectional clinic-based studies in Africa, prevalence of stroke ranged from 2.9% to 16.9%,[272]

whereas another group reported an overall prevalence of 4.2% from a meta-analysis.[6] In a North American study in which the overall incidence of childhood stroke was 1.29 per 100,000 per year, the most common cause was SCD (39%), with an incidence of 285 to 310 per 100,000 per year.[273] However, in older adults with SCD, the rate may be 3 times as high.[274] In a large population study, the biggest risk factor for stroke in children with SCD was hypertension, whereas in adults with SCD, the biggest risk factors included not only hypertension, but also diabetes mellitus, hyperlipidemia, atrial fibrillation, and renal disease.[274] The prevalence of stroke in a cohort of children with hemoglobin C who had been neonatally screened was 0.2%.[275]

One population study found the risk of hemorrhagic stroke to be highest during the period (age 20-29 years) in which risk of ischemic stroke was lowest, potentially indicating different underlying mechanisms or progressive vasculopathy.[2] In a recent cohort study, 10% of SCD patient deaths were attributable to stroke.[276] Although ischemic stroke is rarely fatal, death may occur following 26% of hemorrhagic cases.[2] Recurrence rates of up to 70% have been reported for ischemic stroke,[14] with risk of recurrence greatest within 36 months of the initial event.[14] Both types of stroke are associated with significant long-term morbidity, including seizures, physical disability, and cognitive impairment.[1]

Seizures

Between 7% and 10% of individuals with SCD will experience at least one seizure.[277] In a meta-analysis of studies from Africa, the prevalence of seizures was 4.4%.[6] In the Jamaican Cohort Study of Sickle Cell Disease, the 5-year cumulative incidence of febrile convulsions was 2.2%.[277]

Abnormal and Conditional TCD

The prevalence of abnormal TCD was considered to be around 10% in the United States at the time of the STOP trial, although recent studies suggest a lower prevalence. In an African meta-analysis, the prevalence of abnormal and conditional TCD was 10.6% and 6.1%, respectively.[6]

Silent Cerebral Infarction

Silent cerebral infarction may occur as early as the sixth month of life.[200,201] There is evidence that prevalence reaches 25% by 6 years of age,[149] 39% by 18 years of age,[57] and 53% by adulthood,[68] with no reports of a plateau. Of note, prevalence estimates may vary not only with age, but also with scanner magnet strength and voxel size.[1] Although clinically "silent," evidence of progression was first provided by the CSSCD, where silent cerebral infarction was associated with a 14-fold increase in risk of ischemic stroke, and 25% of children with silent cerebral infarction presented with new or enlarged lesions at follow-up.[278] In the CSSCD, silent cerebral infarction was also associated with cognitive decline.[18] These findings have been replicated in more recent work, including in a study where silent cerebral infarctions in patients younger than 5 years old were shown to be associated with later progressive ischemia, vasculopathy, academic difficulties, and a higher risk of stroke.[201] Further indicative of progressive ischemia, a recent clinical review of 60 unselected adult cases found that 37% of patients with silent cerebral infarction had >1 lesion.[68]

Headache

Headache affects between 20%[6] and 45%[37] of patients with SCD and may occur at any age, including in young children.[66]

Cognitive Impairment

Studies rarely report formal diagnoses of cognitive impairment, which makes meaningful comment on the prevalence challenging. The overwhelming majority of studies also report sample-level mean performance on cognitive tests, rather than the proportion of patients with scores that fall into established clinical categories. However, in one study, 28% of patients had processing speed scores that fell in the borderline to extremely low categories (ie, scores of <80) compared to 6% of controls, indicating that, although there is significant variability within SCD populations, patients are at greater risk of clinically significant cognitive impairment.[16]

Screening

Stroke Risk

Vasculopathy

Seminal studies in the 1990s established the value of TCD for prediction of stroke risk in SCD.[279] The results from the landmark STOP and STOP2 trials formed the basis for the current gold standard of care for primary stroke prevention in SCD: yearly TCD screening with chronic blood transfusion therapy for children with cerebral blood flow velocity >200 cm/s and close monitoring of those with conditional velocities (>170-200 cm/s).[9,66,76,279,280] TCD screening has substantially decreased incidence of stroke,[9] with one center reporting a decline from 0.67 to 0.006 per 100 patient-years,[177] but there are false positives[279] and false negatives.[62,281] There are few data on the utility of TCD screening in adults, in whom time-averaged mean of the maximum velocity is rarely >200 cm/s[282] despite high and probably increasing stroke rates.[283] It is possible that screening with Doppler ultrasound of the neck vessels[63] would allow prediction of stroke in adults, but prospective studies are required.

Silent Stroke

Screening for presence of silent cerebral infarction with MRI is feasible, and recent guidelines recommend that it is undertaken at least once in childhood.[10] However, there are no well-established or validated protocols for screening for risk of silent cerebral infarction.

Cognitive Difficulties

Neurodevelopmental screening using questionnaires and relatively simple tools is recommended in the recent guidelines, particularly in early childhood.[10]

Treatment Options

Blood Transfusion

Mechanism

There is evidence that transfusion has immediate hemodynamic effects, reflected by reductions in cerebral blood flow[284] and cerebral blood volume.[285] Posttransfusion reductions in oxygen extraction fraction[171,286] and increases in cerebrovascular reactivity[108] have also been reported. These findings suggest that reduction in hemodynamic stress, involving normalization of hyperemia, along with restoration of vascular response mechanisms, may contribute to the efficacy of transfusion in reducing the effects of acute ischemia and the risk of future initial or recurrent stroke. Of note, transfusion appears to reduce, but not completely normalize, cerebral blood flow and oxygen extraction fraction in SCD patients, with watershed regions continuing to exhibit "at-risk" regions.[286] There is also evidence that oxygen extraction fraction and cerebral blood flow responses to transfusion are blunted in adult SCD patients.[171] These factors could contribute to continuing risk of morbidity in some patients.

Interestingly, posttransfusion reductions in oxygen extraction fraction and cerebral blood flow are independently associated with improvement in overall hemoglobin levels, but not HbS fraction.[171,286] These findings may suggest that a reduction in vascular instability is primarily achieved via improvement in oxygen delivery rather than red blood cell rheology. However, given their interdependency, these effects are difficult to disentangle. Both the compensatory global increases and posttransfusion reductions in cerebral blood flow are greater than expected by hemoglobin levels alone in SCD.[287] These findings are consistent with a model of vascular instability and hemodynamic stress in which both hemolytic and vaso-occlusive/rheologic processes may play a role.[284]

Role of Blood Transfusion in the Primary Prevention of Stroke in Children With Abnormal TCD

Despite a lack of high-quality evidence,[288] blood transfusion, ideally erythrocytapheresis because of the lower rate of iron accumulation, has been the mainstay for secondary stroke prevention.

In the landmark STOP trial, patients with abnormal cerebral blood flow velocities (>200 cm/s) randomized to monthly blood transfusion showed a 92% reduction in risk of stroke compared to patients randomized to standard care.[279] In the STOP2 follow-up trial, patients who discontinued transfusion after 30 months of treatment demonstrated reoccurrence of abnormal cerebral blood flow velocities.[280] Both trials were stopped early due to higher rates of adverse events in the nontransfused arms. As mentioned earlier, the results formed the basis for the current gold standard of care for primary stroke prevention in SCD: yearly TCD screening with chronic transfusion therapy for children with abnormal velocities (>200 cm/s) and close monitoring of those with conditional velocities (>170-200 cm/s).[66]

Although this strategy has substantially decreased the incidence of stroke,[177] there are several drawbacks. First, up to 60% of children with abnormal TCD screening results may not go on to have a stroke.[279] Second, TCD screening may miss a subset of children in whom blood velocities are very low or undetectable, but in whom risk of stroke may be high.[62,281] Third, even with chronic blood transfusion therapy, up to 45% of children with prior stroke will have silent or overt stroke recurrence,[59,180,289] often in association with worsening vasculopathy.[180] Fourth, for children with silent cerebral infarction, the number needed to treat to prevent one infarct (overt or silent) is as high as 13 over a 3-year period.[12] These findings are particularly significant given that transfusion therapy is burdensome and costly,[290] and there is a lack of clarity on the most optimal transfusion strategy, particularly in terms of treatment length.[291] In addition to the burden of monthly transfusions in terms of school and work absences, there are a number of associated side effects, including iron overload, alloimmunization, and infection transmission.[292,293] The number needing indefinite transfusion to prevent one stroke is 7,[179,280] but the strategy has dramatically reduced the stroke rate. However, patients and their families may feel that the risk-benefit ratio is unfavorable and therefore opt out of treatment.[294] These practical issues mean that regular blood transfusions are rarely available in low income countries.

Role of Blood Transfusion to Prevent Further Infarction in Children With Silent Cerebral Infarction

The SIT trial was conducted to determine whether blood transfusion therapy for 36 months prevents progression of infarct recurrence (stroke or silent cerebral infarction) in children with SCA (5-15 years of age) and preexisting silent cerebral infarction. In participants receiving regular blood transfusion, there was 58% relative risk reduction in cerebral infarct recurrence (stroke or new or progressive silent cerebral infarcts) when compared to the children in the observation arm.[12] The evidence is of moderately good quality,[288] but the number of children with SCA and silent cerebral infarction who need to be transfused to prevent one recurrent infarct is 13. Uncertainty remains over whether there is benefit of clinical relevance to patients (eg, in cognitive function), and again, the high burden of regular blood transfusion may decrease enthusiasm for this management strategy.

Role of Blood Transfusion in Secondary Prevention of Stroke

Although there have been no randomized controlled trials and the definition of primary and secondary stroke was not consistent in the pre–CT scan era when the natural history data were acquired,[182] there appeared to be a substantial reduction in the incidence of recurrent stroke if patients with stroke were regularly transfused long term.[295-297] However, further infarction, both overt and silent, does continue to occur even when the blood transfusion regimen is optimized.[180]

Hydroxyurea for Secondary and Primary Stroke Prevention

Hydroxyurea is in principle a less invasive treatment strategy based on stimulation of fetal hemoglobin (HbF), although if pushed to maximum-tolerated dose, it does require frequent full blood counts. The Stroke With Transfusions Changing to Hydroxyurea (SWiTCH) trial was a noninferiority trial conducted in children undergoing chronic transfusion for previous stroke, with a composite primary end point allowing increased stroke risk (<10%) on hydroxyurea but decreased iron chelation requirement in the context of phlebotomy; it was stopped early for futility because liver iron did not decrease.[298]

The available evidence shows that hydroxyurea is associated with a reduction in time-averaged mean maximum velocity.[299] Noninferiority of hydroxyurea was demonstrated in the TWiTCH trial, a primary stroke prevention trial for SCD children who had received at least 12 months of blood transfusion for TCD velocities >200 cm/s.[11] Standard therapy was continuation with blood transfusion therapy and chelation, and experimental therapy was hydroxyurea therapy and phlebotomy, although there was a median overlap of approximately 6 months. The primary outcome was TCD velocity; after the first interim analysis, the trial was ended early because noninferiority was demonstrated. Trial design limitations included the short period of time on hydroxyurea therapy at maximum-tolerated dose, approximately 18 months, and the exclusion of approximately 10% of children with abnormal TCD *and* MRA, meaning that management for this group cannot be determined from the TWiTCH trial, but it does appear that hydroxyurea is effective in maintaining a lower TCD in those with normal MRA. Hydroxyurea may be an option for primary[300] and secondary[301] prevention in low-income settings if safe blood transfusion is not available or is too expensive; the results of ongoing trials in northern Nigeria are likely to clarify the position.[302,303]

Revascularization

Moyamoya syndrome is associated with an increased risk of stroke recurrence, which appears to be reduced by revascularisation.[304] There are relatively few data on the efficacy of cerebral revascularization procedures (encephalo-duro-arterio-synangiosis [EDAS], encephalo-duro-arterio-myo-synangiosis [EDAMS], pial synangiosis, direct anastomosis, or burr holes) when moyamoya syndrome, a risk factor for recurrent stroke despite transfusion, is diagnosed on MRA or formal arteriography.[305] Studies have compared the incidence of strokes before and after revascularization surgery, but follow-up is relatively short and outcomes have not been compared with patients remaining on chronic blood transfusion. A multidisciplinary team including a hematologist, neurologist, neuroradiologist, and neurovascular surgeon should make the decision on whether surgery is a reasonable option[10] and should consider strategies to prevent neurologic complications before, during, and after surgery.

Bone Marrow Transplantation

Bone marrow transplantation (BMT) is established as an option for secondary stroke prevention if there is an human leukocyte antigen–matched sibling.[306] Primary stroke prevention for children with abnormal TCD is feasible; a French multicenter study recently established that cerebral blood flow velocities were reduced more after BMT than on standard treatment with regular blood transfusion.[307] The majority of patients have stable findings on neuroimaging after hematopoietic stem cell transplant, but although some improve, around 1 in 6 deteriorate.[308] Posterior reversible encephalopathy syndrome is a relatively common complication in the immediate post-transplant period, related to the requirement for immunosuppression as well as fluctuations in blood pressure, while acute and chronic graft-versus-host disease may compromise quality of life.[309]

Cognition

Despite the evidence base for prevention of neurologic complications and the lower average IQ in those with overt or silent stroke, there are currently no evidence-based strategies for management of cognitive impairment or structural injury. Given the mixed and inconclusive findings, larger trials on treatment of cognitive impairment are required.[310] Studies that include more homogeneous patient samples, particularly in terms of age, may enable clearer conclusions to be drawn.

Effect of Blood Transfusion on Cognitive Impairment

In the SIT trial, 196 children (aged 5-15 years) with silent cerebral infarction were randomly assigned to observation or transfusion therapy with a primary end point of recurrent infarction. Despite a statistically significant reduction in recurrent infarction on transfusion (6%) versus observation (14%), there was no effect of transfusion on FSIQ, performance IQ, verbal IQ, or parent-rated executive function following a median treatment period of 3 years.[12] However, transfused patients demonstrated improvement in executive abilities near transfusion compared to far from transfusion.[311] Because this study did not follow patients prospectively and there is no mention of whether time between assessment and closest transfusion were controlled in the SIT trial, the jury is still out on the effect of transfusion on cognition in SCD.

Effect of Hydroxyurea on Cognitive Impairment

There is cross-sectional evidence indicating an association between hydroxyurea use and improved visuospatial and global cognitive functioning in children with SCD.[312] In a small prospective trial in which 21 hydroxyurea-treated and 11 untreated children (aged 7-18 years) were followed for 12 months, there was a small (<1 standard deviation) but significant improvement in FSIQ scores in treated patients.[310] However, although mean change was positive in the treated group and negative in the untreated group, there were no statistically significant between-group differences in change. A recent study showed that, after adjusting for socioeconomic status, adolescents with SCD who had been exposed to hydroxyurea had significantly higher scores on nonverbal IQ, reaction speed, sustained attention, working memory, and verbal memory when compared to those who had not been exposed to hydroxyurea.[313] Longer duration of treatment was associated with better verbal memory and reading in those with homozygous SCD.

Effect of BMT on Cognitive Impairment

One study from France found an improvement in IQ after BMT, despite a reduction in processing speed.[314] Another study found that mean scores for processing speed were significantly greater after transplant, although there were no significant differences in verbal reasoning, perceptual reasoning, working memory, and full-scale IQ.[315] Differences in follow-up time may account for these discrepancies.

Novel Treatments

New approaches to the prevention of acute and chronic complications in SCD include treatment with antioxidants (eg, L-glutamine), drugs to prevent polymerization (eg, voxelotor), and monoclonal antibodies to reduce cellular adhesion and inflammation. Gene therapy approaches include increasing HbF via gene editing strategies or replacing the abnormal gene via lentiviral vectors; both require BMT. Those developing these options are keen to have a CNS end point,[13] which might include TCD, MRI, MRA, or cognitive testing.

"How I Treat" Expert Perspective

The priorities in a child presenting with a focal neurologic deficit, reduced level of consciousness, seizures, or severe headache is to stop any seizures to avoid status epilepticus (using a local protocol), to crossmatch for an emergency top-up or exchange transfusion, and to obtain emergency neuroimaging, either by CT scan to exclude hemorrhage or ideally by MRI, with susceptibility-weighted imaging to exclude hemorrhage and fat embolism. MRI will also allow the diagnosis of acute focal or generalized pathology and help determine whether there is a vascular basis for the pathology. The MRI scan should include diffusion-weighted imaging to determine the timing of any ischemia, FLAIR, MRV, and MRA of the intra- and extracranial vessels.

Conclusion

Overt stroke, silent cerebral infarction, and vasculopathy may represent only the tip of the iceberg in terms of the causes of neurological complications in SCD. Quantitative MRI studies have revealed cerebral hemodynamic, metabolic, volumetric, and microstructural abnormalities that may be more prevalent, widespread, and potentially also more functionally significant. However, findings have been mixed, identified changes are non-specific, mechanisms are poorly understood, and neurodevelopment has largely been neglected. Management strategies are therefore inadequate, with a limited evidence base.

Along with larger and more comprehensive randomized clinical trials with structural and cognitive end points, one of the most pressing needs for patients with SCD and the clinicians tasked with treating them is better methods for prediction of individual risk of neurologic morbidity. This would enable selection of patients who are sufficiently high risk for burdensome and costly treatment, as well as ongoing monitoring of risk so that treatment is not necessarily lifelong. At present, risk-benefit analyses are subject to substantial uncertainty in SCD. Risk stratification of patients likely to benefit from transfusion for primary or secondary stroke prevention versus those unlikely to need prevention for primary stroke or likely to fail secondary prevention is a pivotal next step that would increase the benefit-to-burden ratio. In the future, early identification of risk of structural abnormalities and associated cognitive impairment may enable implementation of preventative strategies before delay/decline occurs. To this end, novel quantitative hemodynamic and oxygen-sensitive MRI techniques hold promise, although significant validation work is required, along with longitudinal cohort studies.

Case Studies

Case 1. This teenager with HbSS had recently arrived in the United Kingdom from an African country and thus had not been in the transcranial Doppler screening program. He developed a severe headache after acute chest syndrome. Nonimaging transcranial Doppler was abnormal on the right (R) and conditional on the left (L) (**A**). Magnetic resonance angiography (MRA) showed signal dropout (**B**) that was worse on the right, but T2-weighted magnetic resonance imaging (MRI) (**C**), diffusion-weighted imaging (**D**), and apparent diffusion coefficient (**E**) were normal. Gadolinium perfusion showed reduced perfusion (**F**) and increased mean transit time (**G**) throughout the right hemisphere and posteriorly on the left, although cerebral blood volume was normal (**H**). He was transfused monthly and 1 year later had normal MRI, MRA, and perfusion. MCA, middle cerebral artery.

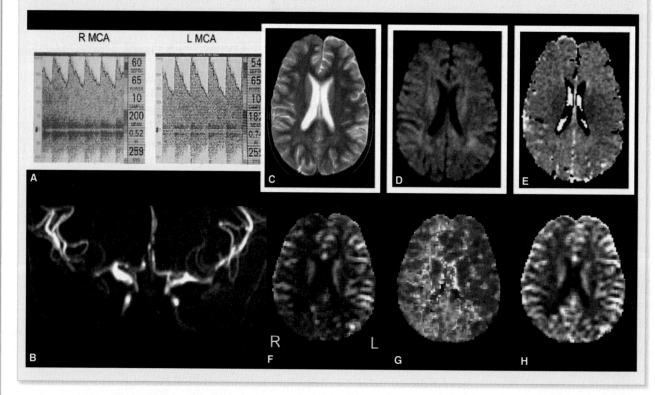

Case Studies: Continued

Case 2. This young child who is a compound heterozygote had a left hemiparesis at the age of 6 months, before transcranial Doppler screening was mandated. Prior to that, the child had had a cold on and off for the past few months and tended to breathe rather heavily and to snore on and off. On T2/fluid-attenuated inversion recovery magnetic resonance imaging, there was patchy hyperintensity within the right superomedial striatocapsular region (**A**), with associated diffusion restriction (not shown), consistent with acute evolving infarction. Magnetic resonance angiography was normal (**B**), as was transcranial Doppler imaging (**C**). A patent foramen ovale was demonstrated on bubble contrast echocardiography (**D1-3** shows appearance of the bubbles after the injection of agitated saline), but venography of the legs (**E**) and pelvis did not demonstrate clot. Treatment was with aspirin as well as regular blood transfusion.

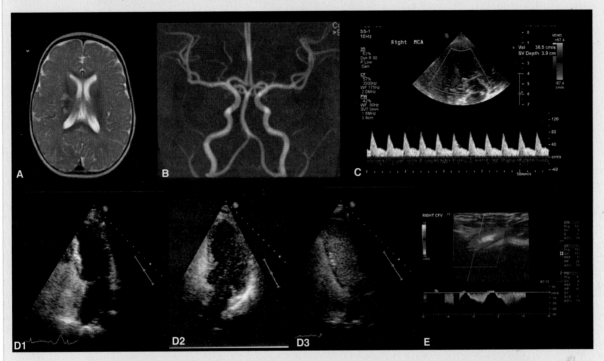

Case 3. This patient with HbSS presented with pneumococcal meningitis as a toddler in the era before pneumococcal vaccination. A sagittal sinus thrombosis was diagnosed because there was an empty delta sign (**A**, blue arrow) on computed tomography. Epilepsy persisted throughout childhood, was associated with residual focal brain damage on magnetic resonance imaging (**B**), and was resistant to several anticonvulsants but eventually ceased on tiagabine.

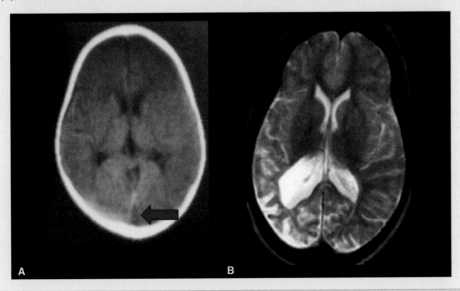

Case Studies: Continued

Case 4. This schoolchild with HbSC disease had had unexplained hydrocephalus in infancy but had not required a shunt. He presented with headache and seizures, but the straight sinus thrombosis (**A**, yellow arrow) visible on the computed tomography scan was not diagnosed until his conscious level had deteriorated with widespread cerebral edema on magnetic resonance imaging (**B**). Despite intensive care and neuroprotection, he fulfilled the criteria for brain stem death.

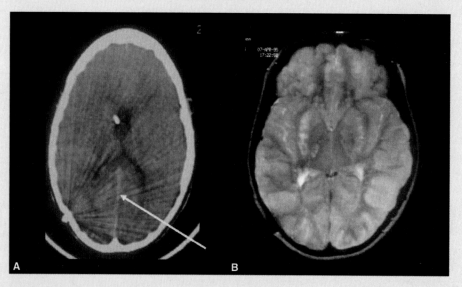

Case 5. This teenager presented with sudden onset of blindness and seizures soon after acute chest syndrome. There is occipital and frontal swelling on T2-weighted magnetic resonance imaging (**A**, **B**), consistent with posterior reversible encephalopathy syndrome, and susceptibility-weighted imaging (SWI) revealed hemorrhage in the parafalcine (**C**) and left frontal (**D**) regions. The patient returned to mainstream school but developed epilepsy.

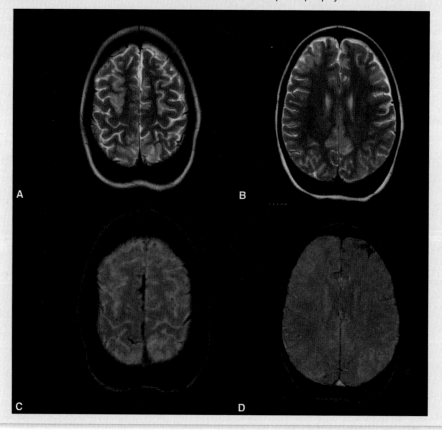

Case Studies: Continued

Case 6. This schoolchild with HbSS had normal transcranial Doppler on screening and an IQ of 100, the same as an identical twin, until the developed a facial infection with seizures. T2- and T1-weighted magnetic resonance imaging (**A, B**) showed bilateral border zone infarction. There was no motor disability, but there were visuoperceptual problems and IQ was 70 at follow-up, although the child continued in mainstream school with support.

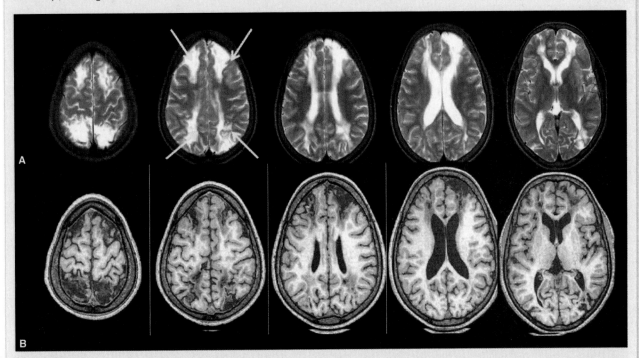

Case 7. Imaging transcranial Doppler screening was normal (**A**) prior to presentation with fever, reduced consciousness, and neck stiffness in this patient with HbSS. Lumbar puncture revealed 16 lymphocytes, and fluid-attenuated inversion recovery magnetic resonance imaging (**B**) shows symmetrical abnormality in the brain stem consistent with rhombencephalitis. The magnetic resonance venogram was normal (**C**). Outcome was good with return to mainstream school.

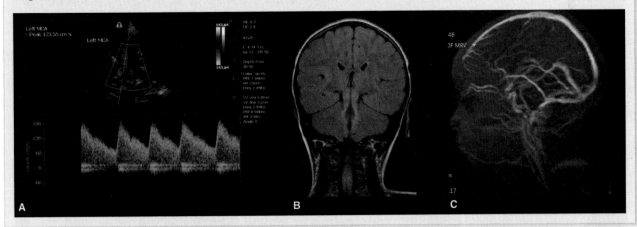

Case Studies: Continued

Case 8. Intracranial transcranial Doppler (TCD) imaging in this patient with HbSS was normal, but extracranial TCD (not shown) suggested bilateral carotid stenosis confirmed on magnetic resonance angiography (**A**), although there were no silent infarcts (**B**). Three years later, the patient developed a left hemiparesis. The carotid abnormality persisted (**C**), and bilateral focal ischemia was seen on diffusion-weighted imaging (**D**) and T2/fluid-attenuated inversion recovery (coronal, **E**, and axial, **F**). The patient had an educational health care plan for 2 years after the event.

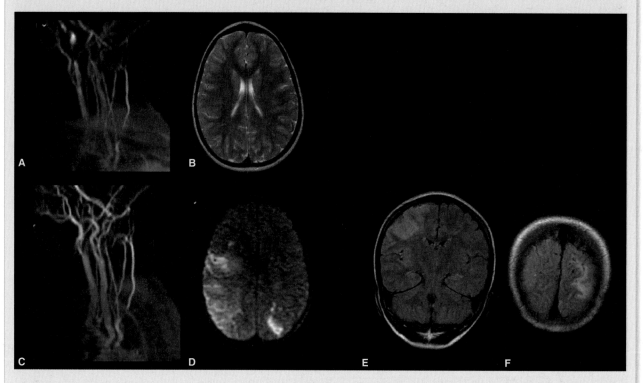

Case 9. This patient with HbSS developed a severe headache after acute chest syndrome. There is intraparenchymal and intraventricular hemorrhage on computed tomography (CT) scan (**A**), but the CT angiogram (**B**) did not reveal an aneurysm, so a digital subtraction arteriogram (**C**) was performed, which showed narrowing of the internal carotid and anterior cerebral arteries but no evidence of an aneurysm. After neurorehabilitation, the patient returned to mainstream school.

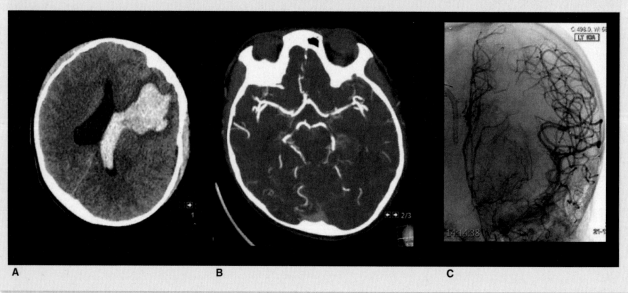

Case Studies: Continued

Case 10. This patient with HbSS had had an adenotonsillectomy 5 years previously and had started hydroxyurea 3 years before undergoing extracranial transcranial Doppler screening, which was considered to be abnormal. Although asymptomatic, the patient underwent magnetic resonance imaging, which showed a small silent infarct (**A**, short arrow). There was tortuosity of the extracranial carotid arteries (**B**) and a small aneurysm (**C**, long arrow). Magnetic resonance angiography a year later showed an increase in the size of the aneurysm, which, in view of the risk of hemorrhage, was successfully clipped at surgery after multidisciplinary discussion.

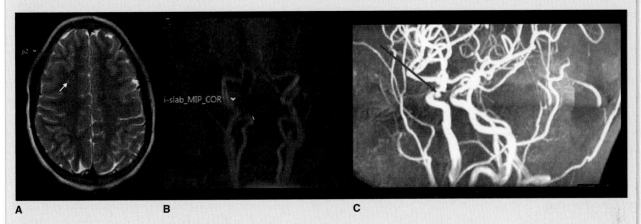

Case 11. This patient with HbSS had no history of trauma but presented with acute headache and was found to have extradural and subarachnoid hemorrhage (**A, B**). After surgery, there was intraparenchymal hemorrhagic contusion (**C**, blue arrow), and the subarachnoid hemorrhage persisted (**C**, white arrow). Occasional focal seizures were seen at follow-up in association with residual parenchymal damage at the site of the contusion (**D, E**).

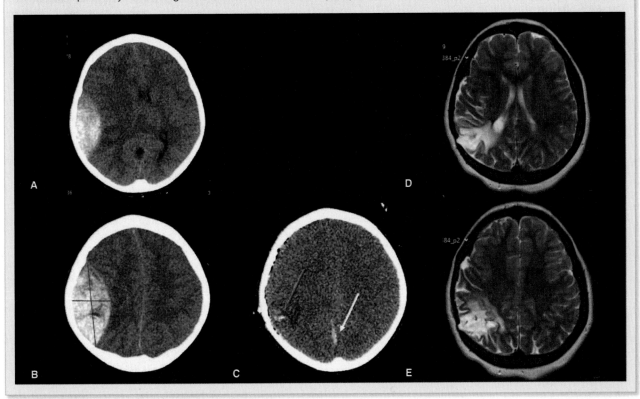

High-Yield Facts

◆ Neurologic complications, including overt and silent stroke, micro- and macrostructural injury, and cognitive impairment, are among the most common causes of morbidity in sickle cell disease (SCD), but are poorly understood.

◆ Increasing evidence points to a role for chronic and acute hemodynamic stress, which is associated with exposure to anemia and hypoxia and is likely exacerbated by pathologies related to these exposures and infection/immune dysregulation, including large-vessel vasculopathy and thromboemboli.

◆ Although there are evidence-based strategies for stroke prevention in children, treatment is often burdensome, the specificity of screening is poor, and many patients continue to suffer progressive vasculopathy and/or recurrent insults.

◆ In the quest for improved neurologic risk stratification strategies, novel quantitative hemodynamic and oxygen-sensitive magnetic resonance imaging (MRI) techniques hold promise, but significant validation work is required.

◆ Despite the increasing evidence for significant microstructural tissue injury and associated cognitive impairment, there are no evidence-based strategies for prevention and/or management, underscoring the need for future randomized controlled trials with structural MRI and cognitive end points.

References

1. DeBaun MR, Kirkham FJ. Central nervous system complications and management in sickle cell disease. *Blood.* 2016;127(7):829-838.

2. Ohene-Frempong K, Weiner SJ, Sleeper LA, et al. Cerebrovascular accidents in sickle cell disease: rates and risk factors. *Blood.* 1998;91(1):288-294.

3. Helton KJ, Adams RJ, Kesler KL, et al. Magnetic resonance imaging/angiography and transcranial Doppler velocities in sickle cell anemia: results from the SWiTCH trial. *Blood.* 2014;124(6):891-898.

4. Hirtz D, Kirkham FJ. Sickle cell disease and stroke. *Pediatr Neurol.* 2019;95:34-41.

5. Kirkham FJ. Therapy insight: stroke risk and its management in patients with sickle cell disease. *Nat Clin Pract Neurol.* 2007;3(5):264-278.

6. Noubiap JJ, Mengnjo MK, Nicastro N, Kamtchum-Tatuene J. Neurologic complications of sickle cell disease in Africa: a systematic review and meta-analysis. *Neurology.* 2017;89(14):1516-1524.

7. Kija EN, Saunders DE, Munubhi E, et al. Transcranial Doppler and magnetic resonance in Tanzanian children with sickle cell disease. *Stroke.* 2019;50(7):1719-1726.

8. Dowling MM, Noetzel MJ, Rodeghier MJ, et al. Headache and migraine in children with sickle cell disease are associated with lower hemoglobin and higher pain event rates but not silent cerebral infarction. *J Pediatr.* 2014;164(5):1175-1180.e1.

9. Kwiatkowski JL, Kanter J, Fullerton HJ, et al. Ischemic stroke in children and young adults with sickle cell disease in the post-STOP era. *Am J Hematol.* 2019;94(12):1335-1343.

10. DeBaun M, Jordan L, King A, et al. American Society of Hematology 2020 guidelines for management of cerebrovascular disease in children and adults with sickle cell disease. *Blood Adv.* 2020;4(8):1554-1588.

11. Ware RE, Davis BR, Schultz WH, et al. Hydroxycarbamide versus chronic transfusion for maintenance of transcranial doppler flow velocities in children with sickle cell anaemia—TCD With Transfusions Changing to Hydroxyurea (TWiTCH): a multicentre, open-label, phase 3, non-inferiority trial. *Lancet.* 2016;387(10019):661-670.

12. DeBaun MR, Gordon M, McKinstry RC, et al. Controlled trial of transfusions for silent cerebral infarcts in sickle cell anemia. *N Engl J Med.* 2014;371(8):699-710.

13. Adams RJ, Barber T, Bauer DE, et al. Endpoints for sickle cell disease clinical trials: patient-reported outcomes, pain, and the brain and central nervous system. *Blood Adv.* 2019;3(23):3982-4001.

14. Kirkham FJ, Angiobi E, Ganesan V. Preventing the recurrence of stroke in children. *Expert Rev Neurother.* In press.

15. Kawadler JM, Clayden JD, Clark CA, Kirkham FJ. Intelligence quotient in paediatric sickle cell disease: a systematic review and meta-analysis. *Dev Med Child Neurol.* 2016;58(7):672-679.

16. Stotesbury H, Kirkham FJ, Kölbel M, et al. White matter integrity and processing speed in sickle cell anemia. *Neurology.* 2018;90(23):e2042-e2050.

17. Prussien KV, Jordan LC, DeBaun MR, Compas BE. Cognitive function in sickle cell disease across domains, cerebral infarct status, and the lifespan: a meta-analysis. *J Pediatr Psychol.* 2019;44(8):948-958.

18. Wang W, Enos L, Gallagher D, et al. Neuropsychologic performance in school-aged children with sickle cell disease: a report from the Cooperative Study of Sickle Cell Disease. *J Pediatr.* 2001;139(3):391-397.

19. Hogan AM, Kirkham FJ, Isaacs EB, Wade AM, Vargha-Khadem F. Intellectual decline in children with moyamoya and sickle cell anaemia. *Dev Med Child Neurol.* 2007;47(12):824-829.

20. Guilliams KP, Fields ME, Dowling MM. Advances in understanding ischemic stroke physiology and the impact of vasculopathy in children with sickle cell disease. *Stroke.* 2019;50(2):266-273.

21. DeBaun MR, Armstrong FD, McKinstry RC, Ware RE, Vichinsky E, Kirkham FJ. Silent cerebral infarcts: a review on a prevalent and progressive cause of neurologic injury in sickle cell anemia. *Blood.* 2012;119(20):4587-4596.

22. Choudhury NA, DeBaun MR, Rodeghier M, King AA, Strouse JJ, McKinstry RC. Silent cerebral infarct definitions and full-scale IQ loss in children with sickle cell anemia. *Neurology.* 2018;90(3):e239-e246.

23. Rothman SM, Fulling KH, Nelson JS. Sickle cell anemia and central nervous system infarction: a neuropathological study. *Ann Neurol.* 1986;20(6):684-690.

24. Koshy M, Thomas C, Goodwin J. Vascular lesions in the central nervous system in sickle cell disease (neuropathology). *J Assoc Acad Minor Phys.* 1990;1(3):71-78.

25. Merkel KH, Ginsberg PL, Parker JC, Post MJ. Cerebrovascular disease in sickle cell anemia: a clinical, pathological and radiological correlation. *Stroke.* 1978;9(1):45-52.

26. Oyesiku NM, Barrow DL, Eckman JR, Tindall SC, Colohan AR. Intracranial aneurysms in sickle-cell anemia: clinical features and pathogenesis. *J Neurosurg.* 1991;75(3):356-363.

27. van der Land V, Zwanenburg JJM, Fijnvandraat K, et al. Cerebral lesions on 7 tesla MRI in patients with sickle cell anemia. *Cerebrovasc Dis.* 2015;39(3-4):181-189.

28. Kimmelstiel P. Vascular occlusion and ischemic infarction in sickle cell disease. *Am J Med Sci.* 1948;216:11-19.

29. Garcia JH. Thrombosis of cranial veins and sinuses: brain parenchymal effects. In: Einhaupl KM, Kempski O, Baethmann A, eds. *Cerebral Sinus Thrombosis: Experimental and Clinical Aspects.* Plenum Press; 1990.

30. Di Roio C, Jourdan C, Yilmaz H, Artru F. [Cerebral deep vein thrombosis: three cases]. *Rev Neurol (Paris).* 1999;155(8):583-587.

31. Stotesbury H, Kawadler JM, Hales PW, Saunders DE, Clark CA, Kirkham FJ. Vascular instability and neurological morbidity in sickle cell disease: an integrative framework. *Front Neurol.* 2019;10:871.

32. Connes P, Verlhac S, Bernaudin F. Advances in understanding the pathogenesis of cerebrovascular vasculopathy in sickle cell anaemia. *Br J Haematol.* 2013;161(4):484-498.

33. Detterich JA, Kato R, Bush A, et al. Sickle cell microvascular paradox-oxygen supply-demand mismatch. *Am J Hematol.* 2019;94(6):678-688.

34. Kaushal M, Byrnes C, Khademian Z, et al. Examination of reticulocytosis among chronically transfused children with sickle cell anemia. *PLoS One.* 2016;11(4):e0153244.

35. Jacob M, Saunders DE, Sangeda RZ, et al. Cerebral infarcts and vasculopathy in Tanzanian children with sickle cell anemia. *Pediatr Neurol.* 2020;107:64-70.

36. Majumdar S, Webb S, Norcross E, et al. Stroke with intracranial stenosis is associated with increased platelet activation in sickle cell anemia. *Pediatr Blood Cancer.* 2013;60(7):1192-1197.

37. Dowling MM, Quinn CT, Ramaciotti C, et al. Increased prevalence of potential right-to-left shunting in children with sickle cell anaemia and stroke. *Br J Haematol.* 2017;176(2):300-308.

38. Dowling MM, Kirkham FJ. Stroke in sickle cell anaemia is more than stenosis and thrombosis: the role of anaemia and hyperemia in ischaemia. *Br J Haematol.* 2017;176(2):151-153.

39. Gavins FNE, Russell J, Senchenkova EL, et al. Mechanisms of enhanced thrombus formation in cerebral microvessels of mice expressing hemoglobin-S. *Blood.* 2011;117(15):4125-4133.

40. Wang H, Luo W, Wang J, et al. Paradoxical protection from atherosclerosis and thrombosis in a mouse model of sickle cell disease. *Br J Haematol.* 2013;162(1):120-129.

41. Cui M-H, Suzuka SM, Branch NA, et al. Brain neurochemical and hemodynamic findings in the NY1DD mouse model of mild sickle cell disease. *NMR Biomed.* 2017;30(5):e3692.

42. Hyacinth HI, Sugihara CL, Spencer TL, Archer DR, Shih AY. Higher prevalence of spontaneous cerebral vasculopathy and cerebral infarcts in a mouse model of sickle cell disease. *J Cereb Blood Flow Metab.* 2019;39(2):342-351.

43. Cahill LS, Gazdzinski LM, Tsui AKY, et al. Functional and anatomical evidence of cerebral tissue hypoxia in young sickle cell anemia mice. *J Cereb Blood Flow Metab.* 2017;37(3):994-1005.

44. Wang L, Almeida LEFF, de Souza Batista CM, et al. Cognitive and behavior deficits in sickle cell mice are associated with profound neuropathologic changes in hippocampus and cerebellum. *Neurobiol Dis.* 2016;85:60-72.

45. Tsitsikas DA, Gallinella G, Patel S, Seligman H, Greaves P, Amos RJ. Bone marrow necrosis and fat embolism syndrome in sickle cell disease: increased susceptibility of patients with non-SS genotypes and a possible association with human parvovirus B19 infection. *Blood Rev.* 2014;28(1):23-30.

46. Adams RJ, Nichols FT, McKie V, McKie K, Milner P, Gammal TE. Cerebral infarction in sickle cell anemia: mechanism based on CT and MRI. *Neurology.* 1988;38(7):1012-1017.

47. Ford AL, Ragan DK, Fellah S, et al. Silent infarcts in sickle cell disease occur in the border zone region and are associated with low cerebral blood flow. *Blood.* 2018;132(16):1714-1723.

48. Guilliams KP, Fields ME, Ragan DK, et al. Large-vessel vasculopathy in children with sickle cell disease: a magnetic resonance imaging study of infarct topography and focal atrophy. *Pediatr Neurol.* 2017;69:49-57.

49. Kawadler JM, Kirkham FJ. Neurological complications and MRI. In: Inusa BPD, ed. *Sickle Cell Disease: Pain and Common Chronic Complications.* InTech; 2016.

50. Kirkham FJ, Kawadler JM, Saunders DE, Stotesbury H. MRI detection of brain abnormality in sickle cell disease. *Expert Rev Hematol.* In press.

51. Kim JA, Leung J, Lerch JP, Kassner A. Reduced cerebrovascular reserve is regionally associated with cortical thickness reductions in children with sickle cell disease. *Brain Res.* 2016;1642:263-269.

52. Balci A, Karazincir S, Beyoglu Y, et al. Quantitative brain diffusion-tensor MRI findings in patients with sickle cell disease. *AJR Am J Roentgenol.* 2012;198(5):1167-1174.

53. Sun B, Brown RC, Hayes L, et al. White matter damage in asymptomatic patients with sickle cell anemia: screening with diffusion tensor imaging. *AJNR Am J Neuroradiol.* 2012;33(11):2043-2049.

54. Steen RG, Emudianughe T, Hankins GM, et al. Brain imaging findings in pediatric patients with sickle cell disease. *Radiology.* 2003;228(1):216-225.

55. Buch K, Arya R, Shah B, et al. Quantitative analysis of extracranial arterial tortuosity in patients with sickle cell disease. *J Neuroimaging.* 2017;27(4):421-427.

56. Stockman JA, Nigro MA, Mishkin MM, Oski FA. Occlusion of large cerebral vessels in sickle-cell anemia. *N Engl J Med.* 1972;287(17):846-849.

57. Bernaudin F, Verlhac S, Arnaud C, et al. Chronic and acute anemia and extracranial internal carotid stenosis are risk factors for silent cerebral infarcts in sickle cell anemia. *Blood.* 2015;125(10):1653-1661.

58. Thangarajh M, Yang G, Fuchs D, et al. Magnetic resonance angiography-defined intracranial vasculopathy is associated with silent cerebral infarcts and glucose-6-phosphate dehydrogenase mutation in children with sickle cell anaemia. *Br J Haematol.* 2012;159(3):352-359.

59. Dobson SR, Holden KR, Nietert PJ, et al. Moyamoya syndrome in childhood sickle cell disease: a predictive factor for recurrent cerebrovascular events. *Blood.* 2002;99(9):3144-3150.

60. Dlamini N, Saunders DE, Bynevelt M, et al. Nocturnal oxyhemoglobin desaturation and arteriopathy in a pediatric sickle cell disease cohort. *Neurology.* 2017;89:2406–2412.

61. Telfer PT, Evanson J, Butler P, et al. Cervical carotid artery disease in sickle cell anemia: clinical and radiological features. *Blood.* 2011;118(23):6192-6199.

62. Arkuszewski M, Krejza J, Chen R, et al. Sickle cell anemia: intracranial stenosis and silent cerebral infarcts in children with low risk of stroke. *Adv Med Sci.* 2014;59(1):108-113.

63. Deane CR, Goss D, Bartram J, et al. Extracranial internal carotid arterial disease in children with sickle cell anemia. *Haematologica.* 2010;95(8):1287-1292.

64. Jacob M, Stotesbury H, Kawadler JM, et al. White matter integrity in Tanzanian children with sickle cell anemia: a diffusion tensor imaging study. *Stroke.* 2020;51(4):1166-1173.

65. Powars D, Adams RJ, Nichols FT, Milner P, Charache S, Sarnaik S. Delayed intracranial hemorrhage following cerebral infarction in sickle cell anemia. *J Assoc Acad Minor Phys.* 1990;1(3):79-82.

66. Kassim AA, Galadanci NA, Pruthi S, DeBaun MR. How I treat and manage strokes in sickle cell disease. *Blood.* 2015;125(22):3401-3410.

67. Yao Z, Li J, He M, You C. Intracranial aneurysm in patients with sickle cell disease: a systematic review. *World Neurosurg.* 2017;105:302-313.

68. Kassim AA, Pruthi S, Day M, et al. Silent cerebral infarcts and cerebral aneurysms are prevalent in adults with sickle cell anemia. *Blood.* 2016;127(16):2038-2040.

69. Birkeland P, Gardner K, Kesse-Adu R, et al. Intracranial aneurysms in sickle-cell disease are associated with the hemoglobin SS genotype but not with moyamoya syndrome. *Stroke.* 2016;47(7):1710-1713.

70. Preul MC, Cendes F, Just N, Mohr G. Intracranial aneurysms and sickle cell anemia: multiplicity and propensity for the vertebrobasilar territory. *Neurosurgery.* 1998;42(5):971-977.

71. Kossorotoff M, Brousse V, Grevent D, et al. Cerebral haemorrhagic risk in children with sickle-cell disease. *Dev Med Child Neurol.* 2015;57(2):187-193.

72. Adams RJ, Nichols FT, Aaslid R, et al. Cerebral vessel stenosis in sickle cell disease: criteria for detection by transcranial Doppler. *Am J Pediatr Hematol Oncol.* 1990;12(3):277-282.

73. Wang WC, Gallagher DM, Pegelow CH, et al. Multicenter comparison of magnetic resonance imaging and transcranial Doppler ultrasonography in the evaluation of the central nervous system in children with sickle cell disease. *J Pediatr Hematol Oncol.* 2000;22(4):335-339.

74. Abboud MR, Cure J, Granger S, et al. Magnetic resonance angiography in children with sickle cell disease and abnormal transcranial Doppler ultrasonography findings enrolled in the STOP study. *Blood.* 2004;103(7):2822-2826.

75. Mazzucco S, Diomedi M, Qureshi A, Sainati L, Padayachee ST. Transcranial Doppler screening for stroke risk in children with sickle cell disease: a systematic review. *Int J Stroke.* 2017;12(6):580-588.

76. Adams RJ, McKie VC, Carl EM, et al. Long-term stroke risk in children with sickle cell disease screened with transcranial Doppler. *Ann Neurol.* 1997;42(5):699-704.

77. Prussien KV, Salihu A, Abdullahi SU, et al. Associations of transcranial Doppler velocity, age, and gender with cognitive function in children with sickle cell anemia in Nigeria. *Child Neuropsychol.* 2019;25(6):705-720.

78. Prussien KV, Siciliano RE, Ciriegio AE, et al. Correlates of cognitive function in sickle cell disease: a meta-analysis. *J Pediatr Psychol.* 2020;45(2):145-155.

79. Adler K, Reghunathan A, Hutchison LH, Kalpatthi R. Dural venous sinus diameters in children with sickle cell disease:

80. Novelli EM, Elizabeth Sarles C, Jay Aizenstein H, et al. Brain venular pattern by 7T MRI correlates with memory and haemoglobin in sickle cell anaemia. *Psychiatry Res.* 2015;233(1):18-22.

81. Wang MK, Shergill R, Jefkins M, Cheung J. A sickle cell disease patient with dural venous sinus thrombosis: a case report and literature review. *Hemoglobin.* 2019;43(3):193-197.

82. Sébire G, Tabarki B, Saunders DE, et al. Cerebral venous sinus thrombosis in children: risk factors, presentation, diagnosis and outcome. *Brain.* 2005;128(Pt 3):477-489.

83. Choi S, Bush AM, Borzage MT, et al. Hemoglobin and mean platelet volume predicts diffuse T1-MRI white matter volume decrease in sickle cell disease patients. *Neuroimage Clin.* 2017;15:239-246.

84. Baldeweg T, Hogan AM, Saunders DE, et al. Detecting white matter injury in sickle cell disease using voxel-based morphometry. *Ann Neurol.* 2006;59(4):662-672.

85. Kawadler JM, Clayden JD, Kirkham FJ, Cox TC, Saunders DE, Clark CA. Subcortical and cerebellar volumetric deficits in paediatric sickle cell anaemia. *Br J Haematol.* 2013;163(3):373-376.

86. Kirk GR, Haynes MR, Palasis S, et al. Regionally specific cortical thinning in children with sickle cell disease. *Cereb Cortex.* 2009;19(7):1549-1556.

87. Steen RG, Emudianughe T, Hunte M, et al. Brain volume in pediatric patients with sickle cell disease: evidence of volumetric growth delay? *AJNR Am J Neuroradiol.* 2005;26(3):455-462.

88. Chen R, Arkuszewski M, Krejza J, Zimmerman RA, Herskovits EH, Melhem ER. A prospective longitudinal brain morphometry study of children with sickle cell disease. *AJNR Am J Neuroradiol.* 2015;36(2):403-410.

89. Darbari DS, Eigbire-Molen O, Ponisio MR, et al. Progressive loss of brain volume in children with sickle cell anemia and silent cerebral infarct: a report from the silent cerebral infarct transfusion trial. *Am J Hematol.* 2018;93(12):E406-E408.

90. Kawadler JM, Clark CA, McKinstry RC, Kirkham FJ. Brain atrophy in paediatric sickle cell anaemia: findings from the silent infarct transfusion (SIT) trial. *Br J Haematol.* 2017;177(1):151-153.

91. Nitkunan A, Lanfranconi S, Charlton RA, Barrick TR, Markus HS. Brain atrophy and cerebral small vessel disease. *Stroke.* 2011;42(1):133-138.

92. Mackin RS, Insel P, Truran D, et al. Neuroimaging abnormalities in adults with sickle cell anemia: associations with cognition. *Neurology.* 2014;82(10):835-841.

93. Kawadler JM, Kirkham FJ, Clayden JD, et al. White matter damage relates to oxygen saturation in children with sickle cell anemia without silent cerebral infarcts. *Stroke.* 2015;46(7):1793-1799.

94. Chai Y, Coloigner J, Qu X, et al. Tract specific analysis in patients with sickle cell disease. *Proc SPIE Int Soc Opt Eng.* 2015;9681:968108.

95. Wheeler-Kingshott CAM, Cercignani M. About "axial" and "radial" diffusivities. *Magn Reson Med.* 2009;61(5):1255-1260.

96. Kumar R, Stanek J, Creary S, Dunn A, O'Brien SH. Prevalence and risk factors for venous thromboembolism in children with sickle cell disease: an administrative database study. *Blood Adv.* 2018;2(3):285-291.

97. Razdan S, Strouse JJ, Naik R, et al. Patent foramen ovale in patients with sickle cell disease and stroke: case presentations and review of the literature. *Case Rep Hematol.* 2013;2013:516705.

98. Dowling MM, Lee N, Quinn CT, et al. Prevalence of intracardiac shunting in children with sickle cell disease and stroke. *J Pediatr.* 2010;156(4):645-650.

99. Razdan S, Strouse JJ, Reddy A, et al. Patent foramen ovale in adults with sickle cell disease and stroke. *Am J Hematol.* 2016;91(9):E358-E360.

100. Nathan CL, Aamodt WW, Yalamarti T, Dogon C, Kinniry P. Cerebral fat embolism syndrome in sickle cell disease without evidence of shunt. *eNeurologicalSci.* 2019;14:19-20.

101. Targueta EP, Hirano AC de G, de Campos FPF, Martines JA dos S, Lovisolo SM, Felipe-Silva A. Bone marrow necrosis and fat embolism syndrome: a dreadful complication of hemoglobin sickle cell disease. *Autops Case Rep.* 2017;7(4):42-50.

102. Gangaraju R, Reddy VVB, Marques MB. Fat embolism syndrome secondary to bone marrow necrosis in patients with hemoglobinopathies. *South Med J.* 2016;109(9):549-553.

103. Ford AL, Ragan DK, Fellah S, et al. Silent infarcts in sickle cell disease occur in the border zone region and are associated with low cerebral blood flow. *Blood.* 2018;132(16):1714-1723.

104. Hulbert ML, Ford AL. Understanding sickle cell brain drain. *Blood.* 2014;124(6):830-831.

105. Bladin CF, Chambers BR, Donnan GA. Confusing stroke terminology: watershed or borderzone infarction? *Stroke.* 1993;24(3):477-478.

106. Behpour AM, Shah PS, Mikulis DJ, Kassner A. Cerebral blood flow abnormalities in children with sickle cell disease: a systematic review. *Pediatr Neurol.* 2013;48(3):188-199.

107. Nur E, Kim Y-S, Truijen J, et al. Cerebrovascular reserve capacity is impaired in patients with sickle cell disease. *Blood.* 2009;114(16):3473-3478.

108. Kosinski PD, Croal PL, Leung J, et al. The severity of anaemia depletes cerebrovascular dilatory reserve in children with sickle cell disease: a quantitative magnetic resonance imaging study. *Br J Haematol.* 2017;176(2):280-287.

109. Václavů L, Meynart BN, Mutsaerts HJMM, et al. Hemodynamic provocation with acetazolamide shows impaired cerebrovascular reserve in adults with sickle cell disease. *Haematologica.* 2019;104(4):690-699.

110. Jordan LC, Gindville MC, Scott AO, et al. Non-invasive imaging of oxygen extraction fraction in adults with sickle cell anaemia. *Brain.* 2016;139(Pt 3):738-750.

111. Fields ME, Guilliams KP, Ragan DK, et al. Regional oxygen extraction predicts border zone vulnerability to stroke in sickle cell disease. *Neurology.* 2018;90(13):e1134-e1142.

112. Kirkham FJ, Hewes DK, Prengler M, Wade A, Lane R, Evans JP. Nocturnal hypoxaemia and central-nervous-system events in sickle-cell disease. *Lancet (London, England).* 2001;357(9269):1656-1659.

113. Rosen CL, Debaun MR, Strunk RC, et al. Obstructive sleep apnea and sickle cell anemia. *Pediatrics.* 2014;134(2):273-281.

114. Pierson DJ. Pathophysiology and clinical effects of chronic hypoxia. *Respir Care.* 2000;45(1):39-51; discussion 51-53.

115. Halphen I, Elie C, Brousse V, et al. Severe nocturnal and postexercise hypoxia in children and adolescents with sickle cell disease. Arez AP, ed. *PLoS One.* 2014;9(5):e97462.

116. Rees DC, Williams TN, Gladwin MT. Sickle-cell disease. *Lancet (London, England).* 2010;376(9757):2018-2031.

117. Rackoff WR, Kunkel N, Silber JH, Asakura T, Ohene-Frempong K. Pulse oximetry and factors associated with hemoglobin oxygen desaturation in children with sickle cell disease. *Blood.* 1993;81(12):3422-3427.

118. Setty BNY, Stuart MJ, Dampier C, Brodecki D, Allen JL. Hypoxaemia in sickle cell disease: biomarker modulation and relevance to pathophysiology. *Lancet (London, England).* 2003;362(9394):1450-1455.

119. Homi J, Levee L, Higgs D, Thomas P, Serjeant G. Pulse oximetry in a cohort study of sickle cell disease. *Clin Lab Haematol.* 1997;19(1):17-22.

120. Fowler NO, Smith O, Greenfield JC. Arterial blood oxygenation in sickle cell anemia. *Am J Med Sci.* 1957;234(4):449-458.

121. Waltz X, Romana M, Lalanne-Mistrih M-L, et al. Hematologic and hemorheological determinants of resting and exercise-induced hemoglobin oxygen desaturation in children with sickle cell disease. *Haematologica.* 2013;98(7):1039-1044.

122. Quinn CT, Ahmad N. Clinical correlates of steady-state oxyhaemoglobin desaturation in children who have sickle cell disease. *Br J Haematol.* 2005;131(1):129-134.

123. Spivey JF, Uong EC, Strunk R, Boslaugh SE, DeBaun MR. Low daytime pulse oximetry reading is associated with nocturnal desaturation and obstructive sleep apnea in children with sickle cell anemia. *Pediatr Blood Cancer.* 2008;50(2):359-362.

124. Kirkham FJ, Datta AK. Hypoxic adaptation during development: relation to pattern of neurological presentation and cognitive disability. *Dev Sci.* 2006;9(4):411-427.

125. Hollocks MJ, Kok TB, Kirkham FJ, et al. Nocturnal oxygen desaturation and disordered sleep as a potential factor in executive dysfunction in sickle cell anemia. *J Int Neuropsychol Soc.* 2012;18(1):168-173.

126. King AA, Strouse JJ, Rodeghier MJ, et al. Parent education and biologic factors influence on cognition in sickle cell anemia. *Am J Hematol.* 2014;89(2):162-167.

127. Hogan AM, Telfer PT, Kirkham FJ, de Haan M. Precursors of executive function in infants with sickle cell anemia. *J Child Neurol.* 2013;28(10):1197-1202.

128. Quinn CT, Sargent JW. Daytime steady-state haemoglobin desaturation is a risk factor for overt stroke in children with sickle cell anaemia. *Br J Haematol.* 2008;140(3):336-339.

129. Sommet J, Alberti C, Couque N, et al. Clinical and haematological risk factors for cerebral macrovasculopathy in a sickle cell disease newborn cohort: a prospective study. *Br J Haematol.* 2016;172(6):966-977.

130. Scheufler K-M. Tissue oxygenation and capacity to deliver O2 do the two go together? *Transfus Apher Sci.* 2004;31(1):45-54.

131. Quinn CT, Variste J, Dowling MM. Haemoglobin oxygen saturation is a determinant of cerebral artery blood flow velocity in children with sickle cell anaemia. *Br J Haematol.* 2009;145(4):500-505.

132. Makani J, Kirkham FJ, Komba A, et al. Risk factors for high cerebral blood flow velocity and death in Kenyan children with sickle cell anaemia: role of haemoglobin oxygen saturation and febrile illness. *Br J Haematol.* 2009;145(4):529-532.

133. Rankine-Mullings AE, Morrison-Levy N, Soares D, et al. Transcranial Doppler velocity among Jamaican children with sickle cell anaemia: determining the significance of haematological values and nutrition. *Br J Haematol.* 2018;181(2):242-251.

134. Baird RL, Weiss DL, Ferguson AD, French JH, Scott RB. Studies in sickle cell anemia. XXI. Clinico-pathological aspects of neurological manifestations. *Pediatrics.* 1964;34:92-100.

135. Herold S, Brozovic M, Gibbs J, et al. Measurement of regional cerebral blood flow, blood volume and oxygen metabolism in patients with sickle cell disease using positron emission tomography. *Stroke.* 1986;17(4):692-698.

136. Bush AM, Borzage MT, Choi S, et al. Determinants of resting cerebral blood flow in sickle cell disease. *Am J Hematol.* 2016;91(9):912-917.

137. Chai Y, Bush AM, Coloigner J, et al. White matter has impaired resting oxygen delivery in sickle cell patients. *Am J Hematol.* 2019;94(4):467-474.

138. Prohovnik I, Hurlet-Jensen A, Adams R, De Vivo D, Pavlakis SG. Hemodynamic etiology of elevated flow velocity and stroke in sickle-cell disease. *J Cereb Blood Flow Metab.* 2009;29(4):803-810.

139. Kim Y-S, Nur E, van Beers EJ, et al. Dynamic cerebral autoregulation in homozygous Sickle cell disease. *Stroke.* 2009;40(3):808-814.

140. Leung J, Duffin J, Fisher JA, Kassner A. MRI-based cerebrovascular reactivity using transfer function analysis reveals temporal group differences between patients with sickle cell disease and healthy controls. *Neuroimage Clin.* 2016;12:624-630.

141. Cottrell JE, Patel P. *Cottrell and Patel's Neuroanesthesia.* Elsevier Health Sciences; 2016. https://books.google.co.uk/books?id=xVboDAAAQBAJ.

142. Busija DW, Leffler CW, Pourcyrous M. Hyperthermia increases cerebral metabolic rate and blood flow in neonatal pigs. *Am J Physiol Circ Physiol.* 1988;255(2):H343-H346.

143. Brown MM, Wade JP, Marshall J. Fundamental importance of arterial oxygen content in the regulation of cerebral blood flow in man. *Brain.* 1985;108(Pt 1):81-93.

144. MacKenzie ET, Farrar JK, Fitch W, Graham DI, Gregory PC, Harper AM. Effects of hemorrhagic hypotension on the cerebral circulation. I. Cerebral blood flow and pial arteriolar caliber. *Stroke.* 1979;10(6):711-718.

145. Lassen NA. Cerebral blood flow and oxygen consumption in man. *Physiol Rev.* 1959;39(2):183-238.

146. Klijn CJM, Kappelle LJ. Haemodynamic stroke: clinical features, prognosis, and management. *Lancet Neurol.* 2010;9(10):1008-1017.

147. Kinney TR, Sleeper LA, Wang WC, et al. Silent cerebral infarcts in sickle cell anemia: a risk factor analysis. The Cooperative Study of Sickle Cell Disease. *Pediatrics.* 1999;103(3):640-645.

148. Henderson JN, Noetzel MJ, McKinstry RC, White DA, Armstrong M, DeBaun MR. Reversible posterior leukoencephalopathy syndrome and silent cerebral infarcts are associated with severe acute chest syndrome in children with sickle cell disease. *Blood.* 2003;101(2):415-419.

149. Kwiatkowski JL, Zimmerman RA, Pollock AN, et al. Silent infarcts in young children with sickle cell disease. *Br J Haematol.* 2009;146(3):300-305.

150. Calvet D, Bernaudin F, Gueguen A, et al. First ischemic stroke in sickle-cell disease: are there any adult specificities? *Stroke.* 2015;46(8):2315-2317.

151. Fridlyand D, Wilder C, Clay ELJ, Gilbert B, Pace BS. Stroke in a child with hemoglobin SC disease: a case report describing use of hydroxyurea after transfusion therapy. *Pediatr Rep.* 2017;9(1):6984.

152. Vichinsky EP, Neumayr LD, Earles AN, et al. Causes and outcomes of the acute chest syndrome in sickle cell disease. National Acute Chest Syndrome Study Group. *N Engl J Med.* 2000;342(25):1855-1865.

153. Kirkham FJ, Calamante F, Bynevelt M, et al. Perfusion magnetic resonance abnormalities in patients with sickle cell disease. *Ann Neurol.* 2001;49(4):477-485.

154. Al-Kandari FA, Owunwanne A, Syed GM, et al. Regional cerebral blood flow in patients with sickle cell disease: study with single photon emission computed tomography. *Ann Nucl Med.* 2007;21(8):439-445.

155. Rodgers GP, Clark CM, Larson SM, Rapoport SI, Nienhuis AW, Schechter AN. Brain glucose metabolism in neurologically normal patients with sickle cell disease. Regional alterations. *Arch Neurol.* 1988;45(1):78-82.

156. Powars DR, Conti PS, Wong WY, et al. Cerebral vasculopathy in sickle cell anemia: diagnostic contribution of positron emission tomography. *Blood.* 1999;93(1):71-79.

157. Deus-Silva L, Bonilha L, Damasceno BP, et al. Brain perfusion impairment in neurologically asymptomatic adult patients with sickle-cell disease shown by voxel-based analysis of SPECT images. *Front Neurol.* 2013;4:207.

158. Parsa MA, Mehregany D, Schulz SC. Psychiatric manifestation of sickle cell disease and findings on single photon emission computed tomography. *Psychosomatics.* 1992;33(2):239-241.

159. Numaguchi Y, Haller JS, Humbert JR, et al. Cerebral blood flow mapping using stable xenon-enhanced CT in sickle cell cerebrovascular disease. *Neuroradiology.* 1990;32(4):289-295.

160. Helton KJ, Paydar A, Glass J, et al. Arterial spin-labeled perfusion combined with segmentation techniques to evaluate cerebral blood flow in white and gray matter of children with sickle cell anemia. *Pediatr Blood Cancer.* 2009;52(1):85-91.

161. Tripette J, Alexy T, Hardy-Dessources M-D, et al. Red blood cell aggregation, aggregate strength and oxygen transport potential of blood are abnormal in both homozygous sickle cell anemia and sickle-hemoglobin C disease. *Haematologica.* 2009;94(8):1060-1065.

162. Detterich J, Alexy T, Rabai M, et al. Low-shear red blood cell oxygen transport effectiveness is adversely affected by transfusion and further worsened by deoxygenation in sickle cell disease patients on chronic transfusion therapy. *Transfusion.* 2013;53(2):297-305.

163. Fieschi C. Cerebral blood flow and energy metabolism in vascular insufficiency. *Stroke.* 1980;11(5):431-432.

164. Baron JC, Bousser MG, Rey A, Guillard A, Comar D, Castaigne P. Reversal of focal "misery-perfusion syndrome" by extra-intracranial arterial bypass in hemodynamic cerebral ischemia. A case study with 15O positron emission tomography. *Stroke.* 1981;12(4):454-459.

165. Baron JC. Pathophysiology of acute cerebral ischemia: PET studies in humans. *Cerebrovasc Dis.* 1991;1(1):22-31.

166. Baird AE, Austin MC, McKay WJ, Donnan GA. Changes in cerebral tissue perfusion during the first 48 hours of ischaemic stroke: relation to clinical outcome. *J Neurol Neurosurg Psychiatry.* 1996;61(1):26-29.

167. Bush AM, Coates TD, Wood JC. Diminished cerebral oxygen extraction and metabolic rate in sickle cell disease using T2 relaxation under spin tagging MRI. *Magn Reson Med.* 2018;80(1):294-303.

168. Croal PL, Serafin MG, Kosinski P, Leung J, Williams S, Kassner A. Quantitative MRI of hemodynamic compromise in children with sickle cell disease: new insights into pathophysiology. *Blood.* 2015;126(23):2168.

169. Vaclavu L, Petersen ET, VanBavel ET, Majoie CB, Nederveen AJ, Biemond BJ. Reduced cerebral metabolic rate of oxygen in adults with sickle cell disease. *Blood.* 2018;132(Suppl 1):11.

170. Watchmaker JM, Juttukonda MR, Davis LT, et al. Hemodynamic mechanisms underlying elevated oxygen extraction fraction (OEF) in moyamoya and sickle cell anemia patients. *J Cereb Blood Flow Metab.* 2018;38(9):1618-1630.

171. Juttukonda MR, Lee CA, Patel NJ, et al. Differential cerebral hemometabolic responses to blood transfusions in adults and children with sickle cell anemia. *J Magn Reson Imaging.* 2019;49(2):466-477.

172. Juttukonda MR, Donahue MJ, Davis LT, et al. Preliminary evidence for cerebral capillary shunting in adults with sickle cell anemia. *J Cereb Blood Flow Metab.* 2019;39(6):1099-1110.

173. Wood JC. Unwinding the path from anemia to stroke. *Blood.* 2018;131(9):950-952.

174. Dowling MM, Quinn CT, Rogers ZR, Buchanan GR. Acute silent cerebral infarction in children with sickle cell anemia. *Pediatr Blood Cancer.* 2010;54(3):461-464.

175. Dowling MM, Quinn CT, Plumb P, et al. Acute silent cerebral ischemia and infarction during acute anemia in children with and without sickle cell disease. *Blood.* 2012;120(19):3891-3897.

176. Quinn CT, McKinstry RC, Dowling MM, et al. Acute silent cerebral ischemic events in children with sickle cell anemia. *JAMA Neurol.* 2013;70(1):58-65.

177. Enninful-Eghan H, Moore RH, Ichord R, Smith-Whitley K, Kwiatkowski JL. Transcranial Doppler ultrasonography and prophylactic transfusion program is effective in preventing overt stroke in children with sickle cell disease. *J Pediatr.* 2010;157(3):479-484.

178. Lee KH, McKie VC, Sekul EA, Adams RJ, Nichols FT. Unusual encephalopathy after acute chest syndrome in sickle cell disease: acute necrotizing encephalitis. *J Pediatr Hematol Oncol.* 2002;24(7):585-588.

179. Adams RJ, McKie VC, Brambilla D, et al. Stroke prevention trial in sickle cell anemia. *Control Clin Trials.* 1998;19(1):110-129.

180. Hulbert ML, McKinstry RC, Lacey JL, et al. Silent cerebral infarcts occur despite regular blood transfusion therapy after first strokes in children with sickle cell disease. *Blood.* 2011;117(3):772-779.

181. Strouse JJ, Hulbert ML, DeBaun MR, Jordan LC, Casella JF. Primary hemorrhagic stroke in children with sickle cell disease is associated with recent transfusion and use of corticosteroids. *Pediatrics.* 2006;118(5):1916-1924.

182. Powars D, Wilson B, Imbus C, Pegelow C, Allen J. The natural history of stroke in sickle cell disease. *Am J Med.* 1978;65(3):461-471.

183. Elmariah H, Garrett ME, De Castro LM, et al. Factors associated with survival in a contemporary adult sickle cell disease cohort. *Am J Hematol.* 2014;89(5):530-535.

184. Prengler M, Pavlakis SG, Boyd S, et al. Sickle cell disease: ischemia and seizures. *Ann Neurol.* 2005;58(2):290-302.

185. Hines PC, McKnight TP, Seto W, Kwiatkowski JL. Central nervous system events in children with sickle cell disease presenting acutely with headache. *J Pediatr.* 2011;159(3):472-478.

186. Henry M, Driscoll MC, Miller M, Chang T, Minniti CP. Pseudotumor cerebri in children with sickle cell disease: a case series. *Pediatrics.* 2004;113(3 Pt 1):e265-e269.

187. Sanger M, Jordan L, Pruthi S, et al. Cognitive deficits are associated with unemployment in adults with sickle cell anemia. *J Clin Exp Neuropsychol.* 2016;38(6):661-671.

188. Hardy SJ, Bills SE, Wise SM, Hardy KK. Cognitive abilities moderate the effect of disease severity on health-related quality of life in pediatric sickle cell disease. *J Pediatr Psychol.* 2018;43(8):882-894.

189. Merkhofer C, Sylvester S, Zmuda M, et al. The impact of cognitive function on adherence to hydroxyurea therapy in patients with sickle cell disease. *Blood.* 2016;128:22.

190. Grant MM, Gil KM, Floyd MY, Abrams M. Depression and functioning in relation to health care use in sickle cell disease. *Ann Behav Med.* 2000;22(2):149-157.

191. Toumi ML, Merzoug S, Boulassel MR. Does sickle cell disease have a psychosomatic component? A particular focus on anxiety and depression. *Life Sci.* 2018;210:96-105.

192. Prussien KV, DeBaun MR, Yarboi J, et al. Cognitive function, coping, and depressive symptoms in children and adolescents with sickle cell disease. *J Pediatr Psychol.* 2018;43(5):543-551.

193. Anie KA, Steptoe A, Bevan DH. Sickle cell disease: pain, coping and quality of life in a study of adults in the UK. *Br J Health Psychol.* 2002;7(3):331-344.

194. Anie KA. Psychological complications in sickle cell disease. *Br J Haematol.* 2005;129(6):723-729.

195. Drazen CH, Abel R, Gabir M, Farmer G, King AA. Prevalence of developmental delay and contributing factors among children with sickle cell disease. *Pediatr Blood Cancer.* 2016;63(3):504-510.

196. Towerman AS, Hayashi SS, Hayashi RJ, Hulbert ML. Prevalence and nature of hearing loss in a cohort of children with sickle cell disease. *Pediatr Blood Cancer.* 2019;66(1):e27457.

197. Rissatto-Lago MR, Fernandes LC, Alves AAG, et al. Dysfunction of the auditory system in sickle cell anaemia: a systematic review with meta-analysis. *Trop Med Int Heal.* 2019;24(11):1264-1276.

198. Bois E, Francois M, Benkerrou M, Van Den Abbeele T, Teissier N. Hearing loss in children with sickle cell disease: a prospective French cohort study. *Pediatr Blood Cancer.* 2019;66(1):e27468.

199. Hogan AM, Pit-Ten Cate IM, Vargha-Khadem F, Prengler M, Kirkham FJ. Physiological correlates of intellectual function in children with sickle cell disease: hypoxaemia, hyperaemia and brain infarction. *Dev Sci.* 2006;9(4):379-387.

200. Wang WC, Langston JW, Steen RG, et al. Abnormalities of the central nervous system in very young children with sickle cell anemia. *J Pediatr.* 1998;132(6):994-998.

201. Cancio MI, Helton KJ, Schreiber JE, Smeltzer MP, Kang G, Wang WC. Silent cerebral infarcts in very young children with sickle cell anaemia are associated with a higher risk of stroke. *Br J Haematol.* 2015;171(1):120-129.

202. Hijmans CT, Fijnvandraat K, Grootenhuis MA, et al. Neurocognitive deficits in children with sickle cell disease: a comprehensive profile. *Pediatr Blood Cancer.* 2011;56(5):783-788.

203. Armstrong FD, Thompson RJ, Wang W, et al. Cognitive functioning and brain magnetic resonance imaging in children with sickle cell disease. Neuropsychology Committee of the Cooperative Study of Sickle Cell Disease. *Pediatrics.* 1996;97(6 Pt 1):864-870.

204. Castro IPS, Viana MB. Cognitive profile of children with sickle cell anemia compared to healthy controls. *J Pediatr (Rio J).* 2019;95(4):451-457.

205. Nunes S, Argollo N, Mota M, Vieira C, Sena EP. Comprehensive neuropsychological evaluation of children and adolescents with sickle cell anemia: a hospital-based sample. *Rev Bras Hematol Hemoter.* 2017;39(1):32-39.

206. Vichinsky EP, Neumayr LD, Gold JI, et al. Neuropsychological dysfunction and neuroimaging abnormalities in neurologically intact adults with sickle cell anemia. *JAMA.* 2010;303(18):1823-1831.

207. Armstrong FD, Elkin TD, Brown RC, et al. Developmental function in toddlers with sickle cell anemia. *Pediatrics.* 2013;131(2):e406-e414.

208. Chua-Lim C, Moore RB, McCleary G, Shah A, Mankad VN. Deficiencies in school readiness skills of children with sickle cell anemia: a preliminary report. *South Med J.* 1993;86(4):397-402.

209. Steen RG, Hu XJ, Elliott VE, Miles MA, Jones S, Wang WC. Kindergarten readiness skills in children with sickle cell disease: evidence of early neurocognitive damage? *J Child Neurol.* 2002;17(2):111-116.

210. Schatz J. Brief report: academic attainment in children with sickle cell disease. *J Pediatr Psychol.* 2004;29(8):627-633.

211. Schatz J, Brown RT, Pascual JM, Hsu L, DeBaun MR. Poor school and cognitive functioning with silent cerebral infarcts and sickle cell disease. *Neurology.* 2001;56(8):1109-1111.

212. Smith KE, Patterson CA, Szabo MM, Tarazi RA, Barakat LP. Predictors of academic achievement for school age children with sickle cell disease. *Adv Sch Ment Health Promot.* 2013;6(1): 5-20.

213. Hood AM, Reife I, King AA, White DA. Brief screening measures identify risk for psychological difficulties among children with sickle cell disease. *J Clin Psychol Med Settings.* 2019;10.1007/ s10880-019-09654-y.

214. Craft S, Schatz J, Glauser TA, Lee B, DeBaun MR. Neuropsychologic effects of stroke in children with sickle cell anemia. *J Pediatr.* 1993;123(5):712-717.

215. Steen RG, Miles MA, Helton KJ, et al. Cognitive impairment in children with hemoglobin SS sickle cell disease: relationship to MR imaging findings and hematocrit. *AJNR Am J Neuroradiol.* 2003;24(3):382-389.

216. Watkins K, Hewes DEM, Connelly A, et al. Cognitive deficits associated with frontal-lobe infarction in children with sickle cell disease. *Dev Med Child Neurol.* 2008;40(8):536-543.

217. Chen R, Krejza J, Arkuszewski M, Zimmerman RA, Herskovits EH, Melhem ER. Brain morphometric analysis predicts decline of intelligence quotient in children with sickle cell disease: a preliminary study. *Adv Med Sci.* 2017;62(1):151-157.

218. Schatz J, Buzan R. Decreased corpus callosum size in sickle cell disease: relationship with cerebral infarcts and cognitive functioning. *J Int Neuropsychol Soc.* 2006;12(1):24-33.

219. Scantlebury N, Mabbott D, Janzen L, et al. White matter integrity and core cognitive function in children diagnosed with sickle cell disease. *J Pediatr Hematol Oncol.* 2011;33(3):163-171.

220. Schatz J, Finke RL, Kellett JM, Kramer JH. Cognitive functioning in children with sickle cell disease: a meta-analysis. *J Pediatr Psychol.* 2002;27(8):739-748.

221. Schatz J, Craft S, Koby M, et al. Neuropsychologic deficits in children with sickle cell disease and cerebral infarction: role of lesion site and volume. *Child Neuropsychol.* 1999;5(2):92-103.

222. Farris N, Branch CA, Zimmerman ME, Suri AK, Billett HH. Lack of association of CNS lesion number with cognitive performance and cerebral blood flow in sickle cell disease. *Blood.* 2015;126:23.

223. Schatz J, White DA, Moinuddin A, Armstrong M, DeBaun MR. Lesion burden and cognitive morbidity in children with sickle cell disease. *J Child Neurol.* 2002;17(12):891-895.

224. Logue SF, Gould TJ. The neural and genetic basis of executive function: attention, cognitive flexibility, and response inhibition. *Pharmacol Biochem Behav.* 2014;123:45-54.

225. Downes M, Kirkham FJ, Berg C, Telfer P, de Haan M. Executive performance on the preschool executive task assessment in children with sickle cell anemia and matched controls. *Child Neuropsychol.* 2019;25(2):278-285.

226. Downes M, Kirkham FJ, Telfer PT, de Haan M. Assessment of executive functions in preschool children with sickle cell anemia. *J Int Neuropsychol Soc.* 2018;24(09):949-954.

227. Anderson P. Assessment and development of executive function (EF) during childhood. *Child Neuropsychol.* 2002;8(2):71-82.

228. Anderson V. Assessing executive functions in children: biological, psychological, and developmental considerations. *Pediatr Rehabil.* 2001;4(3):119-136.

229. Schultz W, Dickinson A. Neuronal coding of prediction errors. *Annu Rev Neurosci.* 2000;23(1):473-500.

230. Gold JI, Mahrer NE, Treadwell M, Weissman L, Vichinsky E. Psychosocial and behavioral outcomes in children with sickle cell disease and their healthy siblings. *J Behav Med.* 2008;31(6): 506-516.

231. Schatz J, Stancil M, Katz T, Sanchez CE. EXAMINER executive function battery and neurologic morbidity in pediatric sickle cell disease. *J Int Neuropsychol Soc.* 2014;20(1):29-40.

232. Bernaudin F, Verlhac S, Fréard F, et al. Multicenter prospective study of children with sickle cell disease: radiographic and psychometric correlation. *J Child Neurol.* 2000;15(5):333-343.

233. Andreotti C, King AA, Macy E, Compas BE, DeBaun MR. The association of cytokine levels with cognitive function in children with sickle cell disease and normal MRI studies of the brain. *J Child Neurol.* 2015;30(10):1349-1353.

234. Baddeley A. The episodic buffer: a new component of working memory? *Trends Cogn Sci.* 2000;4(11):417-423.

235. Schatz J, Roberts CW. Short-term memory in children with sickle cell disease: executive versus modality-specific processing deficits. *Arch Clin Neuropsychol.* 2005;20(8):1073-1085.

236. Wills KE, Nelson SC, Hennessy J, et al. Transition planning for youth with sickle cell disease: embedding neuropsychological assessment into comprehensive care. *Pediatrics.* 2010;126(suppl 3):S151-S159.

237. Berg C, Edwards DF, King A. Executive function performance on the children's kitchen task assessment with children with sickle cell disease and matched controls. *Child Neuropsychol.* 2012;18(5):432-448.

238. Hijmans CT, Grootenhuis MA, Oosterlaan J, Heijboer H, Peters M, Fijnvandraat K. Neurocognitive deficits in children with sickle cell disease are associated with the severity of anemia. *Pediatr Blood Cancer.* 2011;57(2):297-302.

239. Hogan AM, Vargha-Khadem F, Saunders DE, Kirkham FJ, Baldeweg T. Impact of frontal white matter lesions on performance monitoring: ERP evidence for cortical disconnection. *Brain.* 2006;129(8):2177-2188.

240. Brandling-Bennett EM, White DA, Armstrong MM, Christ SE, DeBaun M. Patterns of verbal long-term and working memory performance reveal deficits in strategic processing in children with frontal infarcts related to sickle cell disease. *Dev Neuropsychol.* 2003;24(1):423-434.

241. White DA, Salorio CF, Schatz J, DeBaun M. Preliminary study of working memory in children with stroke related to sickle cell disease. *J Clin Exp Neuropsychol.* 2000;22(2):257-264.

242. Schatz J, Buzan R. Decreased corpus callosum size in sickle cell disease: relationship with cerebral infarcts and cognitive functioning. *J Int Neuropsychol Soc.* 2006;12(1):24-33.

243. Kral MC, Brown RT, Nietert PJ, Abboud MR, Jackson SM, Hynd GW. Transcranial Doppler ultrasonography and neurocognitive functioning in children with sickle cell disease. *Pediatrics.* 2003;112(2):324-331.

244. Ruffieux N, Njamnshi AK, Wonkam A, et al. Association between biological markers of sickle cell disease and cognitive functioning amongst Cameroonian children. *Child Neuropsychol.* 2013;19(2):143-160.

245. Sanchez CE, Schatz J, Roberts CW. Cerebral blood flow velocity and language functioning in pediatric sickle cell disease. *J Int Neuropsychol Soc.* 2010;16(2):326-334.

246. Aron AR. The neural basis of inhibition in cognitive control. *Neuroscientist.* 2007;13(3):214-228.

247. Miller EK, Cohen JD. An integrative theory of prefrontal cortex function. *Annu Rev Neurosci.* 2001;24(1):167-202.

248. Delis DC, Kaplan E, Kramer JH. *Delis-Kaplan Executive Function Scale.* Pearson; 2001.

249. Kral MC, Brown RT, Connelly M, et al. Radiographic predictors of neurocognitive functioning in pediatric sickle cell disease. *J Child Neurol.* 2006;21(1):37-44.

250. Greenberg LM, Waldman ID. Developmental normative data on the test of variables of attention (T.O.V.A.). *J Child Psychol Psychiatry*. 1993;34(6):1019-1030.

251. DeBaun MR, Schatz J, Siegel MJ, et al. Cognitive screening examinations for silent cerebral infarcts in sickle cell disease. *Neurology*. 1998;50(6):1678-1682.

252. Parulekar AD, Diamant Z, Hanania NA. Role of T2 inflammation biomarkers in severe asthma. *Curr Opin Pulm Med*. 2016;22(1):59-68.

253. Jorgensen DR, Metti A, Butters MA, Mettenburg JM, Rosano C, Novelli EM. Disease severity and slower psychomotor speed in adults with sickle cell disease. *Blood Adv*. 2017;1(21):1790-1795.

254. Puffer ES, Schatz JC, Roberts CW. Relationships between somatic growth and cognitive functioning in young children with sickle cell disease. *J Pediatr Psychol*. 2010;35(8):892-904.

255. Montanaro M, Colombatti R, Pugliese M, et al. Intellectual function evaluation of first generation immigrant children with sickle cell disease: the role of language and sociodemographic factors. *Ital J Pediatr*. 2013;39:36.

256. Crawford RD, Jonassaint CR. Adults with sickle cell disease may perform cognitive tests as well as controls when processing speed is taken into account: a preliminary case-control study. *J Adv Nurs*. 2016;72(6):1409-1416.

257. Oluwole OB, Noll RB, Winger DG, Akinyanju O, Novelli EM. Cognitive functioning in children from Nigeria with sickle cell anemia. *Pediatr Blood Cancer*. 2016;63(11):1990-1997.

258. Schatz J, McClellan CB. Sickle cell disease as a neurodevelopmental disorder. *Ment Retard Dev Disabil Res Rev*. 2006;12(3):200-207.

259. Wang WC, Pavlakis SG, Helton KJ, et al. MRI abnormalities of the brain in one-year-old children with sickle cell anemia. *Pediatr Blood Cancer*. 2008;51(5):643-646.

260. Steen RG, Fineberg-Buchner C, Hankins G, Weiss L, Prifitera A, Mulhern RK. Cognitive deficits in children with sickle cell disease. *J Child Neurol*. 2005;20(2):102-107.

261. Thompson RJ, Gustafson KE, Bonner MJ, Ware RE. Neurocognitive development of young children with sickle cell disease through three years of age. *J Pediatr Psychol*. 2002;27(3):235-244.

262. Schatz J, Schlenz AM, Smith KE, Roberts CW. Predictive validity of developmental screening in young children with sickle cell disease: a longitudinal follow-up study. *Dev Med Child Neurol*. 2018;60(5):520-526.

263. Tarazi RA, Grant ML, Ely E, Barakat LP. Neuropsychological functioning in preschool-age children with sickle cell disease: the role of illness-related and psychosocial factors. *Child Neuropsychol*. 2007;13(2):155-172.

264. Aygun B, Parker J, Freeman MB, et al. Neurocognitive screening with the Brigance preschool screen-II in 3-year-old children with sickle cell disease. *Pediatr Blood Cancer*. 2011;56(4):620-624.

265. Glass P, Brennan T, Wang J, et al. Neurodevelopmental deficits among infants and toddlers with sickle cell disease. *J Dev Behav Pediatr*. 2013;34(6):399-405.

266. Hogan AM, Kirkham FJ, Prengler M, et al. An exploratory study of physiological correlates of neurodevelopmental delay in infants with sickle cell anaemia. *Br J Haematol*. 2006;132(1):99-107.

267. Schatz J, McClellan CB, Puffer ES, Johnson K, Roberts CW. Neurodevelopmental screening in toddlers and early preschoolers with sickle cell disease. *J Child Neurol*. 2008;23(1):44-50.

268. Schatz J, Finke R, Roberts CW. Interactions of biomedical and environmental risk factors for cognitive development: a preliminary study of sickle cell disease. *J Dev Behav Pediatr*. 2004;25(5):303-310.

269. Bernaudin F, Verlhac S, Fréard F, et al. Multicenter prospective study of children with sickle cell disease: radiographic and psychometric correlation. *J Child Neurol*. 2000;15(5):333-343.

270. Treadwell MJ, Alkon A, Quirolo KC, Boyce WT. Stress reactivity as a moderator of family stress, physical and mental health, and functional impairment for children with sickle cell disease. *J Dev Behav Pediatr*. 2010;31(6):1.

271. Yarboi J, Compas BE, Brody GH, et al. Association of social-environmental factors with cognitive function in children with sickle cell disease. *Child Neuropsychol*. 2017;23(3):343-360.

272. Marks LJ, Munube D, Kasirye P, et al. Stroke prevalence in children with sickle cell disease in sub-Saharan Africa: a systematic review and meta-analysis. *Glob Pediatr Heal*. 2018;5:2333794X1877497.

273. Earley CJ, Kittner SJ, Feeser BR, et al. Stroke in children and sickle-cell disease: Baltimore-Washington cooperative young stroke study. *Neurology*. 1998;51(1):169-176.

274. Strouse JJ, Jordan LC, Lanzkron S, Casella JF. The excess burden of stroke in hospitalized adults with sickle cell disease. *Am J Hematol*. 2009;84(9):548-552.

275. Rezende PV, Santos MV, Campos GF, et al. Clinical and hematological profile in a newborn cohort with hemoglobin SC. *J Pediatr (Rio J)*. 2018;94(6):666-672.

276. Araujo OMR de, Ivo ML, Ferreira Júnior MA, Pontes ERJC, Bispo IMGP, Oliveira ECL. Survival and mortality among users and non-users of hydroxyurea with sickle cell disease. *Rev Lat Am Enfermagem*. 2015;23(1):67-73.

277. Ali SB, Reid M, Fraser R, MooSang M, Ali A. Seizures in the jamaica cohort study of sickle cell disease. *Br J Haematol*. 2010;151(3):265-272.

278. Pegelow CH, Macklin EA, Moser FG, et al. Longitudinal changes in brain magnetic resonance imaging findings in children with sickle cell disease. *Blood*. 2002;99(8):3014-3018.

279. Adams RJ, McKie VC, Hsu L, et al. Prevention of a first stroke by transfusions in children with sickle cell anemia and abnormal results on transcranial Doppler ultrasonography. *N Engl J Med*. 1998;339(1):5-11.

280. Adams RJ, Brambilla D, Optimizing Primary Stroke Prevention in Sickle Cell Anemia (STOP 2) Trial Investigators. Discontinuing prophylactic transfusions used to prevent stroke in sickle cell disease. *N Engl J Med*. 2005;353(26):2769-2778.

281. Buchanan ID, James-Herry A, Osunkwo I. The other side of abnormal. *J Pediatr Hematol Oncol*. 2013;35(7):543-546.

282. Valadi N, Silva GS, Bowman LS, et al. Transcranial Doppler ultrasonography in adults with sickle cell disease. *Neurology*. 2006;67(4):572-574.

283. Neumayr L, Vichinsky E. Stroke recurrence in adult sickle cell patients: it is time for action! *Transfusion*. 2016;56(5):1001-1004.

284. Hurlet-Jensen AM, Prohovnik I, Pavlakis SG, Piomelli S. Effects of total hemoglobin and hemoglobin S concentration on cerebral blood flow during transfusion therapy to prevent stroke in sickle cell disease. *Stroke*. 1994;25(8):1688-1692.

285. Venketasubramanian N, Prohovnik I, Hurlet A, Mohr JP, Piomelli S. Middle cerebral artery velocity changes during transfusion in sickle cell anemia. *Stroke*. 1994;25(11):2153-2158.

286. Guilliams KP, Fields ME, Ragan DK, et al. Red cell exchange transfusions lower cerebral blood flow and oxygen extraction fraction in pediatric sickle cell anemia. *Blood*. 2018;131(9):1012-1021.

287. Prohovnik I, Pavlakis SG, Piomelli S, et al. Cerebral hyperemia, stroke, and transfusion in sickle cell disease. *Neurology*. 1989;39(3):344-348.

288. Estcourt LJ, Fortin PM, Hopewell S, Trivella M, Wang WC. Blood transfusion for preventing primary and secondary stroke in people with sickle cell disease. *Cochrane Database Syst Rev.* 2017;1(1):CD003146.

289. Brousse V, Hertz-Pannier L, Consigny Y, et al. Does regular blood transfusion prevent progression of cerebrovascular lesions in children with sickle cell disease? *Ann Hematol.* 2009;88(8):785-788.

290. Wayne AS, Schoenike SE, Pegelow CH. Financial analysis of chronic transfusion for stroke prevention in sickle cell disease. *Blood.* 2000;96(7):2369-2372.

291. DeBaun MR, Quirolo K. Chronic transfusion therapy for stroke in sickle cell disease. *J Clin Apher.* 2017;32(5):368-370.

292. Brittenham GM. Iron-chelating therapy for transfusional iron overload. *N Engl J Med.* 2011;364(2):146-156.

293. Adams RJ, McKie VC, Hsu L, et al. Prevention of a first stroke by transfusions in children with sickle cell anemia and abnormal results on transcranial Doppler ultrasonography. *N Engl J Med.* 1998;339(1):5-11.

294. Vichinsky EP, Ohene-Frempong K, Thein SL, et al. Transfusion and chelation practices in sickle cell disease: a regional perspective. *Pediatr Hematol Oncol.* 2011;28(2):124-133.

295. Wilimas J, Goff JR, Anderson HR, Langston JW, Thompson E. Efficacy of transfusion therapy for one to two years in patients with sickle cell disease and cerebrovascular accidents. *J Pediatr.* 1980;96(2):205-208.

296. Russell MO, Goldberg HI, Hodson A, et al. Effect of transfusion therapy on arteriographic abnormalities and on recurrence of stroke in sickle cell disease. *Blood.* 1984;63(1):162-169.

297. Wang WC, Kovnar EH, Tonkin IL, et al. High risk of recurrent stroke after discontinuance of five to twelve years of transfusion therapy in patients with sickle cell disease. *J Pediatr.* 1991;118(3):377-382.

298. Ware RE, Schultz WH, Yovetich N, et al. Stroke With Transfusions Changing to Hydroxyurea (SWiTCH): a phase III randomized clinical trial for treatment of children with sickle cell anemia, stroke, and iron overload. *Pediatr Blood Cancer.* 2011;57(6):1011-1017.

299. Lagunju I, Brown BJ, Sodeinde O. Hydroxyurea lowers transcranial Doppler flow velocities in children with sickle cell anaemia in a Nigerian cohort. *Pediatr Blood Cancer.* 2015;62(9):1587-1591.

300. Lagunju I, Brown BJ, Oyinlade AO, et al. Annual stroke incidence in Nigerian children with sickle cell disease and elevated TCD velocities treated with hydroxyurea. *Pediatr Blood Cancer.* 2019;66(3):e27252.

301. Lagunju IA, Brown BJ, Sodeinde OO. Stroke recurrence in Nigerian children with sickle cell disease treated with hydroxyurea. *Niger Postgrad Med J.* 2013;20(3):181-187.

302. Galadanci NA, Umar Abdullahi S, Vance LD, et al. Feasibility trial for primary stroke prevention in children with sickle cell anemia in Nigeria (SPIN trial). *Am J Hematol.* 2018;93(3):E83.

303. Abdullahi SU, DeBaun MR, Jordan LC, Rodeghier M, Galadanci NA. Stroke recurrence in Nigerian children with sickle cell disease: evidence for a secondary stroke prevention trial. *Pediatr Neurol.* 2019;95:73-78.

304. Hall EM, Leonard J, Smith JL, et al. Reduction in overt and silent stroke recurrence rate following cerebral revascularization surgery in children with sickle cell disease and severe cerebral vasculopathy. *Pediatr Blood Cancer.* 2016;63(8):1431-1437.

305. Aguilar-Salinas P, Hayward K, Santos R, et al. Surgical revascularization for pediatric patients with sickle cell disease and moyamoya disease in the prevention of ischemic strokes: a single-center case series and a systematic review. *World Neurosurg.* 2019;123:435-442.e8.

306. Walters MC, Hardy K, Edwards S, et al. Pulmonary, gonadal, and central nervous system status after bone marrow transplantation for sickle cell disease. *Biol Blood Marrow Transplant.* 2010;16(2):263-272.

307. Bernaudin F, Verlhac S, Peffault de Latour R, et al. Association of matched sibling donor hematopoietic stem cell transplantation with transcranial Doppler velocities in children with sickle cell anemia. *JAMA.* 2019;321(3):266.

308. Bodas P, Rotz S. Cerebral vascular abnormalities in pediatric patients with sickle cell disease after hematopoietic cell transplant. *J Pediatr Hematol Oncol.* 2014;36(3):190-193.

309. Shenoy S, Eapen M, Panepinto JA, et al. A trial of unrelated donor marrow transplantation for children with severe sickle cell disease. *Blood.* 2016;128(21):2561-2567.

310. Wang W, Schreiber J, Kang G, et al. Effects of hydroxyurea (HU) on neurocognitive performance in children with sickle cell disease: a prospective trial. *Blood.* 2017;130(suppl 1).

311. Hood AM, King AA, Fields ME, et al. Blood transfusion acutely improves executive abilities in children and young adults with sickle cell disease. *Pediatr Blood Cancer.* 2019;66(10):e27899.

312. Puffer E, Schatz J, Roberts CW. The association of oral hydroxyurea therapy with improved cognitive functioning in sickle cell disease. *Child Neuropsychol.* 2007;13(2):142-154.

313. Partanen M, Kang G, Wang WC, et al. Association between hydroxycarbamide exposure and neurocognitive function in adolescents with sickle cell disease. *Br J Haematol.* 2020;189(6):1192-1203.

314. Bockenmeyer J, Chamboredon E, Missud F, et al. [Development of psychological and intellectual performance in transplanted sickle cell disease patients: a prospective study from pretransplant period to 5 years after HSCT]. *Arch Pediatr.* 2013;20(7):723-730.

315. Prussien KV, Patel DA, Wilkerson K, et al. Improvement in processing speed following haploidentical bone marrow transplant with posttransplant cytoxan in children and adolescents with sickle cell disease. *Pediatr Blood Cancer.* 2020;67(1):e28001.

Management of Pregnant Women and Newborns With Sickle Cell Disease

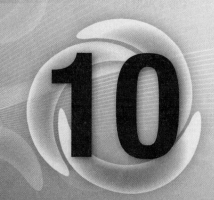

Authors: Samuel A. Oppong, Jodi-Anne Stewart,
Michael R. DeBaun

Chapter Outline

Overview

Pregnant women with sickle cell disease experience significant morbidity and mortality compared to the general population in both low-middle and high-income settings. Women with sickle cell disease are more likely to experience hypertensive emergencies (preeclampsia and eclampsia), intrauterine growth restriction (IUGR), low birth weight, fetal demise, venous thromboembolism, peripartum cardiomyopathy, and maternal death when compared to age-matched healthy pregnant women in both low-middle– and high-income settings.[1-5]

The highest rate of maternal mortality among pregnant women with sickle cell disease occurs in sub-Saharan Africa, where the risk of maternal mortality can be as high as 29 times that of pregnant women without sickle cell disease.[6] The maternal mortality rate of pregnant women with sickle cell disease living in sub-Saharan Africa, without any intervention, is approximately 6000 to 10,000 per 100,000 live births,[2,6-8] as compared to 542 per 100,000 live births in women living in the same environment without sickle cell disease.

In high-income settings, pregnant women with sickle cell disease have an increased risk of pregnancy-related complications compared to those without sickle cell disease, but no evidence of increased mortality.[3] Specifically, in a pooled analysis of published studies, women with sickle cell disease, compared to women without sickle cell disease, had a higher rate of preeclampsia (pooled odds ratio [OR], 1.86; 95% confidence interval [CI], 1.22-2.82), eclampsia (pooled OR, 2.07; 95% CI, 1.43-2.99), cesarean delivery (pooled OR, 1.62; 95% CI, 1.26-2.08), and bacterial infection during pregnancy (pooled OR, 3.03; 95% CI, 1.86-4.92)[3].

Furthermore, in the same analysis, pregnant women with sickle cell disease living in low- and middle-income settings have a statistically significant increased odds ratio of eclampsia, cesarean delivery, and bacterial infection when compared to women without sickle cell disease.[3] Similarly, the analysis showed that pregnancy in women with sickle cell disease had an increased odds of IUGR (OR, 2.79; 95% CI, 1.85-4.21), prematurity (OR, 2.14; 95% CI, 1.56-2.94), and perinatal death (OR, 3.76; 95% CI, 2.34-6.06).[3] The ORs of morbidities in pregnant women with sickle cell disease are summarized in Table 10-1.

Collectively, data from the pooled analyses strongly suggest that mortality in pregnant women is likely related to the gap in medical care between low-middle and high-income settings.[3] Regardless of the setting, there is an increased risk of maternal morbidities.[3] In contrast, an increase in mortality only occurred in women in low-middle–income settings.

TABLE 10-1 Obstetric complications associated with sickle cell disease

Complication	OR	95% CI
Preeclampsia	2.05	1.47-2.85
Eclampsia	3.02	1.20-7.58
Recurrent infections	2.48	1.23-5.01
Cesarean delivery	1.42	1.04-1.93
Maternal mortality	10.91	1.83-65.11
Intrauterine growth restriction	2.79	1.85-4.21
Low birth weight	2.00	1.42-2.83
Preterm birth/prematurity	2.14	1.56-2.95
Stillbirth	4.05	2.59-6.32
Perinatal mortality	3.76	2.34-6.06
Neonatal mortality	2.71	1.41-5.22

Abbreviations: CI, confidence interval; OR, odds ratio.
Data from Boafor et al[3] and Chen et al.[83]

Preconception Care in Women With Sickle Cell Disease

Adequate preconception care in women with sickle cell disease will optimize the opportunity for an improved outcome for both the mother and fetus. Preconception care provides an opportunity for early intervention and the ability to optimize the health of the potential mother. Based on a global consensus in 2012, preconception care was defined as the provision of biomedical, behavioral, and social health interventions to women and couples before conception occurs that aimed at improving their health status and reducing behavioral, individual, and environmental factors that may contribute to poor maternal and fetal outcomes.[9] For the purpose of this review, preconception care will be discussed under the following subheadings: education, screening, counseling, and planning for pregnancy.

Education About Potential Increase in Sickle Cell Disease–Related Morbidity During Pregnancy

Unfortunately, many sickle cell disease–related morbidities occur with higher incidence rates in pregnant women. A significantly higher incidence rate of acute vaso-occlusive pain episodes, acute chest syndrome (ACS), and venous thromboembolism occurs during pregnancy, particularly in the third trimester and puerperium.[10]

The focus on anticipatory guidance improves the future mother's understanding of the intersection between her sickle cell disease and pregnancy. Adequate patient education is expected to improve adherence with contraception, medication, and follow-up schedule and decrease the lag time between onset of symptoms and prompt medical care.[11,12] Critical areas to cover in patient education include signs of pregnancy, early pregnancy symptoms (eg, nausea, vomiting, and loss of appetite), and how changes in appetite may impact oral fluid intake and nutrition. Anticipatory guidance for the management of sickle cell disease–related morbidity should be reviewed carefully.

Screening

Preconception Screening for Sickle Cell Disease in High-Risk Populations

In sub-Saharan Africa, where >85% of the world's newborns with sickle cell disease are delivered,[13] newborn screening is not routine in most countries, and most individuals do not know their hemoglobin phenotype. Premarital screening and counseling for sickle cell disease can be done for couples to make an informed choice. For couples who do not have the opportunity to obtain premarital screening and do not know their hemoglobinopathy trait status, a hemoglobin analysis should be performed for both the mother and father, and, when appropriate, genetic counseling should be provided. In West Africa, where sickle cell trait may occur in 25% of adults, and as many as 15% of the pregnant women with sickle cell disease may have a newborn with sickle cell disease.[14]

Preconception care should include, but not be limited to, screening for immunization status, screening for minor red blood cell antigen alloimmunization, counseling about smoking, and substitution with non teratogenic therapy.[15] Immunizations should be obtained against all encapsulated bacteria—*Neisseria meningitides*, *Streptococcus pneumoniae*, and *Haemophilus influenzae*.[16]

Preconception Counseling and Genetic Testing

Couples who are planning for conception, where the woman has sickle cell disease, require extensive counseling about sickle cell disease, including, but not limited to, mode of inheritance, associated risk to the baby, and common complications in both early and late pregnancy. Culturally sensitive and nondirective support for preconception genetic counseling is preferred.[17]

Screening for End-Organ Damage

The preconception period provides the best opportunity to screen, diagnose, and treat sickle cell disease–related organ disease, particularly heart, lung, and kidney disease, which may cluster and are associated with earlier death in young adults with sickle cell disease.[18]

Cardiovascular disease, as manifested by an elevated tricuspid regurgitant jet velocity (TRJV) >2.5 m/s and brain natriuretic peptide >160 pg/mL or TRJV >3.0 m/s, as a biomarker for pulmonary hypertension, is an established risk factor for premature death in adults with sickle cell disease.[18-20]

Unfortunately, most adults with sickle cell disease do not have symptoms associated with an elevated TRJV. Furthermore, sickle cell disease or obstetric guidelines for management of pregnant women with sickle cell disease do not include screening for an elevated TRJV. Without studies focused on evaluating the clinical utility of echocardiography during pregnancy, we do not advocate screening for elevated TRJV during pregnancy. Rather, we believe that understanding the impact of abnormal heart function in the woman and fetus during pregnancy and postpartum is an ideal circumstance.

Similarly, lung disease, as manifested by a low forced expiratory volume in 1 second (FEV_1) in adults with sickle cell disease, is associated with earlier death and is predictive of ACS.[21] Despite ACS being the major cause of death in pregnant women with sickle cell disease[22] and low FEV_1 being a predictive feature of ACS, current guidelines for pregnant women with sickle cell disease do not include spirometry testing during pregnancy.[21] Without formal studies determining whether abnormal spirometry is associated with adverse maternal and fetal outcomes, we do not advocate screening for a low FEV_1 during pregnancy. However, future research strategies should evaluate the impact of lung disease on the adverse outcome of women and fetuses during pregnancy and postpartum.

Kidney disease is a common complication in adults with sickle cell disease.[23,24] The major manifestations include albuminuria, acute tubular necrosis, and renal failure. The physiologic adaptation of many organ systems, including the kidney, during pregnancy may cause worsening of any such preexisting conditions. The increased plasma volume during pregnancy with an accompanying increase in renal blood flow, increased glomerular filtration rate, and solute delivered to the kidney may worsen a preexisting disease of the kidney.

Pregnancy is associated with basic changes in clinical monitoring of kidney function. In the general population, glomerular filtration rate increases approximately 50% with a concordant decrease in serum creatinine, urea, and uric acid values.[25] Blood pressure also decreases by approximately 10 mm Hg during pregnancy.[25]

Given changes in parameters used to estimate renal function during pregnancy, identifying baseline values and treatment of preexisting renal disease are important interventions prior to pregnancy. Women with preexisting renal disease may also be prone to preeclampsia; however, studies documenting the strength of this association are limited. Before and during early pregnancy, urinalysis should be obtained to screen for albuminuria, blood urea nitrogen, and creatinine. Absolute thresholds for abnormal laboratory and blood pressure measurements should be interpreted cautiously during pregnancy in women with sickle cell disease. Relative increases from baseline in laboratory measures, particularly blood pressures, should be monitored closely and interpreted in the context of the clinical situation.

For the diagnosis of preeclampsia, the classic definition of systolic blood pressure >140 mm Hg or diastolic blood pressure >90 mm Hg with proteinuria has recently been modified to include new onset of hypertension and proteinuria or hypertension and significant end-organ dysfunction with or without proteinuria after 20 weeks of gestation in a previously normotensive woman.[26] Additional clinical features include a protein/creatinine ratio ≥0.3 (30 mg/mmol) in a random urine specimen or dipstick ≥2+ if a quantitative measurement is unavailable, platelet count <100,000/μL, serum creatinine >1.1 mg/dL (97.2 μmol/L) or doubling of the creatinine concentration in the absence of other renal disease, liver transaminases at least twice the upper limit of the normal concentrations for the local laboratory, pulmonary edema, and cerebral or visual symptoms (eg, new-onset and persistent headaches not accounted for by alternative diagnoses and not responding to usual doses of analgesics, blurred vision, flashing lights or sparks, scotomata).[26]

Given the significant overlap between clinical and laboratory features associated with preeclampsia and the preexisting low blood pressure in pregnant women with sickle cell disease,[27] individualized care plans should be considered for clinical actions in pregnant women with sickle cell disease. Specifically, we suggest a multidisciplinary team of obstetricians, hematologists, pediatricians, and individuals with expertise in acute care of pregnant women with sickle cell disease in low-middle– and high-income settings.

Planning for Treatment Modifications

Careful review of the current medications should be employed to determine whether they can be continued throughout pregnancy without any potential risk to the fetus. For women requiring hydroxyurea for strokes, acute pain episode, or life-threatening ACS episodes, strong consideration should be given to regular blood transfusion therapy to keep hemoglobin S levels <30%. The third trimester and puerperium are the intervals with the highest risk of vasoocclusive pain events.[10] Thus, regular transfusion therapy during the third trimester represent the most favorable benefit-risk ratio for secondary prevention of sickle cell disease–related complications.

Adequate planning should be made for optimal chelation therapy in the case of excessive iron stores prior to pregnancy. Diagnosis of excessive iron stores should be based on cardiac T2* values, liver T2* values, and ferritin levels. Iron chelation therapy includes treatment with deferoxamine, deferiprone, or deferasirox. Once pregnancy is confirmed, these medications should be discontinued because they are contraindicated during pregnancy. Deferoxamine is classified as category C by the US Food and Drug Administration because animal reproduction studies have shown an adverse effect on the fetus.[28] Deferiprone is classified as category D by the US Food and Drug Administration because of evidence of human fetal risk.[29] Deferasirox is also classified as category C.[30]

Often women with sickle cell disease will have proteinuria or relative hypertension. However, in the presence of proteinuria or hypertension in women planning to become pregnant,

we would not treat these patients with angiotensin-converting enzyme inhibitors[31] or angiotensin receptor blockers. Both therapies are considered teratogenic.

Nutrition and Micronutrient Supplementation

Nutrition plays a vital role in supporting future pregnancy. Among women with sickle cell disease, there is a strong recommendation for starting daily folic acid at 1 mg at least 3 months before pregnancy. In low-resource settings in sub-Saharan Africa, the combined effects of sickle cell disease, malaria, and malnutrition worsen the risk of anemia. Sickle cell disease has been associated with malnutrition, especially during childhood. The presence of preexisting anemia can result in adverse maternal and fetal outcomes.

Pregnancy in Women With Sickle Cell Disease

Physiologic Adaptation to Pregnancy in Women With Sickle Cell Disease

The normal physiology of pregnancy coupled with chronic anemia associated with sickle cell disease places pregnant women and their fetus at increased risk for complications. Some of the earliest adaptations during the first 2 weeks of pregnancy include cardiovascular and hematologic changes. In the first month of pregnancy, the heart rate and stroke volume increase, causing a proportional increase in cardiac output by 30% to 50%.[32] Additionally, plasma volume increases by 25% to 50%, and excessive erythropoietin production from the kidneys causes a 20% to 30% increase in red blood cell mass (Figure 10-1).[33] As a result, a 1- to 2-g/dL decrease in hemoglobin level occurs and is characterized as physiologic anemia.[34] Another common adaptation is leukocytosis, with a predominance in neutrophils, due to the physiologic stress of pregnancy.[34]

In addition to an increase in cardiac output along with a decrease in hemoglobin levels during pregnancy, lung function parameters change with time. The major changes in lung function during pregnancy are believed to be dependent on diaphragmatic positional change due to the enlarged uterus pushing the diaphragm upward, among other poorly defined influences (Figure 10-2). Static lung functions are generally preserved during pregnancy, except for functional residual capacity, which is decreased by 20% to 30%. This is due to an increase in inspiratory capacity by 5% to 10% and a decrease in residual volume without change in the total lung capacity. Multiple studies have demonstrated that there is a decrease in forced vital capacity and FEV_1 percent predicted when compared to nonpregnant woman, with a significant decrease in the third trimester.[35,36] None of these studies identified the coefficient of variation[37] between pulmonary function tests, which may contribute to the diverging results (Figure 10-3).

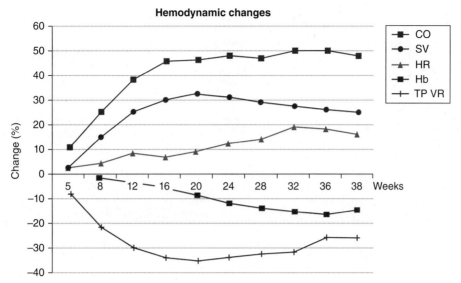

FIGURE 10-1 Hemodynamic changes during pregnancy with gestational age. CO, cardiac output; Hb, hemoglobin; HR, heart rate; SV, stroke volume; TPVR, total peripheral vascular resistance. Reprinted from Ruys TP, Cornette J, Roos-Hesselink JW. Pregnancy and delivery in cardiac disease. *J Cardiol.* 2013;61(2):107-112. Copyright 2013 with permission from Elsevier.

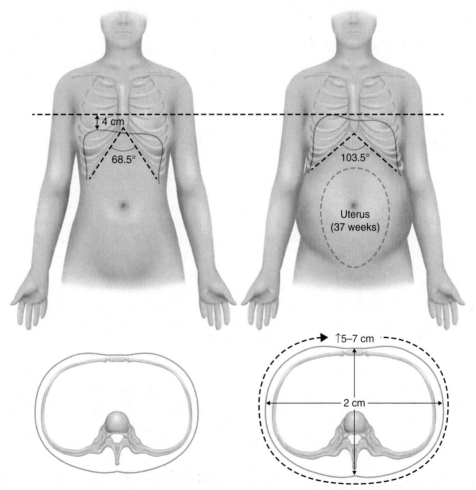

FIGURE 10-2 Changes in chest wall during pregnancy. During pregnancy, there is an increase in the transverse diameter of the chest wall and chest wall circumference but no significant change in total lung capacity. Redrawn from Hegewald MJ, Crapo RO. Respiratory physiology in pregnancy. *Clin Chest Med.* 2011;32(1):1-13. Copyright 2011 with permission from Elsevier.

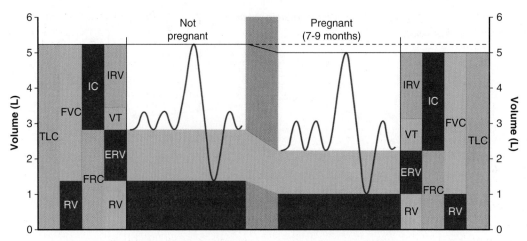

FIGURE 10-3 **Changes in lung volumes during pregnancy.** The changes include a reduction in functional residual capacity (FRC) and increase in inspiratory capacity (IC) and tidal volume (VT). ERV, expiratory reserve volume; FVC, forced vital capacity; IRV, inspiratory reserve volume; RV, residual volume; TLC, total lung capacity. Redrawn from Hegewald MJ, Crapo RO. Respiratory physiology in pregnancy. *Clin Chest Med.* 2011;32(1):1-13. Copyright 2011 with permission from Elsevier.

Women with sickle cell disease experience an increase in metabolic demand and an increase in blood viscosity. This is due to the additive effect of increased coagulation proteins and their sickling effects. This hypercoagulable-hyperviscous state leads to an increase in pain episodes, ACS, osteonecrosis, hepatic necrosis, leg ulcers, and thromboembolic events.[16] Vascular occlusion may occur in the placenta, leading to villous fibrosis, necrosis, and infarction, resulting in decreased uteroplacental circulation. This often manifests as chronic fetal hypoxia, IUGR, and eventually fetal demise.[38]

Antenatal Care

When women with sickle cell disease recognize they are pregnant, they should make an appointment with an obstetrician, and transfer of care to or joint management with a hematologist should occur within the first trimester of pregnancy. The first few visits provide opportunity to reemphasize issues during the preconception care visit and to calibrate early baseline pregnancy laboratory and clinical values. In low-income settings where preconception care is very limited or virtually nonexistent, an early antenatal visit provides the best opportunity to screen for end-organ damage, review and discontinue certain medications, and recommend folic acid supplementation. Early ultrasound confirmation of pregnancy and accurate dating are essential for proper management of pregnant women with sickle cell disease. This early ultrasound examination also provides opportunity for fetal tissue sampling via chorionic villus sampling between 10 and 12 weeks for genetic testing of fetal hemoglobin genotype. Apart from preimplantation testing, this provides the next best opportunity for prenatal diagnosis of sickle cell disease in the fetus.

Strong clinical evidence suggests that pregnant women with sickle cell disease require a multidisciplinary care approach for improved maternal and fetal outcomes.[2,14] If possible, the multidisciplinary care team should include a hematologist, preferably the primary hematologist who managed the woman during the prepregnancy period. Other important members of

the team may include a respiratory physician or pulmonologist, a midwife, and a public health nurse. Before delivery, consultation with the anesthesiologist and neonatologist is essential. At the Korle-Bu Teaching Hospital (KBTH) in Ghana, a multidisciplinary care approach for pregnant women with sickle cell disease reduced maternal death by nearly 90% and perinatal death by 62%[2] In that same institution, major maternal and perinatal outcome measures have been reduced to levels comparable to those of women without sickle cell disease.[14] Essential aspects of antenatal history review, physical assessment, and initial laboratory tests are summarized in Table 10-2.

Schedule of Antenatal Visit

Pregnant women with sickle cell disease are high-risk antenatal patients and therefore often require frequent visits and risk assessments. Due to the risk of sickle cell disease and pregnancy-related complications, we recommend that a multidisciplinary team, including a hematologist or provider with expertise in sickle cell disease, follows the pregnant woman every 2 weeks from the first trimester until 34 weeks and then, thereafter, weekly until delivery.[39,40] We believe that the scheduled visits are particularly important in low-middle–income settings where the sickle cell disease expertise may be limited and the importance of a multidisciplinary team is critical to improving clinical outcomes of both the pregnant woman and fetus.

Antenatal Therapy for Prevention of Pregnancy-Related Complications

Routine *folic acid* supplementation throughout pregnancy is an essential part of the care of pregnant women with sickle cell disease. A daily dose of 1 mg is recommended. In many sub-Saharan African settings where malaria is endemic, a daily dose of folic acid up to 5 mg is often given. The additional burden of malaria-induced red blood cell destruction has been cited as the justification for this higher dose of folic acid during pregnancy.[41]

TABLE 10-2 Antenatal, delivery, and postnatal care plan for management of pregnant women with SCD at the KBTH Comprehensive Obstetric Multidisciplinary Care Program

Review history related to

❏ Symptoms of SCD complications

❏ Hospitalization

❏ Blood transfusion

❏ Steady-state hemoglobin

❏ SCD-associated complications in prior pregnancy including VOC, ACS, AVN, stroke, etc.

❏ Prior OB complications: miscarriages, IUFD, IUGR, cesarean delivery, APH, preeclampsia, eclampsia

❏ Review family history: parents' carrier status, siblings' disease or carrier status

❏ Spouse/partner status (encourage testing of partner, if unknown)

❏ Status of living children (encourage testing, if unknown)

❏ Family planning utilization and experience

Complete physical examination

❏ Pallor, jaundice, hepatosplenomegaly, gait

❏ Blood pressure

❏ BMI

❏ SFH, where appropriate

Diagnosis of pregnancy

❏ Confirm LMP, if known

❏ Review booking USG, if available, and establish viability of fetus

❏ Establish gestational age and confirm EDD

Booking labs

❏ Hb electrophoresis, if genotype in doubt

❏ CBC

❏ Blood film comment

❏ Blood film for malaria parasites

❏ Reticulocyte count

❏ Blood group and Rh factor

❏ G6PD

❏ VDRL/TPHA

❏ HBsAg

❏ HIV serology

❏ Renal function

❏ LFT

❏ Urinalysis, urine CS for ASB

❏ Stool examination for parasites

❏ Iron studies

Initial management after confirmation of pregnancy

❏ Tab folic acid 5 mg daily

❏ Oral iron supplement, 60 mg daily (if no risk of iron overload)

❏ Multivitamin

❏ Commence LDA 75-100 mg daily from 13 weeks

❏ Tetanus toxoid (based on schedule)

❏ Sulfadoxine-pyrimethamine (SP) 3 tabs starting at 16 weeks or after quickening; repeat every 4 weeks until 36 weeks

Antenatal schedule

❏ Visits every 2 weeks until 34 weeks, then weekly until delivery

❏ Repeat CBC every 4-6 weeks

❏ Repeat urine CS every 6 weeks for ASB

❏ Repeat USG at 18-22 weeks for fetal anomaly screening

Fetal surveillance

❏ Fetal growth monitoring

❏ Repeat USG 2-4 times weekly for fetal growth starting at 28 weeks

❏ Request umbilical artery Doppler if signs of IUGR identified

❏ Nonstress test twice weekly if admitted antenatally

Delivery

❏ Deliver at 38-39 weeks and up to 40 weeks for HbSC

❏ IOL and cesarean delivery are based on OB indication

❏ Adequate hydration 40-50 mL/kg in 24 hours, including fluid for augmentation of labor

❏ Labor analgesia: epidural analgesia preferred, parenteral opioid can be given

❏ Maintain Spo_2 above 92% with nasal prongs

❏ Shorten second stage of labor with Ventouse vacuum extraction or forceps delivery

Cesarean delivery:

❏ Use spinal anesthesia and give oxygen supplementation with nasal prongs

❏ Continue oxygen supplementation at recovery and continue for 24 hours after delivery

❏ Start incentive spirometry at the recovery ward

❏ Continue intravenous hydration for 48 hours

❏ Perioperative simple blood transfusion if Hb drops >2 g/dL below the steady state or if Hb <8 g/dL

Abbreviations: ACS, acute chest syndrome; APH, antepartum hemorrhage; ASB, asymptomatic bacteriuria; AVN, avascular necrosis; BMI, body mass index; CBC, complete blood count; CS, culture and sensitivity; EDD, expected date of delivery; G6PD, glucose-6-phosphate dehydrogenase; Hb, hemoglobin; IOL, induction of labor; IUFD, intrauterine fetal demise; IUGR, intrauterine growth restriction; KBTH, Korle-Bu Teaching Hospital; LDA, low-dose aspirin; LFT, liver function test; LMP, last menstrual period; OB, obstetric; SCD, sickle cell disease; SFH, symphysis-fundal height; TPHA, *Treponema pallidum* hemagglutination assay; USG, ultrasonography; VDRL, Venereal Disease Research Laboratory; VOC, vaso-occlusive crisis.

Iron supplementation for pregnant women with sickle cell disease is a source of ongoing debate, with no consensus. In high-income settings pregnant women with sickle cell disease who receive frequent blood transfusion, are not likely to require iron supplementation. In many low-income settings, chronic blood transfusion among women with sickle cell disease is not standard practice due to lack of blood products. Poor nutrition, infestation with malaria, and other helminthic infections may render patients iron deficient. At KBTH, nearly 20% of pregnant women with sickle cell disease who attend the comprehensive sickle cell disease clinic had iron deficiency anemia (unpublished data). In many low-income settings where routine iron studies may be too expensive during the antenatal period, a critical review of the dietary history and medical history that may be enough to initiate iron supplementation during pregnancy.

In malaria-endemic areas, *antimalarial prophylaxis* is recommended for all pregnant women. Antimalarial prophylaxis should start at 16 weeks and continue until 36 weeks. Sulfadoxine-pyrimethamine (25/500 mg) in a fixed-dose combination is given every 4 weeks until 36 weeks to help reduce the risk of IUGR and prevent anemia at term.[42]

Low-dose aspirin is taken for the prevention of preeclampsia. The risk of preeclampsia is increased by about 2- to 3-fold in pregnant women with sickle cell disease compared to women with HbAA.[3,14] Preeclampsia and sickle cell disease combined are associated with a high incidence of preterm birth, low birth weight, IUGR, and an increase in perinatal death among women with sickle cell disease.[14] Even though low-dose aspirin, started between 13 and 17 weeks of pregnancy, has been shown to reduce the risk of preeclampsia in high-risk women, the effectiveness and risks of this intervention in pregnant women with sickle cell disease have not been tested. For women with preexisting renal disease, a case-by-case discussion should be considered for assessment of the risks and benefits of using low-dose aspirin. Despite the lack of evidence of its effectiveness and potential complications, low-dose aspirin is still recommended by the American College of Obstetricians and Gynecologists and United Kingdom National Institute for Health and Care Excellence Guidelines for prevention of preeclampsia in women with sickle cell disease.

Antenatal Therapy for Prevention of Sickle Cell Disease–Related Complications During Pregnancy

No therapy has been established to prevent sickle cell disease–related morbidity in pregnant women. Hydroxyurea is the most commonly prescribed disease-modifying therapy in sickle cell disease, particularly for women with HbSS. In nonpregnant women, hydroxyurea is associated with a decreased rate of acute sickle cell disease–related pain and ACS and decreased use of regular blood transfusion therapy.[43] However, hydroxyurea is teratogenic in rats.[44,45]

Elective blood transfusion during pregnancy is indicated for any acute complications that would otherwise necessitate blood transfusion regardless of pregnancy (eg, ACS, hemoglobin

<7 g/dL or decrease of 2 g/dL below baseline, and stroke).[46,47] Selective prophylactic blood transfusions may be indicated for women with HbSS during the third trimester or high-risk patients with a history of ACS, chronic end-organ dysfunction, stroke, pulmonary hypertension,[48] or a significant number of acute severe pain episodes (at least 3) per year.

Limited evidence supports the efficacy of prophylactic blood transfusion throughout pregnancy. Studies are small and lack a consistent methodology.[46,49] However, some studies have shown that use of prophylactic blood transfusion during pregnancy reduces the incidence of acute pain episodes, ACS, preeclampsia, thromboembolisms, infections, low newborn birth weight, miscarriages, stillbirths, and other complications.[50,51] A randomized controlled trial is required to demonstrate the definitive risks and benefits of prophylactic blood transfusion therapy in pregnant women with sickle cell disease.

Chelation therapy for pregnant women with sickle cell disease and excessive iron stores is typically not performed. In general, iron chelation should be suspended in pregnant women with sickle cell disease. However, the benefits of chelation in pregnant women with excessive iron stores should be weighed against the risks and inconvenience. In women with moderate iron stores with no evidence of organ dysfunction attributable to excessive iron stores, a 6-month course of chelation is not likely to have a dramatic impact on the clinical course. This is especially the case if the patient is not receiving additional iron through routine red blood cell transfusions and there is no evidence of impending organ dysfunction in the liver or heart directly related to excessive iron stores. In women with excessive iron stores and evidence of liver or heart damage directly related to iron deposition, the risk-benefit ratio of chelation therapy should be considered in conjunction with a hematologist. Based on the available data, the risk of chelation-related toxicity to the fetus is far greater than the benefit of 6 months of chelation to the pregnant woman. A summary of a set of recommendations for management of pregnant women with sickle cell disease during the antenatal period is shown in Table 10-3.

Fetal Growth Monitoring and Fetal Surveillance

An obstetric ultrasound assessment of the fetus is critical for an optimal outcome. Early ultrasound assessment to confirm and date the pregnancy in the first trimester is very important. An ultrasound at 18 to 22 weeks for fetal anatomical survey and detection of any gross congenital anomaly is recommended. Regardless of whether the pregnancy occurs in low-middle– or high-income settings, women with sickle cell disease have a higher odds ratio of IUGR when compared to women without sickle cell disease.[3]

Fetal growth monitoring using serial ultrasound to assess multiple fetal biometry is required for fetal growth assessment. Fetal growth assessment every 2 to 4 weeks by ultrasound is recommended from 28 weeks. Patients found to have IUGR (below the tenth percentile of the fetal growth curve) require umbilical artery Doppler studies to assess placental function as a possible cause of growth restriction. Multiple

TABLE 10-3 Summary of recommendations for antenatal care for pregnant women with sickle cell disease

Recommending body/institution	Actions required/activity for antenatal care
NICE, RCOG, ACOG	Multidisciplinary care throughout pregnancy for women with SCD (obstetricians, nurses/midwives, hematologists, etc)
KBTH	Followed biweekly at the outpatient clinic until 34 weeks' gestation and weekly until delivery
NICE, RCOG, ACOG	Serial fetal biometry (fetal growth) every 4 weeks from 24 weeks to detect IUGR
KBTH standard of care	Baseline oxygen saturation measurement and assessment for risk factors associated with asthma.

Abbreviations: ACOG, American College of Obstetricians and Gynecologists; IUGR, intrauterine growth restriction; KBTH, Korle-Bu Teaching Hospital; NICE, National Institute for Health and Care Excellence; RCOG, Royal College of Obstetricians and Gynaecologists; SCD, sickle cell disease.

Doppler assessments combining the umbilical artery and the middle cerebral artery can simultaneously measure blood flow through the placenta as well as the fetal brain.[52]

A comparison of the umbilical artery resistance to that of the cerebral arteries measured by the cerebroplacental ratio measures the brain-sparing effect in fetuses with IUGR.[53] The cerebroplacental ratio has been used in predicting perinatal outcomes in preeclampsia and to postdate pregnancies and fetuses of diabetic mothers,[54] although its use in women with sickle cell disease has not been tested.

Sickle Cell Disease–Related Complications During Pregnancy

ACS

Cardiopulmonary complications and thromboembolism[22] are the most common causes of death in pregnant women with sickle cell disease living in low-middle– and high-income settings, respectively. ACS, the most common manifestation of cardiopulmonary disease, consists of a constellation of clinical findings that include fever, increased respiratory effort, chest pain, drop in hemoglobin oxygen saturation, and new radiodensity on chest roentgenogram.

Critical management important in the diagnosis and multidisciplinary management of ACS includes the following:

1. Early diagnosis of ACS, which is critical for appropriate management (Table 10-4)

   The diagnosis of ACS requires an adequate history, examination, and laboratory evaluation. In pregnant women with sickle cell disease, most ACS presents initially with an acute pain episode,[10,22] which may have been managed

TABLE 10-4 Evidence-based treatment recommendations for acute SCD-related events during pregnancy

Inpatient care for acute SCD-related vaso-occlusive events (pain or ACS)		
NHLBI Expert Committee	Vaso-occlusive pain event	1. Incentive spirometry 2. Rapid parenteral opioid analgesia for severe pain
KBTH standard of care	ACS	The presence of positive chest pain or pulmonary auscultatory finding and at least 2 of the following: 1. Temperature greater than or equal to 38.0°C 2. Increased respiratory rate of greater than the 90th percentile for age or >20 breaths per minute 3. Increased oxygen requirement (Sp_{O2} drop >3% from a documented steady-state value on room air) 4. New radiodensity on chest roentgenogram
NICE, RCOG, NHLBI Expert Committee	ACS management	1. Supplemental oxygen therapy when Spo_2 <95% 2. IV cephalosporin plus an oral macrolide 3. Exchange blood transfusion when rapidly progressive and Spo_2 <90% 4. Simple blood transfusion therapy if clinically stable
NICE, RCOG	Severe anemia	Simple transfusion for acute anemia with hemoglobin <6 g/dL or decrease >2 g/dL from steady-state

Abbreviations: ACS, acute chest syndrome; IV, intravenous; KBTH, Korle-Bu Teaching Hospital; NHLBI, National Heart, Lung, and Blood Institute; NICE, National Institute for Health and Care Excellence; RCOG, Royal College of Obstetricians and Gynaecologists; SCD, sickle cell disease.

with opioids and intravenous fluids. Additionally, ACS can develop after cesarean delivery.

During pregnancy, many women are unlikely to receive a chest roentgenogram in the first and second trimesters, making the detection of ACS more challenging and different from women who are not pregnant. In a low-resource setting, a diagnostic criterion was developed for the early diagnosis of ACS, and this resulted in a drastic reduction in maternal mortality.[2]

Rapidly progressive ACS, a unique clinical presentation of ACS, is a medical emergency in pregnant women with sickle cell disease.[55] The clinical features of rapidly progressive ACS are similar to the clinical presentation of women with HELLP (hemolysis, elevated liver enzymes, and low platelet count) syndrome.[56] The unique clinical phenotype of ACS includes respiratory failure (24 hours after onset of respiratory symptoms) associated with multiorgan failure. Multiorgan failure was defined as dysfunction of ≥2 organs with the following criteria: respiratory failure (respiratory distress and at least 3 L of oxygen to maintain oxygen hemoglobin saturation of at least 90%), acute renal insufficiency (an increase in the serum creatinine concentration of 50% from baseline; or oliguria of 70 U/L, total bilirubin >2 times the upper limit of normal, and direct bilirubin >2 times the upper limit of normal), and prothrombin time prolonged by >3 seconds. On multivariable analysis, a decrease in platelet count (platelet count <150,000/μL) or a 50% decrease from baseline at presentation at the time of onset of increased respiratory symptoms was the only predictor of rapidly progressive ACS (OR, 4.82; 95% CI, 1.20-19.39; $P = .027$).[55]

2. Identifying and correcting the underlying cause

Appropriate treatment should include a third-generation cephalosporin, a macrolide, analgesics (opioids are most often used), and blood transfusion. Incentive spirometry should be prescribed for patients while on admission for acute events and after cesarean delivery to prevent a recurrence.

3. Maintenance of euvolemia

Fluid requirements should be individualized and guided by the patient's fluid balance and cardiopulmonary status. Intake and output should be monitored to prevent fluid overload. Encourage the patient to drink as much fluid as possible.

4. Blood transfusion

Decisions regarding transfusion are based on the clinical status, including hemodynamic instability, oxygen requirement, decrease in hemoglobin from baseline (typically >2 g/dL), and rate of decline of respiratory status.

5. Supplemental oxygen

Supplement oxygen is given to maintain adequate oxygenation, improve oxygen-carrying capacity, and improve tissue oxygen delivery. For severe respiratory failure, mechanical ventilation with positive end-expiratory pressure or continuous positive airway pressure should be considered.

Sickle Cell Disease–Related Acute Pain Episode (Vaso-occlusive Pain)

The most common cause of hospital admissions in pregnant women with sickle cell disease is acute vaso-occlusive pain episodes. The period of time most associated with an increased risk of acute vaso-occlusive pain episodes is the third trimester and 6 weeks postpartum.[10] These episodes can occur in any part of the body, a pain level health care professionals often underestimate. Pregnant women with acute vaso-occlusive pain who present to the emergency department should be given rapid analgesia, most often in the form of opioids. Women who are hypovolemic should be aggressively hydrated (oral hydration preferred to intravenous fluids if the patient can drink) and assessed for sickle cell disease–related comorbidities that may require additional treatment. If acute pain does not abate, the patient should be admitted to the hospital for opioids via intravenous infusion. Generally, we follow the approach outlined in the review article by Brandow and DeBaun.[57]

We do not commonly recommend nonsteroidal anti-inflammatory drugs (NSAIDs) for acute vaso-occlusive pain in pregnant women after 30 weeks of gestation because there is an increased risk of narrowing ductus arteriosus and oligohydramnios. For inpatient management of acute vaso-occlusive pain, no evidence exists that adding NSAIDs to a regimen of intravenous opioids is associated with faster recovery. In a randomized controlled trial, the use of ketoprofen (300 mg/d for 5 days), a nonselective cyclooxygenase inhibitor, plus a morphine derivative was not superior to hasten recovery to baseline when compared to morphine derivatives alone.[58] For mild pain, we recommend acetaminophen in moderation, along with nonmedicinal strategies for mild acute vaso-occlusive pain episodes.

Briefly, for uncomplicated acute vaso-occlusive pain, we titrate the opioid to relieve the pain and then provide a continuous infusion of an opioid with a patient-controlled analgesia. We do not include NSAIDs in the pain regimen before 30 weeks of gestation because of the lack of any evidence that NSAIDs hasten recovery to baseline in individuals. The patient-controlled analgesia is provided such that the patient is only able to increase the dose by 50% above the continuous hourly infusion in an hour when the maximum patient-controlled analgesia is administered. Pregnant women should be prescribed incentive spirometry during acute pain events as prevention of ACS. Specifically, women should be asked to inhale using the spirometer 10 times every 2 hours while awake for 72 hours during acute pain episodes and after surgery. A set of evidence-based recommendations for the management of acute events in sickle cell disease is summarized in Table 10-4.

Unfortunately, optimum management of acute vaso-occlusive pain in pregnancy has not been extensively evaluated and requires further study before evidence-based strategies can be recommended about perceived best practices.

Venous Thromboembolism

Venous thromboembolism is common in pregnant women in general; however, pregnant women with sickle cell disease are at even greater risk. They are 2.5 times more likely to experience deep vein thrombosis compared to healthy age-matched pregnant controls.[59] Monitoring D-dimer levels in this population is not efficacious due to chronic activation of coagulation factors at baseline.[60]

Women with sickle cell disease are also more likely to suffer from a pulmonary embolism. Hospitalized patients should be assessed for known history of venous thromboembolisms. Pregnant women who present with chest pain and respiratory distress with unremarkable chest roentgenogram should be suspected of having a pulmonary embolism.[16] When anticoagulation is indicated, low-molecular-weight heparin should be used,[40] not unfractionated heparin, because of its efficacy and safety profile. The use of new direct oral anticoagulants as a strategy for venous thromboembolism during pregnancy in sickle cell disease has not been evaluated. A discussion on their potential risks and benefits is beyond the scope of this chapter.

Stroke

Cerebral vein thrombosis is almost 5 times more likely in pregnant women with sickle cell disease compared to pregnant women without sickle cell disease.[59] Both acute ischemic and hemorrhagic stroke should be suspected if women are presenting with neurologic impairment.[46] Initial treatment for acute ischemic stroke is blood transfusions, typically followed by regular blood transfusion therapy to prevent infarct recurrence. Hydroxyurea has been used for secondary prevention of ischemic strokes; however, due to its teratogenic potential, hydroxyurea should not be used for secondary prevention of strokes in pregnant women with sickle cell disease.

Anemia

Anemia is the most common complication in women with sickle cell disease during pregnancy. Hemolysis, blood loss, parvovirus B19 infection, and mineral deficiencies increase the risk of anemia in this patient population.[16] Blood transfusions are indicated in the following scenarios: (1) the hemoglobin levels decrease to <7 g/dL and pose a risk of fetal hypoxia; (2) the patient experiences a decrease in hemoglobin of >2 g/dL below the patient's baseline; or (3) the patient is demonstrating pulmonary or hemodynamic compromise.

Labor and Delivery

Timing and Mode of Delivery

The mother and fetus should be closely monitored. Spontaneous vaginal delivery is the preferred mode of delivery in the absence of any contraindication. Delivery should occur between 38 and 40 weeks.[61] If there are indications of imminent complications, a cesarean delivery should be offered. During this time, mothers should be kept warm and hydrated, and pain should be managed with adequate pain medication.[16] Studies have shown that epidural analgesics are particularly efficacious when compared to general anesthesia for operative delivery.[62,63] At the time of delivery, adequate crossmatched blood supply should be available in case it is needed.

Uncomplicated pregnancy with a normally developing fetus in women with sickle cell disease can be carried to 38 weeks before delivery.[39] Unnecessary intervention in such a pregnancy should be avoided in the absence of any complication. Effort must be made to avoid prolonging the pregnancy over 40 weeks of gestation because this increases perinatal complications. Women with sickle cell disease who develop complications such as severe preeclampsia, repeated vaso-occlusive pain episodes, or ACS after 34 weeks should be considered for delivery once they are stabilized. When considering delivery before 37 weeks' gestation, antenatal corticosteroids should be considered for fetal lung maturity, unless there is demonstrable evidence of fetal lung maturity. In offering systemic antenatal corticosteroid therapy, caution must be exercised because this may provoke acute pain episodes in some patients with sickle cell disease.[64,65] To date, there is no randomized trial that tests the optimal mode or timing of delivery for pregnant women with sickle cell disease.

Management of Labor

Labor in women with sickle cell disease is always considered high risk and must be conducted in the setting of specialized care with the requisite resources for timely intervention when necessary. This allows for adequate preparation with effective labor analgesia, intrapartum hydration, prevention of prolonged labor and intrapartum infection, and timely intervention for an emergency cesarean delivery when necessary.

Active management of labor must be employed to prevent prolonged labor, reduce stress, and prevent intrapartum infection. Where necessary, early augmentation of labor with oxytocin should be used, and intensive monitoring of fetal heart rate must be employed. The use of continuous electronic fetal heart monitoring may be necessary for early detection of fetal heart rate abnormality. In low-resource settings where electronic fetal heart monitoring may not be available, the World Health Organization suggests a partograph be used with intermittent auscultation of the fetal heartbeat using the fetal Doppler or Pinard stethoscope. While intermittent auscultation of the fetal heart beat has been shown to be adequate in managing low-risk labor,[66] its utility in managing labor in women with sickle cell disease has not been evaluated.

Where necessary, prompt assistance in the second stage of labor using vacuum extraction or forceps delivery may be recommended. This may be particularly helpful in patients with moderate to severe anemia or other forms of cardiopulmonary complications.

Analgesia During Labor

Pain management and alleviation during labor is a critical part of any labor management. In pregnant women with sickle cell disease, effective labor pain management is crucial for increasing the likelihood of good outcome. Epidural analgesia may be an effective form of labor analgesia that must be offered where available, even though there are only a few reported cases that used this technique for women with sickle cell disease who were in labor.[63,67,68] The skill and resources for epidural analgesia for labor management may not be available in many low-resource settings in sub-Saharan Africa, where most pregnant women with sickle cell disease are managed. In the absence of epidural analgesia, ambulatory spinal analgesia has been used and found to be an effective form of labor analgesia. In both regional techniques, precaution must be taken to avoid hypotension. Alternatively, parenteral opioids may be used in labor where necessary. Short-acting parenteral opioids such as fentanyl at an initial dose of 50 μg slow intravenously (IV) over 3 minutes has been suggested. This may be repeated every 10 minutes with 50 μg slow IV as needed until *either* adequate analgesia is achieved *or* a maximum hourly dose of 300 μg is reached. If adequate analgesia is not attained with these doses, then an alternate pain management plan must be considered.

Prior to any fentanyl administration, assess blood pressure, heart rate, respiratory rate, oxygen saturation by pulse oximetry, fetal heart rate, and pain score as per pain chart. Every effort must be made for continuous vital sign monitoring of the patient and adequate expertise with the appropriate equipment is required to address an emergency if respiratory depression occurs.

Adequate preparation must also be made for resuscitation of the newborn, including the use of opioid antagonists such as naloxone, especially when opioids are administered to mothers in advanced labor.

Cesarean Delivery

There is a high incidence of cesarean delivery among pregnant women with sickle cell disease. Cesarean delivery may be indicated for patients affected by sickle cell disease–specific complications such as pelvic deformity from avascular necrosis of the femoral head. However, we are unaware of any data that suggest routine elective cesarean delivery for pregnant women with sickle cell disease with an uncomplicated pregnancy improves maternal and fetal outcomes when compared to a vaginal delivery. When an elective cesarean delivery is planned, the procedure must be performed between 38 and 39 weeks' gestation.[39] Prior referral for anesthetic consult and planning with the anesthetic team is very important. The choice of anesthesia must be discussed with the obstetric team as well as the patient. The need for preanesthetic blood transfusion must be discussed to determine the best timing for the optimal effect.

Perioperative Care

For pregnant women with sickle cell disease who require cesarean delivery, the best timing of delivery must be decided by the multidisciplinary team together with the patient. The need to correct anemia preoperatively must be discussed. When blood transfusion is required, this should be done 2 hours before delivery. If this is not feasible, then it should be done as quickly after surgery as possible. The goal should be to raise the hemoglobin to approximately 10 g/dl.[69] If they baseline hemoglobin is greater than 9 g/dl then strong consideration should be given to an modified exchange transfusion because of the concern of

hyperviscosity. Oxygen supplementation must be given irrespective of the choice of anesthesia and must be continued after surgery for the next 24 hours. Use of incentive spirometry must be provided to all patients after cesarean delivery and is associated with a 90% relative risk reduction of developing ACS postoperatively.[70] Specifically, women should be asked to inhale with the spirometer 10 times or use balloons every 2 hours while awake for 72 hours after surgery.

Postpartum Care

In all women, regardless of delivery method, close attention should be paid to fluid status, hemoglobin oxygen saturation, hemoglobin level, and renal and liver function. Women who give birth by cesarean section are at increased risk of postoperative complications, such as infections and deep venous thrombosis, when compared to those who have a vaginal delivery. These women should be given low-molecular-weight heparin within 24 hours of delivery, 12 hours after delivery, and as a maintenance dose for 6 weeks after cesarean section. Acute pain episodes occur in 25% of women after delivery, so close attention should be paid to any changes from baseline status such as headaches, respiratory distress, and increased pain.[15,61] For patients who undergo cesarean delivery, the protocol for the prevention of ACS using incentive spirometry must be activated right from the recovery room and maintained until the patient is ready to go home. In women who were taking hydroxyurea before pregnancy, the drug should be held until the patient is no longer breastfeeding.

Immediate Neonatal Care and Concerns

IUGR is 3 times more likely to occur in pregnant women with sickle cell disease compared to pregnant women without sickle cell disease.[3] Neonates born to mothers with sickle cell disease are more likely to be small for gestational age and have low birth weight, and are at an increased risk of fetal demise.[38] Risk factors for small for gestational age include low socioeconomic status, women with HbSS with small body habitus, babies of African descent (babies in the United Kingdom of African descent are 60% more likely to have low birth weight),[71] and placental hypoxia due to chronic vaso-occlusion.[72,73]

Meeks et al[38] recommend regular noninvasive intrauterine monitoring for patients with suspected IUGR. In mothers with preexisting comorbidities, current obstetric recommended guidelines include initiation of fetal surveillance as early as 26 weeks of gestation. In addition, fetal nonstress testing, biophysical profile testing, and umbilical artery Doppler after 28 weeks have been shown to improve fetal outcomes in high-risk pregnancies because they are able to identify infants who may benefit from early interventions such as delivery.

Given the high incidence of IUGR coupled with the challenges of appropriate estimation of gestational age in low-middle–income settings, assessment of IUGR in all pregnancies in women with sickle cell disease should be done preemptively and immediately after delivery. In addition, newborns should be evaluated immediately after delivery, specifically to exclude established complications of IUGR. Obstetric guidelines should be followed for monitoring and treatment of IUGR.[74]

Neonatal abstinence syndrome is seen in babies born to women with substance use disorders, and neonates are at risk of experiencing withdrawal symptoms. Women with sickle cell disease are at increased risk of giving birth to babies with neonatal abstinence syndrome due to chronic opioid treatment to alleviate pain caused by acute pain episodes. The higher rate of acute vaso-occlusive pain episodes during pregnancy and the inability to use hydroxyurea during pregnancy, may increase opioid use.[47,75]

Opioids readily cross the placenta, and their metabolites can be detected in the amniotic fluid, meconium, and neonatal urine.[76,77] Neonatal abstinence syndrome affects multiple organ systems including the gastrointestinal tract (poor feeding, vomiting, diarrhea, and dehydration), the nervous system (seizures, tremors, high-pitched crying, increased muscle tone, hyperreflexia, and increased yawning and sneezing), and the autonomic system (fever, stuffiness, increased sweating, mottling, temperature instability, rapid breathing, and sleep problems). Symptoms generally present within 48 to 72 hours and may even develop after 2 weeks.[78] Neonates experiencing mild withdrawal symptoms may be discharged home with their mothers; however, those with severe symptoms are admitted to the neonatal intensive care unit for a median length of 30 days.[78]

The higher the mean daily dose of opioids during pregnancy in women with sickle cell disease, the higher is the likelihood of neonatal abstinence symptoms.[79] Women who received >200 mg/d of oral morphine equivalent in the last 2 months of pregnancy had a 13-fold increased risk of developing neonatal abstinence syndrome compared to women receiving <200 mg/d.[79] Severe neonatal abstinence syndrome was seen in women receiving approximately 400 mg/d of oral morphine, mild neonatal abstinence syndrome was seen in women receiving approximately 140 mg/d of oral morphine, and no evidence of neonatal abstinence syndrome was seen in women receiving a median of 4 mg/d.[79]

Newborn Screening

The aim of newborn screening for sickle cell disease is to detect sickle cell disease at birth for 2 lifesaving actions: (1) to start penicillin before 4 months of age and (2) to allow the health care providers to educate the parents about anticipatory guidance with evidence-based strategies for preventing mortality and morbidity. The original study demonstrating the benefit of newborn screening in decreasing mortality and morbidity was conducted by Vichinsky et al[80] using 10 years of California state newborn screening data. The overall mortality rate for patients with sickle cell disease who underwent screening along with parental education was 1.8% at 7.2 years of follow-up versus a mortality rate of 8% for those diagnosed after 3 months of age and followed for an average of 9.4 years. Based on these data and sound public health principles, in high-income settings with substantial sickle cell disease populations, 2 major sickle cell disease newborn screening programs have been initiated. The 2 programs include either screening of infants of high-risk

TABLE 10-5 Prevalence of sickle cell disease (SCD) among newborns in the African American population and the Ghanaian population

Population	Incidence of SCD among newborns
African Americans	1 in 400
Ghanaians	7 in 400
Pregnant Ghanaian women with SCD who may have a newborn with SCD	60 in 400

Note. There is a high incidence of Ghanaian women with SCD who give birth to infants with SCD.[14,84-86]

parents or universal testing of all newborns. As of 2008, the US Preventive Services Task Force mandated that all newborns in the United States be screened for sickle cell disease. Laboratory methods used in newborn screening include high-performance liquid chromatography or thin-layer isoelectric focusing.

In low-middle–income settings, particularly in Africa, newborn screening programs are typically absent or of limited scope. Table 10-5 compares the prevalence of sickle cell disease among newborns of different subpopulations. Several barriers must be overcome before newborn screening can be instituted in a low-middle–income settings. These barriers include, but are not limited to, the lack of a formal genetic counseling program, inability to contact the families in both local and rural settings to inform them of the results of the newborn screening, the absence of quality assurance program for newborn screening testing, and lack of a mechanism for sharing accurate and culturally sensitive information about the implementation of the newborn screening between health care professionals, religious, traditional leaders, and family elders. Efforts should also include dispelling myths or strong cultural beliefs regarding screening.[17] Another requirement is for low-cost point-of-care testing for hemoglobinopathy that is both sensitive and specific[81] for newborns.

Since 2015, significant progress has been made in advancing point-of-care testing for newborns at risk for having sickle cell disease in low-income countries. A study by Steele et al[82] demonstrated that point-of-care screening for sickle cell disease was 100% sensitive and specific, with a cost of <$2 per test in low-resource regions with a high sickle cell disease burden.

Despite the increasing advancements in point-of-care testing in low-middle–income settings, these new technologies must be coupled with the sound principles of genetic counseling along with cultural and local public health policies to ensure the highest utility of newborn screening for sickle cell disease. In the absence of a comprehensive approach to newborn screening that takes these other multidisciplinary domains into account, the introduction of point-of-care testing may result in splitting of families and unintended permanent consequences for the mother and infant.

Conclusion

Specific evidence-based strategies for preeclampsia, prematurity, and intrauterine growth restriction are required to determine the optimal approach for the management of pregnant women with sickle cell disease. Over 70% of the world's sickle cell disease population live in sub-Saharan Africa. Despite the high prevalence of sickle cell disease in sub-Saharan Africa, the maternal mortality rate is 10,000 per 100,000 in women with sickle cell disease, as compared to <30 per 100,000 in the United States for women without sickle cell disease. Cardiopulmonary complications are the leading cause of death, with acute chest syndrome responsible for >80% of deaths in pregnant women with sickle cell disease. The majority of vaso-occlusive events, either pain or acute chest syndrome, occur in the third trimester or postpartum. A multidisciplinary team approach and the use of incentive spirometry for every pain episode occurring in the hospital or use of balloons in low-middle–income settings (10 breaths every 2 hours while awake) can significantly decrease the incidence rate of acute chest syndrome after admission to the hospital for pain. Focused sickle cell disease maternal-fetal research in sub-Saharan Africa is likely to improve the overall outcome, not only in low-middle–income settings, but also high-income settings.

High-Yield Facts

- Pregnant women with sickle cell disease experience significant morbidity and mortality compared to the general population in both low-middle– and high-income settings.

- The highest rate of maternal mortality among pregnant women with sickle cell disease occurs in sub-Saharan Africa, where the risk of maternal mortality can be as high as 29 times that of pregnant women without sickle cell disease. The maternal mortality rate in pregnant women without any intervention, is approximately 10,000 per 100,000 live births versus less than 30 per 100,000 live birth in the United States.

- In high-income settings, pregnant women with sickle cell disease have an increased risk of pregnancy-related complications compared to those without sickle cell disease, but no evidence of increased mortality.

- Mortality in pregnant women with sickle cell disease is likely related to the gap in medical care received between patients in low-middle–income versus high-income settings.

- Preconception care should include, but not be limited to, screening for immunization status, screening for minor red blood cell antigen alloimmunization, counseling about smoking and illicit drug use, and preparing for withdrawal and substitution of teratogenic therapy.

- Strong clinical evidence suggests that pregnant women with sickle cell disease require a multidisciplinary care approach for improved maternal and fetal outcomes.

- Pregnant women with sickle cell disease often require frequent visits and risk assessments. Patients should be followed every 2 weeks until 34 weeks and then weekly thereafter until delivery.

- In the first month of pregnancy, the heart rate and stroke volume increase, causing a 30% to 50% increase in cardiac output. In addition, a 25% to 50% increase in plasma volume occurs, and excessive erythropoietin production from the kidneys causes a 20% to 30% increase in red blood cell mass and a 1- to 2g/dL decrease in hemoglobin levels.

- Cardiopulmonary complications and thromboembolism are the most common causes of death in pregnant women with sickle cell disease living in low-middle– and high-income settings, respectively.

- Acute chest syndrome, the most common manifestation of cardiopulmonary disease, consists of a constellation of clinical findings that include fever, increased respiratory effort, chest pain, decrease in hemoglobin oxygen saturation, and new radiodensity on chest roentgenogram.

- Rapidly progressive acute chest syndrome, a unique clinical presentation of acute chest syndrome, is a medical emergency in pregnant women with sickle cell disease. The clinical features of rapidly progressive acute chest syndrome are similar to those of women with HELLP (hemolysis, elevated liver enzymes, and low platelet count) syndrome.

- The most common cause of hospital admissions in pregnant women with sickle cell disease is acute vaso-occlusive pain episodes. The period of time most associated with an increased risk of acute vaso-occlusive pain episodes is the third trimester and 6 weeks postpartum.

- For pregnant women with sickle cell disease who require cesarean delivery, the best timing for delivery must be decided by the multidisciplinary team together with the patient. The need to correct anemia preoperatively must be discussed. When blood transfusion is required, this should be done 2 hours before delivery.

- In all women, regardless of delivery method, close attention to maintaining euvolemia, hemoglobin oxygen saturation, hemoglobin level, and renal and liver function.

- The aim of newborn screening for sickle cell disease is to start penicillin before 4 months of age and for health care providers to initiate evidence-based educational strategies for preventing mortality and morbidity.

References

1. Alayed N, Kezouh A, Oddy L, Abenhaim HA. Sickle cell disease and pregnancy outcomes: population-based study on 8.8 million births. *J Perinatal Med.* 2014;42(4):487-492.

2. Asare EV, Olayemi E, Boafor T, et al. Implementation of multidisciplinary care reduces maternal mortality in women with sickle cell disease living in low-resource setting. *Am J Hematol.* 2017;92(9):872-878.

3. Boafor TK, Olayemi E, Galadanci N, et al. Pregnancy outcomes in women with sickle-cell disease in low and high income countries: a systematic review and meta-analysis. *BJOG.* 2016;123(5):691-698.

4. Boulet SL, Okoroh EM, Azonobi I, Grant A, Craig Hooper W. Sickle cell disease in pregnancy: maternal complications in a Medicaid-enrolled population. *Matern Child Health J.* 2013; 17(2):200-207.

5. Kuo K, Caughey AB. Contemporary outcomes of sickle cell disease in pregnancy. *Am J Obstet Gynecol.* 2016;215(4): 505e501-505.

6. Muganyizi PS, Kidanto H. Sickle cell disease in pregnancy: trend and pregnancy outcomes at a tertiary hospital in Tanzania. *PLoS One.* 2013;8(2):e56541.

7. Dare FO, Makinde OO, Faasuba OB. The obstetric performance of sickle cell disease patients and homozygous hemoglobin C disease patients in Ile-Ife, Nigeria. *Int J Gynaecol Obstet.* 1992;37(3):63-168.

8. Odum CU, Anorlu RI, Dim SI, Oyekan TO. Pregnancy outcome in HbSS-sickle cell disease in Lagos, Nigeria. *West Afr J Med.* 2002;21(1):19-23.

9. World Health Organization. Meeting to develop a global consensus on preconception care to reduce maternal and childhood mortality and morbidity. 2013. https://apps.who.int/iris/handle/10665/78067. Accessed June 22, 2020.

10. Asare EV, Olayemi E, Boafor T, et al. Third trimester and early postpartum period of pregnancy have the greatest risk for ACS in women with SCD. *Am J Hematol.* 2019;94(12):E328-E331.

11. Matsui D. Adherence with drug therapy in pregnancy. *Obstet Gynecol Int.* 2012;2012:796590.

12. Taye B, Abeje G, Mekonen A. Factors associated with compliance of prenatal iron folate supplementation among women in Mecha district, Western Amhara: a cross-sectional study. *Pan Afr Med J.* 2015;20:43.

13. Piel FB, Patil AP, Howes RE, Nyangiri OA, Gething PW, Dewi M, Temperley WH, Williams TN, Weatherall DJ, Hay SI. Global epidemiology of sickle haemoglobin in neonates: a contemporary geostatistical model-based map and population estimates. Lancet. 2013 Jan 12;381(9861):142-51.

14. Oppong SA, Asare EV, Olayemi E, et al. Multidisciplinary care results in similar maternal and perinatal mortality rates for women with and without SCD in a low-resource setting. *Am J Hematol.* 2019;94(2):223-230.

15. Hathaway AR. Sickle cell disease in pregnancy. *South Med J.* 2016;109(9):554-556.

16. Jain D, Atmapoojya P, Colah R, Lodha P. Sickle cell disease and pregnancy. *Mediterr J Hematol Infectious Dis.* 2019;11(1): e2019040.

17. Anie KA, Treadwell MJ, Grant AM, et al. Community engagement to inform the development of a sickle cell counselor training and certification program in Ghana. *J Community Genet.* 2016;7(3):195-202.

18. Nouraie M, Little JA, Hildesheim M, et al. Validation of a composite vascular high-risk profile for adult patients with sickle cell disease. *Am J Hematol.* 2019;94(12):E312-E314.

19. Gladwin MT, Barst RJ, Gibbs JS, et al. Risk factors for death in 632 patients with sickle cell disease in the United States and United Kingdom. *PLoS One.* 2014;9(7):e99489.

20. Gladwin MT, Sachdev V, Jison ML, et al. Pulmonary hypertension as a risk factor for death in patients with sickle cell disease. *N Engl J Med.* 2004;350(9):886-895.

21. Kassim AA, Payne AB, Rodeghier M, Macklin EA, Strunk RC, DeBaun MR. Low forced expiratory volume is associated with earlier death in sickle cell anemia. *Blood.* 2015;126(13):1544-1550.

22. Asare EV, Olayemi E, Boafor T, et al. A case series describing causes of death in pregnant women with sickle cell disease in a low-resource setting. *Am J Hematol.* 2018;93(7):E167-E170.

23. Ataga KI, Orringer EP. Renal abnormalities in sickle cell disease. *Am J Hematol.* 2000;63(4):205-211.

24. Drawz P, Ayyappan S, Nouraie M, et al. Kidney disease among patients with sickle cell disease, hemoglobin SS and SC. *Clin J Am Soc Nephrol.* 2016;11(2):207-215.

25. Cheung KL, Lafayette RA. Renal physiology of pregnancy. *Adv Chronic Kidney Dis.* 2013;20(3):209-214.

26. ACOG Practice Bulletin No. 202: gestational hypertension and preeclampsia. *Obstet Gynecol.* 2019;133(1):e1-e25.

27. Lari NF, DeBaun MR, Oppong SA. The emerging challenge of optimal blood pressure management and hypertensive syndromes in pregnant women with sickle cell disease: a review. *Expert Rev Hematol.* 2017;10(11):987-994.

28. Schunemann HJ, Best D, Vist G, et al. Letters, numbers, symbols and words: how to communicate grades of evidence and recommendations. *CMAJ.* 2003;169(7):677-680.

29. Schunemann HJ, Mustafa R, Brozek J, et al. GRADE Guidelines: 16. GRADE evidence to decision frameworks for tests in clinical practice and public health. *J Clin Epidemiol.* 2016;76:89-98.

30. Guyatt GH, Alonso-Coello P, Schunemann HJ, et al. Guideline panels should seldom make good practice statements: guidance from the GRADE Working Group. *J Clin Epidemiol.* 2016;80:3-7.

31. Yawn BP, Buchanan GR, Afenyi-Annan AN, et al. Management of sickle cell disease: summary of the 2014 evidence-based report by expert panel members. *JAMA.* 2014;312(10):1033-1048.

32. Crapo RO. Normal cardiopulmonary physiology during pregnancy. *Clin Obstet Gynecol.* 1996;39(1):3-16.

33. Heidemann BH, McClure JH. Changes in maternal physiology during pregnancy. *BJA CEPD Rev.* 2003;3(3):65-68.

34. Chandra S, Tripathi AK, Mishra S, Amzarul M, Vaish AK. Physiological changes in hematological parameters during pregnancy. *Indian J Hematol Blood Transfus.* 2012;28(3):144-146.

35. Neeraj SC, Pramod J, Singh J, Kaur V. Effect of advanced uncomplicated pregnancy on pulmonary function parameters of North Indian subjects. *Indian J Physiol Pharmacol.* 2010;54(1): 69-72.

36. Zairina E, Abramson MJ, McDonald CF, et al. A prospective cohort study of pulmonary function during pregnancy in women with and without asthma. *J Asthma.* 2016;53(2):155-163.

37. Willen SM, Cohen R, Rodeghier M, et al. Age is a predictor of a small decrease in lung function in children with sickle cell anemia. *Am J Hematol.* 2018;93(3):408-415.

38. Meeks D, Robinson SE, Macleod D, Oteng-Ntim E. Birth weights in sickle cell disease pregnancies: a cohort study. *PLoS One.* 2016;11(10):e0165238.

39. Howard J, Oteng-Ntim E. The obstetric management of sickle cell disease. *Best Pract Res Clin Obstet Gynaecol.* 2012;26(1):25-36.

40. Royal College of Obstetricians and Gynaecologists. RCOG Green-top Guideline No. 61: Management of sickle cell disease in pregnancy. 2011;1-20. https://www.rcog.org.uk/globalassets/documents/guidelines/gtg_61.pdf. Accessed June 22, 2020.

41. Titaley CR, Dibley MJ, Roberts CL, Agho K. Combined iron/folic acid supplements and malaria prophylaxis reduce neonatal mortality in 19 sub-Saharan African countries. *Am J Clin Nutr.* 2010;92(1):235-243.

42. Steketee RW, Wirima JJ, Slutsker L, Khoromana CO, Heymann DL, Breman JG. Malaria treatment and prevention in pregnancy: indications for use and adverse events associated with use of chloroquine or mefloquine. *Am J Trop Med Hyg.* 1996;55(1 suppl): 50-56.

43. Charache S, Terrin ML, Moore RD, et al. Effect of hydroxyurea on the frequency of painful crises in sickle cell anemia. Investigators of the Multicenter Study of Hydroxyurea in Sickle Cell Anemia. *N Engl J Med.* 1995;332(20):1317-1322.

44. DePass LR, Weaver EV. Comparison of teratogenic effects of aspirin and hydroxyurea in the Fischer 344 and Wistar strains. *J Toxicol Environ Health.* 1982;10(2):297-305.

45. Woo GH, Katayama K, Bak EJ, et al. Effects of prenatal hydroxyurea-treatment on mouse offspring. *Exp Toxicol Pathol.* 2004;56(1-2):1-7.

46. Kassim AA, Galadanci NA, Pruthi S, DeBaun MR. How I treat and manage strokes in sickle cell disease. *Blood.* 2015;125(22): 3401-3410.

47. Naik RP, Lanzkron S. Baby on board: what you need to know about pregnancy in the hemoglobinopathies. *Hematology Am Soc of Hematol Educ Program.* 2012;2012:208-214.

48. Klings ES, Morris CR, Hsu LL, Castro O, Gladwin MT, Mubarak KK. Pulmonary hypertension of sickle cell disease beyond classification constraints. *J Am College Cardiol.* 2014;63(25 Pt A): 2881-2882.

49. Jackson B, Fasano R, Roback J. Current evidence for the use of prophylactic transfusion to treat sickle cell disease during pregnancy. *Transfus Med Rev.* 2018;32(4):220-224.

50. Perseghin P. Erythrocyte exchange and leukapheresis in pregnancy. *Transfus Apher Sci.* 2015;53(3):279-282.

51. Vianello A, Vencato E, Cantini M, et al. Improvement of maternal and fetal outcomes in women with sickle cell disease treated with early prophylactic erythrocytapheresis. *Transfusion.* 2018;58(9): 2192-2201.

52. Odibo AO, Riddick C, Pare E, Stamilio DM, Macones GA. Cerebroplacental Doppler ratio and adverse perinatal outcomes in intrauterine growth restriction: evaluating the impact of using gestational age-specific reference values. *J Ultrasound Med.* 2005;24(9):1223-1228.

53. Flood K, Unterscheider J, Daly S, et al. The role of brain sparing in the prediction of adverse outcomes in intrauterine growth restriction: results of the multicenter PORTO Study. *Am J Obstet Gynecol.* 2014;211(3):288.e281-285.

54. DeVore GR. The importance of the cerebroplacental ratio in the evaluation of fetal well-being in SGA and AGA fetuses. *Am J Obstet Gynecol.* 2015;213(1):5-15.

55. Chaturvedi S, Ghafuri DL, Glassberg J, Kassim AA, Rodeghier M, DeBaun MR. Rapidly progressive acute chest syndrome in individuals with sickle cell anemia: a distinct acute chest syndrome phenotype. *Am J Hematol.* 2016;91(12):1185-1190.

56. Haddad B, Barton JR, Livingston JC, Chahine R, Sibai BM. Risk factors for adverse maternal outcomes among women with HELLP (hemolysis, elevated liver enzymes, and low platelet count) syndrome. *Am J Obstet Gynecol.* 2000;183(2):444-448.

57. Brandow AM, DeBaun MR. Key components of pain management for children and adults with sickle cell disease. *Hematol Oncol Clin North Am.* 2018;32(3):535-550.

58. Bartolucci P, El Murr T, Roudot-Thoraval F, et al. A randomized, controlled clinical trial of ketoprofen for sickle-cell disease vaso-occlusive crises in adults. *Blood.* 2009;114(18):3742-3747.

59. Villers MS, Jamison MG, De Castro LM, James AH. Morbidity associated with sickle cell disease in pregnancy. *Am J Obstet Gynecol.* 2008;199(2):e121-e125.

60. Naik RP, Streiff MB, Lanzkron S. Sickle cell disease and venous thromboembolism: what the anticoagulation expert needs to know. *J Thromb Thrombolysis.* 2013;35(3):352-358.

61. Boga C, Ozdogu H. Pregnancy and sickle cell disease: a review of the current literature. *Crit Rev Oncol Hematol.* 2016;98: 364-374.

62. Bakri MH, Ismail EA, Ghanem G, Shokry M. Spinal versus general anesthesia for cesarean section in patients with sickle cell anemia. *Korean J Anesthesiol.* 2015;68(5):469-475.

63. Winder AD, Johnson S, Murphy J, Ehsanipoor RM. Epidural analgesia for treatment of a sickle cell crisis during pregnancy. *Obstet Gynecol.* 2011;118(2 Pt 2):495-497.

64. Darbari DS, Fasano RS, Minniti CP, et al. Severe vaso-occlusive episodes associated with use of systemic corticosteroids in patients with sickle cell disease. *J Natl Med Assoc.* 2008;100(8):948-951.

65. Strouse JJ, Takemoto CM, Keefer R, Kato GJ, Casella JF. Corticosteroids and increased risk of readmission after acute chest syndrome in children with sickle cell disease. *Pediatr Blood Cancer.* 2008;50(5):1006-1012.

66. Liston R, Sawchuck D, Young D. No.197b-fetal health surveillance: intrapartum consensus guideline. *J Obstet Gynaecol Can.* 2018;40(4):e298-e322.

67. Martin JN Jr, Morrison JC. Managing the parturient with sickle cell crisis. *Clin Obstet Gynecol.* 1984;27(1):39-49.

68. Newhouse BJ, Kuczkowski KM. Uneventful epidural labor analgesia and vaginal delivery in a parturient with Arnold-Chiari malformation type I and sickle cell disease. *Arch Gynecol Obstet.* 2007;275(4):311-313.

69. Howard J, Malfroy M, Llewelyn C, et al. The Transfusion Alternatives Preoperatively in Sickle Cell Disease (TAPS) study: a randomised, controlled, multicentre clinical trial. *Lancet.* 2013;381(9870): 930-938.

70. Bellet PS, Kalinyak KA, Shukla R, Gelfand MJ, Rucknagel DL. Incentive spirometry to prevent acute pulmonary complications in sickle cell diseases. *N Engl J Med.* 1995;333(11):699-703.

71. Kelly Y, Panico L, Bartley M, Marmot M, Nazroo J, Sacker A. Why does birthweight vary among ethnic groups in the UK? Findings from the Millennium Cohort Study. *J Public Health (Oxf).* 2009;31(1): 131-137.

72. Balihallimath RL, Shirol VS, Gan AM, Tyagi NK, Bandankar MR. Placental morphometry determines the birth weight. *J Clin Diagn Res.* 2013;7(11):2428-2431.

73. Thame MM, Osmond C, Serjeant GR. Fetal growth in women with homozygous sickle cell disease: an observational study. *Eur J Obstet Gynecol Reprod Biol.* 2013;170(1):62-66.

74. Vayssiere C, Sentilhes L, Ego A, et al. Fetal growth restriction and intra-uterine growth restriction: guidelines for clinical practice

from the French College of Gynaecologists and Obstetricians. *Eur J Obstet Gynecol Reprod Biol.* 2015;193:10-18.

75. Smith JA, Espeland M, Bellevue R, Bonds D, Brown AK, Koshy M. Pregnancy in sickle cell disease: experience of the Cooperative Study of Sickle Cell Disease. *Obstet Gynecol.* 1996;87(2): 199-204.

76. Finnegan LP, Connaughton JF, Kron RE, Emich JP. Neonatal abstinence syndrome: assessment and management. *Addict Dis.* 1975;2(1-2):141-158.

77. Nnoli A, Seligman NS, Dysart K, Baxter JK, Ballas SK. Opioid utilization by pregnant women with sickle cell disease and the risk of neonatal abstinence syndrome. *J Natl Med Assoc.* 2018;110(2):163-168.

78. Seligman NS, Salva N, Hayes EJ, Dysart KC, Pequignot EC, Baxter JK. Predicting length of treatment for neonatal abstinence syndrome in methadone-exposed neonates. *Am J Obstet Gynecol.* 2008;199(4):396.e391-397.

79. Shirel T, Hubler CP, Shah R, et al. Maternal opioid dose is associated with neonatal abstinence syndrome in children born to women with sickle cell disease. *Am J Hematol.* 2016;91(4): 416-419.

80. Vichinsky E, Hurst D, Earles A, Kleman K, Lubin B. Newborn screening for sickle cell disease: effect on mortality. *Pediatrics.* 1988;81(6):749-755.

81. Diallo AH, Camara G, Lamy JB, et al. Towards an information system for sickle cell neonatal screening in Senegal. *Stud Health Technol Inform.* 2019;258:95-99.

82. Steele C, Sinski A, Asibey J, et al. Point-of-care screening for sickle cell disease in low-resource settings: a multi-center evaluation of HemoTypeSC, a novel rapid test. *Am J Hematol.* 2019;94(1):39-45.

83. Chen C, Grewal J, Betran AP, Vogel JP, Souza JP, Zhang J. Severe anemia, sickle cell disease, and thalassemia as risk factors for hypertensive disorders in pregnancy in developing countries. *Pregnancy Hypertens.* 2018;13:141-147.

84. Hegewald MJ, Crapo RO. Respiratory physiology in pregnancy. *Clin Chest Med.* 2011;32(1):1-13.

85. Lorey FW, Arnopp J, Cunningham GC. Distribution of hemoglobinopathy variants by ethnicity in a multiethnic state. *Genet Epidemiol.* 1996;13(5):501-512.

86. Ohene-Frempong K, Oduro J, Tetteh H, Nkrumah F. Screening newborns for sickle cell disease in Ghana. *Pediatrics.* 2008;121: S120-S121.

The Asthma Conundrum in Sickle Cell Disease

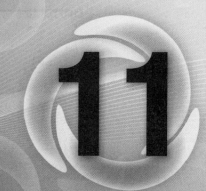

Authors: Natalie R. Shilo, Elizabeth S. Klings, Claudia R. Morris

Chapter Outline

Overview

A comorbid diagnosis of asthma is a negative prognostic factor for patients with sickle cell disease (SCD). It is associated with increased frequency of acute chest syndrome (ACS) episodes in children and adolescents, progression of disease, and an increased mortality rate.[1-8] Given these findings, the concept of asthma as a modifiable risk factor in SCD developed.[3] Simply making an earlier diagnosis of asthma seemed to be an opportunity by which to significantly improve outcomes in SCD. It turns out that the pathophysiology, diagnosis, and treatment of asthma in individuals with SCD is far from straightforward, but recognizing and treating the airway disease in individuals with SCD remains crucial to improving patient outcomes.

Asthma in SCD

An appreciation of the complex interplay of asthma and sickle cell airway pathophysiology begins with a definition of asthma. Yet, asthma itself is not easily defined because it is actually a heterogeneous disease.[9,10] Broadly speaking, asthma involves airway hyperreactivity (AHR) and inflammation in addition to a constellation of recognized signs and symptoms. These signs and symptoms may be persistent or intermittent and even completely absent for months at a time. The consensus put forth by the Global Initiative for Asthma (GINA) is that asthma is characterized by chronic airway inflammation and defined by a history of respiratory symptoms such as wheeze, shortness of breath, chest tightness, and cough, together with variable expiratory airflow limitation.[9] Meanwhile, asthma and airway pathophysiology in SCD are entangled, but not synonymous. Multiple studies have shown that the correlations between symptoms, pulmonary function, and biomarkers typically found in asthma do not uniformly apply to the airway disease that occurs in SCD.[11-15] Although there are numerous overlapping mechanisms common to both classic asthma and SCD, there are also some paradigms unique to SCD (Figure 11-1). Herein lies the diagnostic and therapeutic conundrum that we are confronted with as clinicians.

Epidemiology

Asthma has a significant global disease burden. It is estimated that >300 million individuals worldwide are affected. The existing data show an international asthma prevalence of approximately 5% to 18%.[10,16]

Asthma-Like Condition of Sickle Cell Disease

Normal lung

Asthmatic lung

Normal lining

Subepithelial edema and fibrosis

Relaxed muscle

Excess mucus

Smooth muscle bronchoconstriction

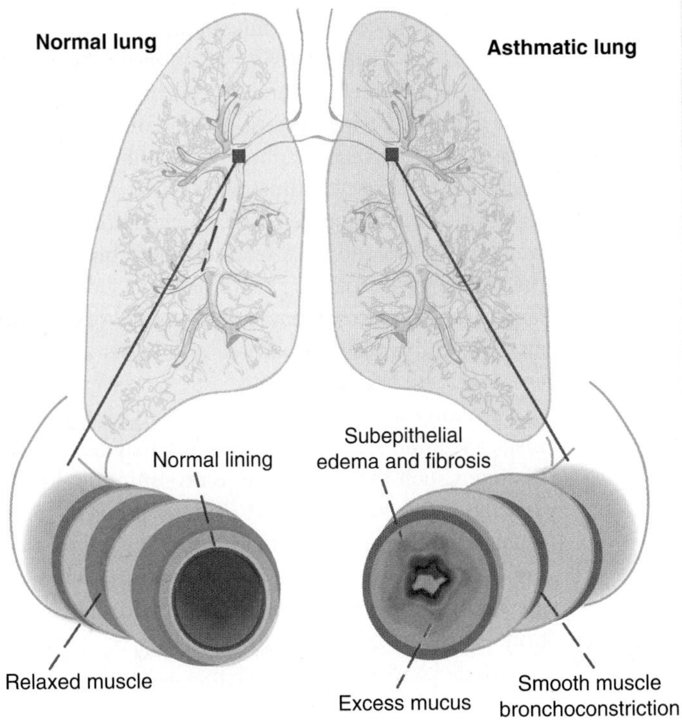

Mechanisms Overlapping With Classic Asthma

Respiratory tract infections

Inhaled aeroallergens

Vitamin D deficiency

Genetic predisposition to asthma
- ADAM33, PHF11, DPP10, GRPA, SPINK5, ORMDL3
- Polymorphisms in β-adrenergic receptor gene

Leukotriene pathway
- ↑ phospholipase A2 (PLA2)
- ↑ cysteinyl leukotrienes (CysLTs)
- ↑ LTB4 → activated neutrophils
- ↑ IL-13
- ↑ cell adhesion molecules
- Airway smooth muscle proliferation and mucus production

Arginine and nitric oxide (NO) dysregulation
- Unopposed reactive oxygen species
- ↑ vasoconstriction
- ↑ hypercoagulability
- ↑ airway remodeling

Hypoxia and ischemia-reperfusion injury
- Endothelial activation
- Leukocyte extravasation
- ↑ iNKTs, ↑ IFN-γ
- ↑ reactive oxygen species → ↑ DAMPs*
- ↑ V/Q mismatch

Autonomic nervous system dysregulation

Sterile inflammation
- Uncoupled NOS
- DAMPs*
- Neutrophil extracellular traps (NETs)
- Toll-like receptors (TLR4)
- ↑ IL-1β, ↑ IL-18

Acetaminophen exposure

Mechanisms Unique to Sickle-Asthma

Hemolysis
- PIGF → ↑ phospholipase A2 (PLA2) → ↑ leukotriene pathway
- ↓ arginine and NO
- ↑ oxidative stress
- ↑ sterile inflammation
- ↑ hypercoagulability

Pulmonary vascular congestion
- ↑ capillary blood volume
- Extrinsic vascular compression of airway

FIGURE 11-1 The Asthma-Like Condition of Sickle Cell Disease. There are numerous overlapping mechanisms in both classic asthma and sickle cell disease. Mechanisms unique to "asthma" in sickle cell disease are also listed. PIGF, placental growth factor; NO, nitric oxide; LTB4, leukotriene B4; IL-13, interleukin-13 (TH2 pathway); iNKTs, invariant natural killer T cells; IFN-gamma, interferon-gamma (pro-inflammatory); DAMPs, damage associated molecular patterns; V/Q, ventilation-to-perfusion ratio; NOS, nitric oxide synthase; IL-1 beta, interleukin-1 beta (pro-inflammatory); IL-18, interleukin-18 (TH1 pathway).

There is not yet a consensus definition of what qualifies as a diagnosis of asthma within the context of SCD, but "asthma" or airway obstruction and hyperreactivity in patients with SCD is interestingly a comorbidity largely limited to pediatric patients. In SCD, the pattern of lung disease appears to change during the transition from childhood to adulthood. When merging data from adult and pediatric cohorts, it seems that there is a decline in the incidence of AHR and obstructive lung disease and a concurrent increase in restrictive lung disease.[17-24] Although one cohort reported no decline in lung function,[24] the average follow-up period in that study was less than in other studies.[23,25,26] Another large cohort study demonstrated a decline of 2% to 3% in forced expiratory volume in 1 second (FEV_1) per year in children with SCD, and this is accompanied by a 2.1% to 2.4% predicted decline in total lung capacity.[26] To lend perspective to the significance of these findings, this rate of decline significantly exceeds that seen in asthma (0%-0.88% per year)[27] and equals that seen in children with cystic fibrosis.[28,29]

Although a number of studies examined the prevalence and incidence of asthma in their respective cohorts, their definitions of asthma varied and often relied on a clinician diagnosis. This was even true in 3 large prospective cohort trials in which an asthma prevalence of 17% to 29% was reported in cohorts that collectively included subjects between the ages of 4 and 20 years.[3,8,30] Overall, the prevalence of a clinician diagnosis of asthma in SCD is estimated to be within the range of 17% to 48%.[1-4,7,31-35]

Because there is variability in clinician diagnosis of asthma and symptoms classically attributed to asthma pathology may independently be due to SCD pathology, clinician-based diagnoses may be a source of error in these prevalence estimates. Yet despite the lack of a clear definition for asthma in SCD, the diagnosis of asthma and/or characteristic features of asthma have been clearly associated with poorer outcomes in people with SCD.[1-7] Increased rates of ACS, stroke, and vaso-occlusive episodes have all been reported.[1-3,7,32,36-41] Asthma is also associated with increased emergency department (ED) visits for both pain and ACS in children with SCD.[42] The increased risk of mortality in SCD patients with asthma that was originally reported by Boyd et al[2] has been subsequently corroborated by others,[38,43] including Knight-Madden et al[38] who reported an increased 10-year mortality rate in SCD patients experiencing "current" asthma, with a hazard ratio of 11.2.

Asthma Pathophysiology

Individuals with asthma differ in their susceptibility to various triggers. However, the unifying pathology is dynamic narrowing of the airway with expiratory airflow limitation either because of inflammation or AHR or a combination of these mechanisms. Airway inflammation occurs secondary to abnormal hypertrophy and proliferation of the airway epithelial cells, smooth muscle cells, endothelial cells, fibroblasts and myofibroblasts. Collagen deposition results in subepithelial fibrosis,[44] and the airways may simultaneously become hypervascularized.[45] Ultimately, this leads to airway remodeling with fixed airway obstruction. Excessive contraction of airway smooth muscle occurs in addition to airway edema as a consequence of microvascular leakage. Overly stimulated sensory nerves add to the pathology with exaggerated bronchoconstriction.[46] The contribution of each of these mechanisms to the airway obstruction observed in SCD patients is not yet clear.

Asthma Management and Treatment

Pulmonary function tests are used to quantify AHR and lower airway obstruction. For home monitoring, peak flow is a measure that may be used; however, it is less frequently used in pediatrics given its variable reliability. It is noteworthy that some patients with long-standing uncontrolled asthma have poor perception of symptoms; in this group, objective measures provide a tool beyond symptomatic complaints by which to determine the degree of asthma control.[47]

Management also entails the control of comorbidities known to exacerbate lower airway inflammation. Upper airway inflammation is associated with lower airway inflammation. Thus, gastroesophageal reflux, rhinitis, and chronic rhinosinusitis need to be addressed, when present, to achieve asthma control. Additionally, obstructive sleep apnea (OSA) is linked to asthma.[9,10] Normally, the nasopharynx functions to filter and humidify inhaled air prior to it entering the lower airways. Patients with upper airway obstruction and OSA tend to mouth breathe. In bypassing the nasopharynx, common airway irritants such as dry air, aeroallergens, and bioaerosols have a direct portal of entry to the lower airways. In this manner, patients with upper airway obstruction are at increased risk for repeated asthma exacerbations.

β_2-Agonists, inhaled corticosteroids, leukotriene antagonists, systemic steroids, intravenous magnesium sulfate, and biologics such as omalizumab (anti–immunoglobulin E [IgE] antibody) and mepolizumab (interleukin [IL]-5 antagonist) are used in the treatment of asthma. The approach to managing and treating asthma in patients with SCD has been largely gleaned from the treatment of asthma in the general population. As we are beginning to better appreciate the airway disease that occurs in the context of SCD, we are tasked with how to better tailor "asthma" therapy for patients with SCD.

Airway Disease in SCD

AHR and Lower Airway Obstruction

What has been clearly identified in pediatric sickle cell patients is that the prevalence of AHR, even in individuals with SCD but without a diagnosis of asthma, is much higher than it is in the general population.[15,17,18,48] With the exception of one study that reported no increased prevalence,[49] multiple studies have shown an increased prevalence ranging from 55% to 77.5% in children.[12,15,17,18] In 2 small studies of <40 adults, the frequency was 31% in adults,[19,20] but this was not confirmed in larger studies,[50,51] which suggested AHR was infrequent in adults.

Recognition of airway disease in patients with SCD is fairly recent. Historically, SCD was associated with restrictive lung disease, as this was the pulmonary physiology most frequently reported in adult patients.[51,52] Although originally reported by Wall et al in 1979,[53] it was only in the 1990s and early 2000s that findings of AHR and lower airway obstruction in children with

SCD increasingly gained attention.[1,6,7,12,17,18,21,22,48,49,53,54] Data accumulated to corroborate that an obstructive pattern is more frequent in children with SCD than is a restrictive pattern.[8,21,48,52,55,56] Estimates of lower airway obstruction in children with SCD range between 13% and 35%.[8,23,37,48] Additionally, one study in infants found an 85% prevalence of lower airway obstruction.[21] Meanwhile, restrictive lung disease is less prevalent, occurring in an estimated 9% to 27% of children with SCD.[8,22,37]

Despite the range of reported prevalence, it is significant that the vast majority of studies demonstrated a higher prevalence for both AHR and lower airway obstruction than the corresponding prevalence estimates of asthma when matched for age and race. Interestingly, many of the patients found to have AHR and/or lower airway obstruction on pulmonary function testing also did not have a preexisting diagnosis of asthma.[1,8,21,48,52,57] Given this finding, questions arose as to the nature of asthma in SCD. What significance did these pulmonary function tests hold in relation to clinical outcomes in SCD? Could it be that asthma was being underdiagnosed in SCD? In people with SCD, might AHR or lower airway obstruction, in the absence of clinical asthma symptoms, suffice for a diagnosis of asthma? The answers to these questions are still somewhat controversial because the studies to date have yielded conflicting observations. After finding an association between a preexisting diagnosis of asthma and increased hospitalization rates in children with SCD,[3] a retrospective study by the same authors found a correlation between lower airway obstruction and higher rates of hospitalization in children with SCD as compared to children with SCD who had normal pulmonary function.[1] However, more recently, a large prospective study found no association between pulmonary function test abnormalities and morbidity.[58] Similarly, another study found that measures of AHR do not predict future pain crises or ACS.[59] Despite the conflicting data in terms of how pulmonary function tests relate to long-term outcomes in SCD, the high prevalence of pulmonary function test abnormalities in SCD patients is striking, and additional research into what exactly these abnormalities may signify is warranted.

Symptomatology

Asthma is a clinical diagnosis. Furthermore, a diagnosis of asthma can be made despite the absence of measured expiratory airflow limitation.[9] A well-controlled (nonsevere) asthmatic patient will have normal pulmonary function at baseline, with abnormalities only developing during an acute exacerbation or during specialized pulmonary function (bronchoprovocation) testing that is used to define the patient's individual threshold for developing bronchoconstriction. As such, asthma-based questionnaires have been employed to gain insights on the symptomatology and clinical presentation of airway disease in SCD. Although questionnaires validated for asthma correlated well with a clinician diagnosis of asthma in some cohorts of patients with SCD,[7,60,61] asthma questionnaires did not correlate well with objective measures of AHR.[12,15] Sensitivity, specificity, negative predictive value, and positive predictive value were all remarkably poor when questionnaires validated for the diagnosis of asthma in the general population were compared to specialized pulmonary function (bronchoprovocation) test results in patients with SCD.[12,15] Why this significant discrepancy between symptomatology and pulmonary function testing exists is still not entirely clear, but it poses a diagnostic and treatment dilemma. Should asymptomatic patients with abnormal pulmonary function findings be treated? It is theorized that the chronic pain and systemic inflammation inherent to SCD may also contribute to symptoms of wheezing, dyspnea, and chest pain, thus blurring the line between what may be attributed to the clinical manifestations of asthma versus those of SCD.[15]

Given the difficulty in applying classic asthma criteria to patients with SCD, interest developed in better characterizing the asthma-like condition in SCD so that it is more easily recognized, diagnosed, and treated. In a cohort of adult patients, Cohen et al[62] provided compelling evidence on the significance of wheezing within the context of SCD. They found no difference in the incidence of pain or ACS, lung function, or mortality risk between adults with and without a clinician diagnosis of asthma. However, they did find that adults with recurrent, severe episodes of wheezing, irrespective of an asthma diagnosis, had twice the rates of pain and ACS, decreased lung function, and increased mortality risk compared to adults without recurrent, severe wheezing.[62] Another study in adults with SCD also linked wheezing to abnormal pulmonary function.[63] Wheezing has thus been identified as an independent risk factor associated with increased morbidity and mortality in adults with SCD.[41,62] The frequent occurrence of diastolic dysfunction of the left ventricle and consequent pulmonary edema in adults with SCD (particularly during vaso-occlusive events) raises the possibility of a nonpulmonary etiology of wheezing in some.[64] In children, wheezing occurs during episodes of ACS,[65] and wheezing is also frequently described outside of an acute illness.[66] A prospective, observational cohort study investigated wheezing as a defining characteristic of airway disease in children with SCD.[67] The investigators reported that the presence of 2 of the following 3 phenotypic characteristics is predictive of an asthma-like condition and increased risk of ACS: wheezing associated with shortness of breath, wheezing after exercise, and/or parental history of asthma. Of interest is the fact that these authors found allergy skin prick testing to be of limited use in making the diagnosis of "asthma" in their cohort, in contrast to reports of atopic asthma and lab findings of elevated total IgE levels correlating with increased morbidity in previous studies. Interestingly, bronchoprovocation testing for AHR did not distinguish between the asthma and nonasthma groups, nor was it helpful in predicting future episodes of ACS.[67] Meanwhile, a more recent study showed an increased decline in lung function associated with wheezing in a pediatric cohort of patients.[68] In summary, although the long-term implications of wheezing in SCD need to be more fully delineated, wheezing has emerged as a distinctive clinical feature of SCD.

Pathophysiobiology

The lungs in SCD are exposed to a chronic, proinflammatory state even at baseline, which is driven by a complex web of pathologic mechanisms that include hypoxia coupled with ischemic-reperfusion injury; oxidative stress; chronic hemolysis; endothelial dysfunction combined with hypercoagulability; arginine and nitric oxide (NO) dysregulation; and genetic susceptibility.[43,52,55,56,69-74] In addition, accumulating evidence of asthma as an unanticipated adverse event associated with acetaminophen use[75,76] establishes plausibility of unforeseen risk in SCD of "asthma-like" symptoms, given the crucial role acetaminophen plays in treatment of both acute and chronic vaso-occlusive pain.

Proinflammatory Mediators

The airways in both SCD and asthma are subject to a proinflammatory state.[52,74] They have chronically elevated levels of the proinflammatory cytokines IL-1β, IL-3, IL-6, IL-8, interferon (IFN)-γ, tumor necrosis factor (TNF)-α, granulocyte-macrophage colony-stimulating factor (GM-CSF), acute-phase proteins (C-reactive protein, platelets, leukocytes), and endothelial cell adhesion molecules.[77-83] Additional proinflammatory markers described in SCD include leukotrienes and prostaglandins. There is also evidence of CD4+ T cells, CD8+ T cells, and regulatory T (Treg) cells contributing to the proinflammatory state.[78] Other data suggest that the airway inflammation is driven by myeloid elements, especially macrophages, as opposed to lymphoid elements.[84] It is also possible that there are varying endotypes of airway inflammation in SCD patients and, thus, variability in the dominant proinflammatory pathways. Because a proinflammatory state already exists at baseline, the inflammatory cascade appears to have a cumulative or exaggerated effect during a vaso-occlusive episode.[77,78,85-88]

Hypoxia and Ischemia-Reperfusion Injury

Hypoxia promotes the polymerization of hemoglobin S, thereby leading to the sickling of red blood cells. Erythrocyte sickling results in impaired blood flow through the microvasculature, setting off a toxic cycle of hypoxia, sickling, hemolysis, and further vaso-occlusive episodes.[52,74] Subsequently, reperfusion injury produces an increased burden of oxidative stress via the generation of reactive oxygen species such as uncoupled NO synthase and NADPH oxidase.[89-92] Kaul and Hebbel[86] explored the concept of ischemia-reperfusion injury triggering an exaggerated inflammatory response in transgenic sickle cell mice.[86] In their study, transgenic sickle cell mice exposed to hypoxia with subsequent reoxygenation demonstrated increased leukocyte extravasation compared to control mice.[88] Subsequently, Wallace et al[93] additionally demonstrated increased levels of invariant natural killer T (iNKT) cells and IFN-γ. Inhibition of iNKT cells via the adenosine A2A receptor agonist regadenoson demonstrated efficacy in reducing pulmonary inflammation in transgenic sickle cell mice.[94] Meanwhile, Field et al[87] demonstrated an increase in activated fibrocytes following hypoxia and reperfusion injury. It is also known that ventilation-perfusion mismatch with transient regional lung hypoxia occurs with AHR, and thus, it is conceivable that outside of ACS, the lungs of a patient with SCD suffer subclinical but repeated insults of transient hypoxia, sickling, intravascular thrombosis, ventilation-perfusion mismatch, and ischemia-reperfusion inj

ury.[55,86,87,91,92] In short, repeated cycles of ischemia and reperfusion injury may occur in the lungs of SCD patients and can lead to both vascular and airway remodeling.[74,87]

Leukotriene Pathway

The leukotriene pathway potentially links the pathologic mechanisms of vaso-occlusion and inflammation in the lungs in SCD. As such, it plays a unique role in SCD, distinct from the role it plays in asthma. The cascade starts with phospholipase A2 and the release of arachidonic acid from membrane phospholipids in the lung, setting off the production of leukotrienes and prostaglandins. Increased levels of free fatty acids result in damage to the alveolar-capillary membrane and the inactivation of surfactant. Interestingly, secretory phospholipase A2 also may serve as a marker for the development of ACS in some patients. Secretory phospholipase A2 activity increases prior to the development of ACS, and its concentration correlates with ACS severity.[95-97]

The leukotrienes are further divided into the cysteinyl leukotrienes (CysLTs; LTC4, LTD4, LTE4) and leukotriene B4 (LTB4). The CysLTs affect both the lungs and the vasculature. In the lungs, CysLTs cause bronchoconstriction, smooth muscle proliferation, mucus production, and airway edema. In the vasculature, CysLTs cause vasoconstriction, vascular leakage, and upregulation of cellular adhesion molecules.[98] In addition, elevated CysLTs have been associated with pain and increase during vaso-occlusive episodes; this may lead to development of vaso-occlusion. A study by Jennings et al[99] examining LTE4 levels found significantly elevated levels of LTE4 at baseline in SCD patients, which correlated with increased frequency of hospitalization for vaso-occlusive episodes. On a different front, LTB4, involved in neutrophil activation, chemotaxis, and adhesion to the endothelium, is elevated at baseline in SCD.[100] Meanwhile, placenta growth factor (PlGF), an erythroblast secreted factor, is another way in which the leukotriene pathway is implicated in the airway pathobiology of SCD. Patel et al[101,102] demonstrated that PlGF is increased in SCD and upregulates the leukotriene pathway by activation of peripheral blood monocytes. A more recent study expanded the role of PlGF in SCD by demonstrating its role in modulating AHR via both TH2 and leukotriene-mediated pathways.[13] In short, the leukotrienes appear to play a significant role in the pathophysiology of airway disease in SCD via mechanisms of inflammation similar to those observed in non-SCD asthma with the contribution of mechanisms related to hemolysis and vaso-occlusion.[103]

Infection

The increased sensitivity to infectious insults in SCD is also corroborated by studies in transgenic sickle cell mice.[85,104] Holtzclaw et al[85] studied the response of transgenic sickle cell mice to an endotoxin challenge. Their results demonstrated a significant increase in mortality, airway tone, TNF-α, IL-1β, and vascular cell adhesion molecule 1 (VCAM1) in the transgenic sickle cell mice. Given these results, the authors argued that SCD is a proinflammatory state that leads to an exaggerated inflammatory response to stress, whether or not hypoxia is part of the inciting stressor.[87]

Allergy

In a study by Nandedkar et al,[77] the effects of ovalbumin sensitization were compared in both wild-type and SCD mice. There was increased mortality in the SCD mice, and the sensitized SCD mice also demonstrated more of an inflammatory response than the sensitized wild-type mice based on inflammatory markers and histopathologic changes. When compared to the wild-type mice, the SCD mice produced significantly higher levels of total IgE, peripheral blood eosinophilia, transforming growth factor (TGF)-β, and fibroblast-specific protein. Histopathology demonstrated airway epithelial desquamation and peribronchial and perivascular collagen deposition observed in a dose-dependent fashion in wild-type mice. In contrast, the SCD mice exhibited maximally increased changes without dose dependency on histopathology regardless of the dose of sensitization with ovalbumin to which they had been exposed. This study supports the theory that there is an exaggerated response to allergen-induced lung inflammation in SCD.[77] Since Nandedkar et al[77] published their findings, other authors have similarly shown an exaggerated inflammatory response to an allergic insult in the transgenic sickle cell mouse model.[78,88]

Taken together, the results of these studies suggest that in SCD, as in asthma, the lungs are exquisitely sensitive to hypoxic, infectious, and allergic insults.[55]

Hemolysis, Arginine, and NO

Hemolysis is central to the pathophysiology of SCD, and it follows that arginine and NO dysregulation play a unique role in sickle cell pulmonary pathology.[72] Intravascular hemolysis leads to both increased consumption and decreased production of NO.[70,105,106] Free hemoglobin released into the plasma from lysed erythrocytes directly scavenges NO and promotes free radicals that consume NO.[105-107] Decreased NO bioactivity is severely problematic in SCD because it compounds some of the key pathologic mechanisms in SCD. Typically, NO functions to counteract endothelial cell activation, transcription of cellular adhesion molecules, platelet activation, and hypoxic vasoconstriction.[107,108] Without the aid of NO as a potent pulmonary vasodilator, the cycle of hypoxia, erythrocyte sickling, hemolysis, endothelial injury, hypercoagulability, and vaso-occlusion continues unabated.[72,74] The lysed erythrocytes also release arginase, which depletes available arginine, the obligate substrate for NO production, and converts it to ornithine.[72,109] Hemolysis thereby directly diminishes the bioavailability of both NO and arginine.[72,105]

As the body's NO stores are depleted, NO synthase (NOS) production is upregulated, but NO production is impaired because erythrocyte arginase competes more effectively than NOS for arginine as substrate.[72] Interestingly, arginase inhibition has been beneficial in allergic asthma, unrelated to underlying hemolysis, and this underscores the central role of arginine and NO in preventing AHR and inflammation.[110] Because reactive oxygen species are formed in the setting of hypoxia, existing NO is consumed and further depleted. Increased reactive oxygen species also occur partially as a consequence of endothelial

NOS being uncoupled when arginine levels are low. Uncoupled NOS will produce the reactive oxygen species nitrite, nitrate, and peroxynitrite instead of NO.[111] Uncoupling of NOS is further driven by increased endogenous NOS inhibitors and decreased availability of NOS cofactors. One endogenous NOS inhibitor in particular, asymmetric dimethylarginine (ADMA), is abnormally elevated in SCD and linked to pathophysiologic mechanisms in both asthma and pulmonary hypertension.[109,112-114] Finally, arginine and ornithine compete for cellular uptake.[107] When ornithine production is favored, downstream production of polyamines and proline is amplified, leading to smooth muscle cell proliferation and peribronchial and perivascular collagen deposition, ultimately resulting in both airway and pulmonary vascular bed remodeling.[52,110]

It is also noteworthy that cellular free heme has pro-oxidant, cytotoxic, and inflammatory effects. Extracellularly, free heme activates the innate immune response and triggers the release of neutrophil extracellular traps (NETs) that promote lung injury. This drives sterile inflammation and endothelial injury through heme toll-like receptor 4 (TLR4) activation.[115] Such hemolysis by-products have become known as damage-associated molecular pattern molecules (DAMPs) and promote systemic inflammation even in the absence of infection.[14]

How NO dysregulation in SCD relates to exhaled NO levels remains unclear. In asthma with some component of airway eosinophilia, levels of exhaled NO are elevated due to increased production by the respiratory epithelium.[116] In SCD, the levels of exhaled NO have been studied with conflicting results. One study initially reported reduced exhaled NO in their cohort of adult patients with SCD, which seemed to fit with the concept of arginine and NO depletion.[117] However, another group reported elevated bronchial NO in a cohort of children with SCD but without a comorbid diagnosis of atopy or asthma. Interestingly, alveolar NO levels were not elevated.[118] Subsequently, another group studying inhaled NO, also in a pediatric cohort, reported opposite findings. Namely, there was no elevation in bronchial NO, whereas alveolar NO was elevated and positively correlated with pulmonary blood flow and negatively correlated with hemoglobin levels. Based on these findings, the authors concluded that the hyperdynamic circulation in SCD and resultant increased pulmonary blood flow were the etiology for elevated levels of alveolar NO.[119] Taken together, these findings suggest that lower airway obstruction in SCD may be reflective of increased pulmonary capillary blood volume and extrinsic airway compression rather than asthma.[120]

Finally, a large, prospective, observational study of 131 children with SCD examined exhaled bronchial NO. The study showed no correlation between exhaled NO levels and pulmonary function test results, which was not surprising given that this correlation is poor even in the asthma population for which it is routinely used. There was also no correlation between exhaled NO and clinician-diagnosed asthma, wheezing, and prior history of ACS, whereas there was a correlation with markers of atopy (total IgE levels, skin prick test positivity, peripheral blood eosinophilia) as well as with future risk of ACS. It is important to note that, at baseline, outside of a vaso-occlusive episode or ACS, plasma arginine concentrations are normal in children but low in adults with SCD.[72,121] However, this still would not explain the discrepancy in findings between the pediatric cohorts. Measurement of exhaled NO is a noninvasive test, and as such, it is an attractive biomarker by which to monitor airway disease; however, further research is needed to determine its true role in monitoring airways disease in SCD.

Genetic Susceptibility, Environmental Risk Factors, and Stress

Environmental factors that trigger expression of asthma in any individual with a genetic predisposition are disproportionately present in individuals with SCD in the United States as a consequence of socioeconomic disparities. Namely, many individuals with SCD live in an environment with significant exposure to indoor allergens, secondhand smoke, indoor and/or outdoor air pollution, and stress.[10,122-128] Stress is a multifaceted environmental factor in that it can be mental, physical, or emotional, and it has also been implicated in the pathophysiology of vaso-occlusive episodes in SCD.[129-131]

Management

Acute Treatment

An asthma exacerbation may easily become ACS because the line between the 2 entities frequently blurs in the pediatric population. Asthma can produce lung atelectasis, which can present as a new opacity on chest radiograph. Bronchodilators are immediately initiated during an acute asthma exacerbation, and patients with SCD need to be treated according to these same asthma guidelines[9,132] (Box 11-1). In fact, there is evidence for bronchodilator therapy specific to ACS. The first large, prospective, multicenter study on ACS reported that 61% of the 531 patients in the study were treated with

---

| **Box 11-1** | **Acute Asthma Management** |

- ◆ Give oxygen to maintain oxygen saturation >90%
- ◆ Start short-acting bronchodilator (short-acting β-agonist [SABA])
- ◆ Start steroids: prednisone 1 mg/kg/d for 3-10 days (maximum, 60 mg/d)
- ◆ If inpatient, give red blood cell transfusion with steroid initiation
- ◆ Add ipratropium for increased severity/poor SABA response
- ◆ Give magnesium sulfate (50 mg/kg intravenously over 15-30 minutes) for moderate to severe exacerbations
- ◆ Consider bilevel positive airway pressure or heliox for severe exacerbations
- ◆ Outpatient follow-up within 4 weeks

---

bronchodilators during an episode of ACS based on a prior clinical diagnosis of reactive airway disease.[133] The authors found a mean improvement in FEV_1 of 27%. The National Acute Chest Syndrome Study Group concluded that AHR should be assumed to be present and all patients with ACS should receive bronchodilator therapy.[65,133]

Meanwhile, systemic steroids compose the core treatment for an asthma exacerbation and, per the GINA/National Heart, Lung, and Blood Institute (NHLBI) guidelines, should be given for 3 to 10 days, pending severity, at a dose of 1 to 2 mg/kg/d of prednisone or methylprednisolone.[9,132] It seems reasonable that systemic corticosteroids should be used for an acute asthma exacerbation in SCD just as they would be for a patient without SCD. Yet, in SCD, the use of systemic steroids is inconsistent.[134] A large, multicenter, retrospective analysis by Sobota et al[134] revealed that only a mean of 48% of patients with ACS, despite a preexisting diagnosis of asthma, received treatment with corticosteroids. The widespread reluctance to use corticosteroids was driven in part by earlier studies[135,136] reporting a possible rebound pain effect after discontinuation of steroids and anecdotal reports of severe vaso-occlusive episodes following systemic corticosteroid use.[137,138] However, the prospective, randomized, double-blinded, placebo-controlled trial by Bernini et al[136] also demonstrated a significant reduction in duration of need for supplemental oxygen, opioid analgesia, need for transfusion, and length of hospitalization. Another study described rebound pain as a phenomenon occurring in both steroid-treated and -untreated patients, suggesting this was not a steroid-specific side effect.[139] Moreover, Isakoff et al[140] looked at the administration of dexamethasone for ACS when given in conjunction with transfusion therapy and found no subsequent readmissions for pain following hospital discharge. Still, a more recent review noted that there is ongoing debate about the usage of systemic steroids in treating an acute asthma exacerbation/ACS episode in patients with SCD.[141] Given that an acute asthma exacerbation can lead to increased hypoxia and thereby promotion of more sickling, hemolysis, and vaso-occlusion in a patient with SCD and that an untreated asthma exacerbation itself can rapidly spiral into acute respiratory failure and death, the reluctance to use steroids in patients with SCD is perplexing.

Although no studies have specifically evaluated intravenous magnesium sulfate for the treatment of asthma in patients with SCD, it is an effective treatment for status asthmaticus and commonly used in the ED setting.[142] Intravenous magnesium sulfate prevented hospitalization when used at a dose of 50 to 75 mg/kg (maximum, 2 g) given over 15 to 30 minutes.[143] It should also be considered for moderate to severe asthma exacerbations in children and adults with SCD. Noninvasive positive-pressure ventilation is inconsistently used for acute asthma; its use has been described in patients with SCD and ACS; however, controlled trials are warranted.[144] Heliox-driven β$_2$-agonist nebulization has shown some benefit for the treatment of acute asthma, decreasing the severity of the exacerbation and risk of hospitalization in a meta-analysis and can be considered in the treatment of patients with SCD

Box 11-2	Chronic Asthma Management in Sickle Cell Disease

◆ Start maintenance low-dose inhaled corticosteroids (ICS) or montelukast

◆ May use short-acting bronchodilator up to once every 4 hours as needed

◆ Wheezing or other respiratory symptoms after exercise?
  • Use short-acting bronchodilator 15 minutes before exercise

◆ Always use a spacer with all metered-dose inhalers

◆ Daily symptoms?
  • Start medium-dose ICS or low-dose ICS plus montelukast
  • Check vitamin D level (goal >30 ng/mL)

◆ Refer all suspected asthma patients to pulmonology

◆ Refer all patients over the age of 6 years for pulmonary function testing

and severe asthma not responding to β_2-agonists and systemic steroids.[145,146]

Chronic Therapies

In the chronic setting, patients with SCD diagnosed with comorbid asthma should be on maintenance therapy with inhaled corticosteroids and/or leukotriene receptor antagonist therapy according to the GINA/NHLBI asthma guidelines[9,132] (Box 11-2). Patients and families also need to be advised and receive counseling and support in avoidance of common environmental triggers (Box 11-3) Comorbidities known to exacerbate asthma should also be addressed (Box 11-4).

Box 11-3	Potential Environmental Triggers

◆ Paint, unvented or wood-burning stove, fireplace

◆ Cleaning agents, perfumes, scented candles

◆ Drapes, rugs, carpets, bed covers

◆ Animal dander

◆ Cockroaches, rodents

◆ Mold

◆ Pollen

Recommendations for those with environmental triggers

◆ Use mattress and pillowcase covers

◆ Wash bedsheets and blankets weekly in hot water

◆ Remove carpets, rugs, and drapes

◆ Avoid exposure to secondhand smoke

◆ Monitor the pattern of allergic symptoms to help localize trigger

Box 11-4	Comorbidities That Exacerbate Asthma

◆ Gastroesophageal reflux

◆ Allergic rhinitis

◆ Chronic nasal congestion

◆ Obstructive sleep apnea

◆ Obesity

What should be done for patients without clear signs and symptoms of asthma remains controversial. Despite the evidence of an unusually high prevalence of pulmonary function test abnormalities that do not correlate with questionnaires validated for asthma, the NHLBI Sickle Cell Management Guidelines do not recommend any routine screening or monitoring for any pulmonary complications of SCD.[147] Meanwhile, a prospective, randomized, double-blinded study by Glassberg et al[148] is compelling in suggesting a possible systemic benefit from inhaled corticosteroid therapy. Low-dose inhaled mometasone resulted in decreased pain scores and levels of soluble vascular cell adhesion molecule (sVCAM) in a cohort of non-asthmatic patients with SCD. This study is intriguing on many levels and offers further insights into sickle cell–related airway disease. Patients enrolled onto the study were aged 15 years and older and had reported wheezing or coughing during the 2 months prior to study enrollment. The authors took care to exclude patients with comorbid asthma not only based on prior clinician diagnosis, but also based on historical risk factors as described in the Sickle Asthma Cohort (SAC) study.[67] Although sVCAM is a biomarker of systemic disease, mometasone is biologically active, locally, in the airways, with minimal systemic absorption. This implies that modulation of airway disease in SCD improves systemic inflammation and thereby vaso-occlusion, especially since the local airway benefits of mometasone occurred in conjunction with a decrease in daily pain diary scores. Interestingly, a marker of hemolytic rate (reticulocyte count) was also decreased in the treatment group when compared to the placebo group. This is significant because it links modulation of airway disease to the hemolytic pathway in SCD. As discussed earlier in this chapter, the leukotriene pathway also appears to link hypercoagulability, vaso-occlusion, and inflammation. The leukotriene receptor antagonist montelukast and the 5-lipoxygenase inhibitor zileuton were both studied in phase I/II trials, but the complete results have not yet been published[149,150] [(NCT01960413, NCT01136941). Meanwhile, clinical trials are ongoing for the adenosine A2A receptor agonist regadenoson given its ability to inhibit iNKT cells and thereby modulate airway inflammation. A phase II study of low-dose regadenoson did not demonstrate efficacy.[151] However, a phase II study using anti-iNKT monoclonal antibody yielded more promising results, and additional studies are planned.[152]

Hydroxyurea

There is some interest as to whether hydroxyurea might directly attenuate airway inflammation in SCD. One study unexpectedly found a relatively increased degree of measured AHR in subjects not on hydroxyurea when compared to subjects who were on therapy.[15] In contrast, another study found no correlation between hydroxyurea and degree of AHR.[12] However, the Pediatric Hydroxyurea Phase III Clinical Trial (BABY HUG) demonstrated decreased rates of ACS in children on hydroxyurea therapy.[153] In addition to its benefits on fetal hemoglobin expression, hydroxyurea is recognized as an NO donor with anti-inflammatory effects that may be beneficial in airway disease.[154-157] One study examined hydroxyurea therapy and its longitudinal impact on lung function in children with SCD.[158] In this study, the rate of pulmonary function decline slowed significantly after hydroxyurea therapy was initiated. If hydroxyurea therapy can modulate the severity of AHR or the progression of lower airway obstruction, optimization of hydroxyurea therapy might be the first-line therapy in patients with SCD who do not exhibit more classic allergic asthma symptomatology or lower airway obstruction.

Vitamin D

Vitamin D is increasingly recognized for its potential immunomodulatory and antimicrobial roles in the lung. Alveolar macrophages, respiratory epithelial cells, dendritic cells, and Treg lymphocytes all have impaired function in the setting of vitamin D deficiency. In numerous respiratory conditions, including asthma, vitamin D deficiency is associated with poorer outcomes.[159] Lee et al[169] extended this finding to patients living with SCD. In their cohort of children with SCD, 77% were vitamin D deficient at baseline. Subjects were randomized into standard-dose cholecalciferol versus high-dose cholecalciferol for a 2-year period. They reported a >50% decrease in respiratory event rate (respiratory infection, asthma exacerbation, ACS) during year 2 of vitamin D supplementation in both groups. Of note, pulmonary function did not decline during the 2-year period, suggesting a possible role for vitamin D in the preservation of pulmonary function in patients with SCD. It is also interesting that the standard-dose group, while demonstrating clinical improvement, did not achieve normal levels of vitamin D.[160]

Allogeneic Hematopoietic Stem Cell Transplantation

Allogeneic hematopoietic stem cell transplantation (aHSCT) has been performed successfully in SCD patients with a matched donor, but it is not without risk. The potential for multisystem adverse effects exists. From a pulmonary perspective, there is concern for graft-versus-host disease, which manifests as bronchiolitis obliterans in the lung. However, one prospective cohort performed from 1991 to 2000[161] found no significant worsening of pulmonary function after transplant. Additionally, nonmyeloablative aHSCT is being increasingly performed in patients

with SCD, and this allows for decreased overall transplant toxicity.[162] It is noteworthy that there is donor-recipient transfer of adaptive immunity with helper T-cell and B-cell clones that have allergen-specific memory. This means that the recipient will be newly atopic and/or asthmatic if the donor was an atopic and/or asthmatic, and this has been demonstrated in long-term follow-up of aHSCT patients.[163] However, this also means that a patient with atopic asthma and SCD who undergoes aHSCT from a nonatopic donor will be cured of both asthma and SCD following transplantation.

Gene Therapy

In 2017, the first successful lentiviral gene therapy was reported in a child with SCD.[164] A phase I/II clinical trial of lentiviral gene therapy in subjects with SCD is ongoing. In addition, CRISPR-Cas9 has been used to edit the DNA sequence in harvested hematopoietic stem cells. After the Cas9 enzyme corrects the DNA mutation, the patient is reinfused with the corrected hematopoietic stem cells. A phase I/II clinical trial is underway.[165-167] Gene therapy for SCD also has the potential to positively impact pulmonary function, but it is too early to draw any conclusions on this outcome.

Outcomes

Asthma is associated with increased morbidity and mortality in SCD and is a modifiable risk factor. What has emerged from a growing body of evidence is that although the asthma observed in the general population may occur in patients with SCD, there is also an airway disease unique to SCD that has overlapping but distinct mechanisms and features. Irrespective of the mechanisms of the airway inflammation, given the gravity of the potential morbidity and mortality in SCD patients, there needs to be a low threshold for the diagnosis and treatment of asthma or an asthma-like condition.

Future Research and Clinical Directions

In contrast to cystic fibrosis, another genetically mediated, multisystem disease with chronic airway inflammation, airway disease in patients with SCD has been underrecognized and underinvestigated for many years. Much of the data pertaining to the pathophysiology and clinical characteristics have been published only within the past 10 years. The interventional studies discussed in this chapter have been even more recent. The current therapeutics under investigation and studies in gene therapy are exciting, but we have only begun to scratch the surface in understanding the airway disease in SCD and much remains to be done. As we have seen, there are conflicting findings about changes in pulmonary function, although the cumulative evidence seems to tilt in the direction of progressive decline and a shift from obstructive disease to restrictive disease. Similarly, there are also conflicting reports regarding whether abnormal pulmonary function tests translate into morbidity in SCD. More longitudinal study of pulmonary function is needed with a clearer delineation of underlying mechanisms driving the observed changes. Similar to asthma, there appears to be more than one phenotype and endotype of airway inflammation in SCD, and these need to be better characterized. Once it is possible to identify and distinguish between the various mechanisms at play, biomarkers and therapeutic interventions will be better tailored to the individual patient. One example is how exhaled NO may be useful for monitoring the airway inflammation in some, but not all, patients with SCD. The mechanisms and therapeutic potential of inhaled corticosteroids, hydroxyurea, and vitamin D all warrant further study. Given the dysregulation of the arginine and NO metabolome in SCD and the significant burden of oxidative stress, the role of antioxidant therapies needs to be explored. Mechanisms of localized pulmonary vasoconstriction in SCD also warrant further study. Because the etiology of airway inflammation in SCD is multifactorial, the ideal therapeutic intervention would target more than one pathway. For instance, modulating inflammatory pathways while also modulating hypercoagulability would likely be more efficacious than targeting either of these individually. In summary, we could be at the brink of exciting developments for airway disease in the SCD, but much remains to be done in this area.

Expert Discussion

Although the mechanisms behind the airway inflammation in SCD are complex, there exists a subset of patients who have classic allergic asthma. As such, all patients with SCD need to be asked about asthma symptoms and wheezing in particular. These patients need to be identified early, monitored closely, and treated in conjunction with a pulmonologist and possibly an allergist to optimize asthma control and prevent unnecessary morbidity and mortality. Skin testing helps with avoidance of triggers, and exhaled NO can be a helpful measure of asthma control in these patients. Patients and families should be counseled in minimizing potential indoor allergens and irritants as much as possible. Minimizing rugs and drapes in the home aids in reducing exposure to dust mites, which are ubiquitous allergens. Similarly, mattress and pillowcase covers are helpful. Organized advocacy in public housing is also needed to avoid patients being exposed to secondhand smoke inhalation, mold, rodents, and cockroaches.

Patients who do not have an atopic phenotype present more of a diagnostic and therapeutic challenge, and risk stratification for screening should be considered. Although wheezing with exercise, wheezing associated with shortness of breath, and parental history of asthma are associated with a clinician diagnosis of asthma, these are also typical questions on validated asthma questionnaires. While validated asthma questionnaires were found to have good sensitivity and specificity with a clinician diagnosis of asthma in SCD patients, this does not hold true when the questionnaires are compared to objective measures of AHR; the lack of correlation may be due to poor perception of symptoms as well as altered pathophysiologic mechanisms in SCD.

The correlation between measures of AHR and lower airway obstruction with increased morbidity in SCD is unclear.[1,3,6,8,11015,17,18,21,48,52,58-60] The growing body of evidence of a proinflammatory state and exaggerated inflammatory response in the lungs of SCD patients is undeniable. When viewed in the context of the histologic, cellular, and molecular findings in the lungs of SCD patients, it is difficult to presume that abnormal pulmonary function testing is benign. Along the same lines, it is difficult to comprehend the NHLBI Guidelines for the Management of Sickle Cell recommending that pulmonary function testing be performed only if there are signs and symptoms suggestive of asthma. Even in uncomplicated asthma, the concept of poor perception of symptoms is recognized and a known risk factor for increased mortality. Furthermore, normal pulmonary function tests in individuals with asthma do not exclude the diagnosis of asthma.

Although beyond the scope of this chapter, patients with SCD may have diffusion abnormalities and restrictive disease on pulmonary function testing. Comprehensive pulmonary function testing is part of a dyspnea evaluation. On average, children can perform pulmonary function testing starting at the age of 6 years. These tests can thus provide a noninvasive screening tool for insidious lung disease in SCD patients, and in an asymptomatic patient, these tests may be performed every 1 to 2 years.

Patients without atopy or classic asthma symptoms may still have risk factors for asthma or other underlying lung pathology. Patients with recurrent ACS, poorly controlled pain, and recurrent vaso-occlusive crises despite adherence to their hematologic therapies may have underlying pulmonary pathology. Other risk factors include a history of prematurity, allergic or chronic rhinitis, gastroesophageal reflux disease, dysphagia with recurrent aspiration, scoliosis, congenital heart disease, obesity, and snoring suggestive of OSA. These patients all warrant referral to a pulmonologist for further evaluation.

Finally, when treating patients for an acute asthma exacerbation, systemic steroids should be used based on NHLBI asthma guidelines. Although some have anecdotally raised concerns about increased risk for rebound vaso-occlusive episodes, this has not been substantiated in subsequent studies. Steroids given in conjunction with red cell transfusion have been shown to be safe, effective, and well tolerated. A steroid taper can also be used as a precaution for mitigating the possibility of rebound pain and vaso-occlusion. Furthermore, not treating an asthma exacerbation means exposing the patient to increased morbidity as the cycle of ongoing hypoxia, sickling, and hemolysis continues without interruption, not to mention that an acute asthma exacerbation itself can be fatal.

Conclusion

In summary, the lungs play an integral role in SCD. The prevention of hypoxia, even subclinical hypoxia, offers a means by which to prevent or at least delay irreversible lung disease in the form of airway remodeling and pulmonary vasculopathy. The challenge remains to better define the mechanisms and subtypes of airway inflammation in the lungs of SCD patients to facilitate diagnosis, monitoring, and the development of targeted therapeutic interventions. Meanwhile, it is essential to monitor and treat comorbid asthma given the severe consequences of untreated asthma in this vulnerable population of patients.

Case Study

A 12-year-old girl with SCD (HbSS) and a history of recurrent ACS presents to the ED with shortness of breath and fever. Symptoms developed earlier in the day. Vital signs are significant for hypoxemia (pulse oximetry 92% on room air), fever to 102°F, tachypnea (respiratory rate in the 40s), and tachycardia (140-150 bpm). On exam, she has subcostal and intercostal retractions and suprasternal tug. Wheezing with prolonged expiratory phase is appreciated bilaterally; aeration to bases is diminished, and aeration to posterior superior aspect of chest wall is also diminished. She is well perfused, with a capillary refill of <2 seconds. She has not complained of pain prior to arrival to the ED but now complains of chest pain, abdominal pain, and back pain that are a 7 on a scale of 0 to 10.

Labs obtained are significant for influenza A–positive direct fluorescent antibody, elevated white blood cell count (17,000/μL), hemoglobin of 6.5 g/dL (baseline, ~8.0 g/dL), and elevated platelets (900,000/μL). Chest x-ray shows a well-delineated homogeneous opacity to the right upper lobe region that is read as an infiltrate by the ED physician.

On further history, she has used bronchodilator therapy during past episodes of ACS, but otherwise, she does not take any inhaled medications at home. She does complain of chest pain when she runs. She is also known to experience seasonal allergies and sometimes wheezes during the spring and fall months. She also has wheezing during ACS. Otherwise, she has no history of coughing and wheezing at rest. She is on hydroxyurea therapy, but adherence has been suboptimal.

She is placed on ceftriaxone and azithromycin therapy in the ED given that she meets the clinical definition for ACS. Accordingly, she is also placed on bronchodilator therapy followed by incentive spirometry every 4 hours while her pain is being controlled with intravenous morphine and ketorolac. Blood is also ordered for simple transfusion. However, both her clinical picture and radiographic findings also fit with status asthmaticus. The chest x-ray interpretation by the pediatric radiologist leans towards right upper lobe atelectasis rather than infiltrate/pneumonia. Typically for status asthmaticus, this would mean that systemic steroids and supplemental oxygen are administered and bronchodilator therapy is given continuously until her respiratory status improves. Discussion ensues as to whether she can be treated for status asthmaticus in the same way that a patient without SCD would be treated.

How to Treat Discussion Points

Q: Supplemental oxygen inhibits hematopoiesis. Is it not better to tolerate a borderline low oxygenation?

A: Low oxygenation promotes regional lung hypoxia that in turn leads to ventilation-perfusion mismatch. When hypoxic regions of lung are perfused, this leads to worsening of the patient's overall oxygenation, and in SCD, the pathologic mechanisms of hemolysis, vaso-occlusion, and hypoxia with reperfusion injury are all amplified. As such, supplemental oxygen should be given liberally, and packed red blood cell (pRBC) transfusions given when needed.

Q: There are reports of systemic steroids leading to rebound pain crises and patients needing to be readmitted. Should systemic steroids be used in this patient's case? Are there scenarios in which patients with SCD should not be given steroids even if the clinical picture is consistent with status asthmaticus?

A: Systemic steroids should be given to a patient with SCD in status asthmaticus just as they should be given to any other patient in status asthmaticus. Risk of rebound pain can be averted if pRBC transfusions are given at the same time that steroids are initiated. In our practice, we also use a steroid taper; however, there remains a paucity of data to define best practice. However, hypoxia that continues unabated will perpetuate vaso-occlusion and hemolysis. In other words, **not** giving steroids may result in recurrent vaso-occlusive episodes.

Q: Should the patient see a pulmonologist as an outpatient once she recovers from her acute illness?

A: Yes; despite the fact that she does not complain of much in the way of persistent asthma symptoms, the story of recurrent ACS in a child with dyspnea and chest pain with exercise raises a red flag. A comorbid diagnosis of asthma increases the risk for recurrent ACS. Meanwhile, many children with SCD do not complain of classic asthma signs and symptoms. In her case, she also has a slightly atopic history, but even if that were not the case, she needs to be assessed with pulmonary function tests when she is at baseline and further history obtained. Given the history of recurrent ACS and her current presentation of status asthmaticus, irrespective of her pulmonary function test results, she has asthma and needs to start a chronic asthma maintenance regimen.

High-Yield Facts

◆ A comorbid diagnosis of asthma in children with sickle cell disease (SCD) is associated with increased morbidity and mortality. Asthma is linked to increased rates of acute chest syndrome (ACS), vaso-occlusive pain crises, and stroke, but it is also a modifiable risk factor. Making the diagnosis of asthma early and achieving good asthma control contributes to improved outcomes.

◆ The incidence of asthma in children with SCD is much higher than that in children without SCD. Asthma is more prevalent in children as opposed to adults with SCD. Adults with SCD more commonly have restrictive lung disease. A significant and progressive yearly decline in lung function is seen in children with SCD.

◆ The diagnosis of asthma in children with SCD can be challenging. Many validated symptom-based questionnaires for the diagnosis of asthma in children have poor sensitivity and specificity in children with SCD. Yet on a cellular and molecular level, just as in asthma, the lungs in SCD are in a proinflammatory state at baseline with exaggerated inflammatory responses to infectious, allergic, and hypoxic insults.

◆ Hemolysis plays a central role in the pathophysiologic mechanisms that drive airway inflammation in SCD. Arginine and nitric oxide dysregulation, hypoxic and ischemic reperfusion injury, and sterile inflammation are all found in asthma but further compounded in SCD due to hemolysis. Hemolysis also uniquely leads to the production of placental growth factor, which augments the leukotriene pathway and promotes neutrophil activation, bronchoconstriction, airway smooth muscle proliferation, and mucus production.

◆ The treatment approach to asthma in patients with SCD is very similar to that used for patients without SCD: inhaled corticosteroids, with or without adjunct anti–leukotriene receptor therapy and β-agonist rescue treatments, and avoidance of asthma triggers should be used for prevention, whereas systemic steroids should be given for moderate and severe exacerbations. A slow steroid taper may be considered, and hospitalized patients should receive a packed red blood cell transfusion during their steroid course to avoid the potential for a rebound pain crisis following discontinuation of steroids.

◆ Vitamin D should be optimized to 30 ng/mL or more. Vitamin D deficiency is associated with poor asthma outcomes, and in children with SCD, it is associated with an increased incidence of respiratory infections and ACS.

◆ Obstructive sleep apnea (OSA) is associated with more difficult to control asthma, and it is also more prevalent in children with SCD. Treatment of OSA leads to better asthma control. Children with snoring, mouth breathing, or other signs and symptoms concerning for OSA should be screened with a sleep study.

References

1. Boyd JH, DeBaun MR, Morgan WJ, et al. Lower airway obstruction is associated with increased morbidity in children with sickle cell disease. *Pediatr Pulmonol.* 2009;44(3):290-296.
2. Boyd JH, Macklin EA, Strunk RC, DeBaun MR. Asthma is associated with increased mortality in individuals with sickle cell anemia. *Haematologica.* 2007;92(8):1115-1118.
3. Boyd JH, Macklin EA, Strunk RC, DeBaun MR. Asthma is associated with acute chest syndrome and pain in children with sickle cell anemia. *Blood.* 2006;108(9):2923-2927.
4. Knight J, Murphy TM, Browning I. The lung in sickle cell disease. *Pediatr Pulmonol.* 1999;28(3):205-216.
5. Sylvester KP, Patey RA, Broughton S, et al. Temporal relationship of asthma to acute chest syndrome in sickle cell disease. *Pediatr Pulmonol.* 2007;42(2):103-106.
6. Sylvester KP, Patey RA, Rafferty GF, et al. Airway hyperresponsiveness and acute chest syndrome in children with sickle cell anemia. *Pediatr Pulmonol.* 2007;42(3):272-276.
7. Knight-Madden JM, Forrester TS, Lewis NA, et al. Asthma in children with sickle cell disease and its association with acute chest syndrome. *Thorax.* 2005;60(3):206-210.
8. Arteta M, Campbell A, Nouraie M, et al. Abnormal pulmonary function and associated risk factors in children and adolescents with sickle cell anemia. *J Pediatr Hematol Oncol.* 2014;36(3):185-189.
9. Global Initiative for Asthma. Pocket guide for health professionals, 2018. https://ginasthma.org/wp-content/uploads/2018/03/wms-GINA-main-pocket-guide_2018-v1.0.pdf. Accessed June 24, 2020.
10. Global Initiative for Asthma. Global strategy for asthma management and prevention, online appendix 2018. https://ginasthma.org/wp-content/uploads/2018/03/WMS-FINAL-GINA-2018-Appendix_v1.3.pdf. Accessed June 24, 2020.
11. Cohen RT, Rodeghier M, ,Kirkham FJ, et al. Exhaled nitric oxide: not associated with asthma, symptoms, or spirometry in children with sickle cell anemia. *J Allergy Clin Immunol.* 2016;138(5):1338-1343.
12. Field JJ, Stocks J, Kirkham FJ, et al. Airway hyperresponsiveness in children with sickle cell anemia. *Chest.* 2011;139(3):563-568.
13. Eiymo Mwa Mpollo MS, Brandt EB, Shanmukhappa SK, et al. Placenta growth factor augments airway hyperresponsiveness via leukotrienes and IL-13. *J Clin Invest.* 2016;126(2):571-584.
14. Gladwin MT, Ofori-Acquah SF. Erythroid DAMPs drive inflammation in SCD. *Blood.* 2014;123(24):3689-3690.
15. Shilo NR, Alawadi A, Allard-Coutu A, et al. Airway hyperreactivity is frequent in non-asthmatic children with sickle cell disease. *Pediatr Pulmonol.* 2016;51(9):950-957.
16. Lai CK, Beasley R, Crane J, et al. Global variation in the prevalence and severity of asthma symptoms: phase three of the International Study of Asthma and Allergies in Childhood (ISAAC). *Thorax.* 2009;64(6):476-483.

17. Leong MA, Dampier C, Varlotta L, et al. Airway hyperreactivity in children with sickle cell disease. *J Pediatr*. 1997;131(2):278-283.

18. Ozbek OY, Malbora B, Sen N, et al. Airway hyperreactivity detected by methacholine challenge in children with sickle cell disease. *Pediatr Pulmonol*. 2007;42(12):1187-1192.

19. Vendramini EC, Vianna EO, De Lucena Ðngulo I, et al. Lung function and airway hyperresponsiveness in adult patients with sickle cell disease. *Am J Med Sci*. 2006;332(2):68-72.

20. Sen N, Kozanoglu I, Karatasli M, et al. Pulmonary function and airway hyperresponsiveness in adults with sickle cell disease. *Lung*. 2009;187(3):195-200.

21. Koumbourlis AC, Hurlet-Jensen A, Bye MR. Lung function in infants with sickle cell disease. *Pediatr Pulmonol*. 1997;24(4):277-281.

22. Koumbourlis AC, Lee DJ, Lee A. Longitudinal changes in lung function and somatic growth in children with sickle cell disease. *Pediatr Pulmonol*. 2007;42(6):483-488.

23. Lunt A, McGhee E, Sylvester K, et al. Longitudinal assessment of lung function in children with sickle cell disease. *Pediatr Pulmonol*. 2016;51(7):717-723.

24. Field JJ, DeBaun MR, Yan Y, et al. Growth of lung function in children with sickle cell anemia. *Pediatr Pulmonol*. 2008;43(11):1061-1066.

25. Willen SM, Cohen R, Rodeghier M, et al. Age is a predictor of a small decrease in lung function in children with sickle cell anemia. *Am J Hematol*. 2018;93(3):408-415.

26. MacLean JE, Atenafu E, Kirby-Allen M, et al. Longitudinal decline in lung volume in a population of children with sickle cell disease. *Am J Respir Crit Care Med*. 2008;178(10):1055-1059.

27. Kupczyk M, Kupryś I, Górski P, et al. Long-term deterioration of lung function in asthmatic outpatients. *Respiration*. 2004;71(3):233-240.

28. Corey M, Edwards L, Levison H, et al. Longitudinal analysis of pulmonary function decline in patients with cystic fibrosis. *J Pediatr*. 1997;131(6):809-814.

29. Konstan MW, Morgan WJ, Butler SM, et al. Risk factors for rate of decline in forced expiratory volume in one second in children and adolescents with cystic fibrosis. *J Pediatr*. 2007;151(2):134-139.

30. Rosen CL, Debaun MR, Strunk RC, et al. Obstructive sleep apnea and sickle cell anemia. *Pediatrics*. 2014;134(2):273-281.

31. Caboot JB, Allen JL. Pulmonary complications of sickle cell disease in children. *Curr Opin Pediatr*. 2008;20(3):279-287.

32. Nordness ME, Lynn J, Zacharisen MC, et al. Asthma is a risk factor for acute chest syndrome and cerebral vascular accidents in children with sickle cell disease. *Clin Mol Allergy*. 2005;3(1):2.

33. Platt OS, Brambilla DJ, Rosse WF, et al. Mortality in sickle cell disease. Life expectancy and risk factors for early death. *N Engl J Med*. 1994;330(23):1639-1644.

34. Miller AC, Gladwin MT. Pulmonary complications of sickle cell disease. *Am J Respir Crit Care Med*. 2012;185(11):1154-1165.

35. Anim SO, Strunk RC, DeBaun MR. Asthma morbidity and treatment in children with sickle cell disease. *Expert Rev Respir Med*. 2011;5(5):635-645.

36. Hagar RW, Michlitsch JG, Gardner J, et al. Clinical differences between children and adults with pulmonary hypertension and sickle cell disease. *Br J Haematol*. 2008;140(1):104-112.

37. Intzes S, Kalpatthi RV, Short R, et al. Pulmonary function abnormalities and asthma are prevalent in children with sickle cell disease and are associated with acute chest syndrome. *Pediatr Hematol Oncol*. 2013;30(8):726-732.

38. Knight-Madden JM, Barton-Gooden A, Weaver SR, et al. Mortality, asthma, smoking and acute chest syndrome in young adults with sickle cell disease. *Lung*. 2013;191(1):95-100.

39. Boyd JH, Moinuddin A, Strunk RC, et al. Asthma and acute chest in sickle-cell disease. *Pediatr Pulmonol*. 2004;38(3):229-232.

40. Paul R, Minniti CP, Nouraie M, et al. Clinical correlates of acute pulmonary events in children and adolescents with sickle cell disease. *Eur J Haematol*. 2013;91(1):62-68.

41. Glassberg JA, Chow A, Wisnivesky J, et al. Wheezing and asthma are independent risk factors for increased sickle cell disease morbidity. *Br J Haematol*. 2012;159(4):472-479.

42. Glassberg JA, Wang J, Cohen R, et al. Risk factors for increased ED utilization in a multinational cohort of children with sickle cell disease. *Acad Emerg Med*. 2012;19(6):664-672.

43. Gomez, E, Morris CR. Asthma management in sickle cell disease. *Biomed Res Int*. 2013;2013:604140.

44. Wenzel SE. Asthma phenotypes: the evolution from clinical to molecular approaches. *Nat Med*. 2012;8(5):716-725.

45. Duong HT, Erzurum SC, Asosingh K. Pro-angiogenic hematopoietic progenitor cells and endothelial colony-forming cells in pathological angiogenesis of bronchial and pulmonary circulation. *Angiogenesis*. 2011;14(4):411-422.

46. Groneberg DA, Quarcoo D, Frossard N, et al. Neurogenic mechanisms in bronchial inflammatory diseases. *Allergy*. 2004;59(11):1139-1152.

47. Killian KJ, Watson R, Otis J, et al. Symptom perception during acute bronchoconstriction. *Am J Respir Crit Care Med*. 2000;162(2 Pt 1):490-496.

48. Koumbourlis AC, Zar HJ, Hurlet-Jensen A, Goldberg MR. Prevalence and reversibility of lower airway obstruction in children with sickle cell disease. *J Pediatr*. 2001;138(2):188-192.

49. Chaudry RA, Rosenthal M, Bush A, et al. Reduced forced expiratory flow but not increased exhaled nitric oxide or airway responsiveness to methacholine characterises paediatric sickle cell airway disease. *Thorax*. 2014;69(6):580-585.

50. Badawy SM, Payne AB, Rodeghier MJ, et al. Exercise capacity and clinical outcomes in adults followed in the Cooperative Study of Sickle Cell Disease (CSSCD). *Eur J Haematol*. 2018;101(4):532-541.

51. Klings ES, Wyszynski DF, Nolan VG, et al. Abnormal pulmonary function in adults with sickle cell anemia. *Am J Respir Crit Care Med*. 2006;173(11):1264-1269.

52. Morris CR. Asthma management: reinventing the wheel in sickle cell disease. *Am J Hematol*. 2009;84(4):234-241.

53. Wall MA, Platt OS, Strieder DJ. Lung function in children with sickle cell anemia. *Am Rev Respir Dis*. 1979;120(1):210-214.

54. Strunk RC, Brown MS, Boyd JH, et al. Methacholine challenge in children with sickle cell disease: a case series. *Pediatr Pulmonol*. 2008;43(9):924-929.

55. Shilo NR, Lands LC. Asthma and chronic sickle cell lung disease: a dynamic relationship. *Paediatr Respir Rev*. 2011;12(1):78-82.

56. De A, Manwani D, Rastogi D. Airway inflammation in sickle cell disease: a translational perspective. *Pediatr Pulmonol*. 2018;53(4):400-411.

57. Graham LM. Sickle cell disease: pulmonary management options. *Pediatr Pulmonol Suppl*. 2004;26:191-193.

58. Cohen RT, Strunk RC, Rodeghier M, et al. Pattern of lung function is not associated with prior or future morbidity in children with sickle cell anemia. *Ann Am Thorac Soc*. 2016;13(8):1314-1323.

59. Willen SM, Rodeghier M, Strunk RC, et al. Airway hyperresponsiveness does not predict morbidity in children with sickle cell anemia. *Am J Respir Crit Care Med.* 2017;195(11):1533-1534.

60. Yadav A, Corrales-Medina FF, Stark JM, et al. Application of an asthma screening questionnaire in children with sickle cell disease. *Pediatr Allergy Immunol Pulmonol.* 2015;28(3):177-182.

61. Sadreameli SC, Alade RO, Mogayzel PJ Jr, et al. Asthma screening in pediatric sickle cell disease: a clinic-based program using questionnaires and spirometry. *Pediatr Allergy Immunol Pulmonol.* 2017;30(4):232-238.

62. Cohen RT, Madadi A, Blinder MA, et al. Recurrent, severe wheezing is associated with morbidity and mortality in adults with sickle cell disease. *Am J Hematol.* 2011;86(9):756-761.

63. Musa BM, Galadanci NA, Rodeghier M, et al. Higher prevalence of wheezing and lower FEV1 and FVC percent predicted in adults with sickle cell anaemia: a cross-sectional study. *Respirology.* 2017;22(2):284-288.

64. Cohen RT, Klings ES, Strunk RC. Sickle cell disease: wheeze or asthma? *Asthma Res Pract.* 2015;1:14.

65. Vichinsky EP, Styles LA, Colangelo LH, et al. Acute chest syndrome in sickle cell disease: clinical presentation and course. Cooperative Study of Sickle Cell Disease. *Blood.* 1997;89(5):1787-1792.

66. Galadanci NA, Liang WH, Galadanci AA, et al. Wheezing is common in children with sickle cell disease when compared with controls. *J Pediatr Hematol Oncol.* 2015;37(1):16-19.

67. Strunk RC, Cohen RT, Cooper BP, et al. Wheezing symptoms and parental asthma are associated with a physician diagnosis of asthma in children with sickle cell anemia. *J Pediatr.* 2014;164(4):821-826.e1.

68. Bendiak GN, Mateos-Corral D, Sallam A, et al. Association of wheeze with lung function decline in children with sickle cell disease. *Eur Respir J.* 2017;50(5):1602433.

69. Potoka KP, Gladwin MT. Vasculopathy and pulmonary hypertension in sickle cell disease. *Am J Physiol Lung Cell Mol Physiol.* 2015;308(4):L314-L324.

70. Morris CR. Mechanisms of vasculopathy in sickle cell disease and thalassemia. *Hematology Am Soc Hematol Educ Program.* 2008:177-185.

71. Newaskar M, Hardy KA, Morris CR. Asthma in sickle cell disease. *ScientificWorldJournal.* 2011;11:1138-1152.

72. Morris CR, Kato GJ, Poljakovic M, et al. Dysregulated arginine metabolism, hemolysis-associated pulmonary hypertension, and mortality in sickle cell disease. *JAMA.* 2005;294(1):81-90.

73. Shilo NR, Morris CR. Pathways to pulmonary hypertension in sickle cell disease: the search for prevention and early intervention. *Expert Rev Hematol.* 2017;10(10):875-890.

74. Gladwin MT, Vichinsky E. Pulmonary complications of sickle cell disease. *N Engl J Med.* 2008;359(21):2254-2265.

75. Holgate ST. The acetaminophen enigma in asthma. *Am J Respir Crit Care Med.* 2011;183(2):147-148.

76. McBride JT. The association of acetaminophen and asthma prevalence and severity. *Pediatrics.* 2011;128(6):1181-1185.

77. Nandedkar SD, Feroah TR, Hutchins W, et al. Histopathology of experimentally induced asthma in a murine model of sickle cell disease. *Blood.* 2008;112(6):2529-2538.

78. Andemariam B, Adami AJ, Singh A, et al. The sickle cell mouse lung: proinflammatory and primed for allergic inflammation. *Transl Res.* 2015;166(3):254-268.

79. Francis RB Jr, Haywood LJ. Elevated immunoreactive tumor necrosis factor and interleukin-1 in sickle cell disease. *J Natl Med Assoc.* 1992;84(7):611-615.

80. Croizat H. Circulating cytokines in sickle cell patients during steady state. *Br J Haematol.* 1994;87(3):592-597.

81. Malave I, Perdomo Y, Escalona E, et al. Levels of tumor necrosis factor alpha/cachectin (TNF alpha) in sera from patients with sickle cell disease. *Acta Haematol.* 1993;90(4):172-176.

82. Graido-Gonzalez E, Doherty JC, Bergreen EW, et al. Plasma endothelin-1, cytokine, and prostaglandin E2 levels in sickle cell disease and acute vaso-occlusive sickle crisis. *Blood.* 1998;92(7):2551-2555.

83. Lanaro C, Franco-Penteado CF, Albuqueque DM, et al. Altered levels of cytokines and inflammatory mediators in plasma and leukocytes of sickle cell anemia patients and effects of hydroxyurea therapy. *J Leukoc Biol.* 2009;85(2):235-242.

84. Langer AL, Kim-Schulze S, Ginzburg Y, et al. Inhaled steroids associated with decreased macrophage markers in nonasthmatic individuals with sickle cell disease in a randomized trial. *Ann Hematol.* 2019;98(4):841-849.

85. Holtzclaw JD, Jack D, Aguayo SM, et al. Enhanced pulmonary and systemic response to endotoxin in transgenic sickle mice. *Am J Respir Crit Care Med.* 2004;169(6):687-695.

86. Kaul DK, Hebbel RP. Hypoxia/reoxygenation causes inflammatory response in transgenic sickle mice but not in normal mice. *J Clin Invest.* 2000;106(3):411-420.

87. Field JJ, Burdick MD, DeBaun MR, et al. The role of fibrocytes in sickle cell lung disease. *PLoS One.* 2012;7(3):e33702.

88. Pritchard KA Jr, Feroah TR, Nandedkar SD, et al. Effects of experimental asthma on inflammation and lung mechanics in sickle cell mice. *Am J Respir Cell Mol Biol.* 2012;46(3):389-396.

89. Aslan M, Freeman BA. Oxidant-mediated impairment of nitric oxide signaling in sickle cell disease: mechanisms and consequences. *Cell Mol Biol.* 2004;50(1):95-105.

90. Granger DN, Kvietys PR. Reperfusion injury and reactive oxygen species: the evolution of a concept. *Redox Biol.* 2015;6:524-551.

91. Osarogiagbon UR, Choong S, Belcher JD, et al. Reperfusion injury pathophysiology in sickle transgenic mice. *Blood.* 2000;96(1):314-320.

92. Pritchard KA Jr, Ou J, Ou Z, et al. Hypoxia-induced acute lung injury in murine models of sickle cell disease. *Am J Physiol Lung Cell Mol Physiol.* 2004;286(4):L705-L714.

93. Wallace KL, Marshall MA, Ramos SI, et al. NKT cells mediate pulmonary inflammation and dysfunction in murine sickle cell disease through production of IFN-gamma and CXCR3 chemokines. *Blood.* 2009;14(3):667-676.

94. Wallace KL, Linden J. Adenosine A2A receptors induced on iNKT and NK cells reduce pulmonary inflammation and injury in mice with sickle cell disease. *Blood* 2010;116(23):5010-5020.

95. Styles LA, Aarsman AJ, Vichinsky EP, et al. Secretory phospholipase A(2) predicts impending acute chest syndrome in sickle cell disease. *Blood.* 2000;96(9):3276-3278.

96. Styles LA, Schalkwijk CG, Aarsman AJ, et al. Phospholipase A2 levels in acute chest syndrome of sickle cell disease. *Blood.* 1996;87(6):2573-2578.

97. Styles L, Wager CG, Labotka RJ, et al. Refining the value of secretory phospholipase A2 as a predictor of acute chest syndrome in sickle cell disease: results of a feasibility study (PROACTIVE). *Br J Haematol.* 2012;157(5):627-636.

98. Peters-Golden M, Henderson WR Jr. Leukotrienes. *N Engl J Med.* 2007;357(18):1841-1854.

99. Jennings JE, Ramkumar T, Jingnan Mao J, et al. Elevated urinary leukotriene E4 levels are associated with hospitalization for pain in children with sickle cell disease. *Am J Hematol.* 2008;83(8):640-643.

100. Setty BN, Stuart MJ. Eicosanoids in sickle cell disease: potential relevance of neutrophil leukotriene B4 to disease pathophysiology. *J Lab Clin Med.* 2002;139(2):80-89.

101. Patel N, Gonsalves CS, Malik P, et al. Placenta growth factor augments endothelin-1 and endothelin-B receptor expression via hypoxia-inducible factor-1 alpha. *Blood.* 2008;112(3):856-865.

102. Patel N, Gonsalves CS, Yang M, et al. Placenta growth factor induces 5-lipoxygenase-activating protein to increase leukotriene formation in sickle cell disease. *Blood.* 2009;113(5):1129-1138.

103. Field JJ, DeBaun MR. Asthma and sickle cell disease: two distinct diseases or part of the same process? *Hematology Am Soc Hematol Educ Program.* 2009;45-53.

104. Karlsson EA, Oguin TH, Meliopoulos V, et al. Vascular permeability drives susceptibility to influenza infection in a murine model of sickle cell disease. *Sci Rep.* 2017;7:43308.

105. Kato GJ, Steinberg MH, Gladwin MT. Intravascular hemolysis and the pathophysiology of sickle cell disease. *J Clin Invest.* 2017;127(3):750-760.

106. Reiter CD, Wang X, Tanus-Santos JE, et al. Cell-free hemoglobin limits nitric oxide bioavailability in sickle-cell disease. *Nat Med.* 2002;8(12):1383-1389.

107. Kato GJ, Gladwin MT, Steinberg MH. Deconstructing sickle cell disease: reappraisal of the role of hemolysis in the development of clinical subphenotypes. *Blood Rev.* 2007;21(1):37-47.

108. Rother RP, Bell L, Hillmen P, Gladwin M. The clinical sequelae of intravascular hemolysis and extracellular plasma hemoglobin: a novel mechanism of human disease. *JAMA.* 2005;293(13):1653-1662.

109. Morris CR. Alterations of the arginine metabolome in sickle cell disease: a growing rationale for arginine therapy. *Hematol Oncol Clin North Am.* 2014;28(2):301-321.

110. Maarsingh H, Zuidhof AB, Bos IS, et al. Arginase inhibition protects against allergen-induced airway obstruction, hyperresponsiveness, and inflammation. *Am J Respir Crit Care Med.* 2008;178(6):565-573.

111. Wood KC, Hsu LL, Gladwin MT. Sickle cell disease vasculopathy: a state of nitric oxide resistance. *Free Radic Biol Med.* 2008;44(8):1506-1528.

112. Kato GJ, Wang Z, Machado RF, et al. Endogenous nitric oxide synthase inhibitors in sickle cell disease: abnormal levels and correlations with pulmonary hypertension, desaturation, haemolysis, organ dysfunction and death. *Br J Haematol.* 2009;145(4):506-513.

113. Schnog JB, Teerlink T, van der Dijs FP, et al. Plasma levels of asymmetric dimethylarginine (ADMA), an endogenous nitric oxide synthase inhibitor, are elevated in sickle cell disease. *Ann Hematol.* 2005;84(5):282-286.

114. Scott JA, North ML, Rafii M, et al. Asymmetric dimethylarginine is increased in asthma. *Am J Respir Crit Care Med.* 2011;184(7):779-785.

115. Chen G, Zhang D, Fuchs TA, et al. Heme-induced neutrophil extracellular traps contribute to the pathogenesis of sickle cell disease. *Blood.* 2014;123(24):3818-3827.

116. Dweik RA, Boggs PB, Erzurum SC, et al. An official ATS clinical practice guideline: interpretation of exhaled nitric oxide levels (FENO) for clinical applications. *Am J Respir Crit Care Med.* 2011;184(5):602-615.

117. Girgis RE, Qureshi MA, Abrams J, et al. Decreased exhaled nitric oxide in sickle cell disease: relationship with chronic lung involvement. *Am J Hematol.* 2003;72(3):177-184.

118. Radhakrishnan DK, Bendiak GN, Mateos-Corral D, et al. Lower airway nitric oxide is increased in children with sickle cell disease. *J Pediatr.* 2012;160(1):93-97.

119. Lunt A, Ahmed N, Rafferty GF, et al. Airway and alveolar nitric oxide production, lung function, and pulmonary blood flow in sickle cell disease. *Pediatr Res.* 2016;79(2):313-317.

120. Lunt A, Desai SR, Wells AU, et al. Pulmonary function, CT and echocardiographic abnormalities in sickle cell disease. *Thorax.* 2014;69(8):746-751.

121. Morris CR, Kuypers FA, Larkin S, et al. Patterns of arginine and nitric oxide in patients with sickle cell disease with vaso-occlusive crisis and acute chest syndrome. *J Pediatr Hematol Oncol.* 2000;22(6):515-520.

122. Miller MK, Lee JH, Miller DP, et al. Recent asthma exacerbations: a key predictor of future exacerbations. *Respir Med.* 2007;101(3):481-489.

123. Raissy HH, Kelly HW, Harkins M, et al. Inhaled corticosteroids in lung diseases. *Am J Respir Crit Care Med.* 2013;187(8):798-803.

124. Wechsler ME, Kelley JM, Boyd IO, et al. Active albuterol or placebo, sham acupuncture, or no intervention in asthma. *N Engl J Med.* 2011;365(2):119-126.

125. Loymans RJ, Honkoop PJ, Termeer EH, et al. Identifying patients at risk for severe exacerbations of asthma: development and external validation of a multivariable prediction model. *Thorax.* 2016;71(9):838-846.

126. Wade S, Weil C, Holden G, et al. Psychosocial characteristics of inner-city children with asthma: a description of the NCICAS psychosocial protocol. National Cooperative Inner-City Asthma Study. *Pediatr Pulmonol.* 1997;24(4):63-76.

127. Klinnert MD, Nelson HS, Price MR, et al. Onset and persistence of childhood asthma: predictors from infancy. *Pediatrics.* 2001;108(4):E69.

128. Kozyrskyj AL, Mai XM, McGrath P, et al. Continued exposure to maternal distress in early life is associated with an increased risk of childhood asthma. *Am J Respir Crit Care Med.* 2008;177(2):142-147.

129. Bhatt RR, Martin SR, Evans S, et al. The effect of hypnosis on pain and peripheral blood flow in sickle-cell disease: a pilot study. *J Pain Res.* 2017;10:1635-1644.

130. Khaleel M, Shah P, Sunwoo J, et al. Individuals with sickle cell disease have a significantly greater vasoconstriction response to thermal pain than controls and have significant vasoconstriction in response to anticipation of pain. *Am J Hematol.* 2017;92(11):1137-1145.

131. Shah P, Khaleel M, Thuptimdang W, et al. Mental stress causes vasoconstriction in sickle cell disease and normal controls. *Haematologica.* 2019;105(1):83-90.

132. Hebbel RP. Extracorpuscular factors in the pathogenesis of sickle cell disease. *Am J Pediatr Hematol Oncol.* 1982;4(3):316-319.

133. Vichinsky EP, Neumayr LD, Earles AN, et al. Causes and outcomes of the acute chest syndrome in sickle cell disease. National Acute Chest Syndrome Study Group. *N Engl J Med.* 2000;342(25):1855-1865.

134. Sobota A, Graham DA, Heeney MM, et al. Corticosteroids for acute chest syndrome in children with sickle cell disease: variation in use and association with length of stay and readmission. *Am J Hematol.* 2010;85(1):24-28.

135. Griffin TC, McIntire D, Buchanan GR. High-dose intravenous methylprednisolone therapy for pain in children and adolescents with sickle cell disease. *N Engl J Med.* 1994;330(11):733-737.

136. Bernini JC, Rogers ZR, Sandler ES, et al. Beneficial effect of intravenous dexamethasone in children with mild to moderately severe acute chest syndrome complicating sickle cell disease. *Blood.* 1998;92(9):3082-3089.

137. Darbari DS, Fasano RS, Minniti CP, et al. Severe vaso-occlusive episodes associated with use of systemic corticosteroids in patients with sickle cell disease. *J Natl Med Assoc.* 2008;100(8):948-951.

138. Couillard S, Benkerrou M, Girot R, et al. Steroid treatment in children with sickle-cell disease. *Haematologica.* 2007;92(3):425-426.

139. Quinn CT, Stuart MJ, Kesler K, et al. Tapered oral dexamethasone for the acute chest syndrome of sickle cell disease. *Br J Haematol.* 2011;155(2):263-267.

140. Isakoff MS, Lillo JA, Hagstrom JN. A single-institution experience with treatment of severe acute chest syndrome: lack of rebound pain with dexamethasone plus transfusion therapy. *J Pediatr Hematol Oncol.* 2008;30(4):322-325.

141. Ogunlesi F, Heeney MM, Koumbourlis AC. Systemic corticosteroids in acute chest syndrome: friend or foe? *Paediatr Respir Rev.* 2014;15(1):24-27.

142. Su Z, Li R, Gai Z. Intravenous and nebulized magnesium sulfate for treating acute asthma in children: a systematic review and meta-analysis. *Pediatr Emerg Care.* 2018;34(6):390-395.

143. Irazuzta JE, Chiriboga N. Magnesium sulfate infusion for acute asthma in the emergency department. *J Pediatr.* 2017;93(suppl 1): 19-25.

144. Korang SK, Feinberg J, Wetterslev J, et al. Non-invasive positive pressure ventilation for acute asthma in children. *Cochrane Database Syst Rev.* 2016;9(9):CD012067.

145. Adisa OA, Gee B, Taylor N, et al. Use of BiPAP in the management of acute chest syndrome (ACS) in children with sickle cell disease (SCD). Presented at the Pediatric Academy Society Annual Meeting, Baltimore, MD, 2016.

146. Rodrigo GJ, Castro-Rodriguez JA. Heliox-driven beta2-agonists nebulization for children and adults with acute asthma: a systematic review with meta-analysis. *Ann Allergy Asthma Immunol.* 2014;112(1):29-34.

147. Hebbel RP, Eaton JW, Steinberg MH, et al. Erythrocyte/endothelial interactions in the pathogenesis of sickle-cell disease: a "real logical" assessment. *Blood Cells.* 1982;8(1):163-173.

148. Glassberg J, Minnitti C, Cromwell C, et al. Inhaled steroids reduce pain and sVCAM levels in individuals with sickle cell disease: a triple-blind, randomized trial. *Am J Hematol.* 2017;92(7):622-631.

149. DeBaun M. Phase 2 study of montelukast for the treatment of sickle cell anemia. https://clinicaltrials.gov/ct2/show/results/NCT01960413?term=montelukast&cond=sickle+cell&rank=1. Accessed June 24, 2020.

150. Malik P. Trial of zileuton CR in children and adults with sickle cell disease (zileuton). https://clinicaltrials.gov/ct2/show/NCT01136941?term=zileuton&cond=sickle+cell&rank=1. Accessed June 24, 2020.

151. Field JJ, Majerus E, Gordeuk VR, et al. Randomized phase 2 trial of regadenoson for treatment of acute vaso-occlusive crises in sickle cell disease. *Blood Adv.* 2017;1(20):1645-1649.

152. Field JJ, Majerus E, Ataga KI, et al. NNKTT120, an anti-iNKT cell monoclonal antibody, produces rapid and sustained iNKT cell depletion in adults with sickle cell disease. *PLoS One.* 2017;12(2):e0171067.

153. Thornburg CD, Files BA, Luo Z, et al. Impact of hydroxyurea on clinical events in the BABY HUG trial. *Blood.* 2012;120(22): 4304-4310.

154. Morris CR, Vichinsky EP, van Warmerdam J, et al. Hydroxyurea and arginine therapy: impact on nitric oxide production in sickle cell disease. *J Pediatr Hematol Oncol.* 2003;25(8):629-634.

155. Pacelli R, Taira J, Cook JA, et al. Hydroxyurea reacts with heme proteins to generate nitric oxide. *Lancet.* 1996;347(9005):900.

156. Cokic VP, Beleslin-Cokic BB, Tomic M, et al. Hydroxyurea induces the eNOS-cGMP pathway in endothelial cells. *Blood.* 2006;108(1):184-191.

157. King SB. Nitric oxide production from hydroxyurea. *Free Radic Biol Med.* 2004;37(6):737-744.

158. McLaren A, Klingel M, Behera S, et al. Effect of hydroxyurea therapy on pulmonary function in children with sickle cell anemia. *Am J Respir Crit Care Med.* 2017;195(5):689-691.

159. Hansdottir S, Monick MM. Vitamin D effects on lung immunity and respiratory diseases. *Vitam Horm.* 2011;86:217-237.

160. Lee MT, Kattan M, Fennoy I, et al. Randomized phase 2 trial of monthly vitamin D to prevent respiratory complications in children with sickle cell disease. *Blood Adv.* 2018;2(9):969-978.

161. Walters MC, Hardy K, Edwards S, et al. Pulmonary, gonadal, and central nervous system status after bone marrow transplantation for sickle cell disease. *Biol Blood Marrow Transplant.* 2010;16(2):263-272.

162. Hsieh MM, Fitzhugh CD, Weitzel RP, et al. Nonmyeloablative HLA-matched sibling allogeneic hematopoietic stem cell transplantation for severe sickle cell phenotype. *JAMA.* 2014;312(1):48-56.

163. Hallstrand TS, Sprenger JD, Agosti JM, et al. Long-term acquisition of allergen-specific IgE and asthma following allogeneic bone marrow transplantation from allergic donors. *Blood.* 2004;104(10):3086-3090.

164. Ribeil JA, Hacein-Bey-Abina S, Payen E, et al. Gene therapy in a patient with sickle cell disease. *N Engl J Med.* 2017;376(9): 848-855.

165. Demirci S, Leonard A, Haro-Mora JJ, et al. CRISPR/Cas9 for sickle cell disease: applications, future possibilities, and challenges. *Adv Exp Med Biol.* 2019;1144:37-52.

166. Dever DP, Bak RO, Reinisch A, et al. CRISPR/Cas9 beta-globin gene targeting in human haematopoietic stem cells. *Nature.* 2016;539(7629):384-389.

167. DeWitt MA, Magis W, Bray NL, et al. Selection-free genome editing of the sickle mutation in human adult hematopoietic stem/progenitor cells. *Sci Transl Med.* 2016;8(360):360ra134.

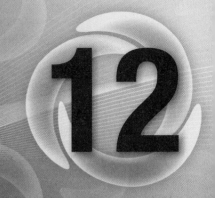

Acute Chest Syndrome

Authors: Armand Mekontso Dessap, Elliott Vichinsky

Chapter Outline

Overview

Sickle cell disease (SCD) is associated with a myriad of complications and great heterogeneity of phenotypic expression between patients and in the same patient over his or her lifetime. Several decades ago, many authors observed that no infection was found in a majority of adult patients with SCD hospitalized with a clinical presentation suggestive of community-acquired pneumonia.[1,2] Thus, they suspected other mechanisms (including vaso-occlusion–driven pulmonary infarction) and the generic term *acute chest syndrome* (ACS) was proposed to account for acute pulmonary complications of SCD.

Epidemiology

Estimates show that half of SCD patients will experience ACS during their lifetime, with an overall incidence >10 per 100 patient-years.[3] ACS is the most common reason for critical care need in SCD, accounting for up to three-quarters of admissions of adults with SCD in intensive care units.[4-6] In fact, ACS may be associated with a need for acute organ support, especially mechanical ventilation, which is required in 5% to 13% of patients with ACS in observational cohorts.[7-9]

The risk of hospital death during ACS also varies across series, ranging from 1.6% to 13%.[6-9] Age may influence the clinical picture of ACS, with a milder disease in children and a more severe disease in adults.[10] ACS is considered one of the leading causes of death from SCD, especially in adulthood.[11-13] Adults with a higher ACS rate also have a higher rate of mortality (from all causes) than those with low ACS rates.[3,11]

Adults are particularly at risk for severe, rapidly progressive ACS, resulting in respiratory failure accompanied by multiorgan dysfunction within 24 hours of onset of pulmonary symptoms. This severe form of ACS may be causally linked to sudden death.[14]

Pathophysiology

Figure 12-1 summarizes the pathophysiology of ACS. Sickling in the pulmonary circulation may be triggered by the polymerization of sickle hemoglobin (HbS) under conditions of hypoxia. The adhesion of sickled red blood cells (RBCs) to the pulmonary vessel endothelium is boosted by inflammation and endothelial dysfunction, notably via the expression of adhesion molecules on the surface of endothelial cells (eg, vascular cell adhesion molecule 1 [VCAM1] endothelial receptor) and RBCs (eg, $\alpha_4\beta_1$ integrin), as well as the alteration of nitric oxide metabolism and lipoprotein oxidation by free hemoglobin and free heme.[15,16] Some experimental studies suggest the relevance of neutrophil-platelet aggregate formation in lung arterioles in promoting lung vaso-occlusion.[17] An enhanced response to inflammatory insults could play a role in the increased susceptibility to pulmonary dysfunction that has been observed clinically in SCD.[18] The dehydration of RBCs (which alters their rheology)[19] and acidosis (which shifts the dissociation curve of hemoglobin to the right, thus promoting its deoxygenation) also play a role in vaso-occlusion.[20]

A vicious cycle has been suggested in the pathogenesis of ACS: as a result of lung injury, ventilation-perfusion mismatches and shunting ensue, with subsequent hemoglobin desaturation and hypoxemia, which in turn triggers further RBC sickling, cellular adhesion, hemolysis, and vaso-occlusion.[21,22] Experiments in SCD mice in vivo suggest a role for neutrophil-platelet aggregate formation in lung arterioles in promoting lung vaso-occlusion during ACS.[17] Several studies suggest a profound alteration of the nitric oxide pathway during ACS, with decreased production, increased consumption, and abnormal metabolism.[23] Intravascular sickling and lysis of RBCs increase cell-free hemoglobin and heme, while the scavenger plasma proteins haptoglobin and hemopexin may be depleted through lipid peroxidation and other mechanisms.[16] All these alterations may favor pulmonary vasoconstriction and endothelial dysfunction. As in other forms of acute lung injury, vasoconstriction may also be enhanced by local hypoxia and hypercapnia; lung edema and atelectasis may also favor some degree of vascular compression.[24]

Etiology: Major Categories

A specific etiology is documented in about half of ACS episodes.[9] Several causes can account for the same episode, with the 3 main causes being fat embolism, pulmonary infarction, and pulmonary infection.

Pulmonary Fat Embolism and Pulmonary Vascular Dysfunction

Pulmonary fat embolism is a distinct cause of ACS and appears to be more common in adulthood ACS than in childhood ACS. Its clinical diagnosis is often missed. Postmortem studies commonly find evidence of fat embolism.[25] It is demonstrated in 8% to 60% of ACS episodes depending on the series,[26-28] upon detection of Oil Red O-stained, lipid-laden macrophages in bronchoalveolar lavage or induced sputum. Compared with infectious etiologies, fat embolism is more often preceded by vaso-occlusive crisis (VOC), which is probably responsible for bone marrow infarction, releasing phospholipids that are then converted into free fatty acids by plasma phospholipase A2. Fat embolism is more often accompanied by thrombocytopenia, hypoxemia, neurologic features, and multiorgan failure. Patients with fat embolism had a statistically higher total white blood cell count, differential cell count of lymphocytes, and polymorphonuclear neutrophil cell count in the bronchoalveolar lavage as compared to their counterparts.[29] Fat microemboli may also enter the arterial circulation through right-to-left shunts, and the systemic release of free fatty acids may cause indirect endothelial damage.[30]

In addition to fat embolism, pulmonary vascular thrombosis and in situ microthromboses are found at autopsy.[25,31,32] Approximately 16% of ACS episodes are attributed to pulmonary infarction resulting from local vaso-occlusion.[9] High-resolution computed tomography (CT) scans often show

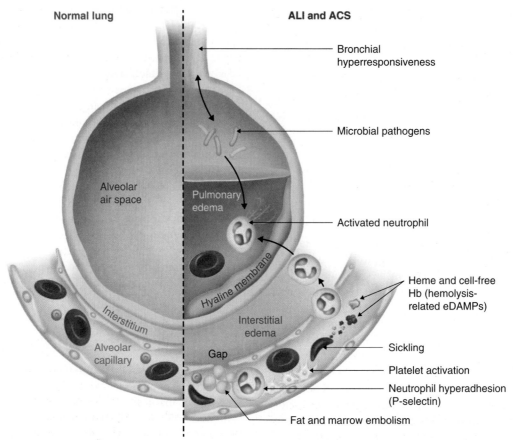

FIGURE 12-1 Pathophysiology of acute chest syndrome (ACS) and acute lung injury (ALI). The main mechanisms leading to ACS include vaso-occlusion, vasoconstriction, alveolitis, and bronchoconstriction. Bronchoconstriction is mostly experienced by children. The neutrophilic alveolitis is secondary to pulmonary infection by microbial pathogens and/or sterile inflammation driven by hemolysis and leads to pulmonary edema. Pulmonary vasoconstriction is also enhanced by hemolysis, in addition to hypoxemia and hypercapnia. Pulmonary vaso-occlusion is driven by fat embolism (from vaso-occlusive crisis–induced bone marrow necrosis), sickling within the pulmonary circulation, neutrophil endothelial hyperadhesion, platelet activation, and hypoxemia and acidosis, leading to in situ thrombosis and pulmonary infarction. eDAMPs, erythrocyte damage-associated molecular pattern molecules; Hb, hemoglobin. Reproduced, with permission, from Sundd P, Gladwin MT, Novelli EM. Pathophysiology of sickle cell disease. *Annu Rev Pathol.* 2019;14:263-292.

paucity or absence of contrast enhancement in small vessels, arterioles, and venules in the lungs of patients with ACS.[33] One study has reported the presence of pulmonary artery thrombosis in approximately 17% of ACS episodes in adults as shown by spiral CT angiography (which explores large elastic vessels >1 mm in diameter).[34] Patients with pulmonary artery thrombosis had more marked thrombocytosis and less hemolysis than those without thrombosis.[34] A clinical risk score for pulmonary artery thrombosis during ACS was proposed, which includes the following 4 factors: baseline hemoglobin >82 g/L, the lack of a triggering factor for ACS, a platelet count >440 × 10^9/L, and a partial pressure of carbon dioxide <38 mm Hg at ACS diagnosis.[35] This score has a good negative predictive value (94%) to identify ACS patients at lower risk of pulmonary artery thrombosis.[35] The hypothesis that these pulmonary thromboses are formed in situ is suggested by their peripheral distribution in the lung vasculature and the low prevalence of concomitant deep venous thrombosis.[34] However, classical pulmonary embolism may also theoretically occur, as patients

with SCD or sickle trait have significantly higher risk for deep venous thrombosis and pulmonary embolism as compared to wild-type individuals.[36,37]

Infection

In the largest study on this subject, an infection was found in one-third of patients with ACS (mostly children).[9] *Chlamydia, Mycoplasma,* and respiratory viruses (eg, respiratory syncytial virus or influenza) each accounted for about one-quarter of the infectious agents, and only 15% of the organisms were pyogenic.[9] The involvement of respiratory viruses partly explains the winter recrudescence of ACS, especially in children.[10] The burden of influenza-related hospitalizations among children with SCD is particularly high, and SCD is considered to be an independent risk factor for severe complications and death from influenza infection.[38-40] Parvovirus B19 can also trigger ACS, with a characteristic anemia due to transient RBC aplasia.[41] In adults, the prevalence of infection during ACS is generally lower than in children (<15%).[7,27,28,34,42]

Atelectasis and Hypoventilation

Chest pain-induced or analgesics-induced hypoventilation, costal infarction, and pleural effusion are likely to promote or aggravate atelectasis and pulmonary consolidation in ACS.[43] However, atelectasis is not typical of ACS by definition and is a rare finding in CT during ACS.[42]

Risk Factors

Age and Previous ACS

The occurrence of ACS is more common during childhood than during adulthood (Table 12-1).[3] Early ACS during the first years of life strongly increases the risk of ACS throughout childhood.[44,45] Among children hospitalized for VOC, those aged 5 to 9 years had 2.59 times higher odds of ACS than those aged 15 to 19 years.[46] In the elderly, the characterization of ACS is complicated by the high prevalence of chronic organ damage, including cardiac diastolic dysfunction, chronic pulmonary hypertension, and chronic lung disease.[47]

Genotype, Polymorphisms, and Laboratory Risk Factors

ACS is more common in SS and S/β^0 thalassemia patients and less common in SC and S/β^+ thalassemia patients.[3] Factors enhancing hyperviscosity (higher baseline concentration of total hemoglobin and/or leukocyte counts) are associated with a higher prevalence of ACS.[3] Conversely, a high concentration of HbF inhibits the polymerization of HbS and reduces the risk of ACS.[3]

ACS is associated with a single nucleotide polymorphism–defined β-globin cluster haplotype in children with SCD.[48] Using a genome-wide association study, a replicated genetic association was found between ACS and rs6141803, a single nucleotide polymorphism located near *COMMD7*, a gene highly expressed in the lung that interacts with nuclear factor-κB signaling.[49] Shorter alleles of a dinucleotide repeat located in the promoter region of heme oxygenase-1 are also associated with decreased rates of hospitalization for ACS.[50] Short alleles of heme oxygenase-1 gene promoter polymorphism are associated with increased activity and inducibility of heme oxygenase-1, the rate-limiting enzyme in the catabolism of heme. As compared with children with longer alleles, those with shorter alleles had lower rates of hospitalization for ACS, after adjustment for other factors influencing ACS occurrence.[50] β^S polymorphism sites across the β-globin locus influence the fetal hemoglobin level and are associated with ACS occurrence.[48]

Environment

Environmental features can be triggering factors of ACS. Patients with SCD exhibit hypersensitivity to thermal but not mechanical stimuli.[51] Winter season, colder temperatures, and higher wind speed were associated with a higher incidence of VOC and/or ACS in children and adults,[52-55] although other reports suggest an association between ACS and the summer and fall seasons.[46] The risk of emergency admission for VOC and/or ACS was also significantly associated with higher values of atmospheric particulate matter and with lower values of carbon monoxide.[55] The latter finding may corroborate the significant impact of carbon monoxide on the RBC life span,[56] vascular inflammation, and organ pathology in SCD.[57]

Comorbid Etiologies

VOC

VOC is considered a prodrome of ACS because it precedes and/or accompanies the majority of ACS episodes.[9,10] ACS secondary to VOC represented 50% of ACS cases in a prospective study, appearing a mean of 2.5 days after admission for VOC.[9] A score predicting ACS in adults with VOC has been proposed; it is based on reticulocyte and leukocyte counts, hemoglobin, and spine and/or pelvis pain.[58]

Surgery and Pregnancy

Pregnancy (especially the postpartum period) poses a high risk of ACS.[59] The risk of developing an ACS episode appears to be increased following surgery. For example, the incidence of ACS after splenectomy in SCD patients has been reported to be around 20%.[60,61] Some authors suggest that laparoscopic surgery promotes a lower postoperative risk of ACS.[61]

Smoking, Asthma, and Bronchoreactive Lung Disease

Children with SCD who are exposed to environmental tobacco smoke have a higher risk of VOC and/or ACS requiring hospitalization than do those not exposed.[62,63] Active smoking is

TABLE 12-1 Risk factors and triggers of acute chest syndrome

Risk factors	Triggers
Age: childhood	VOC episode
Genotype: SS and S/β^0 thalassemia genotypes	Recent surgery
Polymorphisms: *COMMD7*, heme oxygenase-1, and β-globin	Pregnancy and postpartum
Baseline biology: lower HbF, higher total hemoglobin, and/or leukocyte counts	Winter season, colder temperatures, and higher wind speed
Passive or active smoking	Pollution (eg, higher values of atmospheric particulate matter)
Crosslink with asthma/ airway hyperreactivity	

Abbreviations: HbF, fetal hemoglobin; VOC, vaso-occlusive crisis.

also associated with an increased risk of ACS and pain among adolescents and adults.[64,65]

Asthma exacerbation and ACS have overlapping risk factors and symptoms.[66] Bronchial hyperresponsiveness seems more common in children with SCD than in ethnically matched controls.[67] There may be a biologic link between asthma and ACS in SCD. Patients with SCD have elevated plasma arginase activity, decreased nitric oxide, and nitric oxide synthase gene polymorphisms.[68] Asthma (particularly atopic) and obstructive sleep apnea seem to increase the risk of ACS in childhood and adolescence.[45,46,67,69-72] Asthma and wheezing may represent more significant risk factors for the development of ACS in children with hemoglobin SC disease.[73] Documentation of asthma episodes in patients with SCD is poor,[69] and there is a need for baseline spirometry assessment. Smoking and asthma were also found to be independent risk factors for death in young adults with SCD during a 10-year period.[67] Contrary to obstructive lung disease, the correlation of restrictive lung disease with ACS is less obvious.[74]

Pulmonary Edema and Transfusion-Related Acute Lung Injury

There are multiple iatrogenic complications that lead to acute pulmonary disease that may amplify ACS or precipitate it. Pulmonary edema in adults is a relatively common complication of aggressive fluid replacement in older patients.[75] Vigorous fluid replacement may enhance pulmonary edema and lung injury during ACS.[75] Infection and inflammation, as well as underlying cardiopulmonary disease, increase vascular permeability, exacerbating pulmonary disease.[76] In sickle cell patients who have been recently transfused, consideration of transfusion related acute lung injury (TRALI) in the differential diagnosis of ACS is required.[77] TRALI may mimic, exacerbate, or trigger ACS.[77]

Other Cardiopulmonary Comorbidities

The relationship between ACS and chronic pulmonary hypertension during SCD is complex. Elevated tricuspid regurgitant velocity is known to be a physiologic biomarker of severity in adult patients with SCD.[78,79] A higher tricuspid regurgitant velocity was independently associated with history of acute pulmonary events,[45] but other reports found no relationship between ACS and steady-state pulmonary pressures in children[80-82] and adults.[79,83] Low nocturnal oxygen saturation is associated with a higher rate of VOC and potentially secondary risk of ACS.[84]

Definition

The generic term *ACS* was proposed to account for acute pulmonary complications of SCD. The pragmatic definition of ACS is variable in the literature but always includes the association of a clinical symptom and a radiologic criterion.

The clinical symptom is either general (fever) or respiratory (chest pain, dyspnea, polypnea, cough, crepitation, and more rarely sibilant wheezes or hemoptysis). Some patients have a characteristic "golden yellow" expectoration, which is not a cornerstone criterion for the definition and seems to be the result of an intense pulmonary exudative process.[85]

The radiologic criterion is usually a "new opacity on chest x-ray,"[1,26] and some authors add "it should be at least segmental, suggestive of a consolidation, and exclude atelectasis."[9] In general, the latter statement defines more severe patients.[42] Bedside chest x-rays have good sensitivity (>85%) for the radiologic diagnosis of ACS, but with a relatively low specificity (<60%) when compared with chest CT scan as a reference.[42] The parenchymal opacities seen in ACS are typically consolidation (ground-glass pattern is rare and atelectasis is exceptional).[42] Positron emission tomography imaging shows an intense inflammatory activity in the zones of consolidation (see case study, later in this chapter).[86] There is clear basal predominance of consolidations in adults (see case study), and the absence of lower lobe involvement should drive the diagnosis toward ACS in adults.[10,42] This clear basal predominance of consolidations is not found in young children,[10] and its explanation is not straightforward, as it could involve the anatomic distribution of pulmonary vascularization in humans. Moderate pleural effusion is present in a quarter of cases, mostly in severe forms, and generally does not require drainage.[42]

Laboratory Findings

ACS is accompanied by a nonspecific biologic inflammatory syndrome (leukocytosis) and moderate hemolysis (decrease in hemoglobin of ~1 g/dL, increase in lactate dehydrogenase [LDH] and bilirubin).[9] Platelet count is variable, ranging from thrombocytosis, which may increase the risk of pulmonary artery thrombosis, to thrombocytopenia, which may be associated with bone marrow infarction and fat embolism.[26] Hypoxemia affects at least 20% of patients.[10] The partial pressure of carbon dioxide varies from one patient to another: hypercapnia can be precipitated by pain or high-dose morphine-induced hypoventilation, whereas normocapnia/hypocapnia can be caused by hyperventilation associated with acute lung injury and extensive parenchymal involvement.[7,86] The search for extrapulmonary organ failure should be systematic and focused on right heart dysfunction (echocardiography for acute pulmonary hypertension or acute cor pulmonale),[7] as well as liver and kidney dysfunction (liver and renal function tests).[87]

Evaluation and Monitoring

Figure 12-2 depicts the paradigm for overall diagnosis and management of ACS. Close monitoring is necessary given the rapid evolution of ACS in some cases, necessitating a rapid transfer to intensive care unit or tertiary center.

Clinical

Evaluation for diagnosis consists of exclusion of alternative diagnoses (eg, cardiogenic pulmonary edema, TRALI) and careful clinical assessment of the following systems:

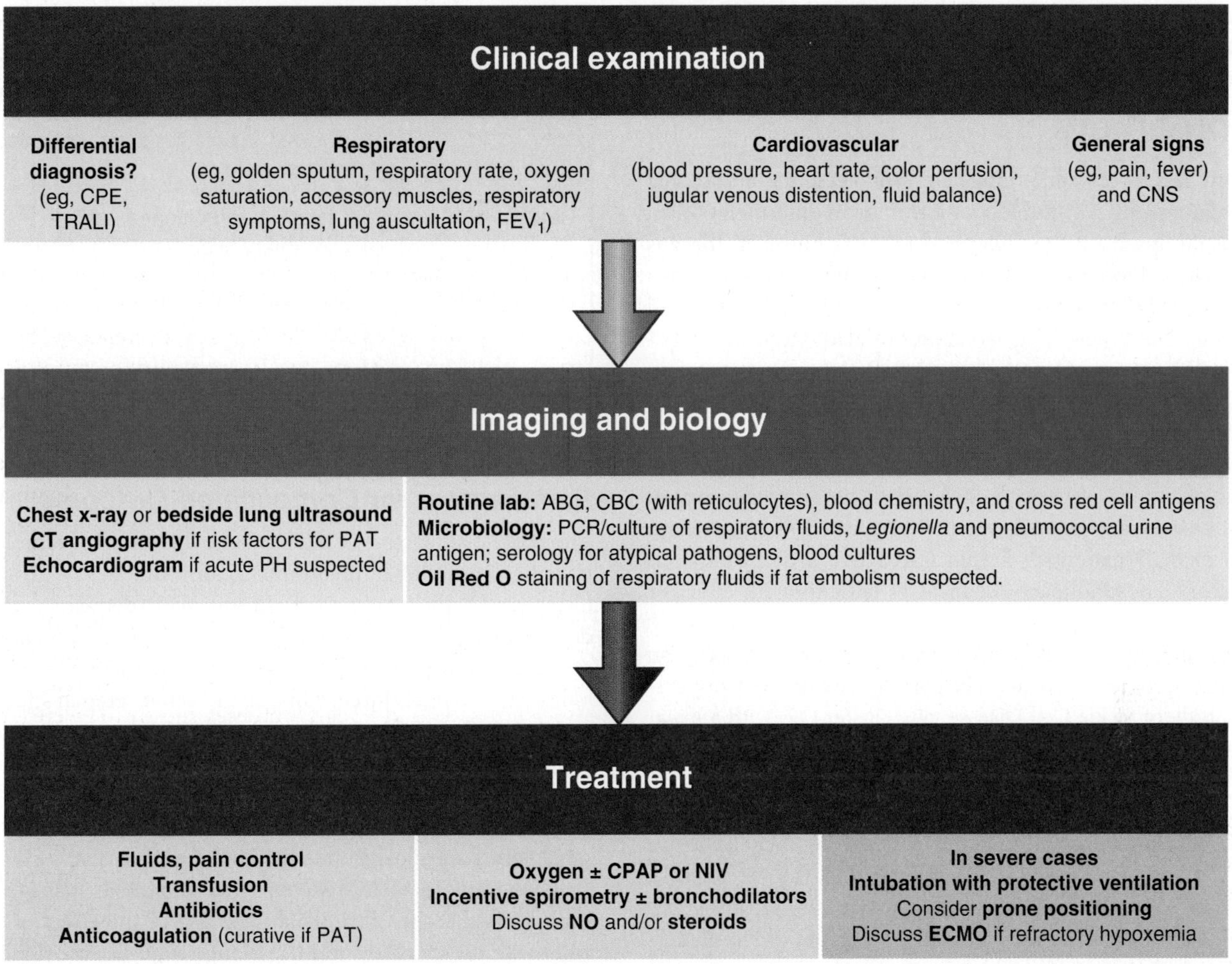

Clinical examination

| **Differential diagnosis?** (eg, CPE, TRALI) | **Respiratory** (eg, golden sputum, respiratory rate, oxygen saturation, accessory muscles, respiratory symptoms, lung auscultation, FEV$_1$) | **Cardiovascular** (blood pressure, heart rate, color perfusion, jugular venous distention, fluid balance) | **General signs** (eg, pain, fever) and CNS |

Imaging and biology

| **Chest x-ray or bedside lung ultrasound** **CT angiography** if risk factors for PAT **Echocardiogram** if acute PH suspected | **Routine lab:** ABG, CBC (with reticulocytes), blood chemistry, and cross red cell antigens **Microbiology:** PCR/culture of respiratory fluids, *Legionella* and pneumococcal urine antigen; serology for atypical pathogens, blood cultures **Oil Red O** staining of respiratory fluids if fat embolism suspected. |

Treatment

| **Fluids, pain control** **Transfusion** **Antibiotics** **Anticoagulation** (curative if PAT) | **Oxygen ± CPAP or NIV** **Incentive spirometry ± bronchodilators** Discuss **NO** and/or **steroids** | **In severe cases** **Intubation with protective ventilation** Consider **prone positioning** Discuss **ECMO** if refractory hypoxemia |

FIGURE 12-2 Paradigm for overall diagnosis and management of acute chest syndrome. ABG, arterial blood gases; CBC, cell blood count; CNS, central nervous system; CPAP, continuous positive airway pressure; CPE, cardiogenic pulmonary edema; CT, computed tomography; ECMO, extracorporeal membrane oxygenation; FEV$_1$, forced expiratory volume in 1 second; NIV, noninvasive ventilation; NO, inhaled nitric oxide; PAT, pulmonary artery thrombosis; PCR, polymerase chain reaction; PH, pulmonary hypertension; TRALI, transfusion-related acute lung injury.

constitutional (eg, fever), respiratory (eg, respiratory rate, transcutaneous oxygen saturation, accessory muscles, respiratory symptoms, lung auscultation, forced expiratory volume in 1 second), cardiovascular (eg, blood pressure, heart rate, color perfusion, jugular venous distention, fluid balance), and central nervous system.

Laboratory Assessment, Imaging, and Procedures

Routine laboratory assessment comprises arterial blood gases, cell blood count (with evaluation of changes in platelets, hemoglobin, and reticulocytes), blood chemistry, and RBC type and crossing.

Chest x-ray is essential to look for the diagnostic criteria of ACS, albeit the diagnostic value of bedside chest x-ray is far from perfect.[42] Lung ultrasonography is a promising avenue for better bedside imaging.[88] Lung ultrasound outperformed chest x-ray for the diagnosis of consolidations and pleural effusion during ACS[88] and seems suitable for daily follow-up. Bedside lung ultrasound is also of interest in case of pulmonary

symptoms with negative initial chest x-ray. Systematic CT angiography to detect pulmonary artery thrombosis poses the risk of cumulative irradiation in young patients who are frequently exposed given the typically high recurrence rate of ACS. A risk score for pulmonary artery thrombosis in ACS has been proposed to select patients for CT angiography.[35]

Investigation of the etiology should include testing for the following:

- Fat embolism (eg, Oil Red O staining of induced sputum or bronchial or pulmonary fluids, but with limited therapeutic implications)[27,28,89]

- Infectious agents (eg, polymerase chain reaction and/or culture of bronchial, nasopharyngeal, or pulmonary specimens for intracellular bacteria, respiratory viruses and pyogenes, *Legionella*, and pneumococcal urine antigen; serology for atypical pathogens; blood cultures)

Other exams comprise electrocardiogram (especially in case of chest pain) and echocardiogram (in case of respiratory distress or venous jugular distention, to assess pulmonary hypertension and cor pulmonale).

Biomarkers

Serum levels of some molecules involved in endothelial adhesion of RBCs (soluble VCAM1)[90] or in lipid metabolism (phospholipase A2)[91] are elevated in ACS; however, there is no definite biomarker for ACS to date. The enzyme secretory phospholipase A2 (sPLA2) cleaves phospholipids and generates fatty acids (eg, arachidonic acid), leading to tissue inflammation. Elevated levels of sPLA2 were detected in patients 24 to 48 hours before the clinical diagnosis of ACS.[91] Increased levels of sPLA2 predicted ACS in some series.[91,92] The degree of sPLA2 elevation in ACS correlated with measures of clinical severity.[93] In a small, randomized clinical trial, blood transfusion lowered sPLA2 levels and prevented ACS in SCD patients.[94] Serum C-reactive protein parallels secretory phospholipase A2 in SCD patients with VOC or ACS.[95]

In a cluster analysis to discover 17 signatures of common circulating biomarkers in 2320 participants of the Cooperative Study of Sickle Cell Disease, one cluster (#2, with a lower hemolytic score) was protective against ACS, whereas another (#6, with a higher hemolytic score) had an increased hazard of ACS.[96]

Tricuspid regurgitant velocities showed significant positive correlations with several cardiac (B-type natriuretic peptide, cardiac troponin) and hepatic (aspartate aminotransferase, alanine aminotransferase, and direct bilirubin) biomarkers during ACS.[7]

High levels of procalcitonin often indicate invasive bacterial infection during VOC.[97] However, a single low procalcitonin level cannot formally confirm or exclude infection during ACS.

Serum LDH levels increase during VOC and ACS and are correlated with plasma free hemoglobin,[98] but it remains ambiguous as to whether elevated levels of LDH are only indicative of enhanced hemolysis, given the variety of isoenzymes.[99]

Overall Clinical Course and Outcome

Overall Clinical Course

ACS is the second leading cause of hospitalization and the leading cause for admission to intensive care units and of death in adult patients with SCD.[3,4,6] Most patients admitted to intensive care are urgent transfers from the floor after being admitted, in initially stable condition, but with rapid deterioration. Clinical deterioration is typically associated with increased respiratory rate and temperature, decreasing hemoglobin and platelet count, and increasing liver function tests and creatinine.[6,100] Hospital mortality of ACS ranges between 1.6% and 13%, depending on the series.[6-9] Table 12-2 summarizes the risk factors for severe ACS.

TABLE 12-2 Risk factors for severe acute chest syndrome

Respiratory	Respiratory distress, extended involvement on chest-x ray or lung ultrasound
Cardiac	Chronic heart disease, acute pulmonary hypertension
Hematologic	Development of thrombocytopenia, profound anemia
Organ failure	Renal failure, acute liver injury, encephalopathy

Risk Factors for Complicated Outcome

The prognostic factors of ACS include the extent of radiologic opacities (multilobar involvement) on chest-x ray[9] or lung ultrasound,[88] the presence of chronic heart disease,[9] and the development of thrombocytopenia.[9,14] Younger age, male gender, and asthma were significantly associated with the comorbidity of ACS in children.[46] In a single-center French study on patients with SCD hospitalized in intensive care units (72% for ACS), the authors found the following risk factors for poor evolution (ie, death or need for vital support): total hemoglobin <7.8 g/dL, respiratory rate ≥32 breaths/min, and acute renal failure on admission to the intensive care unit.[6]

The prognosis of ACS seems better in patients managed by a specialized team,[9,101] probably because of the effect of case volume and expertise and SCD being a rare disease. Referral to a specialized or reference center is therefore highly recommended for the care of these patients.

Respiratory Course

The need for mechanical ventilation may occur in 4.6% to 13% of all admissions, a percentage that may be increasing. Risk factors for mechanical ventilation in children with ACS include obesity, obstructive sleep apnea, cardiac abnormalities, and possibly pulmonary hypertension. Despite a reassuring initial clinical presentation, the course of ACS can quickly evolve toward severe acute respiratory distress syndrome (ARDS).[7] In a large cohort of hospitalized adult patients with ACS, the need for mechanical ventilation predicted higher mortality rates and increased hospital resource utilization.[8]

Cardiovascular Course

Pulmonary artery pressures increase during severe ACS, and this rise is associated with cardiac biomarker elevation and a higher risk of death.[7] Another study confirmed that acute right heart failure was a common finding in almost all deaths in intensive care units.[6] All SCD patients presenting with moderate to severe ARDS as a consequence of ACS experienced pulmonary vascular dysfunction, and >80% of them exhibited acute cor pulmonale.[102] The frequent occurrence of acute cor pulmonale in this context[7] may contribute to circulatory shock and multiorgan failure, involving in particular the liver and kidney.[87,103] For example, acute kidney injury during ACS appears to be confined to patients with pulmonary hypertension, suggesting a pathophysiologic process involving right ventricular dysfunction and venous congestion.[87] Close monitoring of right heart failure signs, using echocardiogram at the slightest doubt, is therefore a keystone in ACS management.

Neurologic Course

High doses of opioids usually contribute to altered consciousness during ACS. However, there is an association between the occurrence of ACS and some brain complications of SCD (eg, ischemic stroke cerebral fat embolism, or posterior reversible encephalopathy syndrome),[104-106] which probably share common pathophysiologic mechanisms.[9]

Hematologic Course

A distinct ACS phenotype associated with multiorgan failure has been proposed; compared to adults without rapidly progressive ACS, adults with rapidly progressive ACS more frequently developed acute kidney injury, hepatic dysfunction, altered mental status, multiorgan failure, and death.[14] This evolution may be ascribable to that of microangiopathic syndromes,[107] is poorly predicted by the severity of the chronic disease, and may occur in otherwise asymptomatic patients.[6,103] ACS is also one of the features of hyperhemolysis syndrome. It is important to diagnose this serious and potentially life-threatening complication of RBC transfusion in order to avoid additional transfusions, because these may exacerbate the hemolysis and worsen the degree of anemia and organ failure.[108]

Treatment

Herein, we summarize the French, United Kingdom, and American recommendations on the management of SCD.[109-111] It is imperative for the clinician to keep in mind that ACS is a serious condition that can decompensate into ARDS with multiple organ failure within a few hours. The transfer to an intensive care unit should therefore be considered in severe forms (eg, those presenting with hypoxemia, multilobar radiologic involvement, extrapulmonary organ failure). Clinical surveillance should pay particular attention to respiratory tolerance and the development of cardiovascular (especially right heart failure) or neurologic disorders. Severe forms of ACS require aggressive, multidisciplinary care.

Fluids

Intravenous fluids (eg, 2 L of crystalloid per 24 hours in adults) reduce dehydration, which may aggravate sickling. However, the risk of volume overload must be borne in mind,[75] especially in patients with heart disease or who develop right heart failure.

Pain Control

Analgesia is a major element in SCD management, especially if there are painful costal infarctions that restrict breathing and promote the formation of atelectasis. Opioids are the cornerstone of analgesia, alone or in combination with adjuvant analgesics (eg, paracetamol, nefopam, or even nitrous oxide or ketamine in hyperalgesic crises). Pain control with parenteral opioids is often necessary, and patient-controlled analgesia should be considered. Nonsteroidal anti-inflammatory drugs have not shown additional clinical efficacy in combination with opioids for the treatment of VOC pain[112]; they should be discussed on an individual basis. Atelectasis secondary to pain or sedation increases the severity of ACS. Incentive spirometry prevents ACS in patients with VOC and is recommended for all hospitalized patients with vaso-occlusive episodes. Standard monitoring, in addition to oxygen saturation and cardiorespiratory vital signs, should include sedation and pain scales.

Transfusion

Figure 12-3 indicates why, when, and how to transfuse during ACS. Transfusion or partial exchange transfusion is effective in improving tissue oxygenation.[113] Despite the absence of a randomized trial on the subject, it is one of the major therapeutic elements for severe forms of ACS.[29] The goal is to lower HbS (and the fraction of sickled RBCs) in order to break the vicious circle of sickling. One study found no difference in efficacy between transfusion and partial transfusion in mild to moderate cases.[9] Because the goal is a return to baseline hemoglobin, simple transfusion is preferred in patients with low total hemoglobin level during ACS. RBC exchange can be performed by manual exchange or by automated exchange using a blood cell separator (erythrocytapheresis). In a small retrospective cohort study, the authors could not detect a difference in the efficacy of exchange transfusion with erythrocytapheresis compared to simple transfusion despite 4-fold higher RBC product usage in the exchange transfusion group.[114] However, in cases of severe or rapidly progressive ACS, erythrocytapheresis is a standard approach.

Transfusion should be considered from the onset of severe signs or after 48 to 72 hours of well-managed symptomatic treatment if no clinical and radiologic improvement is noticed. Transfusion must meet strict compatibility rules (including matching for Rhesus and Kell) in order to minimize the risk of alloimmunization[115] and delayed hemolytic transfusion reaction (DHTR).[116] The latter is suspected if clinical signs suggestive of intravascular hemolysis (with typically porto-colored urine), often with VOC and/or ACS, occur within 5 to 10 days of transfusion, with recurrence of anemia.[117] In such cases, hemoglobin electrophoresis would show a "disproportionate" decrease in the mass of transfused hemoglobin A (HbA). A diagnostic nomogram for DHTR based on HbA as a biologic marker of the survival of transfused RBCs has been proposed.[118] Its use requires the systematic assessment of HbA after RBC transfusion in SCD patients. When ACS is suspected of being a feature of DHTR presentation, further transfusion should be avoided.

The pathophysiology of DHTR is complex and involves reticulocytopenia and hemolysis of autologous RBCs and may occur even when no alloantibodies are detected. The management of patients with a history of alloimmunization or DHTR

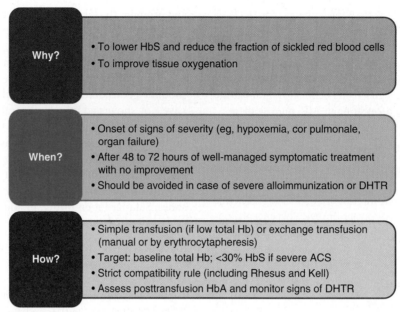

FIGURE 12-3 Rationale, indications, and modalities of transfusion during acute chest syndrome (ACS). DHTR, delayed hemolytic transfusion reaction; Hb, hemoglobin; HbA, hemoglobin A; HbS, sickled hemoglobin.

is best performed in specialized centers in close collaboration with a dedicated blood bank for the implementation of expanded phenotyping. A transfusion error in these patients exposes them to a life-threatening risk of massive intravascular hemolysis with uncontrollable multiorgan failure. Some attempts at immunomodulation (eg, using corticosteroids, immunoglobulins, rituximab, eculizumab) are carried out for the preventive or curative treatment of DHTR[119]; however, the avoidance of any new transfusion, except for life-threatening anemia, remains the most pragmatic approach.

Oxygen and Cardiorespiratory Support

Oxygen therapy is indicated to maintain an overall transcutaneous oxygen saturation (Spo$_2$) of 95%.[109,110] In cases of significant hypoxemia, high-flow oxygen through nasal cannula is routinely administered.[120] The reliability of Spo$_2$ measurements can occasionally be affected by the presence of methemoglobin and carboxyhemoglobin.[121,122]

Retrospective chart reviews suggest that continuous positive airway pressure and noninvasive ventilation can be used to improve oxygenation and decrease the work of breathing among children with ACS.[123,124] However, noninvasive ventilation did not show clear clinical usefulness in a randomized trial in unselected adults with mild ACS.[125] One study tested the effect of inhaled nitric oxide at a high dose (80 ppm) for 3 days in ACS and found a favorable effect only in the subgroup of hypoxemic patients (Pao$_2$/Fio$_2$ ratio <300 mm Hg).[126] When intubation and mechanical ventilation are required, protective ventilation with tidal volume and plateau pressure limitation are essential, as in other forms of ARDS.[127] Right heart failure is often in the foreground[7,102] and requires extra vigilance in controlling cofactors of pulmonary vascular dysfunction (eg, severe hypoxemia, hypercapnia, and elevated

airway pressure).[128] Prone positioning may improve pulmonary vascular dysfunction[129-131] and should be considered early in ARDS complicating ACS. The potential benefit of pulmonary vasodilators other than nitric oxide has not been formally studied. In cases with refractory hypoxemia, venovenous extracorporeal membrane oxygenation should be considered,[132] but membrane-driven hemolysis may be enhanced in the setting of SCD.

Antibiotics

Although the percentage of documented infections in clinical practice is low, especially in adult patients with ACS, the development of functional asplenia in SCD patients raises the risk of infection with encapsulated pathogens (eg, pneumococcus, *Haemophilus influenzae*).[133] However, intracellular germs, which are a common finding in ACS, must also be covered by the treatment.[9] Empiric antibiotics for pneumococcus and intracellular germs (eg, a combination of β-lactams such as amoxicillin or cephalosporin and macrolides) are often initiated, although the level of evidence is low[134] and randomized controlled trials on antibiotic treatment approaches for ACS are lacking.[134] In severely ill patients with progressive pulmonary disease, we may consider the addition of vancomycin to cover resistant bacteria, such as methicillin-resistant *Staphylococcus aureus* in areas where this strain is prevalent. The use of procalcitonin elevation to determine initiation of antibiotic therapy in ACS seems questionable[97]; however, it may serve to stop early, unnecessary antibiotics. Current approaches to antibiotic treatment in children with ACS vary widely, but guideline-adherent therapy appears to result in fewer readmissions compared with non–guideline-adherent therapy.[135]

Increased renal perfusion in patients with SCD[136,137] may lead to augmented clearance of renally cleared antibiotics, including β-lactams[138] and vancomycin.[139] The results of the microbiologic investigation could be useful to adapt or discontinue empiric antibiotic therapy.

Other Medications

Bronchodilators

Despite the lack of randomized trials, bronchodilators are often recommended during ACS in childhood, even in patients who do not have known prior reactive airway disease or obstructive pulmonary symptoms. Over 20% of patients demonstrate clinical improvement with increased mean forced expiratory volume.[9]

Corticosteroid Therapy

Corticosteroids are not standard practice for the management of ACS; they may shorten the duration of ACS but expose the patient to a rebound effect with a higher risk of readmission for VOC.[140,141] However, a brief and tapering course of steroids is often used in the treatment of ACS with an acute asthma event. Steroids are an alternative option for patients with ACS with a known history of severe RBC alloimmunization.

Anticoagulant Therapy

Patients hospitalized for ACS are often confined to bed and require anticoagulants at prophylactic doses for deep vein thrombosis prevention.[109] In our practice, the detection of pulmonary thromboses by CT scan mandates at least a 3-month anticoagulation treatment for which the precise modalities and duration need to be specified in future studies.[34,35]

Prevention

Prophylactic Transfusions

Compliance with aggressive chronic transfusion aimed at reducing the risk of stroke in children also reduces the frequency of ACS episodes.[142] A conservative transfusion regimen was as effective as an aggressive regimen in preventing perioperative complications in patients with sickle cell anemia, and the conservative approach resulted in only half as many transfusion-associated complications.[143] In a more recent study, preoperative transfusion of patients scheduled for low-risk or medium-risk operations was associated with decreased perioperative complications,[144] with a favorable cost-effectiveness ratio.[145] Use of preoperative blood transfusions should be individualized based on the baseline hemoglobin, surgical procedure, anticipated volume of blood loss,[146] and risk of DHTR.[147]

Blunting Evolution From VOC to ACS

sPLA2 levels have been evaluated as a potential biomarker to predict the development of ACS and initiate early transfusion, but their predictive value is low.[94,148] Education programs reduce the incidence of ACS by advocating for early, aggressive management of VOC pain.[149] Incentive spirometry during VOC significantly reduces the risk of secondary ACS[150,151] and is highly recommended.[109,110]

Long-Term Treatments and Measures

Treatment with hydroxyurea reduces the risk of ACS by about a half.[152,153] L-Glutamine has similar effects.[154] In pediatric patients with SCD, monthly oral vitamin D_3 for 2 years was associated with a 50% reduction in the rate of respiratory illness during the second year.[155] Preventive measures should aim at avoiding exposure to certain environmental factors (eg, cold, wind, pollution).[55] Vaccination against infectious agents that may cause ACS (eg, pneumococcus, *Haemophilus*, and influenza) is strongly recommended in SCD patients.[156]

Chronic Transfusion Therapy

Although there are no randomized prospective trials, chronic transfusion therapy likely reduces the incidence of ACS.[157] In children with SCD who have been chronically transfused for stroke prevention, the incidence of ACS was markedly reduced.[142]

Hematopoietic Stem Cell Transplantation

Stem cell transplantation is an accepted indication for children with multiple, serious ACS episodes who have an human leukocyte antigen–matched sibling donor. In the past, stem cell transplantation was not an option for adults with SCD due to the toxicity of myeloablative therapy. Innovative regimens with nonmyeloablative conditioning appear promising in inducing a stable, mixed donor chimerism with improved clinical course. Clinical trials of gene therapy have been initiated, and their success in preventing recurrent pulmonary events is being evaluated.[158]

Conclusion

ACS is a serious and common finding that includes acute pulmonary complications of SCD. Its pathophysiology is complex and its management is essentially symptomatic for the time being. ACS requires close monitoring because of the high risk of rapid deterioration to ARDS, severe pulmonary vascular disease, and multiorgan failure.

Case Study: Imaging of ACS

Figure 12-4 shows a chest x-ray (Figure 12-4A), thoracic computed tomography scan (Figure 12-4B), and echocardiogram (Figures 12-4, C and D) of an adult patient with ACS, showing bilateral basal opacities with consolidation (black arrows on Figure 12-4, A and B) on lung imaging, with a dilatation of the right ventricle (white arrow on Figure 12-4C) and a paradoxical motion of the interventricular septum (white arrow on Figure 12-4D) on echocardiogram, depicting acute cor pulmonale.

Case Study: Continued

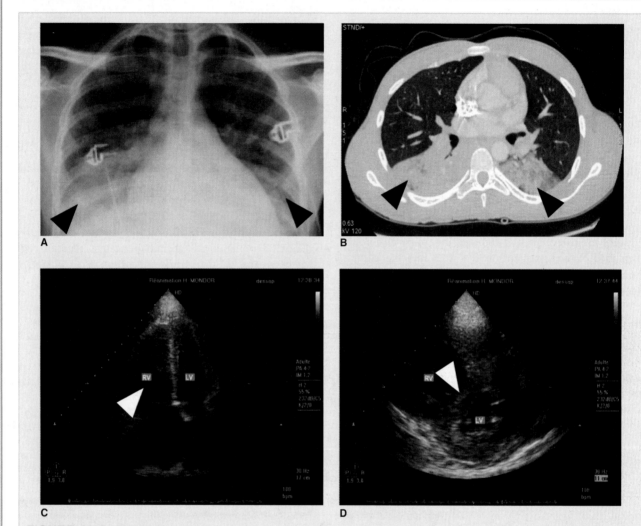

FIGURE 12-4 (A) Chest x-ray, (B) thoracic computed tomography scan, and (C and D) echocardiogram of an adult patient with acute chest syndrome.

High-Yield Facts

Guidelines for acute chest syndrome management:

◆ Monitoring of vital signs and laboratory changes for rapidly progressive ACS and multi-organ failure (MOF)

◆ Oxygen therapy

◆ Morphine and multimodal analgesia

◆ Intravenous hydration/fluid

◆ Transfusion or exchange transfusion in severe forms; to be avoided in case of alloimmunization or delayed hemolytic transfusion reaction; importance of transfusion compatibility

◆ Empirical antibiotic therapy covering pneumococcus and atypical germs

◆ Echocardiography if acute cor pulmonale is suspected; chest computed tomography angiography if pulmonary thrombosis is suspected

◆ Consider noninvasive ventilation or nitric oxide on a case-by-case basis; right ventricle protective ventilation in case of intubation

References

1. Charache S, Scott JC, Charache P. "Acute chest syndrome" in adults with sickle cell anemia: microbiology, treatment, and prevention. *Arch Intern Med.* 1979;139(1):67.

2. Barrett-Connor E. Pneumonia and pulmonary infarction in sickle cell anemia. *JAMA.* 1973;224(7):997-1000.

3. Castro O, Brambilla DJ, Thorington B, et al. The acute chest syndrome in sickle cell disease: incidence and risk factors. the Cooperative Study of Sickle Cell Disease. *Blood.* 1994;84(2):643-649.

4. Gardner K, Bell C, Bartram JL, et al. Outcome of adults with sickle cell disease admitted to critical care: experience of a single institution in the UK. *Br J Haematol.* 2010;150(5):610-613.

5. Tawfic QA, Kausalya R, Al-Sajee D, et al. Adult sickle cell disease: a five-year experience of intensive care management in a university hospital in Oman. *Sultan Qaboos Univ Med J.* 2012;12(2):177-183.

6. Cecchini, J, Lionnet F, Djibré M, et al. Outcomes of adult patients with sickle cell disease admitted to the ICU: a case series. *Crit Care Med.* 2014;42(7):1629-1639.

7. Mekontso Dessap A, Leon R, Habibi A, et al. Pulmonary hypertension and cor pulmonale during severe acute chest syndrome in sickle cell disease. *Am J Respir Crit Care Med.* 2008;177(6):646-653.

8. Allareddy V, Roy A, Lee MK, et al. Outcomes of acute chest syndrome in adult patients with sickle cell disease: predictors of mortality. *PLoS One.* 2014;9(4):e94387.

9. Vichinsky EP, Neumayr LD, Earles AN, et al. Causes and outcomes of the acute chest syndrome in sickle cell disease. national acute chest syndrome study group. *N Engl J Med.* 2000;342(25):1855-1865.

10. Vichinsky P, Styles LA, Colangelo LH, et al. Acute chest syndrome in sickle cell disease: clinical presentation and course. *Blood.* 1997;89(5):1787-1792.

11. Platt OS, Brambilla DJ, Rosse WF, et al. Mortality in sickle cell disease. Life expectancy and risk factors for early death. *N Engl J Med.* 1994;330(23):1639-1644.

12. Powars DR, Chan LS, Hiti A, Ramicone E, Johnson C. Outcome of sickle cell anemia: a 4-decade observational study of 1056 patients. *Medicine (Baltimore).* 2005;84(6):363-376.

13. Fitzhugh CD, Lauder N, Jonassaint JC, et al. Cardiopulmonary complications leading to premature deaths in adult patients with sickle cell disease. *Am J Hematol.* 2010;85(1):36-40.

14. Chaturvedi S, Ghafuri DL, Glassberg J, et al. Rapidly progressive acute chest syndrome in individuals with sickle cell anemia: a distinct acute chest syndrome phenotype. *Am J Hematol.* 2016;91(12):1185-1190.

15. Desai PC, Ataga KI. The acute chest syndrome of sickle cell disease. *Expert Opin Pharmacother.* 2013;14(8):991-999.

16. Yalamanoglu A, Deuel JW, Hunt RC, et al. Depletion of haptoglobin and hemopexin promote hemoglobin-mediated lipoprotein oxidation in sickle cell disease. *Am J Physiol Lung Cell Mol Physiol.* 2018;315(5):L765-L774.

17. Bennewitz MF, Jimenez MA, Vats R, et al. Lung vaso-occlusion in sickle cell disease mediated by arteriolar neutrophil-platelet microemboli. *JCI Insight.* 2017;2(1):e89761.

18. Holtzclaw JD, Jack D, Aguayo SM, et al. Enhanced pulmonary and systemic response to endotoxin in transgenic sickle mice. *Am J Respir Crit Care Med.* 2004;169(6):687-695.

19. Kaul DK, Fabry ME, Windisch P, Baez S, Nagel RL. Erythrocytes in sickle cell anemia are heterogeneous in their rheological and hemodynamic characteristics. *J Clin Invest.* 1983;72(1):22-31.

20. Bartolucci, P, Galacteros F. Clinical management of adult sickle-cell disease. *Curr Opin Hematol.* 2012;19(3):149-155.

21. Jain S, Bakshi N, Krishnamurti L. Acute chest syndrome in children with sickle cell disease. *Pediatr Allergy Immunol Pulmonol.* 2017;30(4):191-201.

22. Novelli EM, Gladwin MT. Crises in sickle cell disease. *Chest.* 2016;149(4):1082-1093.

23. Sullivan KJ, Kissoon N, Gauger C. Nitric oxide metabolism and the acute chest syndrome of sickle cell anemia. *Pediatr Crit Care Med.* 2008;9(2):159-168.

24. Guérin C, Matthay MA. Acute cor pulmonale and the acute respiratory distress syndrome. *Intensive Care Med.* 2016;42(5): 934-936.

25. Graham JK, Mosunjac M, Hanzlick RL, et al. Sickle cell lung disease and sudden death: a retrospective/prospective study of 21 autopsy cases and literature review. *Am J Forensic Med Pathol.* 2007;28(2):168-172.

26. Vichinsky E, Williams R, Das M, et al. Pulmonary fat embolism: a distinct cause of severe acute chest syndrome in sickle cell anemia. *Blood.* 1994;83(11):3107-3112.

27. Lechapt E, Habibi A, Bachir D, et al. Induced sputum versus bronchoalveolar lavage during acute chest syndrome in sickle cell disease. *Am J Respir Crit Care Med.* 2003;168(11):1373-1377.

28. Godeau B, Schaeffer A, Bachir D, et al. Bronchoalveolar lavage in adult sickle cell patients with acute chest syndrome: value for diagnostic assessment of fat embolism. *Am J Respir Crit Care Med.* 1996;153(5):1691-1696.

29. Maitre B, Habibi A, Roudot-Thoraval F, et al. Acute chest syndrome in adults with sickle cell disease. *Chest.* 2000;117(5): 1386-1392.

30. Nathan CL, Aamodt WW, Yalamarti T, et al. Cerebral fat embolism syndrome in sickle cell disease without evidence of shunt. *ENeurologicalSci.* 2018;14:19-20.

31. Haupt HM, Moore GW, Bauer TW, et al. The lung in sickle cell disease. *Chest.* 1982;81(3):332-337.

32. Adedeji MO, Cespedes J, Allen K, Subramony C, Hughson MD. Pulmonary thrombotic arteriopathy in patients with sickle cell disease. *Arch Pathol Lab Med.* 2001;125(11):1436-1441.

33. Bhalla M, Abboud MR, McLoud TC, et al. Acute chest syndrome in sickle cell disease: CT evidence of microvascular occlusion. *Radiology.* 1993;187(1):45-49.

34. Mekontso Dessap A, Deux JF, Abidi N, et al. Pulmonary artery thrombosis during acute chest syndrome in sickle cell disease. *Am J Respir Crit Care Med.* 2011;184(9):1022-1029.

35. Winchenne A, Cecchini J, Deux JF, et al. A clinical risk score for pulmonary artery thrombosis during acute chest syndrome in adult patients with sickle cell disease. *Br J Haematol.* 2017;179(4):627-634.

36. Noubiap JJ, Temgoua MN, Tankeu R, et al. Sickle cell disease, sickle trait and the risk for venous thromboembolism: a systematic review and meta-analysis. *Thromb J.* 2018;16:27.

37. Austin H, Key NS, Benson JM, et al. Sickle cell trait and the risk of venous thromboembolism among blacks. *Blood.* 2007;110(3):908-912.

38. Strouse, JJ, Reller ME, Bundy DG, et al. Severe pandemic H1N1 and seasonal influenza in children and young adults with sickle cell disease. *Blood.* 2010;116(18):3431-3434.

39. Morrison C, Maurtua-Neumann P, Myint MT, Drury SS, Bégué RE. Pandemic (H1N1) 2009 outbreak at camp for children with hematologic and oncologic conditions. *Emerg Infect Dis.* 2011;17(1):87-89.

40. Bundy DG, Strouse JJ, Casella JF, Miller MR. Burden of influenza-related hospitalizations among children with sickle cell disease. *Pediatrics.* 2010;125(2):234-243.

41. Smith-Whitley K, Zhao H, Hodinka RL, et al. Epidemiology of human parvovirus B19 in children with sickle cell disease. *Blood.* 2004;103(2):422-427.

42. Mekontso Dessap A, Deux JF, Habibi A, et al. Lung imaging during acute chest syndrome in sickle cell disease: computed tomography patterns and diagnostic accuracy of bedside chest radiograph. *Thorax.* 2014;69(2):144-151.

43. Kopecky EA, Jacobson S, Joshi P, Koren G. Systemic exposure to morphine and the risk of acute chest syndrome in sickle cell disease. *Clin Pharmacol Ther.* 2004;75(3):140-146.

44. Quinn CT, Shull EP, Ahmad N, et al. Prognostic significance of early vaso-occlusive complications in children with sickle cell anemia. *Blood.* 2007;109(1):40-45.

45. Paul R, Minniti CP, Nouraie M, et al. Clinical correlates of acute pulmonary events in children and adolescents with sickle cell disease. *Eur J Haematol.* 2013;91(1):62-68.

46. Takahashi T, Okubo Y, Handa A. Acute chest syndrome among children hospitalized with vaso-occlusive crisis: a nationwide study in the united states. *Pediatr Blood Cancer.* 2018;65(3):e26885.

47. Thein SL, Howard J. How I treat the older adult with sickle cell disease. *Blood.* 2018;132(17):1750-1760.

48. Bean CJ, Boulet SL, Yang G, et al. Acute chest syndrome is associated with single nucleotide polymorphism-defined beta globin cluster haplotype in children with sickle cell anaemia. *Br J Haematol.* 2013;163(2):268-276.

49. Galarneau G, Coady S, Garrett ME, et al. Gene-centric association study of acute chest syndrome and painful crisis in sickle cell disease patients. *Blood.* 2013;122(3):434-442.

50. Bean CJ, Boulet SL, Ellingsen D, et al. Heme oxygenase-1 gene promoter polymorphism is associated with reduced incidence of acute chest syndrome among children with sickle cell disease. *Blood.* 2012;120(18):3822-3828.

51. Brandow AM, Stucky CL, Hillery CA, Hoffmann RG, Panepinto JA. Patients with sickle cell disease have increased sensitivity to cold and heat. *Am J Hematol.* 2013;88(1):37-43.

52. Amjad H, Bannerman RM, Judisch JM. Letter: sickling pain and season. *Br Med J.* 1974;2(5909):54.

53. Redwood AM, Williams EM, Desal P, Serjeant GR. Climate and painful crisis of sickle-cell disease in Jamaica. *Br Med J.* 1976;1(6001):66-68.

54. Rogovik AL, Persaud J, Friedman JN, et al. Pediatric vasoocclusive crisis and weather conditions. *J Emerg Med.* 2011;41(5):559-565.

55. Mekontso Dessap A, Contou D, Dandine-Roulland C, et al. Environmental influences on daily emergency admissions in sickle-cell disease patients. *Medicine.* 2014;93(29):e280.

56. Beutler E. The effect of carbon monoxide on red cell life span in sickle cell disease. *Blood.* 1975;46(2):253-259.

57. Beckman JD, Belcher JD, Vineyard JV, et al. Inhaled carbon monoxide reduces leukocytosis in a murine model of sickle cell disease. *Am J Physiol Heart Circ Physiol.* 2009;297(4): H1243-H1253.

58. Bartolucci P, Habibi A, Khellaf M, et al. Score predicting acute chest syndrome during vaso-occlusive crises in adult sickle-cell disease patients. *EBioMedicine.* 2016;10:305-311.

59. Oteng-Ntim E, Ayensah B, Knight M, Howard J. Pregnancy outcome in patients with sickle cell disease in the UK: a national cohort study comparing sickle cell anaemia (HbSS) with HbSC disease. *Br J Haematol.* 2015;169(1):129-137.

60. Bonnard A, Masmoudi M, Boimond B, et al. Acute chest syndrome after laparoscopic splenectomy in children with sickle cell disease: operative time dependent? *Pediatr Surg Int.* 2014;30(11):1117-1120.

61. Ghantous S, Al Mulhim S, Al Faris N, et al. Acute chest syndrome after splenectomy in children with sickle cell disease. *J Pediatr Surg.* 2008;43(5):861-864.

62. West DC, Pomeroy JR, Park JK, et al. Impact of environmental tobacco smoke on children with sickle cell disease. *Arch Pediatr Adolesc Med.* 2003;157(12):1197-1201.

63. Sadreameli SC, Eakin MN, Robinson KT, et al. Secondhand smoke is associated with more frequent hospitalizations in children with sickle cell disease: tobacco smoke exposure in sickle cell disease. *Am J Hematol.* 2016;91(3):313-317.

64. Cohen RT, DeBaun MR, Blinder MA, Strunk RC, Field JJ. Smoking is associated with an increased risk of acute chest syndrome and pain among adults with sickle cell disease. *Blood.* 2010;115(18):3852-3854.

65. Young RC Jr, Rachal RE, Hackney RL Jr, et al. Smoking is a factor in causing acute chest syndrome in sickle cell anemia. *J Natl Med Assoc.* 1992;84(3):267-271.

66. DeBaun MR, Strunk RC. The intersection between asthma and acute chest syndrome in children with sickle-cell. anaemia. *Lancet.* 2016;387(10037):2545-2553.

67. Knight-Madden JM, Forrester TS, Lewis NA, Greenough A. Asthma in children with sickle cell disease and its association with acute chest syndrome. *Thorax.* 2005;60(3):206-210.

68. Morris CR. Asthma management: reinventing the wheel in sickle cell disease. *Am J Hematol.* 2009;84(4):234-241.

69. Pahl K, Mullen CA. Original research: acute chest syndrome in sickle cell disease: effect of genotype and asthma. *Exp Biol Med (Maywood).* 2016;241(7):745-758.

70. Bernaudin F, Strunk RC, Kamdem A, et al. Asthma is associated with acute chest syndrome, but not with an increased rate of hospitalization for pain among children in France with sickle cell anemia: a retrospective cohort study. *Haematologica.* 2008;93(12):1917-1918.

71. Boyd JH, Strunk RC, Morgan WJ. The outcomes of sickle cell disease in adulthood are clear, but the origins and progression of sickle cell anemia-induced problems in the heart and lung in childhood are not. *J Pediatr.* 2006;149(1):3-4.

72. Nordness ME, Lynn J, Zacharisen MC, Scott PJ, Kelly KJ. Asthma is a risk factor for acute chest syndrome and cerebral vascular accidents in children with sickle cell disease. *Clin Mol Allergy.* 2005;3(1):2.

73. Poulter EY, Truszkowski P, Thompson AA, Liem RI. Acute chest syndrome is associated with history of asthma in hemoglobin SC disease. *Pediatr Blood Cancer.* 2013;57(2):289-293.

74. Intzes S, Kalpatthi RV, Short R, Imran H. Pulmonary function abnormalities and asthma are prevalent in children with sickle cell disease and are associated with acute chest syndrome. *Pediatr Hematol Oncol.* 2013;30(8):726-732.

75. Haynes J Jr, Allison RC. Pulmonary edema. Complication in the management of sickle cell pain crisis. *Am J Med.* 1986;80(5): 833-840.

76. Karlsson EA, Oguin TH, Meliopoulos V, et al. Vascular permeability drives susceptibility to influenza infection in a murine model of sickle cell disease. *Sci Rep.* 2017;7:43308.

77. Firth PG, Tsuruta Y, Kamath Y, et al. Transfusion-related acute lung injury or acute chest syndrome of sickle cell disease? A case report. *Can J Anaesth.* 2003;50(9):895-899.

78. Anthi A, Machado RF, Jison ML, et al. Hemodynamic and functional assessment of patients with sickle cell disease and pulmonary hypertension. *Am J Respir Crit Care Med.* 2007;175(12):1272-1279.

79. Gladwin MT, Sachdev V, Jison ML, et al. Pulmonary hypertension as a risk factor for death in patients with sickle cell disease. *N Engl J Med.* 2004;350(9):886-895.

80. Chaudry RA, Cikes M, Karu T, et al. Pediatric sickle cell disease: pulmonary hypertension but normal vascular resistance. *Arch Dis Child.* 2011;96(2):131-136.

81. Ambrusko SJ, Gunawardena S, Sakara A, et al. Elevation of tricuspid regurgitant jet velocity, a marker for pulmonary hypertension in children with sickle cell disease. *Pediatr Blood Cancer.* 2006;47(7):907-913.

82. Pashankar FD, Carbonella J, Bazzy-Asaad A, Friedman A. Prevalence and risk factors of elevated pulmonary artery pressures in children with sickle cell disease. *Pediatrics.* 2008;121(4):777-782.

83. Parent F, Bachir D, Inamo J, et al. A hemodynamic study of pulmonary hypertension in sickle cell disease. *N Engl J Med.* 2011;365(1):44-53.

84. Hargrave DR. Nocturnal oxygen saturation and painful sickle cell crises in children. *Blood.* 2003;101(3):846-848.

85. Contou D, Mekontso Dessap A, Carteaux G, et al. Golden tracheal secretions and bronchoalveolar fluid during acute chest syndrome in sickle cell disease. *Respir Care.* 2015;60(4):e73-e75.

86. de Prost N, Sasanelli M, Deux JF, et al. Positron emission tomography with 18F-fluorodeoxyglucose in patients with sickle cell acute chest syndrome. *Medicine (Baltimore).* 2015;94(18):e821.

87. Audard V, Homs S, Habibi A, et al. Acute kidney injury in sickle patients with painful crisis or acute chest syndrome and its relation to pulmonary hypertension. *Nephrol Dial Transplant.* 2010;25(8):2524-2529.

88. Razazi K, Deux JF, de Prost N, et al. Bedside lung ultrasound during acute chest syndrome in sickle cell disease. *Medicine.* 2016;95(7):e2553.

89. Boussat S, Eddahibi S, Coste A, et al. Expression and regulation of vascular endothelial growth factor in human pulmonary epithelial cells. *Am J Physiol Lung Cell Mol Physiol.* 2000;279(2):L371-L378.

90. Stuart MJ, Setty BN. Sickle cell acute chest syndrome: pathogenesis and rationale for treatment. *Blood.* 1999;94(5):1555-1560.

91. Styles LA, Aarsman AJ, Vichinsky EP, Kuypers FA. Secretory phospholipase A(2) predicts impending acute chest syndrome in sickle cell disease. *Blood.* 2000;96(9):3276-3278.

92. Naprawa JT, Bonsu BK, Goodman DG, Ranalli MA. Serum biomarkers for identifying acute chest syndrome among patients who have sickle cell disease and present to the emergency department. *Pediatrics.* 2005;116(3):e420-e425.

93. Styles LA, Schalkwijk CG, Aarsman AJ, Vichinsky EP, Lubin BH, Kuypers FA. Phospholipase A2 levels in acute chest syndrome of sickle cell disease. *Blood.* 1996;87(6):2573-2578.

94. Styles LA, Abboud M, Larkin S, Lo M, Kuypers FA. Transfusion prevents acute chest syndrome predicted by elevated secretory phospholipase A2. *Br J Haematol* 2007;136(2):343-344.

95. Bargoma EM, Mitsuyoshi JK, Larkin SK. Serum C-reactive protein parallels secretory phospholipase A2 in sickle cell disease patients with vasoocclusive crisis or acute chest syndrome. *Blood.* 2005;105(8):3384-3385.

96. Du M, Van Ness S, Gordeuk V, et al. Biomarker signatures of sickle cell disease severity. *Blood Cells Mol Dis.* 2018;72:1-9.

97. Stankovic Stojanovic K, Steichen O, Lionnet F, et al. Is procalcitonin a marker of invasive bacterial infection in acute sickle-cell vaso-occlusive crisis? *Infection.* 2011;39(1):41-45.

98. Kato GJ, McGowan V, Machado RF, et al. Lactate dehydrogenase as a biomarker of hemolysis-associated nitric oxide resistance, priapism, leg ulceration, pulmonary hypertension, and death in patients with sickle cell disease. *Blood.* 2006;107(6):2279-2285.

99. Damanhouri GA, Jarullah J, Marouf S, et al. Clinical biomarkers in sickle cell disease. *Saudi J Biol Sci.* 2015;22(1):24-31.

100. Al Khawaja SA, Ateya ZM, Al Hammam RA. Predictors of mortality in adults with sickle cell disease admitted to intensive care unit in Bahrain. *J Crit Care.* 2017;42:238-242.

101. Jan S, Slap G, Smith-Whitley K, et al. Association of hospital and provider types on sickle cell disease outcomes. *Pediatrics.* 2013;132(5):854-861.

102. Cecchini J, Boissier F, Gibelin A, et al. Pulmonary vascular dysfunction and cor pulmonale during acute respiratory distress syndrome in sicklers. *Shock.* 2016;46(4):358-364.

103. Hassell KL, Eckman JR, Lane PA. Acute multiorgan failure syndrome: a potentially catastrophic complication of severe sickle cell pain episodes. *Am J Med.* 1994;96(2):155-162.

104. Henderson JN, Noetzel MJ, McKinstry RC, et al. Reversible posterior leukoencephalopathy syndrome and silent cerebral infarcts are associated with severe acute chest syndrome in children with sickle cell disease. *Blood.* 2003;101(2):415-419.

105. Ohene-Frempong K, Weiner SJ, Sleeper LA, et al. Cerebrovascular accidents in sickle cell disease: rates and risk factors. *Blood.* 1998;91(1):288-294.

106. Quinn CT, McKinstry RC, Dowling MM, et al. Acute silent cerebral ischemic events in children with sickle cell anemia. *JAMA Neurol.* 2013;70(1):58-65.

107. Shome DK, Ramadorai P, Al-Ajmi A, Ali F, Malik N. Thrombotic microangiopathy in sickle cell disease crisis. *Ann Hematol.* 2013;92(4):509-515.

108. Habibi A, Mekontso-Dessap A, Guillaud C, et al. Delayed hemolytic transfusion reaction in adult sickle-cell disease: presentations, outcomes, and treatments of 99 referral center episodes. *Am J Hematol.* 2016;91(10):989-994.

109. Habibi A, Arlet JB, Stankovic K, et al. Recommandations françaises de prise en charge de la drépanocytose de l'adulte : actualisation 2015. *Rev Méd Interne.* 2015;36(5):5S3-5S84.

110. Yawn BP, Buchanan GR, Afenyi-Annan AN, et al. Management of sickle cell disease: summary of the evidence-based report by expert panel members. *JAMA.* 2014;312(10):1033-1048.

111. Howard J, Hart N, Roberts-Harewood M, et al. Guideline on the management of acute chest syndrome in sickle cell disease. *Br J Haematol.* 2015;169(4):492-505.

112. Bartolucci P, El Murr T, Roudot-Thoraval F, et al. A randomized, controlled clinical trial of ketoprofen for sickle-cell disease vaso-occlusive crises in adults. *Blood.* 2009;114(18):3742-3747.

113. Emre U, Miller ST, Gutierez M, et al. Effect of transfusion in acute chest syndrome of sickle cell disease. *J Pediatr.* 1995;127(6):901-914.

114. Turner JM, Kaplan JB, Cohen HW, Billett HH. Exchange versus simple transfusion for acute chest syndrome in sickle cell anemia adults. *Transfusion.* 2009;49(5):863-868.

115. Vichinsky EP, Earles A, Johnson RA, et al. Alloimmunization in sickle cell anemia and transfusion of racially unmatched blood. *N Engl J Med.* 1990;322(23):1617-1621.

116. Yazdanbakhsh K, Ware RE, Noizat-Pirenne F. Red blood cell alloimmunization in sickle cell disease: pathophysiology, risk factors, and transfusion management. *Blood.* 2012;120(3):528-537.

117. Petz LD, Calhoun L, Shulman IA, Johnson C, Herron RM. The sickle cell hemolytic transfusion reaction syndrome. *Transfusion.* 1997;37(4):382-392.

118. Mekontso Dessap A, Pirenne F, Razazi K, et al. A diagnostic nomogram for delayed hemolytic transfusion reaction in sickle cell disease: diagnostic nomogram in DHTR. *Am J Hematol.* 2016;91(12):1181-1184.

119. Noizat-Pirenne F, Bachir D, Chadebech P, et al. Rituximab for prevention of delayed hemolytic transfusion reaction in sickle cell disease. *Haematologica.* 2007;92(12):e132-e135.

120. Frat JP, Thille AW, Mercat A, et al. High-flow oxygen through nasal cannula in acute hypoxemic respiratory failure. *N Engl J Med.* 2015;372(23):2185-2196.

121. Ahmed S, Siddiqui AK, Sison CP, Shahid RK, Mattana J. Hemoglobin oxygen saturation discrepancy using various methods in patients with sickle cell vaso-occlusive painful crisis. *Eur J Haematol.* 2005;74(4):309-314.

122. Kress JP, Pohlman AS, Hall JB. Determination of hemoglobin saturation in patients with acute sickle chest syndrome: a comparison of arterial blood gases and pulse oximetry. *Chest.* 115(5):1316-1320.

123. Padman R, Henry M. The use of bilevel positive airway pressure for the treatment of acute chest syndrome of sickle cell disease. *Del Med J.* 2004;76(5):199-203.

124. Heilbronner C, Merckx A, Brousse V, et al. Early noninvasive ventilation and nonroutine transfusion for acute chest syndrome in sickle cell disease in children: a descriptive study. *Pediatr Crit Care Med.* 2018;19(5):e235-e241.

125. Fartoukh M, Lefort Y, Habibi A, et al. Early intermittent noninvasive ventilation for acute chest syndrome in adults with sickle cell disease: a pilot study. *Intensive Care Med.* 2010;36(8):1355-1362.

126. Maitre B, Djibre M, Katsahian S, et al. Inhaled nitric oxide for acute chest syndrome in adult sickle cell patients: a randomized controlled study. *Intensive Care Med.* 2015;41(12):2121-2129.

127. Brower RG, Matthay MA, Morris A, et al. Ventilation with lower tidal volumes as compared with traditional tidal volumes for acute lung injury and the acute respiratory distress syndrome. *N Engl J Med.* 2000;342(18):1301-1308.

128. Mekontso Dessap A, Boissier F, Charron C, et al. Acute cor pulmonale during protective ventilation for acute respiratory distress syndrome: prevalence, predictors, and clinical impact. *Intensive Care Med.* 2016;42(5):862-870.

129. Jozwiak M, Teboul JL, Anguel N, et al. Beneficial hemodynamic effects of prone positioning in patients with acute respiratory distress syndrome. *Am J Respir Crit Care Med.* 2013;188(12):1428-1433.

130. Vieillard-Baron A, Charron C, Caille V, et al. Prone positioning unloads the right ventricle in severe ARDS. *Chest.* 2007;132(5):1440-1446.

131. Guérin C, Reignier J, Richard JC, et al. Prone positioning in severe acute respiratory distress syndrome. *N Engl J Med.* 2013;368(23):2159-2168.

132. Combes A, Hajage D, Capellier G, et al. Extracorporeal membrane oxygenation for severe acute respiratory distress syndrome. *N Engl J Med.* 2018;378(21):1965-1975.

133. Booth C, Inusa B, Obaro SK. Infection in sickle cell disease: a review. *Int J Infect Dis.* 2010;14(1):e2-e12.

134. Martí-Carvajal AJ, Conterno LO, Knight-Madden JM. Antibiotics for treating acute chest syndrome in people with sickle cell disease. *Cochrane Database Syst Rev.* 2019;18;9(9):CD006110.

135. Bundy DG, Richardson TE, Hall M, et al. Association of guideline-adherent antibiotic treatment with readmission of children with sickle cell disease hospitalized with acute chest syndrome. *JAMA Pediatr.* 2017;171(11):1090-1099.

136. Haymann JP, Stankovic K, Levy P, et al. Glomerular hyperfiltration in adult sickle cell anemia: a frequent hemolysis associated feature. *Clin J Am Soc Nephrol.* 2010;5(5):756-761.

137. Lionnet F, Stankovic K, Tharaux PL, et al. Prévalence de l'hyperfiltration glomérulaire chez les patients drépanocytaires homozygotes. *Rev Méd Interne.* 2008;29:S320.

138. Cecchini J, Hulin A, Habibi A, et al. Profound underdosing of β-lactams in patients with sickle-cell disease. *J Antimicrob Chemother.* 2018;73(11):3211-3212.

139. Han J, Zhang X, Oderinde J, et al. Increased vancomycin dosing requirements in sickle cell disease due to hyperfiltration-dependent and independent pathways. *Haematologica.* 2017;102(8):e282-e284.

140. Sobota A, Graham DA, Heeney MM, Neufeld EJ. Corticosteroids for acute chest syndrome in children with sickle cell disease: variation in use and association with length of stay and readmission. *Am J Hematol.* 2010;85(1):24-28.

141. Strouse JJ, Takemoto CM, Keefer JR, et al. Corticosteroids and increased risk of readmission after acute chest syndrome in children with sickle cell disease. *Pediatr Blood Cancer.* 2008;50(5):1006-1012.

142. Miller ST, Wright E, Abboud M, et al. Impact of chronic transfusion on incidence of pain and acute chest syndrome during the stroke prevention trial (STOP) in sickle-cell anemia. *J Pediatr.* 2001;139(6):785-789.

143. Vichinsky EP, Haberkern CM, Neumayr L, et al. A comparison of conservative and aggressive transfusion regimens in the perioperative management of sickle cell disease. The Preoperative Transfusion in Sickle Cell Disease Study Group. *N Engl J Med.* 1995;333(4):206-213.

144. Howard J, Malfroy M, Llewelyn C, et al. The Transfusion Alternatives Preoperatively in Sickle Cell Disease (TAPS) study: a randomised, controlled, multicentre clinical trial. *Lancet.* 2013;381(9870):930-938.

145. Spackman E, Sculpher M, Howard J, et al. Cost-effectiveness analysis of preoperative transfusion in patients with sickle cell disease using evidence from the TAPS trial. *Eur J Haematol.* 2013;92(3):249-255.

146. Adjepong KO, Otegbeye F, Adjepong YA. Perioperative management of sickle cell disease. *Mediterr J Hematol Infect Dis.* 2018;10(1):e2018032.

147. Narbey D, Habibi A, Chadebech P, et al. Incidence and predictive score for delayed hemolytic transfusion reaction in adult patients with sickle cell disease. *Am J Hematol.* 2017;92(12):1340-1348.

148. Styles L, Wager CG, Labotka RJ, et al. Refining the value of secretory phospholipase A2 as a predictor of acute chest syndrome in sickle cell disease: results of a feasibility study (PROACTIVE). *Br J Haematol.* 2012;157(5):627-636.

149. Reagan MM, DeBaun MR, Frei-Jones MJ. Multi-modal intervention for the inpatient management of sickle cell pain significantly decreases the rate of acute chest syndrome. *Pediatr Blood Cancer.* 2011;56(2):262-266.

150. Ahmad FA, Macias CG, Allen JY. The use of incentive spirometry in pediatric patients with sickle cell disease to reduce the incidence of acute chest syndrome. *J Pediatr Hematol Oncol.* 2011;33(6):415-420.

151. Bellet PS, Kalinyak KA, Shukla R, Gelfand MJ, Rucknagel DL. Incentive spirometry to prevent acute pulmonary complications in sickle cell diseases. *N Engl J Med.* 1995;333(11):699-703.

152. Charache S, Terrin ML, Moore RD, et al. Effect of hydroxyurea on the frequency of painful crises in sickle cell anemia. Investigators of the Multicenter Study of Hydroxyurea in Sickle Cell Anemia. *N Engl J Med.* 1995;332(20):1317-1322.

153. Tshilolo L, Tomlinson G, Williams TN, et al. Hydroxyurea for children with sickle cell anemia in sub-Saharan Africa. *N Engl J Med.* 2019;380(2):121-213.

154. Niihara Y, Miller ST, Kanter J, et al. A phase 3 trial of l-glutamine in sickle cell disease. *N Engl J Med.* 2018;379(3):226-235.

155. Lee MT, Kattan M, Fennoy I, et al. Randomized phase 2 trial of monthly vitamin D to prevent respiratory complications in children with sickle cell disease. *Blood Adv.* 2018;2(9):969-978.

156. Davies EG, Riddington C, Lottenberg R, et al. Pneumococcal vaccines for sickle cell disease. *Cochrane Database Syst Rev.* 2004;1:CD003885.

157. Hankins J, Jeng M, Harris S, Li CS, Liu T, Wang W. Chronic transfusion therapy for children with sickle cell disease and recurrent acute chest syndrome. *J Pediatr Hematol Oncol.* 2005;27(3):158-161.

158. Ribeil JA, Hacein-Bey-Abina S, Payen E, et al. Gene therapy in a patient with sickle cell disease. *N Engl J Med.* 2017;376(9):848-855.

Pediatric Sickle Cell Disease

Authors: *John J. Strouse, Nancy S. Green*

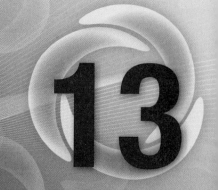

Chapter Outline

Overview

Morbidity and mortality in pediatric sickle cell disease (SCD) in the United States have markedly declined since the 1970s. Initial impact from newborn screening for presymptomatic diagnosis, early initiation of preventative care, and widespread initiation of disease-modifying therapies have led to reduced early mortality and reduced childhood morbidities. Nonetheless, several specific complications remain that are partially or entirely specific to pediatric SCD. Persistence of these complications is related to their early onset and structural and physiologic factors, especially dactylitis and splenic sequestration. Moreover, children with SCD remain especially susceptible to bacterial infections, likely due to early and ongoing decreases in splenic function. Here, we highlight the historical implementation of newborn screening for SCD and disease complications that exclusively or predominantly affect children.

Newborn Screening for SCD

Overview and History

Newborn screening for SCD plays a crucial role in the successful survival of children with SCD in North and South America, Western Europe, and elsewhere.[1-4] Universal screening also enables population surveillance for public health tracking and planning. Here, we review the rationale for, impact of, and opportunities arising from population-based hemoglobinopathy screening, as well as the potential for future research and intervention. In this chapter, we focus primarily on the United States, with limited discussion of the successful efforts to develop newborn SCD screening in sub-Saharan Africa and India, where most children with SCD are born. International progress is described in another chapter.

The foundation of newborn screening is based on the principles that (1) early diagnosis of specific inherited diseases can allow presymptomatic initiation of appropriate therapy during a window of health to safeguard well-being and development and (2) clinical detection in the absence of newborn screening will delay diagnosis and worsen outcomes.[1,5] The model of newborn screening arose in the 1960s and 1970s from the collective efforts of scientists and the public to prevent the developmental effects on infants affected by phenylketonuria (PKU). For PKU, avoiding dietary exposure to phenylalanine led to markedly improved pediatric outcomes. Laboratory screening in centralized laboratories is performed from collected dried bloodspots. Samples are universally obtained prior to discharge from the newborn nursery of birth hospitals.

To reach broad public access to the benefits of newborn screening, testing capacity at state public health laboratories was established. In addition, screening programs developed avenues of rapid communication with birth hospitals, pediatric providers, and parents of infants suspected of being affected by SCD or other screened health condition. To partner with specialists to provide health care for the needs of identified children, each state designates specialty centers at one or more hospitals to provide confirmatory testing and prompt access to treatment. For SCD, each state has identified hemoglobinopathy centers to provide access to expert comprehensive specialized pediatric SCD care. As a public health program, parental consent is not required for routine infant screening.[6]

Population-based newborn screening for SCD began in New York City in 1975, enabling early pediatric referral to specially structured care.[7] As early as 1979, splenic infarction and hypofunction were recognized as common complications of SCD, especially in HbSS and HbS-β[0] thalassemia.[8] In 1986, bacterial sepsis, often caused by *Streptococcus pneumoniae*, had a case mortality rate of 30%. A pivotal randomized trial demonstrated the value of penicillin prophylaxis in reducing risk of invasive pneumococcal infection in infants and young children with SCD.[9] Early introduction of penicillin prophylaxis, usually before clinical symptoms arose, became the standard of care for children with SCD.[10] The combined effects of early penicillin, improved childhood vaccination, parental education, empiric fever therapy, and medical care led to a marked reduction in mortality for children with SCD <10 years of age.[11] In 1993, the predecessor of the current federal Agency for Healthcare Research and Quality (AHRQ) recognized the importance of universal infant screening for SCD, combined with comprehensive health care, for reducing disease-associated infant morbidity and mortality.[12] Pilot experience with selective screening based on perceived ethnicity of parents led to the appreciation of the sensitives surrounding racial self-identification and the importance of universal strategies for screening and care.[13] Selective screening practices were shown to miss a number of cases in the French national screening program, which limited screening to infants of parents of certain geographic descent.[14] Since 2006, universal screening for SCD has been standard in all states in the United States.[11,15]

Laboratory Screening Methods

Newborn hemoglobinopathy screening employs one or more of several possible technologies.[15-18] State public health laboratories need to provide rapid results from large numbers of samples. For example, California and New York test 400,000 and 250,000 babies annually, respectively.[19] Methodologies for screening include isoelectric focusing or high-performance liquid chromatography. More recently, molecular methods and tandem mass spectroscopy have been adapted for use in small pediatric bloodspot samples.[20] As with all screening tests, scaling up requires efficient, inexpensive approaches with high reproducibility and low rates of error or ambiguity.

The Laboratory Quality Assurance is the national reference program for SCD and other newborn disease screening. It is housed at the Centers for Disease Control and Prevention (CDC) and contributes to the public health screening programs through laboratory proficiency testing by and training for state newborn screening personnel.[21]

Results of Screening

Over a 20-year period through 2010, nearly 40,000 babies with SCD were identified through newborn screening. The annual birth prevalence of SCD in the United States was 1 in 1941 live births, totaling approximately 2000 affected births per year.[1] These diagnoses included all major genotypes of SCD, including HbSC and HbS-β+ thalassemia. Less common β-globin chain variants, which, when combined with HbS, can also cause a sickle disease. These, too, are identified through screening, such as compound heterozygous HbS and HbD (HbSD). Each state program reports, newborn sickle screening results, with most states reporting at least one birth affected by SCD per year. Over the same period of time, sickle trait was identified in 1.1 million births. For identification of infants with sickle (HbS) or HbC trait, state newborn screening programs are not uniformly required to directly communicate test results to parents.[1].

Newborn screening data have provided a critical understanding of population prevalence, demographics, clinical outcomes, and complications and use of medical therapies from birth cohorts.[22] Results from state-based screening programs can be associated with child health and mortality data to provide information on the effectiveness of the screening and care of children with SCD.[22-24] Historically, widespread SCD screening and provision of specialty care led to the recognition of a dramatic improvement in mortality among children with SCD <10 years old.[24] Recently, a persistently higher mortality of young children with SCD in New York State, compared to the non-SCD population, was demonstrated.[25] Another application of screening is the tracking of disease complications and the uptake of medical therapies such as hydroxyurea.[26-29]

Population-based screening also provides an opportunity to deliver genetic counseling to families at risk of a genetic condition. Babies found to have sickle trait on neonatal screening will identify families with greatly increased chances of having a future child with SCD. The diagnosis of sickle cell trait thus provides an opportunity to provide targeted genetic counseling, including parental testing for couples at risk. For sickle trait, confirmatory testing and counseling are the primary messages for providers.[22] The awareness and utility of this guidance have not been formally evaluated.

Unfortunately, gaps in SCD detection can still arise.[1,30] For example, hemoglobinopathy status may be lost when infants move to another state. Immigrant children from much of the world have not had hemoglobin screening. These children may not be identified as having SCD until they experience an acute illness and undergo subsequent clinical testing.[1]

Research in Newborn Screening

In addition to the critical assessment of public health and medical outcomes, research to improve understanding of hemoglobin biology and demographics has been a long-standing aspect of newborn hemoglobinopathy screening.[31,32] Unusual α or β gene hemoglobinopathies can be identified and studied to inform about physical properties when combined with HbS that may modify an SCD phenotype. Population-based genomic data can also be identified using stored bloodspot samples from newborn screening.[33]

Worldwide, reliable and robust approaches to hemoglobinopathy detection continue to advance in regions with high burden of SCD.[34-36] Assessment of cost per test and cost-effectiveness of screening overall are critical aspects in support of nascent programs in low-income countries. Innovations in low-cost testing continue to flourish.[4,37-39]

Summary

Newborn screening for SCD has enabled the development of successful clinical programs to provide prompt prospective care to affected children. Standardized regular assessment, parental education, and early introduction of disease-modifying therapies have led to improved outcomes for affected children.[22] These programs have also supported clinical research, leading to testing and evaluation of new therapies.

In the United States, parental attitudes have limited the research testing on newborn screening samples. Such possibilities include screening for an unrelated condition or exploratory DNA sequencing platforms.[40] Many parents appear to place a boundary on utilization of their infant's sample for research testing when results are not directly linked to benefits for their children and their families.

The infrastructure of newborn screening, clinical research, and infant medical care that has evolved over decades has not led to major health advances for migrants or adults who were never screened but were subsequently diagnosed with SCD after clinical presentation.[41-43] Incomplete population-based data on demographics and outcomes of migrating communities or adult care, as well as barriers to medical care, have contributed to difficulties in assessing health status and longitudinal tracking of outcomes.[22] These shortcomings, combined with the demands of adult self-management, accumulating disease-associated morbidities, and limited resources for continuous health care for SCD, contribute to disjointed care and suboptimal outcomes. Nonetheless, opportunities exist to continue to extend the benefits from newborn screening to increasingly cover SCD patients throughout the life span.[44]

Infectious Complications

Definition

Infectious complications, particularly those caused by encapsulated bacteria, are more frequent and severe in children with SCD than in the general population. Common infections include bacteremia, osteomyelitis and septic arthritis, pyelonephritis, and typical childhood viruses causing severe complications.

Prior to the routine implementation of newborn screening, the first recognized complication of SCD was often severe or fatal infection. Young children with SCD are at increased risk of bacteremia from encapsulated organisms including *S pneumoniae* and *Haemophilus influenzae*, osteomyelitis and joint infections with nontyphoidal *Salmonella* species and *Staphylococcus aureus*, and pyelonephritis with fecal coliforms. Both parvovirus B19 and Epstein-Barr virus can cause aplastic crisis, and infection with influenza and respiratory syncytial virus is associated with acute chest syndrome.

Epidemiology

Bacteremia

In the era before routine penicillin prophylaxis and vaccination against encapsulated organisms, bacteremia was a frequent complication in young children with SCD. The Cooperative Study of SCD enrolled 2400 children and >1000 adults in a prospective cohort study between March 1979 and March 1991. There were 178 episodes of bacteremia over 13,771 patient-years of follow-up, with rates as high as 7.98 per 100 person-years in children <3 years old with HbSS and 3.54 for children <3 years old with HbSC. The most common cultured organisms were *S pneumoniae*, *H influenzae*, and gram-negative organisms (50% of bacteremia in children >6 years old).[45] *Neisseria meningitidis* vaccination is recommended for children with decreased splenic function, including those with SCD, although an increased incidence of meningococcal infections has not been demonstrated in children with SCD (Tim McCavitt, personal communication). Urinary tract infection was present during 73% of *Escherichia coli* bacteremias, and 77% of *Salmonella* bacteremias were associated with osteomyelitis, whereas no focus of infection was present in 52% of pneumococcal infections.[45] The incidence of pneumococcal and *H influenzae* infections declined greatly with the routine administration of penicillin prophylaxis to children <5 years of age and conjugate vaccines against *H influenzae* type B (licensed in 1987) and then *S pneumoniae* (7 serotypes, licensed in 2000).[46] Invasive pneumococcal infections were nearly eliminated until 2004, when the incidence of infections began to increase again with predominantly serotypes not included in the conjugate or polysaccharide pneumococcal vaccines.[47] In 2010, a new pneumococcal conjugate vaccine that included 13 serotypes was licensed in the United States.

Even with prophylactic penicillin, in children <5 years old, the risk of invasive pneumococcal infections (1571 per 100,000 children for HbSS and 329 per 100,000 for HbSC) remains 49- and 10-fold higher in children with SCD, respectively, compared with children without SCD (32 per 100,000).[48,49] Many of the infections are with serotypes not covered in the 23-valent polysaccharide and 7-valent conjugate vaccine (7 of 12 cases) or 13-valent conjugate vaccine (5 of 12 cases) and in older children (age >10 years; 4 of 12 cases).[50] Meningitis occurred in 10 of 62 cases of pneumococcal bacteremia in children <10 years old with HbSS in the Cooperative Study of SCD.[51] Invasive *H influenzae* infection remains uncommon, with an incidence rate of 58 per 100,000 person-years for all children with SCD and 160 per 100,000 for those <5 years old.[52] Both infections are severe, with a case fatality rate of 14.5% for pneumococcal bacteremia and 20% for *H influenzae* bacteremia.[51] In contrast, in other cohorts from outside the United States (Saudi Arabia, France), *Salmonella* species are the most frequent cause of bacteremia. These differences may reflect different environmental exposures and the effect of routine penicillin prophylaxis and immunization against *H influenzae* type B and *S pneumoniae*.

Osteomyelitis and Septic Arthritis

Prospective cohort studies of children provide limited data on the incidence of bone infections in children. An incidence of 2.87 per 100 person-years (36 cases) was reported in a French cohort of 299 children and young adults followed from 1987 to 1997 (median age, 9.3 years; mean follow-up, 4.2 years). Half of the infections were in children <5 years old, and 75% occurred in children <10 years old.[53] Several studies reported the cumulative prevalence of osteomyelitis in prospective cohorts of children with SCD hospitalized for suspected infection.[54,55] *Salmonella* species (47%) were the most common causative organism identified by culture, followed by *S aureus* (33%) and other gram-negative enteric bacteria (27%). Other gram-positive organisms such as pneumococcus were uncommon.[56]

Pyelonephritis

The frequency of urinary tract infections is increased in children with SCD based on the more frequent occurrence of *E coli* bacteremia (likely urinary tract source) and an increase in bacteriuria and urinary tract infections in febrile children with SCD. A cohort study in the United States identified 54 urinary infections in 26 children with an incidence rate of 3.5 infections per 100 person-years. The rate of infections was higher in children with HbSS than in HbSC, and two-thirds of the infections were accompanied by fever.[57]

Viral Infections

Infections with respiratory viruses including respiratory syncytial virus (RSV) and influenza have increased severity in children with SCD and are 13 times (RSV) to 56 times (influenza) more likely to lead to hospitalization than in the general population of children.[58,59] The number of cases varies greatly by year (Figure 13-1) and RSV and influenza are diagnosed in 1% to 5% of children with SCD in a typical year. RSV

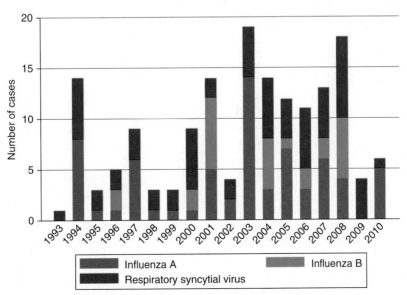

FIGURE 13-1 **Cases by year and virus at Johns Hopkins Hospital, 1993–2010 seasons.** Reproduced with permission from, Sadreameli SC, Reller ME, Bundy DG, Casella JF, Strouse JJ. Respiratory syncytial virus and seasonal influenza cause similar illnesses in children with sickle cell disease. *Pediatr Blood Cancer* 2014;61(5):875-8.

causes admissions for fever and acute chest syndrome (26%), mostly in children <5 years old, whereas influenza causes acute chest syndrome in all ages (15%); in addition, children with SCD had increased risks of intensive care unit admission, mechanical ventilation, and death during the H1N1 epidemic in 2009.[59-61]

Parvovirus B19 infection is the most common cause of aplastic crisis in children with SCD. It consistently causes viremia within 4 to 6 days of infection and is often associated with fever (62%), headache (35%), abdominal pain (32%), upper respiratory infection (29%), and limb pain (21%).[62] Less frequent complications include acute splenic enlargement, acute ischemic stroke, acute chest syndrome, and multiorgan failure syndrome from fat or bone marrow embolism.[63-65] Severe reticulocytopenia develops about 10 days after infection and is often accompanied by mild to moderate neutropenia and thrombocytopenia. The nadir of hemoglobin is after another 5 days, and most children with sickle cell anemia and parvovirus B19 infection have severe anemia requiring transfusion. The anemia is usually less severe in children with HbSC and HbS-β^+ thalassemia, reflecting their longer red cell survival. Bone marrow recovery usually occurs 10 days after viremia and is associated with rash, arthralgia, and sometimes arthritis. In a recent meta-analysis, 42% of children with SCD had evidence of past infection by serology (immunoglobulin G [IgG]).[66]

Other viral infections may also be more severe in children with SCD. There are reports of increased risk of mortality with dengue and Zika infections,[67,68] and Epstein-Barr virus infection can cause severe reticulocytopenia in children with SCD and splenic infarcts in those with sickle cell trait.[69,70]

Pathophysiology

General

There are multiple mechanisms contributing to the increased risk and severity of infections in children with SCD. They can be divided into immune defects and an increased susceptibility to hemolysis and vaso-occlusion in the setting of inflammation and hypoxemia (from pulmonary infections or increased metabolic demand secondary to fever). Defects in both the innate and humoral immune system are seen in children with SCD. Impairments in humoral immunity include decreased phagocytosis of encapsulated bacteria and *Babesia microti* secondary to splenic dysfunction.[71] In addition, hemolysis with circulating heme and increased levels of heme oxygenase impairs macrophage function and causes quantitative defects in the respiratory burst of neutrophils. Iron overload, a common complication of transfusion in children with SCD, contributes to the severity of a large number of infections including those caused by fungi, protozoa, gram-positive and -negative bacteria, and selected viruses.[72] Humoral immunity is also impaired, with defects in IgG leading to impaired opsonization of pneumococcus in children and decreased numbers of memory B cells and CD4$^+$ and CD8$^+$ memory T cells.[73,74]

Bacteremia

Several factors contribute to the frequency and severity of bacteremia. Foremost is loss of splenic function with the development of functional asplenia in many children as vaso-occlusion and infarction cause splenic atrophy. In addition, some children have surgical splenectomy for severe splenic sequestration. Diminished or absent splenic function leads to severe impairment of phagocytosis of encapsulated bacteria. Defects in humoral immunity, specifically impaired opsonization of pneumococcus-dependent IgG, are also present in children with SCD.[73] Finally, iron overload impairs macrophage function and the respiratory burst in granulocytes, contributing to the increased rate and severity of bacteremia with *Salmonella* and other bacteria that thrive in the presence of free heme or iron overload.[72]

Osteomyelitis and Septic Arthritis

Salmonella species (47%) are the most common causative organisms identified by culture in osteomyelitis and septic arthritis, followed by *S aureus* (33%), and other gram-negative enteric bacteria (27%). Other gram-positive organisms, such as pneumococcus, are uncommon. There are several putative mechanisms for the increased susceptibility to bone and joint infections in children with SCD. These include hyposplenism, impairment of the complement system that leads to decreased phagocytosis of *Salmonella*, and impairment of the ingestion and destruction of *Salmonella* by macrophages. In addition, drug- or malaria-induced hemolysis or the administration of hemin causes premature mobilization of granulocytes from the bone marrow with a quantitative defect in oxidative burst and acute fatal bacteremia with high bacterial load in mice.[75]

Urinary Tract Infections

Most urinary tract infections in children with SCD are caused by *E coli* and *Klebsiella pneumoniae*. The risk of infection, particularly upper tract disease, may be increased by the high frequency of renal infarcts. The poorly oxygenated, infarcted tissue may be more susceptible to infection, and pyelonephritis may be more difficult to cure in children with SCD.[57]

Viral Infections

The increased severity of viral infections likely results from the interaction between the virus and the typical pathophysiology of SCD. Viral infections can increase the number of activated monocytes and lymphocytes and contribute to increased levels of cytokines and soluble and endothelial adhesion molecules.[68] Respiratory viruses contribute to pulmonary inflammation, disrupt the respiratory endothelium, and can cause local hypoxia. These viruses can cause acute chest syndrome and other serious pulmonary complications.[59]

Risk Factors

The primary risk factor for bacteremia in children with SCD is impaired splenic function. This correlates strongly with genotype and age, because most children with sickle cell anemia have splenic dysfunction in the first 2 years of life, whereas only 30% of children with HbSC disease and 10% of those with

HbS-β⁺ thalassemia have splenic dysfunction by age 5 years.[76] Penicillin prophylaxis and protein conjugate vaccines against *S pneumoniae* and *H influenzae* are protective. Children with previous bacteremia are at increased risk of recurrent episodes. Another acquired risk factor is the presence of central venous access (temporary central venous catheters, tunneled venous catheters, or percutaneous implanted central venous catheters).

Differential Diagnosis

Fever is the most common presenting symptom of infection in children with SCD. Other symptoms and signs such as localized pain and/or swelling, cough, dyspnea, increased work of breathing, dysuria, urgency or urinary frequency, diarrhea, nausea, and vomiting should help determine the possible diagnosis. Other common causes of fever in children with SCD include noninfectious acute vaso-occlusive events such as bone infarction, dactylitis, and acute chest syndrome. Rare causes of fever include fat emboli syndrome, multiorgan failure syndrome, medications, and autoimmune disorders. Distinguishing bone infarction, joint effusions, and dactylitis from osteomyelitis and joint infections can be very challenging in children with joint or limb swelling and fever. Imaging findings with bone infarction can include periosteal fluid collections and periosteal elevation consistent with osteomyelitis both by magnetic resonance imaging (MRI) and x-ray studies. Nuclear medicine studies of bone infarction initially show decreased uptake of the radiotracer, but as the bone infarct evolves, it may lead to increased uptake as seen with infectious processes.[77,78]

Prognostic Impact on Subsequent Disease Course

Children with an initial episode of pneumococcal bacteremia or urinary tract infection are at increased risk of recurrent infections.[45] For this reason, continuing antibiotic prophylaxis against *S pneumoniae* infection throughout childhood is recommended for those with a history of *S pneumoniae* bacteremia. Many adult hematologists and adults with SCD choose to stop the antibiotic prophylaxis. For children with urinary tract infections, evaluation should be considered based on general pediatric guidelines.[79]

Management

Prevention

All children with SCD should receive routine childhood immunizations with attention to the receipt of the conjugate *S pneumoniae* (PCV13) and *H influenzae* type B vaccines and influenza vaccine (Table 13-1). PCV13 is administered starting at age 2 months, with 3 doses given 8 weeks apart; a fourth dose is given at age 12 to 15 months. Children with SCD should receive the pneumococcal polysaccharide vaccine (PPSV23) at age 2 years (at least 8 weeks after the last dose of PCV13), with a second dose of PPSV23 5 years later. The CDC Advisory Committee on Immunization Practices also recommends the meningococcal groups C and Y and *Haemophilus* B conjugate

TABLE 13-1 Prevention of infections

Intervention	Children	Adults
Antibiotics	Penicillin 125/250 mg BID	Rarely used
Avoid exposures	Reptiles, amphibians, raw egg, and chicken Influenza vaccine for family members	
Evaluate temperature >101.3°F or 38.5°C emergently	CBC with differential, reticulocytes, blood culture Sometimes chest x-ray, urine culture Empiric IV antibiotics	
Vaccination	Per ACIP: PCV13, PPSV23 series (see text) *Haemophilus influenzae* and meningococcal series (individually or HibMenCY combination) Influenza vaccine annually	

Abbreviations: ACIP, Advisory Committee on Immunization Practices, Centers for Disease Control and Prevention; BID, twice a day; CBC, complete blood count; IV, intravenous.

vaccine (HibMenCY) at 2, 4, and 6 months of age, and again at 12 through 15 months. In addition, children <5 years old with sickle cell anemia should receive prophylactic penicillin 125 mg orally every 12 hours from age 3 months to 3 years and then 250 mg orally every 12 hours until age 5 years. In children allergic to penicillin, erythromycin may be substituted. The most recent guidelines do not recommend prophylaxis for children with milder genotypes of SCD, although many pediatric sickle cell providers prescribe penicillin for all of their patients with SCD.[80] Some providers choose to continue penicillin prophylaxis in some or all of their patients with sickle cell anemia throughout childhood, especially if they have had prior invasive pneumococcal infections, have had a surgical splenectomy, or have not received the recommended pneumococcal vaccinations.

Empiric Management of Fever

Fever is often the first recognized manifestation of infection in a child with SCD, and therefore, a temperature of 38.5°C (101.5°F) or higher should be evaluated emergently with a blood culture, complete blood count with differential, and reticulocyte count. In children with urinary symptoms or who are <3 years of age, urinalysis and urine culture are also recommended. All children with respiratory symptoms or signs and those <10 years of age being discharged from the emergency department should have a chest x-ray. The decision to obtain stool studies (fecal leukocytes or lactoferrin and stool culture) or a lumbar puncture should be based on symptoms and signs of gastroenteritis or meningitis. A focal finding of joint or bone pain with swelling should be evaluated by imaging and, if clinically indicated, arthrocentesis or biopsy.

TABLE 13-2 Children appropriate for the outpatient management of fever

Age	>1 year (6 months in initial study)
White blood cell count	5000-30,000/μL
Temperature	<40°C (104°F)
Chest x-ray	No pulmonary infiltrates
Bacteremia	No prior bacteremia
Urinalysis	No pyuria or nitrites
Hemoglobin	>5 g/dL, no reticulocytopenia
Other	No dehydration or severe pain

After the blood culture is obtained, parenteral antibiotics with activity against pneumococcus and enteric gram-negative bacteria should be administered (typically a second- or third-generation cephalosporin). Children at low risk of serious bacterial infection (Table 13-2) can safely be treated as an outpatient with ceftriaxone 50 mg/kg (maximum, 2 g) daily for 48 hours. All children who appear unwell or may be unable to obtain transportation to return to the hospital should be admitted. If no bacterial infection is identified, parenteral antibiotics may be discontinued after 48 hours.[81]

Treatment of Specific Infections

Bacteremia

Treatment depends on the organism. Typically, *Salmonella* bacteremia is treated with a third-generation cephalosporin initially and then based on sensitivities because antimicrobial resistance has been increasing to cephalosporins and fluoroquinolones. The duration of treatment should be at least 2 weeks and longer if there is a focus of infection such as osteomyelitis or septic arthritis.[82] *S pneumoniae* bacteremia without a focus of infection should be treated for 14 days. The antibiotics to complete the course can be given orally once the fever has resolved and repeat blood cultures show no growth after 48 hours.

Osteomyelitis and Septic Arthritis

The optimal duration of treatment for osteomyelitis in SCD is not defined because there have been no randomized controlled trials.[83] *Salmonella* infections can be challenging to eradicate, and some patients received extended treatment with antibiotics (up to 10 months). Empiric treatment is typically a parenteral third-generation cephalosporin until antimicrobial susceptibility testing is available. Treatment of other causes of infections (gram-negative bacteria and *S aureus*) also should be guided by antimicrobial susceptibility testing, with empiric therapy with vancomycin and then a switch to oxacillin or a first-generation cephalosporin if

methicillin resistance is excluded. The minimum duration of treatment with parenteral antibiotics should be 6 weeks, until symptoms and laboratory tests of inflammation have improved. Consultation with an infectious disease specialist is recommended.

Urinary Tract Infections

Treatment depends on the site of infection. Upper tract disease (pyelonephritis) should be treated for 14 days as a complicated disease. This is necessary because of the high frequency of renal infarction and poorly perfused kidney areas that can contribute to treatment failure. A third-generation cephalosporin is typical empiric therapy while awaiting the results of culture and antimicrobial susceptibility testing. Oral antibiotics can be used to complete the course once clinical improvement is seen (resolution of fever, decreasing white blood cell count). Cystitis can be treated for 5 days, typically with a second- or third-generation oral cephalosporin with a change in therapy once susceptibility testing is complete.

Viral Infections

Treatment of children with SCD and suspected or confirmed influenza is recommended given the low rate of significant adverse effects with currently recommended therapies (oseltamivir) and evidence of greatly increased risk of severe influenza in children with SCD. Dosing is 3 mg/kg every 12 hours for infants <8 months old and 3.5 mg/kg every 12 hours for infants ≥9 months old. The dose is 30 mg every 12 hours for children who weigh <15 kg, 45 mg every 12 hours for those who weigh 15 to 23 kg, 60 mg every 12 hours for those who weight 23 to 40 kg, and 75 mg every 12 hours for those who weight >40 kg. Treatment is recommended regardless of the duration of symptoms in those with SCD.[84]

Summary

Infections were the most common cause of death in children with SCD in the United States before 1990. With early diagnosis of SCD by newborn screening, initiation of prophylactic penicillin by 3 months of age, vaccination against encapsulated organisms, and emergency evaluation of fever with empiric parenteral antibiotics, childhood mortality from infections has been greatly reduced. However, children with SCD continue to have increased risk of bacteremia, osteomyelitis, and urinary tract infections and more severe manifestations of both bacterial and viral infections.

Splenic Complications

Definition

Common splenic complications in children with SCD include decreased splenic function (discussed in detail in the infectious complications section), acute splenic sequestration, splenomegaly, and splenic infarct. Splenic complications occur from the unique interaction between the spleen and the sickle erythrocyte. Acute splenic sequestration results from the acute retention of red blood cells in the spleen with a sudden decrease in hemoglobin concentration, often accompanied by a decrease in the platelet count and symptoms or signs of hypovolemia. Formal diagnostic criteria require a decrease in the hemoglobin or hematocrit by 20% or greater from baseline, increased erythropoiesis such as a markedly elevated reticulocyte count, and acute enlargement of the spleen (≥2 cm) by clinical exam or imaging. Episodes are classified as severe if transfusion is required and mild otherwise.[85] Splenomegaly is defined as abnormal enlargement of the spleen. This can be determined by clinical exam by palpation or percussion of the spleen below the left costal margin or by ultrasound or computed tomography imaging with specific values based on the age and height of the child. Normal ranges in healthy children by ultrasound are well defined.[86] A subset of patients will develop hypersplenism, defined as splenomegaly with worsening anemia, thrombocytopenia (platelets <100,000/μL), and/or leukopenia (leukocytes <4000/μL).[87] Acute splenic infarction occurs after venous or arterial occlusion of blood flow in the spleen, and multiple episodes contribute to hyposplenism and functional asplenia in children with SCD. Formal diagnostic criteria require acute left upper quadrant pain that may be referred to the shoulder and visualization of necrotic or ischemic splenic parenchyma by imaging studies, direct visualization during surgery, or pathology examination.[88] Massive splenic infarction involves at least 50% of the spleen.[87]

Epidemiology

Acute Splenic Sequestration

The epidemiology of acute splenic sequestration varies by genotype and age. In the infant cohort of the Cooperative Study of SCD, 43 of 427 participants with HbSS had 61 episodes of acute splenic sequestration with a peak incidence of 5.7 per 100 person-years between 6 months and 2.99 years of age. Sixteen of the 43 children had splenectomies. Seven of 221 children with HbSC had 10 episodes of acute splenic sequestration with a peak incidence of 1.9 per 100 person-years between 3 and 6.99 years of age. No children with HbSC had splenectomy.[51] A more recent French study of a national newborn screening cohort from 2000 to 2009 identified 190 (12.6%) of 1095 children with HbSS or HbS-β[0] thalassemia, with 437 episodes of acute splenic sequestration. Acute splenic sequestration was associated with male sex and glucose-6-phosphate dehydrogenase deficiency, and 91 (48%) of 190 patients presented with fever (isolated in 43 and with evidence of localized infection in 48). Most children had recurrent events (n = 127, 67%), and recurrence was more common in children who had their first episode before age 2 years. Splenectomy occurred in 37% of children and typically after a second episode (97%) at a median age of 4 years.[89]

Splenomegaly

Chronic splenomegaly is an uncommon finding in children with sickle cell anemia, with only 8 (8%) of 100 unselected patients from the United States having splenomegaly.[90]

Hypersplenism was present in 18 (10.4%) of 173 Saudi children.[87] A retrospective review of right upper quadrant ultrasound in patients <21 years old identified splenomegaly in 13 (15%) of 86 patients with HbSS disease and 12 (57%) of 21 patients with HbSC disease. Only 5 of the 25 patients with splenomegaly required splenectomy. In all cases, the indication was acute splenic sequestration, and splenectomy was usually performed within a few months of ultrasound.[91] A retrospective study of medical records identified palpable splenomegaly in 34 (34%) of 100 children age ≥2 years with HbSC. Splenomegaly was often associated with mild worsening of anemia and mild thrombocytopenia.[92]

Splenic Infarct

Splenic infarctions secondary to vaso-occlusion are common in children with SCD but are usually small and asymptomatic. Symptomatic splenic infarct is the least common of the 3 major splenic complications. In a cohort of 173 children with sickle cell anemia treated in Saudi Arabia, 3 children had massive splenic infarct (1.7%) in the setting of preexisting splenomegaly. The largest series of children with massive splenic infarction is from Saudi Arabia. All 15 children presented with severe left upper quadrant pain and tender splenomegaly, 9 with nausea and vomiting, and 3 with fever. Three children required emergency splenectomy for abscess formation, and another 11 underwent splenectomy for persistent abdominal pain. Splenic infarction may be more common in children with HbSC and HbS-β[+] thalassemia.

Pathophysiology

Acute Splenic Sequestration

The hypoxic and acidic splenic environment contributes to increased polymerization of hemoglobin and thereby sickling of the red blood cells, in addition to increased vaso-occlusion, through upregulation of adhesion molecules. Intrasplenic vaso-occlusion is often acute in young children and leads to rapid enlargement of the spleen.[85] The vaso-occlusion leads to worsening hypoxemia with further sickling and vaso-occlusion. Transfusion of sickle-negative blood can often reverse this process, but must be undertaken judiciously because upon resolution of sequestration, autotransfusion of sequestered red blood cells can cause a rapid increase in hemoglobin and hyperviscosity.[91] Fever and infections likely increase the risk of splenic sequestration by stimulating the immune system and triggering inflammation that increases cell adhesion molecule levels.

Splenomegaly

The mechanisms of splenomegaly include splenic congestion, splenic regeneration nodules (most commonly seen after beginning chronic transfusions and sometimes with hydroxyurea), and fibrosis secondary to episodes of vaso-occlusion and acute splenic sequestration. Common findings on pathology include splenic congestion, fibrosis, and hemosiderin deposition.[91]

Splenic Infarct

The exact mechanisms of splenic infarct in children with SCD are not known. Based on the other diseases associated with splenic infarction (myeloproliferative disorders, other hemolytic anemias, and thrombophilic conditions), splenic infarction is likely secondary to vaso-occlusion or thrombosis. Splenomegaly may increase the risk of splenic infarction by the volume of tissue outgrowing the supply of blood.

Risk Factors

Acute Splenic Sequestration

Risk factors for acute splenic sequestration include age, genotype, and acute infections. Children with sickle cell anemia (HbSS and HbS-β^0 thalassemia) have a higher rate than those with HbSC disease, and younger children (<3 years old with HbSS, 3-6.99 years old for HbSC) have a higher rate than older children. Acute splenic sequestration occurs in older children with sickle cell anemia in Saudi Arabia (mean age, 7.6 years; range, 1.8-13), likely secondary to higher levels of fetal hemoglobin (mean, 20.5%; range, 9.2%-36.9%).[87]

Splenomegaly

Risk factors for splenomegaly include certain genotypes of SCD (HbSC, HbS-β^+ thalassemia) and perhaps regular blood transfusion and higher levels of fetal hemoglobin.[92]

Splenic Infarct

Proposed risk factors for splenic infarction include hypoxemia (from high altitude, obstructive sleep apnea, and acute chest syndrome) and activation of the coagulation system and/or cell adhesion (sepsis, severe vaso-occlusive episodes).[87]

Management

Acute Splenic Sequestration

The management of acute splenic sequestration is addressed in the National Heart, Lung, and Blood Institute (NHLBI) Expert Panel Report, which indicates a strong recommendation (based on low-quality evidence) to provide intravenous fluid resuscitation for children with hypovolemia. The expert panel also recommended transfusion for acute splenic sequestration and severe anemia to raise the hemoglobin to a stable level while avoiding overtransfusion (strong recommendation, low-quality evidence). From a practical standpoint, this means transfusion of smaller aliquots of blood, typically 5 to 10 mL/kg based on the degree of anemia, and then checking the hemoglobin. The final recommendation is to address the performance and timing of splenectomy with recurrent acute splenic sequestration in consultation with a sickle cell expert.[93] The decision of when to recommend splenectomy varies among experts. One commonly used strategy is to recommend splenectomy after the first episode of splenic sequestration if it was life threatening or after the second episode. Most children have laparoscopic splenectomies, although conversion to open procedures is occasionally required. The decision between partial and total splenectomy often depends on the experience of the surgeon. A multi-institutional registry comparing these 2 approaches in 50 children with SCD demonstrated similar outcomes between partial (n = 16) and total splenectomy (n = 34). Splenic volume after partial splenectomy was stable for the first year.[94] The length of stay was longer after partial splenectomy (4.1 ± 1.7 days) than after total splenectomy (2.4 ± 1.2 days).[95] In one study of 54 children undergoing splenectomy at a single center for acute splenic sequestration, the rates of acute chest syndrome (0.06-0.22 per person-year) and acute painful episodes (0.6-1.0 per person-year) increased after splenectomy.[96] This may be an effect of splenectomy or the expected age-related increase in acute painful episodes.

Splenomegaly

The NHLBI Expert Panel Report recommends addressing the performance and timing of splenectomy for symptomatic hypersplenism in consultation with a sickle cell expert (moderate recommendation, low-quality evidence).[93] The decision should be made based on symptoms of hypersplenism (pain, early satiety, fatigue from worsening anemia) or cytopenias that limit treatment with hydroxyurea (typically thrombocytopenia or neutropenia).

Splenic Infarct

The management of acute splenic infarction is mostly supportive and should include pain management with both nonsteroidal anti-inflammatory drugs (NSAIDs; if no contraindications) and opiates (usually parenteral) as well as consideration of nerve blocks for severe pain. Incentive spirometry is important to reduce the risk of atelectasis and the development of acute chest syndrome. If fever is present, evaluation for splenic abscess is recommended. In children with large or massive splenic infarction, severe persistent pain may be relieved by splenectomy, although the severe pain generally may resolve gradually over weeks without surgery.

Dactylitis

Definition

Dactylitis defines a clinical entity or occurrence of inflammation of a finger(s) or toe(s). Several medical entities share features and may be called dactylitis. In SCD, an episode of dactylitis may be bilateral and involve both the hands and feet. For this reason, it is also known as hand-foot syndrome.[97-100] It is an early and characteristic manifestation of SCD among young children, especially those with the more severe genotypes of HbSS and HbS-β^0 thalassemia. See Figure 13-2.

Dactylitis is commonly the first pain manifestation of SCD.[51,101,102] Young children experience painful swelling of one or both hands or feet. Tender, erythematous swelling is especially apparent in the dorsum of the hands and/or feet.

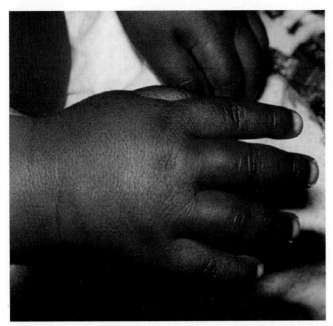

FIGURE 13-2 Child with dactylitis. Photo courtesy of Tom D. Thacher, MD.

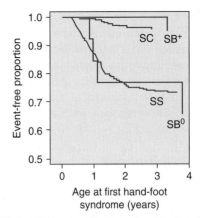

FIGURE 13-3 **Within the Cooperative Study of Sickle Cell Disease, 694 infants with confirmed sickle cell disease were enrolled at <6 months of age.**[51] The graph shows that those with HbSS and HbS-β[0] thalassemia were more likely to develop hand-foot syndrome (dactylitis). Gill FM, Sleeper LA, Weiner SJ, et al. Clinical events in the first decade in a cohort of infants with sickle cell disease. Cooperative Study of Sickle Cell Disease. *Blood.* 1995;86(2):776-783.

Symptomatic areas include the palm or foot and the associated digits. Episodes of dactylitis frequently involve >1 extremity and are accompanied by low to moderate fever, irritability, and voluntary immobility of the affected areas. Episodes typically begin with children refusing to walk, bear weight, or use their hands. Children may have accompanying leukocytosis. An episode can last for several days and may last as long as 2 weeks.[99] Onset can be gradual or acute, and children within the age of risk may have multiple episodes.[97,99]

Affected children typically self-immobilize to minimize pain.[97,98,100] Treatment requires symptomatic relief with hydration, analgesia, and antipyretics, as needed. Analgesia with NSAIDs such as ibuprofen alone may be effective. At times, opioids and/or intravenous NSAIDs may be needed for adequate analgesia. Children may also benefit from intravenous fluids, especially when poor oral intake can be a consequence of pain.

Epidemiology

During early childhood, episodes of dactylitis are characteristic, especially in children younger than age 2 years. Many affected children are younger than 12 months of age. Some children may manifest dactylitis as early as 4 months of age. In a large Jamaican cohort of newborns with HbSS, first episodes of dactylitis occurred at a median age of 1.6 years (range, 0.3-9.4 years), and 21% occurred prior to age 1 year.[101] In a smaller sample of young children with sickle cell anemia in the United States, the incidence of dactylitis was 12%, with it being the first manifestation of SCD in half of these patients.[99] Curiously, first episodes of dactylitis uncommonly occur after age 3 years.[51,97] Other SCD genotypes such as HbSC and HbS-β[+] thalassemia have a lower risk of developing dactylitis. Children with these genotypes may experience the first episode within an older age range[51] (Figure 13-3).

Prior to routine newborn hemoglobinopathy screening in the United States, an episode of dactylitis in a young child raised the suspicion of a diagnosis of SCD, most commonly HbSS.[99] In most of sub-Saharan Africa, large-scale population-based early screening for SCD is not currently being performed.[102,103] There, the onset of dactylitis usually identifies a child with SCD. For example, in a retrospective clinic-based sample of >400 children with SCD in Nigeria, the median age of diagnosis was 2.0 years (range, 2.5 months-14.0 years). Median age at diagnosis was younger for those with HbSS compared to HbSC ($P = .01$). The child's sex does not appear to affect the age of diagnosis.[103]

Pathophysiology

The physical characteristics of SCD dactylitis have much in common with acute SCD painful crises regarding the acute localized inflammation. Histologically, dactylitis in its most severe form is viewed as representing medullary bone infarction, accompanied by periosteal bone formation.[99] Ultrasonography and MRI evaluation of both finger and toe dactylitis has demonstrated a more subtle flexor tenosynovitis.

Longitudinal clinical studies have not provided strong clues as to the trigger of dactylitis and why it ceases to affect children older than age 4 years.[51,97] Speculation about risk being attributable to the size of capillary space in the digits of young children has not been supported by data. Reports of dactylitis among the existing murine models were not found. Additional insights may need virtual modeling or other approaches for understanding why this occurs as an early disease manifestation.

Risk Factors

Beyond the importance of SCD genotype,[51] major risk factors for dactylitis have been identified. These factors are the same as those for disease-associated mortality, pain crises, and other clinically evident complications, namely fetal hemoglobin (HbF) concentration and α thalassemia trait.[11,104-107]

A recent systematic review studied the impact of folic acid treatment on various complications of SCD.[108] One randomized trial suggested a reduced risk of dactylitis with folic acid supplementation. However, the level of evidence was deemed as low quality.

Differential Diagnoses

Clinically, it is critical to distinguish dactylitis from other acute localized processes that may occur in young children with SCD and require prompt intervention such as antibiotics for osteomyelitis or juvenile arthritis. The soft tissue associated with SCD dactylitis, although red, warm, and swollen, is generally not readily confused with cellulitis such as from streptococcal infection, herpetic whitlow, tuberculosis, or congenital syphilis.[100] The diagnosis of SCD, especially HbSS or HbS-β⁰ thalassemia, the age of the child, the diffuse inflammation and pain, and the self-limited nature of the episode often suffice to make the correct diagnosis. SCD findings are most commonly bilateral, symmetric, and not restricted to a single digit. Invasive instrumentation is generally not needed and is counterproductive.[100]

Despite these general differences, an infectious etiology, especially osteomyelitis, sometimes needs to be excluded. Difficulties in diagnosis may more commonly arise if dactylitis is unilateral. Infections need to be considered in the differential diagnosis, especially because these children are more likely to develop osteomyelitis or soft tissue infections with bacterial pathogens, particularly encapsulated organisms such as *Salmonella*, *Streptococcus*, or *Staphylococcus*.[109] Unless there is a specific indication on examination and imaging, invasive instrumentation should not be attempted.

Prognostic Impact on Subsequent Disease Course

Some longitudinal studies had identified a history of dactylitis during early childhood as a marker for subsequent severe clinical disease, while other studies found no such association. In the newborn cohort of the US-based Cooperative Study of SCD, dactylitis, leukocytosis, and low baseline hemoglobin between the ages of 1 and 2 years were identified as markers of clinically severe disease later in life. Outcomes of interest were death, stroke, frequent pain, and recurrent acute chest syndrome.[110,111] However, analysis of a more recent newborn cohort in Dallas, Texas, did not find dactylitis to be predictive for stroke and death later in life. Perhaps differences in the evolved patterns of standard care in the United States have mitigated the association between early and later complications.

A study from India also found no significant differences in prevalence of dactylitis or most other early acute complications between those with HbSS and HbS-β⁰ thalassemia.[112]

In contrast, the decades-long follow-up assessment of the Jamaica newborn cohort of >300 hydroxyurea-naïve patients with SCD reported a shorter survival in those who had ever had a history of dactylitis. Impact of dactylitis on mortality was similar to survival risks such as lower hemoglobin at 1 year or higher total nucleated cell count at 1 year.[101] A smaller retrospective study in Portugal also identified a strong association between dactylitis in the first year of life and hospitalizations or chronic complications.[113] Finally, among candidates for hematopoietic stem cell transplantation in Brazil based on a history of severe disease complications, dactylitis was noted as more common compared to patients lacking these clinical histories.[114]

Overall, outcomes seem to depend on treatment era, as well as the variables of environmental and genomic conditions. These differences may reflect the more recent standardized clinical approaches to interventions in these children, as well as sample sizes.

Management

Dactylitis is often the first presentation of pain in children with SCD. In the absence of newborn hemoglobinopathy screening, this complication may be the sentinel event.[51,97,102] In sub-Saharan Africa, management should be identical to that provided in high-income countries. This involves supportive care that includes hydration, NSAIDs, and/or opioid analgesics and assessment for occult infection, especially bacteremia and malaria.

Disease-Modifying Therapy for Prevention of Dactylitis

Based on at least 2 randomized controlled trials of hydroxyurea therapy in young children, strong evidence exists for prevention of multiple SCD complications, including dactylitis. The US-based BABY HUG study, a randomized, controlled, 24-month trial of hydroxyurea in children approximately 1 year of age, demonstrated a 5-fold reduction in dactylitis in patients receiving hydroxyurea.[115] Similarly, early use of hydroxyurea also reduced the risk of dactylitis in a separate randomized controlled trial of young children (mean age, 2 years) in Uganda.[116]

Hydroxyurea may prevent dactylitis by induction of HbF.[115] This hypothesis is consistent with the paucity of this complication within the first few months of childhood. Effects of hydroxyurea on other SCD-related complications, such as inflammation, may also mitigate this complication.

Summary

As a virtually pathognomonic symptom in young children with severe genotypes of SCD, dactylitis is commonly seen in pediatric care. The associated pain, inflammation, and transient disability are unique manifestations of disease. Why it largely affects very young children and how even children with ≥1 episode will "outgrow" their risk remain part of the pathophysiologic puzzle. With earlier and more widespread initiation of hydroxyurea or perhaps other effective disease-modifying therapies,[44,117] its incidence may decrease over time.[51] This challenge remains to be assessed.

Conclusion

Over the past several decades in the United States and other high-income countries, newborn screening for sickle cell disease and the institution of standardized preventative measures and early interventions for specific disease complications among pediatric patients have led to significant strides in reduced childhood morbidity and mortality.[11] Most of the reduction in mortality has come from the near-elimination of the early deaths from infection and severe splenic sequestration. Nonetheless, a 2015 US report documented that mortality among US-born children with the most severe form of SCD, homozygous HbSS and HbS-β^0 thalassemia, remained several-fold higher than that of non-SCD children aged 1 to 9 years matched for ethnicity and race.[25] Hence, despite early linkage to standardized SCD care, the health of some children with severe SCD remains at risk. Recent evaluations of guideline implementation have revealed incomplete uptake of preventative and disease-modifying therapies both by providers and families.[118-120] Children with SCD in middle- and low-resource countries (described in Chapter 31) likely remain at even higher increased risk from early childhood complications. Barriers to early continuous specialty care include movement between countries, states, and/or districts; distance to care; and inadequate communication among providers and families. These barriers could be better addressed through robust community-based programs and national registries or other means of tracking children identified with SCD through newborn screening.

Case Study: How I Treat

A 6-year-old male with HbSS presented to the emergency department with headache, fever, and decreased activity. His mother reported that he went to school the day prior but was very tired when school ended, and he slept 3 hours in the afternoon until dinner. He drank but ate no solid food and returned to bed immediately after dinner. He awoke at 1:00 AM with fever and headache and was immediately brought to the emergency department. Examination and testing revealed the following:

- Vital signs: temperature 38.5°C; heart rate 163 bpm; respiratory rate 26 breaths/min; blood pressure 87/38 mm Hg; oxygen saturation 96% on room air
- Lethargy
- Moderate scleral icterus and photophobia
- Neck stiffness
- Lungs clear to auscultation
- Capillary refill of 3 seconds
- White blood cell count, 33,000/μL; hemoglobin, 6.8 g/dL (baseline 8 g/dL); platelets, 129,000/μL; reticulocytes, 7.5% (baseline 13%); differential: 76% neutrophils, 12% bands, 1% metamyelocytes, 8% lymphocytes, 3% monocytes

   Management and outcome: The patient had a blood culture drawn and received lactated Ringer's 20 mL/kg bolus × 3 with heart rate to 120 bpm and blood pressure of 103/48 mm Hg.

- Lumbar puncture showed 653 nucleated cells, 95% neutrophils, and 5% monocytes; Gram stain showed gram-positive cocci in pairs.
- Initially treated with ceftriaxone 50 mg/kg every 12 hours and vancomycin 15 mg/kg every 6 hours. The blood and cerebrospinal fluid culture grew S pneumoniae sensitive to ceftriaxone and penicillin. Once this information was available, vancomycin was stopped, and the patient completed 14 days of ceftriaxone. He was transfused with red blood cells 10 mL/kg on day 4 for a hemoglobin of 5 g/dL with reticulocytes of 7%. He had a complete recovery and was discharged home after 8 days with a peripherally inserted central catheter to complete his parenteral antibiotics. He did not receive dexamethasone because of risk for triggering sickle cell pain and unclear benefit versus risks for pneumococcal meningitis.

High-Yield Facts

◆ Despite vaccinations and prophylactic antibiotics, children with sickle cell disease remain at increased risk of life-threatening bacterial and viral infections.

◆ All children with fever ≥38.5°C (101.3°F) should have emergency evaluation (complete blood count with differential; reticulocyte count; blood culture; ± chest x-ray; urinalysis and urine culture; stool evaluation; lumbar puncture based on age, symptoms, and signs) and empiric parenteral antibiotics with activity against pneumococcus and enteric gram-negative bacteria.

◆ Acute splenic sequestration is life threatening and often recurs.

◆ Children with splenic sequestration and hypovolemia should be treated with intravenous fluid bolus until red blood cells are available.

References

1. Therrell BL Jr, Lloyd-Puryear MA, Eckman JR, Mann MY. Newborn screening for sickle cell diseases in the United States: a review of data spanning 2 decades. *Semin Perinatol.* 2015;39(3): 238-251.

2. Huttle A, Maestre GE, Lantigua R, Green NS. Sickle cell in Latin America and the United States [corrected]. *Pediatr Blood Cancer.* 2015;62(7):1131-1136.

3. Lobitz S, Telfer P, Cela E, et al. Newborn screening for sickle cell disease in Europe: recommendations from a Pan-European Consensus Conference. *Br J Haematol.* 2018;183(4):648-660.

4. Kuznik A, Habib AG, Munube D, Lamorde M. Newborn screening and prophylactic interventions for sickle cell disease in 47 countries in sub-Saharan Africa: a cost-effectiveness analysis. *BMC Health Serv Res.* 2016;16:304.

5. Lieberman L, Kirby M, Ozolins L, Mosko J, Friedman J. Initial presentation of unscreened children with sickle cell disease: the Toronto experience. *Pediatr Blood Cancer.* 2009;53(3): 397-400.

6. Botkin JR. Ethical issues in pediatric genetic testing and screening. *Curr Opin Pediatr.* 2016;28(6):700-704.

7. Grover R, Shahidi S, Fisher B, Goldberg D, Wethers D. Current sickle cell screening program for newborns in New York City, 1979-1980. *Am J Public Health.* 1983;73(3):249-252.

8. Pearson HA, McIntosh S, Ritchey AK, Lobel JS, Rooks Y, Johnston D. Developmental aspects of splenic function in sickle cell diseases. *Blood.* 1979;53(3):358-365.

9. Gaston MH, Verter JI, Woods G, et al. Prophylaxis with oral penicillin in children with sickle cell anemia. A randomized trial. *N Engl J Med.* 1986;314(25):1593-1599.

10. Consensus conference. Newborn screening for sickle cell disease and other hemoglobinopathies. *JAMA.* 1987;258(9):1205-1209.

11. Meier ER, Rampersad A. Pediatric sickle cell disease: past successes and future challenges. *Pediatr Res.* 2017;81(1-2):249-258.

12. Smith JA, Kinney TR. Sickle cell disease: screening and management in newborns and infants. Agency for Health Care Policy and Research. *Am Fam Physician.* 1993;48(1):95-102.

13. Panepinto JA, Magid D, Rewers MJ, Lane PA. Universal versus targeted screening of infants for sickle cell disease: a cost-effectiveness analysis. *J Pediatr.* 2000;136(2):201-208.

14. Thuret I, Sarles J, Merono F, et al. Neonatal screening for sickle cell disease in France: evaluation of the selective process. *J Clin Pathol.* 2010;63(6):548-551.

15. Benson JM, Therrell BL Jr. History and current status of newborn screening for hemoglobinopathies. *Semin Perinatol.* 2010; 34(2):134-144.

16. Hertzberg VS, Hinton CF, Therrell BL, Shapira SK. Birth prevalence rates of newborn screening disorders in relation to screening practices in the United States. *J Pediatr.* 2011;159(4): 555-560.

17. Helmich F, van Dongen JL, Kuijper PH, Scharnhorst V, Brunsveld L, Broeren MA. Rapid phenotype hemoglobin screening by high-resolution mass spectrometry on intact proteins. *Clin Chim Acta.* 2016;460:220-6.

18. APHL Hemoglobinopathy Laboratory Workgroup. Hemoglobinopathies: Current Practices for Screening, Confirmation, and Follow-up [Internet]. 2015 Dec [cited 2018 Jul 25]. Available from: https://www.aphl.org/aboutAPHL/publications/Documents/NBS_HemoglobinopathyTesting_122015.pdf.

19. From the Centers for Disease Control and Prevention. Update: newborn screening for sickle cell disease–California, Illinois, and New York, 1998. *JAMA.* 2000;284(11):1373-1374.

20. Boemer F, Cornet Y, Libioulle C, Segers K, Bours V, Schoos R. 3-years experience review of neonatal screening for hemoglobin disorders using tandem mass spectrometry. *Clin Chim Acta.* 2011;412(15-16):1476-1479.

21. De Jesus VR, Mei JV, Cordovado SK, Cuthbert CD. The Newborn Screening Quality Assurance Program at the Centers for Disease Control and Prevention: thirty-five year experience assuring newborn screening laboratory quality. *Int J Neonatal Screen.* 2015;1(1):13-26.

22. Hinton CF, Homer CJ, Thompson AA, et al. A framework for assessing outcomes from newborn screening: on the road to measuring its promise. *Mol Genet Metab.* 2016;118(4): 221-229.

23. Paulukonis ST, Eckman JR, Snyder AB, et al. Defining sickle cell disease mortality using a population-based surveillance system, 2004 through 2008. *Public Health Rep.* 2016;131(2):367-375.

24. Yanni E, Grosse SD, Yang Q, Olney RS. Trends in pediatric sickle cell disease-related mortality in the United States, 1983-2002. *J Pediatr.* 2009;154(4):541-545.

25. Wang Y, Liu G, Caggana M, et al. Mortality of New York children with sickle cell disease identified through newborn screening. *Genet Med.* 2015;17(6):452-459.

26. Anders DG, Tang F, Ledneva T, et al. Hydroxyurea use in young children with sickle cell anemia in New York State. *Am J Prev Med.* 2016;51(1 suppl 1):S31-S38.

27. Reeves SL, Jary HK, Gondhi JP, Raphael JL, Lisabeth LD, Dombkowski KJ. Hydroxyurea use among children with sickle cell anemia. *Pediatr Blood Cancer.* 2019;66(6):e27721.

28. Reeves SL, Madden B, Freed GL, Dombkowski KJ. Transcranial Doppler screening among children and adolescents with sickle cell anemia. *JAMA Pediatr.* 2016;170(6):550-556.

29. Sobota A, Sabharwal V, Fonebi G, Steinberg M. How we prevent and manage infection in sickle cell disease. *Br J Haematol.* 2015;170(6):757-767.

30. Hinton CF, Neuspiel DR, Gubernick RS, et al. Improving newborn screening follow-up in pediatric practices: quality improvement innovation network. *Pediatrics.* 2012;130(3): e669-e675.

31. Hooven TA, Hooper EM, Wontakal SN, Francis RO, Sahni R, Lee MT. Diagnosis of a rare fetal haemoglobinopathy in the age of next-generation sequencing. *BMJ Case Rep.* 2016;2016:10 1136/bcr-2016-215193.

32. Lozar-Krivec J, Stepic M, Hovnik T, Krsnik M, Paro-Panjan D. Neonatal cyanosis due to hemoglobin variant: Hb F-Sarajevo. *J Pediatr Hematol Oncol.* 2016;38(7):e267-e270.

33. Kiyaga C, Hernandez AG, Ssewanyana I, et al. Building a sickle cell disease screening program in the Republic of Uganda: the Uganda Sickle Surveillance Study (US3) with 3 years of follow-up screening results. *Blood Adv.* 2018;2(suppl 1):4-7.

34. Mvundura M, Kiyaga C, Metzler M, et al. Cost for sickle cell disease screening using isoelectric focusing with dried blood spot samples and estimation of price thresholds for a point-of-care test in Uganda. *J Blood Med.* 2019;10:59-67.

35. Detemmerman L, Olivier S, Bours V, Boemer F. Innovative PCR without DNA extraction for African sickle cell disease diagnosis. *Hematology.* 2018;23(3):181-186.

36. Nnodu O, Isa H, Nwegbu M, et al. HemoTypeSC, a low-cost point-of-care testing device for sickle cell disease: promises and challenges. *Blood Cells Mol Dis.* 2019;78:22-28.

37. Bond M, Hunt B, Flynn B, Huhtinen P, Ware R, Richards-Kortum R. Towards a point-of-care strip test to diagnose sickle cell anemia. *PLoS One.* 2017;12(5):e0177732.

38. Piety NZ, George A, Serrano S, et al. A paper-based test for screening newborns for sickle cell disease. *Sci Rep.* 2017;7: 45488.

39. McGann PT, Schaefer BA, Paniagua M, Howard TA, Ware RE. Characteristics of a rapid, point-of-care lateral flow immunoassay for the diagnosis of sickle cell disease. *Am J Hematol.* 2016;91(2):205-210.

40. Genetti CA, Schwartz TS, Robinson JO, et al. Parental interest in genomic sequencing of newborns: enrollment experience from the BabySeq Project. *Genet Med.* 2019;21(3):622-630.

41. Kunz JB, Cario H, Grosse R, Jarisch A, Lobitz S, Kulozik AE. The epidemiology of sickle cell disease in Germany following recent large-scale immigration. *Pediatr Blood Cancer.* 2017;64:7.

42. Corriveau-Bourque C, Bruce AA. The changing epidemiology of pediatric hemoglobinopathy patients in northern Alberta, Canada. *J Pediatr Hematol Oncol.* 2015;37(8):595-599.

43. Cortes-Castell E, Palazon-Bru A, Pla C, et al. Impact of prematurity and immigration on neonatal screening for sickle cell disease. *PLoS One.* 2017;12(2):e0171604.

44. Yawn BP, Buchanan GR, Afenyi-Annan AN, et al. Management of sickle cell disease: summary of the 2014 evidence-based report by expert panel members. *JAMA.* 2014;312(10):1033-1048.

45. Zarkowsky HS, Gallagher D, Gill FM, et al. Bacteremia in sickle hemoglobinopathies. *J Pediatr.* 1986;109(4):579-585.

46. Gill F, Sleeper L, Weiner S, et al. Clinical events in the first decade in a cohort of infants with sickle cell disease. Cooperative Study of Sickle Cell Disease [see comments]. *Blood.* 1995;86(2): 776-783.

47. McCavit TL, Quinn CT, Techasaensiri C, Rogers ZR. Increase in invasive *S. pneumoniae* infections in children with sickle cell disease since pneumococcal conjugate vaccine licensure. *J Pediatr.* 2011;158(3):505-507.

48. Oligbu G, Collins S, Sheppard C, et al. Risk of invasive pneumococcal disease in children with sickle cell disease in england: a national observational cohort study, 2010-2015. *Arch Dis Child.* 2018;103(7):643-647.

49. Oligbu G, Fallaha M, Pay L, Ladhani S. Risk of invasive pneumococcal disease in children with sickle cell disease in the era of conjugate vaccines: a systematic review of the literature. *Br J Haematol.* 2019;185(4):743-751.

50. Ellison AM, Ota KV, McGowan KL, Smith-Whitley K. Pneumococcal bacteremia in a vaccinated pediatric sickle cell disease population. *Pediatr Infect Dis J.* 2012;31(5):534-536.

51. Gill FM, Sleeper LA, Weiner SJ, et al. Clinical events in the first decade in a cohort of infants with sickle cell disease. Cooperative Study of Sickle Cell Disease. *Blood.* 1995;86(2):776-783.

52. Yee ME, Bakshi N, Graciaa SH, et al. Incidence of invasive *H. influenzae* infections in children with sickle cell disease. *Pediatr Blood Cancer.* 2019;66(6):e27642.

53. Neonato MG, Guilloud-Bataille M, Beauvais P, et al. Acute clinical events in 299 homozygous sickle cell patients living in France. French Study Group on Sickle Cell Disease. *Eur J Haematol.* 2000;65(3):155-164.

54. Morrissey BJ, Bycroft TP, Almossawi O, Wilkey OB, Daniels JG. Incidence and predictors of bacterial infection in febrile children with sickle cell disease. *Hemoglobin.* 2015;39(5): 316-319.

55. de Montalembert M, Guilloud-Bataille M, Feingold J, Girot R. Epidemiological and clinical study of sickle cell disease in France, French Guiana and Algeria. *Eur J Haematol.* 1993;51(3): 136-140.

56. Burnett MW, Bass JW, Cook BA. Etiology of osteomyelitis complicating sickle cell disease. *Pediatrics.* 1998;101(2):296-297.

57. Tarry WF, Duckett JW Jr, Snyder HM 3rd. Urological complications of sickle cell disease in a pediatric population. *J Urol.* 1987;138(3):592-594.

58. Bundy DG, Strouse JJ, Casella JF, Miller MR. Burden of influenza-related hospitalizations among children with sickle cell disease. *Pediatrics.* 2010;125(2):234-243.

59. Sadreameli SC, Reller ME, Bundy DG, Casella JF, Strouse JJ. Respiratory syncytial virus and seasonal influenza cause similar illnesses in children with sickle cell disease. *Pediatr Blood Cancer.* 2014;61(5):875-878.

60. Strouse JJ, Reller ME, Bundy DG, et al. Severe pandemic H1N1 and seasonal influenza in children and young adults with sickle cell disease. *Blood.* 2010;116(18):3431-3434.

61. Louie JK, Acosta M, Winter K, et al. Factors associated with death or hospitalization due to pandemic 2009 influenza A (H1N1) infection in California. *JAMA.* 2009;302(17):1896-1902.

62. Goldstein AR, Anderson MJ, Serjeant GR. Parvovirus associated aplastic crisis in homozygous sickle cell disease. *Arch Dis Child.* 1987;62(6):585-588.

63. Wierenga KJ, Serjeant BE, Serjeant GR. Cerebrovascular complications and parvovirus infection in homozygous sickle cell disease. *J Pediatr.* 2001;139(3):438-442.

64. Nguyen H, Le C. Multi-organ failure associated with acute parvovirus infection and exercise in a patient with sickle beta thalassemia. *South Med J.* 2004;97(11):1139-1140.

65. Quek L, Sharpe C, Dutt N, et al. Acute human parvovirus B19 infection and nephrotic syndrome in patients with sickle cell disease. *Br J Haematol.* 2010;149(2):289-291.

66. Obeid Mohamed SO, Osman Mohamed EM, Ahmed Osman AA, Abdellatif MohamedElmugadam FA, Abdalla Ibrahim GA. A meta-analysis on the seroprevalence of parvovirus B19 among patients with sickle cell disease. *Biomed Res Int.* 2019; 2019:2757450.

67. Arzuza-Ortega L, Polo A, Perez-Tatis G, et al. Fatal sickle cell disease and Zika virus infection in girl from Colombia. *Emerg Infect Dis.* 2016;22(5):925-927.

68. Wilder-Smith A, Leong WY. Risk of severe dengue is higher in patients with sickle cell disease: a scoping review. *J Travel Med.* 2019;26:1.

69. Chernoff AI, Josephson AM. Acute erythroblastopenia in sickle-cell anemia and infectious mononucleosis. *Am J Dis Child.* 1951;82(3):310-322.

70. Symeonidis A, Papakonstantinou C, Seimeni U, et al. Non hypoxia-related splenic infarct in a patient with sickle cell trait and infectious mononucleosis. *Acta Haematol.* 2001;105(1):53-56.

71. Tonnetti L, Eder AF, Dy B, et al. Transfusion-transmitted *Babesia microti* identified through hemovigilance. *Transfusion.* 2009; 49(12):2557-2563.

72. Khan FA, Fisher MA, Khakoo RA. Association of hemochromatosis with infectious diseases: expanding spectrum. *Int J Infect Dis.* 2007;11(6):482-487.

73. Bjornson AB, Lobel JS, Magnafichi PI, Lampkin BC. Restoration by normal human immunoglobulin G of deficient serum opsonization for *S. pneumoniae* in sickle cell disease. *Infect Immun.* 1981;33(2):636-640.

74. Nagant C, Barbezange C, Dedeken L, et al. Alteration of humoral, cellular and cytokine immune response to inactivated influenza vaccine in patients with sickle cell disease. *PLoS One.* 2019;14(10): e0223991.

75. Cunnington AJ, de Souza JB, Walther M, Riley EM. Malaria impairs resistance to *Salmonella* through heme- and heme oxygenase-dependent dysfunctional granulocyte mobilization. *Nat Med.* 2011;18(1):120-127.

76. Pearson HA, Gallagher D, Chilcote R, et al. Developmental pattern of splenic dysfunction in sickle cell disorders. *Pediatrics.* 1985;76(3):392-397.

77. Inusa BP, Oyewo A, Brokke F, Santhikumaran G, Jogeesvaran KH. Dilemma in differentiating between acute osteomyelitis and bone infarction in children with sickle cell disease: the role of ultrasound. *PLoS One.* 2013;8(6):e65001.

78. Fontalis A, Hughes K, Nguyen MP, et al. The challenge of differentiating vaso-occlusive crises from osteomyelitis in children with sickle cell disease and bone pain: a 15-year retrospective review. *J Child Orthop.* 2019;13(1):33-9.

79. Jacobson DL, Shannon R, Cheng EY, et al. Adherence to the 2011 American Academy of Pediatrics urinary tract infection guidelines for voiding cystourethrogram ordering by clinician specialty. *Urology.* 2019;126:180-186.

80. National Heart, Lung, and Blood Institute: Evidence-based management of sickle cell disease: expert panel report 2014. https://www.nhlbi.nih.gov/sites/default/files/media/docs/sickle-cell-disease-report%20020816_0.pdf. Accessed June 28, 2020.

81. Wilimas JA, Flynn PM, Harris S, et al. A randomized study of outpatient treatment with ceftriaxone for selected febrile children with sickle cell disease. *N Engl J Med.* 1993;329(7): 472-476.

82. Al Fawaz T, Alzumar O, Al Shahrani D, Alshehri M. Severity of *Salmonella* infection among sickle cell diseases pediatric patients: description of the infection pattern. *Int J Pediatr Adolesc Med.* 2019;6(3):115-117.

83. Martí-Carvajal AJ, Agreda-Pérez LH. Antibiotics for treating osteomyelitis in people with sickle cell disease. *Cochrane Database Syst Rev.* 2019;10:CD007175.

84. Committee on Infectious Diseases. Recommendations for prevention and control of influenza in children, 2019-2020. *Pediatrics.* 2019;144(4):e20192478.

85. Ballas SK, Lieff S, Benjamin LJ, et al. Definitions of the phenotypic manifestations of sickle cell disease. *Am J Hematol.* 2010;85(1):6-13.

86. Calle-Toro JS, Back SJ, Viteri B, Andronikou S, Kaplan SL. Liver, spleen, and kidney size in children as measured by ultrasound: a systematic review. *J Ultrasound Med.* 2020;39(2):223-230.

87. Al-Salem AH. Splenic complications of sickle cell anemia and the role of splenectomy. *ISRN Hematol.* 2011;2011:864257.

88. Ballas SK. Neurocognitive complications of sickle cell anemia in adults. *JAMA.* 2010;303(18):1862-1863.

89. Brousse V, Elie C, Benkerrou M, et al. Acute splenic sequestration crisis in sickle cell disease: cohort study of 190 paediatric patients. *Br J Haematol.* 2012;156(5):643-648.

90. Adekile AD, McKie KM, Adeodu OO, et al. Spleen in sickle cell anemia: comparative studies of Nigerian and U.S. patients. *Am J Hematol.* 1993;42(3):316-321.

91. Gale HI, Bobbitt CA, Setty BN, et al. Expected sonographic appearance of the spleen in children and young adults with sickle cell disease: an update. *J Ultrasound Med.* 2016;35(8):1735-1745.

92. Zimmerman SA, Ware RE. Palpable splenomegaly in children with haemoglobin SC disease: haematological and clinical manifestations. *Clin Lab Haematol.* 2000;22(3):145-150.

93. US Department of Health and Human Services. *Evidence-Based Management of Sickle Cell Disease: Expert Panel Report.* US Department of Health and Human Services; 2014.

94. Rice HE, Englum BR, Rothman J, et al. Clinical outcomes of splenectomy in children: report of the splenectomy in congenital hemolytic anemia registry. *Am J Hematol.* 2015;90(3): 187-192.

95. Mouttalib S, Rice HE, Snyder D, et al. Evaluation of partial and total splenectomy in children with sickle cell disease using an Internet-based registry. *Pediatr Blood Cancer.* 2012;59(1): 100-104.

96. Kalpatthi R, Kane ID, Shatat IF, Rackoff B, Disco D, Jackson SM. Clinical events after surgical splenectomy in children with sickle cell anemia. *Pediatr Surg Int.* 2010;26(5):495-500.

97. Stevens MC, Padwick M, Serjeant GR. Observations on the natural history of dactylitis in homozygous sickle cell disease. *Clin Pediatr (Phila).* 1981;20(5):311-317.

98. da Silva Junior GB, Daher Ede F, da Rocha FA. Osteoarticular involvement in sickle cell disease. *Rev Bras Hematol Hemoter.* 2012;34(2):156-164.

99. Worrall VT, Butera V. Sickle-cell dactylitis. *J Bone Joint Surg Am.* 1976;58(8):1161-1163.

100. Olivieri I, Scarano E, Padula A, Giasi V, Priolo F. Dactylitis, a term for different digit diseases. *Scand J Rheumatol.* 2006;35(5): 333-340.

101. Serjeant GR, Chin N, Asnani MR, et al. Causes of death and early life determinants of survival in homozygous sickle cell disease: the Jamaican cohort study from birth. *PLoS One.* 2018;13(3):e0192710.

102. Brown BJ, Akinkunmi BF, Fatunde OJ. Age at diagnosis of sickle cell disease in a developing country. *Afr J Med Med Sci.* 2010;39(3):221-225.

103. Kambasu DM, Rujumba J, Lekuya HM, Munube D, Mupere E. Health-related quality of life of adolescents with sickle cell disease in sub-Saharan Africa: a cross-sectional study. *BMC Hematol.* 2019;19:9.

104. Platt OS, Brambilla DJ, Rosse WF, et al. Mortality in sickle cell disease. Life expectancy and risk factors for early death. *N Engl J Med.* 1994;330(23):1639-1644.

105. Thein SL. Genetic basis and genetic modifiers of beta-thalassemia and sickle cell disease. *Adv Exp Med Biol.* 2017; 1013:27-57.

106. Brousse V, El Hoss S, Bouazza N, et al. Prognostic factors of disease severity in infants with sickle cell anemia: a comprehensive longitudinal cohort study. *Am J Hematol.* 2018;93(11):1411-1419.

107. Powars DR, Meiselman HJ, Fisher TC, Hiti A, Johnson C. Beta-S gene cluster haplotypes modulate hematologic and hemorheologic expression in sickle cell anemia. Use in predicting clinical severity. *Am J Pediatr Hematol Oncol.* 1994;16(1):55-61.

108. Dixit R, Nettem S, Madan SS, et al. Folate supplementation in people with sickle cell disease. *Cochrane Database Syst Rev.* 2018; 3:CD011130.

109. Sinkin JC, Wood BC, Sauerhammer TM, Boyajian MJ, Rogers GF, Oh AK. *Salmonella* osteomyelitis of the hand in an infant with sickle cell disease. *Plast Reconstr Surg Glob Open.* 2015;3(1):e298.

110. Meier ER, Wright EC, Miller JL. Reticulocytosis and anemia are associated with an increased risk of death and stroke in the newborn cohort of the Cooperative Study of Sickle Cell Disease. *Am J Hematol.* 2014;89(9):904-906.

111. Quinn CT. Minireview: clinical severity in sickle cell disease: the challenges of definition and prognostication. *Exp Biol Med (Maywood).* 2016;241(7):679-688.

112. Jain D, Warthe V, Dayama P, et al. Sickle cell disease in central India: a potentially severe syndrome. *Indian J Pediatr.* 2016;83(10): 1071-1076.

113. Silva IV, Reis AF, Palare MJ, Ferrao A, Rodrigues T, Morais A. Sickle cell disease in children: chronic complications and search of predictive factors for adverse outcomes. *Eur J Haematol.* 2015;94(2):157-161.

114. Flor-Park MV, Kelly S, Preiss L, et al. Identification and characterization of hematopoietic stem cell transplant candidates in a sickle cell disease cohort. *Biol Blood Marrow Transplant.* 2019;25(10):2103-2109.

115. Wang WC, Ware RE, Miller ST, et al. Hydroxycarbamide in very young children with sickle-cell anaemia: a multicentre, randomised, controlled trial (BABY HUG). *Lancet.* 2011;377(9778): 1663-1672.

116. Opoka RO, Ndugwa CM, Latham TS, et al. Novel use Of Hydroxyurea in an African Region with Malaria (NOHARM): a trial for children with sickle cell anemia. *Blood.* 2017;130(24):2585-2593.

117. Reeves SL, Jary HK, Gondhi JP, Raphael JL, Lisabeth LD, Dombkowski KJ. Hydroxyurea initiation among children with sickle cell anemia. *Clin Pediatr (Phila).* 2019;58(13): 1394-1400.

Pulmonary Hypertension and Heart Disease in Patients With Sickle Cell Disease

14

Authors: *Mark T. Gladwin, Kenneth I. Ataga, Roberto Machado*

Chapter Outline

Overview

Sickle cell disease (SCD) is an autosomal recessive disease caused by a single point mutation in the gene encoding the β-globin chain of hemoglobin.[1] The most common form of SCD is caused by the inheritance of homozygous mutant hemoglobin S (HbSS; occurring in up to 75% of patients), whereas approximately 25% of patients have compound heterozygosity of hemoglobin S with another β-globin chain variant (ie, hemoglobin C, D-Punjab, O-Arab, and E).[1-4] The mutant sickle cell hemoglobin polymerizes within the erythrocyte during deoxygenation, altering erythrocyte rheology and causing microvascular obstruction and hemolytic anemia.[1-4] As described in early chapters on mechanisms of disease and summarized in Figure 14-1, the pathogenesis is determined upstream by the extent of hemoglobin S polymerization, which leads to the following 2 major downstream pathologic events: microvascular occlusion (vaso-occlusion) with ischemia-reperfusion

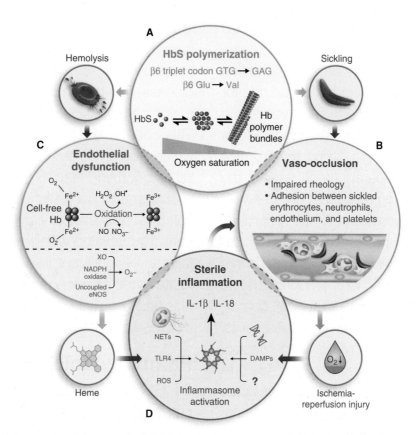

FIGURE 14-1 **Molecular pathophysiology of sickle cell disease. A.** HbS polymerization. **B.** Vaso-occlusion. **C.** Hemolytic anemia and endothelial dysfunction. **D.** Sterile inflammation and inflammasome activation. Hb, hemoglobin; IL, interleukin; NETs, neutrophil extracellular traps; ROS, reactive oxygen species; XO, xanthine oxidase. Other abbreviations are defined in the text. Modified from Sundd P, Gladwin MT, Novelli EM. Pathophysiology of Sickle Cell Disease. *Annu Rev Pathol.* 2019;14:263-292.

tissue injury and infarction,[5,6] and hemolytic anemia, which releases cell free hemoglobin and other erythrocytic products, such as adenosine diphosphate (ADP) and arginase 1, from the red blood cells, reducing nitric oxide (NO) signaling and generating reactive oxygen species.[7-11] These pathobiologic processes may act in concert to activate inflammatory pathways involving selectin-mediated adhesion and inflammasome-mediated sterile inflammation.[4] For example, oxidation of hemoglobin leads to heme release and downstream activation of P-selectin–dependent platelet-neutrophil interactions and toll-like receptor 4 (TLR4)-dependent and -independent sterile inflammation signaling pathways.[12-15] Cycles of ischemia-reperfusion tissue injury and infarction likely also release damage-associated molecular proteins (DAMPs), such as mitochondrial DNA, that can also activate toll-like receptor and **NLRP**

(Nucleotide-binding oligomerization domain, Leucine rich Repeat and Pyrin domain containing), also abbreviated as **NALP** (NACHT, LRR, and PYD domains–containing protein) inflammasome-dependent sterile inflammation. Furthermore, steady-state intravascular hemolysis releases erythrocyte DAMPs (eDAMPs) that may activate the innate immune system, priming it for a second hit, such as infection or trauma, that activates severe inflammation and vaso-occlusive events.[4,16] During acute episodes of pain crisis, the intensity of both vaso-occlusion and hemolytic anemia may increase dramatically, leading to severe acute organ injury and severe pain, sometimes culminating in acute lung injury (called the acute chest syndrome), cor pulmonale, multiorgan dysfunction and failure, and death.[2,4] See Figure 14-1 for an overview of the major pathophysiologic mechanisms that drive SCD.

In the current era, the epidemiology of SCD can be characterized by 2 divergent outcomes, one good and the other quite ominous. The first involves dramatic improvement in outcomes for children with SCD, with rapid improvement in both morbidity and mortality. Although mortality rates remain extremely high during the first few years of life in sub-Saharan Africa, where the prevalence of SCD is highest, most children with SCD now survive to adulthood.[3,17] The improved outcomes are likely related to extended newborn screening to identify children with SCD for more intensive observation and therapy, improvements in public health infrastructure that limit comorbid infections that trigger vaso-occlusive events, vaccination, penicillin prophylaxis in childhood, effective red blood cell transfusions to prevent stroke in high-risk children and treat acute vaso-occlusive complications, and hydroxyurea therapy.[3,17] Red blood cell transfusions and hydroxyurea therapy have had major effects on the reduction of childhood stroke and other complications of SCD.[18-21] These interventions have resulted in increased survival and reduced morbidity for patients with SCD.[22]

Despite improved outcomes, many patients surviving to adulthood are developing chronic neuropathic pain syndromes and chronic systemic vasculopathy, leading to chronic organ dysfunction and failure.[23-35] Despite advances in the care of patients with SCD, the median age of survival is approximately 48 years in patients with sickle cell anemia, even in the post-hydroxyurea era.[36,37] Cardiopulmonary organ dysfunction and chronic kidney injury have a significant effect on patient morbidity and premature mortality in adulthood.[27,37] It is now increasingly clear that sustained intravascular red blood cell hemolysis and anemia over decades, compounded by episodic vascular occlusion and organ ischemia, directly injure the cardiovascular and renal system.[4,28,35,38,39]

This culminates in the development of pulmonary hypertension (PH), left ventricular diastolic heart disease, albuminuria and chronic kidney disease, dysrhythmia, and sudden death, all major cardiovascular complications of SCD.[35] This chapter will focus on the mechanisms by which hemolysis and anemia impair endothelial function and lead to progressive proliferative vasculopathy, particularly in the pulmonary vasculature. The clinical cardiovascular complications that develop with advancing age that have the most significant impact on patient survival relate to the development of PH and left ventricular diastolic dysfunction, both of which will be discussed in detail.

Pathophysiologic Effects of Anemia and Hemolysis on the Cardiopulmonary Vascular System

Hemolysis, Impaired NO Signaling, and Endothelial Dysfunction

Normal blood vessels maintain vasodilation via the elaboration of a number of critical vasodilators from the endothelium, including NO and prostaglandins.[40] The endothelium and smooth muscle also releases vasoconstrictor molecules, such as endothelin-1 and reactive oxygen species.[41] The balance of these factors maintains redox homeostasis and vasomotor tone. One of the major vasodilators, NO, is produced enzymatically by the endothelial NO synthase (eNOS) enzyme via the 5-electron oxidation of L-arginine to form citrulline and NO. NO is also produced via the reduction of nitrite (NO_2^-) by hemoglobin and molybdopterin enzymes.[42] NO diffuses from endothelium to smooth muscle to bind to the heme group of the enzyme soluble guanylate cyclase (sGC), which, once activated, converts guanosine triphosphate (GTP) to cyclic guanosine monophosphate (cGMP), a secondary messenger that signals smooth muscle relaxation and vasodilation. The NO-sGC-cGMP signaling pathway is regulated by the control of eNOS activity (phosphorylation, glutathionylation, calcium binding, and other modifications), the bioavailability of NO (reduced by scavenging reactions with hemoglobin or superoxide), the oxidation state of sGC (reduced enzyme binds NO, whereas oxidized enzyme does not bind NO), and the activity of phosphodiesterases that metabolize cGMP (phosphodiesterases 5 and 9 in particular).[40,41] In SCD, this signaling axis is impaired via a number of mechanisms described later in this chapter.

Although it is well appreciated that hemoglobin can react with and scavenge NO, this reaction is limited when hemoglobin is compartmentalized within the red blood cell. The intact erythrocyte creates a number of barriers for NO diffusion and reaction with the compartmentalized hemoglobin. Laminar flowing erythrocytes align centripetally and form a cell-free zone along the endothelium, which reduces the scavenging of endothelially formed NO.[43-45] Other barriers include an intrinsic diffusion barrier at the red cell membrane and an unstirred layer around the membrane.[43-45] With hemolysis, these barriers are disrupted, and the hemoglobin in plasma can enter the unstirred and cell-free zones to react more rapidly with NO.[7,8,45] Furthermore, it is now appreciated that cell-free hemoglobin will dimerize and can diffuse between endothelial cells and smooth muscle, further impairing endothelial to smooth muscle paracrine NO signaling, a process that is normally limited by haptoglobin binding to plasma hemoglobin.[46] Most patients with homozygous hemoglobin S disease have undetectable haptoglobin levels, limiting the ability to clear the hemoglobin released during active hemolysis.[7,47]

The reaction of oxyhemoglobin with NO is very fast, occurring at a near diffusion limited rate constant of about 10^7 $M^{-1}s^{-1}$ (Equation 1).[41]

Equation 1: NO + oxyhemoglobin (Fe^{2+}-O_2) → nitrate (NO_3^-) + methemoglobin (Fe^{3+})

The methemoglobin can be reduced by plasma reductants, such as urate and ascorbate, back to oxyhemoglobin to catalytically scavenge NO.[48,49] A number of studies have validated this proposed mechanism, with plasma hemoglobin levels in both patients with SCD and in humanized transgenic mouse models of SCD (in addition to mouse, rat, and dog models) correlating with impaired blood flow responses to infused NO donors.[7,38,45,48,50] High plasma hemoglobin levels of cell-free hemoglobin or red blood cell lactate dehydrogenase (an enzyme released during red cell hemolysis) correlate with impairments in flow-mediated vasodilation, an eNOS-dependent vasodilation event.[38] The infusion of cell-free hemoglobin intravenously in mice and dogs produces vasoconstriction and NO scavenging.[45,48] As described later, the development of PH and other vascular complications of SCD is epidemiologically associated with more severe steady-state hemolytic anemia.

In addition to NO scavenging by cell-free hemoglobin, the NO signaling axis is impaired by the generation of reactive oxygen species, such as superoxide, that can react with NO to form peroxynitrite.[51] In SCD, both the xanthine oxidase and NADPH oxidase enzyme systems are upregulated and appear to contribute to vascular dysfunction.[51-53] In addition to direct scavenging of NO, the production of NO is limited in SCD. Arginase 1 is an enzyme that is expressed in red blood cells and released into plasma during hemolysis.[9] This enzyme catabolizes arginine to form ornithine, thus limiting arginine bioavailability for de novo NO synthesis. The eNOS enzyme has also been shown to be oxidized and "uncoupled" in SCD,

such that it produces superoxide rather than NO.[11] Finally, studies suggest that the enzymatic target for NO, sGC, can be oxidized to an NO-insensitive ferric state.[54,55] These deleterious effects on the NO signaling axis are compounded by increased production of endothlin-1, a potent vasoconstrictor molecule that has also been shown to activate the endothelin receptor B in the erythrocyte membrane to activate the Gardos channel and increase erythrocyte dehydration.[56,57] These concerted mechanisms produce a state of deficient NO signaling and endothelial dysfunction, particularly in patients who have more severe hemolytic anemia in steady state and during more severe vaso-occlusive crisis (recently reviewed in Kato et al[47]) (Figure 14-2).

The pulmonary vasculature maintains tonic NO-mediated vasodilation and is rich in eNOS, sGC, and phosphodiesterase 5.[41,58] This vascular system appears to be particularly sensitive to the effects of hemolysis and hemoglobin-mediated NO scavenging, with a number of studies showing that infusions of cell-free hemoglobin or the transfusion of aged stored blood into normal volunteers and animal models produces hemolysis and concomitant PH.[59,60] The intrinsic rate of hemolysis is relatively stable within an individual in steady state, largely determined by the hemoglobin genotype and fetal hemoglobin levels, and can be estimated by steady-state levels of total hemoglobin and reticulocyte and/or plasma levels of cell-free hemoglobin, red cell microparticles, bilirubin, and lactate dehydrogenase.[10,61] As will be described in more detail later on the epidemiology of PH in patients with SCD, these biomarkers of the severity of hemolytic anemia are significantly associated with measures of the presence and severity of PH. The prevalence of PH is higher in patients with hemoglobin SS disease, compared with patients with SC or Sβ+ disease or SS with α thalassemia who have lower steady-state rates of hemolysis. In fact, patients with higher rates of hemolysis are more likely to develop vascular injury and dysfunction and vasculopathic complications that increase with age, including PH, cutaneous leg ulceration, and renal dysfunction (proteinuria, albuminuria, and chronic kidney dysfunction).[27,29,30,35,62] These clinical complications may represent an endophenotype of SCD caused by decades of steady-state hemolytic anemia.

Effects of Anemia on the Heart and Systemic Vasculature

Anemia is a major cause of stress to the cardiovascular system, leading to a chronically elevated cardiac output, caused largely by increased stroke volume, and ventricular dilation and wall stress.[63-65] Dilation of the left ventricle secondary to chronic anemia results in increased systolic wall stress and compensatory hypertrophy.[64,66] Highlighting the effects of chronic anemia on cardiac output, right heart catheterization studies in homozygous SS disease in steady state reveal a basal cardiac output of 10.9 ± 0.6 L/min (range, 7.6-13.7 L/min), with a mean hemoglobin level of 8.1 ± 0.3 g/dL (range, 4.7-10 g/dL).[67] Correction of anemia with transfusions increases systemic vascular resistance and reduces cardiac output to normal.[65] In 2 large echocardiographic studies of patients with SCD, left

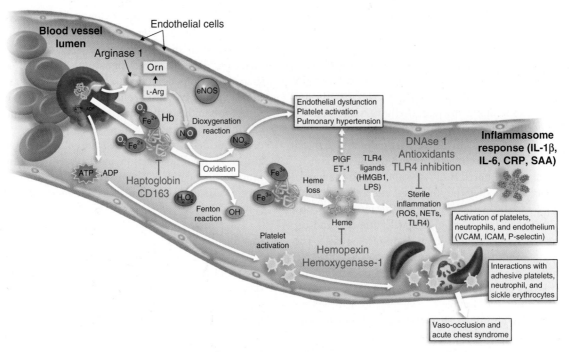

FIGURE 14-2 Effects of hemolysis on the vasculature. Hemolysis releases cell-free oxyhemoglobin and arginase 1 into plasma, both of which inhibit nitric oxide (NO) signaling and can lead to endothelial dysfunction and pulmonary hypertension. Adenosine triphosphate (ATP) and adenosine diphosphate (ADP) released from red cells, in addition to hemoglobin (Hb), can activate platelets. When oxyhemoglobin oxidizes to ferric (Fe^{3+}) methemoglobin, it can release the heme group, which can activate the toll-like receptor 4 (TLR4) and drive sterile inflammation. This causes reactive oxygen species (ROS) and DNA net release from neutrophils and the activation of the inflammasome signaling pathway, all of which drive the P-selectin–dependent adhesion of neutrophils, platelets, and red blood cells to promote vaso-occlusion. Haptoglobin and hemopexin can bind and limit the toxicity of hemoglobin and heme, respectively. CRP, C-reactive protein; eNOS, endothelial nitric oxide synthase; ET-1, endothelin-1; HMGB1, high mobility group box 1; ICAM, intercellular adhesion molecule; IL, interleukin; LPS, lipopolysaccharide; NETs, neutrophil extracellular traps; PIGF, placental growth factor; SAA, serum amyloid A; VCAM, vascular cell adhesion molecule. Modified from Kato GJ, Steinberg MH, Gladwin MT. Intravascular hemolysis and the pathophysiology of sickle cell disease. *J Clin Invest.* 2017;127(3):750-760.

ventricular chamber size and mass both increased with anemia, without changes in systolic function and heart rate.[10,28] The increased left ventricular mass likely contributes to the development of diastolic left heart disease, now referred to as heart failure with preserved ejection fraction (HFpEF). This is thought to be caused by the impaired relaxation of the dilated left ventricle, the chronic increased work (wall stress) required to maintain a high stroke volume, and the increased afterload of a "stiff" vasculature. Consistent with vascular stiffness, patients with SCD develop an increased pulse pressure in both the systemic and pulmonary circulations. This is the result of severe anemia, which lowers vascular resistance and diastolic pressures, accompanied by increases in stroke volume and vascular stiffness, which increase systolic pressures.[32] Elevated systemic systolic blood pressures have been identified as an independent risk factor for the development of PH, hypoxemia, diastolic heart dysfunction, chronic kidney injury, silent infarcts, and infarctive stroke.[28,32,68,69] Both anemia and increases in blood pressure are risk factors for the development of left ventricular diastolic dysfunction in patients with SCD.[28,66] As an example, in a study of 415 patients with SCD, a higher natural log left ventricular lateral E/e′ ratio, reflecting diastolic left ventricular dysfunction, was independently associated with lower hemoglobin concentration (P <.0001) and higher systolic blood pressures

(P <.007).[64] These effects of anemia on the cardiovascular system have been recently reviewed.[39]

In addition to the stress imposed by anemia, recent studies evaluating the transgenic humanized mouse models of SCD suggest that microvascular infarction and fibrosis of the heart develop with age[70] and that the expression of interleukin-18, a well-characterized proinflammatory and fibrotic cytokine associated with development of heart failure and cardiac hypertrophy as well as increased mortality in heart failure patients, is increased in the hearts of these mice.[71] These findings in mice are supported by findings in patients of increased myocardial extracellular matrix detected by magnetic resonance imaging (MRI).[72,73] Whether the fibrosis occurs as a result of increased wall stress, effects of hemolysis and heme on the myocardium, or subclinical vaso-occlusion remains to be determined.

Concerted Effect of Hemolysis and Anemia on the Heart and Systemic and Pulmonary Vasculature

Mechanistic studies in aggregate suggest a concerted effect of hemolysis and anemia on the heart and systemic and pulmonary vasculature (Figure 14-3).[39] Chronic anemia leads to cardiac hypertrophy, chamber dilation, and diastolic heart dysfunction, and hemolysis produces endothelial dysfunction,

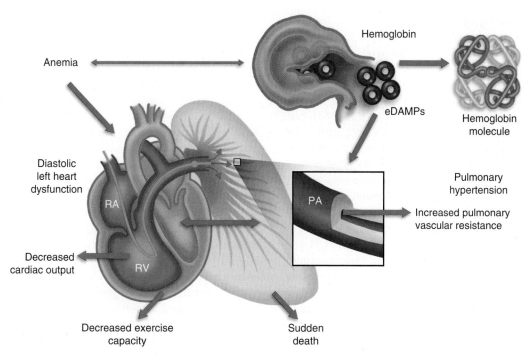

FIGURE 14-3 Concerted effects of hemolysis and anemia on the cardiovascular system. Anemia is associated with the development of diastolic left heart disease, whereas hemolysis releases hemoglobin and heme, which drive endothelial dysfunction, vascular injury, and increased pulmonary vascular resistance (PVR). Both intrinsic pulmonary vascular disease and diastolic left heart disease lead to pulmonary hypertension, reduced exercise tolerance, and increased risk of sudden death. CO, cardiac output; eDAMPs, erythroid damage-associated molecular patterns; PA, pulmonary artery; RA, right atrium; RV, right ventricle. Modified from The Lancet. Gladwin MT. Cardiovascular complications and risk of death in sickle-cell disease. *Lancet.* 2016;387(10037):2565-2574. Copyright 2016, with permission from Elsevier.

pulmonary vascular disease, PH, high pulse pressures, and systemic vascular stiffness. As patients age, the prevalence of pulmonary vascular disease, right heart failure, and diastolic left heart disease increases, all of which are associated with a high risk of death in the SCD adult population.

Thromboembolism and PH

From a mechanistic perspective, hemolysis promotes platelet and hemostatic activation,[74-77] and chronic inflammation is another factor potentially contributing to a hypercoagulable state (see Chapter 22 on hypercoagulability in SCD).[78] Within this context, SCD is associated with an increased risk for thrombotic complications including pulmonary embolism[79] and, consequently, chronic thromboembolic PH (CTEPH). Although 2 published studies suggested that pulmonary thrombi are uncommon in SCD patients with elevated tricuspid regurgitant jet velocity (TRV),[80,81] another study reported high-probability ventilation-perfusion scans for thromboemboli but negative helical spiral computed tomography (CT) scans in 6 of 26 patients with PH.[67] Autopsy studies also suggest the possibility of a contribution of thromboembolism in some cases of SCD-associated PH because microthrombotic and/or thromboembolic lesions are common findings at postmortem examination in patients with SCD.[82,83] Acute or organizing thrombi in the pulmonary arteries, predominantly distal, were a common fining at autopsy in a series of 11 SCD patients with the diagnosis of PH.[84] A significant association was found

between the postmortem diagnosis of PH and thromboembolism in another autopsy series.[85] Furthermore, most hemoglobin SS patients have autosplenectomy, and splenectomy is a recognized risk factor for thrombosis and CTEPH.[86]

Hypoxia, Genetic Variation, and PH

Chronic hypoxia and normoxic activation of hypoxia-inducible factor (HIF)-related pathways are involved in the etiology of various forms of PH.[87-92] Erythropoietin expression sensitively reflects tissue oxygenation status,[93] and HIF-1α, the master regulator of the body's response to hypoxia, regulates its expression.[94] SCD is characterized by high circulating erythropoietin concentrations under steady-state conditions,[95] suggesting that this chronic hemolytic anemia is accompanied by chronic upregulation of the hypoxic response. To test this hypothesis, Xu and colleagues compared clinical characteristics and peripheral blood mononuclear cell (PBMC) genomic profiles of subjects with SCD to those of subjects with Chuvash polycythemia, a monogenic disorder where homozygosity for VHL^{R200W} leads to posttranslational stabilization of the α subunits of HIF at normoxia and increased levels of HIF-1 and HIF-2, leading to altered transcription of a number of genes and elevated systolic pulmonary artery pressures.[96-98] The study observed a strong correlation of altered gene expression profiles in hemoglobin SS subjects and *VHL*[R200W] homozygote polycythemic subjects, suggesting that >50% of PBMC gene expression variation in hemoglobin SS patients may be related to the hypoxic response.[99] Interestingly, *MAPK8*, a hypoxia downregulated gene that has a prominent role in promoting apoptosis,[100] appeared to play an important role in hypoxic gene regulation, and an expression quantitative trait locus of this gene (rs10857560) that further downregulated expression was associated with right heart catheterization–documented precapillary PH in SCD. In addition, in another study, elevated levels of placental growth factor, which activates HIF-1α in normoxia, have been shown to be elevated and associated with elevated systolic pulmonary artery pressures in SCD mice and patients.[101,102]

The phenotypic heterogeneity in the rate of development of acute and chronic complications of SCD, including PH, is well documented. This suggests that other genetic modifiers could play a role in these complications. In fact, single nucleotide polymorphisms for genes in the transforming growth factor-β superfamily, including activin A receptor, type II-like 1 (*ACVRL1*), bone morphogenetic protein receptor 2 (*BMPR2*), bone morphogenetic protein 6 (*BMP6*), the β₁-adrenergic receptor (*ADRB1*),[103] and thrombospondin-1 (*THBS1*),[104] have been associated with an elevated pulmonary artery systolic pressure in patients with SCD. Desai et al[105] explored the usefulness of PBMC-derived gene signatures as biomarkers for PH in SCD. Genome-wide gene and microRNA (miRNA) expression profiles were correlated against estimated right ventricular systolic pressure (RVSP), yielding 631 transcripts and 12 miRNAs correlating with RVSP. Biologic pathway analysis of these 631 genes revealed that pathways that have been associated with pulmonary vascular remodeling such as Wnt signaling, calcium signaling, vascular smooth muscle contraction, and cancer pathways were significantly overrepresented in patients with elevated RVSP. Support vector machine analysis identified a 10-gene signature including *GALNT13* (encoding polypeptide *N*-acetylgalactosaminyltransferase 13, a glycosyltransferase enzyme responsible for the synthesis of O-glycan) that distinguished patients with and without increased RVSP with 100% accuracy. This finding was then validated in a separate cohort of patients who had SCD without or with PH documented by right heart catheterization, with an overall accuracy of 90%. Increased RVSP-related miRNAs revealed strong in silico binding predictions of miR-301a to *GALNT13*, which was corroborated by microarray analyses demonstrating an inverse correlation between their expression. A genetic association study comparing patients with elevated versus normal RVSP revealed 5 significant single nucleotide polymorphisms within *GALNT13* associated with an elevated RVSP.

Clinical Classification and Definitions

PH is a relatively common complication in patients with SCD, particularly with advancing age, and comes in a number of hemodynamic patterns. As defined later, patients with SCD

have been shown to develop PH with primary involvement of the pulmonary vasculature (World Health Organization group 1 PH or pulmonary arterial hypertension [PAH]), secondary to left heart disease (group 2 PH), secondary to interstitial lung disease or pulmonary fibrosis (group 3 PH), and secondary to chronic thromboembolic disease (CTEPH or group 4 PH). Because of the different presentations, PH in the setting of SCD is currently listed in group 5 (a miscellaneous category that includes the hemolytic anemias).[106]

PH is defined by an increase in the mean pulmonary artery pressure (mPAP) measured by right heart catheterization. A value ≥25 mm Hg is about 3 standard deviations above the population mean and has been used to define PH.[107] However, multiple studies in patients with many diseases suggest that even borderline values between 20 and 24 mm Hg also increase risk of death and exercise intolerance, suggesting a new definition of borderline PH.[108,109] In fact, the Sixth World Symposium in Pulmonary Hypertension has proposed to define all forms of precapillary PH as an mPAP >20 mm Hg and a pulmonary vascular resistance (PVR) ≥3 Wood units.[110] This new definition is quite important because it would lead to reclassification of a substantial number of patients with SCD as having PH. PH can occur secondary to isolated pathologic remodeling of the pulmonary arterioles, starting with vasoconstriction and intimal and smooth muscle hyperplasia, and finally leading to severe angioproliferation, occlusion, and recanalization, referred to as the plexogenic lesion.[107] When the disease is restricted to the pulmonary arterioles, the mean pulmonary pressures increase, but the left ventricular end-diastolic pressures (measured by pulmonary artery occlusion pressure [PAOP]) are normal (<15 mm Hg). This is called pulmonary arterial hypertension (PAH; previously referred to as primary PH) and is defined as group 1 PH. Because there is a gradient between the pulmonary arterioles and the left ventricular and atrial pressures (measured by PAOP), there is a high transpulmonary pressure gradient (mPAP-PAOP >12 mm Hg) and an elevated PVR (>3 Wood units).[110]

PH can also arise secondary to left heart disease (defined as group 2 PH) as a result of chronic backpressure elevations from the left heart, secondary to either HFpEF (also referred to as diastolic dysfunction of the left heart) or heart failure with reduced ejection fraction (HFrEF). In this case, the mPAP >20 mm Hg is associated with a PAOP that is ≥15 mm Hg and there is no elevation in the PVR.[110]

A new hemodynamic phenotype of PH has been described in the setting of group 2 PH from left heart disease, but in which the pulmonary vasculature is thought to remodel and the transpulmonary gradient and PVR rise.[111,112] In this case, the mPAP is >20 mm Hg and the PAOP is ≥15 mm Hg, consistent with group 2, but at the same time, the resistance increases to >3 Wood units.[110] This is now referred to as combined pre- and postcapillary PH (CpcPH), and in the setting of both HFpEF and HFrEF, this carries a worse prognosis, with increased risk of hospitalization and death, compared with HFpEF or HFrEF without a high PVR.[113]

Right heart catheterization studies in patients with SCD suggest that approximately 10% of adult patients develop PH with an mPAP ≥25 mm Hg. Approximately half of these patients have group 1 hemodynamics with a PAOP ≤15 mm Hg, and half have group 2 hemodynamics with a PAOP >15 mm Hg.[31,114-117] Most patients with group 2 have normal left ventricular ejection fractions and thus have PH secondary to HFpEF, and many also have an increased transpulmonary gradient consistent with CpcPH. Indeed, the increase in transpulmonary gradient in patients with SCD strongly predicts worse mortality.[31]

Although most patients with SCD have hemodynamics consistent with groups 1 and 2, there are cases of severe advanced lung disease and pulmonary fibrosis with PH (group 3) and CTEPH. CTEPH is a form of PH (group 4) caused by pulmonary thromboemboli followed by secondary fibrotic remodeling of the occluded pulmonary vasculature.[107] CTEPH is particularly important to diagnose because patients require anticoagulation and there are approved drugs such as riociguat and surgical treatment approaches (pulmonary artery balloon angioplasty and pulmonary artery thromboendarterectomy).[118-122] Riociguat is a small-molecule activator of the sGC enzyme and has been approved for the treatment of PAH and CTEPH.[120]

It is important to note that the "normal" PVR is very low in patients with severe anemia.[123,124] This occurs because anemia causes a decrease in the oxygen content of blood, which leads to increases in cardiac output to maintain oxygen delivery. In addition, anemia produces a reduction of blood viscosity.[124] According to Ohm's law, the PVR is equal to the mPAP-PAOP (the transpulmonary gradient) divided by the cardiac output. Thus, even if mPAP increases, as the cardiac output rises with anemia, the calculated PVR decreases. Because of this effect, the PVR in patients with SCD without PH ranges from 68 to 74 dyn·s·cm^{-5}, as compared with the measured values in nonanemic healthy volunteers of 80 to 120 dyn·s·cm^{-5} (or about 1 Wood unit).[123] Thus, anemia increases cardiac output and lowers blood viscosity and may lead to an underestimation of the severity of pulmonary vascular disease.[124] To correct for this effect, a PVR of >160 dyn·s·cm^{-5} has been proposed as abnormal in a patient with SCD.[123]

Clinical Presentation, Diagnostic Studies, and Epidemiology of PH in Adult Patients With SCD

Progressive increases in PVR or left heart pressures lead to PH. As the right heart begins to fail, patients become symptomatic with progressive dyspnea on exertion and signs of right heart failure, which include an elevated jugular venous pressure often with hepatojugular reflux, a loud P_2 heart sound, and peripheral edema.[107,123] Laboratory studies reveal an increase in plasma levels of brain natriuretic peptide (BNP) or N-terminal pro-brain natriuretic peptide (NT-proBNP), which have been studied extensively in patients with sickle

cell disease.[125] Cardiac ultrasound can be used to screen for PH and right heart failure, and the pulmonary artery systolic pressure can be estimated by measuring the tricuspid regurgitant jet velocity (TRV).[29] Backflow of blood from the right ventricle to the right atrium across a leaky tricuspid valve can be measured by Doppler echocardiography. The velocity of this regurgitant flow is converted to pressure according to the equation $4V^2$, where V is the regurgitant velocity in meters per second.[126] Thus, a TRV value of 3.0 m/s produces an estimated RVSP (which equals the pulmonary artery systolic pressure) of $4 \times 3 \times 3$ ($4V^2$), which equals 36 mm Hg. For context, a TRV value ≥2.5 m/s is abnormal and is 2 standard deviations higher than the mean for patients aged 35 to 40 years. A value ≥3.0 m/s is 3 standard deviations above the population mean (Figure 14-4). The cardiac ultrasound can also be used to evaluate right ventricular size and function. Dilation of the right ventricle and a decrease in the tricuspid annular systolic excursion suggest right ventricular dysfunction.[127] Left ventricular systolic and diastolic function can also be measured to diagnose HFpEF and HFrEF. CT scanning can identify right ventricular and atrial chamber enlargement and enlargement of the pulmonary arteries, consistent with PH and right heart dysfunction.[128,129] A mosaic lung parenchymal perfusion pattern is often observed, with areas of hypoattenuation caused by oligemia where the vasculature is obstructed, resulting in less blood volume, in proximity to patches of normal lung with more blood flow (see case example in Figure 14-7 panel B). Finally, cardiac MRI is an increasingly used diagnostic modality that can assess right and left ventricular cardiac output and function and left ventricular extracellular matrix volume.[72,130]

It is clear that PH develops as a common complication during aging in patients with SCD and is a major cause of early death. Right heart catheterization studies show that for every increase of 10 mm Hg in the mPAP there is an associated 1.7-fold increase in the hazard ratio of death (95% confidence interval [CI], 1.1-2.7; $P = .028$).[131] Three large prospective screening studies have been performed in adult patients with SCD with evaluation of PH severity using the gold standard of right heart catheterization.[31,115-117] Prevalence estimates could be underestimated in all of these studies because not all patients agreed to right heart catheterization. Studies at the National Institutes of Health (NIH) evaluated 531 patients followed for a median of 4.4 years, with 84 catheterizations performed.[31,115] Fifty-five (10.4%) of the 531 screened patients had a mPAP ≥25 mm Hg, consistent with a diagnosis of PH. About half (56.4%) had precapillary PAH (PAOP ≤15 mm Hg), and the remainder had group 2 pulmonary venous hypertension with a PAOP >15 mm Hg. As mentioned earlier, the transpulmonary gradient, which is the difference between mPAP and PAOP and indicative of pulmonary vascular disease, was increased (21 ± 10). Cardiac output and mixed venous oxygen saturations were lower in the patients with PH compared to the group without PH, and 6-minute walk distance was also reduced (358 ± 115 m vs 437 ± 108 m; $P = .004$).[31] Multivariate analysis of hemodynamic variables

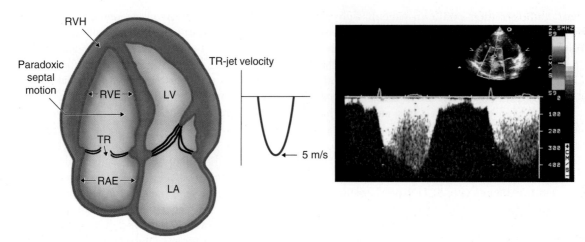

FIGURE 14-4 Use of Doppler echocardiography to estimate pulmonary artery systolic pressure. A 4-chamber illustration of the heart is shown with features of pulmonary hypertension: right ventricular enlargement (RVE), right atrial enlargement (RAE), paradoxical septal motion with septal wall movement from right side of the heart to the left during early ventricular diastole, and a high tricuspid regurgitant jet (TR-jet) velocity. The TR-jet velocity (TRV) is shown as a cartoon Doppler envelope, and next to it is an actual measurement of the TRV from a patient with severe pulmonary hypertension (a TRV value of 400 cm/s or 4 m/s). In this patient, the estimated right ventricular and pulmonary artery systolic pressure is determined by 4 times the TRV value squared, or $4 \times 4 \times 4$, or 64 mm Hg. In patients with sickle cell disease, a TRV value ≥2.5 m/s is abnormal and is 2 standard deviations higher than the mean for patients aged 35 to 40 years. A value ≥3.0 m/s is 3 standard deviations above the population mean. LA, left atrium; LV, left ventricle; RVH, right ventricular hypertrophy.

identified systolic pulmonary artery pressure, pulmonary pulse pressure, transpulmonary gradient, and PVR as predictors of mortality.[31]

Mortality was significantly higher in patients with PH defined by right heart catheterization, with a 6-year mortality of 37%, compared with 13% in the group catheterized and found not to have PH, and a median survival time for patients with PH of only 6.8 years.[115] Table 14-1 lists the hemodynamic characteristics of patients who died in follow-up versus those who survived. Importantly, even in the patients who did not have a right heart catheterization but who had low estimated pulmonary artery systolic pressures by Doppler echocardiographic screening (TRV <2.5 m/s), the 6-year mortality rate was 17%, suggesting that a normal Doppler ultrasound helps rule out significant PH. Death certificates were available for 65% of patients who died, and 80% of these patients were reported to have had right heart failure or sudden cardiac death stated as a cause of death.

Similar to these findings, Fonseca et al[117] found that 10% of 80 screened patients with SCD had PH confirmed by right heart catheterization, and these patients had worse survival as compared to the remaining patients ($P = .0005$). Parent et al[116] reported that 6% of all screened adults with SCD had PH (46% precapillary PH and 54% postcapillary PH), with an observed increased prospective mortality. The latter study excluded patients with a number of known risk factors for PH, including low lung volumes, renal insufficiency, and liver disease, likely underestimating the prevalence of PH.

Consistent with mechanisms of disease discussed earlier, patients with PH in these studies had evidence of more severe hemolytic anemia, a higher prevalence of prior leg ulcers and chronic kidney disease, older age, lower exercise capacity, and increased mortality (Figure 14-5).

Screening for Cardiovascular Disease and Mortality Risk in Patients With SCD

Over the past 2 decades, important risk factors have been validated that identify patients at higher risk of having PH measured by right heart catheterization, reductions in exercise capacity (lower 6-minute walk distance and high New York Heart Association functional class), and mortality.[123] These risk factors also identify patients with systemic vasculopathy in addition to pulmonary vasculopathy. These risk factors are reviewed in this chapter and include (1) the diagnosis of PH, both pre- and postcapillary disease, by right heart catheterization; (2) an elevated TRV-based estimated pulmonary artery systolic pressure measured by Doppler echocardiography; (3) echocardiographic evidence of diastolic left heart dysfunction; (4) an elevated plasma NT-proBNP level; and (5) macroalbuminuria and chronic kidney disease. Other risk factors include long QT on electrocardiogram and a high extracellular matrix volume on MRI.

Guidelines have been developed by the American Thoracic Society recommending that adult sickle cell patients undergo screening echocardiography and/or NT-proBNP testing to assess the risk of death and of having PH for further diagnosis and intensification of sickle cell–specific therapies (see Figure 14-6).[123] Patients with a TRV value of 2.5 to 2.9 m/s are further risk stratified by 6-minute walk testing and plasma NT-proBNP testing, with abnormal values suggesting need for right heart catheterization. Patients with values >2.9 m/s, especially with evidence of right heart dysfunction, should undergo right heart catheterization to determine the hemodynamic classification of PH. Patients with precapillary PH should be

TABLE 14-1 Hemodynamic data from patients with right heart catheterization who survived or died during follow-up

Characteristic	Survivors (n = 32)	Nonsurvivors (n = 23)	P value
sPAP, mm Hg	53 ± 13	64 ± 16	.015
dPAP, mm Hg	22 ± 6	30 ± 7	<.001
dPAP-PCWP, mm Hg	7 ± 6	14 ± 8	<.001
mPAP, mm Hg	33 ± 7	41 ± 9	<.001
CVP, mm Hg	10 ± 5	11 ± 6	.34
PCWP, mm Hg	16 ± 5	16 ± 6	.33
TPG, mm Hg	17 ± 8	25 ± 10	.003
Cardiac output, L/min	8.4 ± 2.3	8.3 ± 2.6	.66
Cardiac index, L/min/m²	4.8 ± 1.5	4.3 ± 1.3	.31
PVR, dyn·s·cm⁻⁵	189 ± 127	279 ± 164	.017
PVRI, dyn·s·cm⁻⁵/m²	339 ± 229	526 ± 276	.009
TRV, m/s	3.3 ± 0.6	3.4 ± 0.4	.37
6-MWD, m	407 ± 79	282 ± 121	<.001
WHO FC III or IV, No. (%)	7 (22)	11 (48)	.08

Abbreviations: 6-MWD, 6-minute walk distance; CVP, central venous pressure; dPAP, diastolic pulmonary artery pressure; mPAP, mean pulmonary artery pressure; PCWP, pulmonary capillary wedge pressure; PVR, pulmonary vascular resistance; PVRI, pulmonary vascular resistance index; sPAP, systolic pulmonary artery pressure; TPG, transpulmonary gradient; TRV, tricuspid regurgitant velocity; WHO FC, World Health organization functional class.

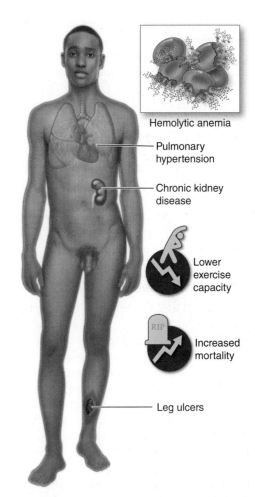

FIGURE 14-5 Pulmonary hypertension subphenotype. Patients with sickle cell disease who have pulmonary hypertension tend to have more severe hemolytic anemia, a higher prevalence of prior leg ulcers and chronic kidney disease, older age, lower exercise capacity, and increased mortality.

evaluated to exclude CTEPH and can be considered for specific vasodilator therapy, such as prostacyclin medications.[132] There is currently insufficient long-term follow-up data in children to ascertain the risk of elevated pulmonary pressures on mortality.[123] Guidelines developed by the National Heart, Lung, and Blood Institute and the American Society of Hematology do not make recommendations for or against screening for PH in asymptomatic patients with SCD.[133] However, they suggest that patients with symptoms suggestive of PH (eg, exercise intolerance, fatigue, chest pain, peripheral edema, etc.) may be evaluated initially by echocardiography, with confirmation of PH by right heart catheterization.

Tricuspid Regurgitant Jet Velocity ≥2.5 m/s

Gladwin et al[29] initially performed a screening study for PH using noninvasive Doppler echocardiography of 195 sickle cell outpatients in steady state in the Washington, DC, and Baltimore region. Borderline PH was prospectively defined by a TRV value of 2.5 to 2.9 m/s because this range is 2 standard deviations above the population mean for 35- to 40-year-old healthy volunteers, and more severe PH was defined by a TRV ≥3.0 m/s (3 standard deviations above the mean). Approximately 33% of the adult sickle cell patients had a TRV value ≥2.5 m/s, and 9% had a value ≥3.0 m/s. An elevated TRV ≥2.5 m/s was associated with a relative risk of death of 10.1 (95% CI, 2.2-47; P <.001), and even borderline values were associated with a high risk of death. In this study, a high TRV was associated with biomarkers of the severity of hemolytic anemia (low hemoglobin and high lactate dehydrogenase levels), mild renal insufficiency, iron overload, advancing age, and cholestatic liver dysfunction.[29]

TRV as an important risk factor for mortality in adults with SCD has been evaluated and validated in numerous studies since this initial cohort study. Consistently, even mild increases ≥2.5 m/s are associated with increased risk of death.[2,23,64,123,134,135] In a meta-analysis of 45 screening studies from 15 countries and including >6000 patients, the average prevalence of elevated TRV ≥2.5 m/s was 21%

(range, 17%-26%) in children and 30% (range, 26%-35%) in adults.[136] An elevated TRV ≥2.5 m/s was associated with a reduction of 30.4 m (range, 6.9-53.9 m) in the 6-minute walk distance and a mortality hazard ratio of 4.9 (range, 2.4-9.7). In a large cohort study from Créteil, France, a TRV ≥2.5 m/s was associated with a hazard ratio of death of 6.81 in multivariate analysis (P <.001), and the risk rose linearly above 2.5 m/s such that patients with a TRV of 3.2 m/s had a 50% probability of death within 3 years.[137] Interestingly, a value of 2.5 m/s was identified by receiver operator analysis as the best cutoff value to predict mortality. A high TRV value also identifies patients at higher risk of having PH by right heart catheterization: in the NIH studies, approximately 40% of patients with a TRV value of 2.5 to 2.9 m/s have PH, whereas 75% of patients with a value ≥3.0 m/s have PH.[31]

Diastolic Heart Disease or HFpEF

Although systolic heart failure is relatively rare in patients with SCD, diastolic left heart disease (HFpEF) is much more common and also defines risk of death, independent of increases in pulmonary pressures.[64,66] While the exact definitions of diastolic dysfunction in SCD have not been established, Doppler echocardiography measurements estimate that 18% of adult patients with SCD have mild to severe diastolic heart disease.[66] Most cases, however, are classified as mild, and even in patients with moderate dysfunction, the E/A ratio is only 1.2 ± 0.2, and only 1 case of severe dysfunction was observed in 141 screened subjects.[66] Proportional hazards regression analysis showed that most diastolic parameters are associated with increased mortality, including E/A (P <.001), peak E velocity (P = .002), deceleration time (P = .002), and tissue Doppler septal Em/Am ratio (P = .026).[66] In fact, a low E/A ratio is associated with high mortality even after adjustment for TRV (risk ratio, 3.5; 95% CI, 1.5-8.4; P <.001).[66] Similar high prevalence of mild diastolic dysfunction has been reported in pediatric studies, but mortality in all pediatric patients is exceedingly low, and it is not clear if these patient progress with age to more severe disease.[138-140] In the largest study conducted to date, 437 patients were evaluated using Doppler echocardiographic assessments of the ratio of early diastolic left ventricular inflow velocity to lateral mitral annular velocity (left ventricular lateral E/e′) to estimate left ventricular filling pressures and diastolic function.[64] Both the left ventricular lateral E/e′ ratio and TRV were found to be independent predictors of a shorter 6-minute walk distance and mortality.[64] Remarkably, the presence of both diastolic dysfunction and an elevated TRV synergistically increased the risk ratio for death (risk ratio, 12.0; 95% CI, 3.8-38.1; P <.001).[66]

Elevated NT-proBNP

NT-proBNP is a pre-pro hormone released from cardiomyocytes of the left and right ventricle subjected to pressure overload and wall stress. This biomarker identifies patients with SCD at higher risk of PH, with lower exercise capacity, and

at increased mortality risk.[27,125,141] The levels of NT-proBNP can also be used to risk stratify patients with borderline elevations in estimated pulmonary artery systolic pressures by Doppler echocardiography (TRV values of 2.5-2.9 m/s). In these cases, a high plasma level of NT-proBNP (>164 pg/mL) or a low 6-minute walk distance (<333 m) identifies 62% of screened patients with PH by subsequent right heart catheterization.[116]

Combined Risk Factor Analysis Identifies Adults With SCD at High Risk for Hospitalization and Death (Table 14-2)

To identify a subgroup of patients with SCD who are at very high risk of death and hospitalization, we analyzed data from both the NIH-PH screening study of >500 patients[29,31,142] and the Walk-PHASST cohort of >600 patients.[10,27,64,114] We used TRV and NT-proBNP values because these are noninvasive screening tests that have been widely validated in large cohort registries of patients with SCD. Elevation of both of these parameters improves the positive predictive value of the echocardiogram to diagnose PH by right heart catheterization to approximately 62%[116] and identifies a group at higher risk of death. The prevalence of TRV ≥2.5 m/s *and* an NT-proBNP ≥160 pg/mL is 19.2% in adults screened in the Walk-PHASST trial (n = 527 patients with both TRV *and* BNP data). This prevalence was 19.4% in the 407 adult patients in the NIH-PH screening cohort. In the Walk-PHASST study, the 12-month mortality rate was 7.9% in this group versus 0.5% in patients with normal TRV or NT-proBNP values. In the NIH-PH cohort, these rates were 8.6% and 0.7%, respectively. This patient population is also at higher risk of hospitalization, with a risk ratio for hospitalization of 1.73. For example, in the Walk-PHASST cohort, 12-month

TABLE 14-2 Burden of TRV ≥2.5 m/s and NT-proBNP ≥160 pg/mL (high-risk group) in adults with SCD[27,29]

	Walk-PHASST n = 527	NIH-PH n = 407
Prevalence of high-risk group	19.2%	19.4%
12-month mortality risk		
High-risk group	7.9%	8.6%
Low-risk group	0.5%	0.7%
12-month hospitalization risk[a]		
High-risk group	78%	NA
Low-risk group	45%	NA

[a]Relative risk of 1.73 for high-risk group.

Abbreviations: NA, not available; NIH-PH, National Institutes of Health Pulmonary Hypertension cohort; NT-proBNP, N-terminal pro-brain natriuretic peptide; SCD, sickle cell disease; TRV, tricuspid regurgitant velocity; Walk-PHASST, Pulmonary Hypertension and Sickle Sildenafil Therapy Trial.

hospitalization risk was 78% for patients with abnormal TRV and NT-proBNP values (high-risk group) compared with 45% for patients with normal TRV or BNP values (low-risk group). This analysis suggests that a simple screening profile of TRV and NT-proBNP can identify patients with SCD at the highest risk of death and hospitalization. Previous studies have also demonstrated that this group has a higher prevalence of PH measured by right heart catheterization, a lower exercise capacity, and more severe renal proteinuria and albuminuria.[116] See Table 14-2.

Macroalbuminuria, Chronic Kidney Disease, and Risk of PH and Death

Macroalbuminuria and chronic kidney disease have been identified as risk factors for PH and have also been associated with hemolytic anemia, likely reflecting the injurious effects of cell-free hemoglobin and heme (see Figure 14-5).[134,143] Stage 3 chronic kidney disease is defined by an estimated glomerular filtration rate <60 mL/min/1.73 m^2, and macroalbuminuria is defined as urine albumin >300 mg/g creatinine. The kidneys are among the most commonly affected organs in patients with SCD, and the presence of chronic kidney disease is an independent predictor of pulmonary vascular disease and of early mortality in adults with SCD.[35,134,143-146] Proposed mechanisms for sickle cell nephropathy include hemoglobinuria, ischemia-reperfusion injury, hyperfiltration, and hypertension.[147] Interestingly, urine dipstick and microscopy-defined hemoglobinuria is present in >20% of adults with SCD, is associated with markers of hemolysis, and is a predictor of chronic kidney disease stage and progression, supporting a deleterious role of hemoglobin or heme in kidney injury.[35]

Sudden Death in SCD

Right heart failure and sudden death appear to be common causes of death in patients with PH.[31,83,115] Fitzhugh et al[26] evaluated the causes of death in patients at Duke University Medical Center and found that cardiac and pulmonary etiologies accounted for 45% of deaths. The causes of death included arrhythmias and pulseless electrical activity, multiorgan failure, pulmonary emboli, stroke, acute chest syndrome or pneumonia, PH, systemic hypertension, congestive heart failure, and myocardial infarction.[26] The pulmonary pressures estimated by TRV were significantly higher in deceased versus alive patients (3.1 m/s vs 2.6 m/s, respectively; P <.001), whereas the hemoglobin value was lower in deceased patients.[26] A study of SCD patients hospitalized with acute chest syndrome identified acute right heart failure as a common comorbidity, which was associated with a very high risk of death during that hospitalization and after discharge.[148]

Of potential relevance to the risk of cardiac arrhythmia and sudden death, the QTc interval is increased in patients with elevated pulmonary artery systolic pressures[149] and associated with increased mortality (hazard ratio, 8.3; 95% CI, 2.8-24.6; P <.001).[150] In a recent regression analysis including QTc measures, TRV (P = .005), acute chest syndrome (P <.001), and prolonged QTc (P = .004) were independently associated with increased mortality.[150] Atrial and ventricular arrhythmias occur commonly in hospitalized patients during vaso-occlusive pain crisis.[151] The cause and prevention of prolonged QT and arrhythmia are not clear and deserve additional study. Although myocardial infarction has been observed in patients with SCD, in most cases, coronary angiography is normal.[152-157] During vaso-occlusive pain crisis, patients may develop elevated troponin levels[156] and cardiac nuclear perfusion[158-160] and MRI abnormalities,[154,157,161] all consistent with myocardial infarction.[156] Reversal of the cardiac abnormalities is typically observed with resolution of the painful crisis.[153,156,162,163] Preclinical models and patient studies have found that intrinsic cardiac fibrosis develops over time, possibly related to chronic episodes of microvascular infarction; this may contribute to QT prolongation and a propensity to develop arrhythmia.[72,73]

These studies in aggregate suggest that the development of PH and intrinsic cardiac conduction disease increases the risk of sudden death in adult patients with SCD.

Specific Management and Therapy

As mentioned earlier, the American Thoracic Society guidelines recommend that adult patients undergo screening echocardiography to assess the risk of death and of having PH for further diagnosis and intensification of sickle cell–specific therapies.[123] Figure 14-6 outlines the screening and evaluation approach for patients at risk for PH and elevated mortality.[123] All patients with TRV ≥2.5 m/s are at increased risk of death and should be considered for more aggressive treatment of their underlying hematologic condition with hydroxyurea therapy, and if hydroxyurea is not tolerated, a chronic transfusion program should be considered, particularly if the TRV is ≥3.0 m/s. Additional screening and treatment for iron overload, oxygen desaturations with exercise or sleep, sleep apnea, and occult thromboembolic disease (CTEPH) may be indicated. Specific treatment recommendations are currently based on expert opinion due to lack of definitive randomized clinical trial data.[114,123] Patients with PAH defined by right heart catheterization (group 1 precapillary disease) and increased PVR of ≥160 dyn·s·cm^{-5} can be considered for treatment with a US Food and Drug Administration–approved PH medication and/or more aggressive transfusion therapy.[123,132,164] Regarding specific therapies, sildenafil has been shown to improve pulmonary pressures and 6-minute walk distance in phase II studies,[165] but increased painful crises in a larger, randomized, double-blind, placebo-controlled trial.[114] Sildenafil should therefore only be considered in patients with well-controlled pain, for example, those responding well to hydroxyurea or on chronic transfusion therapy.[114] Bone marrow and lung

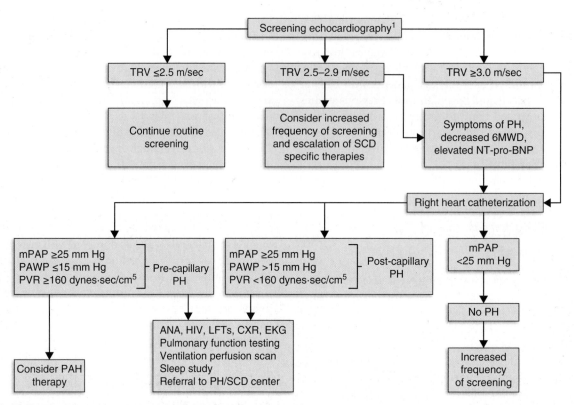

FIGURE 14-6 **Summary of the American Thoracic Society guidelines for screening echocardiography for adult patients with sickle cell disease (SCD) to assess the risk of death and of having pulmonary hypertension for further diagnosis and intensification of sickle cell–specific therapies.** [1]Note: The use of the term *screening* refers to mortality risk assessment. Echocardiography should be performed while patients are clinically stable. Patients with a mean pulmonary artery pressure (mPAP) between 20 and 25 mm Hg need further study as they may be at increased mortality risk. 6MWD, 6-minute walk distance; ANA, antinuclear antibody; CXR, chest x-ray; EKG, electrocardiogram; LFTs, liver function tests; NT-pro-BNP, N-terminal pro-brain natriuretic peptide; PAWP, pulmonary artery wedge pressure; PH, pulmonary hypertension; PVR, pulmonary vascular resistance; TRV, tricuspid regurgitant jet velocity. Reproduced from Klings ES, Machado RF, Barst RJ, et al. An official American Thoracic Society clinical practice guideline: diagnosis, risk stratification, and management of pulmonary hypertension of sickle cell disease. *Am J Respir Crit Care Med.* 2014;189(6):727-740.

transplantations have been shown to normalize pulmonary pressures and to improve short-term outcome measures.[166,167] Prostacyclin-based therapy and chronic red blood cell transfusions have both been shown to reduce pulmonary pressures and increase 6-minute walk distance and functional classification in patients with SCD and PH.[132,164] The National Heart, Lung, and Blood Institute is currently conducting a large multicenter trial of erythrocytopheresis for adult patients at high risk of death, defined by a high TRV value, a high NT-proBNP plasma level, and the development of early chronic kidney disease with macroalbuminuria (ClinicalTrials.gov Identifier: NCT04084080).

echocardiographic measures of TRV, early chronic kidney disease, and prolonged QTc.[39] Chronic transfusion therapy and stem cell transplantation would be expected to both control hemolytic anemia and reduce vaso-occlusive sickling episodes, with open-label studies suggesting benefit.[38,164] For patients with PAH and CTEPH, more specific therapies can be considered based on clinical indications. The identification of clear markers of cardiovascular risk now opens the door to larger population interventions targeting this subgroup of SCD patients using new cardiovascular medications and more traditional and experimental hematologic therapies, such red blood cell exchange transfusion and bone marrow transplantation.

Conclusion

With the aging of the SCD patient population, the prevalence and impact of cardiovascular disease are increasing. We now have a clear understanding of the prevalence and impact of PH, diastolic left ventricular dysfunction, and associated measures of risk, such as the plasma levels of NT-proBNP, Doppler

Acknowledgment

Dr. Gladwin receives research support from National Institutes of Health grants 5R01HL098032-11, 2R01HL125886-05, 5P01HL103455-09, and 5T32HL110849-08; the Burroughs Wellcome Foundation; the Institute for Transfusion Medicine; and the Hemophilia Center of Western Pennsylvania.

Case Studies: How I Treat

Case 1. An 18-year-old male patient with homozygous hemoglobin SS disease was referred for evaluation of progressive severe dyspnea on exertion, lower extremity edema, evident weight loss thought to be secondary to "cardiac cachexia," and PH diagnosed by right heart catheterization, for possible lung transplantation (this case was previously presented as an online supplement in Gladwin[39]). Since childhood, he had been treated with regular transfusions for stroke and had rare episodes of vaso-occlusive painful crisis and only used as-needed nonsteroidal anti-inflammatory medications. Laboratory testing was notable for severe hemolytic anemia despite effective exchange transfusion, with a hemoglobin level of 11.8 g/dL and HbS levels <30%, but with 18% reticulocytes and high lactate dehydrogenase (LDH) levels. His CT scan (Figures 14-7, A and B) showed a large pulmonary artery, which had a greater diameter than his aorta, and a mosaic perfusion pattern, typical

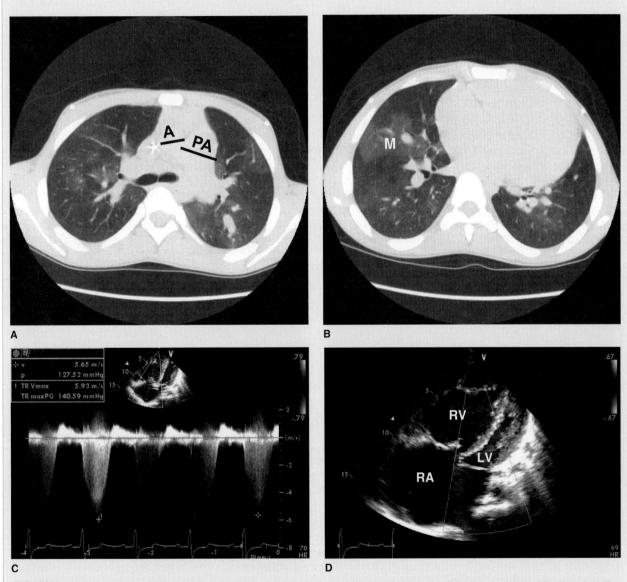

FIGURE 14-7 Imaging studies from an 18-year-old male patient with homozygous hemoglobin SS disease. The patient was referred for evaluation of progressive severe dyspnea on exertion, lower extremity edema, weight loss, and pulmonary hypertension diagnosed by right heart catheterization. (This case was previously presented as an online supplement in Gladwin[39]). **A-B.** Computed tomography scan shows a large pulmonary artery (PA), which has a greater diameter than his aorta (A), and a mosaic perfusion pattern (M), typical for pulmonary arterial hypertension. **C.** Doppler echocardiographic study records a very high tricuspid regurgitant jet velocity (TRV) of 5.93 m/s. **D.** A 4-chamber view of his heart shows a dilated right ventricle (RV) and right atrium (RA) with a compressed left ventricle (LV).

Case Studies: **Continued**

for PAH. The mosaic pattern is caused by areas of higher radiodensity where the blood flow is high (more white), next to areas where the pulmonary arterioles are narrowed or obliterated and blood flow is reduced, leading to lower attenuation or radiodensity (more dark). His Doppler echocardiographic study (Figure 14-7C) recorded a very high TRV of 5.93 m/s, which estimated a pulmonary artery systolic pressure of >140 mm Hg. A 4-chamber view of his heart (Figure 14-7D) showed a dilated right ventricle and right atrium with a compressed left ventricle. This is an example of severe paradoxical septal motion from the right ventricle into the left ventricle. The patient's right heart catheterization revealed a pulmonary artery pressure of 147/49 mm Hg (mean pressure, 82 mm Hg), right atrial pressure of 40 mm Hg, pulmonary capillary wedge pressure of 17 mm Hg, and a transpulmonary gradient of 65 mm Hg.

Management and outcome: In a severe case such as this, we advocate maximally aggressive therapy. The patient underwent CT angiography and ventilation-perfusion scanning to assess for operable CTEPH. He was evaluated for supplemental oxygen therapy. The patient was maintained on monthly erythrocytapheresis to maintain a low HbS level after transfusion of <20% and was treated sequentially with sildenafil, ambrisentan (an endothelin receptor antagonist), and subcutaneous treprostenil. At the same time, he was evaluated for lung transplantation. After aggressive vasodilator therapy, his dyspnea had improved, and he had gained 10 kg of weight and was able to go back to school and graduate from high school. He declined lung transplantation and went to college, despite our stated concerns over his high-risk status. Unfortunately, over his winter break, he developed an acute upper respiratory viral illness and rapidly decompensated. He was admitted to an emergency department near his home and developed cardiac arrest. The emergency department providers were unable to resuscitate him, which is typical for patients with severe PH.

Case 2. A 43-year-old man with HbSC was self-referred after noticing increasing dyspnea while running up and down the sidelines coaching his son's football team. A screening Doppler echocardiogram showed an enlarged right ventricle and right atrium (Figure 14-8A) with a TRV of 4.48 m/s (estimated pulmonary artery systolic pressure of 80 mm Hg; Figure 14-8B). A supine CT scan of the chest (Figure 14-8, C-E) showed a mosaic perfusion pattern, typical for PAH or CTEPH, with clear areas of low attenuation consistent with limited perfusion (see arrow to left upper lobe). A ventilation-perfusion scan was performed showing normal ventilation (not shown) but multiple large segmental perfusion defects throughout the right and left lung (Figure 14-8F). Note the lack of perfusion (arrow in Figure 14-8F) to the left upper lobe that corresponds to the low attenuation of the left upper lobe on the CT scan (Figure 14-8C). A pulmonary angiogram was performed, and the left

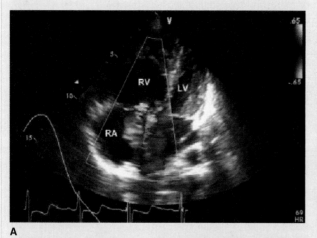

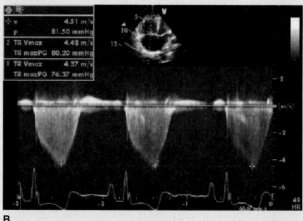

A **B**

FIGURE 14-8 A 43-year-old man with HbSC was self-referred after noticing increasing dyspnea on exertion. A screening Doppler echocardiogram showed an enlarged right ventricle (RV) and right atrium (RA; **A**) with a tricuspid regurgitant jet velocity (TRV) of 4.48 m/s (estimated pulmonary artery systolic pressure of 80 mm Hg; **B**). A supine computed tomography (CT) scan of the chest (**C-E**) shows a mosaic perfusion pattern, typical for pulmonary arterial hypertension or chronic thromboembolic pulmonary hypertension (CTEPH), with clear areas of low attenuation consistent with limited perfusion (see arrow to left upper lobe). A ventilation-perfusion scan was performed showing normal ventilation (not shown) but multiple large segmental perfusion defects throughout the right and left lung (**F**). Note the lack of perfusion (arrow in **F**) to the left upper lobe that corresponds to the low attenuation of the left upper lobe on the CT scan (**C**). A pulmonary angiogram was performed, and the left side study is shown in panels **G-I**. The study shows the enlarged proximal pulmonary artery with loss of peripheral vascularity. Virtually no blood flow goes to the left upper lobe (**I**). Panel **J** shows the typical pathology of a recanalized pulmonary vascular lesion from a different patient with sickle cell disease and severe CTEPH who was cared for by our group at the National Institutes of Health. These findings were all consistent with a diagnosis of CTEPH. LAO, left anterior oblique; LPO, left posterior oblique; LTLAT, left lateral; LV, left ventricle; RAO, right anterior oblique; RPO, right posterior oblique; RTLAT, right lateral.

Case Studies: Continued

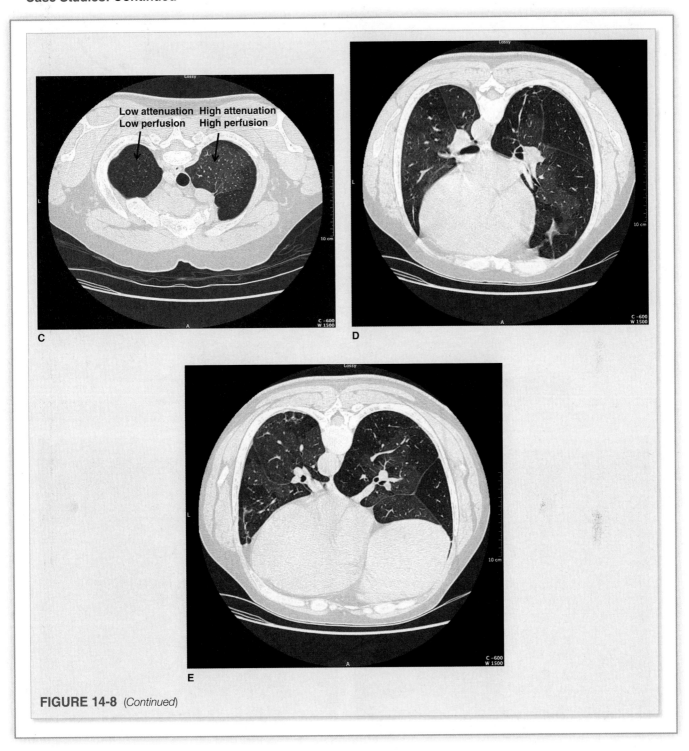

FIGURE 14-8 *(Continued)*

Case Studies: Continued

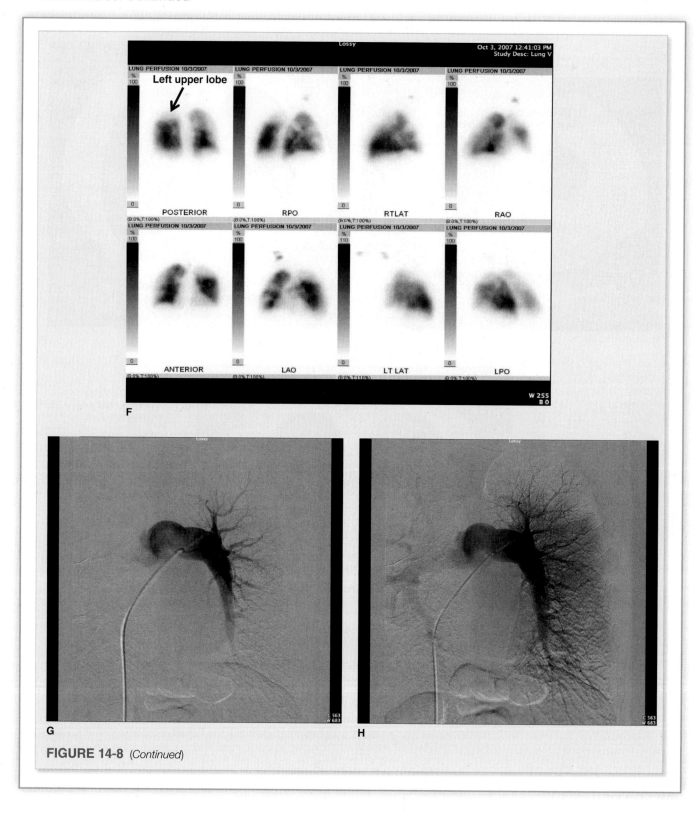

FIGURE 14-8 (Continued)

Case Studies: Continued

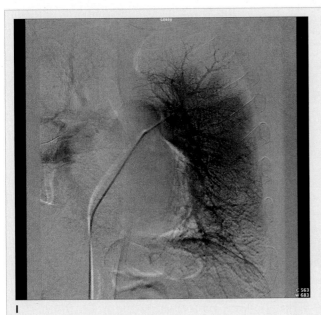

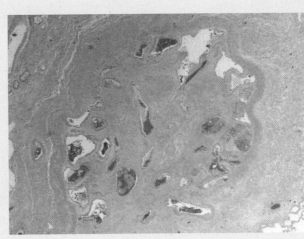

FIGURE 14-8 *(Continued)*

side study is shown in Figures 14-8, G-I. The study showed an enlarged proximal pulmonary artery with loss of peripheral vascularity. Virtually no blood flow went to the left upper lobe (Figure 14-8I). Figure 14-8J shows the typical pathology of a recanalized pulmonary vascular lesion from a different patient with sickle cell and severe CTEPH who was cared for by our group at the NIH. These findings were all consistent with a diagnosis of CTEPH.

Management and outcome: The diagnosis of CTEPH requires the initiation of chronic oral anticoagulation therapy and evaluation to determine if the CTEPH is operable. There is now an approved medical treatment for CTEPH, the sGC stimulator medication riociguat. The patient should also be evaluated for surgical approaches to treatment, which include the less invasive pulmonary artery balloon angioplasty and more invasive but more definitive surgical pulmonary artery thromboendarterectomy.[118-122]

Case 3. A 35-year-old patient with HbSS disease was screened for PH and found to have a TRV of 3.3 m/s. The patient suffered from frequent vaso-occlusive events requiring hospitalization. He also had systemic hypertension and stage 2 chronic kidney disease, requiring antihypertensive medications. His laboratory testing revealed severe steady-state hemolytic anemia, with a hemoglobin value of 8.6 g/dL and 525,000 reticulocytes/μL of blood. His lactate dehydrogenase was reported as "hemolyzed," and bilirubin levels were elevated (total, 6.6 mg/dL; direct, 1.0 mg/dL). He also had iron overload from frequent transfusions, with a ferritin level of 1657 ng/mL.

Management and outcome: This patient was managed initially with hydroxyurea but was later started on chronic exchange transfusions based on increasing admissions with vaso-occlusive crisis, acute chest syndrome, and increasing dyspnea on exertion, thought to be related to his PH, which had been confirmed by right heart catheterization. He was treated during his course with sildenafil while on transfusions to prevent vaso-occlusive pain crisis. His TRV value had improved on exchange transfusion to 2.7 m/s, but then he developed a catheter-related infection and stopped chronic transfusion therapy. His mother was at home with him and heard him fall upstairs in his bedroom and found him in unresponsive. Emergency Medical Services was called to the house, and they could not resuscitate him. He underwent autopsy, which revealed unexpectedly severe pulmonary vascular changes as described by the pathologist: "Widespread vascular changes, medial and intimal hypertrophy with plexiform lesions. Severe PH. Markedly restricted luminal capacity." Selected vascular lesions are shown in Figure 14-9.

Case Studies: Continued

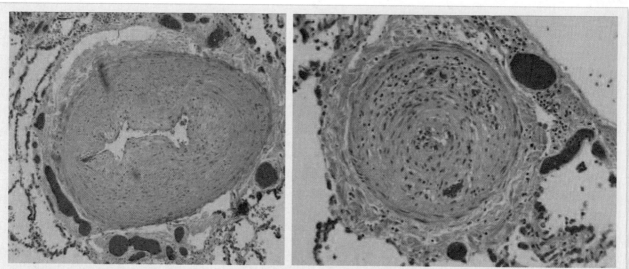

FIGURE 14-9 **Lung tissue obtained from autopsy of a 35-year-old patient with HbSS disease.** The biopsy revealed unexpectedly severe pulmonary vascular changes as described by the pathologist: "Widespread vascular changes, medial and intimal hypertrophy with plexiform lesions. Severe pulmonary hypertension. Markedly restricted luminal capacity."

High-Yield Facts

◆ More severe hemolytic anemia is associated with a number of clinical complications in patients with sickle cell disease, including pulmonary hypertension, diastolic left heart disease, stroke, chronic kidney disease, and cutaneous leg ulcerations.

◆ Patients with sickle cell disease and pulmonary hypertension are older and have severe hemolytic anemia, a higher prevalence of prior leg ulcers and chronic kidney disease, lower exercise capacity, and increased mortality.

◆ A number of risk factors identify patients with sickle cell disease at higher risk of death: (1) the diagnosis of pulmonary hypertension, both pre- and postcapillary disease, by right heart catheterization; (2) an elevated tricuspid regurgitant jet velocity (TRV)-based estimated pulmonary artery systolic pressure measured by Doppler echocardiography; (3) echocardiographic evidence of diastolic left heart dysfunction; (4) an elevated plasma level of N-terminal prohormone of brain natriuretic peptide (NT-proBNP); (5) macroalbuminuria and chronic kidney disease; (6) long QT on electrocardiogram; and (7) a high ventricular extracellular matrix volume on magnetic resonance imaging.

◆ The American Thoracic Society guidelines recommend that adult patients undergo screening echocardiography to assess the risk of death and of having pulmonary hypertension for further diagnosis and intensification of sickle cell–specific therapies.[123]

◆ All patients with TRV ≥2.5 m/s are at increased risk of death and should be considered for more aggressive treatment of their underlying hematologic condition with hydroxyurea therapy. If hydroxyurea is not tolerated, a chronic transfusion program should be considered, particularly if the TRV is ≥3.0 m/s.

◆ Patients with sickle cell disease and pulmonary hypertension should undergo additional screening and treatment for iron overload, oxygen desaturations with exercise or sleep, sleep apnea, and occult thromboembolic disease (chronic thromboembolic pulmonary hypertension).

◆ Patients with pulmonary arterial hypertension defined by right heart catheterization (group 1 precapillary disease) and increased pulmonary vascular resistance of ≥160 dyn·s·cm⁻⁵ can be considered for treatment with a US Food and Drug Administration–approved pulmonary hypertension medication and/or more aggressive transfusion therapy.[123,132,164]

High-Yield Facts (Cont.)

◆ Sildenafil has been shown to improve pulmonary pressures and 6-minute walk distance in phase II studies,[165] but it increased painful crises in a larger, randomized, double-blind, placebo-controlled trial.[114] Therefore, sildenafil should only be considered in patients with well-controlled pain, such as patients who respond well to hydroxyurea or who are on chronic transfusion therapy.[114]

◆ Bone marrow and lung transplantations have been shown to normalize pulmonary pressures and to improve short-term outcome measures.[166,167]

◆ Prostacyclin-based therapy and chronic red blood cell transfusions have both been shown to reduce pulmonary pressures and increase 6-minute walk distance and functional classification in patients with sickle cell disease and pulmonary hypertension.[132,164]

◆ The National Heart, Lung, and Blood Institute is currently conducting a large multicenter trial of erythrocytopheresis for adult patients at high risk of death, defined by a high TRV value, a high NT-proBNP plasma level, and the development of early chronic kidney disease with macroalbuminuria.

References

1. Bunn HF. Pathogenesis and treatment of sickle cell disease. *N Engl J Med.* 1997;337(11):762-769.

2. Gladwin MT, Vichinsky E. Pulmonary complications of sickle cell disease. *N Engl J Med.* 2008;359(21):2254-2265.

3. Rees DC, Williams TN, Gladwin MT. Sickle-cell disease. *Lancet.* 2010;376(9757):2018-2031.

4. Sundd P, Gladwin MT, Novelli EM. Pathophysiology of sickle cell disease. *Annu Rev Pathol.* 2019;14:263-292.

5. Belcher JD, Bryant CJ, Nguyen J, et al. Transgenic sickle mice have vascular inflammation. *Blood.* 2003;101(10):3953-3959.

6. Osarogiagbon UR, Choong S, Belcher JD, Vercellotti GM, Paller MS, Hebbel RP. Reperfusion injury pathophysiology in sickle transgenic mice. *Blood.* 2000;96(1):314-320.

7. Reiter CD, Wang X, Tanus-Santos JE, et al. Cell-free hemoglobin limits nitric oxide bioavailability in sickle-cell disease. *Nat Med.* 2002;8(12):1383-1389.

8. Rother RP, Bell L, Hillmen P, Gladwin MT. The clinical sequelae of intravascular hemolysis and extracellular plasma hemoglobin: a novel mechanism of human disease. *JAMA.* 2005;293(13):1653-1662.

9. Morris CR, Kato GJ, Poljakovic M, et al. Dysregulated arginine metabolism, hemolysis-associated pulmonary hypertension, and mortality in sickle cell disease. *JAMA.* 2005;294(1):81-90.

10. Nouraie M, Lee JS, Zhang Y, et al. The relationship between the severity of hemolysis, clinical manifestations and risk of death in 415 patients with sickle cell anemia in the US and Europe. *Haematologica.* 2013;98(3):464-472.

11. Hsu LL, Champion HC, Campbell-Lee SA, et al. Hemolysis in sickle cell mice causes pulmonary hypertension due to global impairment in nitric oxide bioavailability. *Blood.* 2007;109(7):3088-3098.

12. Ghosh S, Adisa OA, Chappa P, et al. Extracellular hemin crisis triggers acute chest syndrome in sickle mice. *J Clin Invest.* 2013;123(11):4809-4820.

13. Belcher JD, Chen C, Nguyen J, et al. Heme triggers TLR4 signaling leading to endothelial cell activation and vaso-occlusion in murine sickle cell disease. *Blood.* 2014;123(3):377-390.

14. Almeida CB, Souza LE, Leonardo FC, et al. Acute hemolytic vascular inflammatory processes are prevented by nitric oxide replacement or a single dose of hydroxyurea. *Blood.* 2015;126(6):711-720.

15. Bennewitz MF, Jimenez MA, Vats R, et al. Lung vaso-occlusion in sickle cell disease mediated by arteriolar neutrophil-platelet microemboli. *JCI Insight.* 2017;2(1):e89761.

16. Gladwin MT, Ofori-Acquah SF. Erythroid DAMPs drive inflammation in SCD. *Blood.* 2014;123(24):3689-3690.

17. Piel FB, Hay SI, Gupta S, Weatherall DJ, Williams TN. Global burden of sickle cell anaemia in children under five, 2010-2050: modelling based on demographics, excess mortality, and interventions. *PLoS Med.* 2013;10(7):e1001484.

18. Alvarez O, Yovetich NA, Scott JP, et al. Pain and other non-neurological adverse events in children with sickle cell anemia and previous stroke who received hydroxyurea and phlebotomy or chronic transfusions and chelation: results from the SWiTCH clinical trial. *Am J Hematol.* 2013;88(11):932-938.

19. Ware RE, Helms RW, SWiTCH Investigators. Stroke With Transfusions Changing to Hydroxyurea (SWiTCH). *Blood.* 2012;119(17):3925-3932.

20. Tshilolo L, Tomlinson G, Williams TN, et al. Hydroxyurea for children with sickle cell anemia in sub-Saharan Africa. *N Engl J Med.* 2019;380(2):121-131.

21. Kinney TR, Helms RW, O'Branski EE, et al. Safety of hydroxyurea in children with sickle cell anemia: results of the HUG-KIDS study, a phase I/II trial. Pediatric Hydroxyurea Group. *Blood.* 1999;94(5):1550-1554.

22. Steinberg MH, Barton F, Castro O, et al. Effect of hydroxyurea on mortality and morbidity in adult sickle cell anemia: risks and benefits up to 9 years of treatment. *JAMA.* 2003;289(13):1645-1651.

23. Ataga KI, Moore CG, Jones S, et al. Pulmonary hypertension in patients with sickle cell disease: a longitudinal study. *Br J Haematol.* 2006;134(1):109-115.

24. Bartolucci P, Brugnara C, Teixeira-Pinto A, et al. Erythrocyte density in sickle cell syndromes is associated with specific clinical manifestations and hemolysis. *Blood.* 2012;120(15):3136-3141.

25. Day TG, Drasar ER, Fulford T, Sharpe CC, Thein SL. Association between hemolysis and albuminuria in adults with sickle cell anemia. *Haematologica.* 2012;97(2):201-205.

26. Fitzhugh CD, Lauder N, Jonassaint JC, et al. Cardiopulmonary complications leading to premature deaths in adult patients with sickle cell disease. *Am J Hematol.* 2010;85(1):36-40.

27. Gladwin MT, Barst RJ, Gibbs JS, et al. Risk factors for death in 632 patients with sickle cell disease in the United States and United Kingdom. *PLoS One.* 2014;9(7):e99489.

28. Gladwin MT, Sachdev V. Cardiovascular abnormalities in sickle cell disease. *J Am Coll Cardiol.* 2012;59(13):1123-1133.

29. Gladwin MT, Sachdev V, Jison ML, et al. Pulmonary hypertension as a risk factor for death in patients with sickle cell disease. *N Engl J Med.* 2004;350(9):886-895.

30. Kato GJ, McGowan V, Machado RF, et al. Lactate dehydrogenase as a biomarker of hemolysis-associated nitric oxide resistance, priapism, leg ulceration, pulmonary hypertension, and death in patients with sickle cell disease. *Blood.* 2006;107(6):2279-2285.

31. Mehari A, Alam S, Tian X, et al. Hemodynamic predictors of mortality in adults with sickle cell disease. *Am J Respir Crit Care Med.* 2013;187(8):840-847.

32. Novelli EM, Hildesheim M, Rosano C, et al. Elevated pulse pressure is associated with hemolysis, proteinuria and chronic kidney disease in sickle cell disease. *PLoS One.* 2014;9(12):e114309.

33. Platt OS, Brambilla DJ, Rosse WF, et al. Mortality in sickle cell disease. Life expectancy and risk factors for early death. *N Engl J Med.* 1994;330(23):1639-1644.

34. Powars DR, Elliott Mills DD, Chan L. Chronic renal failure in sickle cell disease: risk factors, clinical course, and mortality. *Ann Intern Med.* 1991;115:614-620.

35. Saraf SL, Zhang X, Kanias T, et al. Haemoglobinuria is associated with chronic kidney disease and its progression in patients with sickle cell anaemia. *Br J Haematol.* 2014;164(5):729-739.

36. DeBaun MR, Ghafuri DL, Rodeghier M, et al. Decreased median survival of adults with sickle cell disease after adjusting for left truncation bias: a pooled analysis. *Blood.* 2019;133(6):615-617.

37. Maitra P, Caughey M, Robinson L, et al. Risk factors for mortality in adult patients with sickle cell disease: a meta-analysis of studies in North America and Europe. *Haematologica.* 2017;102(4):626-636.

38. Detterich JA, Kato RM, Rabai M, Meiselman HJ, Coates TD, Wood JC. Chronic transfusion therapy improves but does not normalize systemic and pulmonary vasculopathy in sickle cell disease. *Blood.* 2015;126(6):703-710.

39. Gladwin MT. Cardiovascular complications and risk of death in sickle-cell disease. *Lancet.* 2016;387(10037):2565-2574.

40. Lundberg JO, Gladwin MT, Weitzberg E. Strategies to increase nitric oxide signalling in cardiovascular disease. *Nat Rev Drug Discov.* 2015;14(9):623-641.

41. Tejero J, Shiva S, Gladwin MT. Sources of vascular nitric oxide and reactive oxygen species and their regulation. *Physiol Rev.* 2019;99(1):311-379.

42. Lundberg JO, Weitzberg E, Gladwin MT. The nitrate-nitrite-nitric oxide pathway in physiology and therapeutics. *Nat Rev Drug Discov.* 2008;7(2):156-167.

43. Azarov I, Huang KT, Basu S, Gladwin MT, Hogg N, Kim-Shapiro DB. Nitric oxide scavenging by red blood cells as a function of hematocrit and oxygenation. *J Biol Chem.* 2005;280(47):39024-39032.

44. Azarov I, Liu C, Reynolds H, et al. Mechanisms of slower nitric oxide uptake by red blood cells and other hemoglobin-containing vesicles. *J Biol Chem.* 2011;286(38):33567-33579.

45. Donadee C, Raat NJ, Kanias T, et al. Nitric oxide scavenging by red blood cell microparticles and cell-free hemoglobin as a mechanism for the red cell storage lesion. *Circulation.* 2011;124(4):465-476.

46. Schaer CA, Deuel JW, Schildknecht D, et al. Haptoglobin preserves vascular nitric oxide signaling during hemolysis. *Am J Respir Crit Care Med.* 2016;193(10):1111-1122.

47. Kato GJ, Steinberg MH, Gladwin MT. Intravascular hemolysis and the pathophysiology of sickle cell disease. *J Clin Invest.* 2017;127(3):750-760.

48. Minneci PC, Deans KJ, Zhi H, et al. Hemolysis-associated endothelial dysfunction mediated by accelerated NO inactivation by decompartmentalized oxyhemoglobin. *J Clin Invest.* 2005;115(12):3409-3417.

49. Wang X, Tanus-Santos JE, Reiter CD, et al. Biological activity of nitric oxide in the plasmatic compartment. *Proc Natl Acad Sci USA.* 2004;101(31):11477-11482.

50. Kaul DK, Liu XD, Chang HY, Nagel RL, Fabry ME. Effect of fetal hemoglobin on microvascular regulation in sickle transgenic-knockout mice. *J Clin Invest.* 2004;114(8):1136-1145.

51. Wood KC, Granger DN. Sickle cell disease: role of reactive oxygen and nitrogen metabolites. *Clin Exp Pharmacol Physiol.* 2007;34(9):926-932.

52. Aslan M, Ryan TM, Adler B, et al. Oxygen radical inhibition of nitric oxide-dependent vascular function in sickle cell disease. *Proc Natl Acad Sci USA.* 2001;98(26):15215-15220.

53. Wood KC, Hebbel RP, Granger DN. Endothelial cell NADPH oxidase mediates the cerebral microvascular dysfunction in sickle cell transgenic mice. *FASEB J.* 2005;19(8):989-991.

54. Gladwin MT. Deconstructing endothelial dysfunction: soluble guanylyl cyclase oxidation and the NO resistance syndrome. *J Clin Invest.* 2006;116(9):2330-2332.

55. Potoka KP, Wood KC, Baust JJ, et al. Nitric oxide-independent soluble guanylate cyclase activation improves vascular function and cardiac remodeling in sickle cell disease. *Am J Respir Cell Mol Biol.* 2018;58(5):636-647.

56. Rivera A. Reduced sickle erythrocyte dehydration in vivo by endothelin-1 receptor antagonists. *Am J Physiol Cell Physiol.* 2007;293(3):C960-C966.

57. Rivera A, Jarolim P, Brugnara C. Modulation of Gardos channel activity by cytokines in sickle erythrocytes. *Blood.* 2002;99(1):357-603.

58. Potoka KP, Gladwin MT. Vasculopathy and pulmonary hypertension in sickle cell disease. *Am J Physiol Lung Cell Mol Physiol.* 2015;308(4):L314-L324.

59. Berra L, Pinciroli R, Stowell CP, et al. Autologous transfusion of stored red blood cells increases pulmonary artery pressure. *Am J Respir Crit Care Med.* 2014;190(7):800-807.

60. Rezoagli E, Ichinose F, Strelow S, et al. Pulmonary and systemic vascular resistances after cardiopulmonary bypass: role of hemolysis. *J Cardiothorac Vasc Anesth.* 2017;31(2):505-515.

61. Milton JN, Rooks H, Drasar E, et al. Genetic determinants of haemolysis in sickle cell anaemia. *Br J Haematol.* 2013;161(2):270-278.

62. Kato GJ, Gladwin MT, Steinberg MH. Deconstructing sickle cell disease: reappraisal of the role of hemolysis in the development of clinical subphenotypes. *Blood Rev.* 2007;21:37-47.

63. Poludasu S, Ramkissoon K, Salciccioli L, Kamran H, Lazar JM. Left ventricular systolic function in sickle cell anemia: a meta-analysis. *J Card Fail.* 2013;19(5):333-341.

64. Sachdev V, Kato GJ, Gibbs JS, et al. Echocardiographic markers of elevated pulmonary pressure and left ventricular diastolic

dysfunction are associated with exercise intolerance in adults and adolescents with homozygous sickle cell anemia in the United States and United Kingdom. *Circulation.* 2011;124(13): 1452-1460.

65. Roy SB, Bhatia ML, Mathur VS, Virmani S. Hemodynamic effects of chronic severe anemia. *Circulation.* 1963;28:346-356.

66. Sachdev V, Machado RF, Shizukuda Y, et al. Diastolic dysfunction is an independent risk factor for death in patients with sickle cell disease. *J Am Coll Cardiol.* 2007;49(4):472-479.

67. Anthi A, Machado RF, Jison ML, et al. Hemodynamic and functional assessment of patients with sickle cell disease and pulmonary hypertension. *Am J Respir Crit Care Med.* 2007;175(12): 1272-1279.

68. DeBaun MR, Armstrong FD, McKinstry RC, Ware RE, Vichinsky E, Kirkham FJ. Silent cerebral infarcts: a review on a prevalent and progressive cause of neurologic injury in sickle cell anemia. *Blood.* 2012;119(20):4587-4596.

69. Ohene-Frempong K, Weiner SJ, Sleeper LA, et al. Cerebrovascular accidents in sickle cell disease: rates and risk factors. *Blood.* 1998;91(1):288-294.

70. Bakeer N, James J, Roy S, et al. Sickle cell anemia mice develop a unique cardiomyopathy with restrictive physiology. *Proc Natl Acad Sci USA.* 2016;113(35):E5182-E5191.

71. Duarte JD, Desai AA, Sysol JR, et al. Genome-wide analysis identifies IL-18 and FUCA2 as novel genes associated with diastolic function in African Americans with sickle cell disease. *PLoS One.* 2016;11(9):e0163013.

72. Niss O, Fleck R, Makue F, et al. Association between diffuse myocardial fibrosis and diastolic dysfunction in sickle cell anemia. *Blood.* 2017;130(2):205-213.

73. Niss O, Quinn CT, Lane A, et al. Cardiomyopathy with restrictive physiology in sickle cell disease. *JACC Cardiovasc Imaging.* 2016;9(3):243-252.

74. Villagra J, Shiva S, Hunter LA, Machado RF, Gladwin MT, Kato GJ. Platelet activation in patients with sickle disease, hemolysis-associated pulmonary hypertension, and nitric oxide scavenging by cell-free hemoglobin. *Blood.* 2007;110(6): 2166-2172.

75. Hu W, Jin R, Zhang J, et al. The critical roles of platelet activation and reduced NO bioavailability in fatal pulmonary arterial hypertension in a murine hemolysis model. *Blood.* 2010;116(9):1613-1622.

76. Qin X, Hu W, Song W, et al. Balancing role of nitric oxide in complement-mediated activation of platelets from mCd59a and mCd59b double-knockout mice. *Am J Hematol.* 2009;84(4): 221-227.

77. Ataga KI, Moore CG, Hillery CA, et al. Coagulation activation and inflammation in sickle cell disease-associated pulmonary hypertension. *Haematologica.* 2008;93(1):20-26.

78. Wakefield TW, Myers DD, Henke PK. Mechanisms of venous thrombosis and resolution. *Arterioscler Thromb Vasc Biol.* 2008;28(3):387-391.

79. Lim MY, Ataga KI, Key NS. Hemostatic abnormalities in sickle cell disease. *Curr Opin Hematol.* 2013;20(5):472-477.

80. van Beers EJ, van Eck-Smit BL, Mac Gillavry MR, et al. Large and medium-sized pulmonary artery obstruction does not play a role of primary importance in the etiology of sickle-cell disease-associated pulmonary hypertension. *Chest.* 2008;133(3):646-652.

81. Field JJ, Madadi AR, Siegel MJ, Narra V. Pulmonary thrombi are not detected by 3D magnetic resonance angiography in adults with sickle cell anemia and an elevated triscuspid regurgitant jet velocity. *Am J Hematol.* 2009;84(10):686-688.

82. Graham JK, Mosunjac M, Hanzlick RL, Mosunjac M. Sickle cell lung disease and sudden death: a retrospective/prospective study of 21 autopsy cases and literature review. *Am J Forensic Med Pathol.* 2007;28(2):168-172.

83. Manci EA, Culberson DE, Yang YM, et al. Causes of death in sickle cell disease: an autopsy study. *Br J Haematol.* 2003;123(2):359-365.

84. Haque AK, Gokhale S, Rampy BA, Adegboyega P, Duarte A, Saldana MJ. Pulmonary hypertension in sickle cell hemoglobinopathy: a clinicopathologic study of 20 cases. *Hum Pathol.* 2002;33(10):1037-1043.

85. Darbari DS, Kple-Faget P, Kwagyan J, Rana S, Gordeuk VR, Castro O. Circumstances of death in adult sickle cell disease patients. *Am J Hematol.* 2006;81(11):858-863.

86. Frey MK, Alias S, Winter MP, et al. Splenectomy is modifying the vascular remodeling of thrombosis. *J Am Heart Assoc.* 2014;3(1):e000772.

87. Bonnet S, Michelakis ED, Porter CJ, et al. An abnormal mitochondrial-hypoxia inducible factor-1alpha-Kv channel pathway disrupts oxygen sensing and triggers pulmonary arterial hypertension in fawn hooded rats: similarities to human pulmonary arterial hypertension. *Circulation.* 2006;113(22):2630-2641.

88. Fijalkowska I, Xu W, Comhair SA, et al. Hypoxia inducible-factor1alpha regulates the metabolic shift of pulmonary hypertensive endothelial cells. *Am J Pathol.* 2010;176(3):1130-1138.

89. Archer SL, Weir EK, Wilkins MR. Basic science of pulmonary arterial hypertension for clinicians: new concepts and experimental therapies. *Circulation.* 2010;121(18):2045-2066.

90. Semenza GL. Hypoxia-inducible factors in physiology and medicine. *Cell.* 2012;148(3):399-408.

91. Bailey DM, Bartsch P, Knauth M, Baumgartner RW. Emerging concepts in acute mountain sickness and high-altitude cerebral edema: from the molecular to the morphological. *Cell Mol Life Sci.* 2009;66(22):3583-3594.

92. Shimoda LA, Semenza GL. HIF and the lung: role of hypoxia-inducible factors in pulmonary development and disease. *Am J Respir Crit Care Med.* 2011;183(2):152-156.

93. Ebert BL, Bunn HF. Regulation of the erythropoietin gene. *Blood.* 1999;94(6):1864-1877.

94. Semenza GL, Wang GL. A nuclear factor induced by hypoxia via de novo protein synthesis binds to the human erythropoietin gene enhancer at a site required for transcriptional activation. *Mol Cell Biol.* 1992;12(12):5447-5454.

95. Sachdev V, Kato GJ, Gibbs JS, et al. Echocardiographic markers of elevated pulmonary pressure and left ventricular diastolic dysfunction are associated with exercise intolerance in adults and adolescents with homozygous sickle cell anemia in the United States and United Kingdom. *Circulation.* 2011;124(13):1452-1460.

96. Ang SO, Chen H, Hirota K, et al. Disruption of oxygen homeostasis underlies congenital Chuvash polycythemia. *Nat Genet.* 2002;32(4):614-621.

97. Sable CA, Aliyu ZY, Dham N, et al. Pulmonary artery pressure and iron deficiency in patients with upregulation of hypoxia sensing due to homozygous VHL(R200W) mutation (Chuvash polycythemia). *Haematologica.* 2012;97(2):193-200.

98. Hickey MM, Lam JC, Bezman NA, Rathmell WK, Simon MC. von Hippel-Lindau mutation in mice recapitulates Chuvash polycythemia via hypoxia-inducible factor-2alpha signaling and splenic erythropoiesis. *J Clin Invest.* 2007;117(12):3879-3889.

99. Zhang X, Zhang W, Ma SF, et al. Hypoxic response contributes to altered gene expression and precapillary pulmonary

hypertension in patients with sickle cell disease. *Circulation.* 2014;129(16):1650-1658.

100. Dhanasekaran DN, Reddy EP. JNK signaling in apoptosis. *Oncogene.* 2008;27(48):6245-6251.

101. Sundaram N, Tailor A, Mendelsohn L, et al. High levels of placenta growth factor in sickle cell disease promote pulmonary hypertension. *Blood.* 2010;116(1):109-112.

102. Brittain JE, Hulkower B, Jones SK, et al. Placenta growth factor in sickle cell disease: association with hemolysis and inflammation. *Blood.* 2010;115(10):2014-2020.

103. Ashley-Koch AE, Elliott L, Kail ME, et al. Identification of genetic polymorphisms associated with risk for pulmonary hypertension in sickle cell disease. *Blood.* 2008;111(12):5721-5726.

104. Jacob SA, Novelli EM, Isenberg JS, et al. Thrombospondin-1 gene polymorphism is associated with estimated pulmonary artery pressure in patients with sickle cell anemia. *Am J Hematol.* 2017;92(3):E31-E34.

105. Desai AA, Zhou T, Ahmad H, et al. A novel molecular signature for elevated tricuspid regurgitation velocity in sickle cell disease. *Am J Respir Crit Care Med.* 2012;186(4):359-368.

106. Simonneau G, Gatzoulis MA, Adatia I, et al. Updated clinical classification of pulmonary hypertension. *J Am Coll Cardiol.* 2013;62(25 suppl):D34-D41.

107. Lai YC, Potoka KC, Champion HC, Mora AL, Gladwin MT. Pulmonary arterial hypertension: the clinical syndrome. *Circ Res.* 2014;115(1):115-130.

108. Maron BA, Brittain EL, Choudhary G, Gladwin MT. Redefining pulmonary hypertension. *Lancet Respir Med.* 2018;6(3):168-170.

109. Maron BA, Wertheim BM, Gladwin MT. Under pressure to clarify pulmonary hypertension clinical risk. *Am J Respir Crit Care Med.* 2018;197(4):423-426.

110. Simonneau G, Montani D, Celermajer DS, et al. Haemodynamic definitions and updated clinical classification of pulmonary hypertension. *Eur Respir J.* 2019;53(1):1801913.

111. Lai YC, Wang L, Gladwin MT. Insights into the pulmonary vascular complications of heart failure with preserved ejection fraction. *J Physiol.* 2019;597(4):1143-1156.

112. Levine AR, Simon MA, Gladwin MT. Pulmonary vascular disease in the setting of heart failure with preserved ejection fraction. *Trends Cardiovasc Med.* 2019;29(4):207-217.

113. Vanderpool RR, Saul M, Nouraie M, Gladwin MT, Simon MA. Association between hemodynamic markers of pulmonary hypertension and outcomes in heart failure with preserved ejection fraction. *JAMA Cardiol.* 2018;3(4):298-306.

114. Machado RF, Barst RJ, Yovetich NA, et al. Hospitalization for pain in patients with sickle cell disease treated with sildenafil for elevated TRV and low exercise capacity. *Blood.* 2011;118(4):855-864.

115. Mehari A, Gladwin MT, Tian X, Machado RF, Kato GJ. Mortality in adults with sickle cell disease and pulmonary hypertension. *JAMA.* 2012;307(12):1254-1256.

116. Parent F, Bachir D, Inamo J, et al. A hemodynamic study of pulmonary hypertension in sickle cell disease. *N Engl J Med.* 2011;365(1):44-53.

117. Fonseca GH, Souza R, Salemi VM, Jardim CV, Gualandro SF. Pulmonary hypertension diagnosed by right heart catheterisation in sickle cell disease. *Eur Respir J.* 2012;39(1):112-118.

118. Naik RP, Streiff MB, Haywood C Jr, Segal JB, Lanzkron S. Venous thromboembolism incidence in the Cooperative Study of Sickle Cell Disease. *J Thromb Haemost.* 2014;12(12):2010-2016.

119. Yung GL, Channick RN, Fedullo PF, et al. Successful pulmonary thromboendarterectomy in two patients with sickle cell disease. *Am J Respir Crit Care Med.* 1998;157(5 Pt 1):1690-1693.

120. Ghofrani HA, D'Armini AM, Grimminger F, et al. Riociguat for the treatment of chronic thromboembolic pulmonary hypertension. *N Engl J Med.* 2013;369(4):319-329.

121. Agrawal A, Shah R, Bacchetta MD, Talwar A. Successful pulmonary thromboendarterectomy in a patient with sickle cell disease and associated resolution of a leg ulcer. *Lung India.* 2018;35(1):73-77.

122. Mahesh B, Besser M, Ravaglioli A, et al. Pulmonary endarterectomy is effective and safe in patients with haemoglobinopathies and abnormal red blood cells: the Papworth experience. *Eur J Cardiothorac Surg.* 2016;50(3):537-541.

123. Klings ES, Machado RF, Barst RJ, et al. An official American Thoracic Society clinical practice guideline: diagnosis, risk stratification, and management of pulmonary hypertension of sickle cell disease. *Am J Respir Crit Care Med.* 2014;189(6):727-740.

124. Vanderpool RR, Naeije R. Hematocrit-corrected pulmonary vascular resistance. *Am J Respir Crit Care Med.* 2018;198(3):305-309.

125. Machado RF, Anthi A, Steinberg MH, et al. N-terminal pro-brain natriuretic peptide levels and risk of death in sickle cell disease. *JAMA.* 2006;296(3):310-318.

126. Barnett CF, Hsue PY, Machado RF. Pulmonary hypertension: an increasingly recognized complication of hereditary hemolytic anemias and HIV infection. *JAMA.* 2008;299(3):324-331.

127. Forfia PR, Fisher MR, Mathai SC, et al. Tricuspid annular displacement predicts survival in pulmonary hypertension. *Am J Respir Crit Care Med.* 2006;174(9):1034-1041.

128. Linguraru MG, Pura JA, Gladwin MT, et al. Computed tomography correlates with cardiopulmonary hemodynamics in pulmonary hypertension in adults with sickle cell disease. *Pulm Circ.* 2014;4(2):319-329.

129. Linguraru MG, Pura JA, Van Uitert RL, et al. Segmentation and quantification of pulmonary artery for noninvasive CT assessment of sickle cell secondary pulmonary hypertension. *Med Phys.* 2010;37(4):1522-1532.

130. Nguyen KL, Tian X, Alam S, et al. Elevated transpulmonary gradient and cardiac magnetic resonance-derived right ventricular remodeling predict poor outcomes in sickle cell disease. *Haematologica.* 2016;101(2):e40-e43.

131. Castro O, Hoque M, Brown BD. Pulmonary hypertension in sickle cell disease: cardiac catheterization results and survival. *Blood.* 2003;101(4):1257-1261.

132. Weir NA, Saiyed R, Alam S, et al. Prostacyclin-analog therapy in sickle cell pulmonary hypertension. *Haematologica.* 2017;102(5):e163-e165.

133. Yawn BP, Buchanan GR, Afenyi-Annan AN, et al. Management of sickle cell disease: summary of the 2014 evidence-based report by expert panel members. *JAMA.* 2014;312(10):1033-1048.

134. De Castro LM, Jonassaint JC, Graham FL, Ashley-Koch A, Telen MJ. Pulmonary hypertension associated with sickle cell disease: clinical and laboratory endpoints and disease outcomes. *Am J Hematol.* 2008;83(1):19-25.

135. Lorch D, Spevack D, Little J. An elevated estimated pulmonary arterial systolic pressure, whenever measured, is associated with excess mortality in adults with sickle cell disease. *Acta Haematol.* 2011;125(4):225-229.

136. Caughey MC, Poole C, Ataga KI, Hinderliter AL. Estimated pulmonary artery systolic pressure and sickle cell disease: a meta-analysis and systematic review. *Br J Haematol.* 2015;170(3):416-424.

137. Damy T, Bodez D, Habibi A, et al. Haematological determinants of cardiac involvement in adults with sickle cell disease. *Eur Heart J.* 2016;37(14):1158-1167.

138. Caldas MC, Meira ZA, Barbosa MM. Evaluation of 107 patients with sickle cell anemia through tissue Doppler and myocardial performance index. *J Am Soc Echocardiogr.* 2008;21(10):1163-1167.

139. Hankins JS, McCarville MB, Hillenbrand CM, et al. Ventricular diastolic dysfunction in sickle cell anemia is common but not associated with myocardial iron deposition. *Pediatr Blood Cancer.* 2010;55(3):495-500.

140. Johnson MC, Kirkham FJ, Redline S, et al. Left ventricular hypertrophy and diastolic dysfunction in children with sickle cell disease are related to asleep and waking oxygen desaturation. *Blood.* 2010;116(1):16-21.

141. Machado RF, Hildesheim M, Mendelsohn L, Remaley AT, Kato GJ, Gladwin MT. NT-pro brain natriuretic peptide levels and the risk of death in the cooperative study of sickle cell disease. *Br J Haematol.* 2011;154(4):512-520.

142. Mehari A, Gladwin MT, Tian X, Machado RF, Kato GJ. Mortality in adults with sickle cell disease and pulmonary hypertension. *JAMA.* 2012;307(12):1254-1256.

143. Ataga KI, Brittain JE, Moore D, et al. Urinary albumin excretion is associated with pulmonary hypertension in sickle cell disease: potential role of soluble fms-like tyrosine kinase-1. *Eur J Haematol.* 2010;85(3):257-263.

144. Guasch A, Navarrete J, Nass K, Zayas CF. Glomerular involvement in adults with sickle cell hemoglobinopathies: prevalence and clinical correlates of progressive renal failure. *J Am Soc Nephrol.* 2006;17(8):2228-2235.

145. Powars DR, Chan LS, Hiti A, Ramicone E, Johnson C. Outcome of sickle cell anemia: a 4-decade observational study of 1056 patients. *Medicine.* 2005;84(6):363-376.

146. Platt OS, Brambilla DJ, Rosse WF, et al. Mortality in sickle cell disease. Life expectancy and risk factors for early death. *N Engl J Med.* 1994;330(23):1639-1644.

147. da Silva GB Jr, Liborio AB, Daher Ede F. New insights on pathophysiology, clinical manifestations, diagnosis, and treatment of sickle cell nephropathy. *Ann Hematol.* 2011;90(12):1371-1379.

148. Mekontso Dessap A, Leon R, Habibi A, et al. Pulmonary hypertension and cor pulmonale during severe acute chest syndrome in sickle cell disease. *Am J Respir Crit Care Med.* 2008;177(6):646-653.

149. Akgul F, Seyfeli E, Melek I, et al. Increased QT dispersion in sickle cell disease: effect of pulmonary hypertension. *Acta Haematol.* 2007;118(1):1-6.

150. Upadhya B, Ntim W, Brandon Stacey R, et al. Prolongation of QTc intervals and risk of death among patients with sickle cell disease. *Eur J Haematol.* 2013;91(2):170-178.

151. Maisel A, Friedman H, Flint L, Koshy M, Prabhu R. Continuous electrocardiographic monitoring in patients with sickle-cell anemia during pain crisis. *Clin Cardiol.* 1983;6(7):339-344.

152. Bode-Thomas F, Hyacinth HI, Ogunkunle O, Omotoso A. Myocardial ischaemia in sickle cell anaemia: evaluation using a new scoring system. *Ann Trop Paediatr.* 2011;31(1):67-74.

153. Pannu R, Zhang J, Andraws R, Armani A, Patel P, Mancusi-Ungaro P. Acute myocardial infarction in sickle cell disease: a systematic review. *Crit Pathw Cardiol.* 2008;7(2):133-138.

154. Pavlu J, Ahmed RE, O'Regan DP, Partridge J, Lefroy DC, Layton DM. Myocardial infarction in sickle-cell disease. *Lancet.* 2007;369(9557):246.

155. Deymann AJ, Goertz KK. Myocardial infarction and transient ventricular dysfunction in an adolescent with sickle cell disease. *Pediatrics.* 2003;111(2):E183-E187.

156. Dang NC, Johnson C, Eslami-Farsani M, Haywood LJ. Myocardial injury or infarction associated with fat embolism in sickle cell disease: a report of three cases with survival. *Am J Hematol.* 2005;80(2):133-136.

157. Robard I, Mansencal N, Soulat G, Deblaise J, El Mahmoud R, Dubourg O. Myocardial infarction with normal coronary arteries in double heterozygous sickle-cell disease. *Int J Cardiol.* 2015;180:120-121.

158. Norris S, Johnson CS, Haywood LJ. Sickle cell anemia: does myocardial ischemia occur during crisis? *J Natl Med Assoc.* 1991;83(3):209-213.

159. de Montalembert M, Maunoury C, Acar P, Brousse V, Sidi D, Lenoir G. Myocardial ischaemia in children with sickle cell disease. *Arch Dis Child.* 2004;89(4):359-362.

160. Acar P, Maunoury C, de Montalembert M, Dulac Y. [Abnormalities of myocardial perfusion in sickle cell disease in childhood: a study of myocardial scintigraphy]. *Arch Mal Coeur Vaiss.* 2003;96(5):507-510.

161. Tanner MA, Westwood MA, Pennell DJ. Myocardial infarction following sickle cell chest syndrome. *Br J Haematol.* 2006;134(1):2.

162. Khalique Z, Pavlu J, Lefroy D, Layton M. Erythrocytapheresis in the prevention of recurrent myocardial infarction in sickle cell disease. *Am J Hematol.* 2010;85(1):91.

163. Johnson WH Jr, McCrary RB, Mankad VN. Transient left ventricular dysfunction in childhood sickle cell disease. *Pediatr Cardiol.* 1999;20(3):221-223.

164. Turpin M, Chantalat-Auger C, Parent F, et al. Chronic blood exchange transfusions in the management of pre-capillary pulmonary hypertension complicating sickle cell disease. *Eur Respir J.* 2018;52:1800272.

165. Machado RF, Martyr S, Kato GJ, et al. Sildenafil therapy in patients with sickle cell disease and pulmonary hypertension. *Br J Haematol.* 2005;130(3):445-453.

166. George MP, Novelli EM, Shigemura N, et al. First successful lung transplantation for sickle cell disease with severe pulmonary arterial hypertension and pulmonary veno-occlusive disease. *Pulm Circ.* 2013;3(4):952-958.

167. Pittman C, Hsieh MM, Coles W, Tisdale JF, Weir NA, Fitzhugh CD. Reversal of pre-capillary pulmonary hypertension in a patient with sickle cell anemia who underwent haploidentical peripheral blood stem cell transplantation. *Bone Marrow Transplant.* 2017;52(4):641-642.

Cardiac Complications

Authors: Vandana Sachdev, Punam Malik,
John Wood, Jon Detterich

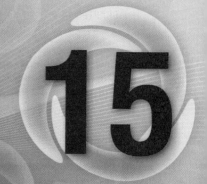

Chapter Outline

Overview

The heart, lungs, and blood vessels represent an integrally coupled system. Sickle cell disease (SCD) is characterized by a diffuse, progressive vascular disease that not only directly damages cardiac microvasculature but also places abnormal mechanical stressors on the heart by increasing preload (anemia) and afterload (peripheral and pulmonary vascular damage). The heart may also be damaged by the sequelae of treatments for SCD, such as chronic transfusions. In this section, we focus on how the primary vascular physiology described in earlier sections impacts the integrated cardiovascular system.

Pathophysiology of Cardiovascular Disease

Cardiac output and pulmonary blood flow are increased in 30% to 60% of SCD patients to compensate for the anemia,[1] comparable to pulmonary blood flow in a moderate atrial septal defect.[2] Although acute increases in systemic and pulmonary blood flow increase wall shear stress, resulting in vasodilation, chronically elevated blood flow produces eccentric arterial remodeling and cardiac dilation.[3] By Laplace's law, arterial and cardiac chamber dilation increases tensile stress, leading to eccentric vascular remodeling and compensatory wall thickening.[4,5] In advanced pulmonary hypertension, arterial dilation ultimately results in decreased wall shear stress, which may impair further shear-mediated nitric oxide signaling.[6] Arterial dilation also causes decreased vascular compliance, increasing the afterload on the right and left ventricles.[2]

    Chemical insults to vascular endothelia result from systemic hypoxia, ischemia-reperfusion injury, vascular inflammation, and products of red cell fragmentation and frank intravascular hemolysis; mechanisms of these processes have been described in previous chapters. Increased erythropoiesis also reinforces these processes, because proerythroblasts release potent chemokines including vascular endothelial growth factor (VEGF) and placenta growth factor (PlGF).[7] In addition, sickle erythrocytes generate a significant amount of reactive oxygen species,[8] which can further potentiate vascular and cardiac toxicity. Free heme may further augment PlGF release through induction of erythroid Krüppel-like factor (EKLF)[9] and Nrf2-mediated antioxidant response.[10] Although VEGF polymorphisms offer some prognostic value with respect to vaso-occlusive risk,[11] a central role for VEGF in chronic vasculopathy has not been defined. In contrast, PlGF overexpression promotes pulmonary hypertension in normal mice by stimulating endothelin release[12,13] and contributes to pulmonary emphysema.[14] PlGF increases airway hyperresponsiveness by stimulating interleukin-13 and leukotriene release.[15] PlGF also promotes vascular leak, edema, and inflammation via endothelial cells and monocytes[16,17] and promotes a procoagulant state by increasing tissue factor and PAI-1 expression.[18] PlGF also modulates adverse vascular remodeling through VEGF release and via prostaglandin mediated pathways.[19-21] The hyperactive erythropoiesis, erythropoietin, free heme, and hypoxia seen in SCD contribute to increased production of PlGF.[9,10,15,22-24]

Thus, sickle hemoglobin (HbS) triggers progressive microvascular damage and vascular dysfunction through multiple interconnected mechanisms. The systemic and pulmonary microvasculature suffers mechanical insults from poorly deformable, adhesive, and sickled erythrocytes, manifesting as microinfarcts in the heart, kidney, spleen, liver, and lungs. Progressive loss of vascular cross-sectional area may contribute to exercise-induced pulmonary hypertension because of impaired capillary recruitment.[25] Rarely, acute microvascular damage can produce an acute myocardial infarction.[26,27] However, cardiac microvascular damage is typically more insidious, producing a restrictive cardiomyopathy mimicking heart failure with preserved ejection fraction (HFpEF).[28] In sickle mice, in situ microvascular thrombosis caused patchy myocyte loss and fibrotic replacement, diastolic dysfunction, eccentric ventricular hypertrophy, and increased risk of sudden death, reflecting the cardiac phenotype observed in humans.[29]

Occasionally, the treatments designed to ameliorate vascular disease can trigger secondary pathology. Some patients with SCD are placed on chronic transfusion therapy to suppress the endogenous HbS percentage to <30%. The indications for chronic transfusion therapy include stroke, abnormal transcranial Doppler velocity, cerebral vasculopathy, and recurrent acute chest syndrome.[30] Each simple transfusion delivers as much iron as would naturally be absorbed by the body in 1 year. The body has no natural mechanisms for iron excretion; iron loss is limited to endothelial sloughing, blood loss, and free hemoglobin filtration in the glomerulus.[31] Iron loading can be ameliorated by using exchange transfusions, which also remove some of the most badly damaged HbS cells and lowers circulating hemolysis products. However, exchange transfusion is resource intensive and requires better vascular access.

Senescent red cells are phagocytosed in the reticuloendothelial system, and recycled ferric iron circulates bound to transferrin.[32] Excess transferrin-bound iron is initially stored in the liver and spleen.[33] The endocrine glands and the heart also uptake transferrin-bound iron but have strict negative feedback systems that prevent excess iron accumulation. However, these organs take up non–transferrin-bound iron constitutively through divalent metal channels such as calcium[34-37] and zinc transporters.[38] Thus, cardiac iron loading only occurs once transferrin has become fully saturated; in SCD, this is rarely before 10 years of chronic transfusion therapy.[39,40]

Transferrin saturation is determined by the balance of iron influx rate (the volume of blood per kilogram per year) compared with the iron utilization rate by the bone marrow.[41] In patients with ineffective erythropoiesis, the iron utilization rate must be estimated by radiolabeled iron studies or by soluble transferrin receptor. However, in SCD, reticulocyte production is a fairly good marker of iron utilization by the bone marrow. Typically, the reticulocyte count is high in SCD patients when they begin chronic transfusion therapy. This keeps transferrin saturation low and is cardioprotective.[40] However, when marrow production of endogenous red blood cells slows, transferrin saturation rises, and the risk of cardiac iron accumulation increases.

Clinical Phenotypes

The evaluation of the cardiac phenotype in SCD is particularly important because epidemiologic studies suggest that over half of deaths are due to cardiovascular and cardiopulmonary causes.[42] Echocardiography is the most widely available method to evaluate cardiac morphology and can provide detailed assessment of systolic and diastolic cardiac function as well as pulmonary pressures. Laboratory markers of hemolysis, hemoglobin F levels, and other hematologic markers have been closely associated with cardiac structural and functional abnormalities.[43] In a large study of sub-Saharan African adolescents and young adults, cardiac morphologic abnormalities (indexed left ventricular [LV] mass, chamber volumes, and cardiac index) were closely associated with extracardiac organ damage (stroke, leg ulcer, priapism, microalbuminuria, and osteonecrosis).[44]

Sickle Cardiomyopathy

The cardiac phenotype of SCD patients has been characterized by chamber dilation, eccentric hypertrophy, normal or increased LV systolic function, and abnormal diastolic filling consistent with anemia and volume overload.[45] In the context of a systemic disease, these types of abnormalities have been called either a secondary[46] or unclassified[47] cardiomyopathy in contemporary classifications. Hereditary hemoglobinopathies other than SCD share some common features with SCD,[48] and the term *rheologic cardiomyopathy* has been used.[49]

Only a small proportion of SCD patients have abnormal LV systolic function,[50] and a recent meta-analysis showed that the ejection fraction (EF) was not significantly different in SCD patients compared with controls. Cardiac dimensions, cardiac mass, and cardiac index were higher in patients with SCD.[51] An abnormal EF of <55 has been seen in approximately 9% of patients, and similar to numerous other cardiovascular conditions, it has been associated with higher mortality.[50,52] Right ventricular (RV) dysfunction is likely to be even more uncommon in SCD patients. In a small study of 41 SCD patients undergoing right heart catheterization for pulmonary hypertension, cardiac magnetic resonance imaging (MRI) showed poor survival for patients with an RVEF <32%.[53]

Because conventional indices of ventricular function are easily affected by loading conditions, speckle-tracking strain echocardiography, a measure of myocardial deformation, has been used to evaluate subclinical changes in ventricular function. The results of strain analysis in SCD patients are mixed, with most studies showing normal myocardial contractility.[54]

Diastolic filling abnormalities are seen frequently in SCD. The guidelines for diagnosis of LV diastolic dysfunction were recently updated[55] and suggest the use of cardiac structural parameters as well as functional information from Doppler imaging when evaluating patients with preserved EF (Figure 15-1 shows echocardiographic evaluation of diastolic dysfunction). This diagnosis includes analysis of 4 main parameters: (1) early mitral inflow (E) velocity and tissue Doppler mitral annular (e′) velocity, (2) ratio of E/e′, (3) left atrial size, and (4) peak tricuspid regurgitant velocity (TRV). A significant limitation of this algorithm is the lack of validation in SCD patients, in whom anemia and pulmonary vascular disease may confound these diagnostic components. SCD patients have a unique compilation of cardiac abnormalities that include both chamber dilation and eccentric hypertrophy; these changes can modify the relationship between noninvasive indices of diastolic function and invasively measured LV filling pressures. Significant anemia, increased metabolic demand, and peripheral vasodilation are known to result in a state of high cardiac output. The anemia also results in compensatory salt and water retention resulting in a volume overload state with increased volume of blood returning to the LV. This high preload can mimic a restrictive Doppler filling pattern seen in other diseases such as coronary artery disease and dilated cardiomyopathy. It is important to distinguish this from the more severe diastolic abnormalities seen in restrictive cardiomyopathies such as amyloidosis and sarcoidosis.[46] Future studies to correlate noninvasive diastolic indices with invasive measures of LV filling pressures are necessary to develop a more accurate algorithm for the diagnosis of diastolic dysfunction in SCD patients.

Several studies have confirmed an association between diastolic abnormalities and exercise limitations. In the Walk-PHaSST (Treatment of Pulmonary Hypertension and Sickle Cell Disease With Sildenafil Therapy) clinical trial, the lateral E/e′ ratio was an independent predictor of a shorter 6-minute walk distance ($P = .014$).[56] Similarly, in a study of 20 SCD patients undergoing cardiopulmonary exercise testing with cycle ergometry, reduced exercise capacity

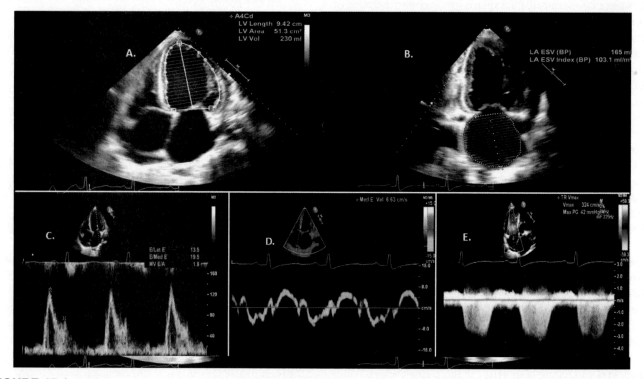

FIGURE 15-1 A 19-year-old man with sickle cell disease (SCD) and diastolic dysfunction. A. The left ventricle is severely dilated, and he has severe eccentric hypertrophy. **B.** The left atrial volume index is severely increased. **C.** Doppler of the mitral inflow shows E, the early filling wave, and A, the atrial contraction wave, with a resulting E/A ratio of 1.8. **D.** Tissue Doppler of the medial (septal) mitral annulus is used to measure the septal e′ wave. This is used to calculate the E/e′ ratio of 19.5. An E/e′ ratio >15 is associated with high left ventricular filling pressure in the non-SCD population. **E.** The peak tricuspid regurgitant velocity is elevated at 3.2 m/s.

was common, and the lateral E/e′ ratio was an independent predictor of this measure.[57]

Diastolic indices have also been used to define high-risk patients.[50,56] In an earlier National Institutes of Health (NIH) cohort, proportional hazards regression analysis found that most echocardiographic parameters of diastolic filling were associated with increased mortality (peak E velocity, $P = .002$; E/A, $P <.001$; deceleration time, $P = .002$). A low E/A ratio had a risk ratio of 3.5 for death (95% confidence interval [CI], 1.5-8.4; $P <.001$) even after adjustment for TRV, and coexisting diastolic dysfunction and a high TRV conferred a risk ratio of 12.0 (95% CI, 3.8-38.1; $P <.001$).[50] The etiology of the diastolic dysfunction is multifactorial, and associations with age, anemia, blood pressure, renal function,[50] and diffuse myocardial fibrosis[58] and contributions of a high-output state have been described.[59]

Left atrial size has been used as a measure of the severity and duration of diastolic dysfunction in the general population; however, it has had mixed results in the SCD population, with some correlation with LV filling pressures seen in children[60] but not adults.[61] Hammoudi et al[61] found that in a large group of young adults with SCD, the majority had left atrial dilation, and it was linked to age, hemoglobin level, and LV remodeling. Left atrial volume index was not a useful predictor of LV diastolic dysfunction.

MRI can be performed to support the diagnosis of cardiac abnormalities. In mouse models, left atrial dilation is absent in juveniles but increases in severity into middle age and senescence.[29] Concentric LV hypertrophy is common and also worsens with age in both mice[29] and humans.[44,62] In humans, left atrial volumes can be accurately measured by MRI using either biplane estimates[63] or multiple-slice planimetry.[64] Normative data must be inferred from 3-dimensional echocardiographic data for children but have been published for adults.[66] LV mass indexed to body surface area and LV diastolic volume represent the best robust markers of ventricular hypertrophy. Norms exist for both children[67] and adults.[68,69]

Recent work suggests that increases in the native T1 value and extracellular volume (ECV) fraction by cardiac MRI, reflecting replacement fibrosis, are sensitive markers of sickle cardiomyopathy.[58] ECV levels are significantly higher in SCD patients than controls and correlate with anemia severity and diastolic filling abnormalities.[58,60] The ECV values in SCD patients are significantly higher than observed in patients with hypertrophic and dilated cardiomyopathy, reaching values observed in the scar regions of myocardial infarction. ECV was also correlated with the logarithm of N-terminal prohormone of brain natriuretic peptide (NT-proBNP) levels ($r = 0.61$, $P <.001$), a known predictor of pulmonary hypertension and mortality in SCD.[58]

Sudden Cardiac Death

Sudden unexplained death is a significant problem in patients with SCD, with one autopsy study finding that 41% of patient deaths were sudden and unexplained. The presumption is that these deaths are due to a fatal arrhythmia or acute pulmonary hypertensive crisis. Pulmonary hypertensive crisis results in an acute and large decrease in pulmonary blood flow due to a rapid increase in pulmonary arterial resistance. This limits venous return to the left heart and causes a rapid decrease in systemic cardiac output.

Fatal arrhythmias have multiple potential etiologies but can be categorized as an automatic rhythm, triggered activity, or a reentrant circuit. Electrocardiograms (ECGs) in the clinical setting tend to demonstrate chamber enlargement and repolarization abnormalities including QTc prolongation and nonspecific ST/T-wave abnormalities.[70] However, a single ECG at one point in time is not very sensitive for arrhythmias.[71] Ambulatory ECG monitoring performed in 30 patients with SCD found arrhythmias in 80% of the patients, and 67% of the arrhythmias found were ventricular in origin.[71]

Myocardial transcriptome analysis in sickle mice shows a dramatic loss of expression of an extensive set of genes associated with maintenance of electrophysiologic integrity of the heart, including key genes whose dysfunction is associated with prolonged QT interval, arrhythmias, and sudden cardiac death.[29] Furthermore, sickle mice developed QTc prolongation and widening of the QRS, which was associated with cardiac ischemic events and fatal arrhythmias with sudden death.[29] Overall, QTc prolongation is a known risk factor for fatal arrhythmias among adults. A systematic review of ECGs and transthoracic echocardiograms of adults with SCD showed that persistently prolonged QTc, besides increased TRV and acute chest syndrome, was independently associated with increased mortality in SCD.[72]

According to the study by Liem et al,[70] QTc prolongation was not associated with LV size or hypertrophy; however, Maisel et al[71] found that ventricular arrhythmias were associated with myocardial dysfunction. QTc prolongation was associated with higher TRV, lactate dehydrogenase, and aspartate aminotransferase values[70] and higher mortality.[72] In the absence of ion channel defects, QTc prolongation and ventricular arrhythmias may be associated with ventricular scarring.

Multiple studies have demonstrated a direct association between myocardial scar and ventricular arrhythmias, which is thought to be related to intraventricular reentrant circuits. Myocardial scarring may lead to reentrant circuits that are established around or through the site of the scar, and arrhythmias do not require a large area of scar to establish a reentrant circuit.[73,74] Therefore, the diffuse fibrosis that was demonstrated by Niss and colleagues[29,58,60,75] may lead to the establishment of arrhythmogenic myocardial fibrosis.

Pulmonary Hypertension

The mechanisms, epidemiology, clinical presentation, and treatment of pulmonary hypertension have been discussed in detail earlier. Severe pulmonary hypertension causes secondary changes in heart morphology (RV hypertrophy, right atrial dilation)[76] and impairment of LV filling through interventricular dependence.[77] These secondary morphologic changes may increase atrial and ventricular arrhythmogenicity and probability of sudden cardiac death.[78]

Echocardiographic guidelines for assessment of the right heart[79] define normal ranges for measures including basal RV diameter, right atrial area, and diameter of the inferior vena cava. Due to the unusual shape of the RV, volumetric quantitation has been challenging; therefore, integration of qualitative and quantitative metrics is now recommended. Visual inspection for a D-shaped curvature of the ventricular septum can help with a diagnosis of RV volume and/or pressure overload. Assessment of pulmonary pressure (or RV systolic pressure [RVSP]) is performed using Doppler-derived peak TRV. The TRV should be acquired in multiple acoustic windows to obtain the technically adequate signals with well-defined borders. As previously described, the highest velocity obtained is converted to a pressure gradient using the simplified Bernoulli equation, and the addition of an estimated right atrial pressure (RAP) is used to derive the RVSP [RVSP = $4 \times$ (peak TRV)^2 + RAP]. In selected patients, the pulmonary artery diastolic pressure may be calculated in a similar manner from the end-diastolic pulmonary regurgitant jet. The mean pulmonary pressure can be derived by adding RAP to the velocity time integral of the tricuspid regurgitant jet. Finally, a simple method of assessing RV function using tricuspid annular motion has emerged, and a tricuspid annular plane systolic excursion cutoff of <17 mm has shown good specificity in identifying abnormal RV function.

Even mild pulmonary systolic hypertension, defined as a TRV between 2.5 and 2.9 m/s, is associated with significant all-cause morbidity and mortality.[45] Increases in TRV are a bellwether of vascular dysfunction and damage across the entire body, correlating with kidney damage,[80,81] stroke,[82] systemic vascular dysfunction,[83] and cardiomyopathy.[58,60] Thus, TRV should be interpreted as a readily accessible surrogate of cardiovascular health (particularly for TRVs <3.0 m/s) rather than a specific indicator of pulmonary arterial hypertension.

Iron Overload

Cardiac iron can be readily imaged and quantified by MRI. Annual screening of liver and heart iron accumulation represents the standard of care in other diseases requiring chronic transfusion therapy.[84] Because patients with SCD have somewhat lower intrinsic cardiac risk, less stringent monitoring can be performed until their transferrin saturation increases to >75% or 80% (the threshold at which non–transferrin-bound iron species begin to appear[85,86]); a review of iron monitoring guidelines can be found in Wood.[87] Cardiac risk is assessed by the MRI relaxation parameter T2*.[88] A cardiac T2* >20 milliseconds indicates no significant cardiac iron deposition. A T2* between 10 and 20 milliseconds reflects detectable cardiac iron with little immediate clinical risk, and a cardiac T2* <10 milliseconds conveys significant risk of developing cardiac arrhythmias or dysfunction. T2* is reciprocally related to cardiac iron concentration, so a T2* of 5 milliseconds indicates double the cardiac iron of a T2* of 10 milliseconds.[89] For perspective, the risk of developing symptomatic heart failure in 1 year is >50%

in thalassemia patients with a T2* <6 milliseconds.[90] Thus, most physicians will aggressively increase iron chelation therapy based on cardiac T2* results alone, rather than waiting for cardiac dysfunction to set in.

Myocardial Infarction

Myocardial infarction is uncommon in SCD, and in most cases, angiography does not show atherosclerotic disease in the coronary arteries. The pathophysiology is thought to be acute and chronic microvascular occlusion, associated increases in inflammatory cytokines, and subsequent thrombosis, as seen in other vascular territories. One autopsy study demonstrated myocardial infarctions in 9.7% of SCD patients.[27] This finding has been supported by more recent work showing troponin elevations[91] during vaso-occlusive episodes, as well as nuclear[92] and MRI[93] perfusion defects. Previous myocardial scarring from either myocardial infarction or myocarditis can also be detected by delayed enhancement imaging.[94]

Valvular Disease

In 1985, Lippman et al[95] reported a greater than expected prevalence of mitral valve prolapse in patients with SCD and postulated that these patients might have a coexisting underlying collagen defect. Subsequent skin biopsies suggested a higher fraction of elastin fibers than the general population but lesser density than observed in pseudoxanthoma elasticum, consistent with a nonspecific underlying elastinopathy.[96] However, several subsequent studies failed to confirm that mitral valve prolapse was increased in SCD patients.[97-99] Thus, although there is considerable literature describing techniques for mitral valve repair and cardiopulmonary bypass in SCD patients, there is no consensus that SCD patients are more prone to valvular disease than the general population.

Systemic Vascular Disease

Vascular endothelia have numerous surface proteins that serve to modulate coagulation/anticoagulation, vascular tone, permeability, cell adhesion, red cell eryptosis, and immune response. Under the influence of mechanical, infectious, or chemical stressors, the vascular endothelium may release these surface proteins. Hence, there has been considerable interest in using circulating endothelial proteins as biomarkers for endothelial damage in infectious disease,[100] cardiovascular disease,[101,102] and SCD.[103-105]

Although nearly every endothelial marker is increased during vaso-occlusive episodes, many are also elevated during steady state, including angiopoietin 1 and 2,[103] the selectins,[104,105] soluble vascular cell adhesion molecule 1 (sVCAM1),[104,105] and soluble intercellular adhesion molecule 1 (sICAM1).[104,105] Levels correlate with other serologic biomarkers (hemoglobin level, liver function tests, blood urea nitrogen, lactate dehydrogenase, platelet count, C-reactive protein) and with mortality.[104] von Willebrand factor and its propeptide are also chronically elevated in SCD, along with thrombin-antithrombin complexes and prothrombin activation fractions, consistent with smoldering activation of coagulation pathways.[106]

The challenge for all these biomarkers has been the dynamic nature of their activation and resolution and the significant overlap between normal subjects and patients with SCD. None of these biomarkers have been validated as surrogates for disease (ie, improvements in biomarkers do not necessarily translate to improvements in vascular disease). Nonetheless, their low cost and their ability to cast some insight on underlying pathophysiology make serum biomarkers attractive research targets.

Systemic hypertension is a traditional marker of peripheral vascular dysfunction. Patients with SCD traditionally have low peripheral vascular resistance to accommodate their chronically elevated cardiac output, leading to low diastolic pressures, low-to-normal systolic pressures, and a wide pulse pressure.[107] Wide pulse pressure is associated with hyperhemolysis, anemia, proteinuria, and chronic kidney disease.[107] However, traditionally defined systemic hypertension (blood pressures >140/90 mm Hg in adults) is relative rare in SCD patients and carries a fairly poor prognosis[80] because it reflects diffuse small-vessel disease. In fact, even "relative hypertension" (blood pressure >120/70 mm Hg but <140/90 mm Hg) conveys increased risk for stroke, pulmonary hypertension, and kidney disease.[80,108,109] Occult (also called masked) systemic hypertension refers to hypertension that is only detected on ambulatory monitoring and not on office monitoring. In a study of 56 children with SCD, only 11 had normal ambulatory blood pressure monitoring, whereas 14 had occult hypertension, 28 had abnormal blood pressure patterns that did not meet criteria for hypertension, and 3 had coincident ambulatory and office-measured hypertension. Thus, ambulatory blood pressure monitoring is probably underutilized in the SCD population and may prove to be a valuable biomarker of vascular disease severity.[110,111]

Systemic endothelial function can be most directly measured by flow-mediated dilation (FMD) of the brachial artery. FMD represents the percent change in the brachial artery after a standardized transient forearm occlusion. FMD is a sensitive and robust assay of shear-mediated vasodilation, which is an endothelial nitric oxide synthase (eNOS)-dependent process. FMD is abnormal in adults with SCD and correlates with the severity of pulmonary hypertension in both SCD[83] and patients with primary pulmonary hypertension.[112] Figure 15-2A demonstrates the relationship between FMD and TRV in nontransfused and chronically transfused SCD patients. Three distinct groups can be seen, supranormal FMD (>9%), normal FMD (5%-9%), and markedly impaired FMD (<5%). All of the patients with supranormal FMD have normal TRV, but the probability of abnormal TRV increases with worsening FMD. Impaired FMD is also observed in children with primary pulmonary hypertension, suggesting that endothelial dysfunction plays a role in increased pulmonary vascular resistance.[112]

FMD is decreased in children with SCD[113,114] and associated with frequency of vaso-occlusive episodes in some studies,[114] but not others,[115] potentially reflecting variations in disease severity and disease-modifying therapies. Although shear-mediated vasodilation is impaired, vasodilatory response to nitroprusside administration appears to be preserved.[116,117] Forearm plethysmography studies suggest that high tonic eNOS activity maintains resting flow but that shear transduction is markedly impaired.[116] Interestingly, acetylcholine-mediated vasodilation was maintained or even exaggerated, suggesting either increased eNOS activity or prostacyclin production. FMD is inversely correlated with cell-free hemoglobin[83] (Figure 15-2B), and plasma from SCD patients inhibits forearm vasodilatory response in normal controls,[118] suggesting that plasma products of red blood cell damage or destruction may be disrupting shear-mediated vasodilation and may contribute to endothelial dysfunction and increased TRV.

Although FMD represents the gold standard for assessing endothelial reactivity, its complexity precludes clinical use. Several fully automated fingertip plethysmography devices

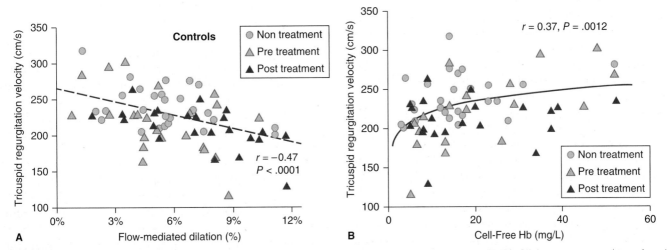

FIGURE 15-2 A. Plot of tricuspid regurgitation velocity (TRV) as a function of flow-mediated dilation (FMD). Circles represent nontransfused sickle cell disease (SCD) patients, triangles represent chronically transfused SCD patients (open symbol indicates pretransfusion, closed symbol indicates posttransfusion). **B.** Plot of TRV against cell-free hemoglobin (Hb) concentration. Same symbol convention as panel A. Tx, treatment (transfusion).

have been marketed as biomarkers of endothelial function (EndoPat, Itamar Medical; Enodthelix, Vendys2) for use in coronary artery disease. Although both devices detect aspects of vascular reactivity, they are not surrogate biomarkers of FMD and are unvalidated in SCD.

Although SCD is thought to primarily affect the microvasculature, there are contradictory data on carotid arteriopathy in adults. A small retrospective study suggested that carotid stiffness was increased in SCD patients compared with controls and was increased in SCD patients who had suffered a stroke.[119] Another study suggested increased carotid distensibility in SCD patients; however, there was decreased diastolic wall stress and no association with other clinical parameters.[115] Carotid intima-media thickness (CIMT) is known to be a surrogate marker of atherosclerosis and has been evaluated as a marker of sickle cell vasculopathy. CIMT is increased in SCD patients compared with controls and is correlated with higher cystatin C levels[120] and a higher number of vascular events.[121]

Because the microvasculature represents a primary target of sickle arteriopathy, there has been some interest in contrast-based microvascular perfusion in SCD.[122-125] An early study using this technique demonstrated abnormal myocardial perfusion reserve and a correlation with indices of systolic function.[122] Another study showed higher myocardial flow in SCD patients treated with hydroxyurea compared with untreated patients.[124] Although promising, further work is necessary to characterize the prognostic value of these techniques.

The human vascular system stiffens with age, but the rate of stiffening is accelerated by many traditional vascular stressors (eg, poor glucose control, hyperlipidemia, systemic hypertension). Increased vascular stiffness is a strong biomarker of poor cardiovascular and cerebrovascular outcomes. Vascular stiffness is commonly inferred by pulse wave propagation velocity, measured by applanation tonography, ultrasound, or MRI. In the general population, increased vascular stiffness results in a wide pulse pressure. In SCD, however, wide pulse pressures result from a large cardiac stroke volume being delivered into a normally compliant aortic arch. Wide pulse pressure is associated with poor renovascular and cerebrovascular outcomes in both control[126-128] and SCD subjects[107,129]; however, the underlying pathophysiology may be different. Most studies have demonstrated that pulse wave velocity is decreased in SCD patients[130,131] because of their low peripheral vascular resistance and diastolic blood pressures. Pulse wave velocity increases with age with SCD but remains lower than for normal subjects. In contrast, the augmentation index is initially lower than in controls[130,131] but increases much more rapidly with age.[130] Paradoxically, aortic radial stiffness is reportedly higher in SCD patients and correlates with LV mass.[117] Similarly, abnormal carotid radial stiffness is highly predictive of stroke in SCD patients.[119] The interaction between radial distensibility and pulse wave propagation velocity is governed by vessel radius and stroke volume, which are significantly larger in SCD patients. Thus, care must be made not to equate the 2 methods or to use risk thresholds defined in control populations.

Epidemiology

The prevalence of sickle cardiomyopathy is not well known. In a study of 134 children and young adults with SCD, >70% had abnormal blood and tissue Doppler filling indices by the age of 18.[60] The diagnosis of diastolic dysfunction is particularly challenging in the pediatric population because of the strong dependence of filling parameters on patient age and heart rate. Anemia further confounds the diagnosis because of increased resting heart rate and cardiac output. In adults with SCD, there is dramatic variation based on criteria used to diagnose diastolic dysfunction. With more stringent criteria, the prevalence of diastolic dysfunction ranges from 14% to 20%.[50,60,61]

In a another study, 25 of 25 SCD patients had abnormally high ECV fraction by cardiac MRI.[58] These data suggest that sickle cardiomyopathy is common, if not universal. Hemodynamic measurements have shown that approximately half of SCD patients undergoing right heart catheterization have pulmonary venous hypertension due to left heart disease from sickle cardiomyopathy as the etiology of their increased pulmonary artery pressures.[132]

Iron cardiomyopathy is restricted to patients with chronic transfusion therapy. Patients with SCD do not spontaneously develop iron overload, unlike those with severe forms of thalassemia. Cardiac iron overload is rare unless somatic iron overload is severe and prolonged,[133] with a prevalence between 2% and 5% of chronically transfused patients.[40]

Systemic vascular disease is common in SCD. Figure 15-3 demonstrates that <20% of children and young adults with SCD have normal FMD and postocclusive hyperemia.[134] Tissue oxygenation, a surrogate for microvascular health, worsened with age, cell-free hemoglobin, red cell deformability, and resting microvascular flow.[134]

The greatest challenge in characterizing the prevalence of cardiovascular complications is the rapid evolution of SCD practice guidelines. Future studies are required to determine the impact of therapies such as chronic transfusions, early hydroxyurea introduction, and L-glutamine on both cardiomyopathy and progressive arteriopathy.

Treatment of Cardiac Complications

Cardiac Screening and Risk Stratification

Cardiovascular disease has been a concern in patients with sickle cell anemia since the recognition of the disease.[135] As our knowledge of chronic cardiovascular disease has improved, cardiac screening guidelines have been developed. In 2014, the National Heart, Lung, and Blood Institute (NHLBI) established management guidelines with some recommendations for cardiac screening.[136] Routine ECG screening was not recommended. Due to the controversy surrounding TRV as a strong predictor of mortality, echocardiographic screening for pulmonary hypertension was neither encouraged nor discouraged by the NHLBI consensus document. In contrast, the

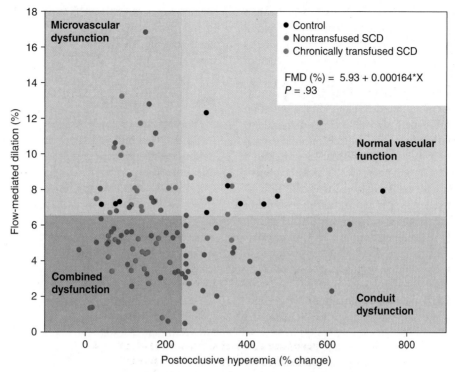

FIGURE 15-3 **Plot of flow-mediated dilation (FMD) versus postocclusive hyperemia by laser Doppler flow measurements.** The green area represents the region where both conduit vessel (FMD) and microvascular (Doppler) vessel function are normal, and the red area represents the region where both are abnormal. SCD, sickle cell disease. Detterich JA, Kato R, Bush A, et al. Sickle cell microvascular paradox—oxygen supply-demand mismatch. *Am J Hematol.* 2019; 94: 678-688. Republished with permission from John Wiley & Sons.

American Thoracic Society (ATS) recommends either surveillance echocardiography or NT-proBNP measurements.[137] There were no recommendations for ambulatory ECG monitoring for arrhythmias despite early data on arrhythmias in SCD. T1 mapping technology was not available in 2014, and thus, there were no recommendations for cardiac MRI screening to determine the presence or absence of diffuse myocardial fibrosis. Single-center recommendations for MRI surveillance of iron overload in SCD patients on chronic transfusions have been previously published, but consensus guidelines only exist for thalassemia and other rare anemias.[84]

Despite the lack of consensus guidelines, strong arguments can be made for routine ECG, arrhythmia monitoring, echocardiography, and ambulatory blood pressure monitoring. Longitudinal monitoring of QT interval by ECG is simple and inexpensive. Changes in QT interval or morphology raises concerns for ventricular arrhythmias and sudden death and should prompt referral to an electrophysiologist. Cardiac arrhythmias, even potentially lethal ones, may be clinically silent. Fortunately, wearable ambulatory ECG technologies are more broadly available and easier to use. As previously discussed, ATS practice guidelines for SCD recommend screening echocardiography and/or NT-proBNP for risk stratification and adjustment of therapies.[137] Valuable information on left atrial and ventricular remodeling, LV hypertrophy, and diastolic parameters can be obtained during screening echocardiograms. Previous attempts to integrate large amounts of phenotypic data for risk stratification have included a network model for prediction of mortality.[138] Biomarker signatures have been associated with different risk levels for disease complications and mortality.[139] Prognostic tools derived from newer analytic models are needed to risk stratify patients and triage emerging therapies. Ambulatory blood pressure monitoring detects occult hypertension in SCD patients[110,111] and is probably underutilized.

Critics of routine screening argue that abnormal results are unactionable because the links between abnormal screening results and outcomes remain murky and there is a paucity of therapeutic agents. Unfortunately, this argument is circular because failure to collect disease biomarkers cripples observational and clinical efficacy studies. Furthermore, dozens of novel therapeutic agents in clinical development will need postmarket validation.

Prophylactic Therapies

Clinical practice regarding hydroxyurea initiation has changed dramatically over the past 2 decades. NIH guidelines first recommended early hydroxyurea initiation (9 months of age) 5 years ago.[140] L-Glutamine supplementation in pharmacologic doses has recently been demonstrated to decrease frequency of vaso-occlusive episodes and hospitalization rate,[141] leading to its approval by the US Food and Drug Administration (FDA). Therefore, it is a key open question whether current aggressive hydroxyurea management, glutamine, or the use of chronic blood transfusions can prevent sickle cardiomyopathy, pulmonary hypertension, and peripheral vascular disease. Because microvascular destruction is central to most SCD end-organ damage, it is likely that any therapies that improve red blood cell flexibility and longevity will ameliorate the myocardial disease by decreasing vaso-occlusion and lowering the burden of circulating red cell debris.

A number of peripheral vascular therapies have demonstrated potential in SCD mouse models, either on the initiation or resolution of ischemia-reperfusion injury. Vascular inflammation can be incited directly by free radicals released during ischemia-reperfusion injury or as a result of toll-like receptor 4 (TLR4) activation by circulating heme.[142,143] TLR4 antagonists can therefore potentially be explored to reduce acute inflammation, especially acute chest syndrome. Tumor necrosis factor (TNF) plays a central role in amplifying vascular inflammation after an inciting stimulus. TNF blockers have been essential tools in managing chronic inflammatory diseases such as rheumatoid arthritis, ankylosing spondylitis, psoriasis, and inflammatory bowel disease. In 3 separate SCD mouse models, etanercept decreased circulating markers of vascular inflammation, pulmonary endothelial expression of tissue factor and VCAM1, and coagulative necrosis of the liver.[144]

Recent work also suggests that modulating recovery from ischemia-reperfusion can be beneficial in SCD. Resolvins are specialized proresolving lipid mediators that are metabolites of omega-3 fatty acids produced in response to systemic inflammation. Resolvins serve a counterregulatory role, shortening the duration of the inflammatory stimulus. Administration of exogenous 17R-RvD1 blunted adverse pulmonary, renal, and peripheral vascular remodeling during repeated hypoxia-reperfusion stress.[145] Simple replacement of polyunsaturated fatty acids (precursors of 17R-RvD1) demonstrated no benefit.

The pathophysiology of microvascular disease in SCD is similar across different organs. Consequently, treatment of peripheral vascular disease has significant overlap with treatment of vascular disease in the brain, lungs, and kidney. In particular, therapies such as hydroxyurea and chronic blood transfusions that improve red cell mechanical properties and survival are likely to ameliorate peripheral vascular disease.

With that caveat, some therapies are uniquely suited to peripheral vascular disease. Selectins are ubiquitously expressed in the peripheral vasculature and essential for initiation of vascular inflammation. A pan-selectin inhibitor, rivipansel, reduced leukocyte adhesion and improved survival in SCD mice exposed to TNF and surgical challenge.[146] Phase I and II trials of rivipansel[147,148] suggested a good safety profile and 83% reduction of intravenous opioid use during hospitalizations for vaso-occlusive episodes. The phase III RESET trial of rivipansel for acute vaso-occlusive episodes was completed in early 2019. Although one would expect primarily peripheral vascular benefit from selectin blockade (because cerebral vasculature is selectin poor[149]), decreased systemic vascular inflammation is likely to decrease toxic circulating red cell fragments, decellularized hemoglobin, and activated platelets. In TNF-treated Townes SCD mice, laser Doppler

from the cerebral cortex demonstrated marked improvement in microvascular flow after rivipansel treatment.[150] Unfortunately, the phase III RESET study failed to meet either the primary or secondary end points.

Rescue Therapies

Prophylaxis is absolutely essential because restrictive cardiomyopathies are difficult to treat in their advanced stages. Gentle diuresis is often employed to improve symptomatology but does not offer a survival benefit and may worsen renal function. Clinical trials of β-blockers, angiotensin receptor blockers, and angiotensin inhibitors in nonsickle HFpEF have been negative to date on meta-analysis.[151] Mineralocorticoid inhibition appears to produce modest benefit,[151,152] primarily in patients with low serologic evidence of collagen cross-linking.[153] A number of novel, targeted approaches for interrupting cardiac fibrosis have been demonstrated in animal models and are in various stages of human translation.[154]

Even in the best of hands, symptomatic iron cardiomyopathy is perilous, despite the potential for full recovery.[155] With the availability of reliable monitoring, iron cardiomyopathy should never come as a surprise. Oral iron chelation is widely available and can be tailored to a patient's lifestyle. Chronically transfused patients with SCD should always be followed by a hematologist with experience in managing iron overload. Iron loading can also be limited by the use of exchange transfusions rather than simple transfusions. Exchange transfusions also offer benefits by removing aged and damaged red blood cells, thereby limiting circulating toxic cell-free hemoglobin. In fact, exchange transfusions may be preferable to simple transfusions but are resource intensive and require better intravenous access than simple transfusions.

Although cardiac T2* thresholds were developed primarily from thalassemia patients, there is no indication that patients with SCD behave differently once cardiac hemosiderosis has developed. In a similar vein, there is no indication that the treatment of symptomatic iron cardiomyopathy is different in SCD compared with thalassemia. In that regard, the American Heart Association guidelines developed for managing iron cardiomyopathy in thalassemia represent an excellent resource for clinicians managing iron cardiomyopathy in SCD.[84] Iron chelation represents the cornerstone of rescue therapy. Immediate initiation of continuous deferoxamine therapy at 60 to 100 mg/kg/d with concomitant deferiprone therapy represents the standard of care. Iron cardiomyopathy is completely reversible if the patient can be sustained long enough for iron chelation to work.[155,156] Stabilization of the toxic intracellular iron pool requires weeks to months, and complete heart iron clearance requires years of therapy. However, symptomatic and functional improvement follows the labile intracellular iron, and patients can typically be transitioned to outpatient management within weeks.

Stabilizing cardiac function during decompensation can be challenging. Cardiac pressors worsen oxidative stress and should be avoided unless absolutely necessary to maintain mentation or urinary output. Comorbid nutritional and endocrine deficiencies often impact cardiac function and need to be corrected.[84,157,158] Amiodarone is the drug of choice for rhythm control because of its broad scope of action and because long-term management is rarely required, thus reducing the risk of iatrogenic complications. Typical heart failure medications such as β-blockers, angiotensin-converting enzyme (ACE) inhibitors, angiotensin blockers, and spironolactone can play a role in the convalescent phase following acute stabilization but are rarely required for lifelong support. Calcium channel blockers may inhibit influx of non–transferrin-bound iron species into the heart through L-type calcium channels.[36,37] They do not play a role in acute heart failure but could potentially be useful during convalescence or for primary prophylaxis.

There is limited information on management of acute myocardial infarction in SCD because patients have atypical presentations and clinical findings that may delay guideline-directed therapy. The most common presentation is that of a non–ST-segment elevation myocardial infarction, and established therapies including anticoagulation, aspirin, nitroglycerin, β-blockers, and ACE inhibitors are often used.[159] Data from the National Inpatient Sample database show that SCD patients hospitalized with either a primary or secondary diagnosis of acute MI had worse outcomes than non-SCD patients when matched for age, sex, race, and year of admission.[160] SCD patients with acute myocardial infarction had an in-hospital mortality of 18%, 3 times that of non-SCD patients, and were more likely to have systemic complications such as pneumonia, respiratory failure, and acute renal failure. Whether transfusions to alleviate the anemia-related myocardial hypoxia will help improve outcomes in the acute setting needs to be explored. A simple transfusion has certainly changed the outcome of acute chest syndrome in SCD.[161]

SCD patients admitted with acute chest syndrome may develop complications such as respiratory failure and right heart failure or cor pulmonale. Sudden increases in pulmonary pressure are seen during episodes of vaso-occlusive crises, and one study of SCD patients admitted to an intensive care unit found that 13% of patients developed cor pulmonale; all of these patients had a peak TRV >3 m/s.[162] Management of these patients with limited cardiopulmonary reserve is difficult and may require sequential volume expansion, red blood cell transfusion, and careful diuretic therapy due to their hemodynamically compromised state.[163]

One of the most painful and vexing peripheral vascular complications in SCD is chronic leg ulcers. Leg ulcers occur in 8% to 10% of SCD patients in North America, heal poorly, and have a high recurrence rate.[164] The underlying microvascular disease is complex and has overlapping pathophysiology with hemolysis-associated pulmonary hypertension.[165] Leg ulcers and pulmonary hypertension also coexist in thalassemia intermedia, particularly in splenectomized patients,[166] suggesting a role for circulating microparticles or other vasoactive cell remnants. Circulating cell-free hemoglobin is equally high in thalassemia and SCD,[167] even though the locations of red cell turnover differ. Studies in mice demonstrate decreased

endothelial progenitor cells and angiogenic cytokines.[168] There have been 2 small studies of successful transdermal oxygen delivery,[169,170] an approach used in diabetic and venous stasis ulceration. A recent phase I dose-finding study of topical sodium nitrite in 18 SCD patients suggested a dose-dependent reduction in ulcer size, accompanied by improvement in pain scores.[171] Topical nitrite increased local skin temperature and blood flow with no detectable systemic effects.

Cardiothoracic Surgery

Patients with sickle cell anemia require cardiopulmonary bypass to repair congenital heart disease or acquired valvular disease at a similar rate as the general population. There are numerous case reports and case series documenting that cardiopulmonary bypass can be performed safely in SCD patients. Most centers have performed preoperative exchange transfusion to lower HbS concentration to <30 or 40%,[172,173] although a single African center reported that preoperative exchange transfusion was unnecessary.[174]

Data from lower risk surgical procedures have documented that simple transfusion is beneficial.[175] Simple transfusion to raise the preoperative hemoglobin level above 10 g/dL appears to be equally effective as exchange transfusion[176,177]; however, these data cannot be generalized to cardiopulmonary bypass with hypothermia. Thus, in the absence of a randomized trial, preoperative exchange transfusion to lower HbS to <30 is recommended prior to cardiopulmonary bypass.

Future Research

All of the cardiovascular complications of SCD, except iron overload cardiomyopathy, share a common pathophysiology, namely the progressive microvascular disease caused by sickle erythrocytes. Thus, measures aimed at improving red cell survival, decreasing vascular adhesion and inflammation, and improving microvascular oxygen delivery are likely to ameliorate cardiac, peripheral vascular, and pulmonary vascular damage. Currently, FDA-approved therapies are limited to transfusion therapy,[178,179] hydroxyurea,[180,181] and L-glutamine supplementation.[182] Many questions with current therapies remain unanswered. For example, does early and aggressive intervention with hydroxyurea (within the first year of life) prevent or slow progression of sickle cardiomyopathy and pulmonary hypertension? Early hydroxyurea initiation often elicits more robust fetal hemoglobin induction compared with hydroxyurea therapy in adults. Given the morbidity and mortality associated with pulmonary hypertension, renal disease, and cardiomyopathy, should abnormalities in any of these organs be sufficient justification for simple or exchange transfusions? There is also a paucity of data using combinations of FDA-approved therapies.

A number of novel therapies are currently in clinical trials. Table 15-1 summarizes all clinical trials in SCD (ClinicalTrials.gov) using experimental therapies (excluding curative and gene therapies) that are enrolling or expecting to enroll

TABLE 15-1 Current SCD trials in ClinicalTrials.gov

ClinicalTrials.gov identifier	Agent	Phase	Mechanism
03285178	IW-1701	II	sGC stimulator (vasoreactivity)
02633397	Riociguat	II	sGC stimulator (vasoreactivity)
03615924	Ticagrelor	III	P2Y$_{12}$ antagonist (platelet inhibition)
03814746	Crizanlizumab	III	Antibody to P-selectin (adhesion, inflammation)
03474965	Crizanlizumab	II	Antibody to P-selectin (adhesion, inflammation)
04000165	AG348	I	Allosteric activator of PK-R (Hb dissociation)
02850406	GBT440	II	Stabilize R-state of Hb (Hb dissociation)
02380079	SCD101	IB	Unknown
02373241	Losartan	II	Angiotensin 2 inhibitor
03719729	Rifaximin	II	Antibiotic (lower circulating activated neutrophils)
02536170	Arginine	II	Improve eNOS coupling (vasoreactivity)
03599609	Simvastatin	I, II	Rho kinase inhibition (adhesion, inflammation)
03401112	IMR-687	IIA	PDE9 inhibition (increase cGMP, vasoreactivity)
03815695	FT-4202	I	Agonist of PK-R (Hb dissociation)
02712346	Ambrisentan	I	Endothelin antagonist
03247218	Memantine	II	NMDA inhibitor (RBC stabilization)
02515838	Sevuparin	II	Polysaccharide (adhesion, inflammation)
03653676	Exercise	II	Unspecified
02961218	Canakinumab	II	Antibody to IL-1β (inflammation)
02433158	Rivipansel	II	Pan selectin inhibitor (adhesion, inflammation)
03758950	Mometasone	II	Inhaled steroid (adhesion, inflammation)
02981329	Metformin	II	FOXO3-dependent hemoglobin F induction
02604368	SC411	III	Increase DHA (adhesion, RBC stabilization)

Abbreviations: cGMP, cyclic guanosine monophosphate; DHA, docosahexaenoic acid; eNOS, endothelial nitric oxide synthase; Hb, hemoglobin; IL-1β, interleukin-1β; NMDA, N-methyl-D-aspartate; PDE9, phosphodiesterase 9; PK-R, protein kinase R; RBC, red blood cell; sGC, soluble guanylate cyclase.

patients. Several agents (AG348, GBT440, FT-4202, and metformin) act by increasing the oxygen affinity of hemoglobin, decreasing the probability of oxygen desaturation and HbS polymerization in the capillary bed. The unanswered question with this approach is whether observed improvements in red cell survival and oxygen-carrying capacity with therapy are sufficient to overcome the impaired oxygen unloading caused by the hemoglobin left shift.

Given the known derangements of eNOS coupling and nitric oxide scavenging by hemoglobin, there are 2 trials of arginine supplementation for acute vaso-occlusive episodes and soluble guanylate cyclase (sGC) stimulators to modify chronic vasculopathy. These agents overcome the nitric oxide depletion caused by circulating hemoglobin and heme by signaling upstream of nitric oxide transduction. However, it is not yet known whether chronic, global sGC stimulation will have long-term vascular benefits. Several other agents strive to decrease vascular adhesion (crizanlizumab, sevuparin, rivipansel) or otherwise modify vascular inflammation (rifaximin, canakinumab, mometasone, simvastatin). Although initial studies suggest amelioration of vaso-occlusive episodes, the role of these agents for chronic vascular prophylaxis needs to be defined.

Further work is also ongoing in the renin-angiotensin-aldosterone-endothelin axis. Current studies are focusing on renovascular implications, but these therapies may also be of benefit in slowing the progression of cardiovascular and cerebrovascular disease. ACE inhibition appears to slow the decline in glomerular function over time,[183] and angiotensin blockade improved proteinuria in 2 recent studies.[184,185] Endothelin blockade[186] improves renal function and decreases neutrophil adhesion to activated vascular endothelia.[187] Endothelin also appears to reinforce chronic pain pathways, with endothelin blockage improving pain thresholds in SCD mice.[188] Despite the preclinical efficacy, there has been only one human trial of endothelin blockade (NCT02712346), which was stopped prematurely due to lack of enrollment.

Finally, it is important to remember that interventions slowing vascular aging in non-SCD patients may ameliorate the chronic vasculopathy of SCD. Fish oil supplementation is protective against hypoxic-ischemic injury in mice,[189] is safe, and improves vascular biomarkers in humans.[190,191] Similarly, statins represent a mainstay of adult cardiovascular medicine in the general population. Even though SCD patients have low total cholesterol, the rho kinase modulation and other anti-inflammatory effects appear to offer vascular protection in SCD patients.[192] Moderate exercise prescriptions are safe[193] and decrease vascular inflammation. There has not been strong evidence indicating that antiplatelet agents prevent vaso-occlusive events,[194] but there have been no studies examining long-term risk and benefits. Thus, although both patients and providers continue to hope for curative and "magic bullet" therapies, multidrug strategies with established medications and lifestyle modifications could go a long way in supporting patients.

Conclusion

In SCD, the heart and vascular system are exposed to a lifetime of anemia and mechanical and chemical insults that produce hypoxia-ischemia, oxidant stress, microvascular damage, abnormal vascular remodeling, cardiac fibrosis, and pulmonary and renal dysfunction. The net result is impaired diastolic function, increased vascular tone, lung disease, thrombotic disease, and progressive pulmonary venous and then arterial hypertension. Renovascular disease and systemic endothelial damage contribute to systemic hypertension that can be cryptic, particular in children. Cardiac microvascular disease and fibrosis produce abnormal repolarization and leave SCD patients vulnerable to sudden cardiac death. Transfusion therapy ameliorates the chronic vascular disease but introduces secondary cardiovascular toxicity through iron overload. The most effective cardiovascular therapies are targeted toward the primary red blood cell defect; however, traditional cardiovascular therapies such as ACE and angiotensin inhibitors, endothelin blockers, and β-blockers, can play a role in select individuals. Curative therapies such as bone marrow transplant and gene therapy are likely to offer significant cardiovascular benefits if initiated before irreversible cardiac damage occurs. However, these benefits must be weighed against the therapy's toxicity, since the reversibility of existing cardiovascular disease is unknown. Studies aimed at identifying mechanistic pathways that are upregulated secondary to SCD and instigate cardiac pathology will result in targeted therapies that can prevent, delay, or ameliorate the cardiac pathophysiology in SCD.

Case Study

A lifelong patient of Children's Hospital Los Angeles with HbSS disease was placed on chronic transfusion therapy in 1996 (at the age of 6 years) because of recurrent acute chest syndrome. Iron chelation with deferoxamine was prescribed 1 year later with poor compliance. In 2002, routine MRI screening of liver and cardiac iron was initiated; pancreas R2* screening was added in 2005. The patient was converted to oral chelation with the advent of deferasirox in 2006. Figure 15-4A summarizes the course of his liver iron concentration (LIC, blue curve), cardiac R2* (green curve), and pancreas R2* (red curve). Despite his poor compliance and high liver iron (averaging 40 mg/g, nearly 40 times normal), his pancreas and heart remained free from iron for almost a decade. In 2011, high pancreas iron was abruptly detected (red squares) followed by abnormal cardiac iron in 2012 (green triangles).

Some insights into the timing of the pancreatic and cardiac iron deposition can be inferred from Figure 15-4B, which plots the reticulocyte counts over the same time intervals. The reticulocyte counts were consistently >10% for the first 10 years. In 2011, the average reticulocyte count decreased to 7% to 8% for approximately 4 to 5 years, corresponding with the period of pancreatic and cardiac iron loading. The reason for this decrease is unclear but could represent iron toxicity in the bone marrow itself. Blood transfusion intensity was unchanged throughout the observation interval. Because transferrin saturation and circulating free iron represent the balance between transfusion intensity and effective iron utilization by the bone marrow, it is not surprising that impaired reticulocytosis could reflect cardiac iron risk.

After diagnosis, the patient was placed on compassionate-use deferiprone and later converted to deferasirox when it was approved in 2015. The patient was much better able to tolerate oral medications, compared with subcutaneous deferoxamine, and his organ iron indices all dramatically improved. Interestingly, his reticulocyte count rebounded after his iron overload was corrected, consistent with iron poisoning of the bone marrow as the inciting stimulus for extrahepatic iron deposition.

Case Study: Continued

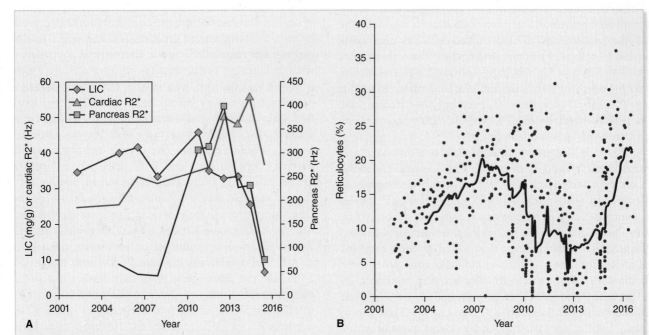

FIGURE 15-4 A. Plot of liver iron concentration (LIC) in milligrams per gram (blue curve), pancreas R2* in hertz (red curve), and cardiac R2* (green curve) in hertz versus date of magnetic resonance imaging examination in the case study. Discrete symbols are used when the value is above the normal range. **B.** Plot of pretransfusion reticulocyte count as a function of exam date over the same study interval. Individual values are displayed as dots, whereas the solid line represents a running average.

High-Yield Facts

- Sickle cell cardiomyopathy is characterized by LV dilation, eccentric hypertrophy, diffuse cardiac fibrosis, normal to increased systolic function, diastolic dysfunction, ventricular arrhythmias, and sudden death.

- Extracardiac complications associated with sickle cell cardiomyopathy include pulmonary hypertension, endothelial dysfunction, systemic hypertension, renal disease, leg ulcers, and stroke.

- Both cardiac and extracardiac complications reflect diffuse, small-vessel disease resulting from vascular endothelial stress caused by chronic hypoxia, abnormal mechanical forces, vascular inflammation, and heme-mediated oxidative damage.

- ATS guidelines call for routine surveillance echocardiography and/or NT-proBNP assessment, although this point remains controversial.[140] Increased TRV is a powerful predictor of mortality in adults because it reflects both left heart disease (fibrosis and diastolic dysfunction) and pulmonary arterial hypertension.

- No guidelines exist for screening ECG, ambulatory arrhythmia monitoring, ambulatory blood pressure monitoring, or cardiac MRI assessment of extracellular fibrosis; however, each of these tests offers actionable information to guide therapy.

- SCD patients are at risk for sudden cardiac death. Prolonged QTc has been associated with sudden cardiac death in SCD. Because pain medications and electrolyte disturbances may affect the QTc, serial ECGs and telemetry monitoring may be considered during acute events and routine monitoring of adults with SCD.

- Diastolic dysfunction contributes to increased pulmonary artery pressures and is an independent predictor of mortality.

- The impact of hydroxyurea, chronic transfusion therapy, and glutamine supplementation on sickle cardiomyopathy is currently unknown.

- Small-vessel disease in the lung (pulmonary hypertension), heart (sickle cardiomyopathy), brain (silent stroke), and kidney (renal disease) are all correlated with one another. Monitoring vascular dysfunction in the cardiopulmonary system can be performed noninvasively by echocardiogram and TRV, akin to abnormal transcranial Doppler velocity for brain vasculopathy.

High-Yield Facts (Cont.)

◆ Large- and small-vessel endothelial dysfunction are extremely common in SCD patients; contribute to renal disease, cardiomyopathy, pulmonary hypertension, and silent stroke; and correlate with cell-free hemoglobin concentration and anemia severity.

◆ Noninvasive monitoring by cardiac MRI and ECV quantification can help detect focal and diffuse fibrosis and quantitate cardiac chamber volumes and function.

◆ Chronic, nontransfused anemia may be associated with nonspecific elastin defects, increasing probability of mitral valve insufficiency. Mitral valve repair and replacement surgeries can be performed safely in SCD patients with appropriate preoperative management.

◆ Iron cardiomyopathy is rare in SCD and not the cause of the sickle cardiomyopathy. Iron cardiomyopathy only occurs in SCD patients with chronic transfusion exposure of at least a decade.

◆ MRI can be used to measure cardiac, pancreatic, and liver iron loading in SCD patients.

◆ Treatment of iron overload and heart failure is similar in sickle cell and thalassemia patients.

References

1. Meloni A, Detterich J, Berdoukas V, et al. Comparison of biventricular dimensions and function between pediatric sickle-cell disease and thalassemia major patients without cardiac iron. *Am J Hematol*. 2013;88:213-218.

2. Schafer M, Kheyfets VO, Schroeder JD, et al. Main pulmonary arterial wall shear stress correlates with invasive hemodynamics and stiffness in pulmonary hypertension. *Pulm Circ*. 2016;6:37-45.

3. Linguraru MG, Pura JA, Gladwin MT, et al. Computed tomography correlates with cardiopulmonary hemodynamics in pulmonary hypertension in adults with sickle cell disease. *Pulm Circ*. 2014;4:319-329.

4. Liu SQ. Alterations in structure of elastic laminae of rat pulmonary arteries in hypoxic hypertension. *J Appl Physiol (1985)*. 1996;81:2147-2155.

5. Ben Driss A, Devaux C, Henrion D, et al. Hemodynamic stresses induce endothelial dysfunction and remodeling of pulmonary artery in experimental compensated heart failure. *Circulation*. 2000;101:2764-2770.

6. Song S, Yamamura A, Yamamura H, et al. Flow shear stress enhances intracellular Ca2+ signaling in pulmonary artery smooth muscle cells from patients with pulmonary arterial hypertension. *Am J Physiol Cell Physiol*. 2014;307:C373-C383.

7. Tordjman R, Delaire S, Plouet J, et al. Erythroblasts are a source of angiogenic factors. *Blood*. 2001;97:1968-1974.

8. George A, Pushkaran S, Konstantinidis DG, et al. Erythrocyte NADPH oxidase activity modulated by Rac GTPases, PKC, and plasma cytokines contributes to oxidative stress in sickle cell disease. *Blood*. 2013;121:2099-2107.

9. Wang X, Mendelsohn L, Rogers H, et al. Heme-bound iron activates placenta growth factor in erythroid cells via erythroid Kruppel-like factor. *Blood*. 2014;124:946-954.

10. Kapetanaki MG, Gbotosho OT, Sharma D, Weidert F, Ofori-Acquah SF, Kato GJ. Free heme regulates placenta growth factor through NRF2-antioxidant response signaling. *Free Radic Biol Med*. 2019;143:300-308.

11. Redha NA, Mahdi N, Al-Habboubi HH, Almawi WY. Impact of VEGFA -583C > T polymorphism on serum VEGF levels and the susceptibility to acute chest syndrome in pediatric patients with sickle cell disease. *Pediatr Blood Cancer*. 2014;61:2310-2312.

12. Sundaram N, Tailor A, Mendelsohn L, et al. High levels of placenta growth factor in sickle cell disease promote pulmonary hypertension. *Blood*. 2010;116:109-112.

13. Patel N, Gonsalves CS, Yang M, Malik P, Kalra VK. Placenta growth factor induces 5-lipoxygenase-activating protein to increase leukotriene formation in sickle cell disease. *Blood*. 2009;113: 1129-1138.

14. Tsao PN, Su YN, Li H, et al. Overexpression of placenta growth factor contributes to the pathogenesis of pulmonary emphysema. *Am J Respir Crit Care Med*. 2004;169:505-511.

15. Eiymo Mwa Mpollo MS, Brandt EB, Shanmukhappa SK, et al. Placenta growth factor augments airway hyperresponsiveness via leukotrienes and IL-13. *J Clin Invest*. 2016;126:571-584.

16. Selvaraj SK, Giri RK, Perelman N, Johnson C, Malik P, Kalra VK. Mechanism of monocyte activation and expression of proinflammatory chemokines by placenta growth factor. *Blood*. 2003;102:1515-1524.

17. Oura H, Bertoncini J, Velasco P, Brown LF, Carmeliet P, Detmar M. A critical role of placental growth factor in the induction of inflammation and edema formation. *Blood*. 2003;101:560-567.

18. Patel N, Sundaram N, Yang M, Madigan C, Kalra VK, Malik P. Placenta growth factor (PlGF), a novel inducer of plasminogen activator inhibitor-1 (PAI-1) in sickle cell disease (SCD). *J Biol Chem*. 2010;285:16713-16722.

19. Ma C, Wang Y, Shen T, et al. Placenta growth factor mediates angiogenesis in hypoxic pulmonary hypertension. *Prostaglandins Leukot Essent Fatty Acids*. 2013;89:159-168.

20. Ahmed A, Dunk C, Ahmad S, Khaliq A. Regulation of placental vascular endothelial growth factor (VEGF) and placenta growth factor (PlGF) and soluble Flt-1 by oxygen: a review. *Placenta*. 2000;21(suppl A):S16-S24.

21. Carmeliet P, Moons L, Luttun A, et al. Synergism between vascular endothelial growth factor and placental growth factor

contributes to angiogenesis and plasma extravasation in pathological conditions. *Nat Med.* 2001;7:575-583.

22. Green CJ, Lichtlen P, Huynh NT, et al. Placenta growth factor gene expression is induced by hypoxia in fibroblasts: a central role for metal transcription factor-1. *Cancer Res.* 2001;61:2696-2703.

23. Perelman N, Selvaraj SK, Batra S, et al. Placenta growth factor activates monocytes and correlates with sickle cell disease severity. *Blood.* 2003;102:1506-1514.

24. Kalra VK, Zhang S, Malik P, Tahara SM. Placenta growth factor mediated gene regulation in sickle cell disease. *Blood Rev.* 2018;32:61-70.

25. de Lima-Filho NN, Figueiredo MS, Vicari P, et al. Exercise-induced abnormal increase of systolic pulmonary artery pressure in adult patients with sickle cell anemia: an exercise stress echocardiography study. *Echocardiography.* 2016;33:1880-1890.

26. Chacko P, Kraut EH, Zweier J, Hitchcock C, Raman SV. Myocardial infarction in sickle cell disease: use of translational imaging to diagnose an under-recognized problem. *J Cardiovasc Transl Res.* 2013;6:752-761.

27. Martin CR, Johnson CS, Cobb C, Tatter D, Haywood LJ. Myocardial infarction in sickle cell disease. *J Natl Med Assoc.* 1996;88:428-432.

28. Wood JC. The heart in sickle cell disease, a model for heart failure with preserved ejection fraction. *Proc Natl Acad Sci U S A.* 2016;113:9670-9672.

29. Bakeer N, James J, Roy S, et al. Sickle cell anemia mice develop a unique cardiomyopathy with restrictive physiology. *Proc Natl Acad Sci U S A.* 2016;113:E5182-E5191.

30. Vichinsky EP, Ohene-Frempong K, Thein SL, et al. Transfusion and chelation practices in sickle cell disease: a regional perspective. *Pediatr Hematol Oncol.* 2011;28:124-133.

31. Inati A, Musallam KM, Wood JC, Taher AT. Iron overload indices rise linearly with transfusion rate in patients with sickle cell disease. *Blood.* 2010;115:2980-2981; author reply 2981-2982.

32. Wood JC. Estimating tissue iron burden: current status and future prospects. *Br J Haematol.* 2015;170:15-28.

33. Wood JC, Cohen AR, Pressel SL, et al. Organ iron accumulation in chronically transfused children with sickle cell anaemia: baseline results from the TWiTCH trial. *Br J Haematol.* 2016;172(1):122-130.

34. Crowe S, Bartfay WJ. Amlodipine decreases iron uptake and oxygen free radical production in the heart of chronically iron overloaded mice. *Biol Res Nurs.* 2002;3:189-197.

35. Oudit GY, Sun H, Trivieri MG, et al. L-type Ca(2+) channels provide a major pathway for iron entry into cardiomyocytes in iron-overload cardiomyopathy. *Nat Med.* 2003;9:1187-1194.

36. Eghbali A, Kazemi H, Taherahmadi H, Ghandi Y, Rafiei M, Bagheri B. A randomized, controlled study evaluating effects of amlodipine addition to chelators to reduce iron loading in patients with thalassemia major. *Eur J Haematol.* 2017;99:577-581.

37. Fernandes JL, Loggetto SR, Verissimo MP, et al. A randomized trial of amlodipine in addition to standard chelation therapy in patients with thalassemia major. *Blood.* 2016;128:1555-1561.

38. Liuzzi JP, Aydemir F, Nam H, Knutson MD, Cousins RJ. Zip14 (Slc39a14) mediates non-transferrin-bound iron uptake into cells. *Proc Natl Acad Sci U S A.* 2006;103:13612-13617.

39. Wood JC, Tyszka JM, Ghugre N, Carson S, Nelson MD, Coates TD. Myocardial iron loading in transfusion-dependent thalassemia and sickle-cell disease. *Blood.* 2004;103:1934-1936.

40. Meloni A, Puliyel M, Pepe A, Berdoukas V, Coates TD, Wood JC. Cardiac iron overload in sickle-cell disease. *Am J Hematol.* 2014;89:678-683.

41. Garbowski MW, Evans P, Vlachodimitropoulou E, Hider R, Porter JB. Residual erythropoiesis protects against myocardial hemosiderosis in transfusion-dependent thalassemia by lowering labile plasma iron via transient generation of apotransferrin. *Haematologica.* 2017;102(10):1640-1649.

42. Hamideh D, Alvarez O. Sickle cell disease related mortality in the United States (1999-2009). *Pediatr Blood Cancer.* 2013;60:1482-1486.

43. Damy T, Bodez D, Habibi A, et al. Haematological determinants of cardiac involvement in adults with sickle cell disease. *Eur Heart J.* 2016;37:1158-1167.

44. Menet A, Ranque B, Diop IB, et al. Subclinical cardiac dysfunction is associated with extracardiac organ damages. *Front Med (Lausanne).* 2018;5:323.

45. Gladwin MT. Cardiovascular complications and risk of death in sickle-cell disease. *Lancet.* 2016;387:2565-2574.

46. Maron BJ, Towbin JA, Thiene G, et al. Contemporary definitions and classification of the cardiomyopathies: an American Heart Association Scientific Statement from the Council on Clinical Cardiology, Heart Failure and Transplantation Committee; Quality of Care and Outcomes Research and Functional Genomics and Translational Biology Interdisciplinary Working Groups; and Council on Epidemiology and Prevention. *Circulation.* 2006;113:1807-1816.

47. Elliott P, Andersson B, Arbustini E, et al. Classification of the cardiomyopathies: a position statement from the European Society of Cardiology Working Group on Myocardial and Pericardial Diseases. *Eur Heart J.* 2008;29:270-276.

48. Farmakis D, Triposkiadis F, Lekakis J, Parissis J. Heart failure in haemoglobinopathies: pathophysiology, clinical phenotypes, and management. *Eur J Heart Fail.* 2017;19:479-489.

49. Sachdev V, Hsieh MM, Jeffries N, et al. Reversal of a rheologic cardiomyopathy following hematopoietic stem cell transplantation for sickle cell disease. *Blood Adv.* 2019;3(19):2816-2824.

50. Sachdev V, Machado RF, Shizukuda Y, et al. Diastolic dysfunction is an independent risk factor for death in patients with sickle cell disease. *J Am Coll Cardiol.* 2007;49:472-479.

51. Poludasu S, Ramkissoon K, Salciccioli L, Kamran H, Lazar JM. Left ventricular systolic function in sickle cell anemia: a meta-analysis. *J Card Fail.* 2013;19:333-341.

52. Damy T, Bodez D, Habibi A, et al. Haematological determinants of cardiac involvement in adults with sickle cell disease. *Eur Heart J.* 2016;37:1158-1167.

53. Nguyen KL, Tian X, Alam S, et al. Elevated transpulmonary gradient and cardiac magnetic resonance-derived right ventricular remodeling predict poor outcomes in sickle cell disease. *Haematologica.* 2016;101:e40-e43.

54. Barbosa MM, Vasconcelos MC, Ferrari TC, et al. Assessment of ventricular function in adults with sickle cell disease: role of two-dimensional speckle-tracking strain. *J Am Soc Echocardiogr.* 2014;27:1216-1222.

55. Nagueh SF, Smiseth OA, Appleton CP, et al. Recommendations for the evaluation of left ventricular diastolic function by echocardiography: an update from the American Society of Echocardiography and the European Association of Cardiovascular Imaging. *J Am Soc Echocardiogr.* 2016;29:277-314.

56. Sachdev V, Kato GJ, Gibbs JS, et al. Echocardiographic markers of elevated pulmonary pressure and left ventricular diastolic dysfunction are associated with exercise intolerance in adults and adolescents with homozygous sickle cell anemia in the United States and United Kingdom. *Circulation.* 2011;124:1452-1460.

57. Alsaied T, Niss O, Powell AW, et al. Diastolic dysfunction is associated with exercise impairment in patients with sickle cell anemia. *Pediatr Blood Cancer*. 2018;65:e27113.

58. Niss O, Fleck R, Makue F, et al. Association between diffuse myocardial fibrosis and diastolic dysfunction in sickle cell anemia. *Blood*. 2017;130:205-213.

59. Reddy YNV, Borlaug BA. High-output heart failure in sickle cell anemia. *JACC Cardiovasc Imaging*. 2016;9:1122-1123.

60. Niss O, Quinn CT, Lane A, et al. Cardiomyopathy with restrictive physiology in sickle cell disease. *JACC Cardiovasc Imaging*. 2016;9:243-252.

61. Hammoudi N, Charbonnier M, Levy P, et al. Left atrial volume is not an index of left ventricular diastolic dysfunction in patients with sickle cell anaemia. *Arch Cardiovasc Dis*. 2015;108:156-162.

62. Covitz W, Espeland M, Gallagher D, Hellenbrand W, Leff S, Talner N. The heart in sickle cell anemia. The Cooperative Study of Sickle Cell Disease (CSSCD). *Chest*. 1995;108:1214-1219.

63. Li W, Coates T, Wood JC. Atrial dysfunction as a marker of iron cardiotoxicity in thalassemia major. *Haematologica*. 2008;93:311-312.

64. Nacif MS, Barranhas AD, Turkbey E, et al. Left atrial volume quantification using cardiac MRI in atrial fibrillation: comparison of the Simpson's method with biplane area-length, ellipse, and three-dimensional methods. *Diagn Interv Radiol*. 2013;19:213-220.

65. Ghelani SJ, Brown DW, Kuebler JD, et al. Left atrial volumes and strain in healthy children measured by three-dimensional echocardiography: normal values and maturational changes. *J Am Soc Echocardiogr*. 2018;31:187-193.e1.

66. Hudsmith LE, Cheng AS, Tyler DJ, et al. Assessment of left atrial volumes at 1.5 Tesla and 3 Tesla using FLASH and SSFP cine imaging. *J Cardiovasc Magn Reson*. 2007;9:673-679.

67. Buechel EV, Kaiser T, Jackson C, Schmitz A, Kellenberger CJ. Normal right- and left ventricular volumes and myocardial mass in children measured by steady state free precession cardiovascular magnetic resonance. *J Cardiovasc Magn Reson*. 2009;11:19.

68. Hudsmith LE, Petersen SE, Francis JM, Robson MD, Neubauer S. Normal human left and right ventricular and left atrial dimensions using steady state free precession magnetic resonance imaging. *J Cardiovasc Magn Reson*. 2005;7:775-782.

69. Alfakih K, Plein S, Thiele H, Jones T, Ridgway JP, Sivananthan MU. Normal human left and right ventricular dimensions for MRI as assessed by turbo gradient echo and steady-state free precession imaging sequences. *J Magn Reson Imaging*. 2003;17:323-329.

70. Liem RI, Young LT, Thompson AA. Prolonged QTc interval in children and young adults with sickle cell disease at steady state. *Pediatr Blood Cancer*. 2009;52:842-846.

71. Maisel A, Friedman H, Flint L, Koshy M, Prabhu R. Continuous electrocardiographic monitoring in patients with sickle-cell anemia during pain crisis. *Clin Cardiol*. 1983;6:339-344.

72. Upadhya B, Ntim W, Brandon Stacey R, et al. Prolongation of QTc intervals and risk of death among patients with sickle cell disease. *Eur J Haematol*. 2013;91:170-178.

73. Spach MS, Boineau JP. Microfibrosis produces electrical load variations due to loss of side-to-side cell connections: a major mechanism of structural heart disease arrhythmias. *Pacing Clin Electrophysiol*. 1997;20:397-413.

74. Spach MS, Josephson ME. Initiating reentry: the role of non-uniform anisotropy in small circuits. *J Cardiovasc Electrophysiol*. 1994;5:182-209.

75. De Muro P, Faedda R, Fresu P, et al. Urinary transforming growth factor-beta 1 in various types of nephropathy. *Pharmacol Res*. 2004;49:293-298.

76. Schafer M, Ivy DD, Barker AJ, et al. Characterization of CMR-derived haemodynamic data in children with pulmonary arterial hypertension. *Eur Heart J Cardiovasc Imaging*. 2017;18:424-431.

77. Schafer M, Browning J, Schroeder JD, et al. Vorticity is a marker of diastolic ventricular interdependency in pulmonary hypertension. *Pulm Circ*. 2016;6:46-54.

78. Rajdev A, Garan H, Biviano A. Arrhythmias in pulmonary arterial hypertension. *Prog Cardiovasc Dis*. 2012;55:180-186.

79. Rudski LG, Lai WW, Afilalo J, et al. Guidelines for the echocardiographic assessment of the right heart in adults: a report from the American Society of Echocardiography endorsed by the European Association of Echocardiography, a registered branch of the European Society of Cardiology, and the Canadian Society of Echocardiography. *J Am Soc Echocardiogr*. 2010;23:685-713; quiz 786-788.

80. Gordeuk VR, Sachdev V, Taylor JG, Gladwin MT, Kato G, Castro OL. Relative systemic hypertension in patients with sickle cell disease is associated with risk of pulmonary hypertension and renal insufficiency. *Am J Hematol*. 2008;83:15-18.

81. Parent F, Bachir D, Inamo J, et al. A hemodynamic study of pulmonary hypertension in sickle cell disease. *N Engl J Med*. 2011;365:44-53.

82. Kato GJ, Hsieh M, Machado R, et al. Cerebrovascular disease associated with sickle cell pulmonary hypertension. *Am J Hematol*. 2006;81:503-510.

83. Detterich JA, Kato RM, Rabai M, Meiselman HJ, Coates TD, Wood JC. Chronic transfusion therapy improves but does not normalize systemic and pulmonary vasculopathy in sickle cell disease. *Blood*. 2015;126:703-710.

84. Pennell DJ, Udelson JE, Arai AE, et al. Cardiovascular function and treatment in beta-thalassemia major: a consensus statement from the American Heart Association. *Circulation*. 2013;128:281-308.

85. Pootrakul P, Breuer W, Sametband M, Sirankapracha P, Hershko C, Cabantchik ZI. Labile plasma iron (LPI) as an indicator of chelatable plasma redox activity in iron-overloaded beta-thalassemia/HbE patients treated with an oral chelator. *Blood*. 2004;104:1504-1510.

86. Piga A, Longo F, Duca L, et al. High nontransferrin bound iron levels and heart disease in thalassemia major. *Am J Hematol*. 2009;84:29-33.

87. Wood JC. The use of MRI to monitor iron overload in SCD. *Blood Cells Mol Dis*. 2017;67:120-125.

88. Anderson LJ, Holden S, Davis B, et al. Cardiovascular T2-star (T2*) magnetic resonance for the early diagnosis of myocardial iron overload. *Eur Heart J*. 2001;22:2171-2179.

89. Carpenter JP, He T, Kirk P, et al. On T2* magnetic resonance and cardiac iron. *Circulation*. 2011;123:1519-1528.

90. Kirk P, Roughton M, Porter JB, et al. Cardiac T2* magnetic resonance for prediction of cardiac complications in thalassemia major. *Circulation*. 2009;120:1961-1968.

91. Wagdy R, Suliman H, Bamashmose B, et al. Subclinical myocardial injury during vaso-occlusive crisis in pediatric sickle cell disease. *Eur J Pediatr*. 2018;177:1745-1752.

92. de Montalembert M, Maunoury C, Acar P, Brousse V, Sidi D, Lenoir G. Myocardial ischaemia in children with sickle cell disease. *Arch Dis Child*. 2004;89:359-362.

93. Raman SV, Simonetti OP, Cataland SR, Kraut EH. Myocardial ischemia and right ventricular dysfunction in adult patients with sickle cell disease. *Haematologica*. 2006;91:1329-1335.

94. Niss O, Taylor MD. Applications of cardiac magnetic resonance imaging in sickle cell disease. *Blood Cells Mol Dis*. 2017;67:126-134.

95. Lippman SM, Ginzton LE, Thigpen T, Tanaka KR, Laks MM. Mitral valve prolapse in sickle cell disease. Presumptive evidence for a linked connective tissue disorder. *Arch Intern Med*. 1985;145:435-438.

96. Lippman SM, Abergel RP, Ginzton LE, et al. Mitral valve prolapse in sickle cell disease: manifestation of a generalized connective tissue disorder. *Am J Hematol*. 1985;19:1-12.

97. Husain A, Ladipo GO, Abdul-Mohsen MF, Knox-Macaulay H. Prevalence of mitral valve prolapse in Saudi sickle cell disease patients in Dammam: a prospective-controlled echocardiographic study. *Ann Saudi Med*. 1995;15:244-248.

98. Ahmed S, Siddiqui AK, Sadiq A, Shahid RK, Patel DV, Russo LA. Echocardiographic abnormalities in sickle cell disease. *Am J Hematol*. 2004;76:195-198.

99. Simmons BE, Santhanam V, Castaner A, Rao KR, Sachdev N, Cooper R. Sickle cell heart disease. Two-dimensional echo and Doppler ultrasonographic findings in the hearts of adult patients with sickle cell anemia. *Arch Intern Med*. 1988;148:1526-1528.

100. Page AV, Liles WC. Biomarkers of endothelial activation/dysfunction in infectious diseases. *Virulence*. 2013;4:507-516.

101. Szmitko PE, Wang CH, Weisel RD, de Almeida JR, Anderson TJ, Verma S. New markers of inflammation and endothelial cell activation: part I. *Circulation*. 2003;108:1917-1923.

102. Szmitko PE, Wang CH, Weisel RD, Jeffries GA, Anderson TJ, Verma S. Biomarkers of vascular disease linking inflammation to endothelial activation: part II. *Circulation*. 2003;108:2041-2048.

103. Antwi-Boasiako C, Frimpong E, Gyan B, et al. Elevated proangiogenic markers are associated with vascular complications within Ghanaian sickle cell disease patients. *Med Sci (Basel)*. 2018;6(3):53.

104. Kato GJ, Martyr S, Blackwelder WC, et al. Levels of soluble endothelium-derived adhesion molecules in patients with sickle cell disease are associated with pulmonary hypertension, organ dysfunction, and mortality. *Br J Haematol*. 2005;130:943-953.

105. Antwi-Boasiako C, Ahenkorah J, Donkor ES, et al. Correlation between soluble endothelial adhesion molecules and nitric oxide metabolites in sickle cell disease. *Med Sci (Basel)*. 2018;7:1.

106. van der Land V, Peters M, Biemond BJ, Heijboer H, Harteveld CL, Fijnvandraat K. Markers of endothelial dysfunction differ between subphenotypes in children with sickle cell disease. *Thromb Res*. 2013;132:712-717.

107. Novelli EM, Hildesheim M, Rosano C, et al. Elevated pulse pressure is associated with hemolysis, proteinuria and chronic kidney disease in sickle cell disease. *PLoS One*. 2014;9:e114309.

108. Lamarre Y, Lalanne-Mistrih ML, Romana M, et al. Male gender, increased blood viscosity, body mass index and triglyceride levels are independently associated with systemic relative hypertension in sickle cell anemia. *PLoS One*. 2013;8:e66004.

109. DeBaun MR, Casella JF. Transfusions for silent cerebral infarcts in sickle cell anemia. *N Engl J Med*. 2014;371:1841-1842.

110. Moodalbail DG, Falkner B, Keith SW, et al. Ambulatory hypertension in a pediatric cohort of sickle cell disease. *J Am Soc Hypertens*. 2018;12:542-550.

111. Shatat IF, Jakson SM, Blue AE, Johnson MA, Orak JK, Kalpatthi R. Masked hypertension is prevalent in children with sickle cell disease: a Midwest Pediatric Nephrology Consortium study. *Pediatr Nephrol*. 2013;28:115-120.

112. Friedman D, Szmuszkovicz J, Rabai M, Detterich JA, Menteer J, Wood JC. Systemic endothelial dysfunction in children with idiopathic pulmonary arterial hypertension correlates with disease severity. *J Heart Lung Transplant*. 2012;31:642-647.

113. de Montalembert M, Aggoun Y, Niakate A, Szezepanski I, Bonnet D. Endothelial-dependent vasodilation is impaired in children with sickle cell disease. *Haematologica*. 2007;92:1709-1710.

114. Teixeira RS, Terse-Ramos R, Ferreira TA, et al. Associations between endothelial dysfunction and clinical and laboratory parameters in children and adolescents with sickle cell anemia. *PLoS One*. 2017;12:e0184076.

115. Hadeed K, Hascoet S, Castex MP, Munzer C, Acar P, Dulac Y. Endothelial function and vascular properties in children with sickle cell disease. *Echocardiography*. 2015;32:1285-1290.

116. Belhassen L, Pelle G, Sediame S, et al. Endothelial dysfunction in patients with sickle cell disease is related to selective impairment of shear stress-mediated vasodilation. *Blood*. 2001;97:1584-1589.

117. Aessopos A, Farmakis D, Tsironi M, et al. Endothelial function and arterial stiffness in sickle-thalassemia patients. *Atherosclerosis*. 2007;191(2):427-432.

118. Reiter CD, Wang X, Tanus-Santos JE, et al. Cell-free hemoglobin limits nitric oxide bioavailability in sickle-cell disease. *Nat Med*. 2002;8:1383-1389.

119. Belizna C, Loufrani L, Ghali A, et al. Arterial stiffness and stroke in sickle cell disease. *Stroke*. 2012;43:1129-1130.

120. Tantawy AAG, Adly AAM, Ismail EAR, Abdelazeem M. Clinical predictive value of cystatin C in pediatric sickle cell disease: a marker of disease severity and subclinical cardiovascular dysfunction. *Clin Appl Thromb Hemost*. 2017;23:1010-1017.

121. Kaddah NA, Saied DA, Alwakeel HA, Hashem RH, Rowizak SM, Elmonem MA. Plasma chitotriosidase and carotid intima-media thickness in children with sickle cell disease. *Int J Hematol*. 2017;106:648-654.

122. Almeida AG, Araujo F, Rego F, David C, Lopes MG, Ducla-Soares J. Abnormal myocardial flow reserve in sickle cell disease: a myocardial contrast echocardiography study. *Echocardiography*. 2008;25:591-599.

123. Belcik JT, Davidson BP, Xie A, et al. Augmentation of muscle blood flow by ultrasound cavitation is mediated by ATP and purinergic signaling. *Circulation*. 2017;135:1240-1252.

124. Sachdev V, Sidenko S, Wu MD, et al. Skeletal and myocardial microvascular blood flow in hydroxycarbamide-treated patients with sickle cell disease. *Br J Haematol*. 2017;179:648-656.

125. Wu MD, Belcik JT, Qi Y, et al. Abnormal regulation of microvascular tone in a murine model of sickle cell disease assessed by contrast ultrasound. *J Am Soc Echocardiogr*. 2015;28:1122-1128.

126. Aribisala BS, Morris Z, Eadie E, et al. Blood pressure, internal carotid artery flow parameters, and age-related white matter hyperintensities. *Hypertension*. 2014;63:1011-1018.

127. Webb AJ, Simoni M, Mazzucco S, Kuker W, Schulz U, Rothwell PM. Increased cerebral arterial pulsatility in patients with leukoaraiosis: arterial stiffness enhances transmission of aortic pulsatility. *Stroke*. 2012;43:2631-2636.

128. Rizzoni D, Rizzoni M, Nardin M, et al. Vascular aging and disease of the small vessels. *High Blood Press Cardiovasc Prev*. 2019;26:183-189.

129. Debaun MR, Sarnaik SA, Rodeghier MJ, et al. Associated risk factors for silent cerebral infarcts in sickle cell anemia: low baseline hemoglobin, sex, and relative high systolic blood pressure. *Blood*. 2012;119:3684-3690.

130. Ranque B, Menet A, Boutouyrie P, et al. Arterial stiffness impairment in sickle cell disease associated with chronic vascular complications: the multinational African CADRE study. *Circulation.* 2016;134:923-933.

131. Lemogoum D, Van Bortel L, Najem B, et al. Arterial stiffness and wave reflections in patients with sickle cell disease. *Hypertension.* 2004;44:924-929.

132. Anthi A, Machado RF, Jison ML, et al. Hemodynamic and functional assessment of patients with sickle cell disease and pulmonary hypertension. *Am J Respir Crit Care Med.* 2007;175:1272-1279.

133. Noetzli LJ, Coates TD, Wood JC. Pancreatic iron loading in chronically transfused sickle cell disease is lower than in thalassaemia major. *Br J Haematol.* 2011;152:229-233.

134. Detterich JA, Kato R, Bush A, et al. Sickle cell microvascular paradox-oxygen supply-demand mismatch. *Am J Hematol.* 2019;94:678-688.

135. Winsor T, Burch G. The electrocardiogram and cardiac state in active sickle-cell anemia. *Am Heart J.* 1945;29:685-696.

136. Yawn BP, Buchanan GR, Afenyi-Annan AN, et al. Management of sickle cell disease: summary of the 2014 evidence-based report by expert panel members. *JAMA.* 2014;312(10):1033-1048.

137. Klings ES, Machado RF, Barst RJ, et al. An official American Thoracic Society clinical practice guideline: diagnosis, risk stratification, and management of pulmonary hypertension of sickle cell disease. *Am J Respir Crit Care Med.* 2014;189:727-740.

138. Sebastiani P, Nolan VG, Baldwin CT, et al. A network model to predict the risk of death in sickle cell disease. *Blood.* 2007;110:2727-2735.

139. Du M, Van Ness S, Gordeuk V, et al. Biomarker signatures of sickle cell disease severity. *Blood Cells Mol Dis.* 2018;72:1-9.

140. Yawn BP, Buchanan GR, Afenyi-Annan AN, et al. Management of sickle cell disease: summary of the 2014 evidence-based report by expert panel members. *JAMA.* 2014;312:1033-1048.

141. Niihara Y, Miller ST, Kanter J, et al. A phase 3 trial of l-glutamine in sickle cell disease. *N Engl J Med.* 2018;379:226-235.

142. Belcher JD, Chen C, Nguyen J, et al. Heme triggers TLR4 signaling leading to endothelial cell activation and vaso-occlusion in murine sickle cell disease. *Blood.* 2014;123:377-390.

143. Ghosh S, Adisa OA, Chappa P, et al. Extracellular hemin crisis triggers acute chest syndrome in sickle mice. *J Clin Invest.* 2013;123:4809-4820.

144. Solovey A, Somani A, Belcher JD, et al. A monocyte-TNF-endothelial activation axis in sickle transgenic mice: therapeutic benefit from TNF blockade. *Am J Hematol.* 2017;92:1119-1130.

145. Matte A, Recchiuti A, Federti E, et al. Resolution of sickle cell disease-associated inflammation and tissue damage with 17R-resolvin D1. *Blood.* 2019;133:252-265.

146. Chang J, Patton JT, Sarkar A, Ernst B, Magnani JL, Frenette PS. GMI-1070, a novel pan-selectin antagonist, reverses acute vascular occlusions in sickle cell mice. *Blood.* 2010;116:1779-1786.

147. Telen MJ, Wun T, McCavit TL, et al. Randomized phase 2 study of GMI-1070 in SCD: reduction in time to resolution of vaso-occlusive events and decreased opioid use. *Blood.* 2015;125:2656-2664.

148. Wun T, Styles L, DeCastro L, et al. Phase 1 study of the E-selectin inhibitor GMI 1070 in patients with sickle cell anemia. *PLoS One.* 2014;9:e101301.

149. Coisne C, Faveeuw C, Delplace Y, et al. Differential expression of selectins by mouse brain capillary endothelial cells in vitro in response to distinct inflammatory stimuli. *Neurosci Lett.* 2006;392:216-220.

150. Jasuja R, Suidan G, Hett S, et al. Rivipansel: a small pan-selection antagonist improves cerebral perfusion and inhibits leukocyte adhesion in a murine sickle cell model. *Blood.* 2016;128:270.

151. Martin N, Manoharan K, Thomas J, Davies C, Lumbers RT. Beta-blockers and inhibitors of the renin-angiotensin aldosterone system for chronic heart failure with preserved ejection fraction. *Cochrane Database Syst Rev.* 2018;6:CD012721.

152. Kapelios CJ, Murrow JR, Nuhrenberg TG, Montoro Lopez MN. Effect of mineralocorticoid receptor antagonists on cardiac function in patients with heart failure and preserved ejection fraction: a systematic review and meta-analysis of randomized controlled trials. *Heart Fail Rev.* 2019;24(3):367-377.

153. Ravassa S, Trippel T, Bach D, et al. Biomarker-based phenotyping of myocardial fibrosis identifies patients with heart failure with preserved ejection fraction resistant to the beneficial effects of spironolactone: results from the Aldo-DHF trial. *Eur J Heart Fail.* 2018;20:1290-1299.

154. de Boer RA, De Keulenaer G, Bauersachs J, et al. Towards better definition, quantification and treatment of fibrosis in heart failure. A scientific roadmap by the Committee of Translational Research of the Heart Failure Association (HFA) of the European Society of Cardiology. *Eur J Heart Fail.* 2019;21(3):272-285.

155. Porter JB, Wood J, Olivieri N, et al. Treatment of heart failure in adults with thalassemia major: response in patients randomised to deferoxamine with or without deferiprone. *J Cardiovasc Magn Reson.* 2013;15:38.

156. Anderson LJ, Westwood MA, Holden S, et al. Myocardial iron clearance during reversal of siderotic cardiomyopathy with intravenous desferrioxamine: a prospective study using T2* cardiovascular magnetic resonance. *Br J Haematol.* 2004;127: 348-355.

157. Claster S, Wood JC, Noetzli L, et al. Nutritional deficiencies in iron overloaded patients with hemoglobinopathies. *Am J Hematol.* 2009;84:344-348.

158. De Sanctis V, De Sanctis E, Ricchieri P, Gubellini E, Gilli G, Gamberini MR. Mild subclinical hypothyroidism in thalassaemia major: prevalence, multigated radionuclide test, clinical and laboratory long-term follow-up study. *Pediatr Endocrinol Rev.* 2008;6(suppl 1):174-180.

159. Amsterdam EA, Wenger NK, Brindis RG, et al. 2014 AHA/ACC guideline for the management of patients with non-ST-elevation acute coronary syndromes: a report of the American College of Cardiology/American Heart Association Task Force on Practice Guidelines. *J Am Coll Cardiol.* 2014;64:e139-e228.

160. Ogunbayo GO, Misumida N, Olorunfemi O, et al. Comparison of outcomes in patients having acute myocardial infarction with versus without sickle-cell anemia. *Am J Cardiol.* 2017;120:1768-1771.

161. Vichinsky EP, Neumayr LD, Earles AN, et al. Causes and outcomes of the acute chest syndrome in sickle cell disease. *N Engl J Med.* 2000;342:1855-1865.

162. Mekontso Dessap A, Leon R, Habibi A, et al. Pulmonary hypertension and cor pulmonale during severe acute chest syndrome in sickle cell disease. *Am J Respir Crit Care Med.* 2008;177:646-653.

163. Novelli EM, Gladwin MT. Crises in sickle cell disease. *Chest.* 2016;149:1082-1093.

164. Connor JL Jr, Sclafani JA, Kato GJ, Hsieh MM, Minniti CP. Brief topical sodium nitrite and its impact on the quality of life in patients with sickle leg ulcers. *Medicine (Baltimore).* 2018;97:e12614.

165. Minniti CP, Eckman J, Sebastiani P, Steinberg MH, Ballas SK. Leg ulcers in sickle cell disease. *Am J Hematol.* 2010;85:831-833.

166. Taher AT, Musallam KM, Karimi M, et al. Overview on practices in thalassemia intermedia management aiming for lowering complication rates across a region of endemicity: the OPTIMAL CARE study. *Blood.* 2010;115:1886-1892.

167. Choi S, O'Neil SH, Joshi AA, et al. Anemia predicts lower white matter volume and cognitive performance in sickle and non-sickle cell anemia syndrome. *Am J Hematol.* 2019;94(10):1055-1065.

168. Nguyen VT, Nassar D, Batteux F, Raymond K, Tharaux PL, Aractingi S. Delayed healing of sickle cell ulcers is due to impaired angiogenesis and CXCL12 secretion in skin wounds. *J Invest Dermatol.* 2016;136:497-506.

169. Massenburg BB, Himel HN. Healing of chronic sickle cell disease-associated foot and ankle wounds using transdermal continuous oxygen therapy. *J Wound Care.* 2016;25:S23-S24, S26-S27.

170. Igwegbe I, Onojobi G, Fadojutimi-Akinsiku MO, et al. Case studies evaluating transdermal continuous oxygen for the treatment of chronic sickle cell ulcers. *Adv Skin Wound Care.* 2015;28:206-210.

171. Minniti CP, Gorbach AM, Xu D, et al. Topical sodium nitrite for chronic leg ulcers in patients with sickle cell anaemia: a phase 1 dose-finding safety and tolerability trial. *Lancet Haematol.* 2014;1:e95-e103.

172. Yousafzai SM, Ugurlucan M, Al Radhwan OA, Al Otaibi AL, Canver CC. Open heart surgery in patients with sickle cell hemoglobinopathy. *Circulation.* 2010;121:14-19.

173. Moutaouekkil el M, Najib A, Ajaja R, Arji M, Slaoui A. Heart valve surgery in patients with homozygous sickle cell disease: a management strategy. *Ann Card Anaesth.* 2015;18:361-366.

174. Edwin F, Aniteye E, Tettey M, et al. Hypothermic cardiopulmonary bypass without exchange transfusion in sickle-cell patients: a matched-pair analysis. *Interact Cardiovasc Thorac Surg.* 2014;19:771-776.

175. Koshy M, Weiner SJ, Miller ST, et al. Surgery and anesthesia in sickle cell disease. Cooperative Study of Sickle Cell Diseases. *Blood.* 1995;86:3676-3684.

176. Vichinsky EP, Haberkern CM, Neumayr L, et al. A comparison of conservative and aggressive transfusion regimens in the perioperative management of sickle cell disease. The Preoperative Transfusion in Sickle Cell Disease Study Group. *N Engl J Med.* 1995;333:206-213.

177. Wali YA, al Okbi H, al Abri R. A comparison of two transfusion regimens in the perioperative management of children with sickle cell disease undergoing adenotonsillectomy. *Pediatr Hematol Oncol.* 2003;20:7-13.

178. Adams RJ, McKie VC, Hsu L, et al. Prevention of a first stroke by transfusions in children with sickle cell anemia and abnormal results on transcranial Doppler ultrasonography. *N Engl J Med.* 1998;339:5-11.

179. Abboud MR, Yim E, Musallam KM, Adams RJ, STOP II Study Investigators. Discontinuing prophylactic transfusions increases the risk of silent brain infarction in children with sickle cell disease: data from STOP II. *Blood.* 2011;118:894-898.

180. Steinberg MH, Barton F, Castro O, et al. Effect of hydroxyurea on mortality and morbidity in adult sickle cell anemia: risks and benefits up to 9 years of treatment. *JAMA.* 2003;289:1645-1651.

181. Ware RE, Davis BR, Schultz WH, et al. Hydroxycarbamide versus chronic transfusion for maintenance of transcranial doppler flow velocities in children with sickle cell anaemia—TCD With Transfusions Changing to Hydroxyurea (TWiTCH): a multicentre, open-label, phase 3, non-inferiority trial. *Lancet.* 2016;387:661-670.

182. Niihara Y, Smith WR, Stark CW. A phase 3 trial of l-glutamine in sickle cell disease. *N Engl J Med.* 2018;379:1880.

183. Thrower A, Ciccone EJ, Maitra P, Derebail VK, Cai J, Ataga KI. Effect of renin-angiotensin-aldosterone system blocking agents on progression of glomerulopathy in sickle cell disease. *Br J Haematol.* 2019;184:246-252.

184. Yee ME, Lane PA, Archer DR, Joiner CH, Eckman JR, Guasch A. Losartan therapy decreases albuminuria with stable glomerular filtration and permselectivity in sickle cell anemia. *Blood Cells Mol Dis.* 2018;69:65-70.

185. Quinn CT, Saraf SL, Gordeuk VR, et al. Losartan for the nephropathy of sickle cell anemia: a phase-2, multicenter trial. *Am J Hematol.* 2017;92(9):E520-E528.

186. Taylor C, Kasztan M, Tao B, Pollock JS, Pollock DM. Combined hydroxyurea and ETA receptor blockade reduces renal injury in the humanized sickle cell mouse. *Acta Physiol (Oxf).* 2019;225:e13178.

187. Koehl B, Nivoit P, El Nemer W, et al. The endothelin B receptor plays a crucial role in the adhesion of neutrophils to the endothelium in sickle cell disease. *Haematologica.* 2017;102:1161-1172.

188. Lutz BM, Wu S, Gu X, et al. Endothelin type A receptors mediate pain in a mouse model of sickle cell disease. *Haematologica.* 2018;103:1124-1135.

189. Kalish BT, Matte A, Andolfo I, et al. Dietary omega-3 fatty acids protect against vasculopathy in a transgenic mouse model of sickle cell disease. *Haematologica.* 2015;100:870-880.

190. Daak AA, Elderdery AY, Elbashir LM, et al. Omega 3 (n-3) fatty acids down-regulate nuclear factor-kappa B (NF-kappaB) gene and blood cell adhesion molecule expression in patients with homozygous sickle cell disease. *Blood Cells Mol Dis.* 2015;55:48-55.

191. Daak AA, Dampier CD, Fuh B, et al. Double-blind, randomized, multicenter phase 2 study of SC411 in children with sickle cell disease (SCOT trial). *Blood Adv.* 2018;2:1969-1979.

192. Hoppe C, Jacob E, Styles L, Kuypers F, Larkin S, Vichinsky E. Simvastatin reduces vaso-occlusive pain in sickle cell anaemia: a pilot efficacy trial. *Br J Haematol.* 2017;177:620-629.

193. Gellen B, Messonnier LA, Galacteros F, et al. Moderate-intensity endurance-exercise training in patients with sickle-cell disease without severe chronic complications (EXDRE): an open-label randomised controlled trial. *Lancet Haematol.* 2018;5:e554-e562.

194. Marti-Carvajal A, Abd El Aziz MA, Marti-Amarista C, Sola I. Antiplatelet agents for preventing vaso-occlusive events in people with sickle cell disease: a systematic review. *Clin Adv Hematol Oncol.* 2019;17:234-243.

Sickle Nephropathy

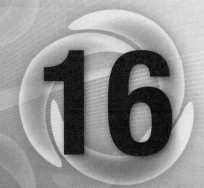

16

Authors: *Santosh L. Saraf, Vimal K. Derebail,*
Victor R. Gordeuk, Jane A. Little

Chapter Outline

Overview

Polymerization of deoxygenated sickle hemoglobin (HbS), resulting in fragile red blood cells (RBCs) and anemia, is the first step in a pathophysiologic cascade that involves the kidney. Damage arises from the cumulative impact of abnormal red cells, hemolysis, and microvascular occlusion. These insults include hyperfiltration in response to anemia, cellular toxicity from plasma and urine cell-free hemoglobin, oxidative stress, inflammation, and potentiation of erythrocyte sickling in the hypoxic and acidotic milieu of the renal medulla. Genetic modifiers of renal disease in sickle cell disease (SCD) include sickle genotype, mutations that modulate HbS polymerization such as α thalassemia and hereditary persistence of fetal hemoglobin (HbF), and haplotypes such as *APOL1* G1 and G2 that increase the risk of kidney disease in the background population.

The effects of kidney disease on the person with SCD include relative hypertension, rapid decrements in glomerular filtration over the life span, depressed erythropoiesis, impaired bone health, altered acid-base homeostasis, and an inability to concentrate urine, which can lead to dehydration. The decreased ability to concentrate urine is present in HbAS trait individuals, in whom it may contribute to an increase in the risk of exercise-related heat stroke. Overall, renal disease is more pronounced in people with homozygous HbSS than HbSC or HbS-β⁺ thalassemia. Most people with SCD living in resource-replete settings, whether homozygous or compound heterozygous, are now surviving into adulthood, and some impairment in kidney function and perturbation in the cardiorenal axis (summarized in Table 16-1)[1-12] is nearly universal with increasing age. Evolution of the clinical phenotype over the life span is affected by recent advances in standard care for SCD. Consideration of these factors is necessary for proper interpretation of historical studies of renal function in SCD.

Pathophysiology of Sickle Cell Nephropathy

In SCD, the unique physiology of the kidney potentiates a vicious cycle of hemoglobin deoxygenation, HbS polymerization, and damage to the exquisitely integrated structures of the kidney. As described later in this chapter, the process is driven by microvascular occlusion with ischemia-reperfusion injury, injurious effects of cell-free hemoglobin and heme, and the chronic stress of hyperfiltration in response to anemia (Figure 16-1). In people with SCD, especially homozygous disease, products of intravascular hemolysis, such as cell-free hemoglobin, arginase, asymmetric dimethylarginine, and adenine nucleotides, together contribute to a widespread vasculopathy of which renal disease is a part.[13] Other manifestations of this vasculopathy include a risk for pulmonary hypertension, leg ulcers, priapism, and stroke.

Cortex/Glomeruli

Histopathologic patterns observed in the glomeruli of SCD patients with kidney disease include glomerular enlargement followed by focal segmental glomerulosclerosis and, uncommonly, immune-mediated membranoproliferative glomerulonephritis or thrombotic microangiopathy due to acute endothelial injury.[14] Other common pathologic features are mesangial proliferation, complement (C3) deposition, and glomerular basement membrane thickening with reduplication.[14-16] In pediatric patients, mesangial hypercellularity is one of the most common findings.[17]

Glomerular hyperfiltration and renal hyperperfusion are common during childhood in SCD, even in infancy.[18,19] While mechanisms driving hyperfiltration are incompletely understood, an underlying "perfusion paradox" has been invoked, wherein hypoperfusion is present in the microcirculatory bed of the renal medulla due to occlusion by erythrocytes containing deoxyhemoglobin polymers while hyperperfusion characterizes

the renal glomeruli.[20] The classic understanding of hyperperfusion is that it is driven by anemia, hypoxic vasodilation with decreased systemic vascular resistance, and, indirectly, renal medullary ischemia. Local vasodilatory substances, including cyclooxygenase-2 (COX-2)-mediated prostaglandins, are released from the ischemic medulla, leading to reduced renal vascular resistance, increased effective renal arterial blood flow, and hyperfiltration.[21] This may result in an excessive sensitivity of glomerular perfusion to nonsteroidal anti-inflammatory drugs (NSAIDs) in people with SCD.[22,23] Although NSAIDs and COX-2 inhibitors may be useful in SCD-mediated pain syndromes,[24,25] these should be used with caution.[26] Recent studies in animal models suggest an additional mechanism that may contribute to hyperfiltration. Increased expression of heme oxygenase-1 (HO-1) in the kidney as a response to oxidative stress and need to process heme leads to increased production of carbon monoxide, which has local vasodilatory properties.[27,28]

Glomerular filtration rate (GFR) is a function of renal plasma flow, the hydraulic pressure gradient across the glomerulus, and the ultrafiltration coefficient, K_f, that reflects glomerular permeability.[29] Renal hyperfiltration in SCD injures the glomerular endothelium, the filtration barrier, and the parietal epithelium of Bowman's capsule. These injuries are thought to produce the characteristic lesion of focal segmental glomerulosclerosis (FSGS) most commonly described in SCD.[14,28,30,31] Early in the life of a patient with homozygous SCD, an increase in renal plasma flow and an increase in glomerular membrane permeability reflected in a high K_f (Table 16-1) result in hyperfiltration but not an increase in capillary hydrostatic pressure. This picture is distinct from the early glomerular hyperperfusion of diabetic nephropathy (from which therapies for SCD-associated renal disease are often adopted), in which hydrostatic pressure does increase. Helal et al[31] posit that, with time, recurrent vaso-occlusion, ischemia, and glomerular dropout cause hyperfiltration at the single-nephron level. This results in histologic glomerulosclerosis, glomerular enlargement, and segmental scarring, which are characteristic of FSGS. Secondary FSGS, seen in SCD, may be more insidious than primary FSGS and may lack its characteristic features, such as full-blown nephrotic syndrome, edema, and hypoalbuminemia. In a cohort of children with SCD, microalbuminuria occurred earlier in those with hyperfiltration, defined as an estimated GFR (eGFR) >180 mL/min/body surface area (BSA) (per serum cystatin C–based formula), than in those without hyperfiltration.[32] Similarly, in SCD adults, the presence of hyperfiltration, defined as a BSA-corrected eGFR >130 mL/min for females and >140 mL/min for males (using the Chronic Kidney Disease Epidemiology Collaboration formula), was associated with a 2.6-fold increased risk for microalbuminuria.[33] In transgenic sickle mice, males demonstrate a rapid onset of hyperfiltration followed by a progressive decline in kidney function over 20 weeks. Females maintain stable kidney function over a similar time period, suggesting a gender-specific protective mechanism from hyperfiltration-mediated nephropathy, at least in mice.[34]

Ongoing hemolysis, vaso-occlusive injury, endothelial dysfunction, and proteinuria contribute to lifelong renal injury.

TABLE 16-1 Cardiorenal physiology: an overview

	Nonanemic controls	Homozygous SCD (HbSS)	Compound heterozygous SCD (HbSC, HbS-β⁺ thalassemia)	P value
Cardiac index	Median, 2.5 L/min/m² (range, 2.3-3.1 L/min/m²), n = 25 adults	Median, 3.7 L/min/m² (range, 3.1-4.3 L/min/m²), n = 656 adults		P <.001, nonanemic vs HbSS[4]
Systemic blood pressure	• NHANES details NA • 144.1 ± 22.9/87.6 ± 13.8 mm Hg (mean, normal creatinine, Jamaica), 30-69 years old, historical controls • UNC (n = 34) details NA	• 110-112/70 mm Hg (median, CSSCD US 1997), 18-24 years old, n = 81 • 114.6 ± 11.0/65.3 ± 5.3 mm Hg (mean, normal creatinine, Jamaica, 1981), 30-69 years old, n = 64 • 122 ± 15/69 ± 10.5 mm Hg (n = 129), UNC	• CSSCD 116 ± 15.5 mm Hg (n = 29 analyzed by UNC) • 131 ± 12 mm Hg (2012)	• P <.05 vs age-, sex-, and race-matched controls from NHANES[5] • P <.01 vs historic controls[6,7] • P = NS vs non-SCD race-matched controls (n = 34)[8]
Pulse pressure		• Median, 45 mm Hg (IQR, 39-55 mm Hg; Ghana 2018), n = 875, SS and SC • Median 50 mm Hg (IQR, 42-59 mm Hg; US), n = 500, HbSS	• Median 48 mm Hg (IQR, 41-55 mm Hg; US), n = 161; HbSC	—[12]
Pulse	Mean ± SD, 75 ± 15 bpm; median age, 24 years; IQR, 14-33 years; n = 943; CADRE, Africa 2016	Mean ± SD, 82 ± 14 bpm; median age, 15 years; IQR, 9-23 years; n = 2456; CADRE, Africa 2016	Mean ± SD, 76 ± 13 bpm; median age, 21 years; IQR, 14-30 years; n = 751; CADRE, Africa 2016	—[1]
Plasma volume	Mean ± SD, 2165 ± 497 mL; mean age ± SD, 25.1 ± 4.3 years, women, n = 19	Mean ± SD, 2714 ± 949 mL; mean age ± SD, 25.1 ± 4.3 years, women, n = 25		P <.005[2]
GFR, measured	Mean ± SD, 120 ± 3 mL/min/BSA; n = 16 young adults	• Mean ± SD, 146 ± 9 mL/min/BSA; n = 14; mean age ± SD, 26.6 ± 1.3 years • Mean ± SD, 112 ± 7 mL/min/BSA; n = 10; median age, 30 years (range, 23-43 years) • Mean ± SD, 97 ± 5 mL/min/BSA; n = 7; median age, 27 years (range, 23-60 years), with albuminuria		P <.01, nonanemic vs HbSS[3]

(continued)

TABLE 16-1 Cardiorenal physiology: an overview (Continued)

	Nonanemic controls	Homozygous SCD (HbSS)	Compound heterozygous SCD (HbSC, HbS-β⁺ thalassemia)	P value
Renal plasma flow	Mean ± SD, 709 ± 38 mL/min/ BSA; n = 16; mean age ± SD, 25.4 ± 1.0 years	• Mean ± SD, 1052 ± 69 mL/min/BSA; n = 14; mean age ± SD, 26.6 ± 1.3 years; mean GFR ± SD, 146 ± 9 mL/min/BSA • Mean ± SD, 734 ± 75 mL/min/BSA; n = 10; median age, 30 years (range, 23-43 years); mean GFR ± SD, 112 ± 7 mL/min/BSA • Mean ± SD, 618 ± 55 mL/min/BSA; n = 7; median age, 27 years (range, 23-60 years); mean GFR ± SD, 97 ± 5 mL/min/BSA		P <.001, nonanemic vs HbSS[3,9]
Ultrafiltration coefficient (K$_f$), measured	Mean ± SD, 25.1 ± 2.6 mL/ min/BSA; n = 16; mean age ± SD, 25.4 ± 1.0 years	• Mean ± SD, 41.3 ± 3.6 mL/min/BSA; n = 14; mean age ± SD, 26.6 ± 1.3 years; mean eGFR ± SD, 146 ± 9 mL/min/BSA • Mean ± SD, 25 ± 3 mL/min/BSA; n = 10; median age, 30 years (range, 23-43 years); mean eGFR ± SD, 112 ± 7 mL/min/BSA • Mean ± SD, 16 ± 3 mL/min/BSA; n = 7; median age, 27 years (range, 23-60 years); mean eGFR ± SD, 97 ± 5 mL/min/BSA		P <.001, nonanemic vs HbSS[3,9]
Creatinine		• Mean ± SD, 0.60 ± 0.2 mg/dL; n = 37; age, 21-30 years • Mean ± SD, 1.3 ± 1.6 mg/dL; n = 39; age >40 years		P <.011, younger vs older[10]
Tubular function				
Serum bicarbonate	Mean ± SD, 24.8 ± 2.9 mEq/dL; n = 4940 adults	Mean ± SD, 23.8 ± 3.4 mEq/dL; n = 367 adults	Mean ± SD, 24.8 ± 3.4 mEq/dL; n = 124 adults	P = .004, HbSS vs HbSC[11]

Abbreviations: BSA, body surface area; CSSCD, Cooperative Study of Sickle Cell Disease; eGFR, estimated glomerular filtration rate; GFR, glomerular filtration rate; IQR, interquartile range; NA, not available; NHANES, National Health and Nutrition Examination Survey; NS, not significant; SCD, sickle cell disease; SD, standard deviation; UNC, University of North Carolina; US, United States.

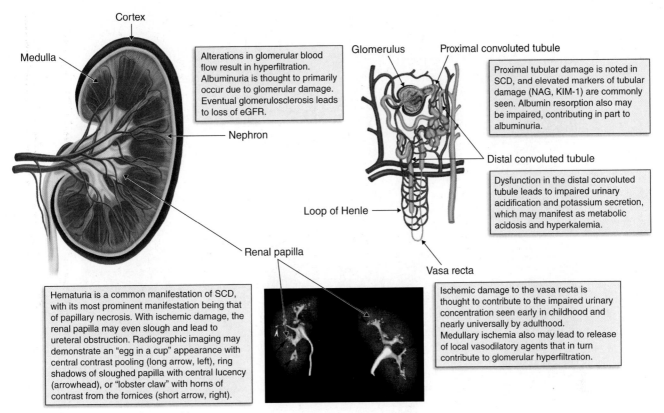

Cortex

Medulla

Alterations in glomerular blood flow result in hyperfiltration. Albuminuria is thought to primarily occur due to glomerular damage. Eventual glomerulosclerosis leads to loss of eGFR.

Nephron

Glomerulus

Proximal convoluted tubule

Proximal tubular damage is noted in SCD, and elevated markers of tubular damage (NAG, KIM-1) are commonly seen. Albumin resorption also may be impaired, contributing in part to albuminuria.

Distal convoluted tubule

Dysfunction in the distal convoluted tubule leads to impaired urinary acidification and potassium secretion, which may manifest as metabolic acidosis and hyperkalemia.

Loop of Henle

Renal papilla

Vasa recta

Hematuria is a common manifestation of SCD, with its most prominent manifestation being that of papillary necrosis. With ischemic damage, the renal papilla may even slough and lead to ureteral obstruction. Radiographic imaging may demonstrate an "egg in a cup" appearance with central contrast pooling (long arrow, left), ring shadows of sloughed papilla with central lucency (arrowhead), or "lobster claw" with horns of contrast from the fornices (short arrow, right).

Ischemic damage to the vasa recta is thought to contribute to the impaired urinary concentration seen early in childhood and nearly universally by adulthood. Medullary ischemia also may lead to release of local vasodilatory agents that in turn contribute to glomerular hyperfiltration.

FIGURE 16-1 Pathology seen in the kidney related to sickle cell disease (SCD). SCD can lead to numerous manifestations in the kidney. The pathology seen in sickle cell-related kidney disease and the various portions of the kidney that may be involved are described above. eGFR, estimated glomerular filtration rate. Radiographic image reproduced from Singanamala S, Krishnamoorthy S, Perazella MA, Dahl NK. Recurrent flank pain from "lobster claw." *NDT Plus.* 2011;4(4):274-275.

Free hemoglobin, arising from intravascular hemolysis (especially in homozygous SCD), is filtered through the glomerulus and is directly toxic to renal tubular epithelial cells.[35] Cell-free hemoglobin may lead to kidney disease by inducing direct oxidative damage and upregulating inflammatory and immune response pathways or by leading to vasculopathy through nitric oxide (NO) depletion.[36,37] A recent study found that hemoglobin competes for reabsorption with filtered albumin by binding to megalin and cubilin in the proximal tubule. Albumin reabsorption can be impaired, leading to tubular proteinuria independent of glomerular damage.[38,39] Kidney biopsy specimens of individuals with SCD demonstrate hemosiderin deposition in glomerular and tubular epithelial cells.[40] Magnetic resonance imaging of the kidney shows increased iron deposition in the cortical regions, which correlates with hemolysis rather than with transfusion burden. This imaging finding suggests that cell-free hemoglobin is being filtered and taken up by the glomeruli and tubules.[41-43] Clinical studies demonstrate an association between markers of hemolysis and albuminuria,[44,45] and between hemoglobinuria and progressive chronic kidney disease (CKD).[46] Free hemoglobin scavenges the endothelial vasodilator NO and contributes to microvascular endothelial dysfunction. Indirect evidence of endothelial dysfunction is noted in multiple studies. Soluble fms-like tyrosine kinase 1 (sFLT-1), a splice variant of vascular endothelial growth factor (VEGF) receptor 1 (VEGFR1), binds circulating VEGF,

prevents its interaction with endothelial cells, and induces endothelial dysfunction. sFLT-1 plays a role in glomerular endothelial damage in preeclampsia and may also do so in SCD. A study of 73 people with SCD demonstrated an association between sFLT-1 and worsening albuminuria.[47] Endothelin-1 (ET-1), a potent vasoconstricting peptide, is produced by endothelial cells in response to various insults including sheer stress, hypoxia, and inflammatory signals. ET-1 mediates endothelial dysfunction by reducing NO bioavailability and by direct injury to podocytes via the endothelin A (ETA) receptor.[48,49] In sickle cell mouse models, ET-1 mediates glomerular injury via reactive oxygen species, and ETA receptor antagonism appears to afford renal protection, as discussed later.[50]

Medulla/Tubules

The renal medulla has an especially low oxygen tension and a low pH, which facilitate hemoglobin deoxygenation, and hyperosmolarity, which lead to dehydration of the RBCs and increased intracellular HbS concentration. These features cumulatively promote HbS polymerization. Repetitive episodes of vaso-occlusion by HbS-containing erythrocytes and associated ischemic injury and microinfarction can destroy the delicate vasculature of the renal medulla (Figure 16-2),[51] resulting in some of the canonical features of SCD-related kidney disease, including impaired urinary concentrating

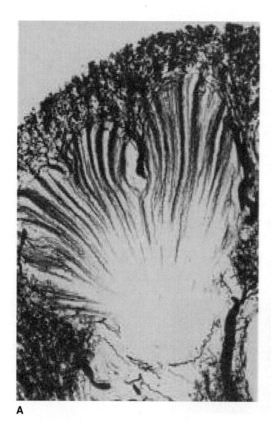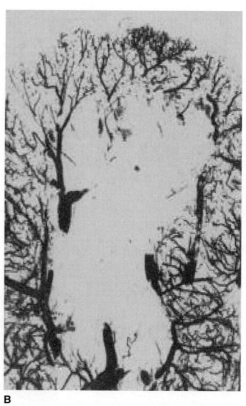

A　　　　　　　　　　　　　　　**B**

FIGURE 16-2 **Renal medullary vasculature in sickle cell disease.** Shown are postmortem microradioangiographic studies of the kidney in people with normal HbA (**A**) and homozygous HbSS (**B**). Note the virtual absence of normal vasa recta in the HbSS kidney.[51]

ability (hyposthenuria), hematuria, and, indirectly, prostacyclin-mediated hyperfiltration.[18,52] In murine models of ischemic renal injury, transgenic sickle mice demonstrate substantially greater renal injury than wild-type mice and even show injury in the kidney contralateral to the induced ischemic insult.[53]

Genetic Predictors of SCD-Related Kidney Disease

Although SCD is considered a monogenetic disorder, the clinical phenotype varies substantially among SCD patients. A number of genetic modifiers may affect the risk of developing sickle cell nephropathy. These include mutations that modulate (1) general SCD severity (eg, coinheritance of α thalassemia), (2) CKD risk in the general population (eg, *APOL1* G1 and G2 CKD risk variants), (3) cell-free hemoglobin processing (*HMOX1* encoding heme oxygenase 1), (4) clearance of inflammatory chemokines (*Fy*), or (5) the transforming growth factor/bone morphogenetic protein inflammatory response pathway (*BMPR1B*) (Table 16-2).

α Thalassemia

Coinheritance of α thalassemia carrier (αα/α–) or trait (α–/α–) is observed in approximately a third of SCD patients and is associated with lower mean corpuscular hemoglobin concentration, less hemolysis, and a higher hemoglobin concentration.[54] In a cohort of HbSS adults from the United States, α thalassemia was observed in 41% of patients and associated with a lower prevalence of macroalbuminuria (13% vs 40% in those without

α thalassemia).[55] The protective effect of α thalassemia from albuminuria has been observed in HbSS cohorts from France, the United Kingdom, and Cameroon.[44,56,57] The association between protection from albuminuria and coinheritance of α thalassemia is not as clear in HbSC patients.[44] An association between coinheritance of α thalassemia and higher eGFR has been observed in one HbSS cohort[58] but not another.[56] α Thalassemia increases the risk of vaso-occlusive events, while decreasing the severity of hemolytic anemia, suggesting that it increases viscosity-related vaso-occlusion.[13] These associations suggest that a dominant mechanism of sickle cell nephropathy may relate to hemolysis and anemia.

APOL1 G1 and G2 Kidney Risk Variants

The *APOL1* G1 (S342G and I384M) and G2 (N388 and T389 deletion) variants are the strongest genetic risk factors of CKD in the general African American population.[59] Similar to the HbS mutation, which in the heterozygote form protects against mortality from malaria, the *APOL1* G1 and G2 variants confer protection from *Trypanosoma brucei rhodesiense* infection by restoring the susceptibility of the parasite to the trypanosome lytic factor.[60,61] The trypanosome lytic factor is a high-density lipoprotein molecule that is composed of APOL1, APOA1, and haptoglobin-related protein. The trypanosome lytic factor is taken up by the trypanosome by a receptor that binds to the hemoglobin-haptoglobin–related protein complex, leading to APOL1 trafficking to the lysosome, activation of an anion

TABLE 16-2 Replicated gene variants implicated in sickle cell nephropathy

Gene	Variants	Gene function	Association with kidney disease phenotype	References
HBA1	α-3.7K deletion α-4.2K deletion	Hemoglobin subunit alpha 1—produces the α-chain component of hemoglobin	α-Globin deletion: reduced albuminuria, higher eGFR, lower risk for CKD progression	55-58
APOL1	G1 (S342G and I384M) G2 (N388 and Y389 deletion)	Apolipoprotein L1—integral component of the trypanosome lytic factor complex	Homozygous or compound heterozygous inheritance of G1 and G2: increased risk for urine dipstick–defined proteinuria, increased albuminuria, lower eGFR, increased CKD stage, CKD progression, ESRD risk	64, 65, 67
HMOX1	1. Promoter GT repeat 2. rs743811	Heme oxygenase-1—rate-limiting, inducible enzyme that metabolizes heme to biliverdin, carbon monoxide, and iron	1. Long GT-tandem repeats (>25): reduced eGFR at baseline and increased risk for AKI 2. rs743811: lower eGFR, greater albuminuria, increased CKD stage, and ESRD risk	56, 64, 72
Fy	rs2814778	Duffy blood group/atypical chemokine receptor 1—Duffy blood group antigen that is the receptor for Plasmodium vivax and serves as a chemokine-scavenging receptor	Fy genotype: increased risk for urine dipstick–defined proteinuria and albuminuria	66, 74

Abbreviations: AKI, acute kidney injury; CKD, chronic kidney disease; eGFR, estimated glomerular filtration rate; ESRD, end-stage renal disease.

channel, and swelling that kills the trypanosome. *T b rhodesiense* evolved to develop a serum-associated resistance (SRA) protein that inhibits APOL1 function. The *APOL1* G1 and G2 mutations prevent binding of SRA, thereby restoring immunity against *T b rhodesiense* in individuals who carry these mutations. Homozygous or compound heterozygous inheritance of the *APOL1* G1/G2 risk variants is observed in approximately 10% to 15% of African Americans and accounts for up to 70% of the CKD risk in nondiabetic African Americans.[59,60,62,63] There is a very high overlap between the distribution of the HbS mutation and the *APOL1* G1 and G2 mutations (Figure 16-3).

Coinheritance of the *APOL1* G1/G2 kidney risk variants has been observed in 7% to 16% of SCD cohorts from the United States, United Kingdom, and Cameroon.[56,64-67] SCD patients who have coinherited the *APOL1* G1/G2 kidney risk variants have an increased risk for hemoglobinuria, albuminuria, and a lower eGFR. In cross-sectional analyses, SCD patients with the *APOL1* G1/G2 kidney risk variants are at a 7- to 30-fold greater risk for end-stage renal disease (ESRD).[64,65] On longitudinal follow-up, the *APOL1* G1/G2 risk variants are associated with a 7-fold higher risk for CKD progression, defined as a 50% decline in eGFR or as requiring renal replacement therapy.[58] How the *APOL1* G1/G2 kidney risk variants lead to kidney disease is not understood. APOL1 binds to haptoglobin-related protein and APOA1 to form the trypanosome lytic factor, a complex that is capable of scavenging cell-free hemoglobin.[68,69] The *APOL1* G1 and G2 variants have been associated with

hemoglobinuria in 2 independent SCD cohorts, and their role in cell-free hemoglobin processing needs further investigation.[64]

Heme Oxygenase 1

HMOX1 is the inducible enzyme responsible for degrading heme to biliverdin, carbon monoxide, and iron. Increased HMOX1 staining has been detected in the renal tubules of a biopsy specimen from a patient with SCD.[27] Gene expression of *HMOX1* is increased in the kidney cortex of HbSS versus HbAA mice.[70] The *HMOX1* rs743811 variant minor allele frequency (MAF 0.14) was associated with lower eGFR, higher urine albumin concentration, progressively worsening CKD, and ESRD in a combined analysis of SCD patients from the United States and United Kingdom.[64] This variant had a borderline association with microalbuminuria and macroalbuminuria in a cohort of SCD patients from Cameroon.[56] Longer GT-tandem repeats in the promoter region of *HMOX1* are associated with reduced *HMOX1* expression in tissue culture cells exposed to hydrogen peroxide.[71] Long GT-tandem repeats (>25) were associated with lower baseline eGFR and a higher risk of acute kidney injury during hospitalizations for vasoocclusive crisis in one SCD cohort,[64,72] although no association with kidney function was observed in a separate cohort.[56] Long GT-tandem repeats of *HMOX1* may be a risk factor for incident episodes of acute chest syndrome, based on findings from a cohort of children with SCD.[73] These observations are

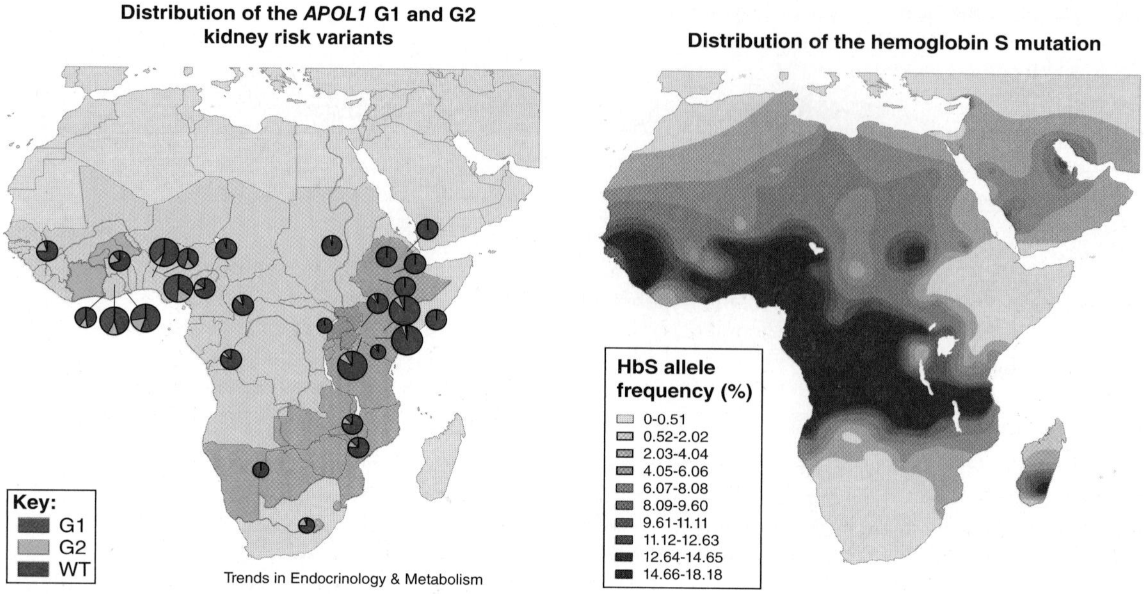

Distribution of the *APOL1* G1 and G2 kidney risk variants

Distribution of the hemoglobin S mutation

HbS allele frequency (%)
- 0–0.51
- 0.52–2.02
- 2.03–4.04
- 4.05–6.06
- 6.07–8.08
- 8.09–9.60
- 9.61–11.11
- 11.12–12.63
- 12.64–14.65
- 14.66–18.18

Key:
- G1
- G2
- WT

Trends in Endocrinology & Metabolism

FIGURE 16-3 Overlapping geographic distributions of the *APOL1* G1 and G2 kidney risk variants with the Hemoglobin S mutation. WT, wild-type. Reprinted by permission of Springer Nature. Piel FB et al. Global distribution of the sickle cell gene and geographical confirmation of the malaria hypothesis. *Nat Commun.* 2010;1:104. Copyright 2010.

consistent with reduced heme metabolism by *HMOX1* in SCD patients with long GT-tandem repeats, leading to increased susceptibility to heme-mediated toxicity in the kidney and vasculature.

Fy

The *FY* rs2814778 polymorphism in the promoter region decreases GATA binding, which is necessary for gene transcription and Duffy antigen expression in RBCs.[74] The Duffy antigen serves as a chemokine sink that may reduce systemic chemokine levels and prevent white blood cell activation. In HbSS adults and children, lack of Duffy antigen expression on RBCs has been associated with a lower white blood cell count and with an increased risk for proteinuria or albuminuria.[66,74] The association of Duffy antigen expression with lower white blood cell counts was reported in SCD patients from Egypt, although no association with kidney dysfunction was observed in this cohort.[75]

Other Genetic Variants

Several other gene variants may be implicated in kidney disease risk in SCD patients. One study focused on variants in the tumor growth factor-β (TGF-β)/bone morphogenetic protein (BMP) pathway, based on its potential role in diabetic nephropathy.[76] In this study of SCD patients from the Cooperative Study of Sickle Cell Disease (CSSCD), an association between variants in the BMP receptor 1B (*BMPR1B*) and eGFR was identified. These variants were tested in another SCD cohort, and although the association of these specific variants with kidney function was not replicated, another *BMPR1B* variant was identified that was associated with eGFR.[67] Mutations in *BMPR1B* have also been implicated in pulmonary arterial hypertension, another hemolysis-related complication of SCD, suggesting overlapping features.[77,78]

Variants in the gene encoding myosin heavy chain 9 (*MYH9*) were initially believed to be associated with CKD risk in African Americans.[79,80] *MYH9* co-segregates with *APOL1*, and most studies have demonstrated that the *APOL1* G1 and G2 risk variants are more strongly associated with CKD risk compared to the *MYH9* variants.[60,81] An autosomal dominant mutation in *MYH9* leads to a genetic disorder characterized by macrothrombocytopenia, cataracts, deafness, and FSGS.[82] In a cohort of SCD patients, *MYH9* rs5750248 and rs11912763, which represent the S-1 and F-1 risk haplotypes that have been linked to kidney disease in the general African American and Hispanic populations,[83] were associated with proteinuria,[67] but this association has not been replicated in other SCD cohorts.[64]

Other potential candidate gene variants have been identified in a cohort of HbSS children.[66] In this cohort, polycystin 1 like 2 (*PKD1L2*) rs76056952, angiogenic factor with G-patch and FHA domains (*AGGF1*) rs72765108, torsin family 2 member A (*TOR2A*) rs114990094, cubulin (*CUBN*) rs111265129, cytochrome P450 family 4 subfamily B member 1 (*CYP4B1*) rs12094024, and *CD163* rs61729510 were associated with measured and estimated GFR. The association of these variants with kidney function should be tested in other SCD cohorts.

Clinical Classification and Definitions

Classification of Kidney Disease

In the general population, creatinine-based estimates of glomerular filtration and albuminuria are used to predict risk of progression of renal disease, of cardiovascular disease, and of all-cause mortality. Detectable proteinuria (1+ or 2+ dipstick-positive proteinuria) and an eGFR <60 mL/min/BSA predict longitudinal risk for progression to ESRD in the general population over decades,[84] with a hazard ratio of 41 for patients with both 2+ proteinuria and a decreased eGFR. Based on these findings, renal damage in the general population has been categorized into 6 stages of eGFR (G classification) and 3 stages of albuminuria (A classification) to better predict risk for adverse renal and cardiovascular outcomes as well as all-cause mortality.[85] In contrast to the general population, SCD is associated with renal injury from infancy and with a phase of hyperfiltration at its outset.[86,87]

Albuminuria[44,88,89] and decreased eGFR[90,91] reflect high-risk disease in homozygous SCD and to a lesser extent in compound heterozygous SCD, with important caveats. First, estimates of GFR in homozygous SCD may be inaccurate, usually overestimating true renal function.[18,92] Some investigators have adopted a cutoff of 90 mL/min/BSA for eGFR[11,52,93] as a definition of CKD in SCD versus the standard cutoff of <60 mL/min/BSA to define stage 3 CKD in the general population. Second, the eGFR inflection below which CKD pathology, including deranged acid-base balance, bone homeostasis, and erythropoietin production, ensues in SCD is not known. Third, eGFR in homozygous SCD needs to be interpreted in context because a high eGFR (hyperfiltration) can reflect abnormal underlying pathophysiology.[33]

We examined 4 manifestations of renal disease in the University of Illinois at Chicago (UIC) SCD cohort: serum bicarbonate, potassium, alkaline phosphatase (perhaps an indicator of bone health), and depressed erythropoiesis (defined as hemoglobin <9 g/dL and absolute reticulocyte count <250 × 10^9/L). We found that an eGFR of 90 mL/min/BSA is a value at which these markers begin to inflect (Figure 16-4A), which may reflect a change in renal function and associated physiology at a higher eGFR than is seen in non–sickle cell populations. These results were replicated in the multicenter Walk-PHaSST cohort (Figure 16-4B).

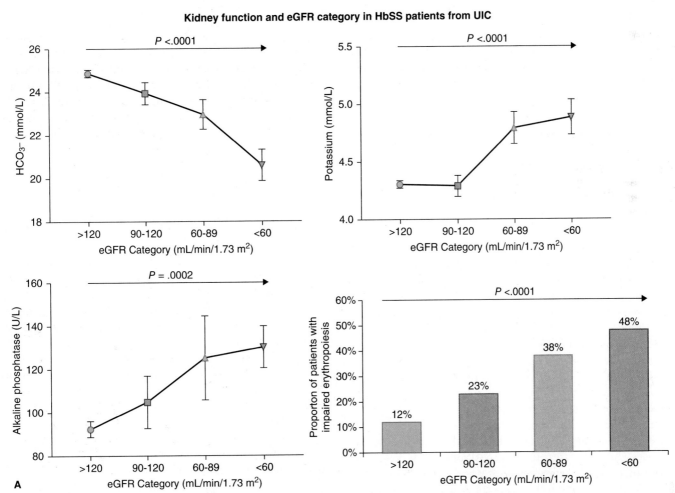

FIGURE 16-4 Progressive kidney dysfunction. A. Progressive kidney dysfunction, assessed by serum bicarbonate (HCO$_3^-$), potassium, alkaline phosphatase, and impaired erythropoiesis (defined as hemoglobin <9 g/dL and absolute reticulocyte count <250 × 10^9/L), was observed with lower estimated glomerular filtration rate (eGFR) categories in sickle cell anemia patients from the University of Illinois at Chicago (UIC). **B.** Progressive kidney dysfunction, assessed by serum HCO$_3^-$, potassium, alkaline phosphatase, and impaired erythropoiesis, was observed in sickle cell anemia patients from the multicenter Walk-PHaSST cohort.

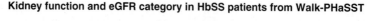

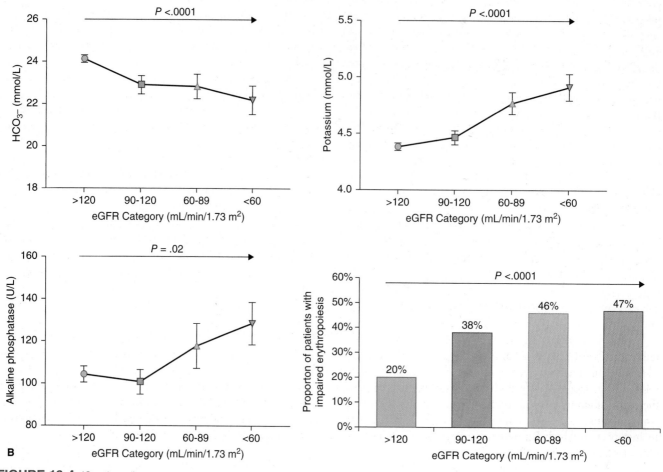

FIGURE 16-4 (*Continued*)

Blood Pressure in SCD

"Normal" blood pressure, like many clinical features of SCD, depends on the stage of life, the type of SCD, and the treatment history. Our understanding of what normal blood pressure is in SCD depends on whether one is talking about a child, in whom a physiologic response to anemia may predominate, or an adult, in whom the cumulative effects of vasculopathy may supervene. Children and young adults historically have had lower blood pressures than normal adults,[6] which then rise to the 'normal range', so-called *relative hypertension*, as the population ages. In the modern era and in resource-replete settings, successful treatments for SCD have aligned the risk factor profile of people with SCD closer to the population as a whole, with rising body mass indices (BMIs), increased predisposition to the metabolic syndrome and diabetes mellitus,[94,95] and true hypertension even in young children.[96,97] These comorbidities occur more commonly in compound heterozygotes such as those with HbSC and HbS-β+ thalassemia or with co-inheritance of α thalassemia, patients who have less hemolysis, and patients with lower metabolic rates, which are associated with more weight gain from Western diets.

Consistently, studies find that blood pressures above the mean for patients with homozygous SCD are associated with age, hemoglobin, pulse pressure, and BMI in the United States[5] and in Africa.[98] Hypertension in people with HbSS is associated with an increased risk for stroke (especially systolic hypertension), renal disease, pulmonary hypertension, and mortality.[5,99,100] Recent modifications in blood pressure goals for the general population, based on analyses published in 2017, resulted in a diagnosis of hypertension at blood pressure values ≥130/80 mm Hg in the general population,[101] with the higher number of the two determining the stage.

Conventional strategies for blood pressure management in the general population include lifestyle modifications (eg, weight loss, salt restriction if excessive, increased physical activity, reduced alcohol consumption, medication review), followed by a stepwise introduction of antihypertensive agents. There is no evidence-based guideline for blood pressure management in SCD. Given the likelihood that physiologic blood pressure is actually lower in many people with homozygous SCD and absent specific studies, recommendations for people with diabetes and albuminuria may be a reasonable surrogate (ie, target <130/80 mm Hg using renin-angiotensin-aldosterone system [RAAS]-acting agents as tolerated).[102] Small studies in SCD suggest that RAAS agents are well tolerated and may slow progression of kidney disease.[103,104] In this young African-American population, one must be mindful of the risks of angioedema and, importantly, the contraindication of RAAS-acting agents during pregnancy. In SCD, hyperkalemia is a risk due to underlying tubular dysfunction and hemolysis, but it has not been seen in small studies to date.

Albuminuria

Albuminuria is defined as the abnormal presence of albumin in the urine. The glomerular filtration barrier typically prevents albumin and other larger serum proteins from passing into the urinary space.[105] In SCD, as in other causes of nephropathy, albuminuria is thought to be an early marker of glomerular injury. The prevalence of albuminuria is age related in sickle cell patients. Approximately 10% to 30% of children with SCD and up to two-thirds of older adults exhibit albuminuria.[11,32,52]

Typical semiqualitative urinalysis dipstick testing for proteinuria primarily detects albumin in the urine but is not sensitive to identify low levels of albuminuria that are still clinically relevant. The albumin excretion rate is most often assessed by the urine albumin-to-creatinine ratio from a spot sample in which albumin and creatinine concentrations are measured. In instances in which laboratory measurement is not possible, qualitative screening with dipstick testing for albumin is a reasonable alternative.[105] Because albumin excretion may have considerable diurnal, temporal, and physiologic variation, positive findings of albuminuria should be confirmed by repeated measurement, particularly at low levels of albuminuria. The Kidney Disease Improving Global Outcomes (KDIGO) grading for albuminuria suggests the following grading system across CKD in general: A1, normal to mildly increased albuminuria (<30 mg/g creatinine); A2, moderately increased (30-300 mg/g creatinine, also known as microalbuminuria); and A3, markedly increased albuminuria (>300 mg/g creatinine, also known as macroalbuminuria).[105]

Albuminuria in SCD likely results from several pathophysiologic pathways. Hyperfiltration has been associated with albuminuria and may precede the development of albuminuria in pediatric patients. Using a definition of hyperfiltration as a BSA-corrected eGFR ≥180 mL/min (cystatin C–based) measured during ages 4 to 10 years, Lebensburger et al[32] demonstrated that hyperfiltration predicted early persistent albuminuria. They suggest that evaluating patients for hyperfiltration by assessment of eGFR early in life may identify those in whom screening for albuminuria might be considered at an earlier age than the current recommendation of 10 years. Similarly, in Jamaican 18- to 23-year-old HbSS patients, those with albuminuria had a higher median eGFR than those without albuminuria (154 vs 126 mL/min/BSA,

respectively; $P <.02$)[93]; this trend was also present in Jamaican children with HbSS.[106]

Albuminuria has been generally considered a marker of glomerular capillary injury and, as such, is associated with a number of additional comorbidities. Albuminuria has been noted in patients who have other manifestations of vascular injury, including elevated pulmonary arterial systolic pressure defined by tricuspid regurgitation jet velocity[88] and change in retinal vasculature hemodynamics.[107] Hemoglobinuria, a marker of intravascular hemolysis-derived cell-free hemoglobin in circulation exceeding scavenging capability and filtering through the glomerulus, may contribute to glomerulopathy in SCD.[46] In 2 independent SCD cohorts, urine dipstick–defined hemoglobinuria (positive for blood with microscopy showing <2 RBCs per high-power field) was observed in 20% to 36% of patients and was associated with higher urine albuminuria categories. Cell-free hemoglobin may contribute to glomerular and tubular damage through direct oxidative damage and upregulation of inflammatory pathways, depletion of NO leading to vasculopathy, or auto-oxidation to ferric hemoglobin with release of free heme, which then leads to increased oxidative stress to podocytes and tubular cells.[37] Flow-mediated brachial artery dilation, a physiologic measure of endothelial dysfunction, and elevated carotid-femoral pulse wave velocity, a measure of vascular stiffness, have been associated with albuminuria in SCD patients.[1,47,108] The pathophysiology of SCD-related nephropathy as described earlier is in line with these findings, as evidenced by the associations of albuminuria with ET-1 and sFLT-1.[47,50,108]

Current management strategies have largely focused on reducing albuminuria with the goal of slowing progression of renal disease, as has been demonstrated in non-SCD nephropathies associated with albuminuria. The mainstay of current therapy has been RAAS blockade (vide supra) and hydroxyurea. The identification of endothelial dysfunction and some of its associated biomarkers offers potential additional therapeutic approaches. 3-Hydroxy-3-methylglutaryl-CoA (HMG-CoA) reductase inhibitors (statins) have pleiotropic effects and improve endothelial function. In a murine model of SCD, 8 weeks of treatment with atorvastatin beginning at age 10 weeks mitigated albuminuria relative to treatment with vehicle.[109] As noted earlier, ET-1 has been associated with albuminuria. Endothelin antagonists have been used for treatment of pulmonary hypertension in SCD. In sickle cell mice treated with ambrisentan, an ET antagonist selective to the ETA receptor, or placebo, proteinuria was attenuated by ambrisentan.[110] In this same series of experiments, treatment with a nonselective ET antagonist (ie, inhibition of both ETA and ETB receptors) did not produce the same protective effects, pointing to the potential importance of ETA receptor blockade. ETA blockade in these mice reduced podocyte injury and tubular damage and preserved eGFR. These additional approaches to managing albuminuria in SCD have yet to be examined in humans but are the subject of current clinical studies.

Epidemiology: Clinical Presentations, Manifestations, and Outcomes

The renal system is among the most commonly affected organ systems in SCD. Renal complications include urinary concentrating defects, hematuria, impaired urine acidification, proteinuria, and renal failure.

Renal Medullary Damage

The urinary concentrating defect is the earliest renal manifestation observed in SCD. In a cohort of HbSS infants between the ages of 8 and 18 months enrolled in the BABY HUG study, decreased ability to concentrate urine was observed in 77% after a limited fluid deprivation test.[111] By childhood, defects in urine concentration are nearly universal. In a cohort of children between 4 and 14 years old, 93% were unable to increase their urine specific gravity to >1.015 after a 15-hour water deprivation test plus the administration of vasopressin. The irreversibility of this defect is observed by the second decade of life, when chronic RBC transfusions are unable to "rescue" urine concentrating ability.[112]

Renal Papillary Necrosis

Renal papillary necrosis is common in patients with SCD. Painless hematuria is the hallmark of this complication and can range from microscopic to gross hematuria. The incidence of renal papillary necrosis is believed to be highest in the third to fourth decade of life.[113] Renal papillary necrosis has been observed in 40% to 65% of patients with SCD who have undergone imaging.[113-115] The possibility of rare urothelial malignancies,[116,117] presenting with hematuria and plausibly linked to medullary ischemia and fibrosis in SCD,[118] should not be overlooked.

Distal Tubular Dysfunction

The manifestations of distal tubular dysfunction in SCD include impaired ability of the distal nephron to acidify the urine and secrete potassium.[28] This may be due to incomplete distal renal tubular acidosis,[21] resistance to aldosterone,[119] and/or hypoaldosteronism,[120] all of which have been described in various SCD cohorts. The prevalence of metabolic acidosis without advanced kidney disease, defined as eGFR ≥60 mL/min/BSA, has been observed in 42% of HbSS SCD patients.[121] In this cohort, 26% of patients had mild acidosis, defined as venous carbon dioxide (CO_2) of 20 to 23 mmol/L, and 16% had more severe acidosis, defined as a venous CO_2 of <20 mmol/L. In a small subset (n = 14), the low serum bicarbonate was associated with an arterial pH of ≤7.36, with evidence for respiratory compensation. A second study reported lower serum bicarbonate levels in all adults with HbSS, regardless of eGFR, compared with people with HbAA or HbSC, and this was associated with a higher potassium level (4.46 mM/L in HbSS compared with 4.24 mM/L in HbSC, P <.001), reticulocytopenic

anemia, and worse renal function.[11] In another cohort, an inability to acidify the urine to pH <5.3 after a $CaCl_2$ load was observed in 38.4% of SCD patients.[122] In the UIC and Walk-PHaSST cohorts of SCD patients, we observed metabolic acidosis, defined by a serum bicarbonate <24 mmol/L, in 30% to 45% of HbSS/S-β⁰ thalassemia patients and in 17% to 31% of HbSC or HbS-β⁺ thalassemia patients without advanced kidney disease (eGFR ≥60 mL/min/BSA).

Chronic Kidney Disease

CKD is a common complication of SCD, as described in worldwide cohorts (Figure 16-5). Glomerular dysfunction, manifested by increased albuminuria, is an early marker of CKD. The prevalence of albuminuria increases with age and is usually in the microalbuminuria range in children. Reports from the United States have demonstrated that abnormal albuminuria is not commonly observed before age 7 years,[123,124] although other pediatric cohorts from Jamaica[106] and the Democratic Republic of Congo[125] have reported microalbuminuria in children as young as 3 and 4 years old, respectively. In 2 cohorts of children with HbSS, microalbuminuria was observed in up to 15% of younger children (<10-12 years old) and in 30% to 46% of older children (10-13 through 20 years old).[123,126] The prevalence of abnormal albuminuria continues to increase in adulthood, with rates ranging between 37% and 69% in HbSS patients.[11,44,46,57,127-132] In these cohorts, microalbuminuria is observed in approximately 28% to 44% and macroalbuminuria in 6% to 29% of HbSS adults. The prevalence rates for abnormal albuminuria are generally lower for non-HbSS genotypes. In children with HbSC or HbS-β⁺ thalassemia, abnormal albuminuria has been reported in 14% to 17%.[126,133] The rates of micro- and macroalbuminuria also increase with older age in the non-HbSS genotypes, ranging from 11% to 32% and 3% to 18%, respectively.[11,127,134]

More advanced stages of CKD are defined by a lower GFR. In children with SCD from the United States, an eGFR between 60 and 89 mL/min/BSA has been observed in 5.3% of HbSS and 21.1% of HbSC or HbS-β⁺ thalassemia patients.[126] These data may not reflect true risk of progression for children with HbSS compared to those with milder disease genotypes because more children with HbSS had hyperfiltration and albuminuria (23.0% vs 16.8%). In a cohort of HbSS children from the Democratic Republic of Congo, an eGFR of <80 mL/min/BSA was observed in 12.3% of children.[135] Although more advanced degrees of CKD are not commonly observed in pediatric cohorts,[126] these have been reported in several adult SCD cohorts. For instance, an eGFR <60 mL/min/BSA has been reported in 11% to 29% of HbSS and 6% of HbSC adults in the United States.[46,127] Lower rates of CKD with an eGFR <60 mL/min/BSA have been reported in cohorts from India (7%)[136] and Jamaica (6%),[130] whereas the prevalence rate is as high as 20% to 46% in adult HbSS cohorts from Nigeria.[137-139]

The rate of kidney function decline is increased in patients with SCD. In cross-sectional studies, GFR measured by ⁵¹Cr-EDTA or ⁹⁹ᵐTc-DTPA clearance increases in childhood

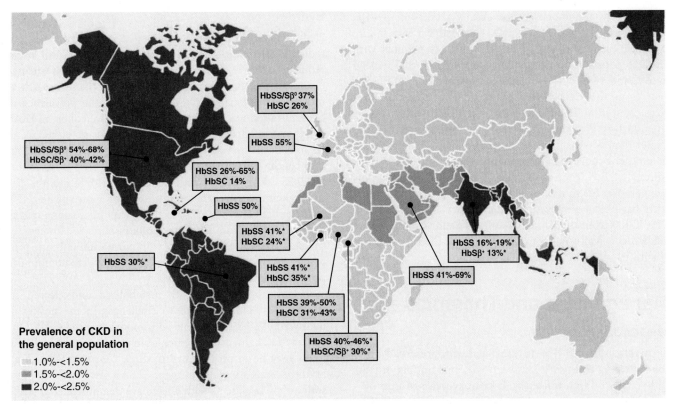

FIGURE 16-5 The global prevalence of chronic kidney disease (CKD) in patients with HbSS and HbSC or HbS-β+ thalassemia.
*Data from combined pediatric and adult cohorts. Figure adapted from Webster AC et al. Chronic Kidney Disease. *Lancet.* 2017;389 (10075): 1238-1252. Copyright 2017, with permission from Elsevier.

and adolescence, peaking between 16 and 29 years, followed by a gradual decline.[140,141] In a cohort of Jamaican adults with SCD, the measured rate of GFR decline was 3.2 ± 2.8 mL/min/BSA per year.[142] In 2 adult African-American SCD cohorts, the estimated rate of GFR decline was between 1.8 and 2.4 mL/min/BSA per year.[143,144] These rates of GFR decline are approximately 2- to 3-fold greater than what is observed in the general African American population.[145] The rates of eGFR decline are steeper in adults with HbSS (2.1 mL/min/BSA per year) versus HbSC (1.2 mL/min/BSA per year) genotypes.[144] Rapid eGFR decline, defined in these cohorts as >3.0 mL/min/BSA per year, has been observed in 31% to 37% of adults with SCD. The prevalence of rapid eGFR decline is greater in those with HbSS (34%) versus HbSC (24%) genotypes.[143,144] SCD patients with preexisting CKD have a more rapid rate of eGFR decline (5.1 mL/min/BSA per year).[143] The slope of eGFR decline accelerates after an acute kidney injury event (β –4.9 ± 1.6 mL/min/BSA per year).[72] In HbSS patients followed over a median of 4 years, clinically significant progression of CKD defined by a 50% reduction in eGFR was observed in 8% of patients and progression defined by requirement for hemodialysis was observed in 2%.[58]

End-Stage Renal Disease

A proportion of SCD patients with CKD will progress to ESRD. In the UIC and Walk-PHaSST cohorts, the prevalence of ESRD is approximately 2% to 5% in HbSS patients. These ESRD rates

are 4- to 9-fold greater than what is observed in the general African-American population.[146] Similar prevalence rates for ESRD have been observed in some HbSS adult cohorts from Jamaica (2%)[130] and Nigeria (4%).[138] The prevalence of ESRD in non-HbSS SCD patients is lower, ranging from 0% to 2% in the UIC and Walk-PHaSST cohorts.

Morbidity and Mortality of Kidney Disease

Several cohorts have demonstrated that kidney disease is an independent predictor for early mortality. Approximately 16% to 20% of deaths in patients with SCD are attributed to kidney failure.[147-149] In the CSSCD, creatinine clearance <100 mL/min was an independent predictor for early death.[147] In another 25-year, prospective, longitudinal cohort study of SCD, kidney disease, defined as a serum creatinine >1.0 mg/dL in children and 1.5 mg/dL in adults, was associated with a median survival of 27 years, compared to 51 years in those without kidney disease.[150] Furthermore, in this cohort, median survival from the time this definition of kidney disease was met was only 4 years. More contemporary SCD cohorts have highlighted the impact of kidney disease on reduced survival. In the Bethesda Sickle Cell Cohort Study, HbSS patients with an eGFR in the lowest quartile had a 2.7-fold increased risk for death compared to those with an eGFR in the top quartile.[151] In another cohort of SCD adults from the United Kingdom, rising serum creatinine was an independent risk factor for early mortality.[152]

Morbidity and mortality are greatly increased in SCD patients who progress to ESRD. Congestive heart failure exacerbations occur in 32% to 41% of SCD patients with ESRD.[153] Sepsis and thrombotic events are reported in 53% to 69% and 14% to 41% of patients, respectively.[153,154] Using data from the Centers for Medicare and Medicaid Services, 26% of SCD patients with ESRD died within 1 year after starting dialysis.[155] This rate was approximately 3-fold higher than what was observed in non-SCD ESRD patients. In another cohort of ESRD patients from France, the 5-year cumulative incidence of mortality was 46% in SCD patients compared to 6% in non-SCD patients.[153] High rates of mortality have been observed in other cohorts of SCD patients with ESRD from the United States and Saudi Arabia, where median survival was 4.5 to 4.9 years from the time dialysis was initiated.[154,156]

Management and Therapies

Medullary Function

In infants, a higher HbF is associated with preserved urine concentrating ability.[111] Consistent with this finding, infants and young children treated with hydroxyurea had improvement in urine osmolality and specific gravity.[157] Chronic RBC transfusion therapy, if offered at age 10 years or younger, may preserve urine concentrating ability. In 4 children <5 years old, chronic RBC transfusion therapy improved maximal urine osmolality from 553 to 682 mOsm/L to 942 to 1042 mOsm/L, but the dysfunction in urine concentrating returned to pretransfusion levels following cessation of transfusion therapy.[112]

Renal Papillary Necrosis

Renal papillary necrosis is typically self-limited and can be managed with conservative therapy, focusing primarily on maintaining a high urine flow rate.[158] Hypotonic fluid at a goal of 4 L/BSA per day has been recommended.[159] Other therapies, such as thiazide or loop diuretics, can help maintain the high urine flow rate but should be used with caution and after the patient is volume replete.[158] In animal models, diuretics reduce medullary osmolality and may help reduce vaso-occlusion in the vasa rectae.[160] Assessing for concurrent urinary tract infections and appropriate antibiotic therapy is recommended during an acute event. In situations that are refractory to hydration, exchange RBC transfusion[113] and arteriographic localization and embolization of the involved renal segment should be considered.[158]

Chronic Kidney Disease

Therapy to treat sickle cell nephropathy has been adopted from interventions that reduce other SCD-related complications (eg, hydroxyurea) or are used to treat other causes of nephropathy such as angiotensin-converting enzyme (ACE) inhibitors and angiotensin receptor blockers (ARBs).

Hydroxyurea

Hydroxyurea is a ribonucleotide reductase inhibitor that can reduce SCD-related complications by increasing HbF levels, reducing white blood cell counts, or increasing NO release during its metabolism and/or via other mechanisms such as reducing inflammation.[161] A reduction in the prevalence of hyperfiltration was observed in a prospective cohort of HbSS children treated with hydroxyurea for 3 years, although no changes in the prevalence of microalbuminuria or urine albumin concentrations were observed.[162] In a prospective cohort of HbSS adults treated with hydroxyurea for 6 months, the urine albumin concentration improved by approximately 43% in the entire cohort, by 72% in those with microalbuminuria, and by 50% in those with macroalbuminuria.[163] However, in this study, 10% of SCD patients with normal albuminuria progressed to microalbuminuria and 4% with microalbuminuria progressed to macroalbuminuria.

Hydroxyurea is primarily metabolized and cleared by the kidneys. This can lead to challenges in the dosing of hydroxyurea in SCD patients with more advanced CKD. One strategy to augment the hemoglobin concentration and HbF levels may be to provide hydroxyurea concurrently with an erythropoiesis-stimulating agent (ESA). Two separate case series of SCD patients with CKD have demonstrated that the combination of hydroxyurea and an ESA leads to improvement in hemoglobin concentration and HbF levels without worsening hypertension or thrombosis risk.[164,165]

ACE Inhibitors and ARBs

Most of the clinical experience with ACE inhibitors and ARBs has been based on small cohorts of SCD patients treated over relatively short periods of time. There is no evidence that the use of these agents in patients with SCD leads to a reduction in CKD progression or in developing ESRD. In a double-blind, placebo-controlled 6-month study, a reduction in albuminuria was observed in HbSS patients treated with captopril (−45 mg/24 h) versus placebo (+18 mg/24 h).[166] One case series of 3 children with HbSS who were treated with enalapril followed by a combination of enalapril plus hydroxyurea demonstrated a reduction in proteinuria with enalapril and near normalization of proteinuria after hydroxyurea therapy was added to the enalapril.[167] Two recent prospective studies have investigated the use of losartan, an ARB, to treat sickle cell nephropathy. The first study treated HbSS patients with losartan for 6 months and demonstrated that the primary end point of a ≥25% reduction in albuminuria from baseline was met in 58% of patients with microalbuminuria and 83% of those with macroalbuminuria.[168] In this cohort, the urine albumin category improved in 50% but worsened in 11% of patients. In the second study, an improvement in the urine albumin excretion rate (median, −134 μg/min; range −327 to −67 μg/min) was observed by 10 weeks of therapy compared to baseline values; with ≥12 months of therapy, this improvement had slowed to −90 μg/min (range, −431 to +19 μg/min).[169]

End-Stage Renal Disease

Mortality in the first year of dialysis is higher in sickle cell patients compared to the general population of dialysis patients. In examining incident ESRD patients from US Renal Data System data from 2005 to 2009, patients with SCD were more likely to die in the first year (hazard ratio, 2.80; 95% confidence interval, 2.31-3.38).[155] The likelihood of death in SCD patients who had established nephrology care prior to dialysis start was markedly attenuated. These data emphasize the importance of pre-ESRD care and early referral to a nephrologist.

Management of renal replacement therapy in the SCD patient with ESRD poses certain unique considerations. Either modality of dialysis, peritoneal dialysis or hemodialysis, is a viable option, each with its own advantages.[170] Hemodialysis offers a readily available vascular access that can be used for transfusions. Establishing and maintaining a permanent vascular access can be challenging in patients with SCD. Volume removal in peritoneal dialysis is performed in a more gradual fashion, and precipitating a vaso-occlusive crisis by causing rapid hemoconcentration is perhaps less likely.

Patients with ESRD and SCD may be particularly resistant to ESAs. Although the optimal hemoglobin target in ESRD patients is unknown, the typical target suggested is between 10 and 11.5 g/dL.[171] In sickle cell patients, this range could precipitate vaso-occlusive crises, so these patients should be excluded from the usual dialysis center algorithms. Targets should be individualized, but a general target of 8 to 9 g/dL may be reasonable, and the target certainly should not exceed 10 g/dL.[170,172]

Other components of hemodialysis treatment may require individualization. Although no data exist to support any recommendation in particular, minimizing volume removal rates and avoiding low-temperature dialysis may reduce the likelihood of precipitating vaso-occlusive crises.

Management of SCD complications in the dialysis patient is somewhat unique. Hydroxyurea can be used in patients on dialysis, but the starting dose should be halved to 7.5 mg/kg/d and should be administered after the dialysis treatment in patients receiving hemodialysis.[170,173] Iron overload in dialysis patients is difficult to manage. The intravenous chelation agent, deferoxamine, can be conveniently administered during the hemodialysis treatment but offers only modest iron chelation at best.[170] Administration of deferoxamine should be avoided between dialysis treatments because the deferoxamine-iron complex, circulating without urinary excretion, increases risk for potentially fatal infections by iron-dependent microorganisms. No studies have been performed specifically evaluating the oral agents deferiprone and deferasirox in patients on dialysis. One report of deferiprone in dialysis patients with aluminum overload included one patient with iron overload. Deferiprone was successful at mobilizing iron removal.[174] Deferasirox, which has primarily fecal clearance, has been reported to be successful in iron chelation in patients on dialysis, although one report indicated that the use of the agent was complicated by hypocalcemia.[170,175] Deferasirox may

have nephrotoxicity and could lead to loss of residual kidney function in ESRD patients. These agents may be useful in sickle cell patients with iron overload but should be used with close monitoring.

Renal Transplantation

Renal transplantation is a viable option for SCD patients who reach ESRD and may reduce mortality, although experience is limited.[158,170,176] Patients with SCD and ESRD are less likely to be listed for transplantation and less likely to receive a transplant compared to ESRD patients with other causes of renal disease. Higher likelihood of sensitization from prior transfusions and an increased burden of comorbidities likely contribute to lower candidacy rates.[170]

Early studies suggested an excess in long-term graft failure for patients with SCD who received a renal transplant.[172,176] A more recent study in the United States was performed in the "modern" transplant era (from 2000-2011) reflecting the current immunosuppressive regimens, specifically tacrolimus and mycophenolate. During this period, 106 SCD patients were identified as having received a renal transplant. Overall, 6-year graft survival tended to be lower in SCD patients compared to non-SCD patients (69.8% vs 80%, respectively; $P = .07$). Compared to subcohorts matched by ESRD cause, 6-year graft survival among SCD patients was similar to that of diabetic transplant recipients.[177] These data suggest an overall improvement in renal allograft survival in SCD patients and support its use in suitable candidates.

Management of renal transplantation in SCD recipients includes considerations specific to this disease. After transplantation, the enhanced erythropoietic stimulus from a healthy kidney can lead to a rise in hematocrit and subsequent hyperviscosity. Patients are at risk for thrombotic events, including renal vein thrombosis and graft infarction, and for an increase in the frequency of vaso-occlusive episodes.[158,172] Recurrence of sickle cell nephropathy may occur in the allograft.[158] A variety of measures have been suggested to improve short- and long-term renal transplant outcomes. Some experts have advocated for preoperative warming of the allograft before implantation, administration of supplemental oxygen, and hydration to lower blood viscosity.[158] Exchange transfusion in the preoperative setting to increase the fraction of HbA may be of benefit.[170] Some centers employ exchange transfusion once a patient has been listed for transplantation and continue this therapy for the life of the allograft.[172] The potential risk for alloimmunization to RBC or human leukocyte antigens should be considered with chronic transfusion therapy. Most of these measures, although reasonable, are based on expert opinion rather than clinical studies given the rare occurrence of renal transplantation in SCD patients.

A future potential therapy of ESRD in SCD patients is that of combined hematopoietic stem cell transplantation (HSCT) and kidney transplantation.[178] A least one report of successful kidney transplant from a living donor to an SCD patient following HSCT from the same donor has been reported.[179]

Such an approach will require careful selection of candidate and donor but could be a feasible approach for treatment of the SCD patient with renal failure.

Conclusion

Kidney disease in SCD is likely to improve as new therapies, gene-based and otherwise, emerge to treat SCD itself. At the present time, optimal management of the patient with SCD on dialysis or after transplantation is poorly understood and understudied.

Potential renal-specific therapeutic targets are likely to expand as our understanding of kidney disease in the contemporary patient with SCD increases in the coming decades.

Haptoglobin and hemopexin have been beneficial in murine models of SCD and in surgical trials in patients without SCD.[180-182] In addition, plasma exchange with fresh frozen plasma, to augment plasma haptoglobin in patients with SCD, has been salutary in small nonrandomized studies and case reports of strategies to manage RBC exchange–resistant multiorgan failure.[183,184]

Future areas of renal-specific therapeutic potential include the use of endothelin receptor blockade (vide supra), free hemoglobin and heme scavengers as organ protection,[180-182] and attention to sickle cell–specific drug toxicity to the kidneys (eg, vascular sensitivity to NSAIDs). Ongoing studies to slow progression of renal disease in SCD should be informative about best practices. .

Case Study

A 42-year-old woman with HbSS SCD and an HbF of 10% (without hydroxyurea), along with obesity, sleep apnea, and intermittent hyperglycemia, was referred for evaluation of an increasing creatinine.

> Teaching Point: Adult people with SCD are increasingly prone to 'Western' complications from obesity, including diabetes and hypertension, which may deleteriously effect kidney disease and its progression.

She had few symptoms and no complications from her disease until 15 years ago, when she experienced significant hematuria and papillary necrosis.

> Teaching Point: 'Point-of-care' hematuria is common in SCD, and may be due to hemoglobinuria from ongoing hemolysis (dipstick positive hemoglobin, without red cells) or true hematuria, which may arise from papillary necrosis. Adults with SCD and gross hematuria should also be evaluated for malignancies.

Ten years ago, she developed multiorgan failure and acute kidney injury. Over the intervening 10 years, she had developed hypertension and progressive renal failure, managed with ACE inhibitors (until her creatinine increased to >2 mg/dL) and β-blockade. Mild pain was managed with NSAIDs, and anemia was managed with blood transfusions. She required >40 RBC transfusions during this interval and was being managed with deferasirox and low-dose (500 mg twice per week) hydroxyurea. She developed new sickle cell pain coincident with initiation of ESAs, titrating to a total hemoglobin of 8 to 9 g/dL.

> Teaching Point: Previous acute kidney injury will increase patient's risk for CKD. Medication management is critical in protecting the kidney. Intravenous contrast should be avoided. Non-steroidal anti-inflammatory agents and oral iron chelation with deferasirox must be managed carefully or avoided, since both can affect rates of progression. Deferoxamine is difficult to administer (subcutaneous infusion or twice-a-day subcutaneous), and it is recommended to decrease dosing by 50-75% with CKD (Lexicomp). Deferiprone does not require renal dosing, but is a three-times-a-day medication, and requires weekly monitoring of blood counts.

On referral, we increased her hydroxyurea, with improvement in symptoms and abrogation in transfusion requirements. NSAIDs were discontinued, as was deferasirox. Symptoms from ESAs disappeared as hydroxyurea was up-titrated.

> Teaching Point: Erythropoiesis-stimulating agents may, unpredictably and non-uniformly, increase pain in patients with CKD.[164-165] Close monitoring and pre-treatment with hydroxyurea for 1-2 weeks may mitigate this.

Her renal function continued to deteriorate over 3 years, from an eGFR of 40 to <10 mL/min/1.73 m^2 BSA, and a peritoneal dialysis catheter was placed. Deferasirox was reinitiated at low dose, and blood pressure control was optimized with β-blockers and calcium channel blockers.

> Teaching Point: All patients with SCD and ESRD should be evaluated for renal transplantation.

She is currently being evaluated for renal transplantation.

High-Yield Facts

◆ To treat the kidney, treat the disease. This is the first principle of managing kidney disease in the patient with SCD. It is clear that hydroxyurea attenuates renal disease in SCD.[163,185,186]

- But it is tricky. As renal disease progresses, erythroid reserve and tolerance for hydroxyurea may wane, requiring concomitant erythropoietin therapy.[164,165]

- Transfusion may help. We and others have initiated transfusion, exchange if possible, to limit iron overload if other management of disease is not possible as renal function deteriorates.

◆ Screen for and manage albuminuria and hypertension.

- Annually monitor albumin-to-creatinine ratios. A sustained urinary albumin-to-creatinine ratio >30 mg/dL should be managed with an ACE inhibitor or ARB, especially if the blood pressure is >120/70 mm Hg.

- Treat hypertension early, especially with concomitant albuminuria. Avoid diuretics. Emphasize ACE inhibitors and ARBs, but remember to monitor potassium. Remember to warn fertile women about the risks of RAAS-acting agents in pregnancy.

◆ Watch for subtle manifestations of renal disease.

- Acidosis warrants treatment. The 2013 KDIGO guidelines suggest that patients with CKD and metabolic acidosis, regardless of comorbid disease such as SCD, be treated with alkali therapy, usually with sodium bicarbonate, to maintain the serum bicarbonate concentration in the normal range (23-29 mEq/L).[187] The serum bicarbonate concentration at which this therapy should be initiated is not well established, and 20 mEq/dL may be a reasonable starting point.

- Manage bone health, including vitamin D supplementation. We simply do not know the impact of a depressed but normal eGFR on bone health in SCD.

◆ Avoid nephrotoxins.

- Minimize use of intravenous contrast, particularly in patients with CKD.

- Beware of NSAIDs at high and prolonged doses. Renal blood flow may be especially dependent on prostaglandin/COX-2 in SCD.[187-189]

- Beware of aminoglycosides.

- Manage chelation carefully. The most commonly used oral chelator in the United States is deferasirox, which can increase creatinine in people with SCD. Expert opinion states that a serum creatinine measured at 2 posttreatment visits that is one-third greater than at 2 pretreatment visits warrants dose adjustment (decrease by 10 mg/kg and close follow-up).[190] In general, we avoid deferasirox in patients with CKD who are not on dialysis. The other oral chelator, deferiprone, is not renally cleared but is a medication that must be taken 3 times a day and rarely can be associated with neutropenia and liver damage.[191]

  Once dialysis is initiated in a patient with SCD, deferasirox can be considered for documented iron overload (by transfusion history and quantitative imaging techniques, as ferritin may be even less useful in these patients than in nondialysis patients). Pharmacokinetic studies suggest that 10 to 15 mg/kg/d may be an appropriate range for these patients,[192] because higher doses may be associated with disabling hypocalcemia.[193] Additional strategies to manage ESRD in SCD include RBC exchanges, which obviate the need for complex hydroxyurea/erythropoietin algorithms and minimize iron overload. Intravenous deferoxamine was used many years ago to manage aluminum toxicity, typically with 1 dose given with dialysis, but this offers very modest iron chelation.[170]

◆ Refer your patients to a nephrologist.

- At the time you recognize renal disease.

- When they are approaching dialysis. Renal transplantation should be discussed with all eligible patients.

References

1. Ranque B, Menet A, Boutouyrie P, et al. Arterial stiffness impairment in sickle cell disease associated with chronic vascular complications: the multinational African CADRE Study. *Circulation.* 2016;134(13):923-933.

2. Afolabi BB, Oladipo OO, Akanmu AS, Abudu OO, Sofola OA, BroughtonPipkin F. Volume regulatory hormones and plasma volume in pregnant women with sickle cell disorder. Journal of the renin-angiotensin-aldosterone system. *J Renin Angiotensin Aldosterone Syst.* 2016;17(3):1470320316670444.

3. Schmitt F, Martinez F, Brillet G, Get al. Early glomerular dysfunction in patients with sickle cell anemia. *Am J Kidney Dis.* 1998;32(2):208-214.

4. Damy T, Bodez D, Habibi A, et al. Haematological determinants of cardiac involvement in adults with sickle cell disease. *Eur Heart J.* 2016;37(14):1158-1167.

5. Pegelow CH, Colangelo L, Steinberg M, et al. Natural history of blood pressure in sickle cell disease: risks for stroke and death associated with relative hypertension in sickle cell anemia. *Am J Med.* 1997;102(2):171-177.

6. Grell GA, Alleyne GA, Serjeant GR. Blood pressure in adults with homozygous sickle cell disease. *Lancet.* 1981;2(8256):1166.

7. Miall WE, Kass EH, Ling J, Stuart KL. Factors influencing arterial pressure in the general population in Jamaica. *Br Med J.* 1962;2(5303):497-506.

8. Desai PC, Deal AM, Brittain JE, Jones S, Hinderliter A, Ataga KI. Decades after the cooperative study: a re-examination of systemic blood pressure in sickle cell disease. *Am J Hematol.* 2012;87(10):E65-E68.

9. Guasch A, Cua M, Mitch WE. Early detection and the course of glomerular injury in patients with sickle cell anemia. *Kidney Int.* 1996;49(3):786-791.

10. McKerrell TD, Cohen HW, Billett HH. The older sickle cell patient. *Am J Hematol.* 2004;76(2):101-106.

11. Drawz P, Ayyappan S, Nouraie M, et al. Kidney Disease among patients with sickle cell disease, hemoglobin SS and SC. *Clin J Am Soc Nephrol.* 2016;11(2):207-215.

12. Benneh-Akwasi Kuma A, Owusu-Ansah AT, Ampomah MA, et al. Prevalence of relative systemic hypertension in adults with sickle cell disease in Ghana. *PloS One.* 2018;13(1):e0190347.

13. Kato GJ, Steinberg MH, Gladwin MT. Intravascular hemolysis and the pathophysiology of sickle cell disease. *J Clin Invest.* 2017;127(3):750-760.

14. Maigne G, Ferlicot S, Galacteros F, et al. Glomerular lesions in patients with sickle cell disease. *Medicine.* 2010;89(1):18-27.

15. Elfenbein IB, Patchefsky A, Schwartz W, Weinstein AG. Pathology of the glomerulus in sickle cell anemia with and without nephrotic syndrome. *Am J Pathol.* 1974;77(3):357-374.

16. Bakir AA, Hathiwala SC, Ainis H, Hryhorczuk DO, et al. Prognosis of the nephrotic syndrome in sickle glomerulopathy. A retrospective study. *Am J Nephrol.* 1987;7(2):110-115.

17. Zahr RS, Yee ME, Weaver J, et al. Kidney biopsy findings in children with sickle cell disease: a Midwest Pediatric Nephrology Consortium study. *Pediatr Nephrol.* 2019;34(8):1435-1445.

18. Becker AM. Sickle cell nephropathy: challenging the conventional wisdom. *Pediatr Nephrol.* 2011;26(12):2099-2109.

19. Chintagari NR, Nguyen J, Belcher JD, Vercellotti GM, Alayash AI. Haptoglobin attenuates hemoglobin-induced heme oxygenase-1 in renal proximal tubule cells and kidneys of a mouse model of sickle cell disease. *Blood Cells Mol Dis.* 2015;54(3):302-306.

20. Bernaudin F, Socie G, Kuentz M, et al. Long-term results of related myeloablative stem-cell transplantation to cure sickle cell disease. *Blood.* 2007;110(7):2749-2756.

21. de Jong PE, Statius van Eps LW. Sickle cell nephropathy: new insights into its pathophysiology. *Kidney Int.* 1985;27(5):711-717.

22. de Jong PE, de Jong-Van Den Berg TW, Sewrajsingh GS, Schouten H, Donker AJ, Statius van Eps LW. The influence of indomethacin on renal haemodynamics in sickle cell anaemia. *Clin Sci.* 1980;59(4):245-250.

23. Allon M, Lawson L, Eckman JR, Delaney V, Bourke E. Effects of nonsteroidal antiinflammatory drugs on renal function in sickle cell anemia. *Kidney Int.* 1988;34(4):500-506.

24. Khasabova IA, Uhelski M, Khasabov SG, Gupta K, Seybold VS, Simone DA. Sensitization of nociceptors by prostaglandin E2-glycerol contributes to hyperalgesia in mice with sickle cell disease. *Blood.* 2019;133(18):1989-1998.

25. Sadler KE, Stucky CL. Blocking COX-2 for sickle cell pain relief. *Blood.* 2019;133(18):1924-1925.

26. Han J, Saraf SL, Lash JP, Gordeuk VR. Use of anti-inflammatory analgesics in sickle-cell disease. *J Clin Pharm Ther.* 2017;42(5):656-660.

27. Nath KA, Grande JP, Haggard JJ, et al. Oxidative stress and induction of heme oxygenase-1 in the kidney in sickle cell disease. *Am J Pathol.* 2001;158(3):893-903.

28. Nath KA, Hebbel RP. Sickle cell disease: renal manifestations and mechanisms. *Nat Rev Nephrol.* 2015;11(3):161-171.

29. Praga M, Morales E, Herrero JC, et al. Absence of hypoalbuminemia despite massive proteinuria in focal segmental glomerulosclerosis secondary to hyperfiltration. *Am J Kidney Dis.* 1999;33(1):52-58.

30. Falk RJ, Scheinman J, Phillips G, Orringer E, Johnson A, Jennette JC. Prevalence and pathologic features of sickle cell nephropathy and response to inhibition of angiotensin-converting enzyme. *N Engl J Med.* 1992;326(14):910-915.

31. Helal I, Fick-Brosnahan GM, Reed-Gitomer B, Schrier RW. Glomerular hyperfiltration: definitions, mechanisms and clinical implications. *Nat Rev Nephrol.* 2012;8(5):293-300.

32. Lebensburger JD, Aban I, Pernell B, et al. Hyperfiltration during early childhood precedes albuminuria in pediatric sickle cell nephropathy. *Am J Hematol.* 2019;94(4):417-423.

33. Vazquez B, Shah B, Zhang X, Lash JP, Gordeuk VR, Saraf SL. Hyperfiltration is associated with the development of microalbuminuria in patients with sickle cell anemia. *Am J Hematol.* 2014;89(12):1156-1157.

34. Kasztan M, Fox BM, Lebensburger JD, et al. Hyperfiltration predicts long-term renal outcomes in humanized sickle cell mice. *Blood Adv.* 2019;3(9):1460-1475.

35. Szabo G, Magyar S, Kocsar L. Passage of haemoglobin into urine and lymph. *Acta Med Acad Sci Hung.* 1965;21(3):349-359.

36. Tracz MJ, Alam J, Nath KA. Physiology and pathophysiology of heme: implications for kidney disease. *J Am Soc Nephrol.* 2007;18(2):414-420.

37. Gladwin MT, Kanias T, Kim-Shapiro DB. Hemolysis and cell-free hemoglobin drive an intrinsic mechanism for human disease. *J Clin Invest.* 2012;122(4):1205-1208.

38. Nielsen R, Christensen EI. Proteinuria and events beyond the slit. *Pediatr Nephrol.* 2010;25(5):813-822.

39. Eshbach ML, Kaur A, Rbaibi Y, Tejero J, Weisz OA. Hemoglobin inhibits albumin uptake by proximal tubule cells: implications for sickle cell disease. *Am J Physiol Cell Physiol.* 2017;312(6):C733-C740.

40. Lusco MA, Fogo AB, Najafian B, Alpers CE. AJKD Atlas of renal pathology: sickle cell nephropathy. *Am J Kidney Dis.* 2016;68(1):e1-e3.

41. Schein A, Enriquez C, Coates TD, Wood JC. Magnetic resonance detection of kidney iron deposition in sickle cell disease: a marker of chronic hemolysis. *J Magn Reson Imaging.* 2008;28(3):698-704.

42. Vasavda N, Gutierrez L, House MJ, Drasar E, St Pierre TG, Thein SL. Renal iron load in sickle cell disease is influenced by severity of haemolysis. *Br J Haematol.* 2012;157(5):599-605.

43. Donnola SB, Piccone CM, Lu L, et al. Diffusion tensor imaging MRI of sickle cell kidney disease: initial results and comparison with iron deposition. *NMR Biomed.* 2018;31(3):10.1002/nbm.3883.

44. Day TG, Drasar ER, Fulford T, Sharpe CC, Thein SL. Association between hemolysis and albuminuria in adults with sickle cell anemia. *Haematologica.* 2012;97(2):201-205.

45. Hamideh D, Raj V, Harrington T, et al. Albuminuria correlates with hemolysis and NAG and KIM-1 in patients with sickle cell anemia. *Pediatr Nephrol.* 2014 Oct;29(10):1997-2003.

46. Saraf SL, Zhang X, Kanias T, et al. Haemoglobinuria is associated with chronic kidney disease and its progression in patients with sickle cell anaemia. *Br J Haematol.* 2014;164(5):729-739.

47. Ataga KI, Brittain JE, Moore D, et al. Urinary albumin excretion is associated with pulmonary hypertension in sickle cell disease: potential role of soluble fms-like tyrosine kinase-1. *Eur J Haematol.* 2010;85(3):257-263.

48. Ramzy D, Rao V, Tumiati LC, et al. Elevated endothelin-1 levels impair nitric oxide homeostasis through a PKC-dependent pathway. *Circulation.* 2006;114(1 suppl):I319-I326.

49. De Miguel C, Speed JS, Kasztan M, Gohar EY, Pollock DM. Endothelin-1 and the kidney: new perspectives and recent findings. *Curr Opin Nephrology Hypertens.* 2016;25(1):35-41.

50. Ataga KI, Derebail VK, Caughey M, et al. Albuminuria is associated with endothelial dysfunction and elevated plasma endothelin-1 in sickle cell anemia. *PloS One.* 2016;11(9):e0162652.

51. Statius van Eps LW, Pinedo-Veels C, de Vries GH, de Koning J. Nature of concentrating defect in sickle-cell nephropathy. Microradioangiographic studies. *Lancet.* 1970;1(7644):450-452.

52. Ataga KI, Derebail VK, Archer DR. The glomerulopathy of sickle cell disease. *Am J Hematol.* 2014;89(9):907-914.

53. Nath KA, Grande JP, Croatt AJ, et al. Transgenic sickle mice are markedly sensitive to renal ischemia-reperfusion injury. *Am J Pathol.* 2005;166(4):963-972.

54. Higgs DR, Aldridge BE, Lamb J, et al. The interaction of alpha-thalassemia and homozygous sickle-cell disease. *N Engl J Med.* 1982;306(24):1441-1446.

55. Guasch A, Zayas CF, Eckman JR, Muralidharan K, Zhang W, Elsas LJ. Evidence that microdeletions in the alpha globin gene protect against the development of sickle cell glomerulopathy in humans. *J Am Soc Nephrol.* 1999;10(5):1014-1019.

56. Geard A, Pule GD, Chetcha Chemegni B, et al. Clinical and genetic predictors of renal dysfunctions in sickle cell anaemia in Cameroon. *Br J Haematol.* 2017;178(4):629-639.

57. Nebor D, Broquere C, Brudey K, et al. Alpha-thalassemia is associated with a decreased occurrence and a delayed age-at-onset of albuminuria in sickle cell anemia patients. *Blood Cells Mol Dis.* 2010;45(2):154-158.

58. Saraf SL, Shah BN, Zhang X, et al. APOL1, alpha-thalassemia, and BCL11A variants as a genetic risk profile for progression of chronic kidney disease in sickle cell anemia. *Haematologica.* 2017;102(1):e1-e6.

59. Parsa A, Kao WH, Xie D, et al. APOL1 risk variants, race, and progression of chronic kidney disease. *N Engl J Med.* 2013;369(23):2183-2196.

60. Genovese G, Friedman DJ, Ross MD, et al. Association of trypanolytic ApoL1 variants with kidney disease in African Americans. *Science.* 2010;329(5993):841-845.

61. Pays E, Vanhollebeke B, Uzureau P, Lecordier L, Perez-Morga D. The molecular arms race between African trypanosomes and humans. *Nat Rev Microbiol.* 2014;12(8):575-584.

62. Freedman BI, Kopp JB, Langefeld CD, et al. The apolipoprotein L1 (APOL1) gene and nondiabetic nephropathy in African Americans. *J Am Soc Nephrol.* 2010;21(9):1422-1426.

63. Friedman DJ, Pollak MR. Genetics of kidney failure and the evolving story of APOL1. *J Clin Invest.* 2011;121(9):3367-3374.

64. Saraf SL, Zhang X, Shah B, et al. Genetic variants and cell-free hemoglobin processing in sickle cell nephropathy. *Haematologica.* 2015;100(10):1275-1284.

65. Kormann R, Jannot AS, Narjoz C, et al. Roles of APOL1 G1 and G2 variants in sickle cell disease patients: kidney is the main target. *Br J Haematol.* 2017;179(2):323-335.

66. Schaefer BA, Flanagan JM, Alvarez OA, et al. Genetic modifiers of white blood cell count, albuminuria and glomerular filtration rate in children with sickle cell anemia. *PloS One.* 2016;11(10):e0164364.

67. Ashley-Koch AE, Okocha EC, Garrett ME, et al. MYH9 and APOL1 are both associated with sickle cell disease nephropathy. *Br J Haematol.* 2011;155(3):386-394.

68. Nielsen MJ, Petersen SV, Jacobsen C, et al. Haptoglobin-related protein is a high-affinity hemoglobin-binding plasma protein. *Blood.* 2006;108(8):2846-2849.

69. Widener J, Nielsen MJ, Shiflett A, Moestrup SK, Hajduk S. Hemoglobin is a co-factor of human trypanosome lytic factor. *PLoS Pathog.* 2007;3(9):1250-1261.

70. Saraf SL, Sysol JR, Susma A, et al. Progressive glomerular and tubular damage in sickle cell trait and sickle cell anemia mouse models. *Transl Res.* 2018;197:1-11.

71. Yamada N, Yamaya M, Okinaga S, et al. Microsatellite polymorphism in the heme oxygenase-1 gene promoter is associated with susceptibility to emphysema. *Am J Human Genet.* 2000;66(1):187-195.

72. Saraf SL, Viner M, Rischall A, et al. HMOX1 and Acute kidney injury in sickle cell anemia. *Blood.* 2018;132(15):1621-1625.

73. Bean CJ, Boulet SL, Ellingsen D, et al. Heme oxygenase-1 gene promoter polymorphism is associated with reduced incidence of acute chest syndrome among children with sickle cell disease. *Blood.* 2012;120(18):3822-3828.

74. Afenyi-Annan A, Kail M, Combs MR, Orringer EP, Ashley-Koch A, Telen MJ. Lack of Duffy antigen expression is associated with organ damage in patients with sickle cell disease. *Transfusion.* 2008;48(5):917-924.

75. Farawela HM, El-Ghamrawy M, Farhan MS, Soliman R, Yousry SM, AbdelRahman HA. Association between Duffy antigen receptor expression and disease severity in sickle cell disease patients. *Hematology.* 2016;21(8):474-479.

76. Nolan VG, Ma Q, Cohen HT, et al. Estimated glomerular filtration rate in sickle cell anemia is associated with polymorphisms of bone morphogenetic protein receptor 1B. *Am J Hematol.* 2007;82(3):179-184.

77. Takeda M, Otsuka F, Nakamura K, et al. Characterization of the bone morphogenetic protein (BMP) system in human pulmonary arterial smooth muscle cells isolated from a sporadic case of primary pulmonary hypertension: roles of BMP type IB receptor (activin receptor-like kinase-6) in the mitotic action. *Endocrinology.* 2004;145(9):4344-4354.

78. Chida A, Shintani M, Nakayama T, et al. Missense mutations of the BMPR1B (ALK6) gene in childhood idiopathic pulmonary arterial hypertension. *Circ J.* 2012;76(6):1501-1508.

79. Kao WH, Klag MJ, Meoni LA, et al. MYH9 is associated with nondiabetic end-stage renal disease in African Americans. *Nat Genet.* 2008;40(10):1185-1192.

80. Kopp JB, Smith MW, Nelson GW, et al. MYH9 is a major-effect risk gene for focal segmental glomerulosclerosis. *Nat Genet.* 2008;40(10):1175-1184.

81. Tzur S, Rosset S, Shemer R, et al. Missense mutations in the APOL1 gene are highly associated with end stage kidney disease

risk previously attributed to the MYH9 gene. *Hum Genet.* 2010;128(3):345-350.

82. Balduini CL, Pecci A, Savoia A. Recent advances in the understanding and management of MYH9-related inherited thrombocytopenias. *Br J Haematol.* 2011;154(2):161-174.

83. Behar DM, Rosset S, Tzur S, et al. African ancestry allelic variation at the MYH9 gene contributes to increased susceptibility to non-diabetic end-stage kidney disease in Hispanic Americans. *Hum Mol Genet.* 2010;19(9):1816-1827.

84. Ishani A, Grandits GA, Grimm RH, et al. Association of single measurements of dipstick proteinuria, estimated glomerular filtration rate, and hematocrit with 25-year incidence of end-stage renal disease in the multiple risk factor intervention trial. *J Am Soc Nephrol.* 2006;17(5):1444-1452.

85. Levey AS, de Jong PE, Coresh J, et al. The definition, classification, and prognosis of chronic kidney disease: a KDIGO Controversies Conference report. *Kidney Int.* 2011;80(1):17-28.

86. Ware RE, Rees RC, Sarnaik SA, et al. Renal function in infants with sickle cell anemia: baseline data from the BABY HUG trial. *J Pediatr.* 2010;156(1):66-70 e1.

87. Alvarez O, Miller ST, Wang WC, et al. Effect of hydroxyurea treatment on renal function parameters: results from the multi-center placebo-controlled BABY HUG clinical trial for infants with sickle cell anemia. *Pediatr Blood Cancer.* 2012;59(4): 668-674.

88. Forrest S, Kim A, Carbonella J, Pashankar F. Proteinuria is associated with elevated tricuspid regurgitant jet velocity in children with sickle cell disease. *Pediatr Blood Cancer.* 2012;58(6): 937-940.

89. Novelli EM, Hildesheim M, Rosano C, et al. Elevated pulse pressure is associated with hemolysis, proteinuria and chronic kidney disease in sickle cell disease. *PloS One.* 2014;9(12): e114309.

90. Paulukonis ST, Eckman JR, Snyder AB, et al. Defining sickle cell disease mortality using a population-based surveillance system, 2004 through 2008. *Pub Health Rep.* 2016;131(2):367-375.

91. Powars DR, Chan LS, Hiti A, Ramicone E, Johnson C. Outcome of sickle cell anemia: a 4-decade observational study of 1056 patients. *Medicine.* 2005;84(6):363-376.

92. Yee MEM, Lane PA, Archer DR, Joiner CH, Eckman JR, Guasch A. Estimation of glomerular filtration rate using serum cystatin C and creatinine in adults with sickle cell anemia. *Am J Hematol.* 2017;92(10):E598-E599.

93. Thompson J, Reid M, Hambleton I, Serjeant GR. Albuminuria and renal function in homozygous sickle cell disease: observations from a cohort study. *Arch Intern Med.* 2007;167(7): 701-708.

94. Ogunsile FJ, Bediako SM, Nelson J, et al. Metabolic syndrome among adults living with sickle cell disease. *Blood Cells Mol Dis.* 2019;74:25-29.

95. Zhou J, Han J, Nutescu EA, et al. Similar burden of type 2 diabetes among adult patients with sickle cell disease relative to African Americans in the U.S. population: a six-year population-based cohort analysis. *Br J Haematol.* 2019;185(1): 116-127.

96. Lebensburger JD, Cutter GR, Howard TH, Muntner P, Feig DI. Evaluating risk factors for chronic kidney disease in pediatric patients with sickle cell anemia. *Pediatr Nephrol.* 2017;32(9):1565-1573.

97. Bodas P, Huang A, O'Riordan MA, Sedor JR, Dell KM. The prevalence of hypertension and abnormal kidney function in children with sickle cell disease: a cross sectional review. *BMC Nephrol.* 2013;14:237.

98. Makubi A, Mmbando BP, Novelli EM, et al. Rates and risk factors of hypertension in adolescents and adults with sickle cell anaemia in Tanzania: 10 years' experience. *Br J Haematol.* 2017;177(6):930-937.

99. Gordeuk VR, Sachdev V, Taylor JG, Gladwin MT, Kato G, Castro OL. Relative systemic hypertension in patients with sickle cell disease is associated with risk of pulmonary hypertension and renal insufficiency. *Am J Hematol.* 2008;83(1):15-18.

100. Ohene-Frempong K, Weiner SJ, Sleeper LA, et al. Cerebrovascular accidents in sickle cell disease: rates and risk factors. *Blood.* 1998;91(1):288-294.

101. Whelton PK, Carey RM, Aronow WS, et al. 2017 ACC/AHA/ AAPA/ABC/ACPM/AGS/APhA/ASH/ASPC/NMA/PCNA guideline for the prevention, detection, evaluation, and management of high blood pressure in adults: executive summary: a report of the American College of Cardiology/American Heart Association Task Force on Clinical Practice Guidelines. *Circulation.* 2018;138(17):e426-e483.

102. Wu HY, Huang JW, Lin HJ, et al. Comparative effectiveness of renin-angiotensin system blockers and other antihypertensive drugs in patients with diabetes: systematic review and bayesian network meta-analysis. *BMJ.* 2013;347:f6008.

103. Thrower A, Ciccone EJ, Maitra P, Derebail VK, Cai J, Ataga KI. Effect of renin-angiotensin-aldosterone system blocking agents on progression of glomerulopathy in sickle cell disease. *Br J Haematol.* 2019;184(2):246-252.

104. Haymann JP, Hammoudi N, Stankovic Stojanovic K, et al. Renin-angiotensin system blockade promotes a cardio-renal protection in albuminuric homozygous sickle cell patients. *Br J Haematol.* 2017;179(5):820-828.

105. Levey AS, Becker C, Inker LA. Glomerular filtration rate and albuminuria for detection and staging of acute and chronic kidney disease in adults: a systematic review. *JAMA.* 2015;313(8):837-846.

106. King L, MooSang M, Miller M, Reid M. Prevalence and predictors of microalbuminuria in Jamaican children with sickle cell disease. *Arch Dis Child.* 2011;96(12):1135-1139.

107. Kord Valeshabad A, Wanek J, Saraf SL, et al. Changes in conjunctival hemodynamics predict albuminuria in sickle cell nephropathy. *Am J Nephrol.* 2015;41(6):487-493.

108. Audard V, Bartolucci P, Stehle T. Sickle cell disease and albuminuria: recent advances in our understanding of sickle cell nephropathy. *Clin Kidney J.* 2017;10(4):475-478.

109. Zahr RS, Chappa P, Yin H, Brown LA, Ataga KI, Archer DR. Renal protection by atorvastatin in a murine model of sickle cell nephropathy. *Br J Haematol.* 2018;181(1):111-121.

110. Kasztan M, Fox BM, Speed JS, et al. Long-term endothelin-a receptor antagonism provides robust renal protection in humanized sickle cell disease mice. *J Am Soc Nephrol.* 2017;28(8):2443-2458.

111. Miller ST, Wang WC, Iyer R, et al. Urine concentrating ability in infants with sickle cell disease: baseline data from the phase III trial of hydroxyurea (BABY HUG). *Pediatr Blood Cancer.* 2010;54(2): 265-268.

112. Itano HA, Keitel HG, Thompson D. Hyposthenuria in sickle cell anemia: a reversible renal defect. *J Clin Invest.* 1956;35(9): 998-1007.

113. Henderickx M, Brits T, De Baets K, et al. Renal papillary necrosis in patients with sickle cell disease: How to recognize this 'forgotten' diagnosis. *J Pediatr Urol.* 2017;13(3):250-256.

114. Pandya KK, Koshy M, Brown N, Presman D. Renal papillary necrosis in sickle cell hemoglobinopathies. *J Urol.* 1976;115(5):497-501.

115. Odita JC, Ugbodaga CI, Okafor LA, Ojogwu LI, Ogisi OA. Urographic changes in homozygous sickle cell disease. *Diagnost Imaging.* 1983;52(5):259-263.

116. Alvarez O, Rodriguez MM, Jordan L, Sarnaik S. Renal medullary carcinoma and sickle cell trait: a systematic review. *Pediatr Blood Cancer.* 2015;62(10):1694-1699.

117. Shah AY, Karam JA, Malouf GG, et al. Management and outcomes of patients with renal medullary carcinoma: a multicentre collaborative study. *BJU Int.* 2017;120(6):782-792.

118. Msaouel P, Tannir NM, Walker CL. A model linking sickle cell hemoglobinopathies and SMARCB1 loss in renal medullary carcinoma. *Clin Cancer Res.* 2018;24(9):2044-2049.

119. DeFronzo RA, Taufield PA, Black H, McPhedran P, Cooke CR. Impaired renal tubular potassium secretion in sickle cell disease. *Ann Intern Med.* 1979;90(3):310-316.

120. Batlle D, Itsarayoungyuen K, Arruda JA, Kurtzman NA. Hyperkalemic hyperchloremic metabolic acidosis in sickle cell hemoglobinopathies. *Am J Med.* 1982;72(2):188-192.

121. Maurel S, Stankovic Stojanovic K, Avellino V, et al. Prevalence and correlates of metabolic acidosis among patients with homozygous sickle cell disease. *Clin J Am Soc Nephrol.* 2014;9(4):648-653.

122. Silva Junior GB, Vieira AP, Couto Bem AX, et al. Renal tubular dysfunction in sickle cell disease. *Kidney Blood Pressure Res.* 2013;38(1):1-10.

123. Dharnidharka VR, Dabbagh S, Atiyeh B, Simpson P, Sarnaik S. Prevalence of microalbuminuria in children with sickle cell disease. *Pediatr Nephrol.* 1998;12(6):475-478.

124. McBurney PG, Hanevold CD, Hernandez CM, Waller JL, McKie KM. Risk factors for microalbuminuria in children with sickle cell anemia. *J Pediatr Hematol Oncol.* 2002;24(6):473-477.

125. Aloni MN, Mabidi JL, Ngiyulu RM, et al. Prevalence and determinants of microalbuminuria in children suffering from sickle cell anemia in steady state. *Clin Kidney J.* 2017;10(4):479-486.

126. McPherson Yee M, Jabbar SF, Osunkwo I, et al. Chronic kidney disease and albuminuria in children with sickle cell disease. *Clin J Am Soc Nephrol.* 2011;6(11):2628-2633.

127. Guasch A, Navarrete J, Nass K, Zayas CF. Glomerular involvement in adults with sickle cell hemoglobinopathies: prevalence and clinical correlates of progressive renal failure. *J Am Soc Nephrol.* 2006;17(8):2228-2235.

128. Maier-Redelsperger M, Levy P, Lionnet F, et al. Strong association between a new marker of hemolysis and glomerulopathy in sickle cell anemia. *Blood Cells Mol Dis.* 2010;45(4):289-292.

129. Abo-Zenah H, Moharram M, El Nahas AM. Cardiorenal risk prevalence in sickle cell hemoglobinopathy. *Nephron Clin Pract.* 2009;112(2):c98-c106.

130. Asnani MR, Reid ME. Renal function in adult Jamaicans with homozygous sickle cell disease. *Hematology.* 2015;20(7):422-428.

131. Bolarinwa RA, Akinlade KS, Kuti MA, Olawale OO, Akinola NO. Renal disease in adult Nigerians with sickle cell anemia: a report of prevalence, clinical features and risk factors. *Saudi J Kidney Dis Transpl.* 2012;23(1):171-175.

132. Ephraim RK, Osakunor DN, Cudjoe O, et al. Chronic kidney disease is common in sickle cell disease: a cross-sectional study in the Tema Metropolis, Ghana. *BMC Nephrol.* 2015;16:75.

133. Becton LJ, Kalpatthi RV, Rackoff E, et al. Prevalence and clinical correlates of microalbuminuria in children with sickle cell disease. *Pediatr Nephrol.* 2010;25(8):1505-1511.

134. Asnani MR, Fraser RA, Reid ME. Higher rates of hemolysis are not associated with albuminuria in Jamaicans with sickle cell disease. *PloS One.* 2011;6(4):e18863.

135. Aloni MN, Ngiyulu RM, Gini-Ehungu JL, et al. Renal function in children suffering from sickle cell disease: challenge of early detection in highly resource-scarce settings. *PloS One.* 2014;9(5):e96561.

136. Lakkakula B, Verma HK, Choubey M, Patra S, Khodiar PK, Patra PK. Assessment of renal function in Indian patients with sickle cell disease. *Saudi J Kidney Dis Transpl.* 2017;28(3):524-531.

137. Arogundade FA, Sanusi AA, Hassan MO, Salawu L, Durosinmi MA, Akinsola A. An appraisal of kidney dysfunction and its risk factors in patients with sickle cell disease. *Nephron Clin Pract.* 2011;118(3):c225-c231.

138. Bukar AA, Sulaiman MM, Ladu AI, et al. Chronic kidney disease amongst sickle cell anaemia patients at the University of Maiduguri Teaching Hospital, Northeastern Nigeria: a study of prevalence and risk factors. *Mediterr J Hematol Infect Dis.* 2019;11(1):e2019010.

139. Aneke JC, Adegoke AO, Oyekunle AA, et al. Degrees of kidney disease in nigerian adults with sickle-cell disease. *Med Princ Pract.* 2014;23(3):271-274.

140. Barros FB, Lima CS, Santos AO, et al. 51Cr-EDTA measurements of the glomerular filtration rate in patients with sickle cell anaemia and minor renal damage. *Nucl Med Commun.* 2006;27(12):959-962.

141. Aygun B, Mortier NA, Smeltzer MP, Hankins JS, Ware RE. Glomerular hyperfiltration and albuminuria in children with sickle cell anemia. *Pediatr Nephrol.* 2011;26(8):1285-1290.

142. Asnani M, Serjeant G, Royal-Thomas T, Reid M. Predictors of renal function progression in adults with homozygous sickle cell disease. *Br J Haematol.* 2016;173(3):461-468.

143. Xu JZ, Garrett ME, Soldano KL, et al. Clinical and metabolomic risk factors associated with rapid renal function decline in sickle cell disease. *Am J Hematol.* 2018;93(12):1451-1460.

144. Derebail VK, Ciccone EJ, Zhou Q, Kilgore RR, Cai J, Ataga KI. Progressive decline in estimated GFR in patients with sickle cell disease: an observational cohort study. *Am J Kidney Dis.* 2019;74(1):47-55.

145. Young BA, Katz R, Boulware LE, et al. Risk factors for rapid kidney function decline among African Americans: the Jackson Heart Study (JHS). *Am J Kidney Dis.* 2016;68(2):229-239.

146. US Renal Data System. 2013 Atlas of CKD & ESRD. https://www.usrds.org/atlas.aspx. Accessed July 6, 2020.

147. Platt OS, Brambilla DJ, Rosse WF, et al. Mortality in sickle cell disease. Life expectancy and risk factors for early death. *N Engl J Med.* 1994;330(23):1639-1644.

148. Hamideh D, Alvarez O. Sickle cell disease related mortality in the United States (1999-2009). *Pediatr Blood Cancer.* 2013;60(9):1482-1486.

149. Cruz IA, Hosten AO, Dillard MG, Castro OL. Advanced renal failure in patients with sickle cell anemia: clinical course and prognosis. *J Natl Med Assoc.* 1982;74(11):1103-1109.

150. Powars DR, Elliott-Mills DD, Chan L, et al. Chronic renal failure in sickle cell disease: risk factors, clinical course, and mortality. *Ann Intern Med.* 1991;115(8):614-620.

151. Darbari DS, Wang Z, Kwak M, et al. Severe painful vaso-occlusive crises and mortality in a contemporary adult sickle cell anemia cohort study. *PloS One.* 2013;8(11):e79923.

152. Gardner K, Douiri A, Drasar E, et al. Survival in adults with sickle cell disease in a high-income setting. *Blood.* 2016;128(10): 1436-1438.

153. Nielsen L, Canoui-Poitrine F, Jais JP, et al. Morbidity and mortality of sickle cell disease patients starting intermittent haemodialysis: a comparative cohort study with non-sickle dialysis patients. *Br J Haematol.* 2016;174(1):148-152.

154. Viner M, Zhou J, Allison D, et al. The morbidity and mortality of end stage renal disease in sickle cell disease. *Am J Hematol.* 2019;94(5):E138-E141.

155. McClellan AC, Luthi JC, Lynch JR, et al. High one year mortality in adults with sickle cell disease and end-stage renal disease. *Br J Haematol.* 2012;159(3):360-367.

156. Alkhunaizi AM, Al-Khatti AA, Al-Mueilo SH, Amir A, Yousif B. End-stage renal disease in patients with sickle cell disease. *Saudi J Kidney Dis Transpl.* 2017;28(4):751-757.

157. Wang WC, Ware RE, Miller ST, et al. Hydroxycarbamide in very young children with sickle-cell anaemia: a multicentre, randomised, controlled trial (BABY HUG). *Lancet.* 2011;377(9778):1663-1672.

158. Scheinman JI. Sickle cell disease and the kidney. *Nat Clin Pract Nephrol.* 2009;5(2):78-88.

159. Osegbe DN. Haematuria and sickle cell disease. A report of 12 cases and review of the literature. *Trop Geogr Med.* 1990;42(1): 22-27.

160. Sabatini S. Pathophysiologic mechanisms of abnormal collecting duct function. *Semin Nephrol.* 1989;9(2):179-202.

161. Platt OS. Hydroxyurea for the treatment of sickle cell anemia. *N Engl J Med.* 2008;358(13):1362-1369.

162. Aygun B, Mortier NA, Smeltzer MP, Shulkin BL, Hankins JS, Ware RE. Hydroxyurea treatment decreases glomerular hyperfiltration in children with sickle cell anemia. *Am J Hematol.* 2013;88(2):116-119.

163. Bartolucci P, Habibi A, Stehle T, et al. Six months of hydroxyurea reduces albuminuria in patients with sickle cell disease. *J Am Soc Nephrol.* 2016;27(6):1847-1853.

164. Little JA, McGowan VR, Kato GJ, et al. Combination erythropoietin-hydroxyurea therapy in sickle cell disease: experience from the National Institutes of Health and a literature review. *Haematologica.* 2006;91(8):1076-1083.

165. Han J, Zhou J, Kondragunta V, et al. Erythropoiesis-stimulating agents in sickle cell anaemia. *Br J Haematol.* 2018;182(4): 602-605.

166. Foucan L, Bourhis V, Bangou J, Merault L, Etienne-Julan M, Salmi RL. A randomized trial of captopril for microalbuminuria in normotensive adults with sickle cell anemia. *Am J Med.* 1998;104(4):339-342.

167. Fitzhugh CD, Wigfall DR, Ware RE. Enalapril and hydroxyurea therapy for children with sickle nephropathy. *Pediatr Blood Cancer.* 2005;45(7):982-985.

168. Quinn CT, Saraf SL, Gordeuk VR, et al. Losartan for the nephropathy of sickle cell anemia: a phase-2, multicenter trial. *Am J Hematol.* 2017;92(9):E520-E528.

169. Yee ME, Lane PA, Archer DR, Joiner CH, Eckman JR, Guasch A. Losartan therapy decreases albuminuria with stable glomerular filtration and permselectivity in sickle cell anemia. *Blood Cells Mol Dis.* 2018;69:65-70.

170. Boyle SM, Jacobs B, Sayani FA, Hoffman B. Management of the dialysis patient with sickle cell disease. *Semin Dial.* 2016;29(1):62-70.

171. Kidney Disease: Improving Global Outcomes (KDIGO) Work Group. KDIGO clinical practice guideline for evaluation and management of chronic kidney disease. *Kidney Int Suppl.* 2013;3:1-163.

172. Sharpe CC, Thein SL. How I treat renal complications in sickle cell disease. *Blood.* 2014;123(24):3720-3726.

173. Yan JH, Ataga K, Kaul S, et al. The influence of renal function on hydroxyurea pharmacokinetics in adults with sickle cell disease. *J Clin Pharmacol.* 2005;45(4):434-445.

174. Kontoghiorghes GJ, Barr J, Baillod RA. Studies of aluminium mobilization in renal dialysis patients using the oral chelator 1,2-dimethyl-3-hydroxypyrid-4-one. *Arzneimittelforschung.* 1994;44(4):522-526.

175. Yusuf B, McPhedran P, Brewster UC. Hypocalcemia in a dialysis patient treated with deferasirox for iron overload. *Am J Kidney Dis.* 2008;52(3):587-590.

176. Ojo AO, Govaerts TC, Schmouder RL, et al. Renal transplantation in end-stage sickle cell nephropathy. *Transplantation.* 1999;67(2):291-295.

177. Huang E, Parke C, Mehrnia A, et al. Improved survival among sickle cell kidney transplant recipients in the recent era. *Nephrol Dial Transpl.* 2013;28(4):1039-1046.

178. Hosoya H, Levine J, Abt P, Henry D, Porter DL, Gill S. Toward dual hematopoietic stem-cell transplantation and solid-organ transplantation for sickle-cell disease. *Blood Adv.* 2018;2(5): 575-585.

179. Knuppel E, Medinger M, Stehle G, et al. Haploidentical hematopoietic bone marrow transplantation followed by living kidney transplantation from the same donor in a sickle cell disease patient with end-stage renal failure. *Ann Hematol.* 2017;96(4): 703-705.

180. Belcher JD, Chen C, Nguyen J, et al. Haptoglobin and hemopexin inhibit vaso-occlusion and inflammation in murine sickle cell disease: role of heme oxygenase-1 induction. *PloS One.* 2018;13(4):e0196455.

181. Kubota K, Egi M, Mizobuchi S. Haptoglobin administration in cardiovascular surgery patients: its association with the risk of postoperative acute kidney injury. *Anesth Analg.* 2017;124(6):1771-1776.

182. Schaer DJ, Buehler PW, Alayash AI, Belcher JD, Vercellotti GM. Hemolysis and free hemoglobin revisited: exploring hemoglobin and hemin scavengers as a novel class of therapeutic proteins. *Blood.* 2013;121(8):1276-1284.

183. Nader E, Connes P, Lamarre Y, et al. Plasmapheresis may improve clinical condition in sickle cell disease through its effects on red blood cell rheology. *Am J Hematol.* 2017;92(11):E629-E630.

184. Louie JE, Anderson CJ, Fayaz MFK, et al. Case series supporting heme detoxification via therapeutic plasma exchange in acute multiorgan failure syndrome resistant to red blood cell exchange in sickle cell disease. *Transfusion.* 2018;58(2):470-479.

185. Laurin LP, Nachman PH, Desai PC, Ataga KI, Derebail VK. Hydroxyurea is associated with lower prevalence of albuminuria in adults with sickle cell disease. *Nephrol Dial Transpl.* 2014;29(6):1211-1218.

186. Tehseen S, Joiner CH, Lane PA, Yee ME. Changes in urine albumin to creatinine ratio with the initiation of hydroxyurea therapy among children and adolescents with sickle cell disease. *Pediatr Blood Cancer.* 2017;64:12.

187. Kaul DK, Liu XD, Chang HY, Nagel RL, Fabry ME. Effect of fetal hemoglobin on microvascular regulation in sickle transgenic-knockout mice. *J Clin Invest*. 2004;114(8):1136-1145.

188. Kaul DK, Zhang X, Dasgupta T, Fabry ME. Arginine therapy of transgenic-knockout sickle mice improves microvascular function by reducing non-nitric oxide vasodilators, hemolysis, and oxidative stress. *Am J Physiol Heart Circ Physiol*. 2008;295(1): H39-H47.

189. de Jong PE, de Jong-van den Berg LT, Schouten H, Donker AJ, Statius van Eps LW. The influence of indomethacin on renal acidification in normal subjects and in patients with sickle cell anemia. *Clin Nephrol*. 1983;19(5):259-264.

190. Vichinsky E. Clinical application of deferasirox: practical patient management. *Am J Hematol*. 2008;83(5):398-402.

191. Kontoghiorghes GJ. New concepts of iron and aluminium chelation therapy with oral L1 (deferiprone) and other chelators. A review. *Analyst*. 1995;120(3):845-851.

192. Maker GL, Siva B, Batty KT, Trengove RD, Ferrari P, Olynyk JK. Pharmacokinetics and safety of deferasirox in subjects with chronic kidney disease undergoing haemodialysis. *Nephrology*. 2013;18(3):188-193.

193. Tsai CW, Yang FJ, Huang CC, Kuo CC, Chen YM. The administration of deferasirox in an iron-overloaded dialysis patient. *Hemodial Int*. 2013;17(1):131-133.

Sickle Cell Trait

Authors: Philippe Connes, Hyacinth I. Hyacinth, Rakhi P. Naik

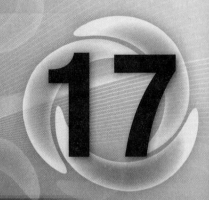

Chapter Outline

Overview

Sickle cell trait (SCT), defined as the heterozygous inheritance of sickle hemoglobin (HbS), is one of the most common hemoglobin mutations in the world. Prevalence estimates suggest that SCT is found in approximately 300 million individuals worldwide and nearly 3 million individuals in the United States. The rates of SCT are highest among populations living in sub-Saharan Africa and parts of the Mediterranean, the Middle East, and India, as well as among individuals whose ancestors come from these areas, such as people of African descent living in Europe or the Americas. Prevalence of SCT ranges from 7% to 9% in the African American population in the United States, and rates may exceed 25% in regions of malarial endemicity such as Nigeria and tribal India.[1] Evidence of the evolutionary advantage of SCT in conferring protection against severe malaria is profound and undisputed. Consistent studies have demonstrated a 90% risk reduction of severe and cerebral malaria among SCT carriers.[1]

Basic Biological and Physiological Aspects of SCT

Blood Rheology

Blood rheologic properties are severely affected in the context of sickle cell disease (SCD) and play a key role in the pathophysiology of acute painful vaso-occlusive crises and chronic complications.[2-4] Blood is a shear-thinning fluid, which means that its viscosity decreases with increasing shear rates.[5] For instance, blood viscosity is higher in veins than in arteries, arterioles, or capillaries. Blood viscosity is highly dependent on hematocrit, with viscosity being more affected by hematocrit at a low shear rate than at a high shear rate. However, the non-Newtonian property of the blood is mainly related to the red blood cell (RBC) rheologic properties (ie, RBC deformability and RBC aggregation). While a reduction in RBC deformability mainly affects blood viscosity at high shear rate, increased RBC aggregation is responsible for a rise in blood viscosity at low shear rate.[5] Several studies have characterized the blood rheologic properties of SCT carriers. Although RBC deformability is severely decreased in patients with SCD,[5] SCT carriers have a slight reduction in RBC deformability compared to non-SCT carriers.[6-9]

More recently, 2 studies investigated the changes in RBC deformability[6-9] and RBC fragility[10] during deoxygenation and after reoxygenation in SCT carriers. Using ektacytometry, Rab et al[11] described a slight but significant reduction in RBC deformability (~4%-5% compared to normoxic conditions) during the deoxygenation procedure, mainly at low oxygen pressure, which was due to HbS polymerization and sickling of few RBCs. Tarasev et al[10] found that RBC fragility increased during hypoxic stress in SCT carriers, and recovery at reoxygenation was observed only in half of the cases. When compared to what happens in SCD, the magnitude of changes is very low in SCT carriers,[10,11] but these studies demonstrate that RBC deformability measured in normoxic or hypoxic conditions is not completely normal in SCT carriers compared to noncarriers, even if the differences between the 2 populations seem marginal. Few studies also focused on RBC aggregation properties, and none of them found differences between SCT and non-SCT carriers.[12,13] In contrast, it seems that blood viscosity may reach high values in one-third of SCT carriers compared to control individuals.[12,13] Blood viscosity of SCT carriers falls between the values observed in healthy individuals and the values observed in HbSC patients, who are usually marked by blood hyperviscosity and sometimes need phlebotomy. A recent study showed that dehydration occurring in Ramadan practitioners further increased blood viscosity in SCT carriers.[14] Another situation where blood viscosity can be changed is acute exercise. It was demonstrated that blood viscosity increased to higher levels in SCT carriers compared to control individuals in response to a short progressive and maximal exercise or to a prolonged submaximal exercise.[8,9,15,16] However, adequate hydration during exercise has been demonstrated to offset these changes and to normalize blood viscosity of SCT carriers.[16,17]

Oxidative Stress, Inflammation, and Adhesion Molecules

Oxidative stress, inflammation, and vascular adhesion of circulating blood cells are involved in the pathophysiology of several acute and chronic complications of SCD.[18-20] Several studies focused on oxidative stress markers in SCT carriers. van den Berg et al[21] compared the RBC oxidative stress response to cumene hydroperoxide among normal individuals, SCT carriers, and patients with SCD. Although the oxidation of parinaric acid was enhanced in the latter group, the control and SCT groups exhibited the same level of parinaric acid oxidation. More recently, Diaw et al[22] reported no difference in advanced oxidation protein products, malondialdehyde, nitrotyrosine, nitric oxide end products, ferric-reducing antioxidant power, and interleukin-1β levels between SCT and non-SCT carriers, which confirms

previous studies.[13,23,24] Two studies also compared oxidative stress responses to a short and intense exercise between SCT and non-SCT carriers and found no difference.[13,23] In contrast, results obtained on soluble adhesion molecules showed differences between SCT and non-SCT carriers at rest and in response to exercise. For instance, Monchanin et al[25] reported higher concentrations of plasma soluble vascular cell adhesion molecule 1 (VCAM1)—a super immunoglobulin involved in the adhesion and transmigration of circulating monocytes and eosinophils to the vascular wall—in SCT carriers than in non-SCT carriers in resting condition and after a short and maximal exercise test. Tripette et al[26] found that plasma soluble P-selectin was increased during a strenuous exercise in SCT carriers but not in a control group. P-selectin is highly involved in the pathophysiology of several acute vaso-occlusive complications of SCD.[27,28] However, it seems that regular training would normalize the levels of plasma soluble VCAM1 and P-selectin in SCT carriers.[29]

Coagulation

Increased coagulation due to increased tissue factor expression, phosphatidylserine externalization, platelet activity, and thrombin generation has been reported in SCD.[30] Several studies have also demonstrated that the amount of circulating microparticles released by RBCs, platelets, white blood cells, and endothelial cells is increased in sickle cell patients and would promote a hypercoagulable state because they express tissue factor and phosphatidylserine.[31] Few studies also looked at coagulation activity in SCT carriers. Westerman et al[32] reported intermediate levels of D-dimers, thrombin-antithrombin complexes, and prothrombin fragment 1.2 in SCT carriers, compared with sickle cell patients (highest) and control individuals (lowest), suggesting relatively increased coagulation activity. The finding of higher plasma D-dimers and thrombin-antithrombin complexes than in controls was confirmed in a recent study.[33] In addition, it was found that plasma microparticle tissue factor activity tended to be higher in SCT carriers than in non-SCT carriers.[33]

In a large group of SCT carriers (n = 241), Naik et al[34] reported increased D-dimer levels compared to non-SCT carriers (n = 2630). The authors also reported that 54% of the SCT group had D-dimer levels >0.5 μg/mL (vs 33% in non-SCT carriers), which corresponds to the cutoff commonly used to predict venous thromboembolism.[34] Of note, co-inheritance of α thalassemia (which is known to decrease the percentage of HbS in SCT) decreased D-dimer levels in SCT carriers. Sickle RBCs trapped in clotted blood confer resistance to fibrinolysis by tissue plasminogen activator in vitro, and SCT RBCs produce the same effect to a smaller degree.[30] A meta-analysis reported that the risks of both venous thromboembolism and pulmonary embolism could be higher in SCT carriers than in the general population, suggesting that increased coagulation activity in SCT carriers may be clinically deleterious.[35] The effects of exercise on blood coagulation markers have been rarely investigated, and the results are insufficiently clear to draw definitive conclusions.[36,37]

Vascular Function

The effects of enhanced hemolysis on vascular function are well documented in SCD.[19] The release of free hemoglobin and RBC arginase into the plasma causes a decrease in nitric oxide bioavailability. In addition, increased circulating free heme enhances oxidative stress, which promotes the formation of peroxynitrite from nitric oxide.[19] The increased nitrosative stress also participates in the pathophysiology of vascular dysfunction in SCD.[38] Etyang et al[39] reported no difference in pulse wave velocity, a marker of arterial stiffness, between adolescents with SCT and those without. The same findings have been reported in SCT adults compared to non-SCT carriers.[22,40] However, vascular function assessed by flow-mediated dilation technique was found to be slightly but significantly decreased in SCT carriers compared to non-SCT carriers, but the level of impairment was less than in diabetic patients.[22]

No study has looked at the microvascular reactivity in SCT carriers, but an interesting study reported that SCT carriers had a reduced number of small microvessels (<5 μm) but a higher percentage of broader microvessels (>10 μm) compared to non-SCT carriers.[41] Whether the microvascular remodeling is the consequence of the increased blood viscosity (and wall shear stress) in SCT carriers remains unknown. Nevertheless, this study was performed on a small sample size of SCT carriers, and further studies are needed to investigate microcirculatory function in this population. A recent study performed on a murine model with an intermediate phenotype between AA and SS (heterozygous Townes mice) showed no difference in pressure-induced cutaneous vasodilation with non-SCT mice, suggesting no alteration of microvascular reactivity.[42]

Clinical Presentations and Manifestations

Exercise Physiology and Exercise-Related Complications

Both epidemiologic and laboratory studies have been conducted in the past to characterize the exercise physiologic responses of SCT carriers. SCT is not a limiting factor for sport participation, even at the highest level.[43,44] However, although it has been suggested that SCT carriers are not excluded from participation in endurance activities,[43,44] several epidemiologic studies demonstrated that SCT could limit individuals from reaching very high performance in aerobic exercises.[43,45] This finding is surprising because maximal oxygen consumption and ventilatory/lactate thresholds determined during a short progressive and maximal exercise test did not differ between SCT and non-SCT carriers,[46-48] even when the exercise tests were performed in hypoxic conditions.[49-52]

Nevertheless, a study demonstrated higher magnitude of the oxygen consumption slow component during a prolonged exercise performed at 70% maximal aerobic power in SCT carriers compared with a control group, which suggested slightly lower exercise tolerance during this submaximal exercise.[48] Data obtained on muscle biopsies demonstrated lower cytochrome C oxidase activity in muscle fibers from SCT carriers compared to non-SCT carriers that could partly support the slightly lower aerobic capacity of this population.[53] In contrast, a large epidemiologic study conducted in Ivory Coast demonstrated a higher percentage of SCT carriers in the track and field throw-and-jump champions, as compared with the percentage in the general population.[54] This is in agreement with small laboratory studies showing higher anaerobic power in SCT carriers than in noncarriers.[55,56] The underlying mechanisms are unknown, but it was reported that SCT carriers are characterized by a higher cross-sectional surface area of IIx fibers, which are muscle fibers involved in explosive forms of exercise.[53]

Although the exercise physiologic responses of SCT carriers have been well characterized, the question of the medical risks of SCT carriers during exercise has been, and is still very much being, debated.[57-59] Numerous case studies have reported exercise-related death in subjects with SCT over the past 5 decades. One of the earliest reports described metabolic acidosis, hyperkalemia, and a kind of "sickle cell crisis" in an SCT carrier that occurred abruptly after running only 1 mile at slightly elevated altitude.[60] Since that time, several case reports have been published on medical complications (eg, rhabdomyolysis, intravascular disseminated coagulation, sudden death) in exercising SCT carriers,[61-68] but it is difficult to prove that SCT was the original or only cause of these adverse events. Most of the studies lack prospective screening for SCT and make assumptions about the prevalence of SCT in the study populations. However, one large epidemiologic study conducted by Kark et al[69] in US Armed Forces recruits over a 5-year period showed that the relative risk of exercise-related death unexplained by preexisting disease was 28 for SCT carriers. Approximately 50% of these deaths occurred during heat illness from overexertion, whereas the remaining cases were classified as "idiopathic." Harmon et al[70] reviewed the causes of all cases of sudden death in student-athletes from the National Collegiate Athletic Association (NCAA) in the United States over a 5-year period and found a 22-fold higher relative risk of exertional death in African American Division I football players with SCT than in those without SCT. A more recent study performed on 47,944 black soldiers who had undergone testing for the presence of SCT over a period of 4 years demonstrated that SCT recruits were at a higher risk of exertional rhabdomyolysis than non-SCT recruits.[71] Further studies are clearly needed to identify factors that could predispose SCT carriers to develop adverse events during exercise, but it seems that low physical fitness, incomplete recovery during the repetition of strenuous exercise, and dehydration may be involved.[59,72]

Renal Manifestations

Renal manifestations are the most commonly reported complications of SCT, ranging from asymptomatic hematuria and impaired urinary concentrating ability to chronic kidney disease (CKD) and, rarely, renal medullary carcinoma. The unique physiologic environment of the kidney, and specifically the renal medulla, is thought to underlie renal injury in sickle hemoglobinopathies. Compared to other organs, the renal medulla is particularly hypoxic, acidotic, and dehydrated, which can promote RBC sickling, in both SCD and SCT, even under unstressed physiologic conditions. Chronic sickling, in turn, leads to vaso-occlusion and microinfarction, resulting in vascular disruption within the renal medulla. Although these pathophysiologic underpinnings have been most well described in SCD, a similar mechanism likely also underlies renal disease in SCT. Injection microradiographs of the renal medulla have demonstrated significant vascular architectural damage in SCD and, to a lesser degree, in SCT compared to those with normal hemoglobin.[73]

Hematuria is one of the most common renal abnormalities seen in SCT, although few formal studies have been performed to determine the risk. A single hospital-based study of >23,000 African American adults found a 2-fold increased risk of hematuria among patients with SCT compared to those without.[74] Impaired urinary concentrating ability (hyposthenuria) is likely also a common finding and has been observed in childhood in SCT carriers; however, the overall prevalence is unknown. Experimental studies have verified impaired urinary concentrating ability (hyposthenuria) in response to desmopressin challenge in individuals with SCT, a phenomenon that appears to inversely correlate with increasing copy number of α-thalassemia mutations and decreasing percent HbS.[75]

Repetitive vaso-occlusion and ischemic injury in the kidney can lead to progressive glomerular damage. In SCD, glomerular hyperfiltration is observed even as early as infancy. This early lesion is thought to be caused by release of vasodilatory substances that result in increased renal arterial blood flow and hyperperfusion injury. Increased glomerular plasma filtration due to anemia and its compensatory increase in cardiac output also promotes increased renal blood flow and hyperfiltration. Combined with continued vaso-occlusive injury, endothelial dysfunction, and hemolysis, this later progresses to albuminuria, glomerulosclerosis, and CKD. Whether hyperfiltration also occurs in SCT is unknown; however, the association between SCT and albuminuria and CKD has been fairly well established in retrospective analyses. Several large population-based studies, totaling >25,000 African American participants, have demonstrated a 1.5- to 2.0-fold increased risk of CKD among SCT carriers compared to noncarriers.[76,77] Most participants in these studies were >45 years of age; therefore, the degree of renal impairment in younger ages is largely unknown. In addition, the risk of further progression to end-stage renal disease has not been definitively established[78]; however, the risk in SCT does appear to be increased to about 2-fold in a general, unselected African American population.[77]

Based on numerous case reports and series, renal medullary carcinoma is an exceedingly rare complication seen almost exclusively in sickling hemoglobinopathies, namely SCT and SCD.[79] Given the extreme rarity of this highly aggressive tumor, the prevalence is unknown. The median age is approximately 22 years, it affects both children and young adults, and the most common presenting symptoms are hematuria and flank pain. The overall prognosis is poor (95% mortality rate) because most patients are diagnosed with metastatic disease. Although chronic sickling may play a part in the pathophysiology of renal medullary carcinoma, additional genetic predispositions, such as in tumor suppressor genes, undoubtedly also contribute to development.[80]

Cerebral Manifestations

Although it is well known that SCD is a risk factor for cerebrovascular complications and phenotypes, the body of work on SCT provides a mixed picture, with available studies providing in some cases conflicting results, especially with regard to stroke risk. Besides several small-scale studies and case reports,[78] there have been only 4 large-scale studies of the cerebral manifestations of SCT.[81-84] Two of these large-scale studies, published by Caughey et al[82] and Hyacinth et al,[84] reported conflicting findings on whether SCT was an independent risk for incident ischemic stroke. In their study, Caughey et al[82] reported that African Americans with SCT have a significantly higher risk of ischemic stroke. Conversely, Hyacinth et al[84] reported that SCT was not independently associated with a higher risk of ischemic stroke among African Americans with SCT. Besides the sample size differences between these 2 studies, there were reported differences in the analytical models used by both studies. Thus, more studies are needed to properly address this subject, including whether there is ischemic stroke subtype specificity or age specificity in the association between SCT and ischemic stroke. The other 2 recently published studies examined whether SCT was an independent risk factor for cognitive impairment, decline, or dementia.[81,83] Both studies were longitudinal, with follow-up time being longer in the study by Chen et al[83] (>20 years) compared to the one by Cahill et al[81] (~10 years). Overall, both studies concluded that SCT was not an independent risk factor for incident cognitive impairment, cognitive decline, or dementia. Additional analysis reported by Chen et al[83] indicated that individuals with SCT who also inherited the ε4 variant of the *APOE* gene or had diabetes had a modestly higher risk of cognitive decline or dementia, respectively.

All these studies indicate that we still do not know enough about how SCT impacts cerebrovascular health, and thus, more and larger studies are needed.

Venous Thromboembolism and Pulmonary Embolism

Given the evidence of increased coagulation and D-dimer in SCT, several large studies have investigated the association between SCT and venous thromboembolism (VTE). Based on these studies, SCT has been established as a modest risk factor for VTE among African Americans, with an overall 1.5- to 2.0-fold risk of VTE comparing SCT carriers and noncarriers.[85,86] This degree of risk is similar to low-risk thrombophilias, such as those conferred by factor V Leiden and prothrombin gene mutation; therefore, screening for SCT in VTE is not recommended. Interestingly, the VTE risk in SCT appears to be fully accounted for by an increase in risk for pulmonary embolism rather than deep venous thrombosis, a phenomenon that has similarly been observed in SCD and is a pattern opposite of that observed in the general population. While the underlying etiology of this paradoxical observation is unknown, several hypotheses have been proposed, including increased susceptibility of VTE embolization, in situ pulmonary artery thrombosis, and clot stability in the setting of sickled RBCs.[87]

Association of SCT With Diabetes

Type 2 diabetes (T2D) is a highly prevalent metabolic disease with severe cardiovascular consequences in high-income countries. However, the rates of T2D are also already high or on the rise in geographic areas where SCT is highly prevalent. For example, the International Diabetes Federation estimated that >15.9 million people in Africa currently have T2D, and the prevalence is expected to increase to 162% by 2045, a more rapid increase than anywhere else in the world.[88] These data indicate that there is a large and increasing population of individuals with both SCT and T2D. For this reason, multiple studies have been conducted to determine whether SCT may potentiate T2D and whether SCT may affect hemoglobin A1c measurement.[89] A small number of studies have also been carried out to determine whether SCT may exacerbate the vascular dysfunction present in T2D and increase the risk of T2D-related vascular complications.

Diaw et al[22] previously demonstrated that diabetic patients with SCT had impaired flow-mediated dilation and higher blood viscosity compared to diabetic patients without SCT, SCT individuals without diabetes, or a control group with neither of these 2 conditions. Skinner et al[40] recently confirmed the presence of higher vascular dysfunction in individuals with both diabetes and SCT in comparison to subjects with only 1 of these 2 conditions. In addition, retinopathy, hypertension, and reduced renal function were more prevalent in subjects with both conditions. The authors demonstrated that the degree of impaired vascular function was independently associated with the level of advanced glycation end products (AGEs). Incubation of cultured endothelial cells with plasma from diabetic individuals with SCT showed an increase in E-selectin expression, and AGE inhibition reversed this effect. These studies suggest that SCT could potentially increase vascular dysfunction in T2D by exacerbating alterations in blood rheology, increasing coagulation activity, augmenting oxidative stress, and decreasing nitric oxide bioavailability, thereby increasing the risk of developing vascular complications. Nevertheless, more studies are needed to confirm that SCT could exacerbate the cardiovascular complications classically found in diabetes.

Specific Management and Therapy

Although epidemiologic evidence suggests an association between SCT and a small number of complications, no specific treatment or management guidelines for SCT currently exist. Table 17-1 summarizes the major clinical complications found in SCT carriers and the proposed counseling recommendations.[1] Given the widespread concerns about exertion-related injury and sudden death among SCT carriers, specific recommendations regarding both SCT screening and prevention have been made for high-risk populations such as military personnel and competitive athletes.

In 2003, the US Army instituted a protocol of universal precautions to decrease exercise-related injury among all recruits, irrespective of SCT status. This formalized regimen involves advanced assessment of climate factors, adjustment of exertion, consistent hydration, and dedicated recovery time as a prevention strategy for all exertion-related injury. Because a follow-up study of exertional complications after the institution of universal precautions demonstrated no increase in sudden death in SCT,[71] universal precautions have been regarded as an effective prevention strategy for high-risk individuals with SCT, such as those in the military and high-intensity sports.

Given the success of universal precautions, up-front screening for SCT is not required.[1] However, in the United States, screening for SCT among high-risk individuals in the military and college athletes has been controversial. The military initially endorsed screening for SCT among all recruits given concerns about sudden death; however, this policy was later withdrawn in 1985 as unnecessarily stigmatizing.[90] In college athletics, however, SCT screening remains mandatory. In 2010, the NCAA approved mandatory opt-out screening for Division I athletes in 2012 in direct response to lawsuits involving sudden death in SCT, a policy that was later extended to Divisions II and III. However, concerns about stigmatization of athletes with SCT have led several national organizations to recommend against screening for SCT and, instead, endorse a policy of universal precautions to reduce exertional injury among all athletes.[91]

Conclusion

In the era of precision medicine, knowledge regarding the association between SCT and its clinical consequences has become increasingly important. Figure 17-1 summarizes the potential mechanisms involved in the major clinical complications reported in SCT carriers. Given the evidence of the association of SCT with the few complications of CKD, VTE, and exertion-related injury, research into the pathophysiology, gene-gene interactions, and potential treatments are needed.

TABLE 17-1 Major clinical complications of sickle cell trait (SCT) and proposed counseling recommendations

Complication	Recommendations for counseling
Exertion-related injury	The vast majority of individuals with SCT will never experience an exertion-related injury event.
	Even among those involved in high-intensity competitive sports or training, the absolute risk of exertional injury with SCT is low.
	Exertional injury in SCT does not seem to occur with usual exercise or low- to moderate-intensity exertion.
	Modifiable factors such as activity duration/recovery, hydration, and climate acclimation likely influence the risk of exertional injury in SCT.
	Universal precautions, such as those employed by the military, seem to mitigate the risk of exertional injury in all individuals, irrespective of SCT status.
	Screening for SCT, even in high-intensity settings, is not necessary, especially when universal precautions are instituted.
CKD	CKD occurs in ~15%-35% of adults with SCT age >45 years, which is approximately twice the risk of those without SCT.
	The risk of progression to ESRD in carriers of SCT is unknown.
	Not all SCT carriers are at risk for CKD, and those with co-inheritance of α thalassemia mutations may be protected from developing CKD.
	Modifiable factors such as coexisting diabetes may influence the risk of CKD in SCT.
	Therapies for the prevention and treatment of CKD in SCT are unknown.
	Research is needed to determine the benefit of screening SCT carriers for CKD.
RMC	RMC is an exceedingly rare cancer; therefore, the vast majority of individuals with SCT will never develop RMC.
	RMC can occur in children or adults, with ~50% of cases occurring at <21 years of age.
	Hemoglobinopathy testing should be performed in any child or young adult with micro- or macroscopic hematuria.
	Prompt referral to urology or renal imaging should be performed in any individual with SCT and unexplained hematuria.
	Routine screening for RMC among known SCT carriers without concerning symptoms is not recommended given the rarity of the diagnosis.
VTE	SCT is a low-risk thrombophilia, similar to factor V Leiden or prothrombin gene mutation.
	Screening for SCT in individuals with VTE is not recommended, and its presence should not influence anti-coagulation duration.
	D-dimer results in SCT carriers should be interpreted with caution and may not be reliable for guiding anti-coagulation discontinuation or ruling out VTE.
Stroke	SCT does not seem to be a risk factor for ischemic stroke.
	SCT should not be assumed to be the etiology of stroke in an SCT carrier, and additional workup for underlying cause should be pursued.

Abbreviations: CKD, chronic kidney disease; ESRD, end-stage renal disease; RMC, renal medullary carcinoma; VTE, venous thromboembolism.

Reproduced, with permission, from Pecker LH, Naik RP. The current state of sickle-cell trait: implications for reproductive and genetic counseling. *Blood.* 2018;132(22):2331-2338.

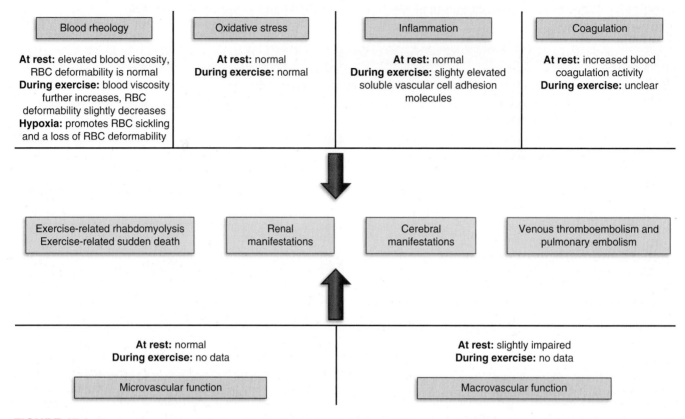

FIGURE 17-1 Mechanisms potentially involved in the major clinical complications of sickle cell trait (SCT). RBC, red blood cell.

High-Yield Facts

◆ Blood viscosity and coagulation activity are increased in SCT.

◆ SCT is a modest risk factor for venous thromboembolic complications, particularly pulmonary embolism, and renal abnormalities such as hematuria, hyposthenuria, and chronic kidney disease.

◆ SCT is also a risk factor for the rare clinical complications of exercise-induced injury and renal medullary carcinoma; however, the absolute risk of these complications is exceedingly low.

◆ High-intensity activity and dehydration modify the risk for exercise-related complications in SCT carriers.

◆ Existing data do not support SCT as an independent risk factor for cerebrovascular or cardiovascular outcomes such as stroke or myocardial infarction.

References

1. Pecker LH, Naik RP. The current state of sickle-cell trait: implications for reproductive and genetic counseling. *Blood.* 2018;132(22):2331-2338.

2. Ballas SK, Larner J, Smith ED, Surrey S, Schwartz E, Rappaport EF. Rheologic predictors of the severity of the painful sickle cell crisis. *Blood.* 1988;72:1216-1223.

3. Connes P, Alexy T, Detterich J, Romana M, Hardy-Dessources MD, Ballas SK. The role of blood rheology in sickle cell disease. *Blood Rev.* 2016;30:111-118.

4. Connes P, Renoux C, Romana M, et al. Blood rheological abnormalities in sickle cell anemia. *Clin Hemorheol Microcirc.* 2018;68:165-172.

5. Baskurt OK, Meiselman HJ. Blood rheology and hemodynamics. *Semin Thromb Hemost.* 2003;29:435-450.

6. Brandao MM, Fontes A, Barjas-Castro ML, et al. Optical tweezers for measuring red blood cell elasticity: application to the study of drug response in sickle cell disease. *Eur J Haematol.* 2003;70:207-211.

7. Connes P, Sara F, Hardy-Dessources MD, Etienne-Julan M, Hue O. Does higher red blood cell (RBC) lactate transporter activity

explain impaired RBC deformability in sickle cell trait? *Jpn J Physiol.* 2005;55:385-387.

8. Connes P, Sara F, Hardy-Dessources MD, et al. Effects of short supramaximal exercise on hemorheology in sickle cell trait carriers. *Eur J Appl Physiol.* 2006;97:143-150.

9. Monchanin G, Connes P, Wouassi D, et al. Hemorheology, sickle cell trait, and alpha-thalassemia in athletes: effects of exercise. *Med Sci Sports Exerc.* 2005;37:1086-1092.

10. Tarasev M, Muchnik M, Light L, Alfano K, Chakraborty S. Individual variability in response to a single sickling event for normal, sickle cell, and sickle trait erythrocytes. *Transl Res.* 2017;181:96-107.

11. Rab MAE, van Oirschot BA, Bos J, et al. Rapid and reproducible characterization of sickling during automated deoxygenation in sickle cell disease patients. *Am J Hematol.* 2019;94:575-584.

12. Tripette J, Alexy T, Hardy-Dessources MD, et al. Red blood cell aggregation, aggregate strength and oxygen transport potential of blood are abnormal in both homozygous sickle cell anemia and sickle-hemoglobin C disease. *Haematologica.* 2009;94:1060-1065.

13. Tripette J, Connes P, Beltan E, et al. Red blood cell deformability and aggregation, cell adhesion molecules, oxidative stress and nitric oxide markers after a short term, submaximal, exercise in sickle cell trait carriers. *Clin Hemorheol Microcirc.* 2010;45: 39-52.

14. Diaw M, Connes P, Samb A, et al. Intraday blood rheological changes induced by ramadan fasting in sickle cell trait carriers. *Chronobiol Int.* 2013;30:1116-1122.

15. Tripette J, Hardy-Dessources MD, Sara F, et al. Does repeated and heavy exercise impair blood rheology in carriers of sickle cell trait? *Clin J Sport Med.* 2007;17:465-470.

16. Tripette J, Loko G, Samb A, et al. Effects of hydration and dehydration on blood rheology in sickle cell trait carriers during exercise. *Am J Physiol Heart Circ Physiol.* 2010;299:H908-H914.

17. Diaw M, Samb A, Diop S, et al. Effects of hydration and water deprivation on blood viscosity during a soccer game in sickle cell trait carriers. *Br J Sports Med.* 2014;48:326-331.

18. Conran N, Belcher JD. Inflammation in sickle cell disease. *Clin Hemorheol Microcirc.* 2018;68:263-299.

19. Kato GJ, Steinberg MH, Gladwin MT. Intravascular hemolysis and the pathophysiology of sickle cell disease. *J Clin Invest.* 2017;127:750-760.

20. van Beers EJ, van Wijk R. Oxidative stress in sickle cell disease; more than a DAMP squib. *Clin Hemorheol Microcirc.* 2018;68:239-250.

21. van den Berg JJ, Kuypers FA, Lubin BH, Roelofsen B, Op den Kamp JA. Direct and continuous measurement of hydroperoxide-induced oxidative stress on the membrane of intact erythrocytes. *Free Radic Biol Med.* 1991;11:255-261.

22. Diaw M, Pialoux V, Martin C, et al. Sickle cell trait worsens oxidative stress, abnormal blood rheology, and vascular dysfunction in type 2 diabetes. *Diabetes Care.* 2015;38:2120-2127.

23. Faes C, Martin C, Chirico EN, et al. Effect of alpha-thalassaemia on exercise-induced oxidative stress in sickle cell trait. *Acta Physiol (Oxf).* 2012;205:541-550.

24. Shimauti EL, Belini Junior E, Baracioli LM, et al. Influence of betaS allele in the lipid peroxidation and antioxidant capacity parameters. *Int J Lab Hematol.* 2014;36:205-212.

25. Monchanin G, Serpero LD, Connes P, et al. Effects of a progressive and maximal exercise on plasma levels of adhesion molecules in athletes with sickle cell trait with or without {alpha}-thalassemia. *J Appl Physiol.* 2007;102:169-173.

26. Tripette J, Connes P, Hedreville M, et al. Patterns of exercise-related inflammatory response in sickle cell trait carriers. *Br J Sports Med.* 2010;44:232-237.

27. Ataga KI, Kutlar A, Kanter J, et al. Crizanlizumab for the prevention of pain crises in sickle cell disease. *N Engl J Med.* 2017;376:429-439.

28. Ghosh S, Flage B, Weidert F, Ofori-Acquah SF. P-selectin plays a role in haem-induced acute lung injury in sickle mice. *Br J Haematol.* 2019;186:329-333.

29. Aufradet E, Monchanin G, Oyonno-Engelle S, et al. Habitual physical activity and endothelial activation in sickle cell trait carriers. *Med Sci Sports Exerc.* 2010;42:1987-1994.

30. Faes C, Ilich A, Sotiaux A, et al. Red blood cells modulate structure and dynamics of venous clot formation in sickle cell disease. *Blood.* 2019;133:2529-2541.

31. Romana M, Connes P, Key NS. Microparticles in sickle cell disease. *Clin Hemorheol Microcirc.* 2018;68:319-329.

32. Westerman MP, Green D, Gilman-Sachs A, et al. Coagulation changes in individuals with sickle cell trait. *Am J Hematol.* 2002;69:89-94.

33. Amin C, Adam S, Mooberry MJ, et al. Coagulation activation in sickle cell trait: an exploratory study. *Br J Haematol.* 2015;171:638-646.

34. Naik RP, Wilson JG, Ekunwe L, et al. Elevated D-dimer levels in African Americans with sickle cell trait. *Blood.* 2016;127:2261-2263.

35. Noubiap JJ, Temgoua MN, Tankeu R, Tochie JN, Wonkam A, Bigna JJ. Sickle cell disease, sickle trait and the risk for venous thromboembolism: a systematic review and meta-analysis. *Thromb J.* 2018;16:27.

36. Beltan E, Chalabi T, Tripette J, Chout R, Connes P. Coagulation responses after a submaximal exercise in sickle cell trait carriers. *Thromb Res.* 2011;127:167-169.

37. Connes P, Tripette J, Chalabi T, et al. Effects of strenuous exercise on blood coagulation activity in sickle cell trait carriers. *Clin Hemorheol Microcirc.* 2008;38:13-21.

38. Mockesch B, Connes P, Charlot K, et al. Association between oxidative stress and vascular reactivity in children with sickle cell anaemia and sickle haemoglobin C disease. *Br J Haematol.* 2017;178:468-475.

39. Etyang AO, Wandabwa CK, Kapesa S, et al. Blood pressure and arterial stiffness in Kenyan adolescents with the sickle cell trait. *Am J Epidemiol.* 2018;187:199-205.

40. Skinner SC, Diaw M, Pialoux V, et al. Increased prevalence of type 2 diabetes-related complications in combined type 2 diabetes and sickle cell trait. *Diabetes Care.* 2018;41:2595-2602.

41. Vincent L, Feasson L, Oyono-Enguelle S, et al. Remodeling of skeletal muscle microvasculature in sickle cell trait and alpha-thalassemia. *Am J Physiol Heart Circ Physiol.* 2010;298:H375-H384.

42. Skinner S, Connes P, Sigaudo-Roussel D, et al. Altered blood rheology and impaired pressure-induced cutaneous vasodilation in a mouse model of combined type 2 diabetes and sickle cell trait. *Microvasc Res.* 2019;122:111-116.

43. Le Gallais D, Prefaut C, Mercier J, Bile A, Bogui P, Lonsdorfer J. Sickle cell trait as a limiting factor for high-level performance in a semi-marathon. *Int J Sports Med.* 1994;15:399-402.

44. Thiriet P, Le Hesran JY, Wouassi D, Bitanga E, Gozal D, Louis FJ. Sickle cell trait performance in a prolonged race at high altitude. *Med Sci Sports Exerc.* 1994;26:914-918.

45. Le Gallais D, Prefaut C, Dulat C, Macabies J, Lonsdorfer J. Sickle cell trait in Ivory Coast athletic champions, 1956-1989. *Int J Sports Med.* 1991;12:509-510.

46. Marlin L, Connes P, Antoine-Jonville S, et al. Cardiorespiratory responses during three repeated incremental exercise tests in sickle cell trait carriers. *Eur J Appl Physiol.* 2008;102:181-187.

47. Marlin L, Sara F, Antoine-Jonville S, Connes P, Etienne-Julan M, Hue O. Ventilatory and lactic thresholds during exercise in subjects with sickle cell trait. *Int J Sports Med.* 2007;28:916-920.

48. Sara F, Connes P, Hue O, Montout-Hedreville M, Etienne-Julan M, Hardy-Dessources MD. Faster lactate transport across red blood cell membrane in sickle cell trait carriers. *J Appl Physiol.* 2006;100:437-442.

49. Martin TW, Weisman IM, Zeballos RJ, Stephenson SR. Exercise and hypoxia increase sickling in venous blood from an exercising limb in individuals with sickle cell trait. *Am J Med.* 1989;87:48-56.

50. Weisman IM, Zeballos RJ, Johnson BD. Effect of moderate inspiratory hypoxia on exercise performance in sickle cell trait. *Am J Med.* 1988;84:1033-1040.

51. Weisman IM, Zeballos RJ, Johnson BD. Cardiopulmonary and gas exchange responses to acute strenuous exercise at 1,270 meters in sickle cell trait. *Am J Med.* 1988;84:377-383.

52. Weisman IM, Zeballos RJ, Martin TW, Johnson BD. Effect of Army basic training in sickle-cell trait. *Arch Intern Med.* 1988;148:1140-1144.

53. Vincent L, Feasson L, Oyono-Enguelle S, et al. Skeletal muscle structural and energetic characteristics in subjects with sickle cell trait, alpha-thalassemia, or dual hemoglobinopathy. *J Appl Physiol (1985).* 2010;109:728-734.

54. Bilé A, Le Gallais D, Mercier J, Bogui P, Prefaut C. Sickle cell trait in Ivory Coast athletic throw and jump champions, 1956-1995. *Int J Sports Med.* 1998;19:215-219.

55. Connes P, Racinais S, Sara F, et al. Does the pattern of repeated sprint ability differ between sickle cell trait carriers and healthy subjects? *Int J Sports Med.* 2006;27:937-942.

56. Hue O, Julan ME, Blonc S, et al. Alactic anaerobic performance in subjects with sickle cell trait and hemoglobin AA. *Int J Sports Med.* 2002;23:174-177.

57. Goldsmith JC, Bonham VL, Joiner CH, Kato GJ, Noonan AS, Steinberg MH. Framing the research agenda for sickle cell trait: building on the current understanding of clinical events and their potential implications. *Am J Hematol.* 2012;87:340-346.

58. Key NS, Connes P, Derebail VK. Negative health implications of sickle cell trait in high income countries: from the football field to the laboratory. *Br J Haematol.* 2015;170:5-14.

59. O'Connor FG, Bergeron MF, Cantrell J, et al. ACSM and CHAMP summit on sickle cell trait: mitigating risks for warfighters and athletes. *Med Sci Sports Exerc.* 2012;44:2045-2056.

60. Jones SR, Binder RA, Donowho EM Jr. Sudden death in sickle-cell trait. *N Engl J Med.* 1970;282:323-325.

61. Anzalone ML, Green VS, Buja M, Sanchez LA, Harrykissoon RI, Eichner ER. Sickle cell trait and fatal rhabdomyolysis in football training: a case study. *Med Sci Sports Exerc.* 2010;42:3-7.

62. Diggs LW, Flowers E. High school athletes with the sickle cell trait (Hb A/S). *J Natl Med Assoc.* 1976;68:492-493.

63. Dincer HE, Raza T. Compartment syndrome and fatal rhabdomyolysis in sickle cell trait. *WMJ.* 2005;104:67-71.

64. Eichner ER. Sickle cell trait in sports. *Curr Sports Med Rep.* 2010;9:347-351.

65. Ferster K, Eichner ER. Exertional sickling deaths in Army recruits with sickle cell trait. *Mil Med.* 2012;177:56-59.

66. Harris KM, Haas TS, Eichner ER, Maron BJ. Sickle cell trait associated with sudden death in competitive athletes. *Am J Cardiol.* 2012;110:1185-1188.

67. Kerle KK, Nishimura KD. Exertional collapse and sudden death associated with sickle cell trait. *Am Fam Physician.* 1996;54:237-240.

68. Zimmerman J, Granatir R, Mummert K, Cioffi R. Sickle crisis precipitated by exercise rhabdomyolysis in a patient with sickle cell trait: case report. *Mil Med.* 1974;139:313-315.

69. Kark JA, Posey DM, Schumacher HR, Ruehle CJ. Sickle-cell trait as a risk factor for sudden death in physical training. *N Engl J Med.* 1987;317:781-787.

70. Harmon KG, Drezner JA, Klossner D, Asif IM. Sickle cell trait associated with a RR of death of 37 times in National Collegiate Athletic Association football athletes: a database with 2 million athlete-years as the denominator. *Br J Sports Med.* 2012;46:325-330.

71. Nelson DA, Deuster PA, Kurina LM. Sickle cell trait and rhabdomyolysis among U.S. Army soldiers. *N Engl J Med.* 2016;375:1696.

72. Tripette J, Hardy-Dessources MD, Romana M, et al. Exercise-related complications in sickle cell trait. *Clin Hemorheol Microcirc.* 2013;55:29-37.

73. Statius van Eps LW, Pinedo-Veels C, de Vries GH, de Koning J. Nature of concentrating defect in sickle-cell nephropathy. Microradioangiographic studies. *Lancet.* 1970;1:450-452.

74. Heller P, Best WR, Nelson RB, Becktel J. Clinical implications of sickle-cell trait and glucose-6-phosphate dehydrogenase deficiency in hospitalized black male patients. *N Engl J Med.* 1979;300:1001-1005.

75. Gupta AK, Kirchner KA, Nicholson R, et al. Effects of alpha-thalassemia and sickle polymerization tendency on the urine-concentrating defect of individuals with sickle cell trait. *J Clin Invest.* 1991;88:1963-1968.

76. Naik RP, Derebail VK, Grams ME, et al. Association of sickle cell trait with chronic kidney disease and albuminuria in African Americans. *JAMA.* 2014;312:2115-2125.

77. Naik RP, Irvin MR, Judd S, et al. Sickle cell trait and the risk of ESRD in blacks. *J Am Soc Nephrol.* 2017;28:2180-2187.

78. Naik RP, Smith-Whitley K, Hassell KL, et al. Clinical outcomes associated with sickle cell trait: a systematic review. *Ann Intern Med.* 2018;169:619-627.

79. Alvarez O, Rodriguez MM, Jordan L, Sarnaik S. Renal medullary carcinoma and sickle cell trait: a systematic review. *Pediatr Blood Cancer.* 2015;62:1694-1699.

80. Beckermann KE, Sharma D, Chaturvedi S, et al. Renal medullary carcinoma: establishing standards in practice. *J Oncol Pract.* 2017;13:414-421.

81. Cahill CR, Leach JM, McClure LA, et al. Sickle cell trait and risk of cognitive impairment in African-Americans: the REGARDS cohort. *EClinicalMedicine.* 2019;11:27-33.

82. Caughey MC, Loehr LR, Key NS, et al. Sickle cell trait and incident ischemic stroke in the Atherosclerosis Risk in Communities study. *Stroke.* 2014;45:2863-2867.

83. Chen N, Caruson C, Alonso A, et al. Association of sickle cell trait with measures of cognitive function and dementia in African Americans. *eNeurologicalSci.* 2019;16:100201.

84. Hyacinth HI, Carty CL, Seals SR, et al. Association of sickle cell trait with ischemic stroke among African Americans: a meta-analysis. *JAMA Neurol.* 2018;75:802-807.

85. Austin H, Key NS, Benson JM, et al. Sickle cell trait and the risk of venous thromboembolism among blacks. *Blood.* 2007;110:908-912.

86. Folsom AR, Tang W, Roetker NS, et al. Prospective study of sickle cell trait and venous thromboembolism incidence. *J Thromb Haemost*. 2015;13:2-9.

87. Faes C, Sparkenbaugh EM, Pawlinski R. Hypercoagulable state in sickle cell disease. *Clin Hemorheol Microcirc*. 2018;68:301-318.

88. Cho NH, Shaw JE, Karuranga S, et al. IDF Diabetes atlas: global estimates of diabetes prevalence for 2017 and projections for 2045. *Diabetes Res Clin Pract*. 2018;138:271-281.

89. Skinner S, Pialoux V, Fromy B, Sigaudo-Roussel D, Connes P. Sickle-cell trait and diagnosis of type 2 diabetes. *Lancet Diabetes Endocrinol*. 2018;6:840-843.

90. Naik RP, Haywood C Jr. Sickle cell trait diagnosis: clinical and social implications. *Hematology Am Soc Hematol Educ Program*. 2015;2015:160-167.

91. Thompson AA. Sickle cell trait testing and athletic participation: a solution in search of a problem? *Hematology Am Soc Hematol Educ Program*. 2013;2013:632-637.

Acute and Chronic Pain

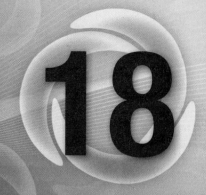

Authors: *Samir K. Ballas, Wally R. Smith*

Chapter Outline

Overview

Sickle cell disease (SCD) is the most common monogenic disease worldwide. Currently, about 250 million people worldwide carry the gene responsible for the various types of sickle hemoglobinopathies. About 300,000 infants are born annually with SCD worldwide, although due to the lack of universal newborn screening in the most affected countries, this number is likely to underestimate the number of infants born with SCD. In the United States, about 1 in every 500 African Americans are born with the disease, and the affected population is expected to increase in the near future.[1-3] The molecular lesion of the sickle hemoglobin (HbS) is a point mutation (GAG → GTG) in exon 1 of the β-globin gene, resulting in the substitution of glutamic acid by valine at position 6 of the β-globin polypeptide chain.[4,5] This single point mutation renders the sickle gene pleiotropic in nature with multiple phenotypic expressions associated with complex genetic interactions and modifiers that are not well understood.[4,5]

Clinically, SCD is a tetrad of (1) pain syndromes, (2) anemia and its sequelae, (3) organ failure, and (4) comorbid conditions. Pain, however, is the major aspect of the disease, and the acute sickle cell painful vaso-occlusive crisis (VOC) is the hallmark of SCD in general and sickle cell anemia (SCA) in particular.[6] VOCs are the most common cause of visits to the emergency department (ED) and/or hospital admissions of patients with SCD.[7] Other types of pain secondary to SCD itself also occur. These include chronic pain syndromes, neuropathic pain, and pain between VOCs. The definition, incidence, frequency, severity, and distinctive features of these pain syndromes are highly controversial and have not been investigated in depth, and except for sporadic anecdotes, the current literature, to the best of our knowledge, is devoid of such reports.

Besides controversy, another major feature of VOCs is heterogeneity, usually latitudinally among patients and less often longitudinally in the same patient. Being aware of this vast heterogeneity will streamline management of affected individuals and avoid stereotyping and faulty accusations of aberrant behavior, as has been described previously.[8]

The purpose of this chapter is to describe the various types of acute and chronic sickle cell pain. This includes their pathophysiology, clinical picture, complications, management, and effect on quality of life.

Acute Pain

Pathophysiology of Pain

Peripheral Pathway

SCD in general and SCA in particular are almost synonymous with pain, and the VOC is its hallmark. Vascular occlusion causes damage (microinfarcts) of the tissues supplied by the occluded vessel. This, in turn, involves interactions with vascular endothelium, as well as contributions from hemolysis, inflammation, and coagulation.[9] Consequently, tissue damage generates a number of inflammatory mediators that initiate an electrical impulse of pain transmitted along peripheral

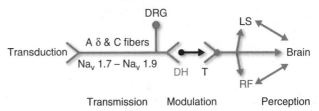

Molecular Mechanism of Pain

FIGURE 18-1 Molecular mechanism of pain. DH, dorsal horn; DRG, dorsal root ganglion; LS, limbic system; RF, reticular formation; T, thalamus. Adapted, with permission, from Ballas SK. Sickle cell disease: current clinical management. *Semin Hematol.* 2001;38(4):307-314.

nerves (Aδ and C fibers) to the dorsal root ganglion (DRG). The sequence of the transmission of painful stimuli from the periphery to the central nervous system (CNS) is shown in Figure 18-1. A series of voltage-gated sodium channels (Na$_{v1.1-1.9}$) are located in peripheral nerves. Na$_{v1.7-1.9}$ are involved in the transmission of the painful stimuli. Transmission of painful stimuli along these nerve fibers is facilitated by glutamate, which is an efficient excitatory neurotransmitter throughout the nervous system. Contrariwise, γ-aminobutyric acid (GABA) is an inhibitor of the transmission of electrical stimuli.[10-13] Excitation by glutamate or inhibition by GABA is achieved either by decreasing the negativity (depolarization) or by increasing the negativity (hyperpolarization), respectively, of the action potential across membranes of nerve cells and nerves.

Central Pathway

The DRG is a relay center that sorts the transition of painful stimuli in different directions. Some stimuli are returned to the periphery, others are directed to the sympathetic nervous system, and the majority are sent to the dorsal horn of the spinal cord where painful stimuli are processed by a number of channels. Most important among these include the α-amino-3-hydroxy-5-methyl-4-isoxazolepropionic acid (AMPA) voltage-gated sodium channels, the N-methyl-D-aspartic acid (NMDA) voltage-gated calcium channel, and the $\alpha2$-δ channel.[14]

The AMPA and NMDA channels function in tandem. Once the AMPA channels are saturated, the NMDA receptors takes over the process of transmission of painful stimuli (Figure 18-2). The $\alpha2$-δ channel[15] is also a voltage-gated calcium channel that facilitates the transmission of painful stimuli that could be inhibited by gabapentins such as pregabalin (Figure 18-3). At the level of the dorsal horn of the spinal cord, the pain stimulus crosses over to the contralateral side and ascends along the spinothalamic tract to the brain stem, hypothalamus, and thalamus, which is a major relay station of the CNS. The thalamus interconnects reversibly with other centers, most notably with the limbic system and reticular formation (mediators of emotion and memory). At the same time, the CNS inhibits the transmission of the painful stimulus at the level of the dorsal horn via a descending pathway that begins in the periaqueductal gray matter of the midbrain.

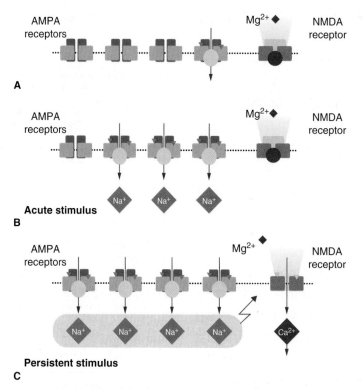

FIGURE 18-2 A diagram of a model synapse showing the α-amino-3-hydroxy-5-methyl-4-isoxazolepropionic acid (AMPA) voltage-gated Na⁺ channel and the *N*-methyl-ᴅ-aspartic acid (NMDA) Ca²⁺-gated channel in the dorsal horn of the spinal cord. **A.** A weak pain stimulus causes weak depolarization by allowing the entry of Na⁺ through 1 of the 4 proteins of the AMPA channel. The NMDA channel is blocked by Mg²⁺. **B.** Continuous weak stimulation allows the entry of Na⁺ through the other proteins of the AMPA channel but keeps the NMDA channel blocked by Mg²⁺. **C.** A continuous strong painful stimulus causes complete depolarization of the membrane secondary to maximal entry of Na⁺ through the 4 components of the AMPA channel. At this point, the NMDA channel is unblocked by the removal of Mg²⁺ allowing the entry of Ca²⁺. Michael Dickinson et al. Histone deacetylase inhibitors: potential targets responsible for their anti-cancer effect. *Invest New Drugs.* 2010;28(Suppl 1): S3-S20.1. Reprinted by permission of Springer Nature. Copyright 2010.

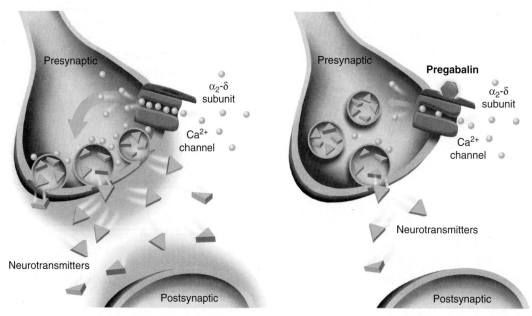

FIGURE 18-3 The mechanism of action of pregabalin. Pregabalin modulates hyperexcited neurons via the following mechanism: pregabalin binds to presynaptic neurons at the α2-δ (a 2-d) subunit of voltage-gated calcium channels. Drug binding reduces calcium influx into presynaptic terminals. Decreased calcium influx reduces excessive release of excitatory neurotransmitters (eg, glutamate, substance P, noradrenaline). Shim, JH. Clinical Application of α2-δ Ligand. Haynyang Med Rev. 2011; 31(2):55-62. Copyright © 2011 Hanyang University School of Medicine.

Eventually, the modified electrochemical impulse that started at the site of vaso-occlusion is sent to the cerebral cortex where it is perceived as pain by the patient. Pain perception is thus a subjective phenomenon and is the result of a complex interplay among enhancing and inhibiting factors at the level of the CNS. Understanding the pathogenesis of acute sickle cell pain and its impact on prognosis and quality of life justifies an aggressive approach to its management at onset.

Classification of Sickle Cell Pain Syndromes

Table 18-1 lists the major types of sickle cell pain syndromes. The following sections will focus on acute pain syndromes, neuropathic pain, and comorbidities. The chronic pain syndromes will be addressed in a later section of this chapter. The pain between VOCs is highly controversial. For some, it is chronic pain superimposed on acute pain or acute pain on chronic pain. For others, it is resolving acute pain, recurrent acute pain, relapsing acute pain, or persistent acute pain similar

TABLE 18-1 Etiologic classification of sickle cell disease pain

Acute pain syndromes
Acute painful vaso-occlusive crisis (VOC)
Acute chest syndrome
Acute abdominal pain syndromes
Right upper quadrant syndrome
Left upper quadrant syndrome
Hand-foot syndrome (dactylitis)
Priapism
Acute multiorgan failure
Neuropathic pain syndromes unique to or common in sickle cell disease
Mental nerve neuropathy
Ischemic optic neuropathy
Spinal cord infarction
Other neuropathies
Pain syndromes due to comorbid conditions
Trauma
Peptic ulcer disease
Migraine headache
Arthritides (septic, rheumatoid, degenerative, collagen)
Other conditions
Chronic pain syndromes
Avascular (aseptic) necrosis
Arthropathies
Vertebral body collapse
Leg ulcers

to what is well described in multiple sclerosis. Each group has their justifications for their consideration. Anecdotally, linking pain between VOCs to chronic pain allowed some ED providers to refuse treating patients with SCD who presented to the ED with uncomplicated VOC, on the assumption that these patients had chronic pain and should be treated as outpatients at home. Some exceptions were made, for example for patients who were severely sick with fever, had difficulty breathing, or had low pulse oximetry value.

Acute Sickle Cell Pain Syndromes

VOC

The acute painful VOC is typically defined as sudden onset of new intense pain lasting ≥ 2 hours that culminates in ED visits and/or hospitalization. It results from vaso-occlusive episodes with ischemia-reperfusion injury involving interactions with vascular endothelium, as well as contributions from hemolysis, inflammation, and coagulation, and may herald the onset of other complications of SCD such as single- or multiple-organ damage.

Genetic Markers

SCD is a complex genetic disorder characterized by intricate genotypic/phenotypic interactions that include correlations among multiple genetic and environmental markers and modifiers. Genetic markers may predict the severity of the disease and the possible or probable incidence of certain complications. This, in turn, allows for the implementation of certain therapeutic measures that may prevent or ameliorate the severity of some of these complications. Traditional approaches to identify genetic markers have included studies of transgenic sickle cell mice and natural history studies and family pedigrees.[16,17] With the advent of the Human Genome Project, novel genetic polymorphisms associated with disease have been identified, thus allowing for the performance of genetic association studies.[17-24]

Genetic markers described to date include 3 categories. The first includes α thalassemia, fetal hemoglobin (HbF) level, and β-globin haplotypes that apply globally to SCD. These are discussed in other chapters. The second category includes markers of complications associated with pain, and the third category includes complications associated with tissue damage not always associated with pain (Figure 18-4).

Although these findings are novel and interesting, their validity and utility in predicting and treating the clinical complications of SCD should be confirmed by large, controlled, multi-institution studies. The studies performed to date are too small to make definitive conclusions.

Predisposing Factors

There are at least 3 sets of predisposing factors that predict the frequency and severity of VOC. These are genetic, cellular, and environmental (or epigenetic) factors. Genetic factors include

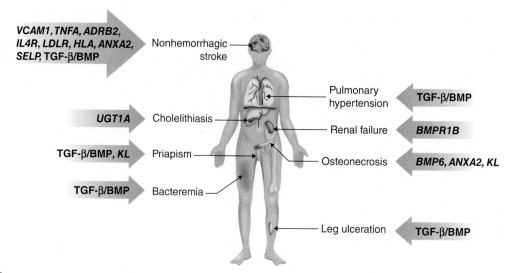

FIGURE 18-4 Genetic modifiers. Single nucleotide polymorphisms in candidate genes suggest associations with subphenotypes of sickle cell anemia. Reproduced, with permission, from Steinberg MS. Genetic etiologies for phenotypic diversity in sickle cell anemia. *ScientificWorldJournal.* 2009;9:46-67.

HbF level, the coexistence of α-gene deletion, β thalassemia, β-haplotypes, and epistatic gene modifiers. They also include sex because males constitute about 60% to 66% of admissions to the hospital.[25,26] Females, however, have longer hospital stays per admission than males.[25] Cellular factors with decreased red blood cell (RBC) deformability and increased number of dense cells in the steady state have a salutary effect, most likely because these are associated with more severe anemia and hence relatively decreased whole blood viscosity.[27,28] Patients with SCA and relatively high hemoglobin level are more likely to experience more frequent crises than those patients with SCA and lower hemoglobin level. A decreased level of vitamin A (<30 µg/dL) and nocturnal hypoxia are environmental factors amenable to preventative therapy.[29,30]

Precipitating Factors

Similar to other acute episodes of illness, VOC has predisposing and precipitating factors. Table 18-2 lists the major factors that precipitate VOCs and their reported effect on the frequency of VOCs. Stress (physical or emotional), infection, acidosis, sleep apnea, and pregnancy are associated with an increased incidence of VOCs. However, one study showed no association between nocturnal oxyhemoglobin desaturation and sleep apnea.[31] Thus, the reason why sleep apnea precipitates VOCs is not clear at present. Nevertheless, most VOCs may not be preceded by an obvious precipitating factor.

Phases of VOC

Extensive review of the literature between 1988 and 2005 pertinent to the clinical description of the painful crisis requiring hospitalization showed that it evolves through distinct phases. These phases were called the prodromal, initial, established, and resolving phases (Figure 18-5). Beyer et al[32] and Jacob et al[33] reported the evolution of painful crises along similar

phases in children. The delineation of phases of VOCs allows providers to monitor the progress of the crisis and manage it according to rational basis and minimize the conflicts that often arise about the authenticity of pain. Figure 18-5 shows a number of changes in objective signs during the evolution of the crisis. These changes can be appreciated if the parameters are determined serially and, more importantly, if they are compared with steady-state values.[34,35]

Acute Chest Syndrome

The current definition of acute chest syndrome (ACS) complicating SCD includes chest pain, fever, hypoxia, dyspnea, cough, leukocytosis, decreasing hemoglobin level, and new infiltrates on chest radiograph.[36-38] Pain is pleuritic in most patients. Abdominal pain may indicate involvement of adjacent diaphragmatic pleura. These signs and symptoms vary from mild to severe or even life threatening. Not all of these signs and symptoms occur in all cases of ACS, with the exception of the new pulmonary infiltrates, which are considered sine qua non for the diagnosis. The presence of new infiltrates with some of the other signs and symptoms is usually enough to make the diagnosis. An infiltrate is new when compared to a previous radiograph with no infiltrate. If a previous radiograph is not available, the infiltrate in question is considered to be new. It is obvious from this description that there are gaps in making an accurate diagnosis. Suffice it to say that ACS, like other syndromes, is a spectrum of clinical manifestations that vary from mild to very severe.[39] Observation and careful monitoring on a daily basis, or more often if needed, are most important in ruling the diagnosis in or out.

The incidence of ACS is age and genotype dependent, with no difference between sexes. It is approximately 3 times more common in young children than in adults but more severe in adults.[37,38] ACS is most common in SCA, sickle β⁰ thalassemia, HbSC disease, and sickle β⁺ thalassemia, in decreasing order of

TABLE 18-2 Precipitating factors of vaso-occlusive crises

Factor	Reported clinical effect
Cold temperature, including cold weather, air conditioning, and swimming in cold water	Associated with increased frequency of pain crises[293-298] No relationship between weather and crises[299-301]
Windy weather and low humidity	Associated with increased frequency of pain crises in children and adults, especially in men[302-304]
Climate and geography	Colder seasons associated with pain intensity but not frequency[305] Higher monthly temperatures associated with lower pain intensity and frequency[305] Higher monthly barometric pressures associated with greater pain intensity and frequency[305] Geographic region of residence not related to pain[305]
Infection	Often precedes painful crises[306-308] Bacteremia common in SS children <4 years old and in SC children <2 years old[309]
Metabolic acidosis	Associated with painful crises[310]
Physical stress	Associated with painful crises[311]
Emotional stress	Associated with painful crises[312]
Menstruation	No clear relationship[313] Contraception with medroxyprogesterone decreased frequency of crises[314]
Pregnancy and postpartum	Associated with increased incidence of vaso-occlusive episodes and increased morbidity and mortality[298,315-317]
Sleep apnea	Associated with painful crises[318-320] No association between nocturnal oxyhemoglobin desaturation and sleep apnea[321]
Alcohol	Decreased frequency of emergency department visits in a study,[322] but increased risk of dehydration

frequency. The incidence of ACS decreases in the presence of high HbF level and severe anemia but is directly proportional to the steady-state white blood cell count.[38] ACS is closely associated with VOCs, especially in adults.[40,41] It occurs in approximately 50% of patients with SCA hospitalized for VOC.[40,42-45] These episodes account for 15% of acute admissions and are potentially fatal.[45-48] Moreover, ACS appears to be the most common cause of death among patients and is second to VOC as the most common cause of hospitalization of patients with SCD.[49-52] Although ACS is usually self-limited and resolves with treatment, it can be associated with respiratory failure, with a mortality rate of 1.8% in children and 4.8% in adults.[40,53]

Causes of ACS include pneumonia, bone marrow fat embolism, pulmonary infarct due to in situ sickling, rib/sternal infarction, infection, and pulmonary embolism.[54-56] Approximately 50% of patients with ACS have no identifiable etiology.[40] Pulmonary bone marrow fat embolism in patients with SCA appears to be more common than previously thought.[40,53] The characteristic clinical picture is that of severe bone pain, usually in long bones, followed by dyspnea, hypoxia, and fever. Tissue infarction of the bone marrow within long bones

appears to generate a source of fat and necrotic tissue that has been demonstrated in the lung on autopsy.

At the same time, the serum level of secretary phospholipase A2 (sPLA2), an inflammatory mediator, increases in patients with ACS,[41,57] liberating free fatty acids from membrane phospholipids of the damaged tissue, which are believed to cause damage to the pulmonary endothelium, culminating in a leak syndrome, which if severe may be similar to adult respiratory distress syndrome. An elevated level of sPLA2 is both a marker and probably a predictor of ACS.

Diagnostic workup should include serial chest radiographs, cultures of sputum and blood, monitoring of arterial blood gases and hemoglobin level, analysis of induced sputum, bronchial washings, analysis of urine for fat globules, and ruling out thrombophlebitis in the pelvis or lower extremities. The diagnosis of fat embolism entails identifying fat-laden macrophages in induced deep sputum or, better, using bronchoalveolar lavage fluid obtained by bronchoscopy.[40,58]

The management of ACS involves multiple modalities to prevent possible catastrophic outcomes. The most important aspect of management is to maintain adequate ventilation. In mild cases, incentive spirometry may be sufficient to achieve this.

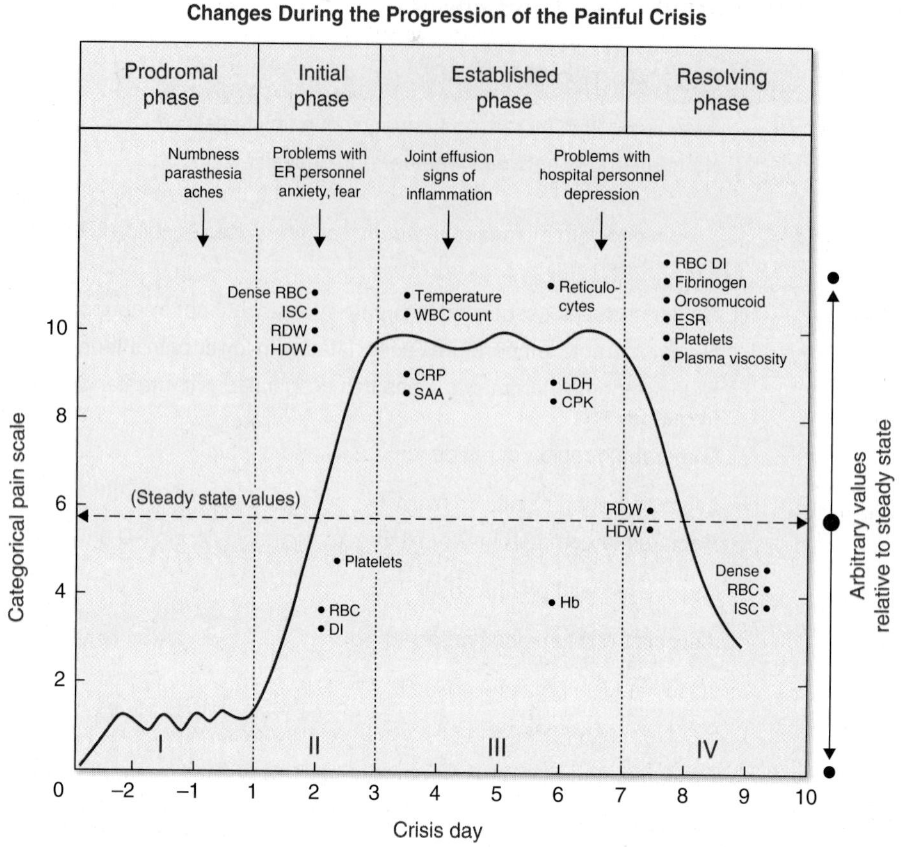

FIGURE 18-5 **A typical profile of the events that develop during the evolution of a severe sickle cell painful crisis in an adult in the absence of overt infection or other complications.** Such events are usually treated in the hospital with an average stay of 9 to 11 days. Pain becomes most severe by day 3 of the crisis and starts decreasing by day 6 or 7. The Roman numerals refer to the phase of the crisis: I indicates prodromal phase; II, initial phase; III, established phase; and IV, resolving phase. Dots on the x-axis indicate the time when changes became apparent; and dots on the y-axis, the relative value of change compared with the steady state indicated by the horizontal line. Arrows indicate the time when certain clinical signs and symptoms may become apparent. Values shown are those reported at least twice by different investigators; values that were anecdotal, unconfirmed, or not reported to occur on a specific day of the crisis are not shown. CPK, creatinine phosphokinase; CRP, C-reactive protein; ESR, erythrocyte sedimentation rate; HDW, hemoglobin distribution width; ISC, irreversibly sickled cells; LDH, lactate dehydrogenase; RBC DI, red cell deformability index; RDW, red cell distribution width; SAA, serum amyloid A. Ballas SK. The sickle cell painful crisis in adults: phases and objective signs. *Hemoglobin.* 1995;19(6):323-33. Reprinted by permission of the publisher Taylor & Francis Ltd, http://www.tandfonline.com.

However, in severe cases, mechanical ventilation in the intensive care unit is essential. Once adequate ventilation is maintained, specific treatment includes oxygen, antibiotics, simple blood transfusion or exchange transfusion, judicious use of analgesics, bronchodilators, careful hydration, and possible vasodilators. Incentive spirometry prevents splinting and atelectasis and may actually prevent ACS in patients with rib infarction.[56] Intravenous antibiotics are indicated because it is difficult to rule out pneumonia or infected lung infarcts. A combination of a third-generation cephalosporin and a macrolide or a quinolone antibiotic should be used to cover typical and atypical pathogens. Simple transfusion or exchange transfusion is indicated in patients with worsening respiratory function.[59] The beneficial effects of blood transfusion may not be due simply to decreasing the proportion of sickled RBCs; other mechanisms may be involved. One mechanism is an immunomodulatory mechanism by which inflammatory cytokines (interleukin-8 in particular) bind to the Duffy antigen present on transfused RBCs but often absent on RBCs of

Africans and African Americans.[60] In another mechanism, the albumin that is present in transfused units or used in blood exchange may bind free fatty acids, thus neutralizing their damaging effect on the pulmonary endothelium.

Acute Multiorgan Failure

Acute multiorgan failure (MOF) is a catastrophic life-threatening complication of SCD that may even occur in patients with otherwise mild SCD.[45,61] Fever, rapid decrease in hemoglobin level and platelet count, nonfocal encephalopathy, and rhabdomyolysis are associated with MOF. Prompt and aggressive simple blood transfusion or blood exchange transfusion could be lifesaving with rapid recovery of organ failure in most cases. MOF may occur in patients with a history of relatively mild disease with little or no evidence of chronic organ damage and may be recurrent. High hemoglobin levels in the steady state may be a predisposing factor. The differential diagnosis of MOF includes ACS and drug overdose. MOF is initially heralded by a rapid decrease in hemoglobin and platelet counts from baseline. Aspartate aminotransferase, alanine aminotransferase, total and direct bilirubin, serum creatinine, and creatine phosphokinase are elevated by the third or fourth day of a VOC.

Right Upper Quadrant Syndromes

Acute pain in the right upper quadrant (RUQ) is common in SCD.[62-64] Differential diagnosis includes VOC, acute cholecystitis, hepatic sequestration, hepatic crisis, and intrahepatic cholestasis.[65] Hemolysis of any etiology results in increased secretion of unconjugated bilirubin that precipitates in the gallbladder, causing cholelithiasis and sludge.

Liver involvement in SCD (sickle hepatopathy) is a spectrum that extends from mild (hepatic sequestration) to severe (intrahepatic cholestasis), with hepatic crisis in between. It is not unusual for the disease to progress from a mild form such as sequestration to severe intrahepatic cholestasis.[66] Detailed history, physical examination, and monitoring of the clinical picture, liver size, and laboratory data will differentiate the components of the spectrum.

Cholelithiasis, Acute Cholecystitis, and Choledocholithiasis

The incidence of gallstones in people with SCD increases with age from 12% in those aged 2 to 4 years to 43% by 15 to 18 years of age.[67,68] In adults with SCD, the prevalence of gallstones can be as high as 70% to 75%.[42,69-71] Although gallstones are usually asymptomatic, they can be associated with acute infection and inflammation involving the gallbladder, and they may also lead to obstruction of the cystic or bile ducts and acute pancreatitis.

Despite the high prevalence of gallstones in people with SCD, acute cholecystitis occurs in <10% of children and adults with SCD. It can occur with or without the presence of gallstones and can present as severe colicky pain in the RUQ with abdominal tenderness on physical exam. Fever, leukocytosis, nausea, and vomiting are also usually present. Nonvisualization of the gallbladder by 60 minutes after cholescintigraphy is a common radiographic finding.

Choledocholithiasis is the presence of gallstones in the common bile duct. Symptoms include dull pain in the RUQ, tender hepatomegaly, and rapidly increasing jaundice. According to a patient survey, choledocholithiasis occurs in <5% of people with SCD who have asymptomatic gallstones.[72,73] In symptomatic people, the rate of choledocholithiasis is higher, affecting 20% to 60% of people with SCD, compared to 15% of those without SCD.[74,75] Endoscopic retrograde cholangiopancreatography and sphincterotomy may be required to remove the offending stones.

Acute Hepatic Sequestration and Acute Intrahepatic Cholestasis

Acute hepatic sequestration is characterized by hepatic enlargement compared to baseline without other explanation and a ≥2 g/dL decline in hemoglobin concentration. Sequestration of RBCs often develops over a few hours to a few days, and the resultant stretching of the hepatic capsule is usually painful. Acute hepatic sequestration appears to be uncommon and may be overlooked unless the size of the liver is closely monitored in cases of acute RUQ pain. About two-thirds of people with SCD have mild baseline hepatomegaly, so change in size should be monitored. In acute hepatic sequestration, liver function tests are only mildly elevated. Acute hemolysis or other causes of hemoglobin decline should be ruled out. Recurrent episodes may occur.[76-79]

Acute intrahepatic cholestasis is characterized by the sudden onset of RUQ pain, increasing jaundice, a progressively enlarging and exquisitely tender liver, light-colored stools, and extreme hyperbilirubinemia usually without urobilinogenuria. Thrombocytopenia and coagulation abnormalities may also be present. The clinical picture suggests cholestatic jaundice or choledocholithiasis but without evidence of common duct obstruction or cholangitis. Acute intrahepatic cholestasis may prove fatal if not recognized and treated promptly.[80-84] Diagnostic evaluation may reveal exquisite tenderness in the RUQ with a total serum bilirubin level >50 mg/dL, hypoalbuminemia, thrombocytopenia, elevated alkaline phosphatase, variable levels of transaminases, coagulopathy with increased prothrombin time, and partial thromboplastin time to values more than twice baseline in the absence of accelerated hemolysis or obstruction of the extrahepatic biliary system.[80-83,85,86]

Left Upper Quadrant Syndrome: Splenic Sequestration

Splenic sequestration is defined as sudden enlargement of the spleen and reduction in hemoglobin concentration by at least 2 g/dL below the baseline value. It is associated with acute anemia. During splenic sequestration, the reticulocyte count and circulating nucleated RBCs are increased, and the platelet count is generally decreased because both RBCs and platelets are trapped in the spleen. Sequestration usually develops without warning or known cause. It may occur as early as several months of age,[87] although it is more typical in children between the ages of 1 and 4 years old. Sequestration events are less common in older children and adults with SCA. In people with SCA, the lifetime prevalence of acute splenic sequestration is 7% to 10%. In patients with HbSC and HbS-β⁺ thalassemia, splenic sequestration often occurs later in childhood or even during the adult years. Splenic sequestration in older patients is often accompanied by severe pain from splenic infarction, which can be documented by imaging studies.[88]

Patients with splenic sequestration must be monitored for recurrences. Thus, parents and patients are instructed to monitor splenic size and immediately report any marked increase above baseline. People with recurrent sequestration or a single life-threatening acute sequestration event most commonly have a splenectomy. Most people with chronic splenic sequestration accompanied by local pain and hypersplenism are also managed with splenectomy. Splenectomy for splenic sequestration does not further increase the risk of death or bacteremia[89] because most patients are already functionally asplenic. Regularly scheduled transfusions aimed at avoiding the need for subsequent splenectomy have not been proven to be beneficial.[90]

Dactylitis (Hand-Foot Syndrome)

Dactylitis is a VOC involving one or often multiple small bones and characterized by swelling and pain in the hands and/or feet, occurring in infants or young children. It is one of the earliest VOCs and may occur as early as 6 months of age.[25,33,91,92]

It is caused by inflammation due to ischemic infarction of the bone of the affected extremity, resulting in swelling, redness, and pain in affected areas. Fever and leukocytosis may be present. The episode is usually self-limited and resolves within 1 week, but recurrent attacks are common. Treatment is symptomatic, and if the attack persists, acute osteomyelitis should be ruled out.[93]

Priapism

Priapism is a sustained, unwanted painful erection lasting ≥4 hours. Stuttering priapism is the occurrence of multiple self-limited episodes of shorter duration (<4 hours) and can be a harbinger of sustained events.[94] Priapism is a common complication of SCD, affecting 35% of boys and men.[95] It is usually of the low-flow ischemic type and characterized by pain and a soft glans. Blood aspirated from the corpora cavernosa of the penis is dark, with a low partial pressure of oxygen, pH, and glucose concentration.[95] Prompt recognition of priapism and initiation of conservative medical management may lead to detumescence and limit the need for more aggressive and invasive intervention. Delayed diagnosis and therapy can result in impotence.

Most episodes of priapism begin during sleep.[96-98] Approximately 75% of priapism episodes occur between midnight and 6 AM or after sexual intercourse.[99]

Management of priapism is highly controversial. Controlled studies are lacking, therapeutic approaches are controversial and often conflicting, and medical and surgical therapies fail in most patients. Minor episodes of priapism and stuttering priapism usually last <4 hours and are often treated at home with analgesics, benzodiazepines, or pseudoephedrine and do not require treatment at the ED or hospital. Patients are advised to report to the ED if an episode lasts >4 hours. Initial treatment in the ED should include hydration and opioid analgesics. Catheterization of the urinary bladder may be indicated to promote emptying. If these measures fail to cause detumescence, penile aspiration and epinephrine irrigation should be performed. Mantadakis et al[100] recommend that aspiration of blood from the corpora cavernosa, followed by irrigation with dilute epinephrine, should be the initial therapy used for patients with SCA and prolonged priapism.

Simple transfusion or exchange transfusion may be performed for patients whose priapism does not respond to aspiration and irrigation procedures and persists for ≥24 hours.[101-103] Siegel et al[104] and Rackoff et al[105] reported significant neurologic complications (the so-called ASPEN syndrome [association of sickle cell disease, priapism, exchange transfusion, and neurologic events]) in patients with priapism who underwent exchange transfusion or partial exchange transfusion. However, analysis of their data shows that the hemoglobin level after blood exchange was much greater than the patient's baseline level. Thus, the neurologic complications were most likely due to transfusion-induced hyperviscosity. A larger study of blood exchange transfusion in patients with priapism, which maintained the postexchange hemoglobin level similar to baseline values, showed no neurologic complication in any of the patients.[106] Patients responding to transfusion therapy usually experience detumescence within 24 to 48 hours after the procedure. If detumescence does not occur within 24 hours after the completion of blood exchange transfusion, surgical intervention should be considered. Surgical intervention includes various shunt procedures between the cavernosa and the spongiosum.[107,108] Without intervention, severe priapism results in impotence in >80% of patients. The combination of transfusions and surgery can decrease this to 25% to 50%. Patients who become impotent may benefit from psychological counseling and the insertion of a prosthetic penile implant.

The treatments for priapism in boys and men with SCD were reviewed in a Cochrane review to assess the benefits and risks of different treatments for stuttering and fulminant priapism in SCD. The review found only one study of 11 participants who met the criteria for inclusion in the study. The study compared diethylstilbestrol to placebo. The only outcome specified in this review was reduction in frequency of stuttering priapism, and there was no significant difference between groups.[109] Three small series reported prophylactic benefit of sildenafil in sickle cell and thalassemia priapism.[110-112] However, it appears unlikely at present that randomized trials of sildenafil versus placebo will be conducted, due to the fact that sildenafil increased the frequency of VOCs in the Treatment of Pulmonary Hypertension and Sickle Cell Disease with Sildenafil Treatment (Walk-PHaSST) trial.[113] Certain medications, such as selective serotonin reuptake inhibitors, tricyclic antidepressants, trazodone, and other antipsychotic drugs, are associated with priapism and hence should not be prescribed to patients with a history of priapism.[114-116]

Neuropathic Pain

Neuropathic pain is usually described as numb, tingling, lancinating, spontaneous, shooting, or paroxysmal in nature, associated with a sensation of pins and needles, hyperalgesia, and allodynia (pain resulting from ambient nonnoxious stimuli).[117,118] Its severity is enhanced by exposure to either cold or heat. Neuropathic pain could be secondary to nerve injury or nerve dysfunction whether peripherally or centrally.

Anecdotally, neuropathic pain in SCD may be the result of tissue damage after vaso-occlusion of blood vessels of nerves (vasa vasorum) and includes mental nerve neuropathy,[119-122] trigeminal neuralgia,[123] acute proximal median mononeuropathy,[124] entrapment neuropathy,[125] acute demyelinating polyneuropathy,[125] ischemic optic neuropathy,[126] orbital infarction,[127] orbital apex syndrome,[128] and spinal cord infarction.[129] Among the peripheral neuropathic pain syndromes in SCD, mental nerve neuropathy was the most commonly reported. Clinically, it is characterized by numbness of the chin with mandibular bone pain speculated to result from nerve ischemia or compression because of mandibular bone infarction. Most of the reported cases occurred during painful sickle crises and resolved after the resolution of the crisis. It is more common in females and was bilateral in 1 patient. Neuropathic pain that is often associated with persistent acute or chronic pain has not been well studied in patients with SCD to date.

Management of Acute Sickle Cell Pain

Table 18-3 lists the major approaches to the management of SCD and its complications. Most important among these include the treatment of pain due to VOCs, prevention of VOCs, and abortive therapy of VOCs.

Pharmacologic Management of Pain

Pharmacologic management of sickle cell pain includes 3 major classes of compounds: nonopioids, opioids, and adjuvants.[11,91,130] Nonopioids include acetaminophen, nonsteroidal anti-inflammatory drugs (NSAIDs), topical agents, and corticosteroids. The most commonly used opioid analgesics include the μ-agonists, although the mixed agonist/antagonist buprenorphine and the partial agonist pentazocine have achieved some popularity, especially in Europe. Adjuvants commonly used in the management of sickle cell pain include antihistamines, antidepressants, anticonvulsants, and phenothiazines.

Benzodiazepines should be avoided. The short-acting opioids are usually used to treat acute pain, whereas controlled-release opioids and long-acting opioids are used in the management of chronic pain.

Preventive Pharmacotherapy

This group includes 3 drugs approved by the US Food and Drug Administration (FDA). Hydroxyurea is an antineoplastic agent that inhibits DNA synthesis through the inhibition of ribonucleotide diphosphate reductase. In addition, it induces the production of HbF. It is believed that HbF decreases the frequency of VOCs, ACS, and blood transfusions. The higher the level of HbF, the better is the frequency of its salutary effects.[93] L-Glutamine was approved by the FDA on July 7, 2017. Its antisickling effect is believed to be due to its antioxidative properties.[131] The P-selectin inhibitor crizanlizumab

TABLE 18-3 Approaches to the management of sickle cell disease (SCD) and its complications

Approach	Definition
Supportive management	Management intended to maintain the essential requirements for good health, such as balanced diet, sleep, hydration, folic acid supplementation, and regular follow-ups.
Symptomatic management	Management targeted to alleviate the symptoms of the disease as they occur. These include blood transfusion for symptomatic anemia, analgesics for pain, and antibiotics for infections, among others.
Preventative management	Approaches to prevent the occurrence of complications of the disease. These include interventions such as vaccination, avoidance of stressful situations, fetal hemoglobin induction with hydroxyurea or other agents, and transfusion to prevent the recurrence of stroke.
Abortive management	The major purpose of this approach is to abort painful crisis, thus preventing them from worsening or precipitating other complications.
Curative therapy	This is the ultimate goal of all inherited disorders. This has been achieved in SCD by stem cell transplantation. Gene therapy remains a challenging goal.

Adapted and used with permission from Ballas SK, Kesen MR, Goldberg MF, et al. Beyond the definitions of the phenotypic complications of sickle cell disease: an update on management. *ScientificWorldJournal*. 2012;2012:949535.

was FDA approved in November 2019 for prophylaxis against vaso-occlusive complications.[132]

Therapeutic or Abortive Pharmacotherapy

These drugs are used to treat VOC during hospitalization with the hope that they may decrease the duration of VOC and decrease the amount of analgesics used to treat pain due to VOC. Rivipansel yielded very promising phase II clinical trial results,[133] but a press release has indicated that the phase III clinical trial results failed to meet the primary end point of the study.

Opioid Treatment Guidelines

Management of outpatients with pain using oral opioids should follow the published recommendations established by the American Pain Society and the American Academy of Pain Medicine[134] and the National Heart, Lung, and Blood Institute guidelines.[135] These recommendations emphasize minimizing the risks associated with prescribing opioids within the framework of optimizing analgesia to achieve adequate pain relief for patients using opioids on a regular and chronic basis.

Optimize Analgesia

Management of patients with sickle cell pain with opioids can be effective if the drug is carefully selected and if the patients are monitored, although there is limited evidence in the literature. Failure to optimize analgesia may cause seemingly aberrant behavior such as pseudoaddiction[136] or serious maladaptive behavior such as the use of illicit street drugs in order to achieve adequate pain relief.[137]

Minimize Risk

Recommended procedures to minimize the risk of abuse, misuse, and diversion include the following[136]: (1) obtain detailed history and physical exam on every patient enrolled in the program; (2) document all subsequent encounters with the patient including progress notes, vital signs, laboratory data, changes in physical examination if any, changes in clinical picture if any, and prescriptions written; (3) establish signed consent and agreement forms and an individualized treatment plan for every patient and revise periodically as needed; (4) prescribe opioids for 1 month at a time; (5) establish a refill policy for every patient; (6) do random urine drug testing using zero cutoffs for opioids; and (7) document all details in the patient's file.

Chronic Sickle Cell Pain

Epidemiology and Definition

Nationally, the prevalence of chronic noncancer pain (CNCP), including SCD pain, is estimated at 14.6%.[138] However, our understanding of chronic pain in SCD is clouded by the epidemiology of pain in SCD, which includes a huge spectrum of pain frequency and severity (Figure 18-6). In addition, SCD pain is unpredictable and may be severe, disabling, and ubiquitous. Pain usually begins in infancy but becomes more frequent and severe with age.[92,139-141] A small proportion of SCD patients

account for a large share of health care utilization and contribute disproportionately to SCD costs and utilization.[142-144] Twenty-nine percent of adults have nearly daily pain.[92] Similarly, 40% of children and adolescents (aged 8-18 years) have chronic pain, and 35% of them report daily pain.[145] Paradoxically, pain is most often treated at home and rarely results in ED or hospital utilization (Figure 18-7). Worsening pain frequency and severity are correlated with more utilization of EDs and inpatient beds, even when compared to other serious hemoglobinopathies,[146] and are also correlated with reduced survival.[6]

In some patients, chronic pain secondary to SCD and its complications develops during adolescence and early adulthood.[117] Thus, there appears to be a continuum linking acute pain and chronic SCD pain. The term *transformation* to chronic pain is meant to describe this link. However, understanding of this link is incomplete. Nonetheless, research consensus definitions of acute and chronic SCD pain have recently been published, allowing a better understanding of each and the relationship between the two. Chronic SCD pain has been defined by national consensus as pain attributable by the patient to SCD, associated with physical findings or features, present on the majority of days, and occurring for at least the previous 6 months.[147,148]

Chronic SCD pain is associated with more functional and psychosocial morbidity,[145,149,150] unemployment, and school[151] and work absenteeism.[149] It may be more prevalent among older patients.[152] The prevalence of chronic SCD pain defined this way in an unselected adult SCD cohort was >50%.[92] In a 4-city cohort, the prevalence of patients presenting with acute SCD pain to either EDs or infusion centers was 68%.[153]

Manifestations, Etiology, and Complications

Chronic pain may manifest from similar syndromes as acute pain. Low back, hip, shoulder, knee, shin, and arm pain all

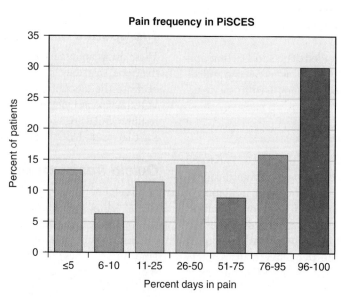

FIGURE 18-6 **Pain histogram.** PiSCES, Pain in Sickle Cell Epidemiology.

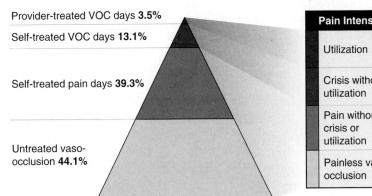

Epidemiology of pain in SCD[a]

Provider-treated VOC days **3.5%**

Self-treated VOC days **13.1%**

Self-treated pain days **39.3%**

Untreated vaso-occlusion **44.1%**

Pain Intensity	Mean	Standard Deviation
Utilization	6.5	2.3
Crisis without utilization	5.5	2.1
Pain without crisis or utilization	4.2	2
Painless vaso-occlusion	0	0

[a]Percentage of days. Utilization indicates utilization with or without crisis or pain; crisis indicates crisis without utilization; pain indicates pain without crisis or utilization.

FIGURE 18-7 Pain iceberg. VOC, vaso-occlusive crisis. Adapted, with permission, from Smith WR, Penberthy LT, Bovbjerg VE, et al. Daily assessment of pain in adults with sickle cell disease. *Ann Intern Med.* 2008;148(2):94-101.

initially result from acute and chronic ischemia. Vertebral body collapse is a nearly universal finding among adults, with its characteristic "rugger-jersey" spine. Symptoms related to avascular necrosis of the hip may be present in >20% of hospitalizations.[154,155] Avascular necrosis may destroy the hip, shoulder, or knee and require surgery in advanced cases. Arthropathies, including osteomyelitis and septic arthritis, comprise a not insignificant portion of SCD morbidity.[156] SCD venous stasis–induced ankle or leg ulcers, when they occur, require significant management resources.[157]

Chronic pain in SCD appears to arise from complex mechanisms, similar to those found in a few other noncancer pain syndromes including fibromyalgia[158,159] and functional bowel disorder.[160] It most commonly manifests in adolescence and adulthood. However, it is believed to originate earlier subclinically as a result of repetitive childhood vaso-occlusive ischemia.[161] Ischemia is sensed by fast-firing nociceptive neurons[11] via elevations of substance P[162] and other neurotransmitters. But pain is maintained by slower, repetitively firing neurons[14] in response to a complicated array of inflammatory and other mechanisms.[152] Berkeley sickle mice studies suggest that ischemia-induced mast cell activation results in release of inflammatory cytokines and neuropeptides, which promote nociceptor activation and enhance neuropeptide release from peripheral nerve terminals, sustaining pain.[163,164] In turn, nociceptor hypersensitivity to mechanical, heat, and cold stimuli may be further exacerbated by the hypoxia-reoxygenation of SCD vaso-occlusion.[165]

Later, central sensitization (CS), defined as nociceptive hyperexcitability known to amplify and maintain clinical pain,[166] likely arises from prior years of nociceptor neuronal injury due to repetitive vaso-occlusive, inflammatory, or other insults from SCD.[167,168] *Centralized pain* or *central neuropathic pain* is thus a subphenotype of chronic pain in SCD that may develop after years of repetitive vaso-occlusive, inflammatory, or other damage from SCD causing nociceptor neuronal injury

and may manifest as prolonged hyperalgesia,[167,168] allodynia (pain due to a stimulus that does not normally provoke pain and that involves a change in the quality of sensation), and loss of function. *Neuroplasticity*[169] is the ability of the brain to remodel or change throughout an individual's life, such that brain activity associated with a given function can be transferred to a different location, the proportion of gray matter can change, and synapses may strengthen or weaken. There may actually be parallel anatomic brain changes in surrounding glia (astrocytes and microglia)—remodeling—that contribute to the maintenance of this central neuropathic phenotype.[167] The most recent grading system for neuropathic pain suggests using the following: (A) a history in accord with neuropathic criteria; (B) clinical examination for the presence of negative (loss of function) and positive (hyperalgesia and/or allodynia) sensory signs; and (C) further diagnostic tests such as imaging or biopsy showing specific underlying neurologic disease or an anatomically corresponding sensory lesion. Patients fulfilling step A have possible neuropathic pain. Those fulfilling A with supporting evidence of type B *or* C are deemed to have probable neuropathic pain. Those fulfilling A with supporting evidence for *both* type B and C have definite neuropathic pain.[170]

The existence of centralized pain is supported by the finding that SCD pain derives from neuropathic mechanisms in as many as 37% of patients aged ≥14 years.[169,171,172] Patients with CS also have more VOCs, acute SCD pain, worse sleep, and more psychosocial disturbances than others.[173]

Research suggests that some SCD patients have acute-on-chronic pain, with mixed mechanisms operative simultaneously.[174,175] In this situation, it may be difficult for patients and clinicians to discern acute versus chronic pain, which mechanism(s) is operative, or whether there is underlying opioid withdrawal or opioid hyperalgesia. This makes SCD perhaps unique among other types of CNCP.

Chronic SCD pain may be complicated by organ failure[176] or by psychosocial overlay such as catastrophizing,[177] somatization,[151] depression and anxiety,[150] kinesiophobia,[178] and disturbed or sleep disordered breathing.[179-184] Fatigue may be severe with severe anemia and correlates significantly not only with pain, but also with sleep quality, anxiety, depression, and stress,[185] as well as neurocognitive function and quality of life.[186] Together, these complications of chronic SCD pain create a vicious cycle of pain, insomnia, fatigue, and psychological overlay that is its own disease.

Treatment

Opioids

Prevalence of Use

Opioid analgesics have long been the mainstay of palliative therapy for SCD pain,[187] and in the past few decades, they have increasingly been used to treat CNCP. However, opioid use is only somewhat prevalent among SCD children. Dampier et al[139,140] studied children and adolescents (aged 6-21 years) with SCD for a total of 18,377 days. Subjects reported sickle pain alone on 8.4% of days (1515 days), whereas other pain occurred on 2.7% of days (490 days) and both sickle pain and other pain occurred on 5.7% of days (1041 days). Analgesic medication (not always opioids) was taken on 88% of the reported pain days and 76% of reported pain nights. A single oral analgesic was used on 58% of pain days. On the remaining pain days, multiple analgesics were used in a variety of combinations. More frequent analgesic dosing was reported on days with more intense pain.[139,140]

In contrast, opioid use is more prevalent among adults with SCD. In the unselected Pain in Sickle Cell Epidemiology (PiSCES) cohort, 104 of 232 patients used opioids at home on >50% of their days (Figure 18-8). The frequency of

home opioid use independently predicted pain, crises, and utilization.[92] In all, patients used opioids on 12,311 (78%) of 15,778 home pain days. Thirty-nine percent of patients used long-acting opioids with or without short-acting opioids, 47% used only short-acting opioids, 9.6% used only nonopioid analgesics, and 4.6% used no analgesics. Both pain intensity and pain frequency were statistically significantly higher among opioid users. Nearly half of the patients used opioids essentially daily (90%-100% of days). Those who used opioids almost daily had the highest frequency of high-pain (intensity ≥4) days (72.4%).[188] High ED utilizers did not use more opioids than non–high utilizers.[189]

In the randomized controlled trial phase of the Multicenter Study of Hydroxyurea (MSH), at-home analgesics were used on 40% of days and 80% of 2-week follow-up periods, with oxycodone and codeine being the most frequently used. Responders to hydroxyurea used analgesics on fewer days. During hospitalization, 96% of patients received parenteral opioids, most often meperidine. Oxycodone was the most frequently used oral agent. Responders to hydroxyurea stayed in the hospital 2 days less than others on average and cumulatively (P <.022). They also had the lowest doses of parenteral opioids during VOC hospitalizations for acute SCD pain (P = .015).[190] The average oral morphine milligram equivalents (MME) per day for males was higher. Opioid use climbed with age until age 36 and varied geographically by 4 regions (Northeast, West, Midwest, and South). However, there was no consistent pattern of variation when oral versus parenteral opioid use and at-home versus facility opioid use were compared. These variations appeared to mirror geographic variations in the number and duration of VOC-related hospitalizations.[191]

Among 203 patients followed in a sickle cell clinic, 75% used opioids over 12 months. Of the 203 patients, 47% took

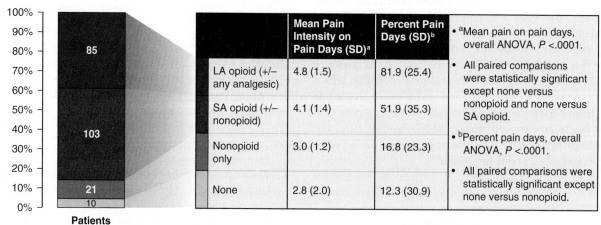

Pain Versus Opioid Use, PiSCES

	Mean Pain Intensity on Pain Days (SD)[a]	Percent Pain Days (SD)[b]	
LA opioid (+/− any analgesic)	4.8 (1.5)	81.9 (25.4)	• [a]Mean pain on pain days, overall ANOVA, P <.0001.
SA opioid (+/− nonopioid)	4.1 (1.4)	51.9 (35.3)	• All paired comparisons were statistically significant except none versus nonopioid and none versus SA opioid.
Nonopioid only	3.0 (1.2)	16.8 (23.3)	• [b]Percent pain days, overall ANOVA, P <.0001.
None	2.8 (2.0)	12.3 (30.9)	• All paired comparisons were statistically significant except none versus nonopioid.

• Fewer patients (38.8%) used LA opioids (with or without analgesics) than used SA opioids (47%; with or without nonopioids).
• 9.6% only used nonopioids; 4.6% used no analgesics.
• Pain intensity and frequency were higher with LA opioids or higher total opioids.

FIGURE 18-8 Opioid use histogram. ANOVA, analysis of variance; LA, long acting; PiSCES, Pain in Sickle Cell Epidemiology; SA, short acting; SD, standard deviation.

short-acting opioids alone, 1% took only long-acting opioids, and 27% took short- and long-acting opioids. The median daily opioid dose of all patients was 2.6 MME (interquartile range [IQR], 0-12.4 MME). Among patients who were prescribed opioids, the median daily opioid dose was 6.1 MME (IQR, 1.7-26.3 MME). Only 13% of patients used >50 mg MME daily. More hospitalizations, a history of avascular necrosis, and some laboratory parameters were correlated with opioid use.[192]

Among 3882 SCD patients identified using a national claims database, the overall prevalence of opioid use was 40% during a 12-month span. The highest use was in the most severely affected patients. The prevalence of any opioid use was highest for 20- to 29-year-old patients (58%). The median daily opioid dose was 1.85 MME (IQR, 0.62-10.68 MME). Only 3% of pediatric patients and 23% of adult patients used >30 MME/d. High-dose opioid use was associated with older age, hydroxyurea therapy, NSAID use, and frequent inpatient hospitalizations, as well as avascular necrosis.[193]

Legal and Social Context

Treatment of chronic pain in SCD with opioids is highly controversial. An uproar of controversy and a wave of conservatism in pain management patterns have occurred in response to a national opioid epidemic. After years of admonitions to use more opioids to treat pain,[194,195] opioid prescribing ballooned,[196,197] and along with it, opioid abuse.[198-202] Both prescribed and street opioid overdose and accidental deaths in the United States skyrocketed from 2009 to 2016.[203-205] Therefore, the Centers for Disease Control and Prevention (CDC) published guidelines in March 2016 that, for the first time, recommended administratively restricting or limiting the dose of chronic opioid therapy (COT). Clinicians were warned against using high doses (>90 MME/d) of opioids because of the increased risk of overdose and were advised to avoid COT, and certainly opioid dose escalation, in CNCP.[206] States and the Drug Enforcement Administration followed suit,[207] with states quickly passing legislation requiring a prescription drug monitoring program (PDMP). Prescribers and pharmacists were urged or required to securely access the PDMP database before prescribing a patient a controlled substance to obtain both their prescription history and their MME in the case of opioids.[208] Regulators suggested or enforced prescribers to conduct urine screening, prescribe naloxone, have patients sign opioid agreements, use statewide prescription monitoring databases, and institute behavioral management for coexisting psychosocial risk factors.[209] This increased scrutiny created a significant challenge for clinicians trying to manage pain adequately but safely. Together, the CDC 2016 guideline, new pharmacy and insurance administrative barriers, and the newly required safe prescribing programs led to substantially reduced opioid use, including discontinuation of opioid use for many providers.[210,211] Undoubtedly, some patients in chronic pain suffered from unjust reduction in prescribing.[212]

This shift toward stricter prescribing recommendations came amid existing skepticism among health care professionals about SCD pain reports or using opioids for SCD pain.[213-216]

A disjointed, mutually distrustful relationship already existed between opioid prescribers and SCD adults in particular.[217,218] High physician mistrust was compounded by social stigma from SCD[219-223] and tied to therapeutic nonadherence,[224,225] including problematic hospital experiences[226] and even hospital self-discharge.[227]

Benefits

Despite their heavy use, opioids appear not to work nearly as well for chronic SCD pain as they do for acute pain. There is little evidence that COT for CNCP is effective.[228,229] The 1999 American Pain Society consensus guidelines for managing SCD pain[91] and similar consensus guidelines from the United Kingdom in 2003[230] found little evidence regarding how to manage SCD-related CNCP,[231] and later evidence only supported short-term (≤12 weeks) efficacy of opioids for reducing pain and improving function in CNCP.[232,233] Surveys of patients receiving opioid therapy for CNCP report some pain relief.[234-236] However, the CDC found little evidence that COT is effective when prescribed for CNCP beyond 12 weeks.[228] Perhaps the first large trial beyond 12 weeks found no superiority of opioids for improving pain-related function. Further, this study found that adverse medication-related symptoms were significantly more common in the opioid group.[237] One review found that for CNCP patients able to continue on opioids without side effects causing discontinuation, the evidence supporting that their pain scores were lower than before therapy and that this relief could be maintained long term (>6 months) was weak. There was also weak evidence that long-term opioid therapy with morphine and transdermal fentanyl not only decreases pain but also improves functioning. However, limited evidence was available for the most commonly used opioids, oxycodone and hydrocodone.[238]

Harms

As a result of repeated or chronic exposure to opioids, SCD patients develop fairly rapid pharmacodynamic tolerance. This reduced analgesic responsiveness creates the need for a higher opioid dose to maintain the analgesic effect.[239] Opioid receptor phosphorylation, which would change the receptor conformation[240]; functional decoupling of receptors from G proteins, leading to receptor desensitization[241]; μ-opioid receptor internalization and/or receptor downregulation (reducing the number of available receptors for morphine to act on); and upregulation of the cyclic adenosine monophosphate (cAMP) pathway (a counterregulatory mechanism to opioid effects) are the mechanisms used to explain tolerance.[242]

In addition, relatively larger doses of opioids are required to treat pain in SCD compared to other conditions, due to increased renal clearance as a result of a urine-concentrating defect in SCD.[243,244]

COT for SCD may also cause opioid physical dependence (ie, adaptive or allostatic changes that modify neuronal circuitry and create an altered normality—the "drug-dependent state"—generally indistinguishable from the drug-naïve state for most overt behaviors, but revealed during opioid withdrawal or administration of an opioid antagonist as the opposite physiologic and psychological effects of acute opioid intoxication). Opioid withdrawal physical symptoms include sweating, shaking, and diarrhea. Mental symptoms such as dysphoria, insomnia, and anxiety can linger for months. Some adaptations, such as learned associations, may be established for life.[245]

Additional risks associated with chronic opioid use are well described and include paradoxical pronociceptive effects,[246] increased mortality,[247] broad endocrine effects,[248] and gastro-intestinal complications.[249]

A review of basic mouse and human studies suggested that morphine might pose other potential harms in SCD, including amplification of endothelial activation and promotion of organ dysfunction, such as retinopathy, strokes, and pulmo-nary hypertension. This review found no human data on the effect of opioid use on or association of opioid use with these outcomes in SCD.[250] However, a Cochrane review of COT for CNCP in adults documented an absolute event rate of 78% for any adverse event with opioids in trials using a placebo as comparison. The absolute event rate for any serious adverse event was 7.5%. However, a number of adverse events that reviewers expected to occur with opioid use were not reported in the included Cochrane reviews.[251] No Cochrane reviews or overviews were found regarding the efficacy and safety of opi-oid doses of ≥200 MME/d (a not uncommon SCD dose) for CNCP.[252]

Of note, a case-control study that selected SCD patients on COT and not on COT found that COT was associated with a paradoxical increase in CS using quantitative sensory testing, with an index of 0.34 versus –0.10. In addition, the expected correlation between CS and levels of noncrisis pain, which was found in the group not on COT, essentially vanished in the COT group. In addition, over 3 months, COT patients reported 3 times greater pain interference with activities on days of non-crisis pain, twice the fatigue, and >3 times higher pain inten-sity. The authors acknowledged these associations were not proof of causation and raised the possibility of confounding by indication for treatment (sicker patients were those who required COT). The authors wondered whether COT for SCD was good (ie, it reduced clinical pain irrespective of the under-lying level of CS), whether it was bad (ie, COT increased CS in a dose-independent manner), or whether their findings could be explained by previous research[217] showing that opioids can produce both anti- and pronociceptive effects.[218]

However, there is little evidence that COT for SCD per se results in higher mortality, despite the evidence of increased mortality for patients with other disorders. A study of a CDC database covering the years 1995 through 2013 found that, despite substantial opioid use, the 95 SCD deaths due to opioid-related mortality (ORM) constituted a low annual rate (0.77%) compared with the ORM rates of 4.4%, 2.1%, and 4.5% for fibromyalgia, low back pain, and migraine, respectively.[220]

Similarly, a study of SCD hospitalizations from the National Inpatient Sample from 1998 to 2013 (n = 1,755,200) demon-strated that in-hospital mortality rates for SCD declined annually by 9.9% from 1998 to 2002 and were flat thereaf-ter. There was no increase in in-hospital SCD mortality dur-ing 1999 to 2013, the period of the opioid epidemic, during which there was a 350% increase in overall ORM.[221] Similarly, a claims-based study of opioid use among SCD patients found no increased opioid use during the period of the opioid epi-demic, although consistently over the years, it was higher for adults than for children.[146]

Misuse

Opioids are well known to be associated with substance use disorder, defined by the *Diagnostic and Statistical Manual of Mental Disorders, Fifth Edition* (DSM-5) in 2013. The rede-fined diagnosis of substance use disorder combines the terms *abuse* and *dependence* into one disorder, arguably an improve-ment. Both are maladaptive patterns of opioid use, leading to clinically significant impairment or distress. However, the old terms *abuse*[253] and *misuse* are still relevant. Misuse of pre-scription opioids is defined by the National Survey on Drug Use and Health as use in any way not directed by a prescrib-ing provider, including using another's prescription or using greater amounts, more often, or longer than directed.[254] Mis-use is a significant risk factors for future or concurrent use of heroin.[255] However, the older terms are being subsumed by a new term, *opioid use disorder*, to determine when problematic use requires treatment by an addictionologist or some other intervention.

The controversial term *pseudoaddiction* has been described as "an abuse of medications driven by unrelieved pain that appears on the surface to be very similar to the behavior pat-terns of addicts."[256] Pseudoaddiction should be extinguishable by adequate prescription of analgesics. However, to profession-ally distinguish pseudoaddiction from opioid use disorder, the gold standard is a time-intensive, resource-intensive interview by a trained addictionologist or mental health professional, using the DSM-5 criteria. If opioid use disorder were con-firmed in SCD patients, they would require cotreatment by an addictionologist, as well as appropriate management of their SCD pain by their provider.[257]

A shift toward stricter prescribing recommendations in response to the recent opioid epidemic has empowered already existing skepticism among health care professionals about SCD pain and reinforced hesitancy to use opioids in SCD.[213-216,258,259] This only exacerbates the disjointed, mutually distrustful rela-tionship that has developed between opioid prescribers and adults with SCD, mentioned earlier.[217,218]

Recommendations

Given the risks, harms, and limited benefit, caution must be exercised when deciding whether to use COT for chronic SCD pain. However, there are few viable alternatives. CNCP care can be fraught with frustration and mutual distrust between patient and provider.[258,259] Using an especially limiting COT in CNCP requires close, open communication, physician empa-thy, and mutual trust.[260]

The ideal management of chronic SCD pain occurs when a multidisciplinary team is available.[261] The team takes into account individual variability in the environment and lifestyles of the patient. It may assess stress and health-related quality of life. Scales include our own Sickle Cell Stress Scale,[188,262,263] the Sickle Cell Self-Efficacy Scale,[264,265] and ASCQ-Me (Adult Sickle Cell Quality of Life Measurement Information System), which are all specific for SCD,[266-268] and the Patient-Reported Outcomes Measurement Information System (PROMIS).[269,270] PROMIS may screen for depression and anxiety, substance misuse, or opioid use disorder. Although little literature supports the efficacy and success of tapering COT or using aids to enable easier tapering,[271] guidelines recommend that if the evaluation suggests chemical coping with opioids or if an initial trial of COT for a few months is unsuccessful, the team should taper and/or stop COT.[206,272] Indicators of successful COT are improved function, improved analgesia, improved health care utilization, and no evidence of misuse or aberrant behavior.

However, the multidisciplinary team and resources necessary for formal psychological or health-related quality of life screening and behavioral therapy are not available to many clinicians caring for SCD patients. In the absence of these resources, opioid prescribers for SCD patients can themselves conduct simple basic screening for opioid safety and appropriateness. It only takes a few seconds to ask a couple of simple, specific psychosocial and other behavioral questions that predict opioid misuse or the risk thereof in general patients: Is there a personal or family history of aberrant alcohol- or drug-related behaviors? Is there a history of physical or sexual abuse? Are there any coexisting psychiatric conditions? Is there a smoking history? Does the patient have difficulty with coping, antisocial personality, and/or impulsivity?[273]

Until evidence is given to the contrary, all pain reports from SCD patients should be believed, and tiered therapy, including opioids, should be applied with the goal of analgesia, using tools such as the World Health Organization's Analgesic Ladder.[274]

The role for screening for recreational drug use and/or presence of prescribed opioids in the practice of pain medicine is mainly regulatory. Screening or monitoring has not been shown to limit use. In 2008, routine screening for illicit drug use was not deemed to be evidence based by many authorities.[275] However, a later expert panel recommended that urine drug screening must be done routinely as part of an overall best practice program in order to prescribe COT.[276] Nonetheless, monitoring for misuse and communicating suspicious results of screening, while continuing to prescribe, may actually enhance trust rather than degrade it. Prescribers may choose one of many candidate screening surveys of opioid misuse or the risk thereof, including the Screener and Opioid Assessment for Patients with Pain–Revised (SOAPP-R)[222]; the Pain Assessment and Documentation Tool (PADT)[223,224]; the Current Opioid Misuse Measure (COMM)[225,226]; the Tobacco, Alcohol, Prescription Medication, and Other Substance Use (TAPS) tool[227]; the CAGE[277] Questions Adapted to Include Drugs (CAGE-AID)[278]; the Prescription CAGE (RxCAGE)[279]; the Prescription Opioid Misuse Index[280,281]; and the Prescription Drug Use Questionnaire (PDUQ)[282] and its companion, the self-administered PDUQp.[283] To date, only the COMM has been used to distinguish among tolerance, physical dependence, recreational drug use, and opioid misuse in SCD patients. These authors calculated a risk behavior subset score from the COMM that excluded questions about utilization or mood and found a higher risk for medication misuse among SCD patients on COT. However, this was a case-control study, rather than a cross-sectional study, so it was not valid evidence from which to quote a misuse prevalence rate.

Other Treatments

Safe and effective therapy for chronic SCD pain means limiting or avoiding the use of opioids when other, less dangerous or abuse-prone therapies will be effective. Multimodal, non-pharmacologic biobehavioral therapies, such as cognitive-behavioral therapy, physical therapy with pain education,[284-286] and mindfulness meditation,[287] and alternative analgesic pain management, such as gabapentin or citalopram, are all recommended, but recent reviews have found little evidence for their long-term efficacy.[288-290] Vitamin D use among SCD patients, who are often vitamin D deficient, has been reported to curb pain, but studies did not measure opioid use.[291,292]

Conclusion

Pain is the hallmark of SCD and the most frequent reason for hospital admissions. Pain sensation results from a very complex and interactive series of mechanisms integrated at all levels of the nervous system—from the peripheral nerve fibers to the higher cerebral cortex where pain is perceived. Recently, there have been major advances in understanding the pathophysiologic mechanisms of pain sensation and its complications, as well as newer approaches that impact the assessment and management of patients with sickle cell pain. Progress in this area may minimize the pain and suffering of patients with SCD and improve their quality of life.

Case Study

A 38-year-old African American woman with SCA was admitted to the gynecologic service with pelvic pain that was not typical of her usual crisis (VOC) pain. The pain was constant, dull, deep, and crampy, with an intensity score of 10 on a scale of 0 to 10. In contrast, her usual VOC pain was throbbing and involved the low back, chest, arms, and legs. Her obstetric history was significant for 1 spontaneous abortion and 1 spontaneous vaginal delivery at 8 months and a dilation and evacuation for retained products of conception. She underwent a laparoscopic tubal ligation and left oophorectomy 2 weeks before admission. Complications of her SCA included >4 severe VOCs per year, which were usually treated with hydromorphone (Dilaudid) 3 to 4 mg parenterally every 2 to 3 hours. Milder episodes of pain were treated at home with oxycodone and acetaminophen (Percocet). Other complications included a history of recurrent pneumonia, ACS, cholecystectomy, and alloimmunization (5 clinically significant alloantibodies) secondary to multiple transfusions for severe anemia. Her baseline hemoglobin level was 5 to 6 g/dL.

Physical examination showed a sick woman complaining of severe low abdominal pain. She had a temperature of 39.2°C (102.6°F), respiratory rate of 26 breaths/min, and pulse of 100 bpm. She had diffuse abdominal tenderness that was most severe in the low abdomen and worse on the right than the left. Pelvic examination was difficult to assess due to guarding. The hemoglobin level decreased to 4.7 g/dL on admission, and the white blood cell count was 36,400/μL.

Management consisted of hydration, antibiotics, and blood transfusion. Pain was initially treated with intramuscular hydromorphone (Dilaudid) 4 mg every 2 hours and then intravenous morphine sulfate 6 mg every 2 hours when venous access became available. She experienced no pain relief with morphine sulfate. Recommendations included increasing the dose of intravenous morphine to 20 mg every 2 hours and continuing pain assessment and monitoring. With 15 to 20 mg of intravenous morphine, she experienced 40% to 50% pain relief, comparable to that experienced with 4 mg of intramuscular hydromorphone. However, she continued to complain of the unusual nature of the pain and insisted that something was wrong with her other than VOC. She continued to have fever and did not respond to antibiotics.

Magnetic resonance imaging of the pelvis showed bilateral adnexal masses suggestive of tubo-ovarian abscesses. Exploratory laparotomy revealed a large pelvic abscess in the cul-de-sac, with multiple bowel adhesions. The abscess was drained, and the adhesions were lysed. Cultures grew *Enterococcus* species. The patient improved gradually after surgery and was afebrile by the third postoperative day. Pain intensity decreased gradually, opioids were tapered gradually, and she began oral acetaminophen and oxycodone (Percocet) 10 days after surgery and was discharged from the hospital 4 days later.

Comments

This case illustrates 2 important points in the management of patients with acute VOCs. The first pertains to equivalent dosing of analgesics. Replacing one opioid with another must consider equianalgesic doses; a 6-mg dose of morphine is not equivalent to 4 mg of hydromorphone, so the morphine dose had to be increased. Alternatively, the same dose of hydromorphone can be administered either intravenously or intramuscularly, although the former is preferable. The second point highlighted by this case is that persistent or worsening pain despite adequate management suggests progression of the nociceptive process.

In addition, the patient's own assessment that the pain was unusual compared to her typical VOCs should provoke an aggressive search for other causes. In this case, pelvic abscesses caused progressive nociception, which was relieved with drainage followed by antibiotic therapy.

High-Yield Facts

◆ The term *sickle cell anemia* (SCA) defines a combination of HbSS and sickle β^0 thalassemia.

◆ The pathophysiology of sickle cell VOC is not simply due to vascular occlusion. Its onset is quickly associated with enhanced hemolysis, cellular interactions with the endothelium, and activation of inflammatory and coagulation parameters.

◆ SCD pain syndromes include acute pain, chronic pain, neuropathic pain, persistent pain, drug-induced pain, or a combination of any 2 or more of these types of pain. The specific definition of the different pain syndromes is highly controversial among the experts.

◆ ACS is 3 times more common in children than in adults but is more severe in adults.

◆ Acute MOF is a potentially catastrophic life-threatening complication of SCD that may even occur in patients with otherwise mild disease.

High-Yield Facts (Cont.)

◆ Opioids are the mainstay of palliative therapy of sickle cell pain, especially in adults, provided they are used wisely. Short-acting opioids are best for acute pain, and long-acting opioids are best for chronic pain.

◆ Hydroxyurea, L-glutamine, and crizanlizumab are approved by the FDA for preventing or decreasing the frequency of VOCs.

◆ Chronic pain secondary to SCD and its complications seems to develop during adolescence and young adulthood, at least in some patients. The link between acute and chronic pain is not well defined.

◆ Chronic SCD pain is associated with more functional and psychosocial morbidity, unemployment, and school and work absenteeism and may be prevalent among older patients.

◆ Central sensitization, defined as nociceptive hyperexcitability known to amplify and maintain clinical pain, likely arises from prior years of nociceptor neuronal injury due to repetitive vaso-occlusive, inflammatory, or other insults from SCD.

◆ Although opioids are the mainstay of treatment of acute pain in SCD, their role in the treatment of chronic pain is highly controversial.

◆ The ideal management of chronic SCD pain occurs when a multidisciplinary team is available.

References

1. Odame I. Developing a global agenda for sickle cell disease: report of an international symposium and workshop in Cotonou, Republic of Benin. *Am J Prev Med.* 2010;38(4 suppl):S571-S575.
2. Piel FB, Hay SI, Gupta S, Weatherall DJ, Williams TN. Global burden of sickle cell anaemia in children under five, 2010-2050: modelling based on demographics, excess mortality, and interventions. *PLoS Med.* 2013;10(7):e1001484.
3. Kato GJ, Piel FB, Reid CD, et al. Sickle cell disease. *Nat Rev Dis Primers.* 2018;4:18010.
4. Ingram VM. A specific chemical difference between the globins of normal human and sickle-cell anaemia haemoglobin. *Nature.* 1956;178(4537):792-794.
5. Ingram VM. Gene mutations in human haemoglobin: the chemical difference between normal and sickle cell haemoglobin. *Nature.* 1957;180(4581):326-328.
6. Platt OS, Thorington BD, Brambilla DJ, et al. Pain in sickle cell disease. Rates and risk factors. *N Engl J Med.* 1991;325(1): 11-16.
7. Ballas SK, Lieff S, Benjamin LJ, et al. Definitions of the phenotypic manifestations of sickle cell disease. *Am J Hematol.* 2010;85(1): 6-13.
8. Ruta NS, Ballas SK. The opioid drug epidemic and sickle cell disease: guilt by association. *Pain Med.* 2016;17(10):1793-1798.
9. Zhang D, Xu C, Manwani D, Frenette PS. Neutrophils, platelets, and inflammatory pathways at the nexus of sickle cell disease pathophysiology. *Blood.* 2016;127(7):801-809.
10. Fields HL. *Pain.* New York: McGraw-Hill; 1987.
11. Fishman SM, Ballantyne JC, Rathmell JP. *Bonica's Management of Pain.* 4th ed. Wolters Kluwer; 2010.
12. McMahon SB, Koltzenburg M. *Wall and Melzack's Textbook of Pain.* 5th ed. Elsevier Churchill Livingstone; 2006.
13. Wall PD, Melzack R. *Textbook of Pain.* 3rd ed. Churchill Livingstone; 1994.
14. Ballas SK. Pathophysiology and principles of management of the many faces of the acute vaso-occlusive crisis in patients with sickle cell disease. *Eur J Haematol.* 2015;95(2):113-123.
15. Shim JH. Clinical application of α2-δ ligand. *Hanyang Med Rev.* 2011;31(2):55-62.
16. Fabry ME. Molecular genetics of the human globin genes. In: Steinberg MH, Forget BG, Higgs D R, Nagel RL, eds. *Disorders of Hemoglobin: Genetics, Pathophysiology and Clinical Management.* Cambridge University Press; 2001:910-940.
17. Thein SL. Genetic modifiers of the beta-haemoglobinopathies. *Br J Haematol.* 2008;141(3):357-366.
18. Ashley-Koch AE, Elliott L, Kail ME, et al. Identification of genetic polymorphisms associated with risk for pulmonary hypertension in sickle cell disease. *Blood.* 2008;111(12):5721-5726.
19. Sebastiani P, Solovieff N, Hartley SW, et al. Genetic modifiers of the severity of sickle cell anemia identified through a genome-wide association study. *Am J Hematol.* 2010;85(1):29-35.
20. Steinberg MH. SNPing away at sickle cell pathophysiology. *Blood.* 2008;111(12):5420-5421.
21. Steinberg MH. Genetic etiologies for phenotypic diversity in sickle cell anemia. *Sci World J.* 2009;9:46-67.
22. Steinberg MH, Adewoye AH. Modifier genes and sickle cell anemia. *Curr Opin Hematol.* 2006;13(3):131-136.
23. Steinberg MH, Sebastiani P. Genetic modifiers of sickle cell disease. *Am J Hematol.* 2012;87(8):795-803.
24. Thein SL. Genetic modifiers of sickle cell disease. *Hemoglobin.* 2011;35(5-6):589-606.
25. Ballas SK, Lusardi M. Hospital readmission for adult acute sickle cell painful episodes: frequency, etiology, and prognostic significance. *Am J Hematol.* 2005;79(1):17-25.
26. Udezue E, Girshab AM. Differences between males and females in adult sickle cell pain crisis in eastern Saudi Arabia. *Ann Saudi Med.* 2004;24(3):179-182.
27. Ballas SK, Larner J, Smith ED, Surrey S, Schwartz E, Rappaport EF. Rheologic predictors of the severity of the painful sickle cell crisis. *Blood.* 1988;72(4):1216-1223.
28. Lande WM, Andrews DL, Clark MR, et al. The incidence of painful crisis in homozygous sickle cell disease: correlation with red cell deformability. *Blood.* 1988;72(6):2056-2059.
29. Schall JI, Zemel BS, Kawchak DA, Ohene-Frempong K, Stallings VA. Vitamin A status, hospitalizations, and other

outcomes in young children with sickle cell disease. *J Pediatr.* 2004;145(1):99-106.

30. Hargrave DR, Wade A, Evans JP, Hewes DK, Kirkham FJ. Nocturnal oxygen saturation and painful sickle cell crises in children. *Blood.* 2003;101(3):846-848.

31. Smith WR, Coyne P, Smith VS, Mercier B. Temperature changes, temperature extremes, and their relationship to emergency department visits and hospitalizations for sickle cell crisis. *Pain Manag Nurs.* 2003;4(3):106-111.

32. Beyer JE, Simmons LE, Woods GM, Woods PM. A chronology of pain and comfort in children with sickle cell disease. *Arch Pediatr Adolesc Med.* 1999;153(9):913-920.

33. Jacob E, Beyer JE, Miaskowski C, Savedra M, Treadwell M, Styles L. Are there phases to the vaso-occlusive painful episode in sickle cell disease? *J Pain Symptom Manage.* 2005;29(4):392-400.

34. Ballas SK. More definitions in sickle cell disease: steady state v base line data. *Am J Hematol.* 2012;87(3):338.

35. Ballas SK, Marcolina MJ. Hyperhemolysis during the evolution of uncomplicated acute painful episodes in patients with sickle cell anemia. *Transfusion.* 2006;46(1):105-110.

36. Charache S, Scott JC, Charache P. "Acute chest syndrome" in adults with sickle cell anemia. Microbiology, treatment, and prevention. *Arch Intern Med.* 1979;139(1):67-69.

37. Vichinsky EP, Styles LA, Colangelo LH, Wright EC, Castro O, Nickerson B. Acute chest syndrome in sickle cell disease: clinical presentation and course. Cooperative Study of Sickle Cell Disease. *Blood.* 1997;89(5):1787-1792.

38. Castro O, Brambilla DJ, Thorington B, et al. The acute chest syndrome in sickle cell disease: incidence and risk factors. The Cooperative Study of Sickle Cell Disease. *Blood.* 1994;84(2):643-649.

39. Miller ST. How I treat acute chest syndrome in children with sickle cell disease. *Blood.* 2011;117(20):5297-5305.

40. Vichinsky EP, Neumayr LD, Earles AN, et al. Causes and outcomes of the acute chest syndrome in sickle cell disease. National Acute Chest Syndrome Study Group. *N Engl J Med.* 2000;342(25):1855-1865.

41. Styles LA, Schalkwijk CG, Aarsman AJ, Vichinsky EP, Lubin BH, Kuypers FA. Phospholipase A2 levels in acute chest syndrome of sickle cell disease. *Blood.* 1996;87(6):2573-2578.

42. Vichinsky EP, Lubin BH. Sickle cell anemia and related hemoglobinopathies. *Pediatr Clin North Am.* 1980;27(2):429-447.

43. Sprinkle RH, Cole T, Smith S, Buchanan GR. Acute chest syndrome in children with sickle cell disease. A retrospective analysis of 100 hospitalized cases. *Am J Pediatr Hematol Oncol.* 1986;8(2):105-110.

44. Ashcroft MT, Serjant GR. Growth, morbidity, and mortality in a cohort of Jamaican adolescents with homozygous sickle cell disease. *West Indian Med J.* 1981;30(4):197-201.

45. Athanasou NA, Hatton C, McGee JO, Weatherall DJ. Vascular occlusion and infarction in sickle cell crisis and the sickle chest syndrome. *J Clin Pathol.* 1985;38(6):659-664.

46. Serjeant G. *Sickle Cell Disease.* 2nd ed. Oxford University Press; 1992.

47. Barrett-Connor E. Acute pulmonary disease and sickle cell anemia. *Am Rev Respir Dis.* 1971;104(2):159-165.

48. Davies SC, Luce PJ, Win AA, Riordan JF, Brozovic M. Acute chest syndrome in sickle-cell disease. *Lancet.* 1984;1(8367):36-38.

49. Gill FM, Sleeper LA, Weiner SJ, et al. Clinical events in the first decade in a cohort of infants with sickle cell disease. Cooperative Study of Sickle Cell Disease. *Blood.* 1995;86(2):776-783.

50. Thomas AN, Pattison C. Causes of death in sickle-cell disease in Jamaica. *Br Med J.* 1982;285(6342):633-635.

51. van Agtmael MA, Cheng JD, Nossent HC. Acute chest syndrome in adult Afro-Caribbean patients with sickle cell disease. Analysis of 81 episodes among 53 patients. *Arch Intern Med.* 1994;154(5):557-561.

52. Vichinsky EP. Comprehensive care in sickle cell disease: its impact on morbidity and mortality. *Semin Hematol.* 1991;28(3):220-226.

53. Claster S, Vichinsky E. Acute chest syndrome in sickle cell disease: pathophysiology and management. *J Intensive Care Med* 2000;15:59-66.

54. Ballas SK, Park CH. Severe hypoxemia secondary to acute sternal infarction in sickle cell anemia. *J Nucl Med.* 1991;32(8):1617-1618.

55. Bellet PS, Kalinyak K. Incentive spirometry to prevent acute pulmonary complications in sickle cell diseases. *N Engl J Med.* 1995;333(11):699-703.

56. Rucknagel DL, Kalinyak KA, Gelfand MJ. Rib infarcts and acute chest syndrome in sickle cell diseases. *Lancet.* 1991;337(8745):831-833.

57. Styles LA, Aarsman AJ, Vichinsky EP, Kuypers FA. Secretory phospholipase A(2) predicts impending acute chest syndrome in sickle cell disease. *Blood.* 2000;96(9):3276-3278.

58. Vichinsky E, Williams R, Das M, et al. Pulmonary fat embolism: a distinct cause of severe acute chest syndrome in sickle cell anemia. *Blood.* 1994;83(11):3107-3112.

59. Alhashimi D, Fedorowicz Z, Alhashimi F, Dastgiri S. Blood transfusions for treating acute chest syndrome in people with sickle cell disease. *Cochrane Database Syst Rev.* 2010(1):CD007843.

60. Abboud MR, Taylor EC, Habib D, et al. Elevated serum and bronchoalveolar lavage fluid levels of interleukin 8 and granulocyte colony-stimulating factor associated with the acute chest syndrome in patients with sickle cell disease. *Br J Haematol.* 2000;111(2):482-490.

61. Hassell KL, Eckman JR, Lane PA. Acute multiorgan failure syndrome: a potentially catastrophic complication of severe sickle cell pain episodes. *Am J Med.* 1994;96(2):155-162.

62. Karayalcin G, Rosner F, Kim KY, Chandra P, Aballi AJ. Sickle cell anemia- clinical manifestations in 100 patients and review of the literature. *Am J Med Sci.* 1975;269(1):51-68.

63. Linklater DR, Pemberton L, Taylor S, Zeger W. Painful dilemmas: an evidence-based look at challenging clinical scenarios. *Emerg Med Clin North Am.* 2005;23(2):367-392.

64. Magid D, Fishman EK, Charache S, Siegelman SS. Abdominal pain in sickle cell disease: the role of CT. *Radiology.* 1987;163(2):325-328.

65. Al-Mulhim AS, Al-Mulhim FM, Al-Suwaiygh AA. The role of laparoscopic cholecystectomy in the management of acute cholecystitis in patients with sickle cell disease. *Am J Surg.* 2002;183(6):668-672.

66. Singh NK, el-Mangoush M. Hepatic sequestration crisis presenting with severe intrahepatic cholestatic jaundice. *J Assoc Phys India.* 1996;44(4):283-284.

67. Sarnaik S, Slovis TL, Corbett DP, Emami A, Whitten CF. Incidence of cholelithiasis in sickle cell anemia using the ultrasonic gray-scale technique. *J Pediatr.* 1980;96(6):1005-1008.

68. Curro G, Iapichino G, Lorenzini C, Palmeri R, Cucinotta E. Laparoscopic cholecystectomy in children with chronic hemolytic anemia. Is the outcome related to the timing of the procedure? *Surg Endosc.* 2006;20(2):252-255.

69. Ballas SK, Lewis CN, Noone AM, Krasnow SH, Kamarulzaman E, Burka ER. Clinical, hematological, and biochemical features of Hb SC disease. *Am J Hematol.* 1982;13(1):37-51.

70. Meshikhes AW, Al-Abkari HA, Al-Faraj AA, Al-Dhurais SA, Al-Saif O. The safety of laparoscopic cholecystectomy in sickle cell disease: An update. *Ann Saudi Med.* 1998;18(1):12-14.

71. Spigelman A, Warden MJ. Surgery in patients with sickle cell disease. *Arch Surg.* 1972;104(6):761-764.

72. McCall IW, Desai P, Serjeant BE, Serjeant GR. Cholelithiasis in Jamaican patients with homozygous sickle cell disease. *Am J Hematol.* 1977;3:15-21.

73. Lee SP, Maher K, Nicholls JF. Origin and fate of biliary sludge. *Gastroenterology.* 1988;94(1):170-176.

74. Cameron JL, Maddrey WC, Zuidema GD. Biliary tract disease in sickle cell anemia: surgical considerations. *Ann Surg.* 1971;174(4):702-710.

75. Lee SP, Nicholls JF, Park HZ. Biliary sludge as a cause of acute pancreatitis. *N Engl J Med.* 1992;326(9):589-593.

76. Ahn H, Li CS, Wang W. Sickle cell hepatopathy: clinical presentation, treatment, and outcome in pediatric and adult patients. *Pediatr Blood Cancer.* 2005;45(2):184-190.

77. Hatton CS, Bunch C, Weatherall DJ. Hepatic sequestration in sickle cell anaemia. *Br Med J (Clin Res Ed).* 1985;290(6470):744-745.

78. Al-Salem AH, Qaisruddin S. The significance of biliary sludge in children with sickle cell disease. *Pediatr Surg Int.* 1998;13(1):14-16.

79. Walker TM, Serjeant GR. Biliary sludge in sickle cell disease. *J Pediatr.* 1996;129(3):443-445.

80. Irizarry K, Rossbach HC, Ignacio JR, et al. Sickle cell intrahepatic cholestasis with cholelithiasis. *Pediatr Hematol Oncol.* 2006;23(2):95-102.

81. Stephan JL, Merpit-Gonon E, Richard O, Raynaud-Ravni C, Freycon F. Fulminant liver failure in a 12-year-old girl with sickle cell anaemia: favourable outcome after exchange transfusions. *Eur J Pediatr.* 1995;154(6):469-471.

82. Shao SH, Orringer EP. Sickle cell intrahepatic cholestasis: approach to a difficult problem. *Am J Gastroenterol.* 1995;90(11):2048-2050.

83. Baichi MM, Arifuddin RM, Mantry PS, Bozorgzadeh A, Ryan C. Liver transplantation in sickle cell anemia: a case of acute sickle cell intrahepatic cholestasis and a case of sclerosing cholangitis. *Transplantation.* 2005;80(11):1630-1632.

84. Costa DB, Miksad RA, Buff MS, Wang Y, Dezube BJ. Case of fatal sickle cell intrahepatic cholestasis despite use of exchange transfusion in an African-American patient. *J Natl Med Assoc.* 2006;98(7):1183-1187.

85. Davies SC, Brozovic M. The presentation, management and prophylaxis of sickle cell disease. *Blood Rev.* 1989;3(1):29-44.

86. Hernandez RJ, Sarnaik SA, Lande I, et al. MR evaluation of liver iron overload. *J Comput Assist Tomogr.* 1988;12(1):91-94.

87. Topley JM, Rogers DW, Stevens MC, Serjeant GR. Acute splenic sequestration and hypersplenism in the first five years in homozygous sickle cell disease. *Arch Dis Child.* 1981;56(10):765-769.

88. Aquino VM, Norvell JM, Buchanan GR. Acute splenic complications in children with sickle cell-hemoglobin C disease. *J Pediatr.* 1997;130(6):961-965.

89. Wright JG, Hambleton IR, Thomas PW, Duncan ND, Venugopal S, Serjeant GR. Postsplenectomy course in homozygous sickle cell disease. *J Pediatr.* 1999;134(3):304-309.

90. Kinney TR, Ware RE, Schultz WH, Filston HC. Long-term management of splenic sequestration in children with sickle cell disease. *J Pediatr.* 1990;117(2 Pt 1):194-199.

91. Benjamin LJ, Dampier CD, Jacox AK. *Guideline for the Management of Acute and Chronic Pain in Sickle Cell Disease.* American Pain Society; 1999.

92. Smith WR, Penberthy LT, Bovbjerg VE, et al. Daily assessment of pain in adults with sickle cell disease. *Ann Intern Med.* 2008;148(2):94-101.

93. Ballas SK. *Sickle Cell Pain.* 2nd ed. International Association for the Study of Pain; 2014.

94. Adeyoju AB, Olujohungbe AB, Morris J, et al. Priapism in sickle-cell disease; incidence, risk factors and complications: an international multicentre study. *BJU Int.* 2002;90(9):898-902.

95. Olujohungbe AB, Adeyoju A, Yardumian A, et al. A prospective diary study of stuttering priapism in adolescents and young men with sickle cell anemia: report of an international randomized control trial—the priapism in sickle cell study. *J Androl.* 2011;32(4):375-382.

96. Rogers ZR. Priapism in sickle cell disease. *Hematol Oncol Clin North Am.* 2005;19(5):917-928, viii.

97. Mantadakis E, Cavender JD, Rogers ZR, Ewalt DH, Buchanan GR. Prevalence of priapism in children and adolescents with sickle cell anemia. *J Pediatr Hematol Oncol.* 1999;21(6):518-522.

98. Hamre MR, Harmon EP, Kirkpatrick DV, Stern MJ, Humbert JR. Priapism as a complication of sickle cell disease. *J Urol.* 1991;145(1):1-5.

99. Emond AM, Holman R, Hayes RJ, Serjeant GR. Priapism and impotence in homozygous sickle cell disease. *Arch Intern Med.* 1980;140(11):1434-1437.

100. Mantadakis E, Ewalt DH, Cavender JD, Rogers ZR, Buchanan GR. Outpatient penile aspiration and epinephrine irrigation for young patients with sickle cell anemia and prolonged priapism. *Blood.* 2000;95(1):78-82.

101. Talacki CA, Ballas SK. Modified method of exchange transfusion in sickle cell disease. *J Clin Apher.* 1990;5(4):183-187.

102. Baron M, Leiter E. The management of priapism in sickle cell anemia. *J Urol.* 1978;119(5):610-611.

103. Seeler RA. Intensive transfusion therapy for priapism in boys with sickle cell anemia. *J Urol.* 1973;110(3):360-363.

104. Siegel JF, Rich MA, Brock WA. Association of sickle cell disease, priapism, exchange transfusion and neurological events: ASPEN syndrome. *J Urol.* 1993;150(5 Pt 1):1480-1482.

105. Rackoff WR, Ohene-Frempong K, Month S, Scott JP, Neahring B, Cohen AR. Neurologic events after partial exchange transfusion for priapism in sickle cell disease. *J Pediatr.* 1992;120(6):882-885.

106. Ballas SK, Lyon D. Safety and efficacy of blood exchange transfusion for priapism complicating sickle cell disease. *J Clin Apher.* 2016;31(1):5-10.

107. Dawson C, Whitfield H. ABC of Urology. Urological emergencies in general practice. *Bmj.* 1996;312(7034):838-840.

108. Gradisek RE. Priapism in sickle cell disease. *Ann Emerg Med.* 1983;12(8):510-512.

109. Chinegwundoh F, Anie KA. Treatments for priapism in boys and men with sickle cell disease. *Cochrane Database Syst Rev.* 2004;4:CD004198.

110. Bialecki ES, Bridges KR. Sildenafil relieves priapism in patients with sickle cell disease. *Am J Med.* 2002;113(3):252.

111. Burnett AL, Bivalacqua TJ, Champion HC, Musicki B. Feasibility of the use of phosphodiesterase type 5 inhibitors in a pharmacologic prevention program for recurrent priapism. *J Sex Med.* 2006;3(6):1077-1084.

112. Tzortzis V, Mitrakas L, Gravas S, et al. Oral phosphodiesterase type 5 inhibitors alleviate recurrent priapism complicating thalassemia intermedia: a case report. *J Sex Med.* 2009;6(7):2068-2071.

113. Machado RF, Barst RJ, Yovetich NA, et al. Hospitalization for pain in patients with sickle cell disease treated with

sildenafil for elevated TRV and low exercise capacity. *Blood.* 2011;118(4):855-864.

114. Compton MT, Miller AH. Priapism associated with conventional and atypical antipsychotic medications: a review. *J Clin Psychiatry.* 2001;62(5):362-366.

115. Hosseini SH, Polonowita AK. Priapism associated with olanzapine. *Pak J Biol Sci.* 2009;12(2):198-200.

116. Songer DA, Barclay JC. Olanzapine-induced priapism. *Am J Psychiatry.* 2001;158(12):2087-2088.

117. Ballas SK, Eckman JR. biology of pain and treatment of the sickle cell pain. In: Steinberg MH, Forget BG, Higgs DR, Nagel RL, eds. *Disorders of Hemoglobin: Genetics, Pathophysiology and Clinical Management.* 2nd ed. Cambridge University Press; 2009:497-524.

118. Benjamin LJ, Payne R. Pain in sickle cell disease: a multidimensional construct. In: Pace B, ed. *Renaissance of Sickle Cell Disease Research in the Genomic Era.* Imperial College Press; 2007:99-118.

119. Konotey-Ahulu FID. Mental nerve neuropathy: a complication of sickle cell crisis. *Lancet.* 1972;2:388.

120. Kirson LE, Tomaro AJ. Mental nerve paresthesia secondary to sickle-cell crisis. *Oral Surg Oral Med Oral Pathol.* 1979;48(6):509-512.

121. Mendes PH, Fonseca NG, Martelli DR, et al. Orofacial manifestations in patients with sickle cell anemia. *Quintessence Int.* 2011;42(8):701-709.

122. Hamdoun E, Davis L, McCrary SJ, Eklund NP, Evans OB. Bilateral mental nerve neuropathy in an adolescent during sickle cell crises. *J Child Neurol.* 2012;27(8):1038-1041.

123. Asher SW. Multiple cranial neuropathies, trigeminal neuralgia, and vascular headaches in sickle cell disease, a possible common mechanism. *Neurology.* 1980;30(2):210-211.

124. Shields RW Jr, Harris JW, Clark M. Mononeuropathy in sickle cell anemia: anatomical and pathophysiological basis for its rarity. *Muscle Nerve.* 1991;14(4):370-374.

125. Ballas SK, Reyes PE. Peripheral neuropathy in adults with sickle cell disease. *Am J Pain Med.* 1997;71:53-58.

126. Salvin ML, Barondes MJ. Ischemic optic neuropathy in sickle cell disease. *Am J Ophthalmol.* 1988;105:221-223.

127. Blank JP, Gill FM. Orbital infarction in sickle cell disease. *Pediatrics.* 1981;67(6):879-881.

128. Al-Rashid RA. Orbital apex syndrome secondary to sickle cell anemia. *J Pediatr.* 1979;95(3):426-427.

129. Rothman SM, Nelson JS. Spinal cord infarction in a patient with sickle cell anemia. *Neurology.* 1980;30(10):1072-1076.

130. Benjamin LJ. Nature and treatment of the acute painful episode in sickle cell disease. In: Steinberg MH, Forget BG, Higgs DR, Nagel RL, eds. *Disorders of Hemoglobin: Genetics, Pathphysiology, and Clinical Management.* Cambridge University Press; 2001:671-710.

131. Niihara Y, Miller ST, Kanter J, et al. A phase 3 trial of l-glutamine in sickle cell disease. *N Engl J Med.* 2018;379(3):226-235.

132. Estepp JH. Voxelotor (GBT440), a first-in-class hemoglobin oxygen-affinity modulator, has promising and reassuring preclinical and clinical data. *Am J Hematol.* 2018;93(3):326-329.

133. Telen MJ, Wun T, McCavit TL, et al. Randomized phase 2 study of GMI-1070 in SCD: reduction in time to resolution of vaso-occlusive events and decreased opioid use. *Blood.* 2015;125(17):2656-2664.

134. Chou R. 2009 clinical guidelines from the American Pain Society and the American Academy of Pain Medicine on the use of chronic opioid therapy in chronic noncancer pain: what are the key messages for clinical practice? *Pol Arch Med Wewn.* 2009;119(7-8):469-477.

135. National Heart, Lung, and Blood Institute. Expert Panel Report. Evidence-Based Management of Sickle Cell Disease. http://www.nhlbi.nih.gov/health-pro/guidelines/sickle-cell-disease-guidelines/. Published 2014. Accessed July 5, 2020.

136. Weissman DE, Haddox JD. Opioid pseudoaddiction: an iatrogenic syndrome. *Pain.* 1989;36(3):363-366.

137. Canfield MC, Keller CE, Frydrych LM, Ashrafioun L, Purdy CH, Blondell RD. Prescription opioid use among patients seeking treatment for opioid dependence. *J Addict Med.* 2010;4(2):108-113.

138. Nahin RL. Estimates of pain prevalence and severity in adults: United States, 2012. *J Pain.* 2015;16(8):769-780.

139. Dampier C, Ely E, Brodecki D, O'Neal P. Home management of pain in sickle cell disease: a daily diary study in children and adolescents. *J Pediatr Hematol Oncol.* 2002;24(8):643-647.

140. Dampier C, Ely B, Brodecki D, O'Neal P. Characteristics of pain managed at home in children and adolescents with sickle cell disease by using diary self-reports. *J Pain.* 2002;3(6):461-470.

141. McClish DK, Smith WR, Dahman BA, et al. Pain site frequency and location in sickle cell disease: the PiSCES project. *Pain.* 2009;145(1-2):246-251.

142. Epstein K, Yuen E, Riggio JM, Ballas SK, Moleski SM. Utilization of the office, hospital and emergency department for adult sickle cell patients: a five-year study. *J Natl Med Assoc.* 2006;98(7):1109-1113.

143. Anie KA, Steptoe A, Ball S, Dick M, Smalling BM. Coping and health service utilisation in a UK study of paediatric sickle cell pain. *Arch Dis Child.* 2002;86(5):325-329.

144. Carroll CP, Haywood C Jr, Fagan P, Lanzkron S. The course and correlates of high hospital utilization in sickle cell disease: evidence from a large, urban Medicaid managed care organization. *Am J Hematol.* 2009;84(10):666-670.

145. Sil S, Cohen LL, Dampier C. Psychosocial and functional outcomes in youth with chronic sickle cell pain. *Clin J Pain.* 2016;32(6):527-533.

146. Lanzkron S, Haywood C, Segal JB, Dover GJ. Hospitalization rates and costs of care of patients with sickle-cell anemia in the state of Maryland in the era of hydroxyurea. *Am J Hematol.* 2006;81(12):927-932.

147. Dampier C, Palermo TM, Darbari DS, Hassell K, Smith W, Zempsky W. AAPT diagnostic criteria for chronic sickle cell disease pain. *J Pain.* 2017;18(5):490-498.

148. Brandow AM, Zappia KJ, Stucky CL. Sickle cell disease: a natural model of acute and chronic pain. *Pain.* 2017;158(suppl 1):S79-s84.

149. Gil KM, Carson JW, Porter LS, Scipio C, Bediako SM, Orringer E. Daily mood and stress predict pain, health care use, and work activity in African American adults with sickle-cell disease. *Health Psychol.* 2004;23(3):267-274.

150. Levenson JL, McClish DK, Dahman BA, et al. Depression and anxiety in adults with sickle cell disease: the PiSCES project. *Psychosom Med.* 2008;70(2):192-196.

151. Sogutlu A, Levenson JL, McClish DK, Rosef SD, Smith WR. Somatic symptom burden in adults with sickle cell disease predicts pain, depression, anxiety, health care utilization, and quality of life: the PiSCES project. *Psychosomatics.* 2011;52(3):272-279.

152. Ballas SK, Gupta K, Adams-Graves P. Sickle cell pain: a critical reappraisal. *Blood.* 2012;120(18):3647-3656.

153. Lanzkron S, Little J, Field J, et al. Increased acute care utilization in a prospective cohort of adults with sickle cell disease. *Blood Adv.* 2018;2(18):2412-2417.

154. Neumayr LD, Aguilar C, Earles AN, et al. Physical therapy alone compared with core decompression and physical therapy for femoral head osteonecrosis in sickle cell disease. Results of a multicenter study at a mean of three years after treatment. *J Bone Joint Surg Am.* 2006;88(12):2573-2582.

155. Aguilar C, Vichinsky E, Neumayr L. Bone and joint disease in sickle cell disease. *Hematol Oncol Clin North Am.* 2005;19(5):929-941, viii.

156. Vanderhave KL, Perkins CA, Scannell B, Brighton BK. Orthopaedic manifestations of sickle cell disease. *J Am Acad Orthop Surg.* 2018;26(3):94-101.

157. Minniti CP, Kato GJ. Critical reviews: how we treat sickle cell patients with leg ulcers. *Am J Hematol.* 2016;91(1):22-30.

158. Staud R, Craggs JG, Perlstein WM, Robinson ME, Price DD. Brain activity associated with slow temporal summation of C-fiber evoked pain in fibromyalgia patients and healthy controls. *Eur J Pain.* 2008;12(8):1078-1089.

159. Williams DA, Gracely RH. Biology and therapy of fibromyalgia. Functional magnetic resonance imaging findings in fibromyalgia. *Arthritis Res Ther.* 2006;8(6):224.

160. Kwan CL, Diamant NE, Pope G, Mikula K, Mikulis DJ, Davis KD. Abnormal forebrain activity in functional bowel disorder patients with chronic pain. *Neurology.* 2005;65(8):1268-1277.

161. Steinberg MH. Mechanisms of vaso-occlusion in sickle cell disease. Updated October 5, 2017. UptoDate.com. https://www.uptodate.com/contents/mechanisms-of-vaso-occlusion-in-sickle-cell-disease. Published 2017. Accessed April 3, 2018.

162. Brandow AM, Wandersee NJ, Dasgupta M, et al. Substance P is increased in patients with sickle cell disease and associated with haemolysis and hydroxycarbamide use. *Br J Haematol.* 2016;175(2):237-245.

163. Kohli DR, Li Y, Khasabov SG, et al. Pain-related behaviors and neurochemical alterations in mice expressing sickle hemoglobin: modulation by cannabinoids. *Blood.* 2010;116(3):456-465.

164. Hillery CA, Kerstein PC, Vilceanu D, et al. Transient receptor potential vanilloid 1 mediates pain in mice with severe sickle cell disease. *Blood.* 2011;118(12):3376-3383.

165. Cain DM, Vang D, Simone DA, Hebbel RP, Gupta K. Mouse models for studying pain in sickle disease: effects of strain, age, and acuteness. *Br J Haematol.* 2012;156(4):535-544.

166. Brandow AM, Stucky CL, Hillery CA, Hoffmann RG, Panepinto JA. Patients with sickle cell disease have increased sensitivity to cold and heat. *Am J Hematol.* 2013;88(1):37-43.

167. Costigan M, Scholz J, Woolf CJ. Neuropathic pain: a maladaptive response of the nervous system to damage. *Annu Rev Neurosci.* 2009;32:1-32.

168. von Hehn CA, Baron R, Woolf CJ. Deconstructing the neuropathic pain phenotype to reveal neural mechanisms. *Neuron.* 2012;73(4):638-652.

169. Brandow AM, Farley RA, Panepinto JA. Early insights into the neurobiology of pain in sickle cell disease: a systematic review of the literature. *Pediatr Blood Cancer.* 2015;62(9):1501-1511.

170. Cruccu G, Sommer C, Anand P, et al. EFNS guidelines on neuropathic pain assessment: revised 2009. *Eur J Neurol.* 2010;17(8):1010-1018.

171. Antunes FD, Propheta VGS, Vasconcelos HA, Cipolotti R. Neuropathic pain in patients with sickle cell disease: a cross-sectional study assessing teens and young adults. *Ann Hematol.* 2017;96(7):1121-1125.

172. Brandow AM, Farley RA, Panepinto JA. Neuropathic pain in patients with sickle cell disease. *Pediatr Blood Cancer.* 2014;61(3):512-517.

173. Campbell CM, Moscou-Jackson G, Carroll CP, et al. An evaluation of central sensitization in patients with sickle cell disease. *J Pain.* 2016;17(5):617-627.

174. Carroll CP. Chronic and noncrisis pain in sickle cell disease. *South Med J.* 2016;109(9):516-518.

175. Smith WR, Scherer M. Sickle-cell pain: advances in epidemiology and etiology. *Hematology Am Soc Hematol Educ Program.* 2010;2010:409-415.

176. Vichinsky E. Chronic organ failure in adult sickle cell disease. *Hematology Am Soc Hematol Educ Program.* 2017;2017(1):435-439.

177. Citero Vde A, Levenson JL, McClish DK, et al. The role of catastrophizing in sickle cell disease: the PiSCES project. *Pain.* 2007;133(1-3):39-46.

178. Pells J, Edwards CL, McDougald CS, et al. Fear of movement (kinesiophobia), pain, and psychopathology in patients with sickle cell disease. *Clin J Pain.* 2007;23(8):707-713.

179. Fisher K, Laikin AM, Sharp KMH, Criddle CA, Palermo TM, Karlson CW. Temporal relationship between daily pain and actigraphy sleep patterns in pediatric sickle cell disease. *J Behav Med.* 2018;41(3):416-422.

180. Katz T, Schatz J, Roberts CW. Comorbid obstructive sleep apnea and increased risk for sickle cell disease morbidity. *Sleep Breath.* 2018;22(3):797-804.

181. Valrie CR, Trout KL, Bond KE, et al. Sleep problem risk for adolescents with sickle cell disease: sociodemographic, physical, and disease-related correlates. *J Pediatr Hematol Oncol.* 2018;40(2):116-121.

182. Whitesell PL, Owoyemi O, Oneal P, et al. Sleep-disordered breathing and nocturnal hypoxemia in young adults with sickle cell disease. *Sleep Med.* 2016;22:47-49.

183. Moscou-Jackson G, Allen J, Kozachik S, Smith MT, Budhathoki C, Haywood C Jr. Acute pain and depressive symptoms: independent predictors of insomnia symptoms among adults with sickle cell disease. *Pain Manag Nurs.* 2016;17(1):38-46.

184. Adegbola M. Sleep quality, pain and self-efficacy among community-dwelling adults with sickle cell disease. *J Natl Black Nurses Assoc.* 2015;26(1):15-21.

185. Ameringer S, Elswick RK Jr, Smith W. Fatigue in adolescents and young adults with sickle cell disease: biological and behavioral correlates and health-related quality of life. *J Pediatr Oncol Nurs.* 2014;31(1):6-17.

186. Anderson LM, Allen TM, Thornburg CD, Bonner MJ. Fatigue in children with sickle cell disease: association with neurocognitive and social-emotional functioning and quality of life. *J Pediatr Hematol Oncol.* 2015;37(8):584-589.

187. Miller ST, Kim HY, Weiner D, et al. Inpatient management of sickle cell pain: a "snapshot" of current practice. *Am J Hematol.* 2012;87(3):333-336.

188. Smith WR, McClish DK, Dahman BA, et al. Daily home opioid use in adults with sickle cell disease: the PiSCES project. *J Opioid Manag.* 2015;11(3):243-253.

189. Aisiku IP, Smith WR, McClish DK, et al. Comparisons of high versus low emergency department utilizers in sickle cell disease. *Ann Emerg Med.* 2009;53(5):587-593.

190. Ballas SK, Bauserman RL, McCarthy WF, Castro OL, Smith WR, Waclawiw MA. Hydroxyurea and acute painful crises in sickle cell anemia: effects on hospital length of stay and opioid utilization during hospitalization, outpatient acute care contacts, and at home. *J Pain Symptom Manage*. 2010;40(6):870-882.

191. Ballas SK, Bauserman RL, McCarthy WF, Castro OL, Smith WR, Waclawiw MA. Utilization of analgesics in the multicenter study of hydroxyurea in sickle cell anemia: effect of sex, age, and geographical location. *Am J Hematol*. 2010;85(8):613-616.

192. Han J, Saraf SL, Zhang X, et al. Patterns of opioid use in sickle cell disease. *Am J Hematol*. 2016;91(11):1102-1106.

193. Han J, Zhou J, Saraf SL, Gordeuk VR, Calip GS. Characterization of opioid use in sickle cell disease. *Pharmacoepidemiol Drug Saf*. 2018;27(5):479-486.

194. The use of opioids for the treatment of chronic pain. A consensus statement from the American Academy of Pain Medicine and the American Pain Society. *Clin J Pain*. 1997;13(1):6-8.

195. Ballantyne JC, Kalso E, Stannard C. WHO analgesic ladder: a good concept gone astray. *BMJ*. 2016;352:i20.

196. Caudill-Slosberg MA, Schwartz LM, Woloshin S. Office visits and analgesic prescriptions for musculoskeletal pain in US: 1980 vs. 2000. *Pain*. 2004;109(3):514-519.

197. Olsen Y, Daumit GL, Ford DE. Opioid prescriptions by U.S. primary care physicians from 1992 to 2001. *J Pain*. 2006;7(4):225-235.

198. Colliver JD, Kroutil LA, Dai L, Gfroerer JC. Misuse of prescription drugs: data from the 2002, 2003 and 2004 national surverys on drug use and health. DHHS publication no. SMA 06-4192, analytic series A-28. Substance Abuse and Mental Health Services Administration, Office of Applied Studies; 2006.

199. Substance Abuse and Mental Health Services Administration, Office of Applied Studies. Emergency department trends from the Drug Abuse Warning Network, final estimates 1995-2002. DAWN series D-24, DHHS publication no. SMA 03-3780. Substance Abuse and Mental Health Services Administration, Office of Applied Studies; 2003.

200. Substance Abuse and Mental Health Services Administration, Office of Applied Studies. Results from the 2005 National Survey on Drug Use and Health: national findings. NSDUH series H-30, DDHS publication no. SMA 06-4194. Substance Abuse and Mental Health Services Administration, Office of Applied Studies; 2006.

201. Substance Abuse and Mental Health Services Administration, Office of Applied Studies. Treatment Episode Data Set (TEDS). Highlights - 2005. National admissions to substance abuse treatment services. DHHS DASIS series: S-36, DHHS publication no. SMA 07-4229. Substance Abuse Mental Health Services Administration, Office of Applied Studies; 2006.

202. Substance Abuse and Mental Health Services Administration, Office of Applied Studies. The NSDUH report. Patterns and trends in nonmedical prescription pain reliever use: 2002 to 2005. https://datafiles.samhsa.gov/study-publication/patterns-and-trends-nonmedical-prescription-pain-reliever-use-2002-2005-nid14247. Published 2007. Accessed July 5, 2020.

203. Rudd RA, Aleshire N, Zibbell JE, Gladden RM. Increases in drug and opioid overdose deaths–United States, 2001-2014. *MMWR Morb Mortal Wkly Rep*. 2016;64(50-51):1378-1382.

204. Centers for Disease Control and Prevention. Opioid painkiller prescribing, where you live makes a difference. http://www.cdc.gov/vitalsigns/opioid-prescribing/. Published 2014. Accessed September 12, 2016.

205. Paulozzi LJ, Strickler GK, Kreiner PW, Koris CM. Controlled substance prescribing patterns—prescription behavior surveillance system, eight states, 2013. *MMWR Surveill Summ*. 2015;64(9):1-14.

206. Centers for Disease Control and Prevention, Prevention Public Health Service, US Department of Health and Human Servicces. Guideline for prescribing opioids for chronic pain. *J Pain Palliat Care Pharmacother*. 2016;30(2):138-140.

207. ASTHO State and Territorial Legislative Tracking. Opioids, use and addiction. http://www.astho.org/state-legislative-tracking/. Published 2018. Accessed April 7, 2018.

208. Centers for Disease Control and Prevention. Prescription drug monitoring programs. https://www.cdc.gov/drugoverdose/pdmp/. Published 2017. Accessed April 22, 2017.

209. Department of Health Provisions. Prescription Monitoring Program PMP Education Toolkit. https://www.dhp.virginia.gov/dhp-programs/pmp/toolkit.htm#Introduction. Published 2017. Accessed July 5, 2020.

210. Garcia MC, Dodek AB, Kowalski T, et al. Declines in opioid prescribing after a private insurer policy change–Massachusetts, 2011-2015. *MMWR Morb Mortal Wkly Rep*. 2016;65(41):1125-1131.

211. Garcia MC, Heilig CM, Lee SH, et al. Opioid prescribing rates in nonmetropolitan and metropolitan counties among primary care providers using an electronic health record system: United States, 2014-2017. *MMWR Morb Mortal Wkly Rep*. 2019;68(2):25-30.

212. Lanzkron S. Opioid backlash threatens sickle cell care. http://dev.physiciansweekly.com/sickle-cell-opioids-backlash/. Published December 19, 2013. Accessed October 30, 2016.

213. Sop DM, Smith WR, Alsalman A, et al. Survey of physician perspective towards management of pain for chronic conditions in the emrgency department. *Mod Clin Med Res*. 2017;1(3):55-70.

214. Shapiro BS, Benjamin LJ, Payne R, Heidrich G. Sickle cell-related pain: perceptions of medical practitioners. *J Pain Symptom Manage*. 1997;14(3):168-174.

215. Labbe E, Herbert D, Haynes J. Physicians' attitude and practices in sickle cell disease pain management. *J Palliat Care*. 2005;21(4):246-251.

216. Lucchesi F, Figueiredo MS, Mastandrea EB, et al. Physicians' perception of sickle-cell disease pain. *J Natl Med Assoc*. 2016;108(2):113-118.

217. Armstrong FD, Pegelow CH, Gonzalez JC, Martinez A. Impact of children's sickle cell history on nurse and physician ratings of pain and medication decisions. *J Pediatr Psychol*. 1992;17(5):651-664.

218. Pack-Mabien A, Labbe E, Herbert D, Haynes J Jr. Nurses' attitudes and practices in sickle cell pain management. *Appl Nurs Res*. 2001;14(4):187-192.

219. Jenerette C, Funk M, Murdaugh C. Sickle cell disease: a stigmatizing condition that may lead to depression. *Issues Ment Health Nurs*. 2005;26(10):1081-1101.

220. Jenerette CM, Brewer C. Health-related stigma in young adults with sickle cell disease. *J Natl Med Assoc*. 2010;102(11):1050-1055.

221. Elander J, Beach MC, Haywood C Jr. Respect, trust, and the management of sickle cell disease pain in hospital: comparative analysis of concern-raising behaviors, preliminary model, and agenda for international collaborative research to inform practice. *Ethn Health*. 2011;16(4-5):405-421.

222. Haywood C Jr, Lanzkron S, Hughes MT, et al. A video-intervention to improve clinician attitudes toward patients with sickle cell

disease: the results of a randomized experiment. *J Gen Intern Med.* 2011;26(5):518-523.

223. Haywood C Jr, Lanzkron S, Ratanawongsa N, et al. The association of provider communication with trust among adults with sickle cell disease. *J Gen Intern Med.* 2010;25(6):543-548.

224. Haywood C Jr, Lanzkron S, Bediako S, et al. Perceived discrimination, patient trust, and adherence to medical recommendations among persons with sickle cell disease. *J Gen Intern Med.* 2014;29(12):1657-1662.

225. Haywood C, Beach MC, Bediako S, et al. Examining the characteristics and beliefs of hydroxyurea users and nonusers among adults with sickle cell disease. *Am J Hematol.* 2011;86(1):85-87.

226. Lattimer L, Haywood C Jr, Lanzkron S, Ratanawongsa N, Bediako SM, Beach MC. Problematic hospital experiences among adult patients with sickle cell disease. *J Health Care Poor Underserved.* 2010;21(4):1114-1123.

227. Haywood C Jr, Lanzkron S, Ratanawongsa N, Bediako SM, Lattimer-Nelson L, Beach MC. Hospital self-discharge among adults with sickle-cell disease (SCD): associations with trust and interpersonal experiences with care. *J Hosp Med.* 2010;5(5): 289-294.

228. Chou R, Deyo R, Devine B, et al. The effectiveness and risks of long-term opioid treatment of chronic pain. Evidence Report/Technology Assessment No. 218. AHRQ Publication No. 14-E005-EF. Agency for Healthcare Research and Quality; 2014.

229. Haroutiunian S, McNicol ED, Lipman AG. Methadone for chronic non-cancer pain in adults. *Cochrane Database Syst Rev.* 2012;11:CD008025.

230. Rees DC, Olujohungbe AD, Parker NE, Stephens AD, Telfer P, Wright J. Guidelines for the management of the acute painful crisis in sickle cell disease. *Br J Haematol.* 2003;120(5):744-752.

231. Savage WJ, Buchanan GR, Yawn BP, et al. Evidence gaps in the management of sickle cell disease: a summary of needed research. *Am J Hematol.* 2015;90(4):273-275.

232. Furlan A, Chaparro LE, Irvin E, Mailis-Gagnon A. A comparison between enriched and nonenriched enrollment randomized withdrawal trials of opioids for chronic noncancer pain. *Pain Res Manag.* 2011;16(5):337-351.

233. American Pain Society, American Academy of Pain Medicine Opioids Guidelines Panel. *Guideline for the Use of Chronic Opioid Therapy in Chronic Noncancer Pain: Evidence Review.* American Pain Society; 2009.

234. Anastassopoulos KP, Chow W, Tapia CI, Baik R, Moskowitz B, Kim MS. Reported side effects, bother, satisfaction, and adherence in patients taking hydrocodone for non-cancer pain. *J Opioid Manag.* 2013;9(2):97-109.

235. Gregorian RS Jr, Gasik A, Kwong WJ, Voeller S, Kavanagh S. Importance of side effects in opioid treatment: a trade-off analysis with patients and physicians. *J Pain.* 2010;11(11): 1095-1108.

236. Thielke SM, Turner JA, Shortreed SM, et al. Do patient-perceived pros and cons of opioids predict sustained higher-dose use? *Clin J Pain.* 2014;30(2):93-101.

237. Krebs EE, Gravely A, Nugent S, et al. Effect of opioid vs nonopioid medications on pain-related function in patients with chronic back pain or hip or knee osteoarthritis pain: the SPACE randomized clinical trial. *JAMA.* 2018;319(9):872-882.

238. Trescot AM, Glaser SE, Hansen H, Benyamin R, Patel S, Manchikanti L. Effectiveness of opioids in the treatment of chronic non-cancer pain. *Pain Physician.* 2008;11(2 suppl): S181-S200.

239. International Association for the Study of Pain. Analgesic tolerance to opioids. pain clinical update. Volume IX, No. 5. https://www.iasp-pain.org/PublicationsNews/NewsletterIssue.aspx?ItemNumber=8090. Published 2001. Accessed July 5, 2020.

240. Klaassen CD. *Casarett & Doull's Toxicology: The Basic Science of Poisons.* 6th ed. McGraw-Hill Professional; 2001:17.

241. Roshanpour M, Ghasemi M, Riazi K, Rafiei-Tabatabaei N, Ghahremani MH, Dehpour AR. Tolerance to the anticonvulsant effect of morphine in mice: blockage by ultra-low dose naltrexone. *Epilepsy Res.* 2009;83(2-3):261-264.

242. Koch T, Hollt V. Role of receptor internalization in opioid tolerance and dependence. *Pharmacol Ther.* 2008;117(2):199-206.

243. Dampier CD, Setty BN, Logan J, Ioli JG, Dean R. Intravenous morphine pharmacokinetics in pediatric patients with sickle cell disease. *J Pediatr.* 1995;126(3):461-467.

244. Darbari DS, Minniti CP, Rana S, van den Anker J. Pharmacogenetics of morphine: potential implications in sickle cell disease. *Am J Hematol.* 2008;83(3):233-236.

245. Evans CJ, Cahill CM. Neurobiology of opioid dependence in creating addiction vulnerability. *F1000Res.* 2016;5.

246. Crofford LJ. Adverse effects of chronic opioid therapy for chronic musculoskeletal pain. *Nat Rev Rheumatol.* 2010;6(4):191-197.

247. Gomes T, Tadrous M, Mamdani MM, Paterson JM, Juurlink DN. The burden of opioid-related mortality in the United States. *JAMA Netw Open.* 2018;1(2):e180217.

248. Brennan MJ. The effect of opioid therapy on endocrine function. *Am J Med.* 2013;126(3 suppl 1):S12-S18.

249. Nee J, Zakari M, Sugarman MA, et al. Efficacy of treatments for opioid-induced constipation: systematic review and meta-analysis. *Clin Gastroenterol Hepatol.* 2018;16(10):1569-1584.e1562.

250. Gupta M, Msambichaka L, Ballas SK, Gupta K. Morphine for the treatment of pain in sickle cell disease. *ScientificWorldJournal.* 2015;2015:540154.

251. Els C, Jackson TD, Kunyk D, et al. Adverse events associated with medium- and long-term use of opioids for chronic non-cancer pain: an overview of Cochrane Reviews. *Cochrane Database Syst Rev.* 2017;10:CD012509.

252. Els C, Jackson TD, Hagtvedt R, et al. High-dose opioids for chronic non-cancer pain: an overview of Cochrane Reviews. *Cochrane Database Syst Rev.* 2017;10:CD012299.

253. Meehan WJ, Adelman SA, Rehman Z, Khoromi S. Opioid abuse. http://www.emedicine.com/med/topic1673.htm. Published 2006. Accessed July 5, 2020.

254. Han B, Compton WM, Blanco C, Crane E, Lee J, Jones CM. prescription opioid use, misuse, and use disorders in U.S. adults: 2015 national survey on drug use and health. *Ann Intern Med.* 2017;167(5):293-301.

255. Jones CM. Heroin use and heroin use risk behaviors among nonmedical users of prescription opioid pain relievers: United States, 2002-2004 and 2008-2010. *Drug Alcohol Depend.* 2013;132(1-2):95-100.

256. Kirsh KL, Whitcomb LA, Donaghy K, Passik SD. Abuse and addiction issues in medically ill patients with pain: attempts at clarification of terms and empirical study. *Clin J Pain.* 2002;18 (4 suppl):S52-S60.

257. Weaver MF, Schnoll SH. Opioid treatment of chronic pain in patients with addiction. *J Pain Palliat Care Pharmacother.* 2002;16(3):5-26.

258. Tobin DG, Andrews R, Becker WC. Prescribing opioids in primary care: safely starting, monitoring, and stopping. *Cleve Clin J Med.* 2016;83(3):207-215.

259. Chen JT, Fagan MJ, Diaz JA, Reinert SE. Is treating chronic pain torture? Internal medicine residents' experience with patients with chronic nonmalignant pain. *Teach Learn Med.* 2007;19(2):101-105.

260. Gallagher RM. Empathy: a timeless skill for the pain medicine toolbox. *Pain Med.* 2006;7(3):213-214.

261. Interagency Pain Research Coordinating Committee. National pain strategy: a comprehensive population health-level strategy for pain. https://iprcc.nih.gov/National-Pain-Strategy/Overview. Published 2018. Accessed July 5, 2020.

262. Smith WR, Bovbjerg VE, Penberthy LT, et al. Understanding pain and improving management of sickle cell disease: the PiSCES study. *J Natl Med Assoc.* 2005;97(2):183-193.

263. McClish DK, Smith WR, Levenson JL, et al. Comorbidity, pain, utilization, and psychosocial outcomes in older versus younger sickle cell adults: the PiSCES project. *Biomed Res Int.* 2017;2017:4070547.

264. Edwards R, Telfair J, Cecil H, Lenoci J. Reliability and validity of a self-efficacy instrument specific to sickle cell disease. *Behav Res Ther.* 2000;38(9):951-963.

265. Clay OJ, Telfair J. Evaluation of a disease-specific self-efficacy instrument in adolescents with sickle cell disease and its relationship to adjustment. *Child Neuropsychol.* 2007;13(2):188-203.

266. Keller S, Yang M, Treadwell MJ, Hassell KL. Sensitivity of alternative measures of functioning and wellbeing for adults with sickle cell disease: comparison of PROMIS(R) to ASCQ-Me. *Health Qual Life Outcomes.* 2017;15(1):117.

267. Keller SD, Yang M, Treadwell MJ, Werner EM, Hassell KL. Patient reports of health outcome for adults living with sickle cell disease: development and testing of the ASCQ-Me item banks. *Health Qual Life Outcomes.* 2014;12:125.

268. Panepinto JA, Torres S, Bendo CB, et al. PedsQL sickle cell disease module: feasibility, reliability, and validity. *Pediatr Blood Cancer.* 2013;60(8):1338-1344.

269. Riley WT, Rothrock N, Bruce B, et al. Patient-reported outcomes measurement information system (PROMIS) domain names and definitions revisions: further evaluation of content validity in IRT-derived item banks. *Qual Life Res.* 2010;19(9):1311-1321.

270. Cella D, Riley W, Stone A, et al. The Patient-Reported Outcomes Measurement Information System (PROMIS) developed and tested its first wave of adult self-reported health outcome item banks: 2005-2008. *J Clin Epidemiol.* 2010;63(11):1179-1194.

271. Windmill J, Fisher E, Eccleston C, et al. Interventions for the reduction of prescribed opioid use in chronic non-cancer pain. *Cochrane Database Syst Rev.* 2013;9:CD010323.

272. Dowell D, Haegerich TM, Chou R. CDC guideline for prescribing opioids for chronic pain–United States, 2016. *JAMA.* 2016;315(15):1624-1645.

273. Chou R, Fanciullo GJ, Fine PG, Miaskowski C, Passik SD, Portenoy RK. Opioids for chronic noncancer pain: prediction and identification of aberrant drug-related behaviors: a review of the evidence for an American Pain Society and American Academy of Pain Medicine clinical practice guideline. *J Pain.* 2009;10(2):131-146.

274. Vargas-Schaffer G. Is the WHO analgesic ladder still valid? Twenty-four years of experience. *Can Fam Physician.* 2010;56(6):514-517, e202-e215.

275. Campos-Outcalt D. Should you screen–or not? The latest recommendations. *J Fam Pract.* 2008;57(7):469-472.

276. Owen GT, Burton AW, Schade CM, Passik S. Urine drug testing: current recommendations and best practices. *Pain Physician.* 2012;15(3 suppl):ES119-133.

277. Ewing JA. Detecting alcoholism. The CAGE questionnaire. *JAMA.* 1984;252(14):1905-1907.

278. Brown RL, Leonard T, Saunders LA, Papasouliotis O. The prevalence and detection of substance use disorders among inpatients ages 18 to 49: an opportunity for prevention. *Prev Med.* 1998;27(1):101-110.

279. Weaver M, Villalobos G, Moore T, et al. Identifying prescription drug misuse in primary care patients: a tale of two instruments. Paper presented at: Annual Meeting of College on Problems of Drug Dependence; June 2014; San Juan, Puerto Rico.

280. Wunsch MJ, Cropsey KL, Campbell ED, Knisely JS. OxyContin use and misuse in three populations: substance abuse patients, pain patients, and criminal justice participants. *J Opioid Manag.* 2008;4(2):73-79.

281. Knisely JS, Wunsch MJ, Cropsey KL, Campbell ED. Prescription Opioid Misuse Index: a brief questionnaire to assess misuse. *J Subst Abuse Treat.* 2008;35(4):380-386.

282. Compton P, Darakjian J, Miotto K. Screening for addiction in patients with chronic pain and "problematic" substance use: evaluation of a pilot assessment tool. *J Pain Symptom Manage.* 1998;16(6):355-363.

283. Compton PA, Wu SM, Schieffer B, Pham Q, Naliboff BD. Introduction of a self-report version of the prescription drug use questionnaire and relationship to medication agreement noncompliance. *J Pain Symptom Manage.* 2008;36(4):383-395.

284. Moseley L. Combined physiotherapy and education is efficacious for chronic low back pain. *Aust J Physiother.* 2002;48(4):297-302.

285. Louw A, Zimney K, Puentedura EJ, Diener I. The efficacy of pain neuroscience education on musculoskeletal pain: a systematic review of the literature. *Physiother Theory Pract.* 2016;32(5):332-355.

286. Blickenstaff C, Pearson N. Reconciling movement and exercise with pain neuroscience education: a case for consistent education. *Physiother Theory Pract.* 2016;32(5):396-407.

287. Williams H, Silva S, Simmons LA, Tanabe P. A telephonic mindfulness-based intervention for persons with sickle cell disease: study protocol for a randomized controlled trial. *Trials.* 2017;18(1):218.

288. Fisher E, Law E, Dudeney J, Palermo TM, Stewart G, Eccleston C. Psychological therapies for the management of chronic and recurrent pain in children and adolescents. *Cochrane Database Syst Rev.* 2018;9:CD003968.

289. Eccleston C, Palermo TM, Williams AC, et al. Psychological therapies for the management of chronic and recurrent pain in children and adolescents. *Cochrane Database Syst Rev.* 2014;5:CD003968.

290. Anie KA, Green J. Psychological therapies for sickle cell disease and pain. *Cochrane Database Syst Rev.* 2012;2:CD001916.

291. Osunkwo I. Complete resolution of sickle cell chronic pain with high dose vitamin D therapy: a case report and review of the literature. *J Pediatr Hematol Oncol.* 2011;33(7):549-551.

292. Soe HH, Abas AB, Than NN, et al. Vitamin D supplementation for sickle cell disease. *Cochrane Database Syst Rev.* 2017;1:CD010858.

293. Addae SK. Mechanism for the high incidence of sickle cell crisis in the tropical cool season. *Lancet.* 1971;2:1256.

294. Amjad H, Bannerman RM, Judisch JM. Sickling pain and season. *Br Med J.* 1974;1:54.

295. Serjeant GR, Serjeant BE, Desai P, Mason KP, Sewell A, England JM. The determinants of irreversibly sickled cells in homozygous sickle cell disease. *Br J Haematol.* 1978;40(3):431-438.

296. Ibrahim AS. Relationship between meterological changes and occurrence of painful sickle cell crises in Kuwait. *Trans R Soc Trop Med Hyg.* 1980;74:159-161.

297. Stevens MC, Padwick M, Serjeant GR. Observations on the natural history of dactylitis in homozygous sickle cell disease. *Clin Pediatr (Phila).* 1981;20(5):311-317.

298. Baum KF, Dunn DT, Maude GH, Serjeant GR. The painful crisis of homozygous sickle cell disease. A study of the risk factors. *Arch Intern Med.* 1987;147(7):1231-1234.

299. Diggs L, Flowers E. Sickle cell anemia in the home environment. *Clin Pediatr.* 1971;10:697-700.

300. Seeler RA. Non-seasonality of sickle-cell crisis. *Lancet.* 1973;2(7831):743.

301. Slovis CM, Talley JD, Pitts RB. Nonrelationship of climatologic factors and painful sickle cell anemia crisis. *J Chronic Dis.* 1986;39(2):121-126.

302. Jones S, Duncan ER, Thomas N, et al. Windy weather and low humidity are associated with an increased number of hospital admissions for acute pain and sickle cell disease in an urban environment with a maritime temperate climate. *Br J Haematol.* 2005;131(4):530-533.

303. Nolan VG, Zhang Y, Lash T, Sebastiani P, Steinberg MH. Association between wind speed and the occurrence of sickle cell acute painful episodes: results of a case-crossover study. *Br J Haematol.* 2008;143(3):433-438.

304. Rogovik AL, Persaud J, Friedman JN, Kirby MA, Goldman RD. Pediatric vasoocclusive crisis and weather conditions. *J Emerg Med.* 2011;41(5):559-565.

305. Smith WR, Bauserman RL, Ballas SK, et al. Climatic and geographic temporal patterns of pain in the Multicenter Study of Hydroxyurea. *Pain.* 2009;146(1-2):91-98.

306. Margolies MP. Sickle cell anemia; a composite study and survey. *Medicine (Baltimore).* 1951;30(4):357-433.

307. Paterson JC, Sprague CC. Observation on the genesis of crises in sickle cell anemia. *Ann Intern Med.* 1959;50(6):1502-1507.

308. Wright CS, Gardner E Jr. A study of the role of acute infections in precipitating crises in chronic hemolytic states. *Ann Intern Med.* 1960;52:530-537.

309. Gill P, Sobeck J, Jarjoura D, Hillier S, Benedetti T. Mortality from early neonatal group B streptococcal sepsis: influence of obstetric factors. *J Matern Fetal Med.* 1997;6(1):35-39.

310. Barreras L, Diggs LW. Bicarbonates, pH and percentage of sickled cells in venous blood of patients in sickle cell crisis. *Am J Med Sci.* 1964;247:710-718.

311. Diggs L. Sickle cell crises. *Am J Clin Pathol.* 1965;44:1-19.

312. Nadel C, Portadin G. Sickle cell crises: psychological factors associated with onset. *N Y State J Med.* 1977;77(7):1075-1078.

313. Samuels-Reid J, Scott RB. Painful crises and menstruation in sickle cell disease. *South Med J.* 1985;78(4):384-385.

314. De Ceulaer K, Gruber C, Hayes R, Serjeant GR. Medroxyprogesterone acetate and homozygous sickle-cell disease. *Lancet.* 1982;2(8292):229-231.

315. Anderson M, Went LN, Maciver JE, Dixon HG. Sickle cell disease in pregnancy. *Lancet.* 1960;2(7149):516-521.

316. Hendrickse JP, Watson-Williams EJ, Luzzatto L, Ajabor LN. Pregnancy in homozygous sickle-cell anaemia. *J Obstet Gynaecol Br Commonw.* 1972;79(5):396-409.

317. Rogers DT, Molokie R. Sickle cell disease in pregnancy. *Obstet Gynecol Clin North Am.* 2010;37(2):223-237.

318. Scharf MB, Lobel JS, Caldwell E, et al. Nocturnal oxygen desaturation in patients with sickle cell anemia. *JAMA.* 1983;249(13):1753-1755.

319. Sidman JD, Fry TL. Exacerbation of sickle cell disease by obstructive sleep apnea. *Arch Otolaryngol Head Neck Surg.* 1988;114(8):916-917.

320. Salles C, Ramos RT, Daltro C, Barral A, Marinho JM, Matos MA. Prevalence of obstructive sleep apnea in children and adolescents with sickle cell anemia. *J Bras Pneumol.* 2009;35(11):1075-1083.

321. Needleman JP, Franco ME, Varlotta L, et al. Mechanisms of nocturnal oxyhemoglobin desaturation in children and adolescents with sickle cell disease. *Pediatr Pulmonol.* 1999;28(6):418-422.

322. Levenson JL, McClish DK, Dahman BA, et al. Alcohol abuse in sickle cell disease: the Pisces Project. *Am J Addict.* 2007;16(5):383-388.

Priapism in Sickle Cell Disease

Authors: *Susan M. MacDonald, Arthur L. Burnett*

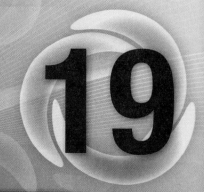

Chapter Outline

Overview

Priapism is defined as a prolonged penile erection, either long beyond sexual stimulation or, more typically, unrelated to sexual stimulation or interest.[1] The condition is relatively uncommon, with a reported incidence of 0.34 to 1.5 cases per 100,000 male patients per year.[2,3] Estimations of incidence are likely to vary by region, however, because the proportion of the population with sickle cell disease or sickle cell trait will vary. Although priapism has many causes, the lifetime risk of a patient with sickle cell disease developing an episode of priapism is between 29% and 42%.[4] In the United States, using the Nationwide Emergency Department Sample, Stein et al[5] estimated a total of 9991 encounters per year, with 27.9% of these encounters leading to admission. They estimated a total cost of $123,860,432 dollars per year in the United States for treatment related to priapism, with 86.8% of these charges stemming from inpatient admission.[5]

In the sickle cell patient population, priapism can be a recurrent issue that severely impairs quality of life in a particularly young group of patients. For a subset of these patients, recurrent ischemic priapism, or stuttering priapism, may occur weekly or even daily.[6,7] In one study, a third of children and adolescents with priapism regard this as the worst complication of the disease.[8] Patients experiencing priapism have reported embarrassment, worry, and social isolation as a consequence of these painful erections.[9] Furthermore, because recurrent ischemic priapism often begins as a nocturnal erection, patients awaken earlier than usual with a painful erection resulting in daytime fatigue that impairs concentration and ability to perform at school or in the workplace.[9] Finally, these patients experience recurrent hospitalizations, significant medical costs, and, in the most devastating cases, erectile dysfunction as a result of priapism.

Priapism is divided into subtypes classified as ischemic (low flow), stuttering (recurrent intermittent), and nonischemic (high flow). The vast majority of patients presenting with priapism present with ischemic priapism, as is the case in patients with sickle cell disease. An estimated 95% of cases are ischemic.[10]

Pathophysiology

Penile Anatomy

The penis is composed dorsally of 2 paired erectile bodies, the corpora cavernosa, and ventrally the corpus spongiosum, which contains the urethra (Figure 19-1A). The glans penis is an extension of the corpus spongiosum.[11] The corpora cavernosa are ensheathed by a thick collagenous connective tissue layer called the tunica albuginea.[11] Within the corpora cavernosa lies the erectile tissue itself, which is a network of smooth muscle bundles forming endothelium-lined sinusoidal spaces (Figure 19-1B).[11] There is a septum between the 2 corpora cavernosa; however, it is freely permeable distally, allowing for communication between these 2 vascular spaces.[11]

The arterial supply for the penis emanates from the internal pudendal artery, which travels and eventually branches into 2 cavernosal arteries that run in the center of each corpora cavernosum as well as the bulbourethral artery that supplies the corpus spongiosum (Figure 19-1C).[12] The venous drainage for these 2 compartments, however, is separate, which provides the rationale for shunt procedures described later in this chapter. Venules within the corpora cavernosa coalesce to form emissary veins that run in the layers of the tunica albuginea. These are compressed during an erection, preventing venous drainage and maintaining the erect state (Figure 19-1B).[12] Emissary veins then drain into circumflex veins that run in paired rows bilaterally between Buck's fascia and the tunica albuginea ultimately draining into the deep dorsal vein.[12] The deep dorsal vein travels with the dorsal neurovascular bundle beneath Buck's fascia in the midline and empties into the periprostatic venous plexus (Figure 19-1D).[12]

Erection Physiology

The smooth muscle comprising the cavernosal sinusoidal tissue as well as that of the penile arterial vessels is tonically contracted. At rest, this allows only a small amount of arterial inflow to the corpora cavernosa, maintaining a flaccid state. This tonic smooth muscle contraction is mediated by sympathetic release of noradrenaline, which maintains penile flaccidity for nearly 23 hours a day.[13] Stimulation of the sacral parasympathetic nerves results in tumescence, an influx of blood flow with resultant penile rigidity, whereas detumescence is regulated by stimulation of the thoracolumbar sympathetic nerves.[12] Direct genital stimulation, psychological arousal, or rapid eye movement sleep can all trigger nerve impulses that inhibit the contractile state, leading to relaxation of the smooth muscle and thus an erection.[14] Studies suggest that the main mediator of smooth muscle relaxation inducing an erection is nitric oxide (NO).[15] Physiologic changes occur once an erection is triggered, including dilation of arterial vessels increasing blood flow, trapping of blood in expanding intracavernosal sinusoidal spaces, compression of venous vessels exiting the tunica albuginea, stretching of the tunica albuginea further compressing venous outflow, and increased intracavernosal pressure and oxygen content.[12]

On a molecular level, stimulation of the cavernous nerves releases NO by neuronal NO synthase (nNOS) (Figure 19-2).[16] This event initiates a penile erection. NO then activates guanylate cyclase generating cyclic guanosine monophosphate (cGMP) (Figure 19-2). cGMP then activates protein kinase G, causing cavernosal smooth muscle relaxation, increased blood flow, and ultimately an erection (Figure 19-2).[14] The increased blood flow by shear activation upregulates serine protein kinase AKT, which then phosphorylates vascular endothelial NO synthase (eNOS) (Figure 19-2). This causes prolonged NO formation, sustaining the penile erection.[17,18]

Phosphodiesterase type 5 (PDE5) is the main enzyme responsible for hydrolysis of cGMP in the penis and ultimately detumescence.[19] Homeostasis is maintained by the generation of cGMP by soluble guanylate cyclases and the degradation by PDE5.[14] New evidence suggests that dysregulation of this homeostasis in the form of downregulation of PDE5 is a molecular basis for priapism.[20]

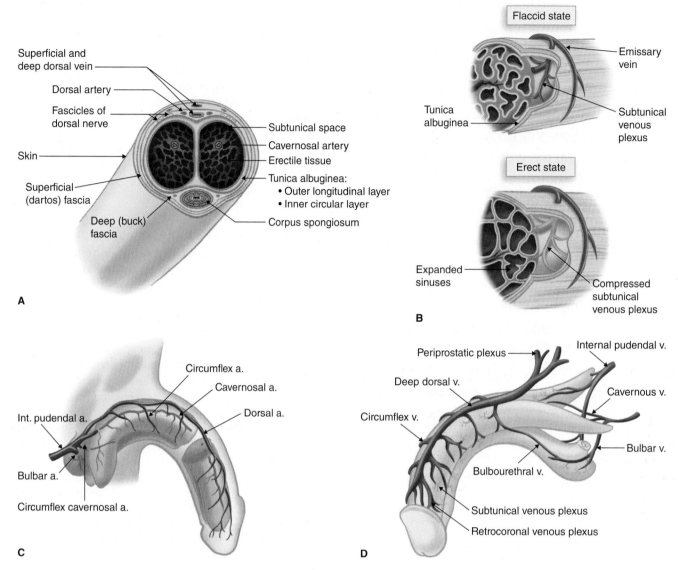

FIGURE 19-1 **Penile anatomy. A.** Cross-sectional illustration demonstrating the layers compromising the penis including the tunica albuginea underlying sinusoidal spaces. **B.** Illustration demonstrating the contracted arteries, arterioles, and sinusoids in the flaccid state contrasted with the expanded sinusoids and compressed emissary veins present in the erect state. **C.** Penile arterial supply. **D.** Penile venous drainage. Panel A reproduced, with permission from Kavoussi PK. Surgical, radiographic, and endoscopic anatomy of the male reproductive system. In: Wein AJ, Kavoussi LR, Partin AW, Peters CA, eds. *Campbell-Walsh Urology*. 11th ed. Elsevier; 2016:498-515. Panels B-D reproduced, with permission, from Lue TF. Physiology of penile erection and pathophysiology of erectile dysfunction. In: Wein AJ, Kavoussi LR, Partin AW, Peters CA, eds. *Campbell-Walsh Urology*. 11th ed. Elsevier; 2016:612-642.

Pathology and Pathophysiology of Ischemic Priapism in Sickle Cell Disease

The same physiology that creates an erection leads to priapism. The pathologic aspect of a priapic erection is the duration of the erection. The longstanding erection leads to the trapping of ischemic blood in intracavernosal spaces due to the compression of the venous outflow system and thus decreased oxygen levels in these tissues. Clinically, ischemic priapism represents a compartment syndrome wherein the high pressure within the corpora cavernosa causes pain and a lack of inflow of oxygenated blood to the erectile tissues. Histologic studies of tissue biopsies from affected corpora cavernosa show time-dependent necrosis.[21,22] Once smooth muscle necrosis occurs,

the ability of the smooth muscle to functionally contract for detumescence is impaired, making longstanding priapism recalcitrant to pharmacologic treatment.

In sickle cell disease, hemoglobin S (HbS) molecules polymerize when deoxygenated, which injures the erythrocyte membrane and causes sickling.[23] A cascade of hemolysis is initiated. The link between hemolysis and priapism in SCD is evidenced by reduced hemoglobin levels and increased reticulocyte count, bilirubin, lactate dehydrogenase, and aspartate aminotransferase, all of which are products of hemolysis, in patients with priapism.[24] Vaso-occlusion has been proposed to occur by increased adhesion of erythrocytes, leukocytes, and platelets to vascular endothelium mediated by immature cell types and cytokines.[23]

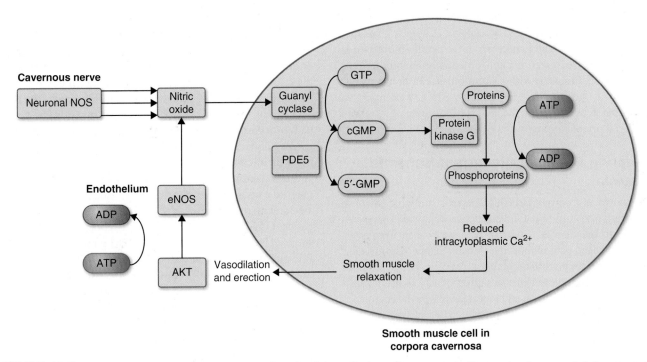

FIGURE 19-2 **Schematic representing the molecular physiology that produces an erection and subsequent detumescence.**
ADP, adenosine diphosphate; ATP, adenosine triphosphate; cGMP, cyclic guanosine monophosphate; eNOS, endothelial nitric oxide synthase; GTP, guanosine triphosphate; NOS, nitric oxide synthase; PDE5, phosphodiesterase type 5.

The presumed etiology of ischemic priapism in patients with sickle cell disease was originally thought to be congestion of viscous blood within the sinusoids of the corpora cavernosa and obstruction of venous outflow secondary to sludging from sickled erythrocytes.[12] This idea was initially supported by the fact that a multitude of hematologic dyscrasias were identified as risk factors for priapism including thalassemia, leukemia, multiple myeloma, hereditary spherocytosis, hemodialysis, and glucose-6-phosphate dehydrogenase deficiency.[25] Recent research suggests a molecular mechanism for priapism, although the aspect of mechanical venous obstruction may still contribute to the pathophysiology of priapism.

In animal studies, mice deficient in eNOS and eNOS/nNOS displayed priapic activity with prolonged erectile responses to direct electrical stimulation of the cavernous nerve.[26] In search of the physiologic basis for this phenomenon, Champion et al[20] measured cGMP levels and found them to be decreased in eNOS knockout and eNOS/nNOS knockout mice. However, once the cavernous nerve was stimulated in both these mouse groups, there was an exaggerated response, with cGMP levels more than double those detected in wild-type mice.[20] To determine whether cGMP production was increased or its catabolism decreased in these mice, PDE5 levels were examined.[20] PDE5, the enzyme responsible for breakdown of cGMP, was shown to be significantly reduced.[20] Additionally, when wild-type mice were incubated with an NOS inhibitor, there was a time-dependent reduction in the expression of the active form of PDE5.[20] This suggests that downregulation of PDE5, secondary to low basal levels of NO, leads to an exaggerated erectile response, resulting in priapism.[20] Paradoxically,

although NO is required for a physiologically normal erection to occur, it is chronic NO deficiency that is thought to lead to priapism.

Chronic NO deficiency is understood to be an underlying molecular basis for PDE5 downregulation.[25] Free hemoglobin released by hemolysis reacts with NO to produce methemoglobin and nitrate.[25] Sickled erythrocytes release arginase I, which converts L-arginine, the substrate for NO production, into ornithine.[25] Taken together, depletion of NO and its substrate results in a state of NO insufficiency referred to as hemolysis-associated endothelial dysfunction, which is thought to promote priapism.[27,28] Several other diseases that induce hemolysis, including thalassemia, hereditary spherocytosis, paroxysmal nocturnal hemoglobinuria, and glucose-6-phosphate dehydrogenase deficiency, have been associated with priapism.[23] Hemolysis-associated endothelial dysfunction is hypothesized to be the underlying cause of priapism in these disease processes. Additionally, data from the Cooperative Study for Sickle Cell Disease show that patients with priapism had lower levels of hemoglobin and higher levels of lactate dehydrogenase, bilirubin, and aspartate aminotransferase, suggesting an association with hemolysis.[29]

Clinical Classifications

Ischemic Priapism (Low Flow)

Ischemic priapism is a persistent erection with rigid erectile bodies causing a compartment syndrome that prevents arterial inflow and thus oxygenation of erectile tissues. The hallmark of major ischemic priapism is a painful erection lasting >4 hours.[1] This is considered a urologic emergency because prolonged episodes lead to necrosis of the penile smooth muscle responsible for erections and potentially lifelong erectile dysfunction.[30] Priapism with a duration of <24 hours results in erectile dysfunction in approximately 50% of patients.[22] No patient has retained spontaneous erections after 36 hours of prolonged priapism in reported case series.[31,32]

Stuttering Priapism (Recurrent Ischemic Priapism)

Also known as recurrent ischemic priapism, stuttering priapism is a pattern of recurrent painful erections traditionally associated with sickle cell disease. Typically, patients awaken from sleep with a prolonged painful morning erection that persists for a few hours but resolves prior to becoming a "major" ischemic priapism episode.[25] These repeated episodes affect quality of life severely, leading to sleep deprivation and repeated visits to the emergency department, in those who are afflicted.[33] Recent research suggests that recurrent ischemic priapism is a predisposing factor for erectile dysfunction, independent of major ischemic priapism episodes.[6] Furthermore, increased duration and frequency of stuttering priapism episodes appear to be a risk factor for erectile dysfunction in the sickle cell disease population.[6] More than 70% of patients with a severe ischemic priapism episode have an antecedent history of stuttering priapism.[34]

Nonischemic Priapism (High Flow)

The classic etiology of nonischemic priapism is blunt trauma to the perineum that causes injury to the cavernosal artery, the main artery coursing through the center of the corpora cavernosa or erectile body.[35] This injury results in the formation of a "high-flow" fistula between the artery and the sinusoidal spaces of the corpora cavernosa.[35] Priapism usually results in a delayed fashion 3 weeks after the initial injury.[35] A "high-flow" priapism erection is a partial or full erection that is persistent for hours to days and classically nonpainful. This type of priapism may resolve spontaneously, whereas ischemic priapism standardly requires intervention. Interestingly, although patients may have prolonged partial erections, they may be unable to attain a rigid erection for sexual activity.[36] Resolution of the fistula by androgen ablation to allow healing, angioembolization, or surgical ligation appears to allow return of natural erectile function in addition to resolution of priapism.[36] High-flow priapism may result from prior interventions to treat ischemic priapism.[37-39] Other reported causes of high-flow priapism include metastatic malignancy to the penis[40,41] and acute spinal cord injury.[42]

Acute Ischemic Priapism: Clinical Presentation

Clinical History

Ischemic priapism associated with sickle cell disease can affect children as well as adults. The typical history is that of a patient awakening from sleep with a rigid erection that becomes progressively more painful with the passage of time. It is important to determine if there have been any similar episodes previously or any precipitating factors, if the patient has tried any relieving maneuvers, and/or if the patient has taken any pertinent medications or erectogenic therapies.[43] Additionally, the clinician should establish the level of erectile function the patient had prior to this episode.[43] A history of prior trauma or spinal cord injury should be ruled out because these are suggestive of nonischemic priapism.

The Priapism Impact Profile (PIP) questionnaire (Figure 19-3) may be a useful adjunct to quickly obtain a comprehensive assessment of the severity of priapism and impact on the patient's quality of life.[44] This patient-reported outcome measure can be completed in <15 minutes by most patients.[44] The PIP questionnaire includes 12 discrete questions that assess the subjective experience of priapism in 3 key domains: quality of life, sexual function, and physical wellness.[44] The PIP questionnaire was validated in a study of 54 patients and warrants further study for widespread use.[44]

Physical Examination

The phallus should be examined and palpated to determine the degree of rigidity as well as any accompanying tenderness. With ischemic priapism, both corpora cavernosa are fully rigid and typically painful to the touch. In comparison, a partially erect phallus with no or minimal tenderness on exam is consistent with nonischemic priapism.

Laboratory Findings

A complete blood count, leukocyte count with differential, and platelet count may expose signs of an active infection or hematologic abnormality.[43] Hemoglobin electrophoresis can identify sickle cell disease as well as other hemoglobin abnormalities. Urine and plasma toxicology screens can be performed if the history is suggestive.[43] Blood should be aspirated directly from the corpora cavernosa and both inspected and sent for blood gas testing. Hypoxic blood appears darkly colored, whereas blood aspirated in nonischemic priapism is bright red secondary to arterial levels of oxygenation. A blood gas measurement will show evidence of hypoxia, hypercarbia, and acidosis. Although values consistent with arterial blood are typically partial pressure of oxygen (Po_2) 90 mm Hg, partial pressure of carbon dioxide (Pco_2) <40 mm Hg, and pH of 7.4, those from an ischemic priapism phallus will be Po_2 <30 mm Hg, Pco_2 >60 mm Hg, and pH <7.25 (Table 19-1).[1]

Penile Imaging

Although penile imaging can provide confirmation of priapism, it is often not crucial to make the diagnosis. Furthermore, because timing is critical in the resolution of ischemic priapism, imaging should not delay treatment. The most readily available imaging study is an ultrasound of the penis using color duplex Doppler. Frog-leg positioning allows for examination of the entire shaft and perineum to identify any evidence of

During the past 2 weeks:

Quality of life	1. Worry about my overall health has been: None = 1 | Minimal = 2 | Slight = 3 | Moderate = 4 | Substantial = 5 | Extreme = 6 | Very extreme = 7						
	2. My distress about my priapism has been: None = 1 | Minimal = 2 | Slight = 3 | Moderate = 4 | Substantial = 5 | Extreme = 6 | Very extreme = 7						
	3. The effect of priapism on my daily activities has been: None = 1 | Minimal = 2 | Slight = 3 | Moderate = 4 | Substantial = 5 | Extreme = 6 | Very extreme = 7						
	4. The negative effect of priapism on my feelings has been: None = 1 | Minimal = 2 | Slight = 3 | Moderate = 4 | Substantial = 5 | Extreme = 6 | Very extreme = 7						
Sexual function	5. The effect of priapism on my sexual satisfaction has been: None = 1 | Minimal = 2 | Slight = 3 | Moderate = 4 | Substantial = 5 | Extreme = 6 | Very extreme = 7						
	6. The effect of priapism on my relationship with my partner has been: None = 1 | Minimal = 2 | Slight = 3 | Moderate = 4 | Substantial = 5 | Extreme = 6 | Very extreme = 7						
	7. The effect of priapism on my sexual confidence has been: None = 1 | Minimal = 2 | Slight = 3 | Moderate = 4 | Substantial = 5 | Extreme = 6 | Very extreme = 7						
	8. Having trouble getting an erection has been: None = 1 | Minimal = 2 | Slight = 3 | Moderate = 4 | Substantial = 5 | Extreme = 6 | Very extreme = 7						
	9. Problems with my sexual desire have been: None = 1 | Minimal = 2 | Slight = 3 | Moderate = 4 | Substantial = 5 | Extreme = 6 | Very extreme = 7						
Physical wellness	10. Physical discomfort caused by my priapism has been: None = 1 | Minimal = 2 | Slight = 3 | Moderate = 4 | Substantial = 5 | Extreme = 6 | Very extreme = 7						
	11. The level of pain in my penis caused by my priapism has been: None = 1 | Minimal = 2 | Slight = 3 | Moderate = 4 | Substantial = 5 | Extreme = 6 | Very extreme = 7						
	12. The abnormal shape of my penis caused by priapism has been: None = 1 | Minimal = 2 | Slight = 3 | Moderate = 4 | Substantial = 5 | Extreme = 6 | Very extreme = 7						

FIGURE 19-3 Priapism Impact Profile questionnaire. Burnett AL, Anele UA, Derogatis LR. Priapism Impact Profile Questionnairre development and initial validation. *Urology.* 2015;85(6):1376-1381. Reprinted with permission from Elsevier.

anatomical malformations or prior trauma.[25,45] The cavernosal arteries are identified at the center of each corpus cavernosum on ultrasound and examined for flow. There will be a lack of inflow, or no arterial wave form, in ischemic priapism. Color Doppler can be used to verify resolution of priapism as well by confirming return of arterial inflow after interventions have been performed. The corporal blood gas measurement can become difficult to interpret with equivocal values after interventions.[25] Corporal fibrosis may also be evident on ultrasound in patients with a prior history of priapism.[25]

Doppler ultrasound may have an application in stuttering priapism as well. Patel et al[46] found higher median peak systolic velocities in the flaccid state in men with sickle cell disease who suffered from stuttering priapism (26 cm/s)

compared with controls (13-16 cm/s). Additionally, these men appeared to have measurable diastolic velocity indicating forward motion during diastole ranging from 2 to 7 cm/s, whereas the diastolic velocity is unmeasurable in the flaccid state.[45] The authors proposed that men with stuttering priapism have reduced and variable smooth muscle tone, predisposing them to uncontrolled erections, as opposed to the typical steady tonic contraction.[46]

Magnetic resonance imaging (MRI) has limited applications with regard to ischemic priapism, especially because it is not often readily attainable in the emergency setting. It has been suggested that MRI may be used to evaluate the degree of tissue thrombosis and smooth muscle necrosis after medical or surgical management has failed in the context of prolonged priapism as part of preoperative planning for an urgent penile prosthesis placement.[30] Alternately, if there is suspicion of nonischemic priapism, MRI may demonstrate an arteriolar-sinusoidal fistula. A penile arteriogram would also demonstrate an established fistula.[10]

TABLE 19-1 Typical corporal blood gas values

Source	Po$_2$ (mm Hg)	Pco$_2$ (mm Hg)	pH
Ischemic priapism (cavernous blood)[3]	<30	>60	<7.25
Normal arterial blood (room air)	>90	<40	7.40
Normal mixed venous blood (room air)	40	50	7.35

Used, with permission, from Montague DK, Jarow J, Broderick GA, et al. American Urological Association guideline on the management of priapism. *J Urol.* 2003;170(4 Pt 1):1318-1324.

Acute Ischemic Priapism: Treatment

Nonoperative

The goal of therapy is to resolve the ischemia as quickly as possible with as minimal morbidity to the patient as possible. Historical treatments have included ice packs, cold baths, cold water enemas, and ejaculation to induce vasoconstriction and thus resolve the priapism episode.[25] Voiding and exercise have also been advised as maneuvers to relieve priapism prior to invasive treatments.[25] Oral hydration may be attempted at home to help resolve priapism in patients with sickle cell disease. Many recurrent ischemic priapism episodes will resolve spontaneously before progressing to a major ischemic episode (erection >4 hours). However, after 4 hours, it is important to seek expeditious medical care to resolve the resultant ischemia. The previously mentioned maneuvers were typically reported in historical literature prior to the widespread use of sympathomimetic medications administered directly into the corpora cavernosa, which reliably induce detumescence in priapism that is not prolonged. Additionally, they were typically recommended with reference to recurrent ischemic priapism (<4 hours) rather than a major ischemic priapism (>4 hours). Due to the unreliable and time-consuming nature of these maneuvers, they are not recommended for the treatment of a major ischemic priapism episode.

For patients with sickle cell disease, there are treatments aimed at treating the underlying systemic disease, but current guidelines advise that directed intracavernosal therapy should be administered concomitantly to reduce any delay in treatment.[1] High-flow oxygen, intravenous hydration, and alkalinization have historically been recommended to reduce HbS polymerization and thus aid in detumescence.[47] Figure 19-4 provides an algorithm for management of priapism. Patients with major ischemic episodes most often present to the emergency department. A consult with urology should be called immediately, intravenous (IV) hydration and high-flow oxygen may be started, and the patient's pain must be addressed. Systemic analgesia is likely needed, and dosing requirements may be elevated in those with recurrent pain crises.

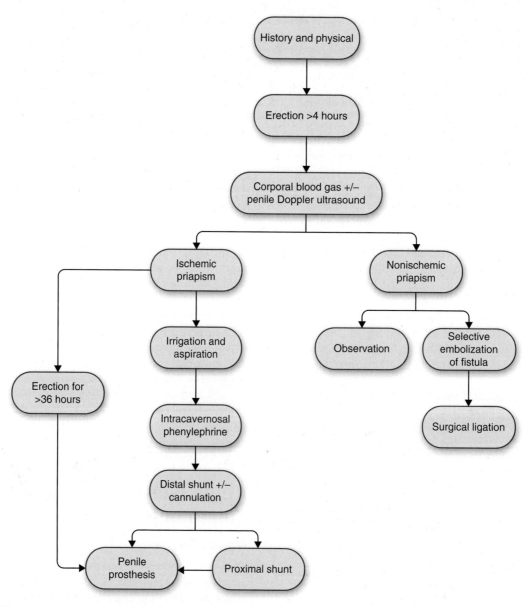

FIGURE 19-4 Algorithm for management of priapism.

Aspiration and Irrigation

A local penile block with anesthetic may be administered to decrease discomfort with insertion of the needle required for aspiration and irrigation. A 16- or 18-gauge needle is inserted through the glands into the corporal body or in the lateral base of the phallus with care to avoid the neurovascular bundle dorsally and the urethra ventrally (Figure 19-5). Viscous dark blood can be aspirated with a large syringe, such as a 60-mL syringe, repeatedly until bright red blood is obtained. Saline instillation through the same needle may help with aspiration of blood. Up to 30% of priapism episodes will be resolved with this treatment alone if they are not prolonged.[1] Aspiration will immediately soften the rigid phallus and reduce the patient's pain.

Sympathomimetics

Sympathomimetic therapy is aimed at causing smooth muscle contraction and thus detumescence. Typically, sympathomimetics are administered intracavernosally as first-line therapy so as not to delay resolution of the priapism.[1,35] As previously discussed, blood within the corpora cavernosa becomes coagulated and viscous in a time-dependent fashion during a priapic episode. For the intracavernosal sympathomimetic to disperse properly, injection is typically preceded by vigorous aspiration of old blood and irrigation with saline. Clearance of coagulated blood then allows for diffusion of the sympathomimetic throughout the corpora.

Historically, oral sympathomimetic medications such as terbutaline (β_2-adrenergic agonist), pseudoephedrine (α-adrenergic agonist), and etilefrine (β-adrenergic agonist) have been shown to have a success rate of approximately 30% in reducing erections lasting >4 hours in duration that were pharmacologically induced.[48] This success rate is modest at best and delays effective therapy. Both European and American urologic guidelines recommend against their use as a treatment for priapism.[1,35]

Although etilefrine, ephedrine, epinephrine, norepinephrine, and metaraminol are all potential options for intracavernosal sympathomimetic therapy, phenylephrine is the medication recommended by the American Urological Association guidelines. Phenylephrine is an α_1-adrenergic agonist primarily that has no indirect neurotransmitter-releasing action.[1] Many of the other options have some degree of β-adrenergic activity, which causes a rapid increase in heart rate through a direct ionotropic effect if acting on β_1 and through an indirect effect secondary to peripheral vasodilation if acting on β_2. Using a selective α-adrenergic agonist avoids these cardiovascular side effects to a large degree.

For intracavernosal injection, phenylephrine is diluted with normal saline to smaller concentrations, and a dose of 100 to 500 µg/mL is injected in 1-mL increments every 3 to 5 minutes for up to an hour.[1] The needle previously placed for aspiration

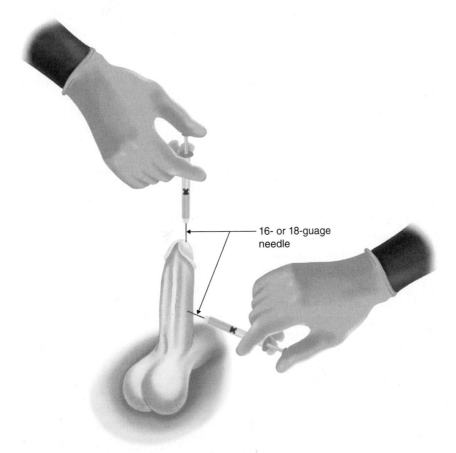

16- or 18-guage needle

FIGURE 19-5 Aspiration and irrigation. Anele UA, Burnett AL. Andrology: Priapism. Decker Medicine LLC. November 9, 2018. Accessed February 17, 2019.

and irrigation can be used to inject directly into the corpora cavernosa. Repeated doses of phenylephrine may induce hypertension and reflexive bradycardia; thus, patients should be on a cardiac monitor as the injections are performed. Caution should be exercised in those particularly susceptible such as children and those with underlying cardiac disease.[1]

Operative Procedures

If sympathomimetic therapy fails, operative intervention is warranted. The objective of shunt surgery is to restore oxygenation to the cavernous smooth muscle. Shunt procedures aim to restore outflow from the corpora cavernosa by creating a connection to the glans, corpus spongiosum, or a vein directly. Without intervention, erectile dysfunction is certain if priapism duration is prolonged, such as for >36 hours. However, some patients may develop erectile dysfunction after shunt creation. Shunt procedures are typically divided into distal and proximal depending on the anatomic level of communication.

Distal Shunting

A simple percutaneous distal shunt involves the use of a needle biopsy device to pierce through the glans cap into the top of the corpora cavernosa underlying it; this is referred to as a Winter shunt.[49] Using a number 11 scalpel blade (Ebbehoj shunt)[50] or a number 10 scalpel blade with a right angle turn upon exiting the glans (T shunt),[51] the same corporoglanular connection can be created. Patency of the shunt is always a concern, and thus, there are distal shunts referred to as "open," as opposed to the previously discussed percutaneous shunts, to more aggressively make this connection. In the al-Ghorab shunt, a small incision (<1 cm) in the dorsal glans is made, and a conical shape of glans tissue is removed from each distal portion of the corpora cavernosa.[52]

In 2009, Burnett and Pierorazio[53] described a "corporal snake" modification of the al-Ghorab shunt and Brant et al[51] described intracavernous "tunneling," both of which involve cannulating the corpora cavernosa with a metal dilator retrogradely to assist with evacuation of clotted blood as well as to ensure patency of the shunt.[53] Segal et al[54] reported priapism resolution in 8 of 10 patients treated with an al-Ghorab shunt and the corporal snake maneuver. Brant et al[51] reported resolution of longstanding priapism (>36 hours) with resumption of cavernosal artery inflow on Doppler ultrasound in 12 of 13 patients with the use of a T shunt and intracavernosal tunneling. Distal shunting with the addition of the corporal snake maneuver and/or intracavernosal tunneling has been demonstrated to be effective in resolving even recalcitrant cases of priapism without significant risk of complications.[51,54] Thus, these procedures are gaining credence, and many surgeons favor them over a proximal shunt procedure.

Proximal Shunting

Proximal shunts are typically more invasive and require an incision in the perineum to access the crus of the corpora cavernosa. Linear incisions are made adjacently in the corpora cavernosa and the spongiosum, and then the edges of these incisions are sutured together, creating an elliptical-shaped shunt.[55] This is referred to as a Sacher or Quackles shunt. Of historical interest, alternative shunt procedures involve direct anastomosis of the proximal cavernosa to either the saphenous vein (Grayhack shunt)[56] or the deep dorsal vein of the penis (Barry shunt).[57]

Penile Implantation

Priapism with a continuous duration of >72 hours will result in certain erectile dysfunction. Although shunt procedures may resolve ischemia for long-standing priapism, ultimately, the patient may undergo a penile implant to restore erectile function, especially if he is young. Extensive corporal fibrosis occurs after long-standing priapism, both making the implant surgery more technically challenging and presenting a higher risk for complications.[30,58] Thus, experts have recently advocated for immediate penile prosthesis placement at the time of priapism or shortly thereafter.[30,59]

Prevention of Stuttering (Recurrent Ischemic) Priapism

The goal of treatment for patients with stuttering priapism is to prevent future episodes and maintain erectile function.[10] By preventing recurrent episodes, the psychological burden and diminished quality of life that result from priapism are lessened. All possible caution is taken to minimize side effects due to treatment for stuttering priapism. In young patients with sickle cell disease, sexual maturation and maintaining future fertility must be considered.

Hydroxyurea

Hydroxyurea, also known as hydroxycarbamide, ameliorates some of the symptoms of sickle cell disease by increasing fetal hemoglobin (HbF).[60] Hydroxyurea is approved for the treatment of sickle cell disease by the US Food and Drug Administrations.[23] Hydroxyurea has been shown to reduce mortality by up to 40% in adult patients who take the drug for >1 year.[61] In one small study, 5 patients were treated with 10 mg/kg/d initially, which was increased to doses of 25 to 30 mg/kg/d until priapism resolved.[62] Four of the 5 patients were successfully treated, with hydroxyurea preventing priapism for several years.[62] In a case report, a 16-year-old patient suffered a major ischemic episode and underwent aspiration and irrigation followed by 6 months of transfusion therapy and hydroxyurea.[63] He was maintained on hydroxyurea, and 18 months after his major ischemic priapism episode, he was noted to regain sexual activity.[63] He was maintained on hydroxyurea for 9 additional years and did not suffer any further ischemic episodes.[63] It is important to note that all patients should be counseled on the potential reproductive implications of hydroxyurea therapy, namely possible azoospermia.[64]

Exchange Transfusion

Exchange transfusion remains controversial as a therapy to treat or prevent priapism. Ideally, it is a chronic therapy designed to target the subset of sickle cell patients with a lower baseline hemoglobin and increased hemolysis markers who have been shown to be susceptible to pulmonary hypertension, leg ulcers, and priapism.[65] Tsitsikas et al[65] reported a 5-year experience with 5 patients suffering from stuttering priapism. Patients received 10 to 14 units of red blood cells per procedure every 8 weeks with a posttransfusion HbS goal of <10%. This group reported an initial resolution of priapism immediately after the first treatment with a recurrence between cycles that diminished as the HbS levels stabilized at low levels with a regular program. No morbidity was reported in this study.[65] In 2016, Ballas and Lyon[66] reported on 10 patients with major ischemic priapism episodes unresponsive to therapy who underwent a total of 239 exchange transfusions with a target postexchange hemoglobin of 10 g/dL and HbS <30%. No significant morbidity or complications were reported. Two patients failed to respond, and 2 patients required exchange transfusion chronically to prevent priapism. However, priapism resolved in the remainder after a variable number of transfusions.[66]

Significant concern has been expressed regarding exchange transfusion as a therapy due to a link between sickle cell disease–associated priapism and severe neurologic events including headache, seizures, focal neurologic deficits, and obtundation.[67,68] The term for this association is ASPEN syndrome, which stands for **a**ssociation of **s**ickle cell disease, **p**riapism, **e**xchange transfusion and **n**eurologic events. Two separate case series report 7 children in total suffering from these symptoms after exchange transfusion.[67,68] This is thought to be due to elevated posttransfusion hemoglobin values (12-13.5 g/dL), and more recently, efforts have been made to avoid transfusion-related hyperviscosity.[66]

Oral Sympathomimetics

Pseudoephedrine is a widely available, inexpensive, and commonly used medication prescribed to prevent stuttering priapism. Unfortunately, the largest randomized trial targeting stuttering priapism failed to demonstrate a difference in the number of weekly episodes of priapism using oral sympathomimetics. The Priapism in Sickle Cell Study (PISCES) compared ephedrine, etilefrine, and placebo.[69] Over a 6-month treatment period, there was no significant difference in the number of stuttering priapism episodes per week in the treatment groups.[69] No significant side effects were reported other than transient tachycardia.[69] These data, however, call into question a common practice.

Intracavernosal Sympathomimetic Self-Injection

Sympathomimetics such as etilefrine and phenylephrine have been prescribed for self-administration by patients with sickle cell disease to prevent stuttering priapism from progressing to a major ischemic episode.[1,70,71] Intracavernosal sympathomimetic injections treat each individual episode of priapism but do not prevent future episodes.

Hormonal Therapy

Spontaneous sleep-related erections are thought to be androgen dependent. In a study of 201 patients, routine sleep-related erections did not occur in subjects with testosterone levels <200 ng/dL.[72] Therefore, suppression of male sex hormones has been one avenue of therapy directed at preventing stuttering priapism. The gonadotropin-releasing hormone analog leuprolide has been used to target the pituitary gland and reduce downstream testosterone production.[73] Diethylstilbestrol has been used to suppress pituitary function through negative feedback.[74] Antiandrogens that inhibit the testosterone receptor directly such as flutamide, bicalutamide, and chlormadinone have demonstrated the ability to inhibit stuttering priapism.[75-77] In case studies of these medications, patients commonly suffered from low libido, erectile dysfunction, and/or gynecomastia while taking the medications, and many had a resumption of stuttering priapism when the medication was discontinued.

Abern and Levine[78] published a small case series on the use of ketoconazole with prednisone supplementation to suppress stuttering priapism. Patients' testosterone levels were decreased from a mean of 468 to 275 ng/dL, and yet no patient reported symptoms of hypogonadism or gynecomastia. After finishing a 6-month course, only 2 of 8 patients experienced a resumption of priapism.[78]

Finasteride, an inhibitor of the conversion of testosterone to dihydrotestosterone via the 5α-reductase enzyme, was administered to 35 patients with stuttering priapism for 120 days.[79] The dosage was 5 mg for the first 40 days, then 3 mg for the next 40 days, and 1 mg for the final 40 days. Rachid-Filho et al[79] found that finasteride was able to prevent priapism in 46% of patients and reduce the overall mean number of episodes per month from 22.7 to 2.1 by the end of the study period.[79] Controversy regarding the existence of a post-finasteride syndrome persists.[80] Symptoms can include chronic fatigue, gynecomastia, muscle atrophy, shrinkage of genitalia, low libido, erectile dysfunction, difficulty with attention, and depression.[80] These reports should be considered carefully before administering finasteride as a treatment because many patients suffering from stuttering priapism are young.

PDE5 Inhibitors

As discussed earlier, eNOS and eNOS/nNOS knockout mice demonstrated exaggerated responses to cavernous nerve stimulation with nearly double the cGMP production.[26] This was shown to be due to decreased levels of the PDE5 enzyme.[20] Thus, modulation of PDE5 levels is a therapeutic objective. Long-term daily administration of a short-acting PDE5 inhibitor, in the absence of any sexual stimulation, has been shown to result in an upregulation of the enzyme.[81,82] The available PDE5 enzyme can then degrade cGMP, which prevents prolonged erections.

Bialecki and Bridges[83] first published a case series in 2002 describing the resolution of priapism in 3 patients with sickle cell disease with the administration of sildenafil citrate 50 mg orally. In this case series, on-demand dosing was used at the time of priapism; however, in all 3 patients, priapism resolved within 90 minutes.[83] Burnett et al[81] supported the efficacy of PDE5 inhibitors in a retrospective study of 4 patients with stuttering priapism and 3 patients with recurrent idiopathic (non–sickle cell disease) priapism. With the administration of 25 to 50 mg of sildenafil citrate daily or 5 to 10 mg of tadalafil every other day, all but 1 patient demonstrated near-complete or complete resolution of stuttering priapism.[81] In a subsequent randomized double-blind study of 13 patients with stuttering priapism, no statistically difference could be demonstrated between sildenafil citrate and placebo.[84] The trial was conducted in 2 phases, however, and during the second open-label phase, there did appear to be a reduction in major priapism episodes for those adherent to sildenafil therapy, which suggests this may be a promising therapy to prevent priapism.[84] Caution should still be exercised, however, because a trial to treat pulmonary hypertension in patients with sickle cell disease was closed early due to more frequent acute pain crises in patients treated with sildenafil versus placebo.[85]

Future Directions

The ultimate goal is to develop a preventive strategy for priapism. The molecular pathophysiology that results in priapism must first be better elucidated. Once key molecules in the pathway are identified, targeted therapies can be developed. The balance of vasodilating and vasoconstricting signals in the penis that maintains flaccidity is one avenue of research. In addition to eNOS and PDE5, several other molecules are being investigated. RhoA/Rho kinase is involved in the signal pathway, causing vasoconstriction that maintains the penis in the flaccid state.[86] Studies conducted on transgenic mice demonstrating a priapism phenotype showed attenuated activity in this pathway.[86] Adenosine, which acts as a vasodilator, is another potential molecular target. Adenosine has been demonstrated to induce penile erection in animal models.[87] Excessive signaling with adenosine due to a lack of the enzyme that catalyzes it, adenosine deaminase, was demonstrated in transgenic sickle cell mice with priapic activity.

Another avenue of research is in preventing the adhesion of erythrocytes, leukocytes, and platelets to either the endothelium or one another to form aggregates that lead to vaso-occlusion. A recent study was published in the *New England Journal of Medicine* examining the effect of crizanlizumab, a monoclonal antibody against the adhesion molecule P-selectin, on the frequency of vaso-occlusive crises in patients with sickle cell disease.[88] P-selectin translocates from storage granules to the cell surface during inflammation and regulates adhesion of activated neutrophils to the endothelium. Activated platelets also bind to neutrophils and aggregate in a P-selectin–dependent fashion.[88] Although the study did not examine priapism in particular, it was considered a vaso-occlusive crisis

event, and the study demonstrated a decrease in the median rate of all crises events per year from 2.98 in the placebo group to 1.63 in the crizanlizumab group (a 45% reduction).[88] A randomized clinical trial of crizanlizumab to prevent priapism is under way.

Many other opportunities for research exist. Opiorphins, pentapeptides found in penile smooth muscle, may have a role in regulating sexual behavior.[87] Oxidative stress and production of free radicals, which are the result of inflammation and ischemia during priapism, could be targeted. Increasing NO availability or eNOS activity to counteract the defect likely responsible for priapism could be examined. Finally, there are animal studies examining the role of antibodies against transforming growth factor-β to prevent fibrosis that results from priapism and future progression to erectile dysfunction.[89] Table 19-2 summarizes potential molecular targets being researched to develop a therapeutic intervention to prevent priapism (Table 19-2).

Conclusion

In patients with an acute episode of ischemic priapism, a thorough history and physical should be performed. A corporal blood gas measurement will confirm ischemia, and Doppler ultrasound may be a useful adjunct. Aspiration and irrigation of the corpora cavernosa should be performed urgently, followed by administration of phenylephrine directly into the corpora cavernosa to resolve priapism. If unsuccessful after

TABLE 19-2 Molecular targets for therapy

Molecular target	Action
Neuronal or endothelial nitric oxide synthase (nNOS/eNOS)	Produces nitric oxide, which initiates or prolongs erection
Phosphodiesterase type 5 (PDE5)	Degrades cyclic GMP to 5′-GMP, resulting in detumescence
RhoA/Rho-associated kinase (ROCK)	Mediator in vasoconstrictive pathway
Adenosine	Vasodilator signal that contributes to erection
Opiorphin	Pentapeptide signal in smooth muscle relaxation prolonging erection
P-selectin	Cell adhesion molecule on endothelium leading to aggregation
TGF-β	Cytokine that induces fibrosis

Abbreviations: GMP, guanosine monophosphate; TGF-β, transforming growth factor-β.

repeated doses in 3- to 5-minute increments for up to 1 hour, then surgical intervention should be performed in the form of a distal shunt. Consideration should be given to performing a bilateral distal corporoglanular shunt with intracavernosal cannulation depending on the clinical situation. Resolution of the priapism can be confirmed clinically in the majority of cases with dissipation of the patient's pain and penile rigidity.

If the exam findings are equivocal, objective data such as a cavernosal blood gas measurement or return of arterial inflow on Doppler ultrasound can confirm that the priapism has resolved. Prevention of future episodes in patients with recurrent ischemic episodes secondary to sickle cell disease may include administration of an antiandrogen or long-term PDE5 inhibitor.

Case Study: How I Treat Priapism

A 17-year-old African American male presented to the emergency department at 9:00 AM. He awoke with a rigid erection 4 hours prior that had not subsided. He had known sickle disease and has had previous painful erections, but never one that lasted this long.

In my practice, patients tend to be young African American men who suffer from recurrent ischemic priapism as well as major ischemic episodes. For a patient such as this, the emergency department physicians usually administer IV hydration, high-flow oxygen, and possibly also terbutaline prior to requesting a urology consult. At this point, time is of the essence. For a major episode, we administer IV antibiotics (1-2 g of cefazolin), a local penile block, and systemic analgesia and expeditiously attempt aspiration and irrigation through an 18-gauge needle placed directly into the lateral base of the phallus. At the time that the 18-gauge needle is inserted, a corporal blood gas is drawn to confirm that this patient truly has ischemic priapism. If priapism still persists after aspiration and irrigation, the patient would be taken immediately for a distal shunt.

In my practice, I perform a bilateral T shunt with the corporal snake maneuver, whereby the corpora cavernosa are dilated with a number 8 Hagar dilator. Timely intervention is the key to maintaining erectile function during a major ischemic episode. Typically, this young man would then be admitted for observation and pain control overnight. Outpatient follow-up is critically important. This patient would be referred to my clinic where a preventative strategy would be employed to avoid recurrent ischemic priapism. A multimodal approach would be used in collaboration with our hematology physicians. Patients are typically already taking hydroxyurea, and I personally prescribe 50 mg of sildenafil taken in the morning with avoidance of sexual stimulus to prevent future episodes. I might also prescribe phenylephrine and injection supplies for self-injection therapy to prevent recurrent ischemic episodes from progressing to a full-blown major ischemic episode.

High-Yield Facts

◆ Priapism, an erection lasting >4 hours, in patients with sickle cell disease is often ischemic. This can be confirmed with a blood gas drawn directly from the corpora cavernosa of the penis. Po_2 should be <30 mm Hg, Pco_2 should be >60 mm Hg, and pH should be <7.25.

◆ Doppler ultrasound can confirm the lack of arterial inflow if the diagnosis is in doubt.

◆ Initial management should include consulting a urologist, high-flow oxygen, and IV hydration.

◆ Aspiration and irrigation should be attempted immediately if unresolved, followed by a distal shunt with intracavernous tunneling.

◆ Without treatment, prolonged priapism results in irreversible erectile dysfunction.

◆ Hydroxyurea, exchange transfusions, antiandrogens, PDE5 inhibitors, and oral sympathomimetics are all therapeutic options for prevention of recurrent ischemic priapism.

References

1. Montague DK, Jarow J, Broderick GA, et al. American Urological Association guideline on the management of priapism. *J Urol.* 2003;170(4 Pt 1):1318-1324.

2. Eland IA, van der Lei J, Stricker BH, Sturkenboom MJ. Incidence of priapism in the general population. *Urology.* 2001;57(5): 970-972.

3. Kulmala RV, Lehtonen TA, Tammela TL. Priapism, its incidence and seasonal distribution in Finland. *Scand J Urol Nephrol.* 1995;29(1):93-96.

4. Emond AM, Holman R, Hayes RJ, Serjeant GR. Priapism and impotence in homozygous sickle cell disease. *Arch Intern Med.* 1980;140(11):1434-1437.

5. Stein DM, Flum AS, Cashy J, Zhao LC, McVary KT. Nationwide emergency department visits for priapism in the United States. *J Sex Med.* 2013;10(10):2418-2422.

6. Anele UA, Burnett AL. Erectile dysfunction after sickle cell disease-associated recurrent ischemic priapism: profile and risk factors. *J Sex Med.* 2015;12(3):713-719.

7. Ekong A, Berg L, Amos RJ, Tsitsikas DA. Regular automated red cell exchange transfusion in the management of stuttering priapism complicating sickle cell disease. *Br J Haematol.* 2018;180(4):585-588.

8. Mantadakis E, Cavender JD, Rogers ZR, Ewalt DH, Buchanan GR. Prevalence of priapism in children and adolescents with sickle cell anemia. *J Pediatr Hematol Oncol.* 1999;21(6):518-522.

9. Addis G, Spector R, Shaw E, Musumadi L, Dhanda C. The physical, social and psychological impact of priapism on adult males with sickle cell disorder. *Chronic Illn.* 2007;3(2):145-154.

10. Broderick GA, Kadioglu A, Bivalacqua TJ, Ghanem H, Nehra A, Shamloul R. Priapism: pathogenesis, epidemiology, and management. *J Sex Med.* 2010;7(1 Pt 2):476-500.

11. Kavoussi PK. Surgical, radiographic, and endoscopic anatomy of the male reproductive system. In: Wein AJ, Kavoussi LR, Partin AW, Peters CA, eds. *Campbell-Walsh Urology.* 11th ed. Elsevier; 2016:498-515.

12. Lue TF. Physiology of penile erection and pathophysiology of erectile dysfunction. In: Wein AJ, Kavoussi LR, Partin AW, Peters CA, eds. *Campbell-Walsh Urology.* 11th ed. Elsevier; 2016:612-642.

13. Anele UA, Burnett AL. Nitrergic mechanisms for management of recurrent priapism. *Sex Med Rev.* 2015;3(3):160-168.

14. Bivalacqua TJ, Musicki B, Kutlu O, Burnett AL. New insights into the pathophysiology of sickle cell disease-associated priapism. *J Sex Med.* 2012;9(1):79-87.

15. Bivalacqua TJ, Burnett AL. Priapism: new concepts in the pathophysiology and new treatment strategies. *Curr Urol Rep.* 2006;7(6):497-502.

16. Hurt KJ, Sezen SF, Lagoda GF, et al. Cyclic AMP-dependent phosphorylation of neuronal nitric oxide synthase mediates penile erection. *Proc Natl Acad Sci U S A.* 2012;109(41):16624-16629.

17. Dimmeler S, Fleming I, Fisslthaler B, Hermann C, Busse R, Zeiher AM. Activation of nitric oxide synthase in endothelial cells by Akt-dependent phosphorylation. *Nature.* 1999; 399(6736):601-605.

18. Hurt KJ, Musicki B, Palese MA, et al. Akt-dependent phosphorylation of endothelial nitric-oxide synthase mediates penile erection. *Proc Natl Acad Sci U S A.* 2002;99(6):4061-4066.

19. Boolell M, Allen MJ, Ballard SA, et al. Sildenafil: an orally active type 5 cyclic GMP-specific phosphodiesterase inhibitor for the treatment of penile erectile dysfunction. *Int J Impot Res.* 1996;8(2):47-52.

20. Champion HC, Bivalacqua TJ, Takimoto E, Kass DA, Burnett AL. Phosphodiesterase-5A dysregulation in penile erectile tissue is a mechanism of priapism. *Proc Natl Acad Sci U S A.* 2005;102(5):1661-1666.

21. Spycher MA, Hauri D. The ultrastructure of the erectile tissue in priapism. *J Urol.* 1986;135(1):142-147.

22. Zacharakis E, Raheem AA, Freeman A, et al. The efficacy of the T-shunt procedure and intracavernous tunneling (snake maneuver) for refractory ischemic priapism. *J Urol.* 2014;191(1):164-168.

23. Kato GJ. Priapism in sickle-cell disease: a hematologist's perspective. *J Sex Med.* 2012;9(1):70-78.

24. Kato GJ, McGowan V, Machado RF, et al. Lactate dehydrogenase as a biomarker of hemolysis-associated nitric oxide resistance, priapism, leg ulceration, pulmonary hypertension, and death in patients with sickle cell disease. *Blood.* 2006;107(6):2279-2285.

25. Broderick GA. Priapism and sickle-cell anemia: diagnosis and nonsurgical therapy. *J Sex Med.* 2012;9(1):88-103.

26. Burnett AL. Nitric oxide regulation of penile erection: biology and therapeutic implications. *J Androl.* 2002;23(5):S20-S26.

27. Rother RP, Bell L, Hillmen P, Gladwin MT. The clinical sequelae of intravascular hemolysis and extracellular plasma hemoglobin: a novel mechanism of human disease. *JAMA.* 2005;293(13):1653-1662.

28. Kato GJ, Gladwin MT, Steinberg MH. Deconstructing sickle cell disease: reappraisal of the role of hemolysis in the development of clinical subphenotypes. *Blood Rev.* 2007;21(1):37-47.

29. Nolan VG, Wyszynski DF, Farrer LA, Steinberg MH. Hemolysis-associated priapism in sickle cell disease. *Blood.* 2005;106(9): 3264-3267.

30. Ralph DJ, Garaffa G, Muneer A, et al. The immediate insertion of a penile prosthesis for acute ischaemic priapism. *Eur Urol.* 2009;56(6):1033-1038.

31. Bennett N, Mulhall J. Sickle cell disease status and outcomes of African-American men presenting with priapism. *J Sex Med.* 2008;5(5):1244-1250.

32. Zheng DC, Yao HJ, Zhang K, et al. Unsatisfactory outcomes of prolonged ischemic priapism without early surgical shunts: our clinical experience and a review of the literature. *Asian J Androl.* 2013;15(1):75-78.

33. Chow K, Payne S. The pharmacological management of intermittent priapismic states. *BJU Int.* 2008;102(11):1515-1521.

34. Adeyoju AB, Olujohungbe AB, Morris J, et al. Priapism in sickle-cell disease; incidence, risk factors and complications: an international multicentre study. *BJU Int.* 2002;90(9):898-902.

35. Salonia A, Eardley I, Giuliano F, et al. European Association of Urology guidelines on priapism. *Eur Urol.* 2014;65(2):480-489.

36. Wu AK, Lue TF. Commentary on high flow, non-ischemic, priapism. *Transl Androl Urol.* 2012;1(2):109-112.

37. Lutz A, Lacour S, Hellstrom W. Conversion of low-flow to high-flow priapism: a case report and review (CME). *J Sex Med.* 2012;9(4):951-954; quiz 955.

38. McMahon CG. High flow priapism due to an arterial-lacunar fistula complicating initial veno-occlusive priapism. *Int J Impot Res.* 2002;14(3):195-196.

39. Mistry NA, Tadros NN, Hedges JC. Conversion of low-flow priapism to high-flow state using T-shunt with tunneling. *Case Rep Urol.* 2017;2017:7394185.

40. Dubocq FM, Tefilli MV, Grignon DJ, Pontes JE, Dhabuwala CB. High flow malignant priapism with isolated metastasis to the corpora cavernosa. *Urology.* 1998;51(2):324-326.

41. Masson-Lecomte A, Rocher L, Ferlicot S, Benoit G, Droupy S. High-flow priapism due to a malignant glomus tumor (glomangiosarcoma) of the corpus cavernosum. *J Sex Med.* 2011;8(12):3518-3522.

42. Todd NV. Priapism in acute spinal cord injury. *Spinal Cord.* 2011;49(10):1033-1035.

43. Burnett AL, Bivalacqua TJ. Priapism: new concepts in medical and surgical management. *Urol Clin North Am.* 2011;38(2):185-194.

44. Burnett AL, Anele UA, Derogatis LR. Priapism Impact Profile questionnaire: development and initial validation. *Urology.* 2015;85(6):1376-1381.

45. LeRoy TJ, Broderick GA. Doppler blood flow analysis of erectile function: who, when, and how. *Urol Clin North Am.* 2011;38(2):147-154.

46. Patel U, Sujenthiran A, Watkin N. Penile Doppler ultrasound in men with stuttering priapism and sickle cell disease: a labile baseline diastolic velocity is a characteristic finding. *J Sex Med.* 2015;12(2):549-556.

47. Baron M, Leiter E. The management of priapism in sickle cell anemia. *J Urol.* 1978;119(5):610-611.

48. Lowe FC, Jarow JP. Placebo-controlled study of oral terbutaline and pseudoephedrine in management of prostaglandin E1-induced prolonged erections. *Urology.* 1993;42(1):51-53; discussion 53-54.

49. Winter CC. Cure of idiopathic priapism: new procedure for creating fistula between glans penis and corpora cavernosa. *Urology.* 1976;8(4):389-391.

50. Ebbehoj J. A new operation for priapism. *Scand J Plast Reconstr Surg.* 1974;8(3):241-242.

51. Brant WO, Garcia MM, Bella AJ, Chi T, Lue TF. T-shaped shunt and intracavernous tunneling for prolonged ischemic priapism. *J Urol.* 2009;181(4):1699-1705.

52. Hanafy HM, Saad SM, El-Rifaie M, Al-Ghorab MM. Early Arabian medicine: contribution to urology. *Urology.* 1976;8(1):63-67.

53. Burnett AL, Pierorazio PM. Corporal "snake" maneuver: corporoglanular shunt surgical modification for ischemic priapism. *J Sex Med.* 2009;6(4):1171-1176.

54. Segal RL, Readal N, Pierorazio PM, Burnett AL, Bivalacqua TJ. Corporal Burnett "snake" surgical maneuver for the treatment of ischemic priapism: long-term followup. *J Urol.* 2013;189(3):1025-1029.

55. Quackels R. [Treatment of a case of priapism by cavernospongious anastomosis]. *Acta Urol Belg.* 1964;32:5-13.

56. Grayhack JT, McCullough W, O'Conor VJ Jr, Trippel O. Venous bypass to control priapism. *Invest Urol.* 1964;1:509-513.

57. Barry JM. Priapism: treatment with corpus cavernosum to dorsal vein of penis shunts. *J Urol.* 1976;116(6):754-756.

58. Zacharakis E, Garaffa G, Raheem AA, Christopher AN, Muneer A, Ralph DJ. Penile prosthesis insertion in patients with refractory ischaemic priapism: early vs delayed implantation. *BJU Int.* 2014;114(4):576-581.

59. Yafi FA, Hellstrom WJG. Immediate placement of penile prosthesis for the management of ischemic priapism as first-line treatment. *Eur Urol Focus.* 2019;5(4):531-532.

60. Steinberg MH. Management of sickle cell disease. *N Engl J Med.* 1999;340(13):1021-1030.

61. Steinberg MH, Barton F, Castro O, et al. Effect of hydroxyurea on mortality and morbidity in adult sickle cell anemia: risks and benefits up to 9 years of treatment. *JAMA.* 2003;289(13):1645-1651.

62. Saad ST, Lajolo C, Gilli S, et al. Follow-up of sickle cell disease patients with priapism treated by hydroxyurea. *Am J Hematol.* 2004;77(1):45-49.

63. Anele UA, Mack AK, Resar LMS, Burnett AL. Hydroxyurea therapy for priapism prevention and erectile function recovery in sickle cell disease: a case report and review of the literature. *Int Urol Nephrol.* 2014;46(9):1733-1736.

64. Nevitt SJ, Jones AP, Howard J. Hydroxyurea (hydroxycarbamide) for sickle cell disease. *Cochrane Database Syst Rev.* 2017;4:CD002202.

65. Tsitsikas DA, Orebayo F, Agapidou A, Amos RJ. Distinct patterns of response to transfusion therapy for different chronic complications of sickle cell disease: a useful insight. *Transfus Apher Sci.* 2017;56(5):713-716.

66. Ballas SK, Lyon D. Safety and efficacy of blood exchange transfusion for priapism complicating sickle cell disease. *J Clin Apher.* 2016;31(1):5-10.

67. Rackoff WR, Ohene-Frempong K, Month S, Scott JP, Neahring B, Cohen AR. Neurologic events after partial exchange transfusion for priapism in sickle cell disease. *J Pediatr.* 1992;120(6):882-885.

68. Siegel JF, Rich MA, Brock WA. Association of sickle cell disease, priapism, exchange transfusion and neurological events: ASPEN syndrome. *J Urol.* 1993;150(5 Pt 1):1480-1482.

69. Olujohungbe AB, Adeyoju A, Yardumian A, et al. A prospective diary study of stuttering priapism in adolescents and young men with sickle cell anemia: report of an international randomized control trial—the Priapism in Sickle Cell Study. *J Androl.* 2011;32(4):375-382.

70. Virag R, Bachir D, Lee K, Galacteros F. Preventive treatment of priapism in sickle cell disease with oral and self-administered intracavernous injection of etilefrine. *Urology.* 1996;47(5):777-781; discussion 781.

71. Teloken C, Ribeiro EP, Chammas M Jr, Teloken PE, Souto CA. Intracavernosal etilefrine self-injection therapy for recurrent priapism: one decade of follow-up. *Urology.* 2005;65(5):1002.

72. Granata AR, Rochira V, Lerchl A, Marrama P, Carani C. Relationship between sleep-related erections and testosterone levels in men. *J Androl.* 1997;18(5):522-527.

73. Steinberg J, Eyre RC. Management of recurrent priapism with epinephrine self-injection and gonadotropin-releasing hormone analogue. *J Urol.* 1995;153(1):152-153.

74. Shamloul R, el Nashaar A. Idiopathic stuttering priapism treated successfully with low-dose ethinyl estradiol: a single case report. *J Sex Med.* 2005;2(5):732-734.

75. Costabile RA. Successful treatment of stutter priapism with an antiandrogen. *Tech Urol.* 1998;4(3):167-168.

76. Dahm P, Rao DS, Donatucci CF. Antiandrogens in the treatment of priapism. *Urology.* 2002;59(1):138.

77. Yamashita N, Hisasue S, Kato R, et al. Idiopathic stuttering priapism: recovery of detumescence mechanism with temporal use of antiandrogen. *Urology.* 2004;63(6):1182-1184.

78. Abern MR, Levine LA. Ketoconazole and prednisone to prevent recurrent ischemic priapism. *J Urol.* 2009;182(4):1401-1406.

79. Rachid-Filho D, Cavalcanti AG, Favorito LA, Costa WS, Sampaio FJ. Treatment of recurrent priapism in sickle cell anemia with finasteride: a new approach. *Urology.* 2009;74(5):1054-1057.

80. Ganzer CA, Jacobs AR, Iqbal F. Persistent sexual, emotional, and cognitive impairment post-finasteride: a survey of men reporting symptoms. *Am J Mens Health.* 2015;9(3):222-228.

81. Burnett AL, Bivalacqua TJ, Champion HC, Musicki B. Feasibility of the use of phosphodiesterase type 5 inhibitors in a pharmacologic prevention program for recurrent priapism. *J Sex Med.* 2006;3(6):1077-1084.

82. Bivalacqua TJ, Musicki B, Hsu LL, Berkowitz DE, Champion HC, Burnett AL. Sildenafil citrate-restored eNOS and PDE5 regulation in sickle cell mouse penis prevents priapism via control of oxidative/nitrosative stress. *PLoS One.* 2013;8(7):e68028.

83. Bialecki ES, Bridges KR. Sildenafil relieves priapism in patients with sickle cell disease. *Am J Med.* 2002;113(3):252.

84. Burnett AL, Anele UA, Trueheart IN, Strouse JJ, Casella JF. Randomized controlled trial of sildenafil for preventing recurrent ischemic priapism in sickle cell disease. *Am J Med.* 2014; 127(7):664-668.

85. Machado RF, Barst RJ, Yovetich NA, et al. Hospitalization for pain in patients with sickle cell disease treated with sildenafil for elevated TRV and low exercise capacity. *Blood.* 2011;118(4):855-864.

86. Bivalacqua TJ, Ross AE, Strong TD, et al. Attenuated RhoA/ Rho-kinase signaling in penis of transgenic sickle cell mice. *Urology.* 2010;76(2):510.e517-512.

87. Anele UA, Morrison BF, Burnett AL. Molecular pathophysiology of priapism: emerging targets. *Curr Drug Targets.* 2015;16(5): 474-483.

88. Ataga KI, Kutlar A, Kanter J, et al. Crizanlizumab for the prevention of pain crises in sickle cell disease. *N Engl J Med.* 2017;376(5): 429-439.

89. Sanli O, Armagan A, Kandirali E, et al. TGF-beta1 neutralizing antibodies decrease the fibrotic effects of ischemic priapism. *Int J Impot Res.* 2004;16(6):492-497.

Ocular Complications in Sickle Cell Disease

Authors: Adrienne W. Scott, Morton F. Goldberg

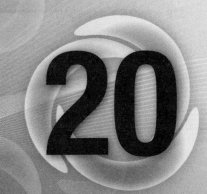

Chapter Outline

Overview

Sickle cell disease (SCD) can affect the vascular bed of any part of the eye, including the conjunctiva, iris and anterior segment, optic nerve, retina, and choroid (Figure 20-1).[1] Fortunately, severe vision loss in patients with SCD is rare. Proliferative sickle cell retinopathy (PSR), in which pathologic preretinal neovascularization occurs, is the most common cause of significant vision loss in patients with SCD.[2-4]

Detection of sickling within the eye can be observed directly by the practitioner using conventional diagnostic instruments (well-illuminated magnifying devices such as the ophthalmoscope and also the slit lamp biomicroscope). Both transient and permanent effects of intraocular sickling are virtually pathognomonic, especially in the white of the eye (conjunctiva) and in the ocular fundus (retina and associated tissues). In the fundus, potentially blinding complications of sickling can be identified and treated. Growth of neovascular tissue in the retina, PSR, is usually treated by laser photocoagulation or by intraocular injection of anti–vascular endothelial growth factor (VEGF) agents (eg, bevacizumab and others). Intraocular blood clots within the vitreous chamber in the rear of the eye can be treated surgically. Blood clots in the front (anterior) chamber of the eye can be treated with surgical evacuation.

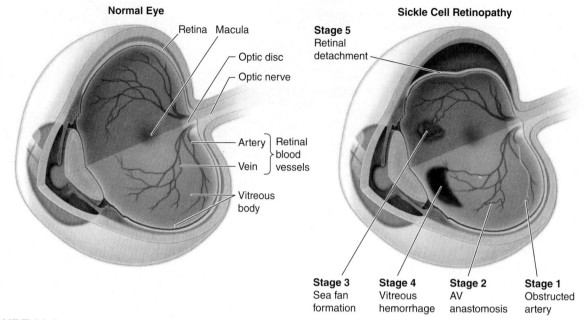

FIGURE 20-1 **Diagram of the eye.** Note the peripheral location of many of the pathological events.

This chapter includes discussions of the following topics: pathophysiology and epidemiology of vision loss in SCD; sickle cell hyphema (blood in the anterior chamber of the eye and its induced ocular hypertension, which can be blinding); natural history of SCD affecting the peripheral and also the central macular portion of the retina; the classification of PSR; imaging modalities for both the front and back portions of the eye; treatment techniques; and screening advice. The chapter concludes with illustrative cases and "High-Yield Facts."

The risk for permanent and severe vision loss is highly correlated with SCD genotype. PSR lesions can be identified through regular dilated fundus exams and may potentially regress with or without treatment. Herein, we discuss how SCD affects the eyes and our recommendations for evaluation, management, and prevention of vision loss related to SCD.

Pathophysiology and Risk Factors for Loss of Vision in SCD

Risk factors for loss of vision in SCD are primarily understood to be those that predispose to PSR, including genotype, age, and systemic SCD therapy. Individuals with the homozygous genotype (HbSS), although more likely to experience higher rates of vaso-occlusive crises and overall morbidity and mortality, are counterintuitively less likely to experience PSR and subsequent loss of vision as compared to individuals with compound heterozygous mutations (eg, HbSC) or those with hemoglobin S (HbS)-β thalassemia. Reasons for this are not fully understood. However, it is likely that in HbSS, small arterioles throughout the retina frequently undergo complete occlusion, causing local retinal infarction and loss of production of vascular growth factors. On the other hand, in HbSC, less complete vascular occlusions may occur, thereby causing relative, but not complete, hypoxia of the surrounding tissue and allowing viable cells to chronically express proangiogenic growth factors, such as VEGF and hypoxia-inducible factor (HIF)-1α. This creates an environment conducive to upregulation of growth factors and pathologic neovascularization.[5,6] In comparison with HbSS patients, individuals with HbSC have higher hematocrit and blood viscosity levels and lower fetal hemoglobin (HbF). These factors in HbSC cause vascular stasis and sludging of the sickled cells throughout the microcirculation of the eye. Decreased blood flow causes poor oxygen delivery to the retina due to, for example, abnormal interaction with cellular adhesion molecules and upregulation of leukokines. In addition, irreversibly sickled HbSS erythrocytes are easily trapped in retinal capillaries and precapillary arterioles under hypoxic conditions.[6] HbSC blood with fewer irreversibly sickled cells, however, regardless of oxygen levels, is less easily trapped in the retinal microvasculature. Thus, HbSC-related vaso-occlusive eye disease may be the result of the complex interaction among cytokines, growth factors, and adhesion molecules. Although individuals with sickle cell trait are typically asymptomatic with a normal ocular phenotype, retinal pathology occasionally has been described[7-9] and may become manifest in conditions conducive to erythrocytic sickling, such as high altitudes, colder climates, or dehydration.[3]

Incident PSR has been noted to increase with increasing age. Downes et al[2] studied a Jamaican cohort of 307 HbSS patients and 201 HbSC sickle cell patients over 20 years. The annual PSR incidence rate was 0.5 cases per 100 in HbSS subjects and 2.5 cases per 100 in HbSC subjects. These authors also described spontaneous regression of PSR lesions in 32% of affected eyes.[2]

Systemic associations with vision loss in SCD have been studied, but it is still incompletely understood which systemic risk factors of SCD are associated with the likelihood of vision loss. In a retrospective study, Duan et al[10] reported older age and male sex to be most associated with loss of vision in HbSS patients and suggested that chronic transfusion therapy may be protective against the need for laser photocoagulation or vitrectomy surgery, the most common therapeutic interventions in PSR.

Hydroxyurea increases HbF and decreases vascular occlusion by lowering expression of endothelial cell adhesion molecules and decreasing the numbers of circulating leukocytes and reticulocytes.[11,12] Use of hydroxyurea has been formally evaluated as a protective agent against development of sickle cell retinopathy. Estepp et al[13] reported decreased odds of incident sickle cell retinopathy in HbSS children with hydroxyurea-induced elevated HbF compared to untreated controls. Overall, children with an HbF level <15% demonstrated increased odds of incident sickle cell retinopathy independent of hydroxyurea use. Mian et al[11] studied adults with sickle cell retinopathy to assess the effect of hydroxyurea on incident retinopathy. These authors reported an overall 50% reduction in odds of retinopathy developing in HbSS adults with an HbF level of at least 15%.[11] The potential protective effect of hydroxyurea use, especially for HbSC patients, remains inconclusive, possibly because patients with HbSC disease are less likely to meet criteria for hydroxyurea therapy.[11] Although these contemporary studies report promising data for hydroxyurea use in decreasing the risk of sickle cell retinopathy, studies to date evaluating this relationship have been retrospective. In addition, reports have described suboptimal adherence to prescribed hydroxyurea therapy in SCD.[14-16] Prospective studies are needed to confirm any relationship between hydroxyurea use and sickle cell retinopathy.

In summary, microvascular occlusions cause impaired oxygen delivery to ocular tissues. Tissue ischemia occurs due to the complex interplay between dehydrated, sickled erythrocytes and activated endothelial cells, reticulocytes, leukocytes, platelets, and cytokines, plus upregulation of pathologic growth factors. These abnormalities within the microcirculation occur throughout the entire body in SCD and can uniquely be observed directly within the eye because of its transparent media.

Clinical Topics

Clinical topics include the following: sickling in the front of the eye (anterior segment and anterior chamber); the conjunctival sign of sickling; natural history of SCD in the retina (both the peripheral retina and the central macular portions of the retina); diagnostic imaging; screening guidelines; and specific management advice.

Anterior Segment and Anterior Chamber

SCD can affect almost every tissue of the eye.

Sickling of erythrocytes within the vasculature of the white of the eye (the conjunctiva) is highly typical for sickling hemoglobinopathy, especially for HbSS (but less common in HbSC).[17,18] This sign is totally absent in sickle cell trait. It is best seen with an illuminated slit lamp (biomicroscope) but can also be detected with a conventional hand-held direct ophthalmoscope with its lens set to +10 to +40 diopters.

The conjunctival sign of sickling is seen as a partially perfused network of tiny, red, comma-shaped and hyphen-shaped capillaries and precapillary arterioles. There are no visual consequences.[17] This specific sign of sickling should not be confused with "box-carring" (sluggish or intermittent flow, which is a nonspecific finding and not diagnostic for sickling). Iris infarcts and atrophy also occur from closure of iris arteries (Figure 20-2).

Sickled Erythrocytes in the Front (Anterior) Chamber of the Eye: Hyphema and Elevation of Intraocular Pressure

Blood within the anterior chamber of the eye is known as *hyphema*. It is always pathologic. Even with nonsickling cells, blood in the anterior chamber often clogs the channels that normally allow outflow of intraocular fluid from the anterior chamber. This phenomenon is exacerbated by the presence of rigid, sickled erythrocytes, which create a logjam in the outflow channels within the anterior segment of the eye. As a result, intraocular pressure increases, a vision-threatening condition called secondary glaucoma. Elevated pressure within the eye reduces blood flow to important tissues, including the optic nerve. Reduced blood flow, which is further worsened by the

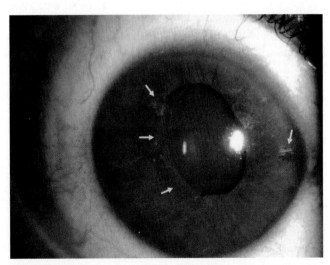

FIGURE 20-2 The iris of a 43-year-old man with HbSC demonstrates patchy iris atrophy (white arrows).

presence of sickled cells within the blood vessels of the optic nerve, can lead to irreversible loss of vision. Thus, hyphema is always a serious event; it deserves urgent, and sometimes immediate, therapeutic intervention, especially when the erythrocytes are capable of sickling. This is true regardless of the etiology of the hemorrhage (eg, blunt or perforating trauma, neovascularization of the iris, hemorrhage following intraocular surgery). This pathophysiologic scenario occurs in all genomic forms of SCD, including sickle cell trait. Although sickle cell trait rarely causes tissue destruction or symptoms elsewhere in the body, it can cause devastating intraocular complications, such as those described earlier. The intraocular biochemical milieu seems tailor-made to induce and also maintain sickling (in both sickle cell trait and in all other more serious sickling variants). The characteristics of the normal anterior chamber that enable and exacerbate sickling include the following: a typically low partial pressure of oxygen, low pH, high partial pressure of carbon dioxide, and an especially high concentration of ascorbate (a reducing agent).[19]

Metabolizing blood within the anterior chamber induces a vicious cycle by contributing to further hypoxia, acidosis, and hypercarbia, which, in turn, may result in further HbS polymerization within erythrocytes. These events can occur even when the amount of blood in the anterior chamber is minimal. Abnormally high intraocular pressure often results, even when only a small percentage of erythrocytes are sickled (eg, 5%-15% of the erythrocytes within the anterior chamber). Unfortunately, clinical inspection of a hyphema (even if magnified and illuminated with a slit lamp) does not reveal whether any erythrocytes are or are not in the sickled configuration. Thus, it is best to assume that the optic nerve is at imminent risk of infarction (with permanent loss of vision) in all sickle cell patients with hyphema, including individuals with sickle cell trait. These patients should therefore have frequent and regular measurements of intraocular pressure (eg, every 6 hours around the clock) until the hyphema disappears and intraocular pressure returns to normal. Whenever the average pressure measurement during any consecutive 24-hour period exceeds 24 mm Hg (easy to remember using the mnemonic "24 for 24") or whenever a pressure spike exceeds 30 mm Hg, some of the blood should immediately be removed by paracentesis of the anterior chamber. This decompresses the eye and improves blood flow within the optic nerve. The following interventions may additionally be used simultaneously: intranasal/face mask oxygen; transcorneal oxygen; eye drops containing β-blockers, corticosteroids, and/or atropine; and oral ε-aminocaproic acid. Because of pharmacologically induced hemoconcentration and/or acidosis, repeated use of drugs such as hyperosmotic agents and carbonic anhydrase inhibitors may be deleterious in sickle cell patients.[19]

Natural History and Epidemiology of the Vasculopathy of the Peripheral Retina and the Central (Macular) Retina

Typically, patients with SCD remain visually asymptomatic; however, as previously noted, rates of vision loss increase with age. What specifically defines the term *retinopathy* differs throughout different studies in the literature and depends on sensitivity of methods of retinal examination, skill of the retinal examiner, and use of adjunctive retinal imaging.[20] Talbot et al[21] evaluated children aged 5 to 13 years among a Jamaican cohort and reported peripheral retinal vessel closure in 50% of children with HbSS and HbSC genotypes at age 6 years. By age 12, 90% of HbSS and HbSC children were noted to have peripheral retinal vessel closure. PSR was rare in children and developed in only 1 boy with HbSC disease at age 8.[21] The incidence of retinopathy, however, increases with patient age, as noted previously.[20,22]

Peripheral Retina

Nonproliferative Sickle Cell Retinopathy

Nonproliferative sickle cell retinopathy (NPSR) findings are extremely common in the retinal periphery of patients with SCD. Retinal changes, such as salmon patch hemorrhages, iridescent spots, and black sunburst lesions, are common sequelae of peripheral retinal nonperfusion, especially in HbSS.[7,23-26]

Salmon patch hemorrhages, named for their pinkish-red color, are transient fundus findings that result from a blowout of a retinal arteriolar wall associated with an arteriolar occlusion (Figure 20-3). These well-defined hemorrhages are located within the superficial inner retina, just external to the internal limiting membrane. As salmon patch hemorrhages resorb, focal retinal thinning, chorioretinal scarring, and/or iridescent spots within a retinoschisis cavity (splitting within the retinal layers) can be observed with an ophthalmoscope. Iridescent spots are refractile yellowish granules and likely represent hemosiderin-laden macrophages.[25] Additionally, dark chorioretinal scars called black sunburst lesions are also commonly observed in NPSR (Figure 20-4). Black sunburst lesions, which are round or ovoid areas of hypertrophy and hyperplasia of the retinal pigment epithelium,[27] are typically located in the retinal periphery abutting an area of retinal nonperfusion. Other common retinal findings include posterior retinal vascular tortuosity, the optic disc sign (dark red spots within the optic nerve head), and angioid streaks (Figure 20-5). Angioid streaks are breaks in Bruch's membrane, the innermost layer of the choroid (Figure 20-1), and are observed as fissures radially emanating from the optic nerve head. They are most commonly seen in the HbSS genotype. Angioid streaks typically follow a benign course in patients with SCD and do not usually result in choroidal neovascularization (abnormal pathologic blood vessel growth under the retina), unlike similar streaks in patients without SCD. Treatment is not usually recommended for NPSR.

Proliferative Sickle Cell Retinopathy

Individuals with SCD may also develop pathologic neovascularization on the internal surface of the peripheral retina, known as PSR. Even those who develop neovascularization from PSR may often remain asymptomatic, at least initially, because this neovascularization commonly occurs in the far

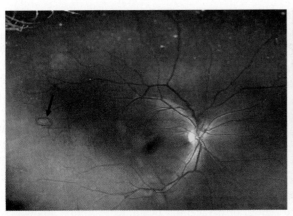
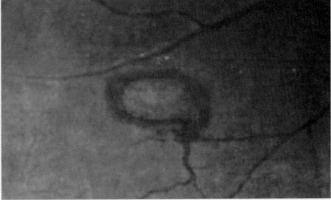

FIGURE 20-3 Ultra-widefield fundus image of a 29-year-old man with HbSS demonstrates a salmon patch hemorrhage (black arrow, left) in the retinal periphery. Salmon patch hemorrhages represent a blowout of a retinal arteriolar wall (magnified image, right).

peripheral retina out of the line of sight. Central visual acuity is therefore not typically affected unless vitreous hemorrhage or retinal detachment occurs. The hallmark of PSR, sea fan neovascularization (Figure 20-6), is named for *Gorgonia flabellum*, a marine animal species with a characteristic fan-shaped appearance.

In 1971, Goldberg[28] described the widely used classification system for PSR, which was based on clinical observations of sequential retinal vascular remodeling. The major stages are as follows: stage 1, peripheral retinal arteriolar occlusions (Figure 20-4); stage 2, arteriolar-venular anastomoses (Figure 20-7); stage 3, neovascular and fibrous proliferations (called sea fan neovascularization); stage 4, vitreous hemorrhage; and stage 5, retinal detachment. Progression of sea fan neovascularization to the vision-threatening stages of PSR has been reported to be most frequent between age 20 and 39 years in HbSS and HbSC patients.[29] Sea fan lesions initially appear as a vascularized complex of red blood vessels. These lesions may autoinfarct and regress spontaneously without visual consequence, thereupon appearing more fibrotic (whitish) and less vascular. Sea fan regression has been reported in up to 30% to 60% of PSR cases.[2,28,30-34] PSR may be more stable in HbSC

patients over 40 years of age. Spontaneous regression of PSR is more commonly noted in HbSS patients, sometimes with progression to complete nonperfusion.[29] The natural history of PSR can be quite variable, even among individuals with the same genotype.

Most peripheral retinal artery occlusions (stage 1) affect the smaller arteriolar branches in the retinal periphery in patients with SCD, particularly those with the HbSS genotype. These peripheral arteriolar occlusions are typically not known to cause vision loss. These vascular occlusions can occur early in life in SCD. For example, a postmortem specimen of a 20-month-old infant with HbSS disease showed retinal vascular occlusion at the capillary and precapillary arteriolar level.[35] Subsequent retinal vascular remodeling (progression

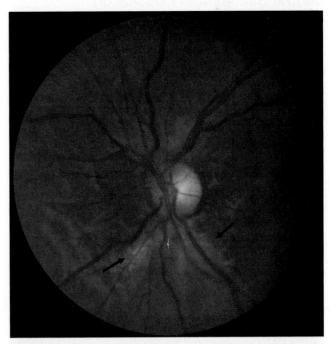

FIGURE 20-4 Ultra-widefield fundus photograph demonstrates a black sunburst lesion (white arrow) and a peripheral arteriolar occlusion (black arrow), consistent with Goldberg stage 1 sickle cell retinopathy.

FIGURE 20-5 A 30-degree fundus image demonstrates angioid streaks, breaks in Bruch's membrane, noted as radial fissures emanating from the optic nerve, in a 61-year-old patient with HbSS (black arrows).

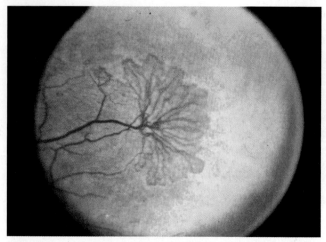

FIGURE 20-6 The 30-degree fundus photograph demonstrates the characteristic sea fan neovascular lesion in proliferative sickle cell retinopathy. Note peripheral nonperfusion of the retina.

to stages 2 through 5) occurs extensively over the lifetime of a patient with SCD, evidenced by occluded vessels, hairpin loops, arteriovenous anastomoses, and formation of sea fan neovascular complexes.[35,36] Whereas the retinal vasculature in children with SCD demonstrates arteriole and capillary occlusions, larger arteries occlude in adults, possibly due to cumulative vascular insults from longer disease duration. Causes of vaso-occlusion are related to sickled erythrocytes in the microcirculation and to repetitive damage to the vascular beds with resultant leukocyte and endothelial activation.[8]

Central Retinal Artery Occlusion

Central retinal artery occlusions occur rarely, but especially in HbSS, and present with sudden, painless, severe loss of vision when the central retinal circulation is affected. These rare occurrences require emergent diagnosis and treatment. In the case of central retinal artery occlusion in SCD, urgent intravenous hydration and oxygen administration are indicated, and acute ocular decompression should be considered in order to maximize blood flow. Hematologic consultation should be promptly obtained for consideration of urgent red cell exchange transfusion and possibly other systemic therapies in these patients.

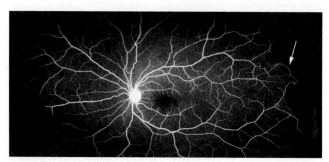

FIGURE 20-7 Ultra-widefield fluorescein angiogram demonstrates arteriolar-venular anastomoses (white arrow), Goldberg stage 2 sickle cell retinopathy.

Macula

The macula is the functional center of the retina. Although primarily known to affect the periphery of the retina, sickle hemoglobinopathies commonly affect the macula as well, evidenced by characteristic vascular abnormalities noted on both fundus exam and macular imaging. The fovea, the small central depression in the macular center, has the highest concentration of cone cells in the retina and is responsible for sharp central visual acuity. A normal foveal center is devoid of blood vessels with a smooth and symmetric pattern of capillaries at its border. This avascular central fovea is termed the *foveal avascular zone*. The macula in SCD shows pathologic thinning and central or paracentral ovoid depression(s), known as the *macular depression sign*. It can be observed on ophthalmoscopy and slit lamp examination. Macular thinning is caused by macular vaso-occlusions in SCD with subsequent atrophy. This macular thinning is characteristically noted in the temporal macula, where there are terminal branches of the retinal vasculature that form a watershed zone. This vascular bed is thought to be anatomically analogous to the vasculature in the far temporal retinal periphery, where sea fans commonly occur.[37] Patients with maculopathy demonstrate irregularities around the foveal avascular zone, microaneurysmal dots, and hairpin loops.[37] The prognostic significance of macular vascular changes in SCD is not completely understood, and their relationship to overall visual function can vary. There is no known treatment for sickle cell maculopathy.

Diagnostic Imaging of the Retina

Novel imaging techniques have greatly enhanced our understanding of the pathophysiology of sickle cell retinopathy. Fluorescein angiography (FA) is a commonly used outpatient clinic test in retinal practice, in which sodium fluorescein dye is injected into a vein in the arm. The various transit phases of the fluorescein dye in the choroidal and retinal circulations are imaged through a specialized blue camera filter. FA has long been used in ophthalmology. Kikai published the first visualization of fluorescein dye in the retinal vessels after fluorescein injection in 1930.[38,39] This is the gold standard test for retinal perfusion, and FA is commonly used in the evaluation and treatment of retinal diseases. However, traditional, or standard, FA captures only 30 degrees of the retina. In order to image the retinal periphery, where sickling changes typically occur, peripheral retinal image "sweeps" must be obtained (the patient is instructed to look in various fields of gaze) so that images of the peripheral retina may be acquired. The initial description of the Goldberg stages of PSR was in part derived from observations of the peripheral retina using standard 30-degree FA images.[28]

Sickle cell vascular pathology, including NPSR and PSR lesions, is most commonly noted in the far retinal periphery, but standard 30-degree FA, even with peripheral sweeps, may only capture up to about 75 degrees of the entire retinal field.[40] Thus, the standard camera may miss many important lesions. Penman et al[41] performed a study in a Jamaican cohort and described a new classification system of PSR based on the appearance of the border of the peripheral vasculature as seen

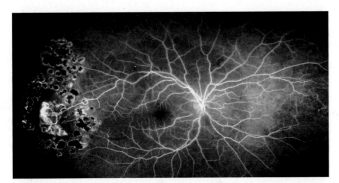

FIGURE 20-8 Ultra-widefield fluorescein angiogram demonstrates sea fan neovascularization (red arrow), Goldberg stage 3 sickle cell retinopathy. The sea fan neovascular lesion is surrounded by laser photocoagulation marks.

on FA. Qualitatively normal vascular borders (type I) versus abnormal vascular borders (type II) were evaluated. Type I borders demonstrated a low likelihood of progression to PSR, whereas type II borders carried a higher risk of conversion to neovascularization over the course of the 12-year follow-up period. The authors note that the peripheral border of the retinal vasculature was too peripheral to be captured in 13 of 24 eyes with only 30-degree FA.[42]

Modern ultra-widefield imaging, in which up to 200 degrees of the retina is captured in a single image, enables the characteristic peripheral retinal changes in SCD to be routinely imaged and is an excellent technique for documenting peripheral retinal disease in both NPSR and PSR (Figures 20-3, 20-4, 20-7, and 20-8; see also later Figure 20-11). The ultra-widefield image may be captured quickly and requires less technical skill from the photographer. It is also less dependent upon patient cooperation than the standard 7 fields of 30-degree FA. Cho and Kiss[42] compared standard FA to ultra-widefield FA in patients with SCD and observed that ultra-widefield FA captured retinal vascular pathology not seen on standard field

imaging. Ultra-widefield FA is also ideal for evaluating peripheral nonperfusion and for detecting or evaluating leakage from PSR lesions. Ultra-widefield FA has also proven to be useful in staging sickle cell retinopathy. Another study evaluated the utility of ultra-widefield FA in sickle cell retinopathy in 70 eyes of 35 patients.[43] Approximately 60% of eyes had no visible retinopathy on dilated fundus exam alone, but with ultra-widefield FA, nearly all eyes showed peripheral retinal vascular changes consistent with Goldberg stage 2 or greater. However, grade 3 PSR, in which preretinal neovascularization is noted, was reliably detected on clinical examination by indirect ophthalmoscopy, without usage of photographic techniques. Therefore, ultra-widefield FA, although helpful in documenting a higher stage of retinopathy than that detected on clinical exam alone, did not impact clinical management of these patients.

Another imaging technique, spectral domain (SD) optical coherence tomography (OCT), has become a vital tool for evaluation and management of most posterior segment ophthalmic diseases and rapidly provides cross-sectional imaging of the retina. SD-OCT is noninvasive, can show detailed retinal structure and quantification of retinal thickness, and is most commonly used to image the macula. Sickle cell maculopathy has been well described with SD-OCT. Sickle cell patients show characteristic thinning patterns (Figure 20-9). SCD patients demonstrate overall retinal thinning in the central macula as compared to healthy controls, particularly in the outer retinal layers of the central macular and parafoveal regions.[44-47] In a prospective study of 513 eyes, Lim and Cao[47] reported increased retinal thinning in the inner retina in HbSS patients compared to HbSC and HbS-β thalassemia patients. Retinal thinning increases with age and with sickle cell retinopathy stage.[47] In addition to generalized retinal thinning, "foveal splay," or a flattening of the foveal contour, is commonly observed in sickle cell maculopathy.[45] Individuals with SCD may also demonstrate characteristic focal macular thinning, frequently noted in the temporal macula, a

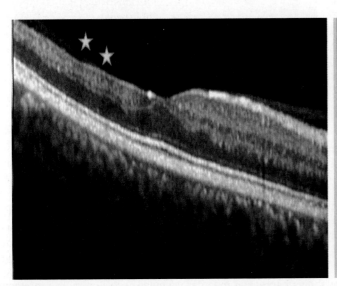

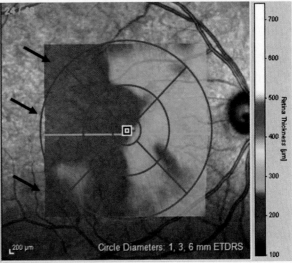

FIGURE 20-9 Spectral domain optical coherence tomography demonstrates flattening and thinning of the temporal macula (stars) in a 29-year-old patient with HbSS. Blue and purple areas of the corresponding macular thickness map (black arrows) depict the macular thinning, which extends into the foveal center.

known watershed zone for the macular microvasculature. Murthy et al[48] described thinning of the temporal fovea on SD-OCT in association with peripheral PSR and posited that SD-OCT may be used as a screening tool; if focal thinning is noted, the clinician should consider ultra-widefield FA to evaluate for PSR lesions in the periphery. However, macular thinning has been known to occur early in SCD and is often present in the absence of the pathologic retinal neovascularization defined as PSR. Paramacular atrophy on SD-OCT was noted to occur in 64% of children in a cohort of 81 children with SCD, whereas only 11% were noted to have PSR.

It is currently unclear what the visual significance is of the macular thinning. Although most patients with SCD have excellent distance vision, there is some evidence that macular thinning may affect near vision, which is not routinely tested. In a small study of 3 HbSS patients with cerebral vasculopathy (each with 20/20 distance visual acuity), temporal macular atrophy noted on SD-OCT corresponded to paracentral scotomas on central visual field testing.[49] A larger series reported significantly decreased retinal sensitivity in areas of temporal macular thinning in a cohort of sickle cell patients with 20/20 distance visual acuity, compared to those without thinning and compared to age-matched healthy controls.[50] In addition to macular thinning, other macular pathology may be observed in SCD, including macular epiretinal membranes (layers of preretinal tissue), vitreomacular traction (abnormal pulling of the vitreous on the macular retina causing anatomic distortion), macular schisis (splitting of retinal layers), and macular holes.

Angiography based on fluorescein dye enables visualization of retinal vasculature and is helpful in evaluating peripheral retinal perfusion in sickle cell retinopathy as well as leakage from lesions of PSR. However, FA has several disadvantages. Venipuncture is required for the procedure, which may be uncomfortable and inconvenient for patients, particularly those with SCD who have to undergo regular venipuncture for management of their systemic disease. Although fluorescein injection is generally well tolerated, patients commonly experience transient nausea and/or vomiting with injection of intravenous fluorescein. A small percentage of individuals may exhibit allergy to fluorescein dye and develop itching or a rash after fluorescein injection. Rarely, cases of anaphylaxis after fluorescein injection have occurred. FA can also be time consuming. Capturing the fluorescein transit may take up to 20 to 30 minutes. Although FA is helpful for in vivo visualization of the superficial capillary plexus of the retinal circulation and for providing 2-dimensional images, it does not image the radial peripapillary capillary plexus or the deep capillary plexus.[39]

OCT angiography (OCT-A) is a newer noninvasive imaging modality proven to be capable of imaging all of the major retinal capillary networks (Figure 20-10). OCT-A uses motion contrast technology and vascular flow characteristics to provide information about the choriocapillaris, radial peripapillary capillaries, and the deep and superficial capillary networks of the retina.[39] OCT-A scans can be acquired in <1 minute in a cooperative patient. No venipuncture or fluorescein dye injection is required.

There are extensive publications evaluating application of OCT-A in patients with SCD.[51] For example, in 2015, Han et al[52] described loss of vascular flow in a small series of patients with SCD. These authors reported that the superficial and deep retinal capillary plexuses both showed characteristic areas of

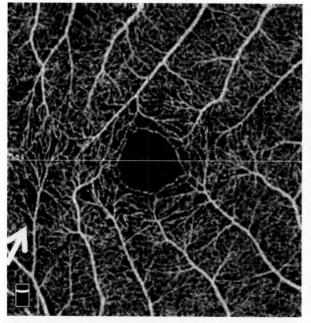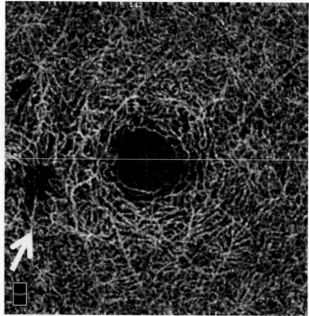

FIGURE 20-10 Optical coherence tomography angiography shows decreased macular vascular perfusion more prominently noted in the deep capillary plexus (white arrow, right) as compared to the analogous area in the superficial vascular plexus (white arrow, left) in a patient with sickle cell disease. The center of the macula (the fovea) normally is avascular (see central dark oval).

decreased flow, with the deep plexus more commonly and severely affected.[53] These findings have been consistently corroborated in larger series.[54] Characteristic areas of decreased blood flow or nonperfusion are commonly noted in the temporal macula (in the terminal capillary beds, which represent a watershed zone for the macular circulation) (Figure 20-10). The areas of decreased vascular flow tend to correspond with the areas of structural thinning noted on conventional SD-OCT. OCT-A is highly sensitive in detection of microangiopathy in SCD, whereas FA may not image some of these areas of vascular nonperfusion. In a study of 18 eyes of 9 SCD patients, OCT-A demonstrated abnormalities in the macular microvasculature in the presence of normal-appearing FA.[53]

Vascular flow voids have also been identified in pediatric and adolescent SCD populations.[40] These areas of nonperfusion on OCT-A may be observed even before the structural thinning becomes manifest on conventional SD-OCT imaging.[51] Repetitive vascular occlusions of the microcirculation due to SCD likely cause the retina to become atrophic and thin over time. A meta-analysis of OCT-A in SCD reported a prevalence of 45.6% with sickle cell maculopathy (defined as any vascular changes in the macular region).[51] Qualitative and quantitative findings of SCD on OCT-A include irregularity and increased size of the foveal avascular zone (Figure 20-10), increased vascular diameter, decreased macular vascular density, and increased vascular tortuosity, typically in the temporal macula.[55] It remains unclear how these microvascular abnormalities relate to overall visual function, but OCT-A shows promise as an imaging tool that provides objective structural and functional information about macular perfusion in SCD.

The microcapillary beds in the temporal macula and those in the peripheral retina are both terminal vascular beds and may have analogous structure and function. Peripheral retinal ischemia on ultra-widefield FA has been correlated with vessel density observed on OCT-A in the temporal subfield of the superficial capillary plexus and in all subfields of the deep capillary plexus.[56] Thus, OCT-A may have future utility in an updated staging classification of sickle cell retinopathy. Further studies are needed to determine the correlation of macular pathology, as demonstrated by OCT-A, with peripheral retinal ischemia or PSR in SCD.

There is no consensus among retinal specialists regarding the ideal baseline imaging techniques to evaluate sickle cell retinopathy during a routine screening visit. Because macular thinning and peripheral nonperfusion are both quite common in SCD patients, even in those with good visual acuity, we routinely obtain SD-OCT and OCT-A macular imaging as well as ultra-widefield FA imaging of the peripheral retina. If venipuncture is difficult or if dye-based angiography is challenging, baseline color widefield retina photographs are obtained in the absence of fluorescein injections.

Treatment

There is no known preventive treatment for microvascular occlusive diseases in sickle cell retinopathy. NPSR lesions are followed expectantly; they may be transient and resolve over time. Scatter laser photocoagulation has been the mainstay of treatment for PSR and is typically considered when preretinal neovascularization occurs (stage 3). Small, flat, or fibrotic areas of sea fan neovascularization can be observed without initial intervention, because they may remain quiescent or involute in the retinal periphery (without progression to vitreous hemorrhage or retinal detachment). Ultra-widefield fundus photographs and FA are particularly helpful in this instance to document lesion size and to monitor progression over time. Laser treatment is recommended in cases of vitreous hemorrhage related to PSR, for large areas of sea fan neovascularization, or when vascularized sea fan neovascularizations have been observed to increase over time, or to demonstrate traction by adherent vitreous. Laser treatment may also be considered if there is concern about a patient with SCD not adhering to close retinal follow-up or if a patient has experienced PSR stage 4 (vitreous hemorrhage) or stage 5 (retinal detachment) in the contralateral eye.

A Cochrane Database analysis evaluated 341 eyes from 2 trials of laser treatment for PSR.[57-59] In the first trial, Jampol et al[58] evaluated feeder vessel photocoagulation laser technique, and in the second trial, Rednam et al[59] employed scatter retinal photocoagulation. The Cochrane Database analysis concluded that laser photocoagulation using scatter laser or feeder vessel coagulation for PSR may prevent the loss of vision at a median follow-up of 21 to 47 months. Another study by the same group corroborated safety and efficacy of scatter laser photocoagulation in PSR, with a decreased incidence of vitreous hemorrhage in treated eyes compared to controls.[60] The findings from these clinical trials evaluating laser treatment in PSR must be interpreted cautiously, because these studies were performed in the 1980s and 1990s and significant advancements in laser treatment technology and technique have occurred since then. The feeder vessel technique is rarely used today.

A recent study in autopsied eyes with PSR confirmed the increased presence of proangiogenic factors (HIF-1α and VEGF) in peripheral nonperfused retina, in the border between nonperfused and perfused retina, and in posterior ischemic retina.[61] Laser photocoagulation of the retina in ischemic retinopathies may work successfully through ablation of ischemic retinal tissue, thereby decreasing production of retinal VEGF. Therefore, targeting laser photocoagulation to ischemic retina in eyes prior to development of neovascularization has been considered.[61] Similar laser applications have been performed in diabetic retinopathy and in retinal vein occlusion in attempts to decrease the risk of neovascularization; however, no substantive evidence supports this prophylactic approach in sickle cell retinopathy.

VEGF is one of the proangiogenic growth factors implicated in pathologic angiogenesis in PSR. It follows that anti-VEGF therapy may be effective in decreasing retinal neovascularization in this disease (Figure 20-11). Anti-VEGF medications are commonly injected intravitreally in several retinal diseases, including age-related macular degeneration, diabetic retinopathy, diabetic macular edema, and retinal vein occlusion. Off-label use of bevacizumab (a widely used anti-VEGF

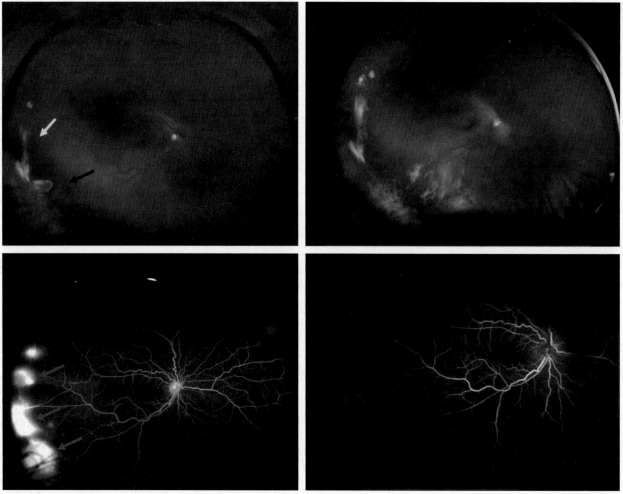

FIGURE 20-11 Ultra-widefield images of Goldberg stage 3 retinopathy before and after treatment with intravitreal bevacizumab. The white arrow shows the fibrotic neovascular complex with preretinal hemorrhage (black arrow, top left). Ultra-widefield fluorescein angiogram shows late leakage (bottom left, red arrows). After scatter laser treatment and intravitreal bevacizumab, the preretinal hemorrhage has regressed (top right), and the peripheral vascular leakage on ultra-widefield fluorescein angiography has resolved (bottom right).

agent) was described in HbSC patients with PSR.[62] In this series, 4 patients with recurrent vitreous hemorrhage and 1 patient with significant sea fan neovascularization were treated with intravitreal bevacizumab injection.[62] Following a single intravitreal bevacizumab injection, all neovascular lesions showed an anatomic response, with decrease in the vascularity and in the leakage on FA. Intravitreal injections were well tolerated in sickle cell patients. Because no large-scale clinical trials have yet evaluated anti-VEGF treatment in PSR, the optimal treatment frequency, dosages, and long-term outcomes have yet to be defined.

Surgical treatment of PSR may be considered for eyes that progress to nonclearing vitreous hemorrhage. Anti-VEGF injections can cause involution of neovascular complexes and facilitate clearing of vitreous hemorrhage. Therefore, anti-VEGF intravitreal injection may be considered as an alternative to vitrectomy surgery for clearing of vitreous hemorrhage and may avoid the risks of surgery in carefully selected cases.[62] Tractional and/or combined tractional-rhegmatogenous retinal detachment (ie, a retinal detachment with a retinal hole

or retinal tear) is usually an indication for surgery. Neovascular complexes in PSR frequently regress spontaneously or undergo autoinfarction without treatment. However, in rare cases, tractional retinal detachment results when the neovascular complexes contract, causing progressive traction on the retina, leading to retinal detachment (defined as separation of the retina from the underlying retinal pigment epithelium) (Figure 20-1). Combined tractional-rhegmatogenous retinal detachment may also occur if the sea fan complex causes traction on the retina, resulting in a retinal hole or a tear. As a result of prior sickle cell–related peripheral nonperfusion, the peripheral retina is often thinned and is thus prone to retinal breaks from progressive atrophy and/or traction.

Retinal surgeons must take care in preoperative, intraoperative, and postoperative planning for patients with PSR. Preoperative consultation with hematologists is suggested because some patients may benefit from red blood cell exchange to minimize the fraction of HbS prior to retina surgery. In addition, coordination with the anesthesiology team is important. General anesthesia is preferred in order to maximize analgesia.

In cases where there are medical contraindications to general anesthesia, sub-Tenon's anesthesia injection is preferred over retrobulbar anesthesia injection in order to avoid the risk of iatrogenic elevation of intraocular pressure and the orbital compression syndrome causing reduced vascular perfusion.[63,64] Hydration status should be optimized with intravenous fluids, and hyperoxygenation of the patient should be done before, during, and after surgery. Special care should be taken to minimize elevations in intraocular pressure spikes during and after surgery in order to decrease the risk of retinal artery occlusion.

The goals of retina surgery are to relieve vitreoretinal traction and to identify and seal all retinal holes or tears. Surgery for retinal detachment associated with PSR is complex and challenging, even in experienced hands. Visual prognosis is guarded. In a retrospective review including 8 cases of retinal detachment associated with PSR, a second surgery was required in 50% of cases due to recurrent retinal detachment.[65] Risk of iatrogenic retinal breaks is significant because surgical dissection of retinal membranes can lead to inadvertent tears of the thin, avascular retina. Preoperative bevacizumab injection may be used to decrease vascularity of sea fan neovascular complexes in order to facilitate their dissection and removal.[66]

Screening Guidelines

To date, there are no large, randomized, prospective, controlled clinical trials to inform screening recommendations for sickle cell retinopathy. Most studies of sickle cell retinopathy are retrospective, observational, or cross-sectional.[67] Current screening guidelines, based on expert consensus, recommend referral of all SCD patients to an ophthalmologist for dilated fundus examination annually or biannually beginning at age 10. These are strong recommendations, but based on low-quality evidence from a 2014 National Heart, Lung, and Blood Institute report.[68]

Although mild NPSR changes are frequently present in young children with SCD, PSR is unlikely to be present in SCD patients under the age of 10.[69] Hematologists or primary medical physicians caring for patients with SCD should ask patients about visual symptoms, such as floaters (often described as moving black dots in the visual field), because an association has been reported between such visual symptoms and necessary intervention such as vitrectomy or laser photocoagulation for PSR.[10] Physicians should take special care to refer SCD patients with HbSC and HbS-β thalassemia, especially those between the ages 20 and 39, for complete dilated eye exams because incidence and rates of progression of PSR lesions have been reported to be highest in these groups. PSR also occurs in HbSS patients but to a lesser extent. It is important that the primary medical team and hematologists emphasize to patients that (1) it is possible to have no visual symptoms but still have potentially sight-threatening PSR that should be monitored or treated, and (2) *dilated* eye exams are necessary to screen for potentially sight-threatening sickle cell retinopathy. Undilated examination (eg, for eyeglasses) is not sufficient for sickle cell retinopathy screening.

Specific Management and Therapy: How We Treat

Consistent, clear communication and efficient referral patterns between ophthalmology and hematology specialists are important to identify and manage patients at risk for vision loss from sickle cell retinopathy. We recommend the following for SCD patients referred to our retinal clinic:

1. At a minimum, all patients should undergo a complete ophthalmic exam, including slit lamp biomicroscopy and dilated indirect ophthalmoscopy annually. Communication to the patient and to the hematology team must occur regarding any recommendations for treatment and follow-up.

2. Patients of all SCD genotypes should receive baseline imaging to include OCT and OCT-A. If NPSR lesions are present, ultra-widefield fundus photos are obtained to document the findings and to facilitate assessment of progression over time. If PSR lesions are noted on dilated fundus exam, barring any medical contraindications, ultra-widefield FA is obtained to evaluate the extent of the PSR lesions and to guide scatter laser photocoagulation if recommended. Annual return is recommended for reassessment if no PSR is present, and more frequent follow-up (typically every 6 months) is recommended if PSR is present.

3. If sea fan neovascular complexes are small, stable, or mostly nonvascularized, observation is recommended with 6-month follow-up (assuming that the patient is likely to follow up). However, (1) if active, vascularized, progressively enlarging sea fan lesions are identified or are under traction; (2) if vitreous hemorrhage is identified; or (3) if the patient will not or cannot comply with follow-up instructions, scatter laser photocoagulation treatment is performed immediately. Scatter laser photocoagulation may also be recommended if the patient has a history of vision loss in the other eye from PSR complications. The ultra-widefield fluorescein angiogram is used as a guide, and scatter laser photocoagulation is performed to surround sea fan neovascular lesions. Scatter laser is also applied to the retinal periphery both anterior and posterior to areas of neovascularization (Figure 20-8).[70] If a patient with PSR has had laser treatment and is experiencing vitreous hemorrhage, additional supplemental laser may be considered. More recently, adjunctive anti-VEGF treatments, such as intravitreal bevacizumab injections, have been considered in these cases to facilitate regression of sea fan neovascular complexes and clearing of vitreous hemorrhage.

Future Research

Novel imaging techniques have revolutionized our understanding of the retinal microvascular circulation in patients with SCD. Almost all patients with SCD will show some evidence of abnormal retinal circulation during their lifetime. It remains as yet unclear which systemic factors related to SCD will influence incidence or progression of sight-threatening retinopathy from sea fan formation or from sudden retinal arterial occlusion. It is difficult to conduct controlled trials of systemic disease-modifying agents because the natural history and clinical course of sickle cell retinopathy can be quite variable, even among patients of the same genotype, and even between the 2 eyes of the same patient. A controlled trial would require large numbers of patients to be followed prospectively over long periods of time. Promising systemic interventions, such as bone marrow transplantation, gene therapy, and pharmacotherapy, have been reported to decrease systemic morbidity from SCD but, as yet, not ocular complications. Coordination among ophthalmologists and hematologists to evaluate the effect of these systemic interventions on retinal findings would be invaluable.

The association between sickle cell maculopathy and peripheral retinal ischemia is still unclear, although there may be an association between decreased vascular flow in the macula and nonperfusion in the peripheral retina. Further study is needed to better define the relationship between these circulatory beds, and an updated classification and staging system should incorporate macular findings as well as the Goldberg classification.

The severe burden of SCD produces challenges in caring for affected patients in areas such as sub-Saharan African countries where prevalence and morbidity of sickle cell retinopathy care are greatest. In developed countries, permanent and severe vision loss from sickle cell retinopathy is uncommon. However, young people of working age in sub-Saharan African countries too often experience blinding sickle cell retinopathy because

interventions such as laser photocoagulation and vitreoretinal surgery are difficult to obtain.[67,71] Tele-ophthalmology technology has been successful in screening for highly prevalent retinal diseases such as diabetic retinopathy and is a promising method of identifying patients who are at risk for vision loss associated with PSR.

Conclusion

Although much is known about SCD and its effects on the eye, there is much information that remains unknown. Severity of sickle cell retinopathy and risk of vision loss are largely dependent on SCD genotype for reasons that are yet unclear. Fortunately, severe vision loss is rare in SCD patients and is most often related to complications from PSR. This primarily affects individuals with the HbSC genotype, likely attributable to higher blood viscosity in these patients. Regular surveillance screening exams are important because PSR can be present even in asymptomatic patients with SCD and can threaten vision. Further research is needed to determine how to better refine screening protocols and to facilitate screening for retinopathy through tele-ophthalmology combined with machine learning approaches. In addition, further study is needed to assess the impact of emerging systemic treatments for SCD, such as gene therapy, bone marrow transplantation, and newer pharmacologic agents, and their impact on sickle cell retinopathy's incidence and progression.

Case Studies

Case 1 (Figure 20-12)
A 31-year-old HbSS patient with a small sea fan neovascular lesion and 20/12 (normal) vision was lost to follow-up for 2 years. He presented urgently with decreased vision down to hand motions from Goldberg stage 4 PSR (vitreous hemorrhage), which cleared without intervention. Scatter laser photocoagulation was then performed.

Case 2 (Figure 20-13)
A 36-year-old HbSC patient with PSR presented acutely to the emergency department with painless severe vision loss down to 20/400 because of central retinal artery occlusion. He required hospital admission for red blood cell exchange transfusion and hydration. Partial visual recovery to 20/250 and partial recovery of retinal perfusion were noted 9 days later.

Case Studies: Continued

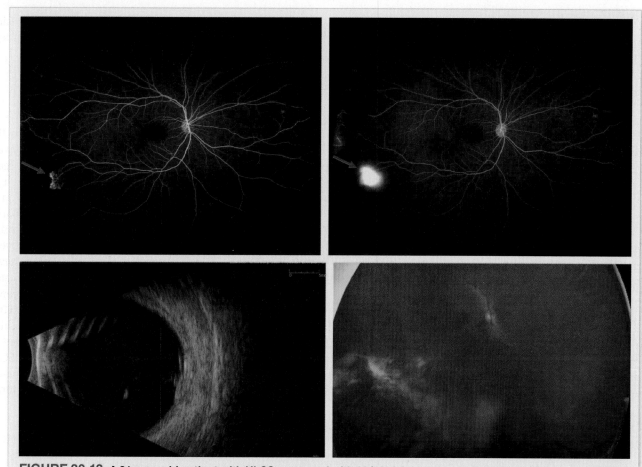

FIGURE 20-12 **A 31-year-old patient with HbSS presented with 20/12 vision and a small sea fan neovascular complex (red arrows; early frame ultra-widefield fluorescein angiogram, top left, late frame ultra-widefield fluorescein angiogram, top right).** Observation and 6-month follow-up were recommended. The patient was lost to follow-up and, 2 years later, suffered a vitreous hemorrhage with drop in vision to counting fingers. The vitreous hemorrhage prevented a view of the fundus. B-scan ultrasound showed hyperreflective vitreous hemorrhage (bottom left). The vitreous hemorrhage cleared with observation (bottom right), and scatter laser was then placed through the retinal periphery.

Case Studies: Continued

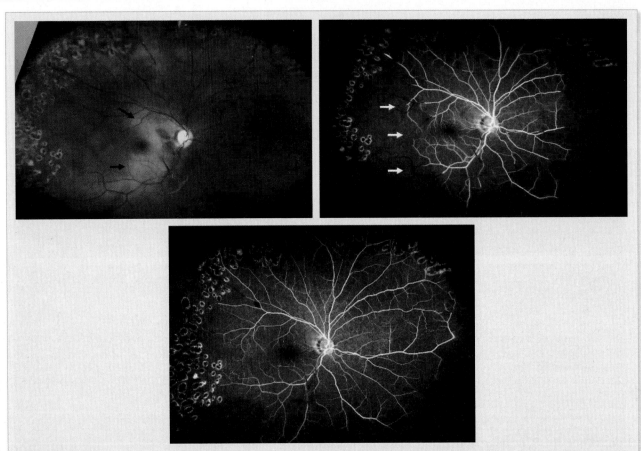

FIGURE 20-13 **A 36-year-old HbSC patient with proliferative sickle cell retinopathy presented with sudden painless vision loss down to 20/400 because of central retinal artery occlusion.** Ultra-widefield fundus image showed retinal whitening through the macula (top left, black arrows). Ultra-widefield fluorescein angiogram on presentation showed decreased retinal vascular perfusion (top right, white arrows). Eleven days later, after red cell exchange transfusion and hydration, ultra-widefield fluorescein angiogram showed partial recovery of retinal perfusion (bottom right). Also note well-healed peripheral circular scars from prior scatter laser therapy.

High-Yield Facts

◆ Sickle cell retinopathy, including sickle cell maculopathy, is prevalent among patients with SCD.

◆ Patients with SCD should have at least annual dilated fundus exams with an ophthalmologist or retinal specialist.

◆ Floaters or other visual symptoms should alert the hematologist or primary medical care team to refer the SCD patient for ophthalmic evaluation.

◆ Newer retinal imaging techniques, including ultra-widefield FA, OCT, and OCT-A are highly sensitive methods of detecting even subtle levels of retinopathy.

◆ Permanent and severe vision loss occurs most commonly from PSR-related vitreous hemorrhage or retinal detachment but is otherwise uncommon in SCD.

◆ PSR is more common in the HbSC genotype; however, HbSS patients can also develop advanced stages of PSR.

◆ Patients with SCD can experience abrupt decreased vision due to acute vascular events such as central or branch retinal artery occlusion. Ophthalmologists and emergency department physicians should be certain to maximize hydration and oxygenation in such SCD patients and to consult hematologists urgently for consideration of red blood cell exchange transfusions or other therapy.

High-Yield Facts (Cont.)

◆ Hyphema in sickle cell patients requires emergency management.
◆ The rate of progression of PSR is greatest between ages 20 and 39.
◆ Reappraisal of clinical staging, with novel imaging, should incorporate macular pathology.

References

1. Cook WC. A case of sickle cell anemia with associated subarachnoid hemorrhage. *Am J Med.* 1930;11:541.

2. Downes SM, Hambleton IR, Chuang EL, et al. Incidence and natural history of proliferative sickle cell retinopathy: observations from a cohort study. *Ophthalmology.* 2005;112(11):1869-1875.

3. Moriarty BJ, Acheson RW, Condon PI, et al. Patterns of visual loss in untreated sickle cell retinopathy. *Eye.* 1988;2(Pt 3):330-335.

4. Fox PD, Dunn DT, Morris JS, et al. Risk factors for proliferative sickle retinopathy. *Br J Ophthalmol.* 1990;74(3):172-176.

5. Gagliano DA, Jampol L, Rabb M, et al. Sickle cell disease. In: Tasman WS, Jaeger E, eds. *Duane's Clinical Ophthalmology.* Lippincott Raven; 1996;vol.3:1-40.

6. Lutty GA, Phelan A, Mcleod DS, et al. A rat model for sickle-cell mediated vaso-occlusion in retina. *Microvasc Res.* 1996;52:270-280.

7. Welch RB, Goldberg MF. Sickle-Cell hemoglobin and its relation to fundus abnormality. *Arch Ophthalmol.* 1966;75(3):353-362.

8. Elagouz M, Jyothi S, Gupta B, et al. Sickle cell disease and the eye: old and new concepts. *Surv Ophthalmol.* 2010;55(4):359-377.

9. Nagpal KC, Asdourian GK, Patrianakos D, et al. Proliferative retinopathy in sickle cell trait. *Arch Intern Med.* 1977;137(3):325-328.

10. Duan XJ, Lanzkron S, Linz MO, et al. Clinical and ophthalmic factors associated with the severity of sickle cell retinopathy. *Am J Ophthalmol.* 2019;197:105-113.

11. Mian UK, Tang J, Allende APM, et al. Elevated fetal hemoglobin levels are associated with decreased incidence of retinopathy in adults with sickle cell disease. *Br J Haematol.* 2018;183(5):807-811.

12. Ware RE. How I use hydroxyurea to treat young patients with sickle cell anemia. *Blood.* 2010;115(26):5300-5311.

13. Estepp JH, Smeltzer MP, Wang WC, et al. Protection from sickle cell retinopathy is associated with elevated HbF levels and hydroxycarbamide use in children. *Br J Haematol.* 2013;161:402-405.

14. Walsh KE, Cutrona SL, Kavanagh PL, et al. Medication adherence among pediatric patients with sickle cell disease: a systematic review. *Pediatrics.* 2014;134(6):1175-1183.

15. Loiselle K, Lee JL, Szulczewski L, et al. Systematic and meta-analytic review: medication adherence among pediatric patients with sickle cell disease. *J Pediatr Psychol.* 2016;41(4):406-418.

16. Badawy SM, Thompson AA, Holl JL, et al. Healthcare utilization and hydroxyurea adherence in youth with sickle cell disease. *Pediatr Hematol Oncol.* 2018;35(5-6):297-308.

17. Paton D. The conjunctival sign of sickle-cell disease. *Arch Ophthalmol.* 1961;66(1):90-94.

18. Roy MS, Rodgers GP, Podgor MJ, et al. Conjunctival sign in sickle cell anaemia: an in vivo correlate of the extent of red cell heterogeneity. *Br J Ophthalmol.* 1985;69(8):629-632.

19. Goldberg MF, Dizon R, Moses VK. Sickled erythrocytes, hyphema, and secondary glaucoma. VI. The relationship between intracameral blood cells and aqueous humor pH, pO2, and pCO2. *Ophthal Surg.* 1979;10(4):78-88.

20. Pahl DA, Green NS, Bhatia M, et al. New ways to detect pediatric sickle cell retinopathy: a comprehensive review. *J Pediatr Hematol Oncol.* 2017;39(8):618-625.

21. Talbot JF, Bird AC, Maude GH, et al. Sickle cell retinopathy in Jamaican children: further observations from a cohort study. *Br J Ophthalmol.* 1988;72:727-732.

22. Leveziel N, Bastugi-Garin S, Lalloum F, et al. Clinical and laboratory factors associated with the severity of proliferative sickle cell retinopathy in patients with sickle cell hemoglobin C (SC) and homozygous sickle cell disease (SS). *Medicine (Baltimore).* 2011;90(6):372-378.

23. Kassim AA, DeBaun MR. Sickle cell disease, vasculopathy, and therapeutics. *Annu Rev Med.* 2013;64:451-466.

24. Ballas SK, Kesen MR, Goldberg MF, et al. Beyond the definitions of the phenotypic complications of sickle cell disease: an update on management. *ScientificWorldJournal.* 2012;2012:949535.

25. Gagliano DA, Goldberg MF. The evolution of salmon-patch hemorrhages in sickle cell retinopathy. *Arch Ophthalmol.* 1989;107(12):1814-1815.

26. Romayananda N, Goldberg MF, Green WR. Histopathology of sickle cell retinopathy. *Trans Am Acad Ophthalmol Otolaryngol.* 1973;77(5):652-676.

27. Asdourian G, Nagpal KC, Goldbaum M, et al. Evolution of the retinal black sunburst in sickling haemoglobinopathies. *Br J Ophthalmol.* 1975;59(12):710-716.

28. Goldberg MF. Natural history of untreated proliferative sickle retinopathy. *Arch Ophthalmol.* 1971;85(4):428-437.

29. Fox PD, Vessey SJR, Forshaw ML, et al. Influence of genotype on natural history of untreated proliferative sickle retinopathy-an angiographic study. *Br J Ophthalmol.* 1991;75(4):229-231.

30. Farber MD, Jampol LM, Fox P, et al. A randomized clinical trial of scatter photocoagulation of proliferative sickle cell retinopathy. *Arch Ophthalmol.* 1991;109(3):363-367.

31. Goldberg MF, Jampol LM. Treatment of neovascularization, vitreous hemorrhage and retinal detachment in sickle cell retinopathy. *Trans New Orleans Acad Ophthalmol.* 1983;31:53-81.

32. Nagpal KC, Patrianakos D, Asdourian GK, et al. Spontaneous regression (autoinfarction) of sickle cell retinopathy. *Am J Ophthalmol.* 1975;80(5):885-892.

33. Condon PI, Serjeant GR. Behaviour of untreated proliferative sickle retinopathy. *Br J Ophthalmol.* 1980;64(6):404-411.

34. McLeod DS, Merges C, Fukushima A, et al. Histopathologic features of neovascularization in sickle cell retinopathy. *Am J Ophthalmol.* 1997;124:455-472.

35. McLeod DS, Goldberg MF, Lutty GA. Dual-perspective analysis of vascular formations in sickle cell retinopathy. *Arch Ophthalmol.* 1993;111(9):1234-1245.

36. Galinos SO, Asdourian GK, Woolf MB, et al. Spontaneous remodeling of the peripheral retinal vasculature in sickling disorders. *Am J Ophthalmol.* 1975;79(5):853-870.

37. Stevens TS, Busse B, Lee CB. Sickling hemoglobinopathies; macular and perimacular vascular abnormalities. *Arch Ophthalmol.* 1974;92(6):455-463.

38. Kikai K. Uber die vitalfarbung des hinteren bulbussabschnittes. *Arch Augenheilkd.* 1930;103:541-553.

39. Spaide RF, Klancnik JM, Cooney MJ. Retinal vascular layers imaged by fluorescein angiography and optical coherence tomography angiography. *JAMA Ophthalmol.* 2015;133(1):45-50.

40. Pahl DA, Green NS, Bhatia M, et al. Optical coherence tomography and ultra-widefield fluorescein angiography for early detection of adolescent sickle retinopathy. *Am J Ophthalmol.* 2017;183:91-98.

41. Penman AD, Talbot F, Chuang EL, et al. New classification of peripheral retinal vascular changes in sickle cell disease. *Br J Ophthlmol.* 1994;78(9):68-69.

42. Cho M, Kiss S. Detection and monitoring of sickle cell retinopathy using ultra wide-field color photography and fluorescein angiography. *Retina.* 2011;31(4):738-747.

43. Han IC, Zhang Y, Liu TYA, et al. Utility of ultra-widefield retinal imaging for staging and management of sickle cell retinopathy. *Retina.* 2019;39(5):836-843.

44. Witkin AJ, Rogers AH, Ko TH, et al. Optical coherence tomography demonstration of macular infarction in sickle cell retinopathy. *Arch Ophthalmol.* 2006;124(5):747-747.

45. Hoang QV, Chau FY, Shahidi M, et al. Central macular splaying and outer retinal thinning in asymptomatic sickle cell patients by spectral-domain optical coherence tomography. *Am J Ophthalmol.* 2011; 151(6):990-994.

46. Cai CX, Han IC, Tian J, et al. Progressive retinal thinning in sickle cell retinopathy. *Ophthalmol Retina.* 2018;2(2):1241-1248.e2.

47. Lim JI, Cao D. Analysis of retinal thinning using spectral-domain optical coherence tomography imaging of sickle cell retinopathy eyes compared to age- and race-matched control eyes. *Am J Ophthalmol.* 2018;192:229-238.

48. Murthy RK, Grover S, Kakarla C. Temporal macular thinning on spectral-domain optical coherence tomography in proliferative sickle cell retinopathy. *Arch Ophthalmol.* 2011;129(2):247-249.

49. Martin GC, Denier C, Zambrowski O, et al. Visual function in asymptomatic patients with homozygous sickle cell disease and temporal macular atrophy. *JAMA Ophthalmol.* 2017;135(10):1100-1105.

50. Chow CC, Genead MA, Anastasakis A, et al. Structural and functional correlation in sickle cell retinopathy using spectral-domain optical coherence tomography and scanning laser ophthalmoscope microperimetry. *Am J Ophthalmol.* 2011;152(4):704-711.e2.

51. Leitão Guerra RL, Leitão Guerra CL, Bastos MG, et al. Sickle cell retinopathy: what we now understand using optical coherence tomography angiography. A systematic review. *Blood Rev.* 2019;35:32-42.

52. Han IC, Tadarati M, Scott AW. Macular vascular abnormalities identified by optical coherence angiography in patients with sickle cell disease. *JAMA Ophthalmol.* 2015;133(11):1337-1340.

53. Mienville W, Caillaux V, Cohen SY, et al. Macular microangiopathy in sickle cell disease using optical coherence angiography. *Am J Ophthalmol.* 2016;164:137-144.

54. Han IC, Tadarati M, Pacheco KD, et al. Macular vascular abnormalities identified by optical coherence tomography angiography in sickle cell disease. *Am J Ophthalmol.* 2017;177:90-99.

55. Alam M, Thapa D, Lim JI, et al. Quantitative characteristics of sickle cell retinopathy in optical coherence tomography angiography. *Biomed Opt Express.* 2017;8(3):1741-1753.

56. Han IC, Linz MO, Liu TYA, et al. Correlation of ultra-widefield fluorescein angiography and OCT angiography in sickle cell retinopathy. *Ophthalmol Retina.* 2018;2(6):599-605.

57. Myint KT, Sahoo S, Thein AW, et al. Laser therapy for retinopathy in sickle cell disease. *Cochrane Database Syst Rev.* 2015;9(10): 14651858.

58. Jampol LM, Condon P, Farber M, et al. A randomized clinical trial of feeder vessel photocoagulation of proliferative sickle cell retinopathy. I. Preliminary results. *Ophthalmology.* 1983;90(5): 540-545.

59. Rednam KR, Jampol LM, Goldberg MF. Scatter retinal photocoagulation for proliferative sickle cell retinopathy. *Am J Ophthalmol.* 1982;93:594-599.

60. Farber MD, Jampol LM, Fox P, et al. A randomized clinical trial of scatter photocoagulation of proliferative sickle cell retinopathy. *Arch Ophthalmol.* 1991;109(3):363-367.

61. Rodrigues M, Kashiwabuchi F, Deshpande M, et al. Expression pattern of HIF-1α and VEGF supports circumferential application of scatter laser for proliferative sickle retinopathy. *Invest Ophthalmol Vis Sci.* 2016;57(15):6739-6746.

62. Cai CX, Linz MO, Scott AW. Intravitreal bevacizumab for proliferative sickle retinopathy: a case series. *J Vitreo Retinal Dis.* 2017;2(1):32-38.

63. Abdalla Elsayed ME, Muro M, Al Dhibi H, et al. Sickle cell retinopathy. A focused review. *Graefes Arch Clin Exp Ophthalmol.* 2019;257(7):1353-1364.

64. Curran EL, Fleming JC, Rice K, et al. Orbital compression syndrome in sickle cell disease. *Ophthalmology.* 1997;104(10):1610-1615.

65. Chen RWS, Flynn HW, Lee W, et al. Vitreoretinal management and surgical outcomes in proliferative sickle retinopathy: a case series. *Am J Ophthalmol.* 2014;157(4):870-875.

66. Moshiri A, Ha NK, Ko FS, Scott AW. Bevacizumab presurgical treatment for proliferative sickle-cell retinopathy-related retinal detachment. *Retin Cases Brief Rep.* 2013;7(3):204-205.

67. Amissah-Arthur KN, Mensah E. The past, present and future management of sickle cell retinopathy within and African context. *Eye.* 2018;32(8):1304-1314.

68. Yawn BP, Buchanan GR, Afenyi-Annan AN, et al. Management of sickle cell disease: summary of the 2014 evidence-based report by expert panel members. *JAMA.* 2014;312(10):1033-1048.

69. Rosenberg JB, Hutcheson K. Pediatric sickle cell retinopathy: correlation with clinical factors. *J AAPOS.* 2011;15(1):49-53.

70. Rodrigues GB, Abe RY, Zangalli C, et al. Neovascular glaucoma: a review. *Int J Retina Vitreous.* 2016;14(2):26.

71. Yorston D, Jalali S. Retinal detachment in developing countries. *Eye Lond Engl.* 2002;16:353-358.

Rare Presentations and Emerging Complications of Sickle Cell Disease

Authors: Oswaldo Castro, Kathryn L. Hassell

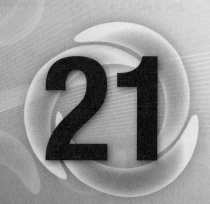

21

Chapter Outline

Overview

This chapter addresses clinical presentations of sickle cell disease that are uncommon or newly emerging or that pose special diagnostic and therapeutic challenges. Many of them are life threatening or can result in severe loss of organ function. Some clinical presentations also illustrate features of sickle cell disease pathophysiology that are not always recognized in the more common complications such as pain crisis and chest syndrome. There are no clinical trials and few published reviews dealing with these issues, their pathogenetic mechanisms, or their treatment. Hence, the diagnostic and management measures suggested here necessarily are based on published single reports and small case series and on clinical experience. Acute multiorgan failure syndrome is summarized first because of its life-threatening potential and also because its clinical features and treatment are similar to some of the other, less common conditions discussed. Information on drug-induced pain episodes (crises) is included primarily to promote awareness of these newly emerging and unexpected complications. The chapter ends with descriptions of how other, nonsickling, red cell disorders affect patients with sickle cell disease, with a special emphasis on the immune hemolysis that characterizes sickle-related hyperhemolysis syndrome.

Acute Multiorgan Failure Syndrome

Definition, Epidemiology, and Putative Pathophysiology

Acute multiorgan failure (MOF) syndrome refers to the acute onset of the failure of at least 2 of 3 vital organ systems in the setting of an acute sickle cell vaso-occlusive episode (VOE). As defined by the initial case series,[1] the syndrome occurs in the absence of sepsis or other comorbidities that might lead to MOF in a patient without sickle cell disease. Furthermore, the syndrome may account for up to 10% of deaths in sickle cell patients.[2] The specific mechanisms whereby acute simultaneous severe injury occurs in the lungs, liver, and/or kidneys have not been defined but may reflect an acute cytokine-mediated systemic inflammatory response that is associated with several subsequent processes including activation of endothelium with diffuse worsening vaso-occlusion and hemolysis. Case reports also document evidence of fat emboli, thought to arise from severe bone marrow necrosis (see later discussion), and the occurrence of MOF in patients with relatively high baseline hemoglobin values and in patients with all types of sickle cell disease including HbSC disease and HbS-β[+] thalassemia.[3]

Clinical Presentation and Diagnosis

MOF most often arises in hospitalized patients 2 to 3 days after presentation for a VOE that is described as more severe or diffuse than is typical for an individual.[1] This complication arises in up to 90% of adults with rapidly progressive acute chest syndrome as manifested by the development of acute severe respiratory failure in <24 hours.[4] Fever and tachycardia are common early signs. The development of somnolence and mental status changes may reflect hypoxia and the effects of acute hepatic and renal failure. Clinical manifestations include acute worsening of anemia, thrombocytopenia, and dysfunction of at least 2 of 3 vital organ systems: evidence for acute chest syndrome, a 2- to 5-fold increase in alanine aminotransferase and total bilirubin, a 2-fold rise in direct bilirubin indicative of hepatic failure, and/or a rise in creatinine indicative of acute kidney injury (AKI).[1] Rhabdomyolysis may occur, with significant increases in creatine kinase contributing to AKI.

The syndrome may be fatal within 24 to 36 hours and refractory to interventions such as transfusion in later stages, but it often responds readily to transfusion when recognized early. Thus, prompt attention to changes in vital signs and mental status that may herald the onset of the process is important. This acute process may progress rapidly, with significant clinical and laboratory changes within 8 to 12 hours. Rapid assessment of organ function is indicated if MOF syndrome is suspected, even if recent prior assessment was not concerning. In addition, full evaluation for and empiric management of other causes of systemic syndromes unrelated to sickle cell disease itself, such as sepsis and thrombotic microangiopathies, are also required because there is no specific diagnostic testing that identifies sickle cell–related MOF from that due to other processes.

Management and Expected Outcomes

The mainstay of therapy of sickle cell–related MOF is transfusion, although extensive evaluation for and management of comorbidities and contributing factors are also important. Exchange transfusion is used most commonly, particularly in individuals without severe anemia or when volume overload or anuria precludes aggressive simple transfusion. The initial case series also described successful reversal using aggressive simple transfusion of 4 or more units when exchange transfusion is not available, targeting and maintaining a hemoglobin of 10 g/dL. Even severe acute end-organ damage can be quickly reversed with effective transfusion therapy.[1] The case fatality rate is unclear but is thought to be quite high without early recognition and rapid initiation of simple or exchange transfusion. A small series noted improved survival with therapeutic plasma exchange in cases refractory to transfusion therapy, which may serve to remove inflammatory proteins and cytokines as well as provide heme-binding proteins.[5]

Fat Embolization Syndrome

Definition and Pathophysiology

When sickling-related microvascular occlusion of the bone marrow results in necrosis,[6] microscopic particles of necrotic marrow and/or marrow fat can embolize to the pulmonary circulation (Figure 21-1). This clinical picture is called pulmonary marrow/fat embolization and causes tissue injury by impairing blood flow and possibly also by the generation of toxic free fatty acids.[7] Clinical severity ranges from a hypoxic chest syndrome picture[8] to acute respiratory failure (acute respiratory distress syndrome).[9] Systemic fat embolization accompanies or follows pulmonary fat embolization when microscopic marrow fat droplets gain access to the systemic circulation through

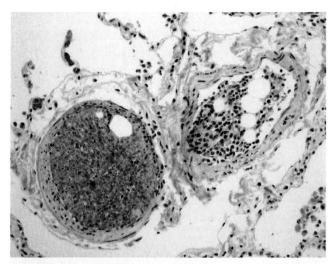

FIGURE 21-1 Microscopic findings in lung of sickle cell disease patient who died of marrow and fat embolization (hematoxylin and eosin stain). The pulmonary blood vessel at the left is occluded by an embolus consisting of necrotic bone marrow. The one at the right shows embolized bone marrow and bone marrow fat. Photomicrograph used with permission from Dr. William Green, Department of Pathology, Howard University College of Medicine.

additional marrow/fat embolization and organ injury and further hypoxia (Figure 21-2).

Frequency and Risk Factors

Fat embolization syndrome (FES) is thought to be a relatively infrequent occurrence. However, because FES can be difficult to diagnose, it is probably more common than the literature would suggest. At a single institution, fat embolization was diagnosed as a circumstance of death in 7% of 141 sickle patients who died between 1974 and 2001.[13] Pulmonary fat emboli were found in about one-third of 19 forensic autopsies of sickle cell disease patients who had sudden unexpected deaths.[14] A 2014 review of FES by Tsitsikas et al[3] included 58 cases, mainly adults, with a median age of 27 years. As earlier case reports and series observed, most of the FES cases were in patients with the milder, non-SS genotypes: 43% had HbSC disease and 20% had sickle-β thalassemia. A follow-up 2019 publication by Tsitsikas et al[15] reviewed 27 additional FES case reports, and 86% of the patients had the mild, non-HbSS genotypes. Marrow necrosis with embolism has been reported in HbSE disease, a rare sickle genotype also characterized by mild hemolysis.[16,17] The reason for the overrepresentation of milder sickle genotypes among FES cases is unknown. It is possible that the higher hematocrit—and higher blood viscosity—in sickle patients with relatively low hemolysis may be involved.[7] Lower hemolytic rates may be associated with less hyperplastic marrow with relatively larger quantities of marrow fat than that of HbSS patients. In up to 33% of the cases recently reviewed,[3] fat embolization was the first manifestation of sickle cell disease in patients with a mild clinical course and in those without

the pulmonary capillaries and veins and embolize to the brain,[10,11] liver, kidneys, and heart.[12] The resulting MOF is life threatening and can be further complicated by disseminated intravascular coagulation through fat droplet activation of the coagulation cascade. Hypoxemia from impaired lung function establishes a vicious cycle characterized by hypoxia-related sickling, which leads to more extensive marrow necrosis with

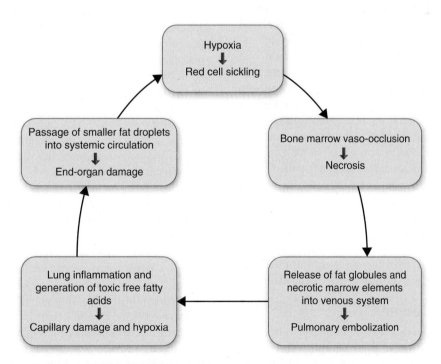

FIGURE 21-2 Pathophysiology of pulmonary and systemic fat embolization syndrome. Gangaraju et al. CME Article: Fat Embolism Syndrome Secondary to Bone Marrow Necrosis in Patients with Hemoglobinopathies. *Southern Medical Journal.* 2016;109:549-53. Reprinted with permission.

a previous hemoglobinopathy diagnosis.[18-20] Pregnancy may be a risk factor for sickle-related FES[21-23]; 8 (25%) of the 32 women with FES in the Tsitsikas review were pregnant at the time.[3]

Systemic fat embolism is often preceded by a severe acute chest syndrome and/or an unusually painful VOE. Concurrent parvovirus B19 infection was documented in 24% of recent FES cases,[3] which might be associated hypothetically with virus-related endothelial injury, causing bone marrow necrosis, and with endothelial injury to the pulmonary vasculature, leading to severe hypoxia.[24] Medications such as corticosteroids[25,26] and prostaglandin[23] also may be triggering factors. Patients with sickle cell disease who are administered granulocyte colony-stimulating factor (G-CSF) can develop life-threatening VOEs and extensive marrow necrosis[27] and may be at risk for FES.

Diagnosis

FES is difficult to document during life, and the correct diagnosis is often made only at autopsy.[28] The development of severe bone pain, hypoxemia, altered mental state, and/or MOF, along with upper body petechiae, should raise the possibility of FES.[7] Laboratory findings that suggest the syndrome are worsening anemia, thrombocytopenia, a leukoerythroblastic blood picture, and increasing serum ferritin and lactate dehydrogenase (LDH) levels. Positive stains for fat within macrophages in induced sputum, in bronchoalveolar lavage,[29] and in cytologic examination of pulmonary capillary wedge blood[30] provide strong evidence of pulmonary fat embolization. Systemic fat embolization can be demonstrated by the finding of fat globules within retinal arteries.[31] Rarely, painful erythematous plaques or papules on the skin of the lower extremities have been described, and histology of these lesions showed superficial vein thrombosis with fat vacuoles within the thrombus.[32] Magnetic resonance images (MRIs) in sickle patients with cerebral fat embolism have shown innumerable foci of susceptibility artifact diffusely throughout the supratentorial and infratentorial brain parenchyma and brainstem with associated restricted diffusion but no enhancement ("starfield" pattern, Figure 21-3).[11,33] The diagnostic sensitivity of these tests in sickle cell patients is unknown. A high index of suspicion is the best strategy for preventing the high mortality and morbidity of FES. The syndrome should be considered in patients with unusually severe and/or widespread bone pain, in patients with worsening acute chest syndrome, in patients with neurologic symptoms,[3] and in all sickle patients with acute MOF (see earlier section). The development of symptoms such as uncontrollable pain, agitation, or changes in level of consciousness could be a manifestation of FES. It is important to avoid routinely ascribing an altered mental state to opioid overdose or to illegal drug use, as this could result in critical delays in FES diagnosis.

Treatment and Outcome

Sickle-related marrow necrosis with pulmonary and/or systemic fat embolism syndrome is a catastrophic illness that often has a fulminant course. Nine of the 24 patients with fat embolization reviewed by Dang et al[34] died within the first 24 hours. Patients usually require intensive care unit

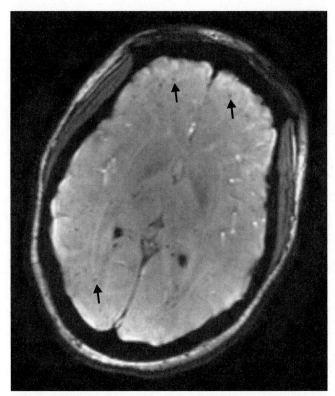

FIGURE 21-3 Magnetic resonance imaging of cerebral fat embolism showing innumerable foci of susceptibility artifact (arrows) in the cortex, gray-white junction, and deep white matter. Used with permission from Case Report 1 kindly provided of Allison Weyer, MD, and Enrico Novelli, MD, MS, University of Pittsburgh Medical Center, Pittsburgh, PA.

monitoring, critical care management, and cardiopulmonary support. Mortality rates are high, and 14% of FES survivors may be left with severe neurologic residual deficits.[3] Survival may be associated with prompt and aggressive transfusion therapy; survival was ≤9% in nontransfused patients, but it was 39% to 50% in those given simple transfusions and 71% to 79% in those treated with red blood cell (RBC) exchange transfusion.[3,15] Hence, many authors stress the need for both a high index of suspicion and prompt institution of transfusion therapy once the diagnosis seems a reasonable possibility. Because it can take some time to arrange for erythrocytapheresis and/or because the patients are often severely anemic, rapid initiation of simple transfusions is appropriate, followed by RBC exchange as needed.

Transfusion therapy is not recommended for treatment of fat embolization due to other etiologies such as bone fractures or adipose tissue trauma. However, in patients with sickle cell disease, transfusions lower the proportion of sickling erythrocytes in the recipient's blood, which may reduce vaso-occlusion and improve blood flow to ischemic tissues surrounding areas of marrow necrosis, halting the progression of the syndrome. Transfusions may also improve tissue oxygenation by promoting better blood flow to ischemic lung and other organs. It is known that in hypoxic acute chest syndrome transfusions rapidly improve arterial blood oxygenation.[35,36]

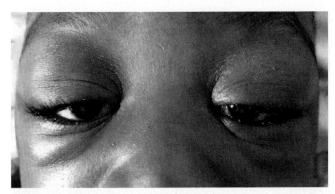

FIGURE 21-4 Proptosis in 8-year old sickle cell anemia patient with bilateral orbital syndrome. Reprinted from Schündeln MM, et al. Orbital compression syndrome in a child with sickle cell disease. *J Pediatr.* 2014;164(3):671, with permission from Elsevier.

Orbital Syndrome

Definition and Pathophysiology

Orbital syndrome, also called orbital wall infarction, is an unusual vaso-occlusive manifestation of sickle cell disease. It is characterized clinically by a painful swelling of the soft tissues within and surrounding the ocular orbit, leading to lid edema, eye protrusion, or exophthalmos (Figure 21-4) and threatening permanent eye injury and vision loss (orbital compression syndrome). Orbital syndrome is generally due to sickle cell–related ischemia and/or infarction of the bones of the orbital wall, with subperiosteal hematoma formation, inflammation, and soft tissue edema. There are, however, also reports of orbital syndrome caused by other mechanisms such as bleeding from hyperplastic bone marrow following minor trauma,[37] cranial bone ischemia/infarction,[38] epidural hematoma,[39] and bulky extramedullary hematopoiesis.[40]

Epidemiology and Risk Factors

A 2008 review by Sokol et al[41] found only 27 previously published case reports of orbital syndrome; 24 additional cases have appeared in the literature from 2007 to 2018.[37-58] Orbital syndrome affects primarily young patients (mean age, 11 years; range, 2-22 years), predominantly males (male-to-female ratio, 4:1), and those with the more severe sickling genotypes (20 of the 24 recent cases had HbSS or "SCD" and 4 had HbS-β thalassemia). The persistence of hyperplastic marrow in the facial and periorbital bones in children and in patients with a greater degree of hemolysis (those with HbSS or HbS-β thalassemia) may contribute to the development of this complication.[59] Only 1 instance of orbital syndrome in a patient with HbSC disease has been reported,[60] and in a case series from Oman, only 1 of 10 orbital syndrome patients from that country had the Arab-Indian βS haplotype,[59] a polymorphism associated with higher fetal hemoglobin (HbF) and lower hemolytic rate.[61] There is no known explanation for the striking preponderance of males among sickle patients with orbital syndrome. Male infants, toddlers, and prepubertal children with HbSS disease are more anemic and tend to have higher reticulocyte counts and lower fetal hemoglobin production than their female counterparts.[62-64] Taken together, these findings suggest a greater degree of hemolysis and marrow compensatory hyperplasia in male children with sickle cell anemia.

Diagnosis

In about 46% of cases, orbital syndrome develops during a VOE and 62% of patients are febrile. Orbital pain is almost always present, decreased ocular motion occurs in 82% of cases, and visual impairment occurs in 43% of patients. In one-third of patients, the syndrome is bilateral. Often it mimics soft tissue swelling caused by other serious conditions such as orbital cellulitis or abscess. Only 10 of the most recent 24 cases reported hematologic values: a mean hemoglobin level of 7.6 ± 0.8 g/dL and mean white blood cell (WBC) count of $16.6 \pm 7.3 \times 10^3/\mu L$. Two additional cases described the WBC as "normal." Orbital examination with computed tomography and, especially, with MRI shows changes suggestive of subperiosteal hemorrhagic fluid collection or hematoma in most cases (71%). MRI can exclude other pathologic orbital processes and detect orbital bone marrow abnormalities helpful in diagnosing bone infarction (Figure 21-5), and it has been recommended as the imaging procedure of choice.[41] Other imaging techniques such as bone and, especially, bone marrow scintigraphy have been used.[39,59]

Treatment and Outcomes

Most sickle patients with orbital syndrome (83%) were treated with intravenous broad-spectrum antibiotics even though there are no case reports in which bacteriologic tests were positive. This reflects inability at the time of presentation to rule

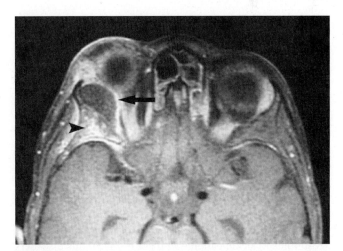

FIGURE 21-5 Axial magnetic resonance imaging with contrast in an 11-year-old sickle cell disease patient with right orbital syndrome. Marrow space involvement (infarction) of the greater wing of sphenoid bone is shown (arrowhead), as well as adjacent subperiosteal fluid collection and surrounding ring enhancement (arrow). Alsuhaibani AH, Marzouk MA. Recurrent infarction of sphenoid bone with subperiosteal collection in a child with sickle cell disease. *Ophthalmic Plast Reconstr Surg.* 2011;27(5):e136-8.

out a primary infectious etiology or a secondary infection of the tissues affected by orbital ischemia, necrosis, or edema. In 42% of cases, short courses of systemic, usually intravenous corticosteroids were also administered because of the threat of orbital compression with loss of vision or damage to ocular muscles. When steroid doses and treatment duration were specified, they ranged from 250 to 1000 mg of methylprednisolone intravenously daily for 1 to 3 days. No instances of steroid-induced VOE (see later section) were described. To address sickling-related vaso-occlusion, simple transfusions or erythrocytapheresis were administered in 7 of 24 recent cases, although only 3 patients received transfusions as the only treatment modality. The paucity of orbital syndrome reports does not allow reliable identification of its most effective treatment, but most cases were treated conservatively. Surgical interventions, mainly orbital aspiration or decompression, were carried out in only 3 of 24 recent cases. In most sickle patients, the orbital syndrome resolves completely, although instances of mild residual visual impairment and bilateral loss of sight have been reported[45,60] and the syndrome can be recurrent.[54,57]

Drug-Induced Pain Episodes (Crises)

Definition

Some sickle cell patients develop typical pain episodes after administration of certain conventional or experimental therapeutic agents. It is difficult to ascertain how frequently drug-induced pain episodes occur because generally only experiences with untoward outcomes tend to be reported. Study of these adverse reactions may allow some insight into the mechanisms triggering acute pain episodes in sickle cell patients when considering the common adverse effects of these drugs.

Corticosteroids

Numerous case reports suggest that the administration of systemic corticosteroids to sickle patients may be followed by adverse events, mainly pain episodes. In 2008, Darbari et al[65] reviewed 30 such cases. Michel et al[66] published their experience in 30 adult sickle cell patients with connective tissue disorders. They reported an increased number of painful crises in 6 of 9 sickle cell patients with systemic lupus erythematosus and in 5 of 10 sickle patients with rheumatoid arthritis treated with corticosteroids. In the same review, 10 of the 11 patients who developed severe infections (and all of the 5 patients with septicemia) were being treated with systemic corticosteroids at the time. The authors recommended avoiding the use of corticosteroids in sickle patients with connective tissue disorders and suggested transfusion therapy for those requiring corticosteroids at doses of ≥10 mg of prednisone or equivalent per day. In a review of 16 sickle cell children with coexisting autoimmune disorders or connective tissue diseases who were treated with corticosteroids,[67] 7 developed more severe or more frequent pain episodes, suggesting poor steroid tolerance in the

pediatric population also. The time interval between start of steroid treatment and the VOE can be as short as 1 day, but most events occur within the first month. It is certainly possible that these patients' pain episodes became more frequent or more severe as a result of both the connective tissue disease's inflammatory state and its treatment with steroids. Some patients with postcorticosteroid crises had been treated with other immunosuppressive agents in addition to steroids, which may have also contributed to an increase in pain episodes. Hemorrhagic stroke is not an acute pain event, but it too could be associated to the use of corticosteroids. A case-control study of pediatric sickle patients with hemorrhagic stroke found that corticosteroid administration and transfusions within the previous 14 days were each much more frequent (odd ratios of 20 and 35, respectively) than in a control group of pediatric sickle cell patients with ischemic stroke.[68]

By contrast, in sickle cell patients who already have a pain episode or acute chest syndrome, corticosteroid treatment shortens the duration of pain and hospital stay.[69-71] However, rebound pain and rehospitalization were associated with steroid use,[69,70,72] and a large retrospective study also suggested longer length of hospital stay in steroid-treated chest syndrome patients.[73] Some clinicians have used both steroids and transfusions to treat acute chest syndrome,[74] but as of yet, there is no evidence that steroid administration adds to the beneficial effect of transfusions in this complication.

Short courses of corticosteroids have been used in the treatment of orbital syndrome (see earlier discussion) and of autoimmune hemolysis in sickle patients with severe delayed transfusion reactions (hyperhemolytic syndrome) and did not trigger painful events.[75-80] Interestingly, 2 transfusion reaction patients in whom corticosteroid treatment was continued for 11 and 14 days and whose hemoglobin level increased to 11 to 12 g/dL did develop severe VOEs.[81] There is a single report of sickle crises precipitated by intra-articular injection of corticosteroids.[82] However, inhaled steroids are prescribed widely to sickle patients with asthma without reports of drug-related pain events in this context. A single-center randomized and placebo-controlled trial in adult sickle patients with history of cough or wheezing (but *without* asthma) found that inhaled corticosteroids decreased self-reported pain scores and also lowered serum levels of soluble vascular cell adhesion molecule, a surrogate biomarker for vascular injury,[83] and of cytokines involved in inflammation.[84]

The mechanism of corticosteroid-induced crises is unknown. Polymorphonuclear leukocytosis readily follows systemic steroid treatment in sickle patients, and there are arguments for and against increased leukocyte count as a potential mechanism for steroid-related crises. There is a well-known association between leukocytosis and vaso-occlusive severity and mortality.[85-87] Recent support for a role of polymorphonuclear leukocyte activity in the pathophysiology of VOEs was provided by the finding that crizanlizumab, a P-selectin inhibitor, decreases crisis frequency in sickle cell patients.[88] P-selectin initiates the process of leukocyte-endothelial adhesion, which promotes slow blood flow and microvascular occlusion.

However, the leukocytosis–clinical severity association also may be explained by sickle-related chronic hemolysis and/or chronic tissue injury causing reactive leukocytosis so that the latter would be a marker rather than a driver of disease severity. In the rare cases of sickle cell disease with coexisting chronic myeloproliferative disorders, there is no consistent relationship between leukocytosis and vaso-occlusive severity.[89-92] Long-term corticosteroid administration to patients without hemoglobinopathy can lead to osteonecrosis, probably related to osteoblast/osteocyte apoptosis and possibly also decreased angiogenesis.[93] However, this is a chronic condition usually developing over many months, whereas steroid-associated pain episodes are acute events.

Until more information becomes available, we believe that the following conclusions about treating sickle cell patients with systemic steroids are reasonable:

- Administration of oral or parenteral corticosteroids has the potential for triggering severe VOEs.

- In patients for whom systemic steroid treatment is judged indispensable, prior or simultaneous transfusions will reduce the proportion of sickle cells in the recipient's blood, which is expected to also lower the vaso-occlusive risk.

- Short-term courses of corticosteroids appear to be a safe option for treating orbital syndrome and also hyperhemolysis during delayed hemolytic transfusion reactions, but steroid use should not be prolonged (see "Immune Hemolysis: Hyperhemolytic Crises" section later in this chapter).

Hematopoietic Stem Cell–Mobilizing Agents

Mobilization of marrow hematopoietic stem cells (HSCs) for collection from peripheral blood has been used in sickle cell patients who require autologous stem cell transplantation during cancer treatment.[94-96] Mobilizing HSC is also crucial for gene therapy protocols.[97] However, administration of the traditional stem cell–mobilizing agent G-CSF to sickle cell patients has been associated with severe pain episodes and 1 death from MOF. In a review of these cases, Fitzhugh et al[98] discussed potential mechanisms for the adverse outcomes and recommended against the use of G-CSF for peripheral blood stem cell collection or for chemotherapy-induced neutropenia. Transfusions or exchange transfusions, when given before G-CSF administration, prevented post–G-CSF sickle pain in 3 of 5 patients. Reports that G-CSF appears to be safe in sickle trait[99-102] suggest that the G-CSF vaso-occlusive effects are specific to sickle cell disease patients.

As in poststeroid pain episodes, neutrophilia may contribute to the pathogenesis of the severe sickle cell complications that follow G-CSF administration. Peak leukocyte counts after G-CSF treatment were as high as $105 \times 10^3/\mu L$, and in 6 of 9 cases in which these values were reported, they were $>50 \times 10^3/\mu L$.[98] Plerixafor is a new HSC-mobilizing agent that acts by inhibiting the interaction of stem cell chemokine receptor CXCR-4 with stromal-derived factor-1α (SDF-1α).[103] In contrast to G-CSF, plerixafor does not act on marrow and peripheral blood polymorphonuclear granulocytes directly, so that the postmobilization peak leukocyte count was $<35 \times 10^3/\mu L$ in all of the 24 sickle patients who received this cytokine.[104-106] None of the 10 pretransfused patients had a postmobilization VOE, and 2 of the 14 patients who were not pretransfused developed pain crises. Thus, although it seems that plerixafor is a safer agent than G-CSF for sickle cell patients, the number of patients so far treated is small, and it would seem prudent to pretransfuse sickle patients prior to plerixafor administration.

Additional insight into the pathogenesis of G-CSF–related VOEs may be gained by considering the mechanism(s) of G-CSF adverse events in patients without hemoglobinopathy. The 2 most frequent side effects of G-CSF administration to normal stem cell donors are mild bone pain, which occurs in 52% to 84% of patients, and asymptomatic splenomegaly detected by ultrasound in most patients.[107] In healthy stem cell donors, post–G-CSF bone pain occurs most frequently in the axial skeleton where hemopoietic marrow is normally distributed[108]: back, hips, pelvis, ribs, and sternum. Hence, post–G-CSF bone pain and splenomegaly may be a consequence of cytokine-induced acute expansion of the hematopoietic bone marrow and spleen.[107,108] This may be problematic in sickle patients because (1) the skeletal areas at risk for hematopoietic marrow expansion would be more widespread, corresponding to the wider distribution of their blood-forming marrow and (2) the microvascular flow to the acutely expanding marrow could become impaired because of the abnormal rheology of sickle hemoglobin (HbS) polymer–containing erythrocytes and lead to marrow ischemia or necrosis, and more severe pain.[27]

Sildenafil

Pulmonary hypertension occurs in about 10% of adult sickle cell disease patients and is associated with increased mortality.[109-111] Sildenafil is an inhibitor of phosphodiesterase 5 that promotes vasodilatation in pulmonary blood vessels and has been used successfully to treat pulmonary hypertension in patients without hemoglobinopathies[112] and also in thalassemia-related pulmonary hypertension.[113] An international, multicenter, placebo-controlled, 16-week trial of sildenafil was implemented to determine its safety and efficacy in 132 sickle cell patients with proven or probable pulmonary hypertension and low 6-minute walk distance test (Walk-PHaSST).[114] The trial was stopped after 74 patients had been enrolled when hospitalizations for painful episodes occurred in a significantly higher proportion of sildenafil-treated patients (13 of 37 patients, 35%) than in those assigned to placebo (5 of 37 patients, 14%). Sildenafil-related pain episodes were not observed and may have been prevented in a prior open-label study in which all 12 subjects received disease-modifying therapy (transfusions in 4 patients and hydroxyurea in 8 patients) before sildenafil was started.[115] In the Walk-PHaSST trial, 5% of patients assigned to sildenafil were on regular transfusions, and 57% were taking hydroxyurea. Sildenafil failed to improve functional capacity or tricuspid regurgitant velocity in Walk-PHaSST study participants, although the study was closed before full enrollment. The mechanism of sildenafil-induced pain crises remains mysterious. It is possible that back pain and myalgias, frequent sildenafil side effects in non–sickle cell patients,[116] may have contributed to the development of episodes of pain in patients treated with the drug.[114] Sildenafil in rats increases the sensitivity to pain, and this mechanism might be relevant to patients with SCD.[117] The most frequent sildenafil side effects in patients without hemoglobinopathy are headaches (12%) and flushing (13%),[118] likely related to vasodilatation, and 35% of sildenafil-treated patients in the Walk-PHaSST study complained of headaches. However, drug-related vasodilatation would not be expected to promote VOEs in sickle cell patients.

Senicapoc

In sickle cell disease, RBC dehydration increases intracellular HbS concentration, which promotes HbS polymerization and shortens RBC intravascular life span. Dense, dehydrated sickle RBCs have a much lower intravascular survival than other less abnormal sickle cells.[119] One of the main mechanisms of RBC dehydration is potassium (and water) efflux through the calcium-activated Gardos membrane channel.[120] Senicapoc is an experimental agent that prevents RBC dehydration by blocking the Gardos channel. A phase III placebo-controlled trial of senicapoc (10 mg/d) was conducted in adult sickle cell patients to determine its efficacy in lowering their pain episode rate. In this 52-week trial, the drug significantly increased the hemoglobin level by about 0.6 g/dL.[121] The increase appeared to be associated with a reduced hemolytic rate as indicated by lowered percent reticulocytes, serum LDH, indirect bilirubin, and percent dense RBCs. Data on mean corpuscular hemoglobin concentration (MCHC) were not reported, so it was not possible to determine to what extent decreased intracellular RBC HbS concentration and lower HbS polymerization were responsible for decreasing the hemolytic rate. Despite hemolysis reduction and improvement of the anemia, senicapoc was also associated with a 36% increase in pain episode rate. However, there was no statistically significant increase in painful events in subjects who were also taking hydroxyurea. If the drug's disease-modifying effect that improved the anemia had simply been too weak to also affect sickle-related vaso-occlusion, senicapoc-treated patients would not have been expected to experience more frequent crises. These results raise interesting hypotheses: the 2 major clinical subphenotypes of sickle cell disease, chronic hemolysis and episodic vascular occlusion,[122] may be in some sort of equilibrium. If so, disease-modifying interventions may improve both the anemia and vaso-occlusive severity (hydroxyurea, transfusion), may improve the anemia but be neutral in regard to vaso-occlusion (voxelotor[123]), may improve VOEs but not the anemia (crizanlizumab[88]), or may improve the anemia and exacerbate vaso-occlusion (senicapoc). The senicapoc experience could have some similarity to that of sickle cell anemia patients with coexisting α thalassemia, in whom hemolysis is less intense but vaso-occlusive severity seems worse than in the more anemic SS patients without α thalassemia.[124]

It is also possible that senicapoc, independently of its anti-hemolysis effect, could act on RBC membrane or vascular endothelium in some way that promotes cell adhesion and sickling.

Sickle Cell Disease With Other RBC Disorders

The combination of sickle cell anemia with other RBC disorders presents unusual diagnostic and therapeutic challenges. This section reviews 2 hemolytic syndromes unrelated to HbS polymerization that can coexist in sickle cell patients: immune hemolysis, a relatively common problem that severely compounds sickle cell–induced hemolysis, and thrombotic microangiopathy, a rare systemic and hemolytic disorder that can be difficult to differentiate from other forms of MOF in sickle cell disease. Also reviewed here is iron deficiency, an RBC production abnormality that would be expected to critically worsen the anemia of sickle cell disease but that usually does not.

Immune Hemolysis: Hyperhemolytic Crises*

Definition and Pathophysiology

Hyperhemolytic crises are episodes of severe, often life-threatening anemia that occur during delayed hemolytic transfusion reactions (DHTRs). In sickle cell patients, the hyperhemolytic syndrome adds acute immune-mediated hemolysis to the chronic anemia of sickle cell disease. Hence, there are 3 mechanisms of RBC destruction in sickle patients with hyperhemolytic crises: (1) the alloantibody(ies) that triggers the DHTR, the specificity of which can be difficult to identify; (2) autoantibodies, which frequently develop during DHTRs, presumably through an innocent bystander process; and (3) chronic HbS polymerization–related hemolysis. The acute anemia can be further compounded by a decrease in compensatory marrow RBC production (relative reticulocytopenia)[125] due mainly to the higher posttransfusion hematocrit immediately before the DHTR. Hemoglobin nadirs in sickle patients with hyperhemolysis are often around 5 g/dL, can be as low as 1.9 to 2.8 g/dL,[80,125] and are associated with mortality rates of up to 9% to 12%.[125,126] The pathogenesis of DHTRs follows these steps:

1. One or more RBC alloantibodies are formed after a transfusion, a primary alloimmunization process resulting in rising antibody titers within 2 to 3 months after transfusion; the process is asymptomatic because in most cases, by the time antibody titers are high enough for clinical hemolysis, the transfused RBCs are no longer in circulation.

2. A subsequent gradual decrease in the alloantibody titer (evanescence) occurs such that it is no longer detectable serologically within about a year after the alloimmunizing transfusion (>50% of alloantibodies are evanescent[127,128]).

---

*For a more extensive discussion of this topic, see Chapter 23 on Transfusion Medicine.

3. There is a failure to detect the evanescent alloantibody before it disappears because no posttransfusion serologic examination is done, or if the antibody *is* detected, the record of its presence is not available at the time of subsequent transfusion.

4. A new transfusion is administered, with RBCs bearing the antigen against which the patient initially developed an antibody; this happens because pretransfusion testing is unable to detect evanescent antibodies and deems the RBC unit to be serologically compatible even though biologically it is not.

5. The transfused incompatible RBCs stimulate a strong secondary, anamnestic, booster-type antibody response, such that after a delay period of about 10 days, immune hemolysis of the transfused RBCs takes place (DHTR).

6. Formation of autoantibodies often accompanies this secondary alloimmune reaction; the autoantibodies also destroy the patient's own RBCs[129,130] and worsen hemolysis and anemia.

This DHTR pathogenesis differs substantially from that of serologic reactions in sickle patients on chronic transfusions, in whom primary—not anamnestic—alloimmunization can, in 30% of cases, also lead to hemolysis.[131] In these cases, patients are often asymptomatic, the serologic reaction is first suspected by finding a lower than expected hemoglobin level on pretransfusion testing (11 to 31 days after the last scheduled transfusion), the anemia is significantly less severe, and there is no life-threatening hyperhemolysis.[131]

Epidemiology

Although this chapter focuses on rare presentations, hyperhemolysis is relatively common in sickle cell disease. Hyperhemolysis and DHTRs occur rarely in the general population[132] and in other hemoglobinopathies.[133,134] The DHTR risk in the general US population is 6.9 per 100,000 transfused RBC units.[135] By comparison, publications in which this metric is reported for sickle patients suggest a higher risk: 9 DHTRs in approximately 11,000 transfused RBC units,[136] 7 in 915 units,[137] 4 in 2674 units,[138] and 23 in 10,585 units.[125] Remarkably, in the subset of sickle patients who are on monthly regular transfusions, the reported DHTR risk is quite low: 2 in 1830 transfused units,[139] 1 in 10,949 units,[140] 0 in 3236 units,[141] and 0 in 10,112 units.[138] Combined data from these reports indicate that the sickle cell disease DHTR risk, expressed as events per 10,000 RBC units transfused, is 25 times higher than in the general US transfused population (17/0.69) but that it is only marginally greater (1.1/0.69) in sickle patients receiving exclusively monthly transfusions. Several papers also have called attention to this association between sporadic transfusions in sickle cell patients and their DHTR risk.[138,142-144] β Thalassemia patients appear to have a very low DHTR risk despite their lifelong RBC transfusion exposure and alloimmunization frequencies of 9.3%,[145] 16.5%,[146] and 18.3%.[147] The proportion of transfused β thalassemia patients who develop hemolytic transfusion reactions is 2.5%,[148] or about half of that

for transfused sickle cell patients (4%-7.7%).[125,136,137] This difference may reflect the fact that most β thalassemia patients receive regular monthly transfusions, whereas many sickle patients receive only sporadic transfusions. The few DHTRs reported in thalassemic patients occurred primarily in patients with β thalassemia intermedia,[134] who are only sporadically transfused.

The reason for the lower DHTR risk in regularly versus sporadically transfused sickle cell patients is not known. Potential explanations are as follows: (1) regular transfusions are usually started during childhood when alloimmunization risk appears to be lower[149]; (2) regular monthly transfusions and exposure to a larger number of donors could have an immunosuppressive effect[138,140]; (3) many sporadic transfusions are given during acute inflammatory conditions, which enhance the likelihood of an immune response[150]; and (4) sickle patients with DHTR history may be less likely to be enrolled or to remain in chronic transfusion programs. There is an additional and perhaps more relevant explanation: patients on monthly transfusions have all their new alloantibodies detected before evanescence by means of their monthly pretransfusion antibody screening. In addition, most chronically transfused patients receive their care at a single institution where information about new antibodies is readily available, avoiding the third crucial step in DHTR pathogenesis (see previous section).

Diagnosis

In 2 recent reviews of DHTR in sickle patients,[125,126] the most frequent presenting symptoms were pain indistinguishable from that of a sickle crisis (89%), fever, and dark or red urine due to hemoglobinuria (94%). The interval between the precipitating transfusion and these symptoms had a mean (± standard deviation) of 10.1 ± 5.5 days[125] and a median of 9.4 days (interquartile range [IQR], 3-22 days).[126] The median hemoglobin level at the onset of the DHTR was 7.8 g/dL, about 2 g/dL lower than hemoglobin levels (9.5-9.8 g/dL)[125,126] immediately after the triggering transfusion. Mean and median nadir hemoglobin values were reported at 5.4 ± 1.4 g/dL and 5.5 g/dL (IQR, 4.5-6.2 g/dL), respectively, and were lower than those before the transfusion that resulted in the DHTR. Serum LDH values were high, consistent with brisk intravascular hemolysis, but reticulocyte counts in most cases were lower than expected for the degree of anemia (relative reticulocytopenia). Five recent case series describe immunologic findings in a total of 162 DHTRs in sickle patients[125,126,134,144,151] (99 of them from Habibi et al[126]). The direct antiglobulin (Coombs) test was positive in 64% of cases; new alloantibodies, frequently multiple, were identified in 35% of cases; and autoantibodies (or positive auto-screen) were demonstrable in 25% of cases. In 41% of cases, however, new antibodies were never found, which illustrates the frequent difficulty in establishing a serologic diagnosis of DHTR. In view of this, any recently transfused sickle cell patient who develops pain crisis, dark urine, and a decreasing hemoglobin level should be suspected of having a DHTR and to be at risk for the hyperhemolytic syndrome. Supporting evidence would be a reduction in the posttransfusion hemoglobin A percentage, a new positive direct Coombs test, or the appearance of any new antibody, including auto-antibody. The reason DHTRs develop in sickle patients without a positive direct Coombs or detectable antibodies is not clear. It could be related to factors such as heme activation of the alternative pathway of complement,[152] antibodies to low-frequency antigens that are not present in reagent RBCs, or antibody-independent macrophage activation.

Management

The following principles for treating DHTR/hyperhemolysis syndrome are based on expert recommendations, particularly those by Danaee et al (2015),[134] Gardner et al (2015),[142] Dean et al (2019),[151] and Pirenne and Yazdanbakhsh (2018).[153]

Most hyperhemolysis/DHTR deaths ultimately are the consequence of severe hemolytic anemia. Therefore, the first management principle is preventing progression to life-threatening anemia while at the same time also avoiding additional transfusions that can make the anemia worse. Clinical judgment is indispensable for defining the degree of anemia that is life threatening for an individual patient. A hemoglobin level decline to <3 g/dL, particularly with circulatory compromise and/or lactic acidosis, has been proposed as a reasonable indication of life-threatening anemia in this group of patients,[153] but clearly, there are cardiopulmonary and other factors that could render the anemia life threatening at a higher hemoglobin level (or allow tolerance of a lower hemoglobin value). It is important to monitor the rapidity of the hemoglobin decline by blood hemoglobin measurements at least twice daily, potentially more often, to allow timely institution of management interventions (eg, intensive care unit transfer, immunosuppression) before life-threatening anemia develops. High dose erythropoietin (300-800 U/kg 3 times per week) can be used to drive RBC production if relative reticulocytopenia (relatively low reticulocyte index) is present. Administration of hematinics such as iron, folic acid, and vitamin B_{12} may support marrow erythropoietic response. First-line immunosuppressive treatment often consists of methylprednisolone, 500 mg intravenously for 2 days, and intravenous γ-globulin (IVIg), 1 g/kg/d for 2 days (0.4 g/kg/d if renal impairment). Episodes that are refractory to these measures may respond to immunosuppression with rituximab.[142,154] Sickle RBCs have increased sensitivity to the effects of complement, and complement-related RBC destruction appears to be a frequent feature of DHTR with hyperhemolysis.[152] The anti-C5 monoclonal antibody eculizumab (900 mg intravenously) also has been used successfully for treating massive hemolysis in sickle patients with DHTRs.[155] There are recent reports of patients with immunosuppression-resistant hyperhemolysis who improved after the administration of tocilizumab, an antibody against soluble and membrane-associated interleukin-6 receptor,[156,157] suggesting a role for macrophage activation in the pathogenesis of the hyperhemolytic syndrome.

If transfusions are deemed essential because the anemia is life threatening, only 1 RBC unit should be transfused before reevaluation of the need for further transfusion. The unit should be as closely matched as possible to the recipient's RBC antigen pattern. Intravenous corticosteroids and IVIg have been used to minimize the immune destruction of the transfused RBCs. The hemoglobin-based oxygen carrier Hemopure (HBOC-201) has been used as an additional therapeutic measure in critically ill sickle patients with a DHTR.[75,158]

There are no specific studies to date to indicate which therapeutic interventions are associated with improved outcomes and survival. It is likely that a national or international registry of DHTRs will be needed to find the answer.

Prevention

Prevention of DHTRs has been attempted along 2 approaches. The first is prevention of alloimmunization (ie, transfusing more closely matched RBC units). Matching for the Rh and Kell blood groups, now the standard at institutions specializing in treatment of sickle patients, has reduced,[159] but unfortunately not eliminated, alloimmunization.[160] More extensive donor-recipient RBC antigen matching will need to also include Rh genotyping to identify this blood group's frequent polymorphisms, many of which are undetectable serologically.[153] Depending on the degree of extended matching, this type of prevention is also likely to reduce the pool of RBC donors for a given patient and could result in delays in finding matched units when emergency transfusions are needed.

An additional approach, pretransfusion prophylactic rituximab administration, has been used successfully for preventing DHTRs in high-risk sickle patients,[161] particularly those with a history of alloimmunization or of previous DHTR.[153,162]

The pathophysiology of DHTRs suggests that a third preventive approach is worthy of consideration. If all sporadically transfused sickle patients were screened for new antibodies 1 to 3 months following each transfusion episode[143] and if this antibody information were available at a central or national repository, then exposure to evanescent antibodies with future transfusion could be avoided. This would also facilitate the currently recommended approach to provide more fully minor antigen–matched units to patients who have formed an alloantibody. The feasibility, cost, and effectiveness of this approach would need to be determined by prospective studies.

Thrombotic Microangiopathy

Thrombotic microangiopathy (TMA) is a group of disorders characterized by formation and accumulation of platelet-rich thrombi in the microvasculature leading to organ dysfunction, particularly central nervous system involvement, thrombocytopenia, and mechanical RBC destruction or microangiopathic hemolytic anemia. Primary TMA, or thrombotic thrombocytopenic purpura, is a rare life-threatening disorder due to a congenital or autoimmune-mediated deficiency of ADAMTS-13, an enzyme that cleaves von Willebrand factor (vWF) multimers.[163,164] With low (<10%) ADAMTS-13 activity, ultra-large, highly adhesive vWF multimers are not cleaved, accumulate in the endothelium, and, in the presence of high shear rates, promote platelet aggregation and formation of platelet-rich microthrombi. Most TMAs are secondary and associated with common conditions such as pregnancy, infection, and malignancy. In secondary TMAs, plasma ADAMTS-13 activity is normal or only mildly decreased, and no autoantibody is detectable.[165] The pathogenesis of secondary TMA probably varies depending on the triggering condition. It has been proposed, for example, that in TMA secondary to inflammation and/or severe sepsis, vWF levels increase to a degree that overwhelms the ability of ADAMTS-13 to prevent an excess of multimer formation.[166]

Although the combination of hemoglobinopathy and TMA would be expected to be quite rare, sickle cell disease was listed as the associated disorder in about 1% of secondary TMAs.[167] Shome et al[168] reviewed plasmapheresis records for a period of 4 years and reported data on 10 adult sickle patients (9 with HbSS and 1 with HbS-β thalassemia) in whom TMA was diagnosed during VOEs with acute chest syndrome. They all developed varying degrees of MOF, and their laboratory results showed a mean hemoglobin level of 7.3 ± 0.8 g/dL, platelet count of $34.6 \pm 13.8 \times 10^3/\mu L$, and LDH of 3274 ± 1442 U/L. All patients initially were transfused to treat acute chest syndrome and MOF but continued to deteriorate despite posttransfusion HbS levels of <30% in most cases. They began to improve only after initiation of daily plasmapheresis sessions (median, 10 sessions; range, 5-17 sessions). All patients recovered, and there was only 1 TMA recurrence during a median follow-up of 77 months (range, 3-100 months).

Table 21-1 summarizes similar clinical and laboratory features in 9 additional single case reports of sickle cell disease and TMA. Initiation of plasmapheresis was sometimes delayed for 3 to 11 days due to the difficulty in diagnosing TMA in sickle patients, who are more likely to have other etiologies, such as FES and/or disseminated intravascular coagulation, as a cause of MOF. Once instituted, most patients survived the episode, although 1 patient died with a recurrence 2 months later. Another patient died after 3 months as a result of immunosuppression- related infection.

The following clinical patterns can be derived from published cases. First, schistocytosis, one of the most helpful laboratory features of TMA, was not initially recognized but became quite evident after transfusion. The phenomenon could be explained if the abnormal sickle RBCs were resistant to schistocyte formation, if schistocyte morphology were altered or obscured by sickle-related poikilocytosis, or if sickle schistocytes were more rapidly removed from circulation. Schistocytes may appear as they develop from normal, transfused RBCs that are exposed to the abnormal TMA environment. Second, as in the FES discussed earlier, there could be an overrepresentation (6 of 19 patients) of the milder, less hemolytic sickle genotypes (SC, sickle thalassemia) among sickle patients with TMA. Perhaps TMA is more difficult to identify correctly when it occurs in the setting of high-level background hemolysis, as is the case in

HbSS patients. Third, sickle cell anemia patients who develop chest syndrome, MOF, or other critical complications and who fail to respond to transfusions should be suspected of TMA, particularly if thrombocytopenic or if their posttransfusion smear shows schistocytes. The differential diagnosis would have to include disseminated intravascular coagulation, but in most TMA episodes, coagulation paraments are normal or not as severely affected as in disseminated intravascular coagulation.

As expected for secondary TMAs, ADAMTS13 activity was normal or only slightly reduced in the 3 patients who had this measurement. In sickle cell disease, there is evidence of chronic endothelial injury[169] and of increased vWF activity and multimers.[170] Higher than normal ADAMTS-13/vWF antigen ratios might be required in sickle cell disease to prevent accumulation and exposure of vWF multimers, but these ratios are lower in sickle patients, particularly during crisis, than in normal subjects.[171]

It is also interesting that the first case of TMA reported in a patient with the HbS gene was in a man with sickle cell trait whose blood smear during the TMA showed typical RBC sickling, leading to the erroneous diagnosis of a sickle cell crisis episode.[172]

Iron Deficiency

In patients without hemoglobinopathy, a degree of iron deficiency severe enough to reduce RBC MCHC to ≤31 g/dL (stage IV iron deficiency[173]) leads to an anemia with blood hemoglobin levels of ≤9 g/dL.[174] This represents a 40% decrease from the normal hemoglobin level of 15 g/dL. In sickle cell anemia patients, a comparable iron deficiency effect would be expected to also decrease their hemoglobin level by about 40% of their steady state level of approximately 8 g/dL (ie, to ≤4.8 g/dL). Because sickle RBCs have a short intravascular life span, maintaining a typical steady-state hemoglobin level of 8 g/dL requires optimal marrow compensatory erythropoiesis. For this reason, an erythropoiesis-limiting process such as iron deficiency would be expected to lead to a much greater degree of hemoglobin reduction in patients with hemolysis than in normal subjects. Parvovirus B19 infection, for example, impairs RBC production and causes a critically severe anemia in sickle patients with an average hemoglobin level of 3.9 g/dL.[175] Based on these considerations, severe iron deficiency in sickle cell subjects should be poorly tolerated and should reduce hemoglobin levels to a range of 3.9 to 4.8 g/dL. Table 21-2, however, shows that in 14 sickle cell patients with severe iron deficiency, the mean blood hemoglobin was not only higher (7.8 g/dL) than the 3.9 to 4.8 g/dL range expected, but that this represented a much less dramatic (18%) decrease from their iron-replete baseline hemoglobin level. The table includes 4 patients with milder degrees of baseline hemolysis (HbSC, HbS thalassemia), but exclusion of these patients from analysis still shows, for HbSS patients only, iron deficiency values with a mean hemoglobin level of 6.9 g/dL or a 20% decrease from baseline. This was the case even though their

TABLE 21-1 Clinical and laboratory features of sickle cell disease patients with thrombotic microangiopathy

Patient No.	Reference	Age (y)/ sex/ genotype	Hemoglobin (g/dL)	LDH (U/L)	Platelet count (× 10³/μL)	Schistocytes	Symptoms	CNS	Treatment	Outcome
1	Chinowsky, 1994[184]	22/F/HbSC	6	3147	56	More apparent after transfusion	Arthralgias, fever	AMS, normal CT and MRI	Exchange transfusion, plasmapheresis (started day 3)	Recovered
2	Geigel and Francis, 1997[185]	23/M/HbSS	*		<25	After transfusion	Pain crisis, melena, acidosis, coagulopathy, renal dysfunction	Lethargy	FFP for coagulopathy, exchange transfusion, improvement only after plasmapheresis (started day 5)	Recovered
3	Bolaños-Meade et al, 1999[186]	44/M/HbSS	5.5	5809	23	Only after transfusion	Dark urine, weakness, vomiting, acute renal failure	Seizures, coma, normal MRI	Simple transfusions, improvement only after plasmapheresis (started day 9)	Recovered but recurrence and death 2 months later
4	Chehal et al, 2002[187]	40/M/HbS thalassemia	7.5	7689	38	Increasing to 3+, 3 days after transfusion when HbS was 11%	Pain crisis, ACS, ARDS improved with treatment, then MOF	Drowsy, unresponsive	Exchange transfusion, plasmapheresis (started day 6)	Recovered
5	Lee et al, 2003[188]	24/M/HbSC	6.6	11,250	55	Occasional; later many	Pain crisis, fever, developed hypoxemia, renal impairment	Lethargy, seizure	Simple transfusions, improvement only after plasmapheresis (started day 1)	Recovered

6	Majjiga et al, 2010[189]	3/M/HbSC	1.5	9418	102	Yes	Fever, hypotension, abdominal pain, renal insufficiency, respiratory distress due to ACS	Lethargy, altered sensorium, Glasgow coma scale 7, normal CT	Intubation, mechanical ventilation, simple transfusions, improvement only after plasmapheresis (started day 1)	Recovered
7	Shelat, 2010[190]	16/F/HbSS	7	6000	~70	1+	Pain crisis, fever, hypoxia, ACS, purpura, ecchymoses	Headache, CT and MRI normal	Exchange transfusion, plasmapheresis (started day 1)	Recovered
8	Vlachaki et al, 2014[191]	30/M/HbS-β+ thalassemia	7.1	2000	7	None initially; appeared after transfusion	Initially diagnosed as ITP; bleeding after dental procedure, later pain crisis	Agitation, headache, CT showed brain hemorrhage	Transfusion, corticosteroids, IVIg, then plasmapheresis (started day 11)	Died of MOF
9	Gangemi and Pickens, 2015[192]	48/F/HbS-β+ thalassemia	6.9	3556	35	Schistocytes, with increase after treatment	Pain crisis, fever, SOB	Altered mental state	Transfusion, FFP, but improvement only after plasmapheresis (started day 3), then steroids and weekly rituximab	Recovered without recurrence but died 3 months later of *Pneumocystis jirovecii* pneumonia

*Hematocrit 17%.

Abbreviations: ACS, acute chest syndrome; AMS, altered mental status; ARDS, acute respiratory distress syndrome; CNS, central nervous system symptoms; CT, computed tomography; F, female; FFP, fresh frozen plasma; ITP, idiopathic thrombocytopenic purpura; IVIg, intravenous immunoglobulin; LDH, lactate dehydrogenase; MRI, magnetic resonance imaging; MOF, multiorgan failure; M, male; SOB, shortness of breath.

TABLE 21-2 Laboratory values in sickle cell disease patients with iron deficiency, including their blood Hb level also during the period without iron deficiency

Patient No.	Reference	Age/sex/genotype	Hb (g/dL) with iron deficiency	Hb (g/dL) without iron deficiency	Change in Hb with iron deficiency (%)	Ferritin (ng/mL)	MCV (fL)	MCHC (g/dL)
1	Castro and Haddy, 1982[193]	53/M/HbSS	6.4	8.7	−26	10	61	29
2	"	6/F/HbSS	3.2	9.4	−66		51	25.6
3	"	45/F/HbSS	6.8	7.7	−12	8.6	65	30.6
4	Rao et al, 1983[194]	46/M/HbSS	7	9	−22	14.5	60	27.9
5	Castro et al, 1994[195]	47/M/HbSS	8.4	9	−7	19	65	30.2
6	"	55/F/HbSS	6.7	7.8	−14	20	67	31.6
7	"	20/M/HbSS	8	9	−11	10	60	30.7
8	"	36/M/HbSS	7.9	8.1	−2	14	63	31.7
9	Bouchair et al, 2000[196]	12/M/HbSS	9.4	10.9	−14	6.7	56	31.6
10	"	15/F/HbSC	9.2	10.8	−15	4.9	61	31
11	Rombos et al, 2002[197]	59/F/HbS-β+ thalassemia	9.4	10.4	−10	21.4	62	31.9
12	"	50/M/HbS-Lepore	9.7	12.6	−23	13	64	31.3
13	Markham et al, 2003[198]	26/M/HbSC	11.1	11.6	−4	18.6	69	31.2
14	Castro et al, 2009[199]	47/F/HbSS	5.4	7.3	−26	4.8	57	31
Mean			7.8	9.5	−18.0	12.7	62	30.4
± SD			2.0	1.6	0.2	5.8	4.7	1.8

Abbreviations: F, female; Hb, hemoglobin; M, male; MCHC, mean corpuscular hemoglobin concentration; MCV, mean corpuscular volume; SD, standard deviation.

ferritin, mean corpuscular volume, and especially MCHC values corresponded to those of severe, stage IV iron deficiency in nonsickle subjects, in whom a 40%, not a 20%, blood hemoglobin level reduction is expected. Additional case series of iron deficiency in sickle cell patients also report relatively mild, 10% to 21% reductions of hemoglobin level.[176,177] In a study of 12 Jamaican sickle cell children with iron deficiency, hemoglobin levels were actually higher (mean, 9.3 g/dL) than in 129 sickle cell disease children without iron deficiency (8.3 g/dL), a difference that was not statistically significant. However, with iron deficiency, the children's reticulocyte counts were significantly lower and their RBC counts significantly higher.[178]

It is difficult to explain the above findings without concluding that iron deficiency decreases hemolytic rate in sickle cell patients. The delay time of HbS polymerization is highly dependent on HbS concentration,[179,180] so that sickle RBCs with low MCHC due to iron deficiency would be expected to have less HbS polymerization and longer intravascular survival. Studies in sickle mice also suggest that iron deficiency lowers hemolysis and improves anemia, although no MCHC values were reported.[181] Increased RBC survival was reported in 1 sickle cell anemia patient during iron deficiency.[182] Phlebotomy programs to induce iron deficiency are already being used to treat patients with HbSC disease.[183] Future efficacy and safety studies may determine also whether there is a degree of iron deficiency at which the hemoglobin level in SS patients remains stable or even increases. If so, iron depletion should be induced in sickle cell anemia patients, at least in adults, and if already present, its cause should be ascertained and addressed, but iron "treatment" should be withheld.

Acknowledgment

Dr. Allison Weyer and Dr. Enrico Novelli, University of Pittsburgh Medical Center, kindly provided the case study and Figure 21-3.

Case Study

Cerebral Fat Embolism in Sickle Cell Disease

A 22-year-old woman with hemoglobin SC disease and a recent history of acute chest syndrome presented to the emergency department with progressive pain in the thighs for 2 days. She was afebrile and had normal pulse oximetry values. Laboratory results showed leukocytosis (WBC 24.1×10^9/L) with a left shift, a hemoglobin level of 11.8 g/dL, and a platelet count of 288×10^9/L. Serum electrolytes were normal, and serum creatinine was 0.9 mg/dL. The initial chest x-ray revealed no acute abnormalities. She was treated with opioids and intravenous (IV) fluids, appeared to improve, and was discharged. However, she returned to the emergency department a few hours later with a new complaint of chest pain, which she described as "similar to that of my acute chest syndrome." At this time, her cardiopulmonary exam, electrocardiogram, and cardiac enzymes were normal, and a chest computed tomography (CT) showed only "minimal bibasilar atelectasis." She received additional IV opioids without relief and was admitted to the hospital with a diagnosis of vaso-occlusive pain crisis. Upon admission, she had a high serum LDH (2976 IU/L), and her creatinine had increased to 1.3 mg/dL, but otherwise, there were no significant laboratory abnormalities. She was treated with hydromorphone, 1 mg IV every 3 hours as needed, and IV fluids with improvement of her pain.

Approximately 24 hours after her initial presentation, the patient became obtunded, hypoxic, and febrile (39.9°C [103.8°F]). Her mental status transiently improved after a dose of naloxone, but she became disoriented shortly thereafter. A repeat chest x-ray showed "new diffuse right lung opacities most compatible with pneumonia, possibly from aspiration," and a noncontrast head CT was normal. She was transferred to the intensive care unit on hospital day (HD) 2. An arterial blood gas showed a normal pH and carbon dioxide, and her partial pressure of oxygen was 73 mm Hg on 1.5 L/min of oxygen via nasal cannula. The patient was hemodynamically stable and had a normal serum lactate level. A presumptive diagnosis of aspiration pneumonia was made, and she was intubated and mechanically ventilated (tidal volume, 550 mL; 40% fraction of inspired oxygen; positive end-expiratory pressure, 5 cm H_2O; respiratory rate, 12 breaths/min) for airway protection and treated with IV antibiotics. A transthoracic echocardiogram revealed a flattened interventricular septum and evidence of right ventricular pressure overload with a tricuspid regurgitant velocity of 3.3 m/s.

On HD3, the sickle cell service was consulted and diagnosed severe acute chest syndrome. Emergency erythrocytapheresis was arranged, which lowered HbS to 12.3% (corresponding to about 24% HbSC red cells, given that these cells have nearly equal amounts of HbS and HbC). The electroencephalogram revealed diffuse severe slowing without seizures or epileptiform discharges. Magnetic resonance imaging (MRI) of the brain with and without contrast showed "innumerable foci of abnormal susceptibility artifact diffusely throughout the supratentorial and infratentorial brain parenchyma and brainstem with associated restricted diffusion but no enhancement" (Figure 21-3). Magnetic resonance angiography and magnetic resonance venography were unremarkable. Lupus anticoagulant and antiphospholipid antibodies and HIV and syphilis serologies were all negative. A diagnosis of FES was entertained. Bronchoalveolar lavage revealed a moderate number of Oil Red O stain–positive, lipid-laden macrophages, consistent with this diagnosis. Given the patient's diagnosis of FES/MOF syndrome, 7 additional RBC units were transfused to minimize the proportion of HbSC erythrocytes and to maintain her total hemoglobin >10 g/dL. Hydroxyurea treatment was started on HD9. She had persistent thrombocytopenia until HD11. Throughout her hospitalization, the patient remained hemodynamically stable and on minimal ventilator support, but her altered mental status remained the principal concern. She experienced multiple febrile spikes to >39°C (102.2°F), prompting several adjustments to her antibiotic regimen, but no infectious agent was ever identified. A tracheostomy was performed on HD9. Two days later, the patient's mental status started to progressively improve and ventilator weaning was initiated. She was discharged on HD31 with a normal mental status and without neurologic sequelae. The patient was then maintained on monthly exchange transfusions and hydroxyurea and returned to work a few months after discharge. A brain MRI obtained approximately 10 months after her illness revealed complete resolution of the lesions.

In summary, this patient was admitted with an uncomplicated pain episode, but 1 to 2 days later, she developed severe acute chest syndrome with evidence of pulmonary and systemic fat embolization. These diagnoses were supported by the typical brain MRI changes, the finding of fat-laden macrophages on bronchoalveolar lavage, and thrombocytopenia without evidence for disseminated intravascular coagulation or thrombotic macroangiopathy. It is quite likely that the early institution of exchange transfusion prevented progressive organ dysfunction and death.

High-Yield Facts

◆ MOF in sickle cell disease can present de novo or during an acute event such as a pain episode or acute chest syndrome.

◆ MOF is life threatening, often due to widespread sickling-related vaso-occlusion or to FES and, rarely, to TMA.

◆ FES disproportionately affects the milder genotypes (HbSC, HbS-β⁺ thalassemia). It can be the first manifestation of sickle cell disease in patients with a benign clinical course and previously undiagnosed hemoglobinopathy.

◆ Prompt treatment with transfusions or exchange transfusions is lifesaving in sickle patients with MOF and/or FES.

◆ In MOF due to TMA, plasma exchanges are effective.

◆ Sickle cell disease–related orbital syndrome occurs primarily in children and adolescents, especially males. It is most often due to orbital bone or bone marrow infarction with subperiosteal hematoma. The syndrome responds to conservative measures, which prevent orbital compression.

◆ Severe episodes of pain can be triggered by administration of systemic corticosteroids, stem cell–mobilizing agents, and sildenafil. When treatment with these agents is essential, this risk may be reduced by transfusions.

◆ Hyperhemolytic syndrome is a common feature of DHTRs, which occur in about 4% of transfused SCD patients, particularly those receiving sporadic transfusions.

◆ Both the transfused RBCs and the patient's own RBCs are destroyed in hyperhemolytic syndrome, the offending antibodies often are undetectable, and anemia is compounded by relative reticulocytopenia. Mortality can be as high as 9% to 12% and is usually due to severe anemia.

◆ In hyperhemolytic syndrome, the critically severe anemia can worsen with transfusions.

◆ Immunosuppression (corticosteroids, rituximab, anticomplement agents) and intravenous immunoglobulin have been reported to improve hyperhemolytic syndrome's severe anemia.

References

1. Hassell KL, Eckman JR, Lane PA. Acute multiorgan failure syndrome: a potentially catastrophic complication of severe sickle cell pain episodes. *Am J Med.* 1994;96(2):155-162.

2. Karacaoglu PK, Asma S, Korur A, et al. East Mediterranean region sickle cell disease mortality trial: retrospective multicenter cohort analysis of 735 patients. *Ann Hematol.* 2016;95(6):993-1000.

3. Tsitsikas DA, Gallinella G, Patel S, Seligman H, Greaves P, Amos RJ. Bone marrow necrosis and fat embolism syndrome in sickle cell disease: increased susceptibility of patients with non-SS genotypes and a possible association with human parvovirus B19 infection. *Blood Rev.* 2014;28(1):23-30.

4. Chaturvedi S, Ghafuri DL, Glassberg J, Kassim AA, Rodeghier M, DeBaun MR. Rapidly progressive acute chest syndrome in individuals with sickle cell anemia: a distinct acute chest syndrome phenotype. *Am J Hematol.* 2016;91(12):1185-1190.

5. Louie JE, Anderson CJ, Fayaz MFK, et al. Case series supporting heme detoxification via therapeutic plasma exchange in acute multiorgan failure syndrome resistant to red blood cell exchange in sickle cell disease. *Transfusion.* 2018;58(2):470-479.

6. Ataga KI, Orringer EP. Bone marrow necrosis in sickle cell disease: a description of three cases and a review of the literature. *Am J Med Sci.* 2000;320(5):342-347.

7. Gangaraju R, Reddy VV, Marques MB. Fat embolism syndrome secondary to bone marrow necrosis in patients with hemoglobinopathies. *South Med J.* 2016;109(9):549-553.

8. Vichinsky E, Williams R, Das M, et al. Pulmonary fat embolism: a distinct cause of severe acute chest syndrome in sickle cell anemia. *Blood.* 1994;83(11):3107-3112.

9. Medoff BD, Shepard JA, Smith RN, Kratz A. Case records of the Massachusetts General Hospital. Case 17-2005. A 22-year-old woman with back and leg pain and respiratory failure. *N Engl J Med.* 2005;352(23):2425-2434.

10. Horton DP, Ferriero DM, Mentzer WC. Nontraumatic fat embolism syndrome in sickle cell anemia. *Pediatr Neurol.* 1995;12(1):77-80.

11. Gibbs WN, Opatowsky MJ, Burton EC. AIRP best cases in radiologic-pathologic correlation: cerebral fat embolism syndrome in sickle cell beta-thalassemia. *Radiographics.* 2012;32(5):1301-1306.

12. Dang NC, Johnson C, Eslami-Farsani M, Haywood LJ. Myocardial injury or infarction associated with fat embolism in sickle cell disease: a report of three cases with survival. *Am J Hematol.* 2005;80(2):133-136.

13. Darbari DS, Kple-Faget P, Kwagyan J, Rana S, Gordeuk VR, Castro O. Circumstances of death in adult sickle cell disease patients. *Am J Hematol.* 2006;81(11):858-863.

14. Graham JK, Mosunjac M, Hanzlick RL, Mosunjac M. Sickle cell lung disease and sudden death: a retrospective/prospective study of 21 autopsy cases and literature review. *Am J Forensic Med Pathol.* 2007;28(2):168-172.

15. Tsitsikas DA, May JE, Gangaraju R, Abukar J, Amos RJ, Marques MB. Revisiting fat embolism in sickle syndromes: diagnostic and emergency therapeutic measures. *Br J Haematol.* 2019;186(4):e112-e115.

16. Eichhorn RF, Buurke EJ, Blok P, Berends MJ, Jansen CL. Sickle cell-like crisis and bone marrow necrosis associated with parvovirus B19 infection and heterozygosity for haemoglobins S and E. *J Intern Med.* 1999;245(1):103-106.

17. Rayburg M, Kalinyak KA, Towbin AJ, Baker PB, Joiner CH. Fatal bone marrow embolism in a child with hemoglobin SE disease. *Am J Hematol.* 2010;85(3):182-184.

18. de Campos FPF, Ferreira CR, Felipe-Silva A. Bone marrow necrosis and fat embolism: an autopsy report of a severe complication of hemoglobin SC disease. *Autops Case Rep.* 2014;4(2):9-20.

19. Adamski J, Hanna CA, Reddy VB, Litovsky SH, Evans CA, Marques MB. Multiorgan failure and bone marrow necrosis in three adults with sickle cell-beta+-thalassemia. *Am J Hematol.* 2012;87(6):621-624.

20. Myers CF, Ipe TS. Bone marrow necrosis in sickle cell-beta thalassemia patient mimicking thrombotic thrombocytopenic purpura. *Ann Clin Lab Sci.* 2018;48(5):670-673.

21. Rizk S, Pulte ED, Axelrod D, Ballas SK. Perinatal maternal mortality in sickle cell anemia: two case reports and review of the literature. *Hemoglobin.* 2017;41(4-6):225-229.

22. Niraimathi M, Kar R, Jacob SE, Basu D. Sudden death in sickle cell anaemia: report of three cases with brief review of literature. *Indian J Hematol Blood Transfus.* 2016;32(suppl 1):258-261.

23. Godeau B, Dhainaut JF, Bachir D, Galacteros F. Pulmonary fat embolism after prostaglandin infusion in sickle cell disease with fatal outcome despite exchange blood transfusion. *Am J Hematol.* 1993;43(4):330-331.

24. Lowenthal EA, Wells A, Emanuel PD, Player R, Prchal JT. Sickle cell acute chest syndrome associated with parvovirus B19 infection: case series and review. *Am J Hematol.* 1996;51(3):207-213.

25. Castro O. Systemic fat embolism and pulmonary hypertension in sickle cell disease. *Hematol Oncol Clin North Am.* 1996;10(6): 1289-1303.

26. Johnson K, Stastny JF, Rucknagel DL. Fat embolism syndrome associated with asthma and sickle cell-beta(+)-thalassemia. *Am J Hematol.* 1994;46(4):354-357.

27. Grigg AP. Granulocyte colony-stimulating factor-induced sickle cell crisis and multiorgan dysfunction in a patient with compound heterozygous sickle cell/beta+ thalassemia. *Blood.* 2001;97(12): 3998-3999.

28. Targueta EP, Hirano ACG, de Campos FPF, Martines J, Lovisolo SM, Felipe-Silva A. Bone marrow necrosis and fat embolism syndrome: a dreadful complication of hemoglobin sickle cell disease. *Autops Case Rep.* 2017;7(4):42-50.

29. Lechapt E, Habibi A, Bachir D, et al. Induced sputum versus bronchoalveolar lavage during acute chest syndrome in sickle cell disease. *Am J Respir Crit Care Med.* 2003;168(11):1373-1377.

30. Castella X, Valles J, Cabezuelo MA, Fernandez R, Artigas A. Fat embolism syndrome and pulmonary microvascular cytology. *Chest.* 1992;101(6):1710-1711.

31. Chmel H, Bertles JF. Hemoglobin S/C disease in a pregnant woman with crisis and fat embolization syndrome. *Am J Med.* 1975;58(4):563-566.

32. Bachmeyer C, Lionnet F, Stojanovic KS, Moguelet P, Aractingi S. Unusual cutaneous lesions indicating fat embolism syndrome in homozygous sickle cell disease. *Am J Hematol.* 2014;89(2):233.

33. Kang JH, Hargett CW, Sevilis T, Luedke M. Sickle cell disease, fat embolism syndrome, and "starfield" pattern on MRI. *Neurol Clin Pract.* 2018;8(2):162-164.

34. Dang NC, Johnson C, Eslami-Farsani M, Haywood LJ. Bone marrow embolism in sickle cell disease: a review. *Am J Hematol.* 2005;79(1):61-67.

35. Vichinsky EP, Neumayr LD, Earles AN, et al. Causes and outcomes of the acute chest syndrome in sickle cell disease. National Acute Chest Syndrome Study Group. *N Engl J Med.* 2000;342(25):1855-1865.

36. Emre U, Miller ST, Gutierez M, Steiner P, Rao SP, Rao M. Effect of transfusion in acute chest syndrome of sickle cell disease. *J Pediatr.* 1995;127(6):901-904.

37. Procianoy F, Brandao Filho M, Cruz AA, Alencar VM. Subperiosteal hematoma and orbital compression syndrome following minor frontal trauma in sickle cell anemia: case report. *Arq Bras Oftalmol.* 2008;71(2):262-264.

38. Tostivint L, Pop-Jora D, Grimprel E, Quinet B, Lesprit E. [Orbital bone infarction in a child with homozygous sickle cell disease]. *Arch Pediatr.* 2012;19(6):612-615.

39. Ilhan N, Acipayam C, Aydogan F, et al. Orbital compression syndrome complicated by epidural hematoma and wide cephalohematoma in a patient with sickle cell disease. *J AAPOS.* 2014;18(2):189-191.

40. Reiersen DA, Mandava M, Jeroudi M, Gungor A. Maxillofacial extramedullary hematopoiesis in a child with sickle cell presenting as bilateral periorbital cellulitis. *Int J Pediatr Otorhinolaryngol.* 2014;78(7):1173-1175.

41. Sokol JA, Baron E, Lantos G, Kazim M. Orbital compression syndrome in sickle cell disease. *Ophthalmic Plast Reconstr Surg.* 2008;24(3):181-184.

42. Ozkavukcu E, Fitoz S, Yagmurlu B, Ciftci E, Erden I, Ertem M. Orbital wall infarction mimicking periorbital cellulitis in a patient with sickle cell disease. *Pediatr Radiol.* 2007;37(4):388-390.

43. Noble J, Schendel S, Weizblit N, Gill HS, Deangelis DD. Orbital wall infarction in sickle cell disease. *Can J Ophthalmol.* 2008;43(5): 603-604.

44. Mueller EB, Niethammer K, Rees D, Partsch CJ. Orbital compression syndrome in sickle cell crisis. *Klin Padiatr.* 2009;221(5): 308-309.

45. Douvoyiannis M, Fakioglu E, Litman N. Orbital compression syndrome presenting as orbital cellulitis in a child with sickle cell anemia. *Pediatr Emerg Care.* 2010;26(4):285-286.

46. Douira-Khomsi W, Jarraya M, Ben Hassine L, et al. [Orbital subperiosteal hematoma in child with sickle cell thalassemia. A case report]. *Arch Pediatr.* 2010;17(8):1174-1177.

47. Ghafouri RH, Lee I, Freitag SK, Pira TN. Bilateral orbital bone infarction in sickle-cell disease. *Ophthalmic Plast Reconstr Surg.* 2011;27(2):e26-e27.

48. Alsuhaibani AH, Marzouk MA. Recurrent infarction of sphenoid bone with subperiosteal collection in a child with sickle cell disease. *Ophthalmic Plast Reconstr Surg.* 2011;27(5): e136-e138.

49. Louati H, Hedhli M, Chebbi A, et al. [Spontaneous orbital hematoma: two case reports]. *J Fr Ophthalmol.* 2012;35(7):e531-e534.

50. Helen OO, Ajite KO, Oyelami OA, Asaleye CM, Adeoye AO. Bilateral orbital infarction and retinal detachment in a previously undiagnosed sickle cell hemoglobinopathy African child. *Niger Med J.* 2013;54(3):200-202.

51. Huckfeldt RM, Shah AS. Sterile subperiosteal fluid collections accompanying orbital wall infarction in sickle-cell disease. *J AAPOS.* 2014;18(5):485-487.

52. Schündeln MM, Ringelstein A, Storbeck T, Kocadag K, Grasemann C. Orbital compression syndrome in a child with sickle cell disease. *J Pediatr.* 2014;164(3):671.

53. Janssens C, Claeys L, Maes P, Boiy T, Wojciechowski M. Orbital wall infarction in child with sickle cell disease. *Acta Clin Belg.* 2015;70(6):451-452.

54. McBride CL, Mai KT, Kumar KS. Orbital infarction due to sickle cell disease without orbital pain. *Case Rep Ophthalmol Med.* 2016;2016:5867850.

55. Sundu C, Dinc E, Sari A, Unal S, Dursun O. Bilateral subperiosteal hematoma and orbital compression syndrome in sickle cell disease. *J Craniofac Surg.* 2017;28(8):e775-e776.

56. Edmunds MR, Butler L. Orbital infarction with haematoma in sickle cell disease. *BMJ.* 2017;356:i6651.

57. Alghamdi A. Recurrent orbital bone sub-periosteal hematoma in sickle cell disease: a case study. *BMC Ophthalmol.* 2018;18(1):211.

58. Stewart CM, Sipkova Z, Hildebrand GD, Norris JH. Acute sickle cell orbitopathy masquerading as orbital cellulitis. *J Pediatr Hematol Oncol.* 2018;40(1):79-80.

59. Ganesh A, Al-Zuhaibi S, Pathare A, et al. Orbital infarction in sickle cell disease. *Am J Ophthalmol.* 2008;146(4):595-601.

60. Seeler RA. Exophthalmos in hemoglobin SC disease. *J Pediatr.* 1983;102(1):90-91.

61. Daar S, Hussain HM, Gravell D, Nagel RL, Krishnamoorthy R. Genetic epidemiology of HbS in Oman: multicentric origin for the betaS gene. *Am J Hematol.* 2000;64(1):39-46.

62. Serjeant GR, Grandison Y, Lowrie Y, et al. The development of haematological changes in homozygous sickle cell disease: a cohort study from birth to 6 years. *Br J Haematol.* 1981;48(4):533-543.

63. West MS, Wethers D, Smith J, Steinberg M. Laboratory profile of sickle cell disease: a cross-sectional analysis. The Cooperative Study of Sickle Cell Disease. *J Clin Epidemiol.* 1992;45(8):893-909.

64. Dover GJ, Smith KD, Chang YC, et al. Fetal hemoglobin levels in sickle cell disease and normal individuals are partially controlled by an X-linked gene located at Xp22.2. *Blood.* 1992;80(3):816-824.

65. Darbari DS, Fasano RS, Minniti CP, et al. Severe vaso-occlusive episodes associated with use of systemic corticosteroids in patients with sickle cell disease. *J Natl Med Assoc.* 2008;100(8):948-951.

66. Michel M, Habibi A, Godeau B, et al. Characteristics and outcome of connective tissue diseases in patients with sickle-cell disease: report of 30 cases. *Semin Arthritis Rheum.* 2008;38(3):228-240.

67. Couillard S, Benkerrou M, Girot R, Brousse V, Ferster A, Bader-Meunier B. Steroid treatment in children with sickle-cell disease. *Haematologica.* 2007;92(3):425-426.

68. Strouse JJ, Hulbert ML, DeBaun MR, Jordan LC, Casella JF. Primary hemorrhagic stroke in children with sickle cell disease is associated with recent transfusion and use of corticosteroids. *Pediatrics.* 2006;118(5):1916-1924.

69. Griffin TC, McIntire D, Buchanan GR. High-dose intravenous methylprednisolone therapy for pain in children and adolescents with sickle cell disease. *N Engl J Med.* 1994;330(11):733-737.

70. Bernini JC, Rogers ZR, Sandler ES, Reisch JS, Quinn CT, Buchanan GR. Beneficial effect of intravenous dexamethasone in children with mild to moderately severe acute chest syndrome complicating sickle cell disease. *Blood.* 1998;92(9):3082-3089.

71. Quinn CT, Stuart MJ, Kesler K, et al. Tapered oral dexamethasone for the acute chest syndrome of sickle cell disease. *Br J Haematol.* 2011;155(2):263-267.

72. Strouse JJ, Takemoto CM, Keefer JR, Kato GJ, Casella JF. Corticosteroids and increased risk of readmission after acute chest syndrome in children with sickle cell disease. *Pediatr Blood Cancer.* 2008;50(5):1006-1012.

73. Sobota A, Graham DA, Heeney MM, Neufeld EJ. Corticosteroids for acute chest syndrome in children with sickle cell disease: variation in use and association with length of stay and readmission. *Am J Hematol.* 2010;85(1):24-28.

74. Isakoff MS, Lillo JA, Hagstrom JN. A single-institution experience with treatment of severe acute chest syndrome: lack of rebound pain with dexamethasone plus transfusion therapy. *J Pediatr Hematol Oncol.* 2008;30(4):322-325.

75. Unnikrishnan A PJ, Bari S, Zumberg M, et al. Anti-N and anti-Do immunoglobulin G alloantibody-mediated delayed hemolytic transfusion reaction with hyperhemolysis in sickle cell disease treated with eculizumab and HBOC-201: case report and review of the literature. *Transfusion.* 2019;59(6):1907-1910.

76. Moya F, Rivera M, Araya F, Donoso J, Sandoval P, Varas P. [Delayed hemolytic reaction to transfusion in sickle cell anemia. Report of one case]. *Rev Med Chil.* 2018;146(11):1347-1350.

77. Cattoni A, Cazzaniga G, Perseghin P, et al. An attempt to induce transient immunosuppression pre-erythrocytapheresis in a girl with sickle cell disease, a history of severe delayed hemolytic transfusion reactions and need for hip prosthesis. *Hematol Rep.* 2013;5(2):36-38.

78. Reyes MA, Illoh OC. Hyperhemolytic transfusion reaction attributable to anti-Fy3 in a patient with sickle cell disease. *Immunohematology.* 2008;24(2):45-51.

79. Cullis JO, Win N, Dudley JM, Kaye T. Post-transfusion hyperhaemolysis in a patient with sickle cell disease: use of steroids and intravenous immunoglobulin to prevent further red cell destruction. *Vox Sang.* 1995;69(4):355-357.

80. de Montalembert M, Dumont MD, Heilbronner C, et al. Delayed hemolytic transfusion reaction in children with sickle cell disease. *Haematologica.* 2011;96(6):801-807.

81. Elenga N, Mialou V, Kebaili K, Galambrun C, Bertrand Y, Pondarre C. Severe neurologic complication after delayed hemolytic transfusion reaction in 2 children with sickle cell anemia: significant diagnosis and therapeutic challenges. *J Pediatr Hematol Oncol.* 2008;30(12):928-930.

82. Gladman DD, Bombardier C. Sickle cell crisis following intraarticular steroid therapy for rheumatoid arthritis. *Arthritis Rheum.* 1987;30(9):1065-1068.

83. Glassberg J, Minnitti C, Cromwell C, et al. Inhaled steroids reduce pain and sVCAM levels in individuals with sickle cell disease: a triple-blind, randomized trial. *Am J Hematol.* 2017;92(7):622-631.

84. Langer AL, Leader A, Kim-Schulze S, Ginzburg Y, Merad M, Glassberg J. Inhaled steroids associated with decreased macrophage markers in nonasthmatic individuals with sickle cell disease in a randomized trial. *Ann Hematol.* 2019;98(4):841-849.

85. Quinn CT, Lee NJ, Shull EP, Ahmad N, Rogers ZR, Buchanan GR. Prediction of adverse outcomes in children with sickle cell anemia: a study of the Dallas Newborn Cohort. *Blood.* 2008;111(2):544-548.

86. Litos M, Sarris I, Bewley S, Seed P, Okpala I, Oteng-Ntim E. White blood cell count as a predictor of the severity of sickle cell disease during pregnancy. *Eur J Obstet Gynecol Reprod Biol.* 2007;133(2):169-172.

87. Sebastiani P, Nolan VG, Baldwin CT, et al. A network model to predict the risk of death in sickle cell disease. *Blood.* 2007;110(7):2727-2735.

88. Ataga KI, Kutlar A, Kanter J, et al. Crizanlizumab for the prevention of pain crises in sickle cell disease. *N Engl J Med.* 2017;376(5):429-439.

89. Chen L, Zhuang M, Shah HQ, Lin JH. Chronic myelogenous leukemia in sickle cell anemia. *Arch Pathol Lab Med.* 2005;129(3):423-424.

90. Sallam MM, Alsuliman AM, Alahmed HE, Alabdulaali MK. Chronic myelogenous leukemia in sickle cell/beta 0-thalassemia. *Indian J Pathol Microbiol.* 2011;54(3):597-598.

91. Phillips G Jr, Hartman J, Kinney TR, Sokal JE, Kaufman RE. Chronic granulocytic leukemia in a patient with sickle cell anemia. *Am J Med.* 1988;85(4):567-569.

92. Baron F, Dresse MF, Beguin Y. Transmission of chronic myeloid leukemia through peripheral-blood stem-cell transplantation. *N Engl J Med.* 2003;349(9):913-914.

93. Weinstein RS. Glucocorticoid-induced osteonecrosis. *Endocrine.* 2012;41(2):183-190.

94. Kamble RT, Tin UC, Carrum G. Successful mobilization and transplantation of filgrastim mobilized hematopoietic stem cells in sickle cell-hemoglobin C disease. *Bone Marrow Transplant.* 2006;37(11):1065-1066.

95. Tormey CA, Snyder EL, Cooper DL. Mobilization, collection, and transplantation of peripheral blood hematopoietic progenitor cells in a patient with multiple myeloma and hemoglobin SC disease. *Transfusion.* 2008;48(9):1930-1933.

96. Onitilo AA, Lazarchick J, Brunson CY, Frei-Lahr D, Stuart RK. Autologous bone marrow transplant in a patient with sickle cell disease and diffuse large B-cell lymphoma. *Transplant Proc.* 2003; 35(8):3089-3092.

97. Hsieh MM, Tisdale JF. Hematopoietic stem cell mobilization with plerixafor in sickle cell disease. *Haematologica.* 2018;103(5): 749-750.

98. Fitzhugh CD, Hsieh MM, Bolan CD, Saenz C, Tisdale JF. Granulocyte colony-stimulating factor (G-CSF) administration in individuals with sickle cell disease: time for a moratorium? *Cytotherapy.* 2009;11(4):464-471.

99. Kang EM, Areman EM, David-Ocampo V, et al. Mobilization, collection, and processing of peripheral blood stem cells in individuals with sickle cell trait. *Blood.* 2002;99(3):850-855.

100. Panch SR, Yau YY, Fitzhugh CD, Hsieh MM, Tisdale JF, Leitman SF. Hematopoietic progenitor cell mobilization is more robust in healthy African American compared to Caucasian donors and is not affected by the presence of sickle cell trait. *Transfusion.* 2016;56(5):1058-1065.

101. De Santis GC, Prado BPA Jr, Dotoli GM, Simoes BP, Covas DT. Mobilizing hematopoietic progenitor cells in donors with sickle cell trait is safe. *Hematol Transfus Cell Ther.* 2019;41(1):101-102.

102. Al-Khabori M, Al-Ghafri F, Al-Kindi S, et al. Safety of stem cell mobilization in donors with sickle cell trait. *Bone Marrow Transplant.* 2015;50(2):310-311.

103. Domingues MJ, Nilsson SK, Cao B. New agents in HSC mobilization. *Int J Hematol.* 2017;105(2):141-152.

104. Boulad F, Shore T, van Besien K, et al. Safety and efficacy of plerixafor dose escalation for the mobilization of CD34(+) hematopoietic progenitor cells in patients with sickle cell disease: interim results. *Haematologica.* 2018;103(9):1577.

105. Esrick EB, Manis JP, Daley H, et al. Successful hematopoietic stem cell mobilization and apheresis collection using plerixafor alone in sickle cell patients. *Blood Adv.* 2018;2(19):2505-2512.

106. Lagresle-Peyrou C, Lefrere F, Magrin E, et al. Plerixafor enables safe, rapid, efficient mobilization of hematopoietic stem cells in sickle cell disease patients after exchange transfusion. *Haematologica.* 2018;103(5):778-786.

107. Tigue CC, McKoy JM, Evens AM, Trifilio SM, Tallman MS, Bennett CL. Granulocyte-colony stimulating factor administration to healthy individuals and persons with chronic neutropenia or cancer: an overview of safety considerations from the Research on Adverse Drug Events and Reports project. *Bone Marrow Transplant.* 2007;40(3):185-192.

108. Pulsipher MA, Chitphakdithai P, Miller JP, et al. Adverse events among 2408 unrelated donors of peripheral blood stem cells: results of a prospective trial from the National Marrow Donor Program. *Blood.* 2009;113(15):3604-3611.

109. Parent F, Bachir D, Inamo J, et al. A hemodynamic study of pulmonary hypertension in sickle cell disease. *N Engl J Med.* 2011;365(1):44-53.

110. Fonseca GH, Souza R, Salemi VM, Jardim CV, Gualandro SF. Pulmonary hypertension diagnosed by right heart catheterisation in sickle cell disease. *Eur Respir J.* 2012;39(1):112-118.

111. Mehari A, Gladwin MT, Tian X, Machado RF, Kato GJ. Mortality in adults with sickle cell disease and pulmonary hypertension. *JAMA.* 2012;307(12):1254-1256.

112. Galie N, Ghofrani HA, Torbicki A, et al. Sildenafil citrate therapy for pulmonary arterial hypertension. *N Engl J Med.* 2005; 353(20):2148-2157.

113. Derchi G, Forni GL, Formisano F, et al. Efficacy and safety of sildenafil in the treatment of severe pulmonary hypertension in patients with hemoglobinopathies. *Haematologica.* 2005;90(4): 452-458.

114. Machado RF, Barst RJ, Yovetich NA, et al. Hospitalization for pain in patients with sickle cell disease treated with sildenafil for elevated TRV and low exercise capacity. *Blood.* 2011; 118(4):855-864.

115. Machado RF, Martyr S, Kato GJ, et al. Sildenafil therapy in patients with sickle cell disease and pulmonary hypertension. *Br J Haematol.* 2005;130(3):445-453.

116. Gong B, Ma M, Xie W, et al. Direct comparison of tadalafil with sildenafil for the treatment of erectile dysfunction: a systematic review and meta-analysis. *Int Urol Nephrol.* 2017;49(10): 1731-1740.

117. Patil CS, Padi SV, Singh VP, Kulkarni SK. Sildenafil induces hyperalgesia via activation of the NO-cGMP pathway in the rat neuropathic pain model. *Inflammopharmacology.* 2006;14(1-2):22-27.

118. Moore RA, Edwards JE, McQuay HJ. Sildenafil (Viagra) for male erectile dysfunction: a meta-analysis of clinical trial reports. *BMC Urol.* 2002;2:6.

119. Franco RS, Yasin Z, Lohmann JM, et al. The survival characteristics of dense sickle cells. *Blood.* 2000;96(10):3610-3617.

120. Lew VL, Bookchin RM. Ion transport pathology in the mechanism of sickle cell dehydration. *Physiol Rev.* 2005;85(1):179-200.

121. Ataga KI, Reid M, Ballas SK, et al. Improvements in haemolysis and indicators of erythrocyte survival do not correlate with acute vaso-occlusive crises in patients with sickle cell disease: a phase III randomized, placebo-controlled, double-blind study of the gardos channel blocker senicapoc (ICA-17043). *Br J Haematol.* 2011;153(1):92-104.

122. Kato GJ, Gladwin MT, Steinberg MH. Deconstructing sickle cell disease: reappraisal of the role of hemolysis in the development of clinical subphenotypes. *Blood Rev.* 2007;21(1):37-47.

123. Vichinsky E, Hoppe CC, Ataga KI, et al. A phase 3 randomized trial of voxelotor in sickle cell disease. *N Engl J Med.* 2019;381(6): 509-519.

124. Steinberg MH, Rosenstock W, Coleman MB, et al. Effects of thalassemia and microcytosis on the hematologic and vasoocclusive severity of sickle cell anemia. *Blood.* 1984;63(6):1353-1360.

125. Vidler JB, Gardner K, Amenyah K, Mijovic A, Thein SL. Delayed haemolytic transfusion reaction in adults with sickle cell disease: a 5-year experience. *Br J Haematol.* 2015;169(5):746-753.

126. Habibi A, Mekontso-Dessap A, Guillaud C, et al. Delayed hemolytic transfusion reaction in adult sickle-cell disease: presentations, outcomes, and treatments of 99 referral center episodes. *Am J Hematol.* 2016;91(10):989-994.

127. Reverberi R. The persistence of red cell alloantibodies. *Blood Transfus.* 2008;6(4):225-234.

128. Harm SK, Yazer MH, Monis GF, Triulzi DJ, Aubuchon JP, Delaney M. A centralized recipient database enhances the serologic safety of RBC transfusions for patients with sickle cell disease. *Am J Clin Pathol.* 2014;141(2):256-261.

129. King KE, Shirey RS, Lankiewicz MW, Young-Ramsaran J, Ness PM. Delayed hemolytic transfusion reactions in sickle cell disease: simultaneous destruction of recipients' red cells. *Transfusion.* 1997;37(4):376-381.

130. Garratty G. Severe reactions associated with transfusion of patients with sickle cell disease. *Transfusion.* 1997;37(4):357-361.

131. Coleman S, Westhoff CM, Friedman DF, Chou ST. Alloimmunization in patients with sickle cell disease and underrecognition of accompanying delayed hemolytic transfusion reactions. *Transfusion.* 2019;59(7):2282-2291.

132. Eberly LA, Osman D, Collins NP. Hyperhemolysis syndrome without underlying hematologic disease. *Case Rep Hematol.* 2015;2015:180526.

133. Dolatkhah R, Esfahani A, Torabi SE, et al. Delayed hemolytic transfusion reaction with multiple alloantibody (Anti S, N, K) and a monospecific autoanti-JK(b) in intermediate beta-thalassemia patient in Tabriz. *Asian J Transfus Sci.* 2013;7(2):149-150.

134. Danaee A, Inusa B, Howard J, Robinson S. Hyperhemolysis in patients with hemoglobinopathies: a single-center experience and review of the literature. *Transfus Med Rev.* 2015;29(4):220-230.

135. Harvey AR, Basavaraju SV, Chung KW, Kuehnert MJ. Transfusion-related adverse reactions reported to the National Healthcare Safety Network Hemovigilance Module, United States, 2010 to 2012. *Transfusion.* 2015;55(4):709-718.

136. Talano JA, Hillery CA, Gottschall JL, Baylerian DM, Scott JP. Delayed hemolytic transfusion reaction/hyperhemolysis syndrome in children with sickle cell disease. *Pediatrics.* 2003;111(6 Pt 1):e661-e665.

137. Cox JV, Steane E, Cunningham G, Frenkel EP. Risk of alloimmunization and delayed hemolytic transfusion reactions in patients with sickle cell disease. *Arch Intern Med.* 1988;148(11):2485-2489.

138. Michot JM, Driss F, Guitton C, et al. Immunohematologic tolerance of chronic transfusion exchanges with erythrocytapheresis in sickle cell disease. *Transfusion.* 2015;55(2):357-363.

139. Vichinsky EP, Luban NL, Wright E, et al. Prospective RBC phenotype matching in a stroke-prevention trial in sickle cell anemia: a multicenter transfusion trial. *Transfusion.* 2001;41(9):1086-1092.

140. Wahl SK, Garcia A, Hagar W, Gildengorin G, Quirolo K, Vichinsky E. Lower alloimmunization rates in pediatric sickle cell patients on chronic erythrocytapheresis compared to chronic simple transfusions. *Transfusion.* 2012;52(12):2671-2676.

141. DeBaun MR, Gordon M, McKinstry RC, et al. Controlled trial of transfusions for silent cerebral infarcts in sickle cell anemia. *N Engl J Med.* 2014;371(8):699-710.

142. Gardner K, Hoppe C, Mijovic A, Thein SL. How we treat delayed haemolytic transfusion reactions in patients with sickle cell disease. *Br J Haematol.* 2015;170(6):745-756.

143. Castro O, Oneal P, Medina A, Onojobi G, Gordeuk VR. Preventing delayed hemolytic transfusion reactions in sickle cell disease. *Transfusion.* 2016;56(11):2899-2900.

144. Narbey D, Habibi A, Chadebech P, et al. Incidence and predictive score for delayed hemolytic transfusion reaction in adult patients with sickle cell disease. *Am J Hematol.* 2017;92(12):1340-1348.

145. Al-Riyami AZ, Al-Muqbali A, Al-Sudiri S, et al. Risks of red blood cell alloimmunization in transfusion-dependent beta-thalassaemia in Oman: a 25-year experience of a university tertiary care reference center and a literature review. *Transfusion.* 2018;58(4):871-878.

146. Thompson AA, Cunningham MJ, Singer ST, et al. Red cell alloimmunization in a diverse population of transfused patients with thalassaemia. *Br J Haematol.* 2011;153(1):121-128.

147. Cheng CK, Lee CK, Lin CK. Clinically significant red blood cell antibodies in chronically transfused patients: a survey of Chinese thalassemia major patients and literature review. *Transfusion.* 2012;52(10):2220-2224.

148. Vichinsky E, Neumayr L, Trimble S, et al. Transfusion complications in thalassemia patients: a report from the Centers for Disease Control and Prevention (CME). *Transfusion.* 2014;54(4):972-981.

149. Murao M, Viana MB. Risk factors for alloimmunization by patients with sickle cell disease. *Braz J Med Biol Res.* 2005;38(5):675-682.

150. Fasano RM, Booth GS, Miles M, et al. Red blood cell alloimmunization is influenced by recipient inflammatory state at time of transfusion in patients with sickle cell disease. *Br J Haematol.* 2015;168(2):291-300.

151. Dean CL, Maier CL, Chonat S, et al. Challenges in the treatment and prevention of delayed hemolytic transfusion reactions with hyperhemolysis in sickle cell disease patients. *Transfusion.* 2019;59(5):1698-1705.

152. Merle NS, Boudhabhay I, Leon J, Fremeaux-Bacchi V, Roumenina LT. Complement activation during intravascular hemolysis: implication for sickle cell disease and hemolytic transfusion reactions. *Transfus Clin Biol.* 2019;26(2):116-124.

153. Pirenne F, Yazdanbakhsh K. How I safely transfuse patients with sickle-cell disease and manage delayed hemolytic transfusion reactions. *Blood.* 2018;131(25):2773-2781.

154. Delmonte L, Cantini M, Olivieri O, De Franceschi L. Immunoglobulin-resistant delayed hemolytic transfusion reaction treated with rituximab in an adult sickle cell patient. *Transfusion.* 2013;53(3):688-689.

155. Dumas G, Habibi A, Onimus T, et al. Eculizumab salvage therapy for delayed hemolysis transfusion reaction in sickle cell disease patients. *Blood.* 2016;127(8):1062-1064.

156. Sivapalaratnam S, Linpower L, Sirigireddy B, et al. Treatment of post-transfusion hyperhaemolysis syndrome in sickle cell disease with the anti-IL6R humanised monoclonal antibody tocilizumab. *Br J Haematol.* 2019;186(6):e212-e214.

157. Lee LE, Beeler BW, Graham BC, Cap AP, Win N, Chen F. Post-transfusion hyperhemolysis is arrested by targeting macrophage activation with novel use of tocilizumab. *Transfusion.* 2020;60(1):30-35.

158. Epstein SS, Hadley TJ. Successful management of the potentially fatal hyperhaemolysis syndrome of sickle cell anaemia with a regimen including bortezomib and Hemopure. *J Clin Pharm Ther.* 2019;44(5):815-818.

159. Compernolle V, Chou ST, Tanael S, et al. Red blood cell specifications for patients with hemoglobinopathies: a systematic review and guideline. *Transfusion.* 2018;58(6):1555-1566.

160. Chou ST, Jackson T, Vege S, Smith-Whitley K, Friedman DF, Westhoff CM. High prevalence of red blood cell alloimmunization in sickle cell disease despite transfusion from Rh-matched minority donors. *Blood.* 2013;122(6):1062-1071.

161. Noizat-Pirenne F, Habibi A, Mekontso-Dessap A, et al. The use of rituximab to prevent severe delayed haemolytic transfusion reaction in immunized patients with sickle cell disease. *Vox Sang.* 2015;108(3):262-267.

162. Pirenne F: Prevention of delayed hemolytic transfusion reaction. *Transfus Clin Biol* 2019;26(2):99-101.

163. Coppo P, Cuker A, George JN. Thrombotic thrombocytopenic purpura: toward targeted therapy and precision medicine. *Res Pract Thromb Haemost.* 2019;3(1):26-37.

164. Knobl P. Thrombotic thrombocytopenic purpura. *Memo.* 2018; 11(3):220-226.

165. Zheng XL. ADAMTS13 and von Willebrand factor in thrombotic thrombocytopenic purpura. *Annu Rev Med.* 2015;66: 211-225.

166. Schwameis M, Schorgenhofer C, Assinger A, Steiner MM, Jilma B. VWF excess and ADAMTS13 deficiency: a unifying pathomechanism linking inflammation to thrombosis in DIC, malaria, and TTP. *Thromb Haemost.* 2015;113(4): 708-718.

167. Bayer G, von Tokarski F, Thoreau B, et al. Etiology and outcomes of thrombotic microangiopathies. *Clin J Am Soc Nephrol.* 2019;14(4):557-566.

168. Shome DK, Ramadorai P, Al-Ajmi A, Ali F, Malik N. Thrombotic microangiopathy in sickle cell disease crisis. *Ann Hematol.* 2013;92(4):509-515.

169. Strijbos MH, Landburg PP, Nur E, et al. Circulating endothelial cells: a potential parameter of organ damage in sickle cell anemia? *Blood Cells Mol Dis.* 2009;43(1):63-67.

170. Chen J, Hobbs WE, Le J, Lenting PJ, de Groot PG, Lopez JA. The rate of hemolysis in sickle cell disease correlates with the quantity of active von Willebrand factor in the plasma. *Blood.* 2011;117(13):3680-3683.

171. Schnog JJ, Kremer Hovinga JA, Krieg S, et al. ADAMTS13 activity in sickle cell disease. *Am J Hematol.* 2006;81(7):492-498.

172. Prichard JG, Clark HG, James RE 3rd. Abdominal pain and sicklemia in a patient with sickle cell trait. *South Med J.* 1988;81(10): 1312-1314.

173. Herbert V. Everyone should be tested for iron disorders. *J Am Diet Assoc.* 1992;92(12):1502-1509.

174. Fairbanks VF, Beutler E. Eyrthrocyte disorders: anemias related to disturbances of hemoglobin synthesis. In: Williams WJ, Beutler E, Erslev AJ, Lichtman MA, eds. *Hematology.* 4th ed. McGraw-Hill; 1990:482-505.

175. Goldstein AR, Anderson MJ, Serjeant GR. Parvovirus associated aplastic crisis in homozygous sickle cell disease. *Arch Dis Child.* 1987;62(6):585-588.

176. Kassim A, Thabet S, Al-Kabban M, Al-Nihari K. Iron deficiency in Yemeni patients with sickle-cell disease. *East Mediterr Health J.* 2012;18(3):241-245.

177. Mohanty D, Mukherjee MB, Colah RB, et al. Iron deficiency anaemia in sickle cell disorders in India. *Indian J Med Res.* 2008;127(4):366-369.

178. King L, Reid M, Forrester TE. Iron deficiency anaemia in Jamaican children, aged 1-5 years, with sickle cell disease. *West Indian Med J.* 2005;54(5):292-296.

179. Ferrone FA. The delay time in sickle cell disease after 40 years: a paradigm assessed. *Am J Hematol.* 2015;90(5):438-445.

180. Eaton WA, Hofrichter J, Ross PD. Editorial: delay time of gelation: a possible determinant of clinical severity in sickle cell disease. *Blood.* 1976;47(4):621-627.

181. Das N, Xie L, Ramakrishnan SK, Campbell A, Rivella S, Shah YM. Intestine specific disruption of HIF-2alpha improves anemia in sickle cell disease. *J Biol Chem.* 2015;290(39):23523-23527.

182. Castro O, Haddy TB. Improved survival of iron-deficient sickle erythrocytes. *N Engl J Med.* 1983;308(9):527.

183. Lionnet F, Hammoudi N, Stojanovic KS, et al. Iron restriction is an important treatment of hemoglobin SC disease. *Am J Hematol.* 2016;91(7):E320.

184. Chinowsky MS. Thrombotic thrombocytopenic purpura associated with sickle cell-hemoglobin C disease. *South Med J.* 1994;87(11):1168-1171.

185. Geigel EJ, Francis CW. Reversal of multiorgan system dysfunction in sickle cell disease with plasma exchange. *Acta Anaesthesiol Scand.* 1997;41(5):647-650.

186. Bolaños-Meade J, Keung YK, Lopez-Arvizu C, Florendo R, Cobos E. Thrombotic thrombocytopenic purpura in a patient with sickle cell crisis. *Ann Hematol.* 1999;78(12):558-559.

187. Chehal A, Taher A, Shamseddine A. Sicklemia with multi-organ failure syndrome and thrombotic thrombocytopenic purpura. *Hemoglobin.* 2002;26(4):345-351.

188. Lee HE, Marder VJ, Logan LJ, Friedman S, Miller BJ. Life-threatening thrombotic thrombocytopenic purpura (TTP) in a patient with sickle cell-hemoglobin C disease. *Ann Hematol.* 2003; 82(11):702-704.

189. Majjiga VS, Tripathy AK, Viswanathan K, Shukla M. Thrombotic thrombocytopenic purpura and multiorgan system failure in a child with sickle cell-hemoglobin C disease. *Clin Pediatr (Phila).* 2010;49(10):992-996.

190. Shelat SG. Thrombotic thrombocytopenic purpura and sickle cell crisis. *Clin Appl Thromb Hemost.* 2010;16(2):224-227.

191. Vlachaki E, Agapidou A, Neokleous N, Adamidou D, Vetsiou E, Boura P. Thrombotic thrombocytopenic purpura or immune thrombocytopenia in a sickle cell/beta+-thalassemia patient: a rare and challenging condition. *Transfus Apher Sci.* 2014;51(2):175-177.

192. Gangemi AJ, Pickens PV. Coagulopathy and functional hyposplenism during an episode of thrombotic thrombocytopenic purpura in a HgbS/beta (+)-thalassemia patient. *Clin Case Rep.* 2015;3(7):521-526.

193. Haddy TB, Castro O. Overt iron deficiency in sickle cell disease. *Arch Intern Med.* 1982;142(9):1621-1624.

194. Rao KR, Patel AR, Honig GR, Vida LN, McGinnis PR. Iron deficiency and sickle cell anemia. *Arch Intern Med.* 1983;143(5):1030-1032.

195. Castro O, Poillon WN, Finke H, Massac E. Improvement of sickle cell anemia by iron-limited erythropoiesis. *Am J Hematol.* 1994;47(2):74-81.

196. Bouchair N, Manigne P, Kanfer A, et al. [Prevention of sickle cell crises with multiple phlebotomies]. *Arch Pediatr.* 2000;7(3):249-255.

197. Rombos Y, Tzanetea R, Kalotychou V, et al. Amelioration of painful crises in sickle cell disease by venesections. *Blood Cells Mol Dis.* 2002;28(2):283-287.

198. Markham MJ, Lottenberg R, Zumberg M. Role of phlebotomy in the management of hemoglobin SC disease: case report and review of the literature. *Am J Hematol.* 2003;73(2):121-125.

199. Castro O, Medina A, Gaskin P, Kato G, Gordeuk V. Iron deficiency decreases hemolysis in sickle cell anemia. *Rev Bras Hematol Hemoter.* 2009;31(1):51-53.

Thrombophilia in Sickle Cell Disease

Authors: *Enrico M. Novelli, Rafal Pawlinski, Sruti Shiva, Nigel Key*

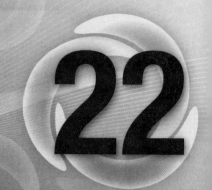

Chapter Outline

Overview

Hemostatic activation is a hallmark of sickle cell disease (SCD). Cellular activation and hyperadhesion, sterile inflammation, hemolysis, and hemostatic activation contribute to a chronic coagulopathy that exacerbates during vaso-occlusive episodes. This chapter will review the main clinical manifestations of thrombophilia in SCD and explore its pathogenic mechanisms, including the role of whole blood cellular components in the activation of the intrinsic and extrinsic coagulation pathways, the main alterations of procoagulant and anticoagulant pathways in SCD, and the role of hemolysis and nitric oxide depletion, with their downstream effects on endothelial and mitochondrial dysfunction. Finally, the role of established and novel therapeutic strategies will be discussed.

The Coagulation Cascade

The coagulation cascade refers to an interactive series of enzymatic reactions mediated by serine proteases and cofactors that collectively maintain hemostasis (the physiologic process of halting bleeding due to vascular injury). However, although these reactions are often presented as a series of sequential protein-protein interactions (Figure 22-1), they are in fact highly dependent on

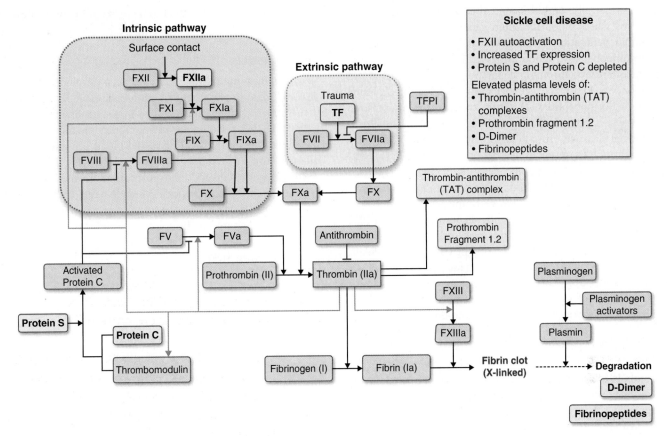

FIGURE 22-1 Abnormalities of the coagulation cascade in sickle cell disease. F, factor; SCD, sickle cell disease; TF, tissue factor; TFPI, tissue factor pathway inhibitor. Used with permission from Lydia Perkins, PhD.

vascular and blood cell–dependent contributions. Exposure of tissue factor (TF), a transmembrane glycoprotein receptor, is considered to be the primary event in activation of coagulation. Under physiologic conditions, TF is expressed at high levels by perivascular cells and is essential for hemostasis. Following blood vessel injury, exposure of blood to TF results in the formation of a complex with circulating factor (F) VIIa that activates both FIX and FX. This is known as the extrinsic pathway of coagulation activation. The ultimate result is thrombin generation; thrombin cleaves soluble fibrinogen to form insoluble fibrin, activates platelets, and thereby results in platelet-fibrin clots that prevent blood loss. However, aberrant expression of TF by circulating blood cells or excessive exposure of perivascular TF resulting from breakdown of the endothelial barrier can promote unwanted intravascular thrombosis that results in impairment or cessation of blood flow.

In addition to the extrinsic pathway, the coagulation cascade can be activated via FXIIa-dependent activation of FXI, with subsequent activation of FIX by FXIa. This mechanism is known as the intrinsic pathway. Although this pathway is readily demonstrable in blood ex vivo, controversy remains whether FXII/XIIa plays any role in thrombosis, although there is little doubt that FXI/FXIa is important. Thrombosis can occur in any vascular bed and may be divided into arterial, venous, or microvascular thrombosis. Arterial thrombosis is frequently the terminal event in myocardial infarction

and ischemic stroke, whereas venous thrombosis results in deep vein thrombosis and may lead to pulmonary embolism. However, in addition to these macrovascular occlusive events, regional or systemic activation of coagulation (that is not in response to bleeding) may contribute in a subtler fashion to end-organ damage in a variety of disease states, such as sepsis, major trauma, or indeed, sickle cell disease (SCD).

Pathophysiology of Thrombosis

The Hypercoagulable State in SCD

A prothrombotic state is one of the hallmarks of SCD.[1-3] Increased levels of various biomarkers of in vivo thrombin generation and ongoing fibrinolysis parallel the increase in thrombotic events observed in both sickle cell patients and in animal models of SCD. Animal models have provided many potential insights into the pathogenesis of vascular disease in SCD, and as a result, a number of possible future therapeutic targets have been suggested. We will review these human and mouse studies separately.

Epidemiology of Venous Thromboembolism in Humans

Chronically increased thrombin generation in sickle cell patients is witnessed by elevated plasma levels of thrombin-antithrombin (TAT) complexes and prothrombin fragment 1.2.[4-7]

When sickle cell blood is examined ex vivo, it is notable that increased whole blood thrombin generation but not plasma thrombin generation is observed, suggesting that the cellular components of blood are essential contributors to the enhanced in vivo thrombin generation in these patients.[8] In addition, SCD patients also have chronically elevated plasma levels of fibrinopeptides, D-dimer, and plasmin-antiplasmin complexes, which indicate ongoing thrombin-dependent fibrinogen cleavage, cross-linked fibrin formation, and subsequent fibrinolysis, respectively.[5,7,9-13]

Consistent with the chronic elevation of these biomarkers, an increased risk of venous thromboembolism (VTE) has now also been well documented in SCD. In the general population, VTE has an overall annual incidence of approximately 1 in 1000 with a marked age-dependent increase, such that in children, the rate is approximately one-tenth of this. VTE may be incidentally discovered in otherwise asymptomatic patients, usually by radiologic studies performed for another reason. VTE is most commonly manifested as deep vein thrombosis (DVT) with or without pulmonary embolism (PE), but at times, other venous circulations may also be affected, such as the splanchnic veins, renal veins, or cerebral venous sinuses. In SCD, autopsy studies have consistently reported high rates of acute and chronic thrombi in the pulmonary vasculature, in addition to other vascular changes such as intimal hyperplasia.[14-17] Clinically, it has been shown that the incidence of PE is higher in the hospitalized SCD population compared to the non-SCD population.[18] Of interest, the usual ratio of clinically apparent DVT to PE (~2:1) appears to be reversed in some studies of VTE in SCD, with a higher incidence of pulmonary thrombosis relative to DVT compared to age- and race-matched non-SCD patients.[19] Indeed, it has been suggested that pulmonary thrombosis occurs as an in situ thrombotic event rather than as a result of embolization from the peripheral vasculature.[20] This hypothesis may be compatible with the high prevalence of angiographically demonstrated pulmonary artery thrombi (17%) in sickle cell patients presenting with acute chest syndrome.[21] Other population-based studies demonstrated that VTE has a cumulative incidence of about 25% in adult SCD patients and is associated with a higher risk of mortality.[18,22,23] In children, the 10-year incidence rate is approximately 2% to 3%, and VTE is also independently associated with mortality.[24,25] Of the deep vein thrombi seen in patients with SCD, upper extremity DVT appears to account for about 50% of the events. As expected, the presence of an indwelling central venous catheter appears to be an associated risk factor (Figure 22-2),[26] and this is also true in children with SCD complicated by upper extremity DVT.[25]

Several studies have suggested that the risk of recurrence is high after a first VTE event in SCD. In a California population-based study of 877 patients with an incident event, the 1- and 5-year cumulative incidences of recurrence were 13.2% and 24.1%, respectively.[27] These high recurrence rates have been corroborated by other studies.[22,23] SCD also appears to be a significant independent risk factor for pregnancy-related VTE, with a 2- to 10-fold increased risk compared to pregnant women unaffected by SCD.[28-30] Finally, the chronic hypercoagulable state

may also be associated with chronic cardiopulmonary complications such as pulmonary hypertension.[5,31-33]

Mouse Models

Several mouse models of SCD have been developed over the past decades. Replacement of mouse hemoglobin genes by their human counterparts resulted in the generation of mice with SCD that recapitulate many clinical manifestations of the disease including sickling of red blood cells, severe anemia, and end-organ damage.[34] So-called Berkeley (BERK) and Townes mice are currently the most commonly used models in SCD research.[35,36] Reduced embryonic lethality and the ability to obtain nonsickle littermate controls provide an advantage of Townes compared to BERK mice. Similar to their human counterparts, plasma levels of TAT complexes are chronically elevated in sickle mice at steady state.[37,38] Furthermore, microthrombi and increased fibrin deposition are observed in multiple organs including lung, liver, kidneys, and brain.[37,39] Exposing sickle cell mice to hypoxic conditions results in further increases in plasma TAT levels and thrombosis within the pulmonary vasculature.[37,40] Importantly, recent data demonstrate that the dynamics of venous thrombosis and the structure of venous clots differ in SCD mice compared with control animals. Specifically, SCD mice developed less compacted venous clots containing a large number of red blood cells undergoing sickling and an increased fibrin content.[41] Whether these qualitative differences help to explain the observation that clinically apparent PE occurs more commonly than DVT in humans with SCD requires further evaluation.

Mechanism of Increased Thrombin Generation in SCD

The underlying hypercoagulable state and thrombotic complications of SCD are well documented.[1,3,42] Dysregulation of the hemostatic system is due to both upregulation of procoagulant and downregulation of natural anticoagulant pathways, together with chronic endothelial dysfunction (Figure 22-1). Potential causes of coagulation activation in SCD are discussed later in this chapter, with the emphasis placed on the contribution of cellular components to activation of the extrinsic and intrinsic coagulation pathways (Figure 22-3).

Activation of the Extrinsic Coagulation Pathway

In contrast to the protective role of TF expressed by perivascular cells, inducible expression of TF observed in vascular and/or hematopoietic cells during pathologic conditions, including SCD, has been linked to a hypercoagulable state.[43-45] Inhibition of TF with anti-TF antibodies during steady-state disease significantly reduced plasma TAT levels in both BERK and Townes mice, indicating that activation of coagulation is TF dependent in these 2 models of SCD.[38]

Leukocyte TF

Sickle cell patients have increased TF expression on circulating monocytes,[46] with elevated whole blood TF procoagulant

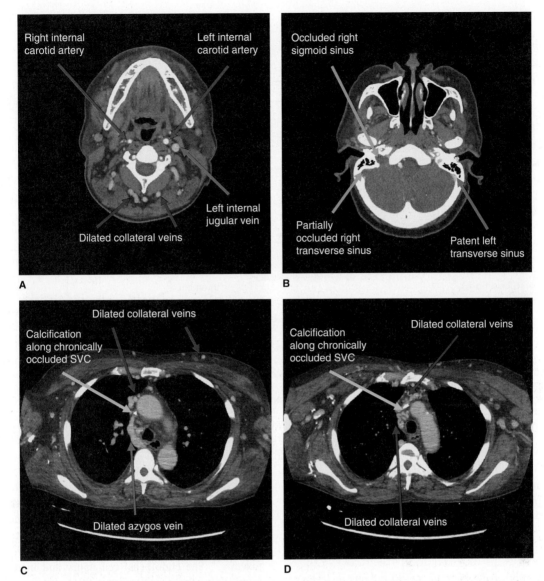

FIGURE 22-2 Chronic superior vena cava (SVC) occlusion in a 64-year-old man with HbS/beta zero thalassemia. The patient had a history of multiple episodes of upper extremity DVT after placement of numerous indwelling, dual lumen intravenous catheters for chronic exchange transfusion, and developed worsening SVC syndrome. CT angiography of the neck and chest revealed lack of contrast filling of the right internal jugular vein and inferior aspect of the right sigmoid sinus. There was some contrast filling of the superior aspect of the right sigmoid sinus and of the right transverse sinus (**A-B**). There was occlusion of the SVC and innumerable well-developed venous collaterals throughout the mediastinum and chest walls (**C-D**). *Courtesy of Allison Weyer, MD.*

activity.[47] Furthermore, circulating endothelial cells isolated from sickle cell patients showed increased levels of TF mRNA, antigen, and activity.[48] TF expression in whole blood and circulating endothelial cells was similarly increased in patients in pain crisis and those with steady-state disease.[47,48] TF expression is also increased in circulating monocytes in mouse models of SCD in the baseline state,[38,49] with a further increase observed after hypoxia-reoxygenation.[49] In addition to monocytes, increased TF expression is also observed in neutrophils isolated from sickle cell mice during steady state.[38] However, it remains doubtful that (nonclonal) human neutrophils express TF.[50] Furthermore, at present, there are no experimental data directly linking monocyte TF expression to thrombin generation in SCD. However, in SCD patients, elevated numbers of

TF-positive monocytes correlated with whole blood TF activity and increased plasma levels of TAT and D-dimer,[46] suggesting that monocyte TF does indeed play a role in the ongoing activation of coagulation. Simvastatin treatment did not attenuate the increased monocyte TF expression in mice,[49] and short-term use of simvastatin in sickle cell patients had only a modest effect on plasma levels of TF antigen.[51] In contrast, hydroxyurea therapy has been shown to reduce monocyte TF mRNA expression and plasma levels of TF protein.[52] Increased TF expression observed on monocytes of sickle cell patients may be induced via activation of toll-like receptor 4 (TLR4) receptors by free heme.[53] Indeed, heme induces coagulation activation in vivo in mice via a TF-dependent pathway.[54] However, neutralizing the toxic level of free heme with hemopexin

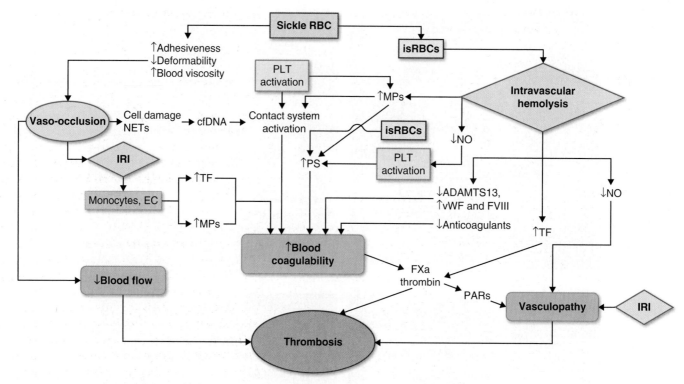

FIGURE 22-3 Pathogenesis of thrombosis in sickle cell disease. cfDNA, cell-free DNA; EC, endothelial cell; FVIII, factor VIII; FXa, activated factor X; IRI, ischemia reperfusion injury; isRBCs, irreversibly sickled red blood cells; MP, microparticles; NETs, neutrophil extracellular traps; NO, nitric oxide; PARs, protease-activated receptors; PLT, platelets; PS, phosphatidylserine; RBC, red blood cells; TF, tissue factor; vWF, von Willebrand factor. *Reprinted from Nobuouossie, D, Key NS, Ataga KI. Coagulation abnormalities of sickle cell disease: Relationship with clinical outcomes and the effect of disease modifying therapies. Blood Rev.* 30(4);2016, 245-256, with permission from Elsevier.

resulted in only partial inhibition of thrombin generation in sickle mice, indicating that heme is not the only activator of coagulation.[54]

Endothelial Cell TF

Activation of endothelial cells by heme (the circulating levels of which are greatly increased in SCD) leads to increased TF expression in vitro.[55] As already noted, circulating endothelial cells from sickle cell patients have increased TF antigen and activity, as well as TF mRNA.[48] Increased endothelial cell TF expression is also observed in mouse models of SCD and has been linked to hypoxia-reoxygenation and extracellular heme.[49,55] Results from mouse models of SCD indicate that increased endothelial TF expression is dependent on the activation of nuclear factor-κB (NF-κB) (p50) in blood mononuclear cells, but not endothelial cells themselves, suggesting that peripheral blood mononuclear cells indirectly promote endothelial TF expression.[56] Furthermore, endothelial TF is negatively regulated by endothelial nitric oxide synthase (eNOS) via nitric oxide (NO) generation[57] and can be reduced by lovastatin[49] as well as histone deacetylase inhibitors.[58] In sickle mice, inhalation of NO not only attenuated the increased endothelial TF expression, but also reduced the number of thrombi in the lung microvasculature after hypoxia-reoxygenation injury,[40,57] suggesting that endothelial cell TF may contribute to microvascular thrombosis in the lung. However, endothelial cell–specific deletion of TF expression had no

effect on thrombin generation.[38] It is possible that endothelial cell TF does not contribute to the thrombin generation because it is expressed on the endothelial cell in its encrypted form. Perivascular cells can also be a source of TF contributing to the activation of coagulation, as shown in a mouse model of endotoxemia.[59] The endothelial cell injury and increased vascular permeability that are observed in SCD could make perivascular TF accessible to circulating clotting factors and thereby lead to activation of coagulation.[60-62]

Activation of the Intrinsic Coagulation Pathway

Autoactivation of FXII, which occurs following exposure to negatively charged surfaces, leads to 2 events: (1) FXIIa-dependent activation of prekallikrein (PK) to kallikrein (PKa) with subsequent cleavage of high-molecular-weight kininogen (HK) to generate bradykinin and other HK cleavage fragments; and (2) FXIIa-dependent activation of FXI, which subsequently leads to the activation of FIX (the intrinsic coagulation pathway). Numerous endogenous activators of FXII have been proposed, including cell-free DNA, misfolded proteins, and polyphosphates.[63-65] Consumption of FXII, PK, and HK has been observed in the plasma of SCD patients compared to healthy controls, which is consistent with activation of the contact pathway[66,67]; however, any contribution of this pathway to the increased thrombin generation in SCD has not been investigated. In contrast, several in vitro studies suggest that red blood cells, as well as microparticles (MPs) released from these cells, contribute to thrombin generation via activation of the intrinsic pathway.[68]

Sickle Red Blood Cells

In normal red blood cells, procoagulant anionic phospholipids, such as phosphatidylserine (PS), are almost completely restricted to the inner leaflet of the cell membrane.[69] Repeated cycles of sickling result in increased exposure of PS on the surface of sickle red blood cells.[70] PS exposure increases procoagulant activity by providing a negatively charged surface that facilitates assembly of the coagulation enzymatic complexes. This process is mediated via an electrostatic interaction between negatively charged PS and positively charged γ-carboxyglutamic acid domains present in the procoagulant proteins FVII, FIX, FX, and prothrombin.[71] Analysis of blood from sickle cell patients demonstrated a positive correlation between PS-positive red blood cells and plasma levels of prothrombin fragment 1.2, D-dimer, and plasmin-antiplasmin complex.[72,73] Interestingly, no correlation has been found between the number of PS-positive platelets and these biomarkers, suggesting that sickle red blood cells, rather than platelets, contribute to the hypercoagulable state in SCD.[73]

Circulating MPs

MPs are small (<1 μm) membrane vesicles released from activated or apoptotic cells. They contribute to thrombin generation by a variety of mechanisms. Their role in SCD was recently reviewed in depth[74] but will be briefly summarized here. The procoagulant properties of MPs are due to the presence of PS with or without TF on their surface.[71] Two recent publications demonstrated that MPs derived from different cellular sources contribute to thrombin and fibrin generation via different mechanisms.[68,75] Platelet- and erythrocyte-derived MPs, which are TF negative, failed to induce thrombin generation in FXII-deficient plasma, and inhibition of FVII had no effect on thrombin generation.[68] The majority of circulating MPs in sickle cell patients originate from erythrocytes and platelets.[76,77] These MPs are TF negative and demonstrate increased exposure of PS on their surface.[78] It has been shown that erythrocyte-derived MPs isolated from the blood of sickle cell patients contribute to thrombin generation via an FXI-dependent but not FVII-dependent mechanism.[79] In contrast, thrombin generation induced by TF-positive monocyte-derived MPs requires FVII but not FXII.[68] SCD patients also have increased plasma levels of TF-positive MPs[1] derived from endothelial cells and monocytes.[78,80,81] However, 2 other studies did not detect monocyte MPs[79] or increased MP-associated TF activity in sickle patients compared to controls.[46] Similarly, there was no correlation between MP TF activity and markers of coagulation activation in clinical[82] or mouse studies.[38] These data suggest that although MPs can contribute to coagulation activation, it is likely through a PS-dependent mechanism that requires the intrinsic coagulation cascade.

Depletion of Natural Anticoagulants

Protein C and protein S are also vitamin K–dependent proteins with anticoagulant functions that are commonly depleted in SCD patients. Overall, several studies have reported lower plasma protein C and protein S levels in adults[8,12,83] and children with SCD.[4,84-88] Furthermore, Tam et al[88] reported greater reduction in protein S and protein C levels in sickle cell children with a history of stroke compared to children with SCD without neurologic sequelae. Chronic transfusion did not seem to reverse the depletion of these natural anticoagulants.[85]

The activation of protein C is triggered by binding to the endothelial protein C receptor (EPCR) through thrombomodulin-bound thrombin. Activated protein C can dissociate from EPCR and acts as an antithrombotic protease by inactivating clotting factors FVa and FVIIIa.[89] It was demonstrated in vitro that red blood cells from sickle cell patients provide a catalytic surface for FVa inactivation by activated protein C.[90] Consequently, chronic or persistent activation of coagulation in SCD may enhance the consumption of protein C. In the standard assays for TF-initiated thrombin generation in platelet-poor plasma, the addition of thrombomodulin reveals the activity of the protein S/C pathway. Thus, in SCD, enhanced endogenous thrombin potential (area under the curve), peak height, and peak velocity compared to race-matched controls are evident.[8,86] In addition, murine protein C and arteriolar EPCR expression were found to be significantly reduced in the cerebral vasculature of sickle mice, suggesting a possible pathogenic role for this pathway in the tendency to develop thrombotic occlusion. This hypothesis was supported by the fact that administration of activated protein C prevented the enhanced thrombosis observed in both the arterioles and venules of sickle mice.[91]

The anticoagulant action of activated protein C is enhanced by several cofactors, such as protein S and PS.[92] Protein S had been shown to bind with high affinity to vesicles and dense irreversibly sickled red blood cells in a calcium-dependent manner.[93] In SCD patients, Whelihan et al[8] demonstrated that lower protein S levels in plasma were inversely correlated with red blood cell PS exposure and confirmed the presence of protein S on the surface of sickle red blood cells by flow cytometry. Thus, as previously suggested,[12] lower protein S in SCD patients may result from accelerated clearance due to protein S binding to exposed negatively charged phospholipid on sickle RBCs. Finally, it has also been suggested that elevated FVIIIa levels in SCD patients may be an additional factor contributing to the depletion of protein C and protein S.[8,94,95]

Interplay Between Hemolysis and Hemostatic Activation

Accumulating studies suggest a strong association between intravascular hemolysis and hemostatic activation (Figure 22-4). In SCD patients, many markers of a prothrombotic phenotype correlate with levels of hemolysis. For example, levels of platelet activation correlate positively with concentrations of cell-free hemoglobin and lactate dehydrogenase in SCD

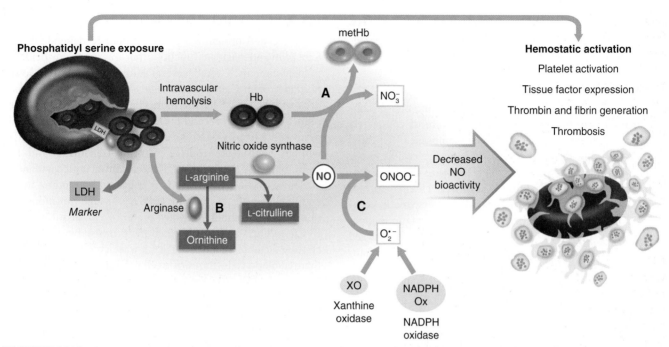

FIGURE 22-4 Hemolysis-associated hemostatic activation. Intravascular hemolysis releases hemoglobin into plasma, which quenches nitric oxide (NO) and generates reactive oxygen species (directly via Fenton chemistry or via induction of xanthine oxidase and nicotinamide adenine dinucleotide phosphate oxidase). In addition, arginase is released from the red blood cell during hemolysis and metabolizes arginine, the substrate for NO synthesis, further impairing NO homeostasis. The depletion of NO is associated with pathologic platelet activation and tissue factor expression. Hemolysis and splenectomy are also associated with enhanced phosphatidylserine exposure on red blood cells, which potentiates expressed tissue factor procoagulant activity and forms a platform for coagulation. Hb, hemoglobin; LDH, lactate dehydrogenase; metHb, methemoglobin.

patients.[96,97] Setty et al[46] showed that TF-positive monocyte numbers correlate significantly with reticulocytes and lactate dehydrogenase levels in children with SCD. Weaker associations were found in this population between TAT complexes or D-dimer and reticulocyte count.[46] The rate of hemolysis in SCD patients has also been shown to correlate with the level of active von Willebrand factor expressed in plasma.[98] Moreover, in vitro studies demonstrate that exposure of platelets to hemolytic components stimulates activation,[96,97,99] and animal models of hemolysis show causality between hemolysis and select markers of hemostatic activation.[98,100,101] Although these studies establish a causal relationship between hemolysis and a prothrombotic phenotype, the molecular mechanisms that underlie this relationship remain unclear.

One challenge in elucidating the molecular underpinnings of how hemolysis causes hemostatic activation is the fact that hemolysis releases a mixture of a number of red blood cell components into the vasculature. Of all the intracellular components released by hemolysis, the most focus has been placed on adenosine diphosphate (ADP), hemoglobin, and arginase as mediators of hemolysis-induced coagulopathy. Perhaps the clearest studies in this regard have investigated the role of ADP. ADP is a known platelet agonist, and infusion of ADP into rat and rabbit models has demonstrated clear platelet activation.[102,103] Mechanistically, ADP is known to bind purinergic P2Y1 and P2Y12 receptors on the surface of platelets to stimulate downstream signaling cascades resulting in activation.[104] However, the mechanisms by

which cell-free hemoglobin activates hemostatic processes is much less clear. In the following sections, we discuss potential molecular mechanisms underlying hemolysis-induced hemostatic activation with a focus on the role of cell-free hemoglobin.

NO Depletion

NO is an integral vasodilator and regulator of hemostasis. The primary source of NO in the vasculature is the endothelial isoform of NO synthase (NOS), which catalyzes the conversion of L-arginine to L-citrulline, yielding 1 molecule of NO in the process. In addition to the endothelium, NOS is also expressed in the platelet, where it is activated by a number of agonists including thrombin.[105-108] Recent studies have also shown that NOS is expressed in red blood cells and that NO generated in the red blood cell contributes to vascular tone[109,110]; however, the role of this isoform in hemostasis remains unclear.

Physiologically, NO maintains hemostasis by a number of mechanisms. NO is a potent inhibitor of platelet activation by stimulating soluble guanylate cyclase within the platelet. This leads to the production of the second messenger cyclic guanosine monophosphate (cGMP), which ultimately, through multiple signaling cascades, decreases fibrinogen binding to glycoprotein IIb/IIIa, modulates phospholipase A2 and C activity, and can attenuate cytosolic free calcium levels induced by thrombotic agonists.[111-113] NO also inhibits the adhesion of platelets and other leukocytes to the endothelium.[114,115] NO-dependent regulation of the transcription factor NF-κB inhibits the expression of key endothelial adhesion molecules including intercellular adhesion molecule 1 (ICAM1), vascular cell adhesion molecule 1 (VCAM1), and E-selectin.[114,115] In addition, NO has been shown to inhibit the exocytosis of Weibel-Palade bodies from the endothelium, preventing the translocation of P-selectin and other mediators of thrombosis.[116,117] Consistent with these roles for NO in hemostasis, blocking endogenous NO production with the NOS inhibitor nitro-L-arginine methyl ester citrate (L-NAME) has been shown to increase leukocyte adhesion to the endothelium as well as increase platelet activation in a number of models,[118-120] and eNOS knockout mice are more susceptible to thrombosis.[121-123]

In SCD patients, intravascular hemolysis leads to a state of NO depletion and resistance. The half-life of NO in blood is very short—on the order of 2 milliseconds—due to its rapid reaction with hemoglobin.[124] NO reacts with oxygenated hemoglobin (oxyHb) within red blood cells through a dioxygenase reaction in which NO is inactivated to nitrate and oxyHb is oxidized to methemoglobin. The physiologic compartmentalization of oxyHb within the red blood cell establishes diffusional barriers, such that NO entry into the red blood cell attenuates the rate at which NO is scavenged by oxyHb.[124] However, intravascular hemolysis abolishes this critical diffusional barrier by releasing free hemoglobin into the plasma, resulting in the scavenging of NO by free oxyHb at a diffusion-limited rate.[125,126] Arginase released from the red blood cell by hemolysis also contributes to diminished NO bioavailability. Arginase catalyzes the conversion of L-arginine to ornithine, thus depleting the plasma availability of L-arginine as a substrate for NOS-dependent NO generation.[127] In addition, the level of asymmetric dimethyl arginine, an endogenously produced inhibitor of NOS, is significantly increased in SCD patients and associated with hemolysis.[128,129] Through these mechanisms of both increased NO scavenging and decreased NO production, hemolysis causes a state of chronic NO depletion, resulting in vasculopathy characterized by endothelial dysfunction and activation, as well as hemostatic activation.[130,131]

A number of studies link hemolysis-dependent NO depletion to a prothrombotic phenotype. In murine models, acute osmotically induced hemolysis upregulates adhesion molecule expression and leukocyte recruitment as well as platelet adhesion, and these effects are attenuated by enhancing NO signaling.[132,133] Transgenic murine models of SCD show characteristics of NO resistance that contributes to vascular dysfunction and the pathogenesis of complications such as pulmonary hypertension and priapism in this model.[134,135] Solovey et al[57] demonstrated in both the NY1DD and BERK murine models of SCD, which express increased levels of TF, that deficiency of eNOS-derived NO contributes to this increased expression. Villagra et al[97] showed that in patients with SCD and pulmonary hypertension, platelet activation is associated with increased hemolysis and the severity of pulmonary hypertension. In addition, administration of sildenafil, a phosphodiesterase 5 inhibitor that potentiates NO signaling,

significantly decreased platelet activation in this cohort.[97] Notably, Ataga et al[5] demonstrated that SCD patients with pulmonary hypertension show increased markers of coagulation and endothelial activation. Although these authors did not investigate the effect of NO supplementation on coagulation markers, this study, taken with that of Villagra et al,[97] suggests an association between hemolysis, NO depletion, and increased coagulopathy in SCD patients.

The previously discussed studies support the concept that hemolysis-dependent decreased NO bioavailability propagates thrombotic activation in SCD and suggests that NO therapeutics could attenuate hemostatic activation in this population. A number of studies have used SCD transgenic mouse models to demonstrate that potentiation of NO production or signaling is beneficial in SCD. For example, NO inhalation increased survival in the SAD mouse exposed to hypoxia[136] and decreased lung injury in another SCD model exposed to hypoxia.[40] L-Arginine supplementation (as a substrate for NOS) improved red cell density in the murine model,[137] and sildenafil prevented priapism in mice that received a bone marrow transplant from SCD mice.[135] Fewer studies have directly assessed the effect of NO therapeutics on hemostatic activation. Wajih et al[133] used dietary sodium nitrite as a donor of NO and showed in humanized SCD mice that nitrite attenuated platelet and leukocyte adhesion. As mentioned earlier, Villagra et al[97] demonstrated that sildenafil decreases platelet activation in SCD patients. A number of ongoing trials using inhaled sodium nitrite and L-arginine supplementation are currently evaluating the effect of these therapeutics on platelet function and coagulation activation, suggesting that the role of NO depletion in SCD-associated hemostatic activation will remain an active area of study for years to come.

Mitochondrial Dysfunction

Although mitochondria are traditionally recognized as the "powerhouse" of the cell, mitochondrial function is not only critical for energy homeostasis in most cell types, but also regulates cellular signaling through the production of oxidants and initiates apoptosis through the release of cytochrome c.[138,139] Unlike red blood cells that lose their mitochondria through mitophagic processes during maturation, platelets and leukocytes contain fully functional mitochondria,[140] and these mitochondria are now known to have distinctive bioenergetic roles in each cell type.[141]

In the platelet, mitochondrial function is essential for providing adenosine triphosphate (ATP) for the energy-consuming processes of coagulation activation and granule secretion. Although quiescent platelets use both glycolysis and oxidative phosphorylation to generate energy, mitochondrial respiration and oxidative phosphorylation are stimulated significantly upon exposure to a platelet agonist.[142,143] Oxidative phosphorylation occurs through a process whereby electron transport complexes I and II, embedded within the inner mitochondrial membrane, receive electrons from NADH and $FADH_2$ and transfer these electrons down the respiratory chain to reduce oxygen at complex IV. In response to electron transfer, protons are pumped from the matrix to the intermembrane space, creating a membrane potential across the inner mitochondrial membrane. This potential drives the reentry of protons into the matrix through ATP synthase (complex V), which converts ADP to ATP. In this way, the proton gradient couples oxygen consumption to ATP production. Upon activation, substrate availability to the platelet mitochondrion is increased, enhancing respiratory rate.[144]

It is important to note that not all electrons that enter the mitochondrial electron transport chain complete the path to reduce oxygen to water. A small proportion of these electrons exit the chain before complex IV and mediate a 1-electron oxidation of oxygen to generate the reactive oxygen species (ROS) superoxide, which is converted to hydrogen peroxide in the mitochondrion (Figure 22-5). The rate of generation of ROS by the electron transport chain is governed by the membrane potential across the inner mitochondrial membrane, with increased membrane potential potentiating ROS generation. Notably, a number of studies in the past decade have demonstrated that these ROS can propagate platelet activation.[145-148] For example, healthy platelets treated with opsonized zymosan A showed mitochondrial hyperpolarization, enhanced ROS production, and platelet activation.[146]

Similarly, Yamagishi et al[148] demonstrated that hyperglycemia induces mitochondrial hyperpolarization in healthy platelets, leading to platelet activation that can be inhibited by a scavenger of ROS.[148]

With respect to SCD, relatively little is known about the role of mitochondria in disease pathogenesis. However, Cardenes et al[96] have shown that platelet mitochondrial ROS generation potentially links hemolysis to platelet activation. A bioenergetic screen of platelets from SCD patients showed a mitochondrial functional alteration characterized by decreased mitochondrial respiratory rate but no change in maximal capacity for oxidative phosphorylation compared to platelets from healthy subjects. This alteration was due to an inhibition of mitochondrial ATPase activity that resulted in increased mitochondrial membrane potential and ROS production. Importantly, these mitochondrial changes were significantly correlated with both hemolysis and platelet activation in this cohort. Consistent with a role for hemolysis in causing platelet mitochondrial changes, exposure of platelets isolated from healthy subjects to free oxyHb recapitulated the mitochondrial alterations observed in platelets from SCD patients and caused platelet activation. Importantly, this platelet activation was significantly attenuated by mitochondria-targeted ROS scavengers.[96]

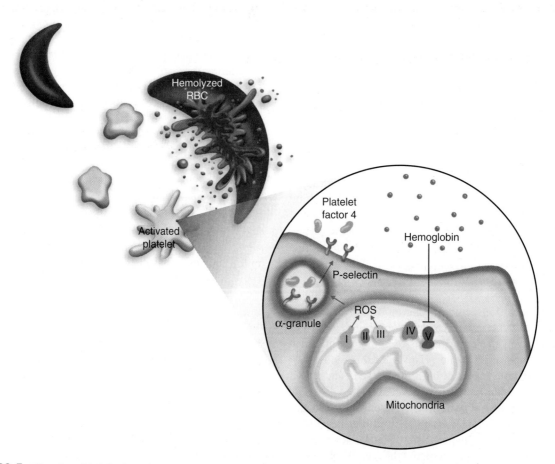

FIGURE 22-5 Mitochondrial dysfunction and platelet activation. Free hemoglobin from hemolytic red blood cells inhibits mitochondrial complex V within the platelet mitochondria, resulting in reactive oxygen species (ROS) production from the electron transport chain, which stimulates platelet activation as shown by α-granule release of P-selectin and platelet factor 4. Used with permission from Lydia Perkins, PhD.

Specific Management and Therapy

Antiplatelet Agents: Clinical Trials and Current Practice

The finding of hemostatic activation and the established role of platelets in vaso-occlusion have spurred clinical research to harness antiplatelet agents for both prevention of thrombosis and control of vaso-occlusion. Clinical studies of antiplatelet agents range from small interventional studies to multicenter randomized case-control studies and are summarized in Table 22-1. In most studies, surrogate outcome measures have typically been used to assess efficacy.[149-152] Although vaso-occlusive crisis (VOC) is common, the lack of objective measures of VOC and pain has also made VOC an unattractive outcome measure for antiplatelet drug studies. Thus, any summary of the existing clinical evidence on antiplatelet drugs will have to contend with a plethora of biomarkers of hemostatic activation and surrogate outcome measures that complicate any generalization on the utility of these drugs. In general, however, most studies have shown a reduction in markers of platelet activation that has correlated poorly with any clinical outcome. The largest and most rigorous studies published to date employed prasugrel, an irreversible antagonist of P2Y12 ADP receptors of the thienopyridine class.

Prasugrel attracted interest because of its potency and lower susceptibility to heterogeneity in metabolism than first-generation thienopyridines. Hopes of an effect on pain were further stoked by the finding that in a randomized, double-blind, 30-day study in adults with SCD, the mean pain intensity score was lower with prasugrel (1.8) compared with placebo (2.4).[153] However, the subsequent phase III DOVE trial in children and adolescents aged 2 to 17 years with SCD failed to show a significant difference in rate of VOC between the prasugrel and placebo groups.[154] These results mirror those subsequently obtained in a similar age group with ticagrelor, a reversible P2Y12 inhibitor; the drug had no effect on diary-reported pain in the HESTIA2 phase IIb, randomized, multicenter clinical trial.[155]

Because of the largely negative results of the clinical trials with antiplatelet drugs, their role in therapy is currently limited. Aspirin use in SCD is typically reserved for prevention of cardiovascular complications in subjects at risk, following the guidelines for the non-SCD population. In particular, low-dose aspirin is typically used as an adjunct to chronic transfusions for the secondary prevention of stroke in children and adults. Nonsteroidal anti-inflammatory drugs and cyclooxygenase-2 inhibitors have also been used to treat mild to moderate pain with limited success,[156] but their cardiovascular risks in the general population and the potential for nephrotoxicity have tempered enthusiasm for their use as analgesics in SCD.[157]

TABLE 22-1 Selected clinical studies of antiplatelets in SCD

Study	Genotype	No. of patients	Drug	Randomization	Duration	Outcome
Osamo et al[151] (1981)	HbSS	100	Aspirin (1.2 g)	Yes vs placebo	6 weeks	Increase in oxygen affinity, Hb levels, and RBC life span
Greenberg et al[150] (1983)	SCD	49	Aspirin (3-6 mg/kg)	Yes vs placebo	21 months	No change in frequency or severity of crises
Semple et al[152] (1984)	HbSS	9	Ticlopidine (250 mg BID)	Yes vs placebo	1 month	Lower platelet activation, but no improved platelet survival or crisis prevention
Desai et al[149] (2013)	HbSS/Sβ⁰ HbSC	12 1	Eptifibatide (2 boluses + infusion)	Yes vs placebo	6 hours	No change in times to crisis resolution or hospital discharge
Wun et al[153] (2013)	HbSS/Sβ⁰ HbSC/Sβ⁺	40 21	Prasugrel (5 mg)	Yes vs placebo	30 days	Lower platelet activation, "trend" for better pain
Heeney et al[154] (2016)	HbSS	341	Prasugrel (0.08 mg/kg)	Yes vs placebo Phase III RCT	9-24 months	Lower platelet reactivity but no effect on crises
Kanter et al[155] (2018)	HbSS/Sβ⁰	87	Ticagrelor (10, 45 mg BID)	Yes vs placebo Phase IIb RCT	12 weeks	No effect on pain

Abbreviations: BID, twice a day; Hb, hemoglobin; RBC, red blood cell; RCT, randomized controlled trial; SCD, sickle cell disease.

Anticoagulants: Clinical Trials and Current Practice

The experience with anticoagulants for the prevention of VOC in SCD has been more promising. Even before P-selectin became a viable therapeutic target,[158] there was hope that heparinoids would reduce cellular adhesion by blocking adhesion to P-selectin. Subsequently, blockade of VLA4 also emerged as another potential mechanism of action because low-molecular-weight heparin has been found to block adhesion of melanoma cells to the endothelial receptor VCAM1.[159] VLA4 is an important adhesion molecule in VOC because it mediates adhesion of red blood cells to the endothelium via VCAM1 and the binding of red blood cell–white blood cell aggregates to the subendothelial matrix via fibronectin in SCD.[160-162] Thus, any strategy that blocks VLA4 holds promise.

Of the studies testing conventional anticoagulants for prevention of VOC to date,[163-168] the largest was a randomized, double-blind study published in 2013 reporting the effect of up to 7 days of tinzaparin on the duration of VOC[164] (Table 22-2). In the arm receiving tinzaparin, the duration of hospitalization was reduced by >40%, with a >25% reduction in days with the most severe pain score, at the expense of 2 minor bleeding episodes. More recently, research efforts on the identification of anticoagulant strategies to prevent VOC have been boosted by the development of direct oral anticoagulants, whose ease of use presents clear advantages in the preventive arena. There is preliminary evidence that direct oral anticoagulants may be at least as effective as warfarin while affording a lower risk of bleeding in SCD patients with VTE.[169] Randomized clinical trials to test the safety and efficacy of rivaroxaban and apixaban in SCD are ongoing.

Although the jury is out on the potential role of anticoagulants in preventing and ameliorating VOC, there is general consensus that VTE should be treated aggressively in SCD. In the absence of SCD-specific guidelines, American College of Chest Physicians[170] and American Society of Hematology guidelines on VTE[171] should be followed when determining the dose and duration of anticoagulation. As previously mentioned, recent evidence on the high risk of VTE recurrence in SCD argues for long-term therapy, but this has to be tempered against the risk of bleeding.[23] Similarly, routine thromboprophylaxis in hospitalized patients with SCD would currently seem to be indicated based on the available evidence of thrombotic risk; once again, however, this decision should be based on established criteria in other populations, specifically an assessment of the risk/benefit profile in each patient. Finally, another situation in which VTE prophylaxis in SCD patients requires prospective randomized clinical trials to inform evidence-based recommendations is in the setting of pregnancy. In particular, a trial evaluating the use of prophylactic anticoagulant versus placebo for 6 to 8 weeks postpartum would be highly informative.

TABLE 22-2 Selected clinical studies of anticoagulants in SCD

Study	Genotype	No. of patients	Drug	Randomization	Duration	Outcome
Salvaggio et al[165] (1963)	HbSS	12	Warfarin	No	12-34 months	Modest decrease in rate of VOC
Chaplin et al[163] (1989)	HbSS	4	Heparin	No	2-6 years	Decreased rate of VOC
Wolters et al[168] (1995)	HbSS HbSC	6 1	Acenocoumarol	No	2 months	Decreased fragment 1.2
Schnog et al[166] (2001)	HbSS HbSC	14 8	Acenocoumarol vs placebo	Yes	14 weeks	Decreased coagulation markers; no decrease in VOC
Qari et al[164] (2007)	HbSS	253	Tinzaparin	Yes vs placebo	7 days	Decrease in days with most severe pain score and duration of VOC hospitalization
Shah et al[167] (2013)	SCD	29	Dalteparin	Yes vs placebo	7 days	No change in coagulation markers but greater decrease in pain scores

Abbreviations: SCD, sickle cell disease; VOC, vaso-occlusive crisis.

Thrombolytics: Is There a Role for Ischemic Stroke in SCD?

Thrombolytics have an established role in the acute treatment of ischemic stroke in the general population[172]; prompt fibrinolysis immediately restores flow and reduces infarct size. However, there has been reluctance to use thrombolytics in SCD, and consequently, their role in reversing or ameliorating stroke in SCD has not been established. The fundamental unanswered question pertains to the relative contribution of acute thrombosis on large-vessel occlusive stroke in SCD. To date, the mechanisms leading to carotid occlusion in SCD are not entirely clear, but its natural history,[173,174] characterized by the onset in early childhood, and the overwhelming importance of anemia imply that stroke in SCD has a distinct pathophysiology and that fibrinolysis may have, at most, an ancillary role. Supporting the role of anemia in the pathogenesis of stroke in SCD is the dramatic improvement of symptoms with red blood cell transfusions, particularly when coupled with rapid dilution of sickle hemoglobin (HbS) levels, as achieved by erythrocytapheresis. Thus, red blood cell exchange remains the treatment modality of choice for pediatric stroke.[175]

In adults, however, it is likely that the contribution of conventional cardiovascular risk factors over SCD-specific risk factors (eg, anemia and the presence of HbS) rises proportionally with age. Thus, aging patients with SCD may be more likely to benefit from the same interventions that are recommended for the general population, including thrombolytic therapy. An additional concern that has stood in the way of researching thrombolytic therapy in SCD has been the propensity to develop hemorrhagic stroke in SCD patients.[176] Intracerebral hemorrhage is particularly common in individuals who have suffered from a prior ischemic stroke and tends to preferentially strike young adults.[177] Consequently, the low therapeutic index of thrombolytic therapy for nonhemorrhagic stroke in the general population may be further reduced in SCD. Countering the concerns about excessive bleeding in SCD, however, a recent retrospective, registry-based study demonstrated that adult patients with SCD with a median age of 50 years (interquartile range, 39-62 years) receiving tissue-type plasminogen activator in the United States did not experience a significantly higher number of intracerebral hemorrhages.[178] A limitation of this study is that the genotype of the patients was unknown, but the relatively high median age suggests that a significant proportion of them may have had HbSC disease. It is likely that in the HbSC group, stroke pathogenesis differs from that of patients with HbSS, who, unlike patients with HbSC, develop stroke in early childhood.

DVT Prophylaxis in the Hospitalized Patient

Beginning in the first decade of the 21st century, a growing body of evidence demonstrated an increased risk of VTE in adults with SCD.[18,20,22,179,180] Currently, most adult patients with SCD receive thromboprophylaxis when hospitalized. In a cross-sectional, single-center study, hospitalization was found to be the sole provoking factor for VTE in 23.7% of patients with SCD.[22] To date, only one retrospective, single-institution study has evaluated the effectiveness and safety of thromboprophylaxis in adult patients with SCD. The results showed that hospitalized patients with SCD receiving thromboprophylaxis had similar outcomes to medically ill patients in historical cohorts.[181] In children, the evidence on the utility of thromboprophylaxis remains limited because most cases of VTE are provoked and typically linked to central venous catheters.[25] Thus, pediatric patients routinely do not receive thromboprophylaxis. In the absence of additional evidence in children, a prudent approach is to use thromboprophylaxis only in those who are hospitalized and have central venous catheters.[182]

Impact of Hydroxyurea on Thrombotic Risk

Hydroxyurea may reduce the risk of thrombosis via multiple mechanisms. Reducing HbS polymerization may prevent red blood cell membrane damage and externalization of PS.[183] Reduction of hemolysis would then limit quenching of NO by free hemoglobin released from hemolyzed red blood cells. Thus, NO-derived platelet activation would be reduced. The beneficial effect on NO metabolism may be compounded by the role of hydroxyurea as an NO donor.[184] A cross-sectional study showed that patients on long-term therapy with hydroxyurea had significant downregulation of TF expression and decreased levels of markers of thrombin generation (TAT and fragment 1.2).[52] Longitudinal prospective studies should be conducted to determine whether hydroxyurea-mediated reduction of prothrombotic markers is associated with VTE prevention.

Impact of Chronic Transfusions on Thrombotic Risk

Red blood cell transfusions have a beneficial effect on reducing the rate of complications in SCD. Improvement of total hemoglobin and reduction of the HbS fraction are common biomarkers used to monitor the response to transfusion therapy in the primary and secondary prevention of stroke.[176,185-187] Transfusions of red blood cells are expected to also affect other blood parameters that reflect endothelial dysfunction, hemolysis, and hemostatic activation by replacing rigid, proadhesive, and irreversibly sickled red blood cells.[188] Although markers of hemostatic activation are not routinely monitored during transfusion therapy, recent observations have shown that they are positively impacted by both simple and exchange transfusions. Stored serum samples from children with high transcranial Doppler velocity in the STOP trial had significantly lower levels of von Willebrand factor, TAT, and D-dimer after transfusion therapy.[189]

Future Research and Clinical Directions

Contribution of Coagulation to the Pathology of SCD

The majority of clinical studies investigating the role of anticoagulation in SCD have primarily focused on the frequency or severity of vaso-occlusive events. Therefore, based on these clinical trials, it remains uncertain whether chronic activation of coagulation contributes to other pathologies associated with SCD.[190] However, several studies from mouse models clearly indicate that the chronic activation of coagulation may contribute to systemic vascular inflammation and end-organ damage. For example, inhibition of TF in sickle mice reduced circulating markers of systemic inflammation and the number of inflammatory cells in the lungs.[38] The TF:FVIIa complex promotes inflammation and end-organ damage either directly or via generation of downstream coagulation proteases, including FXa and thrombin.[191,192] As discussed, endothelial cell–specific deletion of the TF gene reduced plasma levels of interleukin-6 (IL-6) but not TAT complexes.[38] This intriguing observation suggests that endothelial TF contributes to the expression of IL-6 independent of thrombin generation in SCD, most likely via FVIIa- and/or FXa-dependent activation of protease-activated receptor 2 (PAR2).[191,193,194] Inhibition of TF or thrombin abrogated microvascular thrombosis in the cerebral microvasculature of mice expressing the sickle form of hemoglobin.[91] Strikingly, chronic reduction of prothrombin levels (to 10%-15% of baseline) significantly attenuated markers of vascular inflammation and endothelial cell activation and protected SCD mice from multiorgan dysfunction.[195] The authors of this study also demonstrated that targeting prothrombin mRNA with antisense oligonucleotides reduced mortality and reduced vascular congestion in multiple organs.[195] However, it is unclear whether the lower incidence of end-organ damage, including pathologic heart remodeling, was due to a reduction of coagulation activation and/or a secondary reduction in inflammation. Further studies in animal models (and thereafter in humans with SCD) are needed to investigate the mechanism by which TF and downstream coagulation proteases, including FXa and thrombin, contribute to vascular inflammation. Possible mechanisms may involve coagulation protease-dependent activation of PARs or thrombin-dependent fibrin generation, which independently contributes to local tissue inflammation via activation and enhanced diapedesis of leukocytes into inflamed tissues.[196-199]

Potential Role of Selectin Blockade in Thrombosis

It has been known since the 1990s that the adhesion molecule P-selectin promotes binding of leukocytes to activated platelets at the site of thrombosis, which in turn promotes the deposition of fibrin.[200] Subsequently, injected soluble P-selectin was also found to directly mediate thrombosis in mice by inducing fibrin deposition on the luminal face of injured vessels.[201]

Selectin blockade has become a viable strategy to prevent VOC in SCD; however, its effect on thrombotic risk is not known. Clinical trials with the P-selectin inhibitor crizanlizumab[158] and the pan-selectin inhibitor GMI-1070 (rivipansel)[202,203] have shown reduction in VOC, but they were not powered to explore effects on thrombotic complications. One patient receiving crizanlizumab developed intracerebral hemorrhage, but this was not deemed to be related to P-selectin

(the patient was also on ketorolac) and no other hemorrhagic events were observed.[158] In mice, however, selectin blockade reduced venous thrombus formation.[204]

Plasma Exchange in the Critically Ill Patient

Anecdotal reports have shown that plasma exchange is occasionally incorporated in the care of critically ill patients with SCD, particularly in cases of multiorgan failure with features of thrombotic microangiopathy.[205,206] When plasma exchange is used in SCD, it usually follows or accompanies red blood cell exchange, so its relative contribution is difficult to ascertain. However, it can be hypothesized that reduction in ultralarge von Willebrand factor, TSP1, and other prothrombotic proteins known to be elevated in the plasma of patients with SCD[207] may lead to more rapid improvement of the systemic vasculopathy that characterizes the catastrophic complications of SCD.

Prophylactic Anticoagulation in Acute Chest Syndrome

Acute chest syndrome (ACS) is complicated by a high rate of in situ pulmonary thrombosis. In a large single-institution study, 17% (95% confidence interval, 10%-23%) of patients experienced pulmonary thrombosis.[21] Interestingly, in patients with thrombosis, a precipitating factor was less commonly found, suggesting that pulmonary artery thrombosis may have been a trigger for ACS or that, perhaps, thrombosis was misdiagnosed as ACS given the overlap in presentation. In addition, patients with ACS who subsequently developed thrombosis were noted to have higher platelet counts at the onset of ACS (517 [range, 273-729] vs 307 [range, 228-412] × 10^9/L, $P <.01$), thereby potentially implicating platelets in the pathogenesis. This finding begs the question of whether full-dose, therapeutic anticoagulation with or without antiplatelet therapy may have a role in all patients hospitalized with ACS. Clinical trials are ongoing to address this question.

L-Arginine for Mitochondrial Dysfunction and Platelet Activation

The studies in the earlier section titled "NO Depletion" support the concept that hemolysis-dependent decreased NO bioavailability propagates thrombotic activation in SCD and suggests that NO therapeutics could attenuate hemostatic activation in this population. A number of studies have used SCD transgenic mouse models to demonstrate that potentiation of NO production or signaling is beneficial in SCD. For example, NO inhalation increased survival in the SAD mouse exposed to hypoxia[136] and decreased lung injury in another SCD model exposed to hypoxia.[40] L-Arginine supplementation as a substrate for NOS improved red cell density in the murine model,[137] and sildenafil prevented priapism in mice that received a bone marrow transplant from SCD mice.[135] Fewer studies have directly assessed the effect of NO therapeutics on hemostatic activation. Wajih et al[133] used dietary sodium nitrite as a donor of NO and showed in humanized SCD mice that nitrite attenuated platelet and leukocyte adhesion. As mentioned earlier, Villagra et al[97] demonstrated in SCD patients that sildenafil decreases platelet activation. A number of ongoing trials using inhaled sodium nitrite and L-arginine supplementation are currently evaluating the effect of these therapeutics on platelet function and coagulation activation.

Mitochondrial ROS Scavenging

The finding that platelet-enhanced mitochondrial ROS is a potential molecular link between hemolysis and platelet activation raises both mechanistic and therapeutic questions. On a mechanistic level, mitochondrial ROS are known to propagate thrombosis on many levels. For example, mitochondrial ROSs have been shown to activate protease-activated receptors in endothelial cells, resulting in TF induction.[208] In a separate study, endothelial loss of mitochondrial antioxidants augmented mitochondrial ROS levels, leading to a prothrombotic phenotype responsible for the formation of microthrombi in a mouse model of femoral artery ligation.[209] Although it is currently unknown whether hemolysis induces mitochondrial ROS in the endothelium or in other cell types, this is potentially an additional mechanism by which hemolysis activates a thrombotic phenotype in SCD. On a therapeutic level, mitochondria-targeted ROS scavengers are currently in clinical trials for a number of conditions,[210-212] and future studies will test their efficacy in attenuating thrombosis in SCD patients.

Conclusion

There is ample evidence of a prothrombotic state in SCD, as evidenced by testing of primary and secondary hemostasis, and fibrinolysis. Yet the full clinical impact of coagulation abnormalities on the risk of VTE has not been exhaustively assessed, particularly in children. Another gap in knowledge resides in the link between coagulation abnormalities and vaso-occlusive complications. Although it is clear that increases in procoagulant factors translate to a large-vessel prothrombotic phenotype (eg, VTE, stroke), their impact on the individual propensity to vaso-occlusive episodes in the microcirculation is less clear. Importantly, clinical trials of antiplatelet and anticoagulant agents in SCD have largely been disappointing in the prophylaxis and management of pain episodes. The evolving fund of knowledge of how HbS polymerization results in sterile inflammation, activation of coagulation, and an altered redox status, with their downstream effects on endothelial health and vascular adhesion, will result in a more nuanced understanding of the imbalance between procoagulant pathways and natural anticoagulants and to more targeted, precision medicine approaches to antithrombotic therapy.

Case Studies: "How I Treat" Expert Perspective

Case 1: An Adult Patient With SCD and Conventional Cardiovascular Risk Factors Presents With Acute Ischemic Stroke

A 43-year-old woman with HbSS disease and a history of frequent vaso-occlusive episodes presents to the emergency department with the acute onset of dense, left hemiplegia of 2 hours in duration. The history is also significant for a 20-pack-year smoking history, cholecystectomy, and ACS in her 20s. Prior to the onset of neurologic symptoms, she was in her usual state of health. Other than hydroxyurea, she is on oxycodone as needed for pain, folic acid, and a multivitamin. Her vital signs show that she is afebrile and mildly hypertensive. A noncontrast computed tomography (CT) scan of the head is negative for hemorrhage. Laboratory data show a hemoglobin of 7.2 g/dL (baseline, 8-9 g/dL) with appropriate reticulocyte response, leukocytosis with a left shift in the differential, and thrombocytosis. Coagulation indices and serum chemistries are normal except for elevated lactic dehydrogenase and aspartate aminotransferase. Alteplase is immediately administered according to protocol for ischemic stroke. While alteplase is infusing, 2 cross-matched units of red blood cells are procured and administered as soon as available. A dual-lumen large-bore dialysis catheter is placed, and the local transfusion service is contacted for emergent exchange transfusion, which the patient receives the day after presentation with reduction of the HbS to <30%. Magnetic resonance imaging (MRI) shows a right parietal ischemic stroke. Low-dose aspirin, angiotensin-converting inhibitor therapy, and cholesterol-lowering therapy are added. Prior to discharge, the patient is placed on hydroxyurea, and follow-up in the sickle cell clinic is arranged.

Ischemic stroke has a multimodal distribution in SCD, with a peak in childhood and another rise in incidence later in life.[174] Whereas the high incidence in children with homozygous SCD can be explained on the basis of SCD-specific factors alone, it is likely that the lifetime burden of vasculopathy from conventional cardiovascular risk factors (eg, smoking, hypercholesterolemia, sedentary lifestyle) contributes to the pathogenesis of stroke later in life. In our patient, the possibility of a ruptured plaque in the middle cerebral artery territory was entertained, and she received thrombolysis given her presentation during the therapeutic window for alteplase. However, correction of anemia and reduction of HbS have proven valuable in children with HbSS and stroke,[185,186] and data have been extrapolated to the adult population. Because, as in this case, there is usually a delay in procuring blood units for exchange and securing suitable venous access, simple transfusion is an important

Case Studies: Continued

temporizing measure. Alongside medical therapy commonly instituted in the general population (eg, antiplatelet agents, statins, antihypertensives), hydroxyurea has the potential to reduce stroke recurrence, although it is not as effective as transfusion in this regard, based on the pediatric literature. A case could be made to start hydroxyurea earlier in the course of acute stroke due to its potential to improve vasculopathy via its NO donor properties, but there is no support for this strategy in the literature. In summary, we elected to treat this patient aggressively with both thrombolytics and other conventional stroke treatment and transfusion support to address both conventional cardiovascular and SCD-specific pathology.

Case 2: A Hospitalized Patient With ACS Develops Multiorgan Failure Syndrome, Hyperhemolysis, and Schistocytosis

A 14-year-old patient with HbS/β+ thalassemia is hospitalized for a vaso-occlusive episode. On day 2 of the hospitalization, he develops pleuritic chest pain, fever, and an oxygen requirement. A chest x-ray reveals bibasilar infiltrates. He is placed on broad-spectrum antibiotics and 2 L/min of supplemental oxygen with restoration of normal pulse oximetry. At this time, his hemoglobin is 10.6 g/dL (average, 12.0 g/dL), platelet count is 120,000/μL, and chemistries are normal with the exception of his lactate dehydrogenase, which is elevated at 450 U/dL. On day 4, the patient is found to be obtunded, icteric, and toxic appearing with labored respiration. He is transferred to the intensive care unit, where a chest x-ray reveals extension of the infiltrates. A noncontrast head CT is normal; however, he has developed shock liver with severe transaminitis and hyperbilirubinemia and acute kidney injury and his lactate dehydrogenase has risen to 1430 U/dL. Platelets have fallen to 82,000/μL. The most notable findings in the peripheral smear are normoblastosis, polychromasia, schistocytosis, and bandemia. Platelets are reduced in keeping with the blood count. Fibrinogen is low-normal, and coagulation indices are slightly elevated. ADAMTS13 activity is 48%. He is intubated for acute respiratory distress syndrome, and cytology on a bronchoalveolar lavage shows lipid-laden, "foamy" alveolar macrophages. Blood cultures show no growth, but the antibiotic coverage is broadened empirically to cover for common causes of sepsis. Emergent exchange transfusion is instituted, but the patient's condition does not improve 2 days later despite of HbS <15%. A trial of daily therapeutic plasma exchange is then started. On day 8, the patient is successfully extubated, and serum chemistries are normalizing. Plasma exchange is discontinued, and the patient experiences a full recovery.

Multiorgan failure syndrome is an ominous complication of SCD that often follows ACS and occurs in all SCD subtypes.[213] Some studies have reported a higher incidence in patients with HbS/β thalassemia,[214] as was the case in our vignette. Shower embolism from massive bone marrow necrosis is hypothesized to be the cause, and phospholipids trapped in the pulmonary microcirculation may be phagocytized by alveolar macrophages, generating the characteristic, yet nonspecific finding on lipid-laden macrophages. Thrombocytopenia often heralds deterioration and a more severe prognosis in ACS.[215] Some patients also have accompanying schistocytosis, which raises concern for thrombotic microangiopathy. In most cases, ADAMTS13 activity levels are low-normal and not in the range typically observed in autoimmune thrombotic thrombocytopenic purpura (TTP).[207,216] It is possible that circulating inhibitors of ADAMTS13 such as free hemoglobin[98] or TSP1[207] inhibit ADAMTS13 activity in sufficient measure to inhibit degradation of ultralarge von Willebrand factor multimers. Platelet activation and consumption would then follow and potentially precipitate a TTP-like syndrome. Therapeutic plasma exchange has been used in many anecdotal reports and case series with benefit,[188,205,206] and we contend it is a reasonable option in combination with erythrocytapheresis. In these cases, and particularly in patients who do not respond to supportive therapy, it is important to consider a broad differential diagnosis. Conditions whose presentation overlaps with multiorgan failure syndrome include, but are not limited to, sepsis with acute respiratory distress syndrome, hyperhemolysis syndrome in patients with a history of red blood cell alloimmunization, thrombotic microangiopathy, catastrophic antiphospholipid antibody syndrome, disseminated intravascular coagulation, and hemophagocytic lymphohistiocytosis.

High-Yield Facts

◆ A prothrombotic state is a hallmark of SCD and is characterized by increased thrombin generation, particularly during vaso-occlusive episodes.

◆ VTE has a cumulative incidence of 25% in adult SCD patients and a 10-year incidence of 2% to 3% in children.

◆ In SCD, there is a higher incidence of pulmonary thrombosis relative to DVT compared to other populations, with a prevalence of 17% in patients presenting with ACS.

◆ Of the deep vein thrombi seen in SCD patients, upper extremity DVT accounts for about 50% of the events due to the high prevalence of indwelling central venous catheters.

High-Yield Facts (Cont.)

- Whole blood cellular components play a major role in the activation of the intrinsic and extrinsic coagulation pathways in SCD.
- Procoagulant pathways (ie, increased TF expression in vascular, hematopoietic, and endothelial cells; autoactivation of FXII; exposure of PS by sickle red blood cells and circulating MPs) are upregulated, and natural anticoagulants (ie, proteins C and S) are depleted in SCD at steady state, with more pronounced alterations during vaso-occlusive episodes.
- Hemolysis and NO depletion are major mechanisms of hemostatic activation in SCD.
- Platelet mitochondrial dysfunction in SCD leads to platelet activation and the generation of ROSs.
- Clinical trials of antiplatelet agents and anticoagulants have not resulted in robust amelioration of the SCD phenotype, particularly concerning vaso-occlusive episodes.
- DVT prophylaxis is recommended for hospitalized adult patients with SCD and may be beneficial for hospitalized children with indwelling venous catheters.
- Existing treatments (eg, hydroxyurea) and developing treatments (eg, P-selectin blockade) for SCD may reduce thrombotic risk.
- Multiorgan failure syndrome in SCD may be accompanied by schistocytosis and features of TTP.

References

1. Ataga KI, Key NS. Hypercoagulability in sickle cell disease: new approaches to an old problem. *Hematol Am Soc Hematol Educ Program.* 2007:91-96.
2. Ataga KI. Hypercoagulability and thrombotic complications in hemolytic anemias. *Haematologica.* 2009;94(11):1481-1484.
3. De Franceschi L, Cappellini MD, Olivieri O. Thrombosis and sickle cell disease. *Semin Thromb Hemost.* 2011;37(3):226-236.
4. Peters M, Plaat BE, ten Cate H, Wolters HJ, Weening RS, Brandjes DP. Enhanced thrombin generation in children with sickle cell disease. *Thromb Haemost.* 1994;71(2):169-172.
5. Ataga KI, Moore CG, Hillery CA, et al. Coagulation activation and inflammation in sickle cell disease-associated pulmonary hypertension. *Haematologica.* 2008;93(1):20-26.
6. Stuart MJ, Setty BN. Hemostatic alterations in sickle cell disease: relationships to disease pathophysiology. *Pediatr Pathol Mol Med.* 2001;20(1):27-46.
7. van Beers EJ, Spronk HM, Ten Cate H, et al. No association of the hypercoagulable state with sickle cell disease related pulmonary hypertension. *Haematologica.* 2008;93(5):e42-e44.
8. Whelihan MF, Lim MY, Mooberry MJ, et al. Thrombin generation and cell-dependent hypercoagulability in sickle cell disease. *J Thromb Haemost.* 2016;14(10):1941-1952.
9. Adam SS, Key NS, Greenberg CS. D-dimer antigen: current concepts and future prospects. *Blood.* 2009;113(13):2878-2887.
10. Tomer A, Harker LA, Kasey S, Eckman JR. Thrombogenesis in sickle cell disease. *J Lab Clin Med.* 2001;137(6):398-407.
11. Leslie J, Langler D, Serjeant GR, Serjeant BE, Desai P, Gordon YB. Coagulation changes during the steady state in homozygous sickle-cell disease in Jamaica. *Br J Haematol.* 1975;30(2):159-166.
12. Westerman MP, Green D, Gilman-Sachs A, et al. Antiphospholipid antibodies, proteins C and S, and coagulation changes in sickle cell disease. *J Lab Clin Med.* 1999;134(4):352-362.
13. Tomer A, Kasey S, Connor WE, Clark S, Harker LA, Eckman JR. Reduction of pain episodes and prothrombotic activity in sickle cell disease by dietary n-3 fatty acids. *Thromb Haemost.* 2001;85(6):966-974.
14. Oppenheimer EH, Esterly JR. Pulmonary changes in sickle cell disease. *Am Rev Respir Dis.* 1971;103(6):858-859.
15. Kirkpatrick MB, Haynes J. Sickle-cell disease and the pulmonary circulation. *Semin Respir Crit Care Med.* 1994;15(6):473-481.
16. Adedeji MO, Cespedes J, Allen K, Subramony C, Hughson MD. Pulmonary thrombotic arteriopathy in patients with sickle cell disease. *Arch Pathol Lab Med.* 2001;125(11):1436-1441.
17. Carstens GR, Paulino BBA, Katayama EH, et al. Clinical relevance of pulmonary vasculature involvement in sickle cell disease. *Br J Haematol.* 2019;185(2):317-326.
18. Novelli EM, Huynh C, Gladwin MT, Moore CG, Ragni MV. Pulmonary embolism in sickle cell disease: a case-control study. *J Thromb Haemost.* 2012;10(5):760-766.
19. Brunson A, Lei A, Rosenberg AS, White RH, Keegan T, Wun T. Increased incidence of VTE in sickle cell disease patients: risk factors, recurrence and impact on mortality. *Br J Haematol.* 2017;178(2):319-326.
20. Stein PD, Beemath A, Meyers FA, Skaf E, Olson RE. Deep venous thrombosis and pulmonary embolism in hospitalized patients with sickle cell disease. *Am J Med.* 2006;119(10):e897-e911.
21. Mekontso Dessap A, Deux JF, Abidi N, et al. Pulmonary artery thrombosis during acute chest syndrome in sickle cell disease. *Am J Respir Crit Care Med.* 2011;184(9):1022-1029.
22. Naik RP, Streiff MB, Haywood C Jr, Nelson JA, Lanzkron S. Venous thromboembolism in adults with sickle cell disease: a serious and under-recognized complication. *Am J Med.* 2013;126(5):443-449.
23. Naik RP, Streiff MB, Haywood C Jr, Segal JB, Lanzkron S. Venous thromboembolism incidence in the Cooperative Study of Sickle Cell Disease. *J Thromb Haemost.* 2014;12(12):2010-2016.
24. Kumar R, Stanek J, Creary S, Dunn A, O'Brien SH. Prevalence and risk factors for venous thromboembolism in children with sickle cell disease: an administrative database study. *Blood Adv.* 2018;2(3):285-291.

25. Woods GM, Sharma R, Creary S, et al. Venous thromboembolism in children with sickle cell disease: a retrospective cohort study. *J Pediatr.* 2018;197:186-190 e181.

26. Shah N, Landi D, Shah R, Rothman J, De Castro LM, Thornburg CD. Complications of implantable venous access devices in patients with sickle cell disease. *Am J Hematol.* 2012;87(2):224-226.

27. Brunson A, Keegan T, Mahajan A, White R, Wun T. High incidence of venous thromboembolism recurrence in patients with sickle cell disease. *Am J Hematol.* 2019;94(8):862-870.

28. James AH, Jamison MG, Brancazio LR, Myers ER. Venous thromboembolism during pregnancy and the postpartum period: incidence, risk factors, and mortality. *Am J Obstet Gynecol.* 2006;194(5):1311-1315.

29. Boulet SL, Okoroh EM, Azonobi I, Grant A, Craig Hooper W. Sickle cell disease in pregnancy: maternal complications in a Medicaid-enrolled population. *Matern Child Health J.* 2013;17(2):200-207.

30. Villers MS, Jamison MG, De Castro LM, James AH. Morbidity associated with sickle cell disease in pregnancy. *Am J Obstet Gynecol.* 2008;199(2):e121-e125.

31. Chaouat A, Weitzenblum E, Higenbottam T. The role of thrombosis in severe pulmonary hypertension. *Eur Respir J.* 1996;9(2):356-363.

32. De Franceschi L, Platt OS, Malpeli G, et al. Protective effects of phosphodiesterase-4 (PDE-4) inhibition in the early phase of pulmonary arterial hypertension in transgenic sickle cell mice. *FASEB J.* 2008;22(6):1849-1860.

33. Gladwin MT, Sachdev V. Cardiovascular abnormalities in sickle cell disease. *J Am Coll Cardiol.* 2012;59(13):1123-1133.

34. Beuzard Y. Mouse models of sickle cell disease. *Transfus Clin Biol.* 2008;15(1-2):7-11.

35. Paszty C, Brion CM, Manci E, et al. Transgenic knockout mice with exclusively human sickle hemoglobin and sickle cell disease. *Science.* 1997;278(5339):876-878.

36. Wu LC, Sun CW, Ryan TM, Pawlik KM, Ren J, Townes TM. Correction of sickle cell disease by homologous recombination in embryonic stem cells. *Blood.* 2006;108(4):1183-1188.

37. Guo Y, Uy T, Wandersee N, et al. The protein C Pathway in human and murine sickle cell disease: alterations in protein C, thrombomodulin (TM), and endothelial protein C receptor (EPCR) at baseline and during acute vaso-occlusion. *Blood.* 2008;112(11):202.

38. Chantrathammachart P, Mackman N, Sparkenbaugh E, et al. Tissue factor promotes activation of coagulation and inflammation in a mouse model of sickle cell disease. *Blood.* 2012;120(3):636-646.

39. Trudel M, De Paepe ME, Chretien N, et al. Sickle cell disease of transgenic SAD mice. *Blood.* 1994;84(9):3189-3197.

40. de Franceschi L, Baron A, Scarpa A, et al. Inhaled nitric oxide protects transgenic SAD mice from sickle cell disease-specific lung injury induced by hypoxia/reoxygenation. *Blood.* 2003;102(3):1087-1096.

41. Faes C, Ilich A, Sotiaux A, et al. Red blood cells modulate structure and dynamics of venous clot formation in sickle cell disease. *Blood.* 2019;133(23):2529-2541.

42. Singer ST, Ataga KI. Hypercoagulability in sickle cell disease and beta-thalassemia. *Curr Mol Med.* 2008;8(7):639-645.

43. Pawlinski R, Mackman N. Cellular sources of tissue factor in endotoxemia and sepsis. *Thromb Res.* 2010;125(suppl 1):S70-S73.

44. Pawlinski R, Pedersen B, Erlich J, Mackman N. Role of tissue factor in haemostasis, thrombosis, angiogenesis and inflammation: lessons from low tissue factor mice. *Thromb Haemost.* 2004;92(3):444-450.

45. Mackman N, Tilley RE, Key NS. Role of the extrinsic pathway of blood coagulation in hemostasis and thrombosis. *Arterioscler Thromb Vasc Biol.* 2007;27(8):1687-1693.

46. Setty BN, Key NS, Rao AK, et al. Tissue factor-positive monocytes in children with sickle cell disease: correlation with biomarkers of haemolysis. *Br J Haematol.* 2012;157(3):370-380.

47. Key NS, Slungaard A, Dandelet L, et al. Whole blood tissue factor procoagulant activity is elevated in patients with sickle cell disease. *Blood.* 1998;91(11):4216-4223.

48. Solovey A, Gui L, Key NS, Hebbel RP. Tissue factor expression by endothelial cells in sickle cell anemia. *J Clin Invest.* 1998;101(9):1899-1904.

49. Solovey A, Kollander R, Shet A, et al. Endothelial cell expression of tissue factor in sickle mice is augmented by hypoxia/reoxygenation and inhibited by lovastatin. *Blood.* 2004;104(3):840-846.

50. Noubouossie DF, Reeves BN, Strahl BD, Key NS. Neutrophils: back in the thrombosis spotlight. *Blood.* 2019;133(20):2186-2197.

51. Hoppe C, Kuypers F, Larkin S, Hagar W, Vichinsky E, Styles L. A pilot study of the short-term use of simvastatin in sickle cell disease: effects on markers of vascular dysfunction. *Br J Haematol.* 2011;153(5):655-663.

52. Colella MP, De Paula EV, Conran N, et al. Hydroxyurea is associated with reductions in hypercoagulability markers in sickle cell anemia. *J Thromb Haemost.* 2012;10(9):1967-1970.

53. Belcher JD, Chen C, Nguyen J, et al. Heme triggers TLR4 signaling leading to endothelial cell activation and vaso-occlusion in murine sickle cell disease. *Blood.* 2014;123(3):377-390.

54. Sparkenbaugh EM, Chantrathammachart P, Wang S, et al. Excess of heme induces tissue factor-dependent activation of coagulation in mice. *Haematologica.* 2015;100(3):308-314.

55. Setty BN, Betal SG, Zhang J, Stuart MJ. Heme induces endothelial tissue factor expression: potential role in hemostatic activation in patients with hemolytic anemia. *J Thromb Haemost.* 2008;6(12):2202-2209.

56. Kollander R, Solovey A, Milbauer LC, Abdulla F, Kelm RJ Jr, Hebbel RP. Nuclear factor-kappa B (NFkappaB) component p50 in blood mononuclear cells regulates endothelial tissue factor expression in sickle transgenic mice: implications for the coagulopathy of sickle cell disease. *Transl Res.* 2010;155(4):170-177.

57. Solovey A, Kollander R, Milbauer LC, et al. Endothelial nitric oxide synthase and nitric oxide regulate endothelial tissue factor expression in vivo in the sickle transgenic mouse. *Am J Hematol.* 2010;85(1):41-45.

58. Hebbel RP, Vercellotti GM, Pace BS, et al. The HDAC inhibitors trichostatin A and suberoylanilide hydroxamic acid exhibit multiple modalities of benefit for the vascular pathobiology of sickle transgenic mice. *Blood.* 2010;115(12):2483-2490.

59. Pawlinski R, Wang JG, Owens AP 3rd, et al. Hematopoietic and nonhematopoietic cell tissue factor activates the coagulation cascade in endotoxemic mice. *Blood.* 2010;116(5):806-814.

60. Wallace KL, Marshall MA, Ramos SI, et al. NKT cells mediate pulmonary inflammation and dysfunction in murine sickle cell disease through production of IFN-gamma and CXCR3 chemokines. *Blood.* 2009;114(3):667-676.

61. Polanowska-Grabowska R, Wallace K, Field JJ, et al. P-selectin-mediated platelet-neutrophil aggregate formation activates

neutrophils in mouse and human sickle cell disease. *Arterioscler Thromb Vasc Biol.* 2010;30(12):2392-2399.

62. Ghosh S, Tan F, Ofori-Acquah SF. Spatiotemporal dysfunction of the vascular permeability barrier in transgenic mice with sickle cell disease. *Anemia.* 2012;2012:582018.

63. Smith SA, Morrissey JH. Polyphosphate: a new player in the field of hemostasis. *Curr Opin Hematol.* 2014;21(5):388-394.

64. Gould TJ, Vu TT, Swystun LL, et al. Neutrophil extracellular traps promote thrombin generation through platelet-dependent and platelet-independent mechanisms. *Arterioscler Thromb Vasc Biol.* 2014;34(9):1977-1984.

65. Kannemeier C, Liao R, Sun P. The RING finger domain of MDM2 is essential for MDM2-mediated TGF-beta resistance. *Mol Biol Cell.* 2007;18(6):2367-2377.

66. Miller RL, Verma PS, Adams RG. Studies of the kallikrein-kinin system in patients with sickle cell anemia. *J Natl Med Assoc.* 1983;75(6):551-556.

67. Gordon EM, Klein BL, Berman BW, Strandjord SE, Simon JE, Coccia PF. Reduction of contact factors in sickle cell disease. *J Pediatr.* 1985;106(3):427-430.

68. Van Der Meijden PE, Van Schilfgaarde M, Van Oerle R, Renne T, ten Cate H, Spronk HM. Platelet- and erythrocyte-derived microparticles trigger thrombin generation via factor XIIa. *J Thromb Haemost.* 2012;10(7):1355-1362.

69. Connor J, Schroit AJ. Transbilayer movement of phosphatidylserine in erythrocytes. Inhibitors of aminophospholipid transport block the association of photolabeled lipid to its transporter. *Biochim Biophys Acta.* 1991;1066(1):37-42.

70. Franck PF, Bevers EM, Lubin BH, et al. Uncoupling of the membrane skeleton from the lipid bilayer. The cause of accelerated phospholipid flip-flop leading to an enhanced procoagulant activity of sickled cells. *J Clin Invest.* 1985;75(1):183-190.

71. Owens AP 3rd, Mackman N. Microparticles in hemostasis and thrombosis. *Circ Res.* 2011;108(10):1284-1297.

72. Setty BN, Kulkarni S, Rao AK, Stuart MJ. Fetal hemoglobin in sickle cell disease: relationship to erythrocyte phosphatidylserine exposure and coagulation activation. *Blood.* 2000;96(3):1119-1124.

73. Setty BN, Rao AK, Stuart MJ. Thrombophilia in sickle cell disease: the red cell connection. *Blood.* 2001;98(12):3228-3233.

74. Hebbel RP, Key NS. Microparticles in sickle cell anaemia: promise and pitfalls. *Br J Haematol.* 2016;174(1):16-29.

75. Aleman MM, Gardiner C, Harrison P, Wolberg AS. Differential contributions of monocyte- and platelet-derived microparticles towards thrombin generation and fibrin formation and stability. *J Thromb Haemost.* 2011;9(11):2251-2261.

76. Wun T, Paglieroni T, Rangaswami A, et al. Platelet activation in patients with sickle cell disease. *Br J Haematol.* 1998;100(4):741-749.

77. Allan D, Limbrick AR, Thomas P, Westerman MP. Release of spectrin-free spicules on reoxygenation of sickled erythrocytes. *Nature.* 1982;295(5850):612-613.

78. Shet AS, Aras O, Gupta K, et al. Sickle blood contains tissue factor-positive microparticles derived from endothelial cells and monocytes. *Blood.* 2003;102(7):2678-2683.

79. van Beers EJ, Schaap MC, Berckmans RJ, et al. Circulating erythrocyte-derived microparticles are associated with coagulation activation in sickle cell disease. *Haematologica.* 2009;94(11):1513-1519.

80. Kasar M, Boga C, Yeral M, Asma S, Kozanoglu I, Ozdogu H. Clinical significance of circulating blood and endothelial cell

microparticles in sickle-cell disease. *J Thromb Thrombolysis.* 2014;38(2):167-175.

81. Brunetta DM, De Santis GC, Silva-Pinto AC, Oliveira de Oliveira LC, Covas DT. Hydroxyurea increases plasma concentrations of microparticles and reduces coagulation activation and fibrinolysis in patients with sickle cell anemia. *Acta Haematol.* 2015;133(3):287-294.

82. Ataga KI, Brittain JE, Desai P, et al. Association of coagulation activation with clinical complications in sickle cell disease. *PLoS One.* 2012;7(1):e29786.

83. el-Hazmi MA, Warsy AS, Bahakim H. Blood proteins C and S in sickle cell disease. *Acta Haematol.* 1993;90(3):114-119.

84. Bayazit AK, Kilinc Y. Natural coagulation inhibitors (protein C, protein S, antithrombin) in patients with sickle cell anemia in a steady state. *Pediatr Int.* 2001;43(6):592-596.

85. Liesner R, Mackie I, Cookson J, et al. Prothrombotic changes in children with sickle cell disease: relationships to cerebrovascular disease and transfusion. *Br J Haematol.* 1998;103(4):1037-1044.

86. Noubouossie DF, Le PQ, Corazza F, et al. Thrombin generation reveals high procoagulant potential in the plasma of sickle cell disease children. *Am J Hematol.* 2012;87(2):145-149.

87. Piccin A, Murphy C, Eakins E, et al. Protein C and free protein S in children with sickle cell anemia. *Ann Hematol.* 2012;91(10):1669-1671.

88. Tam DA. Protein C and protein S activity in sickle cell disease and stroke. *J Child Neurol.* 1997;12(1):19-21.

89. Griffin JH, Zlokovic BV, Mosnier LO. Activated protein C: biased for translation. *Blood.* 2015;125(19):2898-2907.

90. Bezeaud A, Venisse L, Helley D, Trichet C, Girot R, Guillin MC. Red blood cells from patients with homozygous sickle cell disease provide a catalytic surface for factor Va inactivation by activated protein C. *Br J Haematol.* 2002;117(2):409-413.

91. Gavins FN, Russell J, Senchenkova EL, et al. Mechanisms of enhanced thrombus formation in cerebral microvessels of mice expressing hemoglobin-S. *Blood.* 2011;117(15):4125-4133.

92. Mosnier LO, Zlokovic BV, Griffin JH. The cytoprotective protein C pathway. *Blood.* 2007;109(8):3161-3172.

93. Lane PA, O'Connell JL, Marlar RA. Erythrocyte membrane vesicles and irreversibly sickled cells bind protein S. *Am J Hematol.* 1994;47(4):295-300.

94. Chekkal M, Rahal MCA, Moulasserdoun K, Seghier F. Increased level of factor VIII and physiological inhibitors of coagulation in patients with sickle cell disease. *Indian J Hematol Blood Transfus.* 2017;33(2):235-238.

95. Wright JG, Malia R, Cooper P, Thomas P, Preston FE, Serjeant GR. Protein C and protein S in homozygous sickle cell disease: does hepatic dysfunction contribute to low levels? *Br J Haematol.* 1997;98(3):627-631.

96. Cardenes N, Corey C, Geary L, et al. Platelet bioenergetic screen in sickle cell patients reveals mitochondrial complex V inhibition, which contributes to platelet activation. *Blood.* 2014;123(18):2864-2872.

97. Villagra J, Shiva S, Hunter LA, Machado RF, Gladwin MT, Kato GJ. Platelet activation in patients with sickle disease, hemolysis-associated pulmonary hypertension, and nitric oxide scavenging by cell-free hemoglobin. *Blood.* 2007;110(6):2166-2172.

98. Chen J, Hobbs WE, Le J, Lenting PJ, de Groot PG, Lopez JA. The rate of hemolysis in sickle cell disease correlates with the quantity of active von Willebrand factor in the plasma. *Blood.* 2011;117(13):3680-3683.

99. Annarapu GK, Singhal R, Gupta A, et al. HbS binding to GP1balpha activates platelets in sickle cell disease. *PLoS One.* 2016;11(12):e0167899.

100. Helms CC, Marvel M, Zhao W, et al. Mechanisms of hemolysis-associated platelet activation. *J Thromb Haemost.* 2013;11(12): 2148-2154.

101. Wollny T, Iacoviello L, Buczko W, de Gaetano G, Donati MB. Prolongation of bleeding time by acute hemolysis in rats: a role for nitric oxide. *Am J Physiol.* 1997;272(6 Pt 2): H2875-H2884.

102. Aursnes I, Stenberg-Nilsen H. Low dose infusion of adenosine diphosphate prolongs bleeding time in rats and rabbits. *Thromb Res.* 1992;68(1):67-74.

103. Doni MG, Aragno R. ADP-induced platelet aggregation in vivo after exclusion of different circulatory districts. *Experientia.* 1975;31(10):1224-1225.

104. Foster CJ, Prosser DM, Agans JM, et al. Molecular identification and characterization of the platelet ADP receptor targeted by thienopyridine antithrombotic drugs. *J Clin Invest.* 2001;107(12):1591-1598.

105. Freedman JE, Loscalzo J, Barnard MR, Alpert C, Keaney JF, Michelson AD. Nitric oxide released from activated platelets inhibits platelet recruitment. *J Clin Invest.* 1997;100(2): 350-356.

106. Gambaryan S, Tsikas D. A review and discussion of platelet nitric oxide and nitric oxide synthase: do blood platelets produce nitric oxide from L-arginine or nitrite? *Amino Acids.* 2015;47(9):1779-1793.

107. Mehta JL, Chen LY, Kone BC, Mehta P, Turner P. Identification of constitutive and inducible forms of nitric oxide synthase in human platelets. *J Lab Clin Med.* 1995;125(3):370-377.

108. Radziwon-Balicka A, Lesyk G, Back V, et al. Differential eNOS-signalling by platelet subpopulations regulates adhesion and aggregation. *Cardiovasc Res.* 2017;113(14):1719-1731.

109. Cortese-Krott MM, Rodriguez-Mateos A, Sansone R, et al. Human red blood cells at work: identification and visualization of erythrocytic eNOS activity in health and disease. *Blood.* 2012;120(20):4229-4237.

110. Wood KC, Cortese-Krott MM, Kovacic JC, et al. Circulating blood endothelial nitric oxide synthase contributes to the regulation of systemic blood pressure and nitrite homeostasis. *Arterioscler Thromb Vasc Biol.* 2013;33(8):1861-1871.

111. Makhoul S, Walter E, Pagel O, et al. Effects of the NO/soluble guanylate cyclase/cGMP system on the functions of human platelets. *Nitric Oxide.* 2018;76:71-80.

112. Radomski MW, Moncada S. Regulation of vascular homeostasis by nitric oxide. *Thromb Haemost.* 1993;70(1):36-41.

113. Radomski MW, Moncada S. The biological and pharmacological role of nitric oxide in platelet function. *Adv Exp Med Biol.* 1993;344:251-264.

114. De Caterina R, Libby P, Peng HB, et al. Nitric oxide decreases cytokine-induced endothelial activation. Nitric oxide selectively reduces endothelial expression of adhesion molecules and proinflammatory cytokines. *J Clin Invest.* 1995;96(1):60-68.

115. Radomski MW, Vallance P, Whitley G, Foxwell N, Moncada S. Platelet adhesion to human vascular endothelium is modulated by constitutive and cytokine induced nitric oxide. *Cardiovasc Res.* 1993;27(7):1380-1382.

116. Lowenstein CJ. Nitric oxide regulation of protein trafficking in the cardiovascular system. *Cardiovasc Res.* 2007;75(2): 240-246.

117. Matsushita K, Morrell CN, Cambien B, et al. Nitric oxide regulates exocytosis by S-nitrosylation of N-ethylmaleimide-sensitive factor. *Cell.* 2003;115(2):139-150.

118. Broeders MA, Tangelder GJ, Slaaf DW, Reneman RS, oude Egbrink MG. Endogenous nitric oxide protects against thromboembolism in venules but not in arterioles. *Arterioscler Thromb Vasc Biol.* 1998;18(1):139-145.

119. Stagliano NE, Zhao W, Prado R, Dewanjee MK, Ginsberg MD, Dietrich WD. The effect of nitric oxide synthase inhibition on acute platelet accumulation and hemodynamic depression in a rat model of thromboembolic stroke. *J Cereb Blood Flow Metab.* 1997;17(11):1182-1190.

120. Yao SK, Ober JC, Krishnaswami A, et al. Endogenous nitric oxide protects against platelet aggregation and cyclic flow variations in stenosed and endothelium-injured arteries. *Circulation.* 1992;86(4):1302-1309.

121. Atochin DN, Huang PL. Endothelial nitric oxide synthase transgenic models of endothelial dysfunction. *Pflugers Arch.* 2010;460(6):965-974.

122. Moore C, Tymvios C, Emerson M. Functional regulation of vascular and platelet activity during thrombosis by nitric oxide and endothelial nitric oxide synthase. *Thromb Haemost.* 2010;104(2):342-349.

123. Nakayama T, Sato W, Yoshimura A, et al. Endothelial von Willebrand factor release due to eNOS deficiency predisposes to thrombotic microangiopathy in mouse aging kidney. *Am J Pathol.* 2010;176(5):2198-2208.

124. Lancaster JR Jr. Simulation of the diffusion and reaction of endogenously produced nitric oxide. *Proc Natl Acad Sci U S A.* 1994;91(17):8137-8141.

125. Doherty DH, Doyle MP, Curry SR, et al. Rate of reaction with nitric oxide determines the hypertensive effect of cell-free hemoglobin. *Nat Biotechnol.* 1998;16(7):672-676.

126. Reiter CD, Wang X, Tanus-Santos JE, et al. Cell-free hemoglobin limits nitric oxide bioavailability in sickle-cell disease. *Nat Med.* 2002;8(12):1383-1389.

127. Morris CR, Kato GJ, Poljakovic M, et al. Dysregulated arginine metabolism, hemolysis-associated pulmonary hypertension, and mortality in sickle cell disease. *JAMA.* 2005;294(1):81-90.

128. Landburg PP, Teerlink T, Biemond BJ, et al. Plasma asymmetric dimethylarginine concentrations in sickle cell disease are related to the hemolytic phenotype. *Blood Cells Mol Dis.* 2010;44(4):229-232.

129. Schnog JB, Teerlink T, van der Dijs FP, Duits AJ, Muskiet FA, CURAMA Study Group. Plasma levels of asymmetric dimethylarginine (ADMA), an endogenous nitric oxide synthase inhibitor, are elevated in sickle cell disease. *Ann Hematol.* 2005;84(5):282-286.

130. Kato GJ, Hebbel RP, Steinberg MH, Gladwin MT. Vasculopathy in sickle cell disease: Biology, pathophysiology, genetics, translational medicine, and new research directions. *Am J Hematol.* 2009;84(9):618-625.

131. Morris CR. Mechanisms of vasculopathy in sickle cell disease and thalassemia. *Hematol Am Soc Hematol Educ Program.* 2008;2008:177-185.

132. Almeida CB, Souza LE, Leonardo FC, et al. Acute hemolytic vascular inflammatory processes are prevented by nitric oxide replacement or a single dose of hydroxyurea. *Blood.* 2015;126(6):711-720.

133. Wajih N, Basu S, Jailwala A, et al. Potential therapeutic action of nitrite in sickle cell disease. *Redox Biol.* 2017;12:1026-1039.

134. Hsu LL, Champion HC, Campbell-Lee SA, et al. Hemolysis in sickle cell mice causes pulmonary hypertension due to global impairment in nitric oxide bioavailability. *Blood.* 2007;109(7):3088-3098.

135. Sopko NA, Matsui H, Hannan JL, et al. Subacute hemolysis in sickle cell mice causes priapism secondary to NO imbalance and PDE5 dysregulation. *J Sex Med.* 2015;12(9):1878-1885.

136. Martinez-Ruiz R, Montero-Huerta P, Hromi J, Head CA. Inhaled nitric oxide improves survival rates during hypoxia in a sickle cell (SAD) mouse model. *Anesthesiology.* 2001;94(6):1113-1118.

137. Romero JR, Suzuka SM, Nagel RL, Fabry ME. Arginine supplementation of sickle transgenic mice reduces red cell density and Gardos channel activity. *Blood.* 2002;99(4):1103-1108.

138. Hamanaka RB, Chandel NS. Mitochondrial reactive oxygen species regulate cellular signaling and dictate biological outcomes. *Trends Biochem Sci.* 2010;35(9):505-513.

139. Nunnari J, Suomalainen A. Mitochondria: in sickness and in health. *Cell.* 2012;148(6):1145-1159.

140. Moras M, Lefevre SD, Ostuni MA. From erythroblasts to mature red blood cells: organelle clearance in mammals. *Front Physiol.* 2017;8:1076.

141. Kramer PA, Ravi S, Chacko B, Johnson MS, Darley-Usmar VM. A review of the mitochondrial and glycolytic metabolism in human platelets and leukocytes: implications for their use as bioenergetic biomarkers. *Redox Biol.* 2014;2:206-210.

142. Akkerman JW, Holmsen H. Interrelationships among platelet responses: studies on the burst in proton liberation, lactate production, and oxygen uptake during platelet aggregation and Ca²⁺ secretion. *Blood.* 1981;57(5):956-966.

143. Akkerman JW, Holmsen H, Loughnane M. Simultaneous measurement of aggregation, secretion, oxygen uptake, proton production, and intracellular metabolites in the same platelet suspension. *Anal Biochem.* 1979;97(2):387-393.

144. Slatter DA, Aldrovandi M, O'Connor A, et al. Mapping the human platelet lipidome reveals cytosolic phospholipase A2 as a regulator of mitochondrial bioenergetics during activation. *Cell Metab.* 2016;23(5):930-944.

145. Lopez JJ, Salido GM, Gomez-Arteta E, Rosado JA, Pariente JA. Thrombin induces apoptotic events through the generation of reactive oxygen species in human platelets. *J Thromb Haemost.* 2007;5(6):1283-1291.

146. Matarrese P, Straface E, Palumbo G, et al. Mitochondria regulate platelet metamorphosis induced by opsonized zymosan A: activation and long-term commitment to cell death. *FEBS J.* 2009;276(3):845-856.

147. Pignatelli P, Pulcinelli FM, Lenti L, Gazzaniga PP, Violi F. Hydrogen peroxide is involved in collagen-induced platelet activation. *Blood.* 1998;91(2):484-490.

148. Yamagishi SI, Edelstein D, Du XL, Brownlee M. Hyperglycemia potentiates collagen-induced platelet activation through mitochondrial superoxide overproduction. *Diabetes.* 2001;50(6):1491-1494.

149. Desai PC, Brittain JE, Jones SK, et al. A pilot study of eptifibatide for treatment of acute pain episodes in sickle cell disease. *Thromb Res.* 2013;132(3):341-345.

150. Greenberg J, Ohene-Frempong K, Halus J, Way C, Schwartz E. Trial of low doses of aspirin as prophylaxis in sickle cell disease. *J Pediatr.* 1983;102(5):781-784.

151. Osamo NO, Photiades DP, Famodu AA. Therapeutic effect of aspirin in sickle cell anaemia. *Acta Haematol.* 1981;66(2):102-107.

152. Semple MJ, Al-Hasani SF, Kioy P, Savidge GF. A double-blind trial of ticlopidine in sickle cell disease. *Thromb Haemost.* 1984;51(3):303-306.

153. Wun T, Soulieres D, Frelinger AL, et al. A double-blind, randomized, multicenter phase 2 study of prasugrel versus placebo in adult patients with sickle cell disease. *J Hematol Oncol.* 2013;6:17.

154. Heeney MM, Hoppe CC, Abboud MR, et al. A multinational trial of prasugrel for sickle cell vaso-occlusive events. *N Engl J Med.* 2016;374(7):625-635.

155. Kanter J, Abboud MR, Kaya B, et al. Ticagrelor does not impact patient-reported pain in young adults with sickle cell disease: a multicentre, randomised phase IIb study. *Br J Haematol.* 2019;184(2):269-278.

156. Beiter JL Jr, Simon HK, Chambliss CR, Adamkiewicz T, Sullivan K. Intravenous ketorolac in the emergency department management of sickle cell pain and predictors of its effectiveness. *Arch Pediatr Adolesc Med.* 2001;155(4):496-500.

157. Han J, Saraf SL, Lash JP, Gordeuk VR. Use of anti-inflammatory analgesics in sickle-cell disease. *J Clin Pharm Ther.* 2017;42(5):656-660.

158. Ataga KI, Kutlar A, Kanter J, et al. Crizanlizumab for the prevention of pain crises in sickle cell disease. *N Engl J Med.* 2017;376(5):429-439.

159. Schlesinger M, Schmitz P, Zeisig R, et al. The inhibition of the integrin VLA-4 in MV3 melanoma cell binding by non-anticoagulant heparin derivatives. *Thromb Res.* 2012;129(5):603-610.

160. Brittain JE, Parise LV. The alpha4beta1 integrin in sickle cell disease. *Transfus Clin Biol.* 2008;15(1-2):19-22.

161. Chaar V, Picot J, Renaud O, et al. Aggregation of mononuclear and red blood cells through an {alpha}4{beta}1-Lu/basal cell adhesion molecule interaction in sickle cell disease. *Haematologica.* 2010;95(11):1841-1848.

162. Turhan A, Weiss LA, Mohandas N, Coller BS, Frenette PS. Primary role for adherent leukocytes in sickle cell vascular occlusion: a new paradigm. *Proc Natl Acad Sci U S A.* 2002;99(5):3047-3051.

163. Chaplin H Jr, Monroe MC, Malecek AC, Morgan LK, Michael J, Murphy WA. Preliminary trial of minidose heparin prophylaxis for painful sickle cell crises. *East Afr Med J.* 1989;66(9):574-584.

164. Qari MH, Aljaouni SK, Alardawi MS, et al. Reduction of painful vaso-occlusive crisis of sickle cell anaemia by tinzaparin in a double-blind randomized trial. *Thromb Haemost.* 2007;98(2):392-396.

165. Salvaggio JE, Arnold CA, Banov CH. Long-term anticoagulation in sickle-cell disease. A clinical study. *N Engl J Med.* 1963;269:182-186.

166. Schnog JB, Kater AP, Mac Gillavry MR, et al. Low adjusted-dose acenocoumarol therapy in sickle cell disease: a pilot study. *Am J Hematol.* 2001;68(3):179-183.

167. Shah N, Willen S, Telen MJ, Ortel TL. Prophylactic dose low molecular weight heparin (dalteparin) for treatment of vaso-occlusive pain crisis in patients with sickle cell disease. *Blood.* 2013;122(21):2241.

168. Wolters HJ, ten Cate H, Thomas LL, et al. Low-intensity oral anticoagulation in sickle-cell disease reverses the prethrombotic state: promises for treatment? *Br J Haematol.* 1995;90(3):715-717.

169. Patel A, Williams H, Baer MR, Zimrin AB, Law JY. Use of direct oral anticoagulants in patients with sickle cell disease and venous

thromboembolism is associated with a significant decrease in incidence of bleeding compared to vitamin K antagonists and low-molecular-weight heparins. *Blood.* 2017;130(suppl 1):978.

170. Kearon C, Akl EA, Ornelas J, et al. Antithrombotic therapy for VTE disease: CHEST guideline and expert panel report. *Chest.* 2016;149(2):315-352.

171. Witt DM, Nieuwlaat R, Clark NP, et al. American Society of Hematology 2018 guidelines for management of venous thromboembolism: optimal management of anticoagulation therapy. *Blood Adv.* 2018;2(22):3257-3291.

172. Powers WJ, Rabinstein AA, Ackerson T, et al. 2018 guidelines for the early management of patients with acute ischemic stroke: a guideline for healthcare professionals from the American Heart Association/American Stroke Association. *Stroke.* 2018; 49(3):e46-e110.

173. Ohene-Frempong K, Weiner SJ, Sleeper LA, et al. Cerebrovascular accidents in sickle cell disease: rates and risk factors. *Blood.* 1998;91(1):288-294.

174. Powars D, Wilson B, Imbus C, Pegelow C, Allen J. The natural history of stroke in sickle cell disease. *Am J Med.* 1978;65(3): 461-471.

175. Kassim AA, Galadanci NA, Pruthi S, DeBaun MR. How I treat and manage strokes in sickle cell disease. *Blood.* 2015;125(22): 3401-3410.

176. DeBaun MR, Kirkham FJ. Central nervous system complications and management in sickle cell disease. *Blood.* 2016;127(7):829-838.

177. Dobson SR, Holden KR, Nietert PJ, et al. Moyamoya syndrome in childhood sickle cell disease: a predictive factor for recurrent cerebrovascular events. *Blood.* 2002;99(9):3144-3150.

178. Adams RJ, Cox M, Ozark SD, et al. Coexistent sickle cell disease has no impact on the safety or outcome of lytic therapy in acute ischemic stroke: findings from Get With the Guidelines-Stroke. *Stroke.* 2017;48(3):686-691.

179. Noubiap JJ, Temgoua MN, Tankeu R, Tochie JN, Wonkam A, Bigna JJ. Sickle cell disease, sickle trait and the risk for venous thromboembolism: a systematic review and meta-analysis. *Thromb J.* 2018;16:27.

180. Yu TT, Nelson J, Streiff MB, Lanzkron S, Naik RP. Risk factors for venous thromboembolism in adults with hemoglobin SC or Sbeta(+) thalassemia genotypes. *Thromb Res.* 2016;141: 35-38.

181. Kelley D, Jones LT, Wu J, Bohm N. Evaluating the safety and effectiveness of venous thromboembolism prophylaxis in patients with sickle cell disease. *J Thromb Thrombolysis.* 2017;43(4): 463-468.

182. Morales E, Villanueva GI, Hsu LL, Seleski N. Should sickle cell disease be among the risk factors for use of thromboprophylaxis in adolescents and young adults? *Blood.* 2016;128:4855.

183. Bridges KR, Barabino GD, Brugnara C, et al. A multiparameter analysis of sickle erythrocytes in patients undergoing hydroxyurea therapy. *Blood.* 1996;88(12):4701-4710.

184. Gladwin MT, Shelhamer JH, Ognibene FP, et al. Nitric oxide donor properties of hydroxyurea in patients with sickle cell disease. *Br J Haematol.* 2002;116(2):436-444.

185. Adams RJ, Brambilla D, Optimizing Primary Stroke Prevention in Sickle Cell Anemia Trial I. Discontinuing prophylactic transfusions used to prevent stroke in sickle cell disease. *N Engl J Med.* 2005;353(26):2769-2778.

186. Adams RJ, McKie VC, Hsu L, et al. Prevention of a first stroke by transfusions in children with sickle cell anemia and abnormal

results on transcranial Doppler ultrasonography. *N Engl J Med.* 1998;339(1):5-11.

187. Ware RE, Davis BR, Schultz WH, et al. Hydroxycarbamide versus chronic transfusion for maintenance of transcranial doppler flow velocities in children with sickle cell anaemia-TCD With Transfusions Changing to Hydroxyurea (TWiTCH): a multicentre, open-label, phase 3, non-inferiority trial. *Lancet.* 2016;387(10019):661-670.

188. Louie JE, Anderson CJ, Fayaz MFK, et al. Case series supporting heme detoxification via therapeutic plasma exchange in acute multiorgan failure syndrome resistant to red blood cell exchange in sickle cell disease. *Transfusion.* 2018;58(2):470-479.

189. Hyacinth HI, Adams RJ, Greenberg CS, et al. Effect of chronic blood transfusion on biomarkers of coagulation activation and thrombin generation in sickle cell patients at risk for stroke. *PLoS One.* 2015;10(8):e0134193.

190. Noubouossie D, Key NS, Ataga KI. Coagulation abnormalities of sickle cell disease: relationship with clinical outcomes and the effect of disease modifying therapies. *Blood Rev.* 2016;30(4): 245-256.

191. Sparkenbaugh EM, Chantrathammachart P, Mickelson J, et al. Differential contribution of FXa and thrombin to vascular inflammation in a mouse model of sickle cell disease. *Blood.* 2014;123(11):1747-1756.

192. Sparkenbaugh EM, Chantrathammachart P, Chandarajoti K, Mackman N, Key NS, Pawlinski R. Thrombin-independent contribution of tissue factor to inflammation and cardiac hypertrophy in a mouse model of sickle cell disease. *Blood.* 2016;127(10): 1371-1373.

193. Camerer E, Huang W, Coughlin SR. Tissue factor- and factor X-dependent activation of protease-activated receptor 2 by factor VIIa. *Proc Natl Acad Sci U S A.* 2000;97(10):5255-5260.

194. Rao LV, Pendurthi UR. Tissue factor-factor VIIa signaling. *Arterioscler Thromb Vasc Biol.* 2005;25(1):47-56.

195. Arumugam PI, Mullins ES, Shanmukhappa SK, et al. Genetic diminution of circulating prothrombin ameliorates multi-organ pathologies in sickle cell disease mice. *Blood.* 2015;126(15):1844-1855.

196. Flick MJ, Du X, Degen JL. Fibrin(ogen)-alpha M beta 2 interactions regulate leukocyte function and innate immunity in vivo. *Exp Biol Med (Maywood).* 2004;229(11):1105-1110.

197. Flick MJ, Du X, Witte DP, et al. Leukocyte engagement of fibrin(ogen) via the integrin receptor alphaMbeta2/Mac-1 is critical for host inflammatory response in vivo. *J Clin Invest.* 2004;113(11):1596-1606.

198. Petzelbauer P, Zacharowski PA, Miyazaki Y, et al. The fibrin-derived peptide Bbeta15-42 protects the myocardium against ischemia-reperfusion injury. *Nat Med.* 2005;11(3):298-304.

199. Nasimuzzaman M, Arumugam PI, Mullins ES, et al. Elimination of the fibrinogen integrin alphaMbeta2-binding motif improves renal pathology in mice with sickle cell anemia. *Blood Adv.* 2019;3(9):1519-1532.

200. Palabrica T, Lobb R, Furie BC, et al. Leukocyte accumulation promoting fibrin deposition is mediated in vivo by P-selectin on adherent platelets. *Nature.* 1992;359(6398):848-851.

201. Andre P, Hartwell D, Hrachovinova I, Saffaripour S, Wagner DD. Pro-coagulant state resulting from high levels of soluble P-selectin in blood. *Proc Natl Acad Sci U S A.* 2000;97(25):13835-13840.

202. Telen MJ, Wun T, McCavit TL, et al. Randomized phase 2 study of GMI-1070 in SCD: reduction in time to resolution of vaso-occlusive events and decreased opioid use. *Blood.* 2015;125(17): 2656-2664.

203. Wun T, Styles L, DeCastro L, et al. Phase 1 study of the E-selectin inhibitor GMI 1070 in patients with sickle cell anemia. *PLoS One.* 2014;9(7):e101301.

204. Culmer DL, Dunbar ML, Hawley AE, et al. E-selectin inhibition with GMI-1271 decreases venous thrombosis without profoundly affecting tail vein bleeding in a mouse model. *Thromb Haemost.* 2017;117(6):1171-1181.

205. Boga C, Kozanoglu I, Ozdogu H, Ozyurek E. Plasma exchange in critically ill patients with sickle cell disease. *Transfus Apher Sci.* 2007;37(1):17-22.

206. Geigel EJ, Francis CW. Reversal of multiorgan system dysfunction in sickle cell disease with plasma exchange. *Acta Anaesthesiol Scand.* 1997;41(5):647-650.

207. Novelli EM, Kato GJ, Hildesheim ME, et al. Thrombospondin-1 inhibits ADAMTS13 activity in sickle cell disease. *Haematologica.* 2013;98(11):e132-134.

208. Banfi C, Brioschi M, Barbieri SS, et al. Mitochondrial reactive oxygen species: a common pathway for PAR1- and PAR2-mediated tissue factor induction in human endothelial cells. *J Thromb Haemost.* 2009;7(1):206-216.

209. Kirsch J, Schneider H, Pagel JI, et al. Endothelial dysfunction, and a prothrombotic, proinflammatory phenotype is caused by loss of mitochondrial thioredoxin reductase in endothelium. *Arterioscler Thromb Vasc Biol.* 2016;36(9):1891-1899.

210. Rossman MJ, Santos-Parker JR, Steward CAC, et al. Chronic supplementation with a mitochondrial antioxidant (MitoQ) improves vascular function in healthy older adults. *Hypertension.* 2018;71(6):1056-1063.

211. Snow BJ, Rolfe FL, Lockhart MM, et al. A double-blind, placebo-controlled study to assess the mitochondria-targeted antioxidant MitoQ as a disease-modifying therapy in Parkinson's disease. *Mov Disord.* 2010;25(11):1670-1674.

212. Villalba JM, Parrado C, Santos-Gonzalez M, Alcain FJ. Therapeutic use of coenzyme Q10 and coenzyme Q10-related compounds and formulations. *Expert Opin Investig Drugs.* 2010;19(4):535-554.

213. Hassell KL, Eckman JR, Lane PA. Acute multiorgan failure syndrome: a potentially catastrophic complication of severe sickle cell pain episodes. *Am J Med.* 1994;96(2):155-162.

214. Tedla FM, Friedman EA. Multiorgan failure during a sickle cell crisis in sickle/beta-thalassemia. *Am J Kidney Dis.* 2003;42(2):E6-E8.

215. Vichinsky EP, Styles LA, Colangelo LH, Wright EC, Castro O, Nickerson B. Acute chest syndrome in sickle cell disease: clinical presentation and course. Cooperative Study of Sickle Cell Disease. *Blood.* 1997;89(5):1787-1792.

216. Schnog JJ, Kremer Hovinga JA, Krieg S, et al. ADAMTS13 activity in sickle cell disease. *Am J Hematol.* 2006;81(7):492-498.

PART III
Emerging Therapeutics

Overview

David Rees, Sophie M. Lanzkron

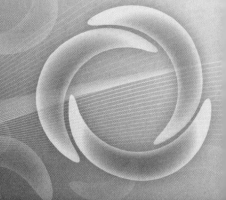

Although sickle cell disease (SCD) is probably the most common severe genetic disorder in the world, there are still only 3 therapeutic interventions that have been convincingly shown to alter the natural history of the condition in clinical trials: penicillin prophylaxis (prevention of invasive pneumococcal disease), hydroxyurea (reduction of acute complications, primary stroke prevention), and regular blood transfusion (primary stroke prevention). Although there are other treatments that are undoubtedly beneficial, including vaccination, analgesia, intermittent blood transfusion for symptomatic anemia, and hematopoietic stem cell transplantation, the treatment options in SCD are currently very limited.

Clinical management has lagged behind molecular discoveries. It was initially considered a form of rheumatism, and the treatment of acute pain in the 1920s, with rest and analgesia, was remarkably similar to its treatment today.[1] In addition, it was believed that SCD was nearly always lethal in childhood until the 1970s when specialist care started to develop, particularly in the United States with the Sickle Cell Anemia Control Act.

Clinical care and research for SCD have historically been underfunded relative to other rare inherited and life-threatening conditions such as cystic fibrosis (CF).[2,3] In a study examining funding per affected individual, funding was 11.4-fold greater for CF than SCD and included 3.5-fold higher National Institutes of Health (NIH) funding and 440-fold higher national foundation funding. NIH career development awards were similar for the 2 diseases despite that there are nearly 3-fold more individuals affected by SCD in the United States. Recent emphasis on SCD by the Department of Health and Human Services[4] and the American Society of Hematology is anticipated to change the landscape of research and access to care in the coming years.

To date, 3 randomized controlled trials have had a major impact on the management and prognosis of sickle cell anemia (SCA) in high-income countries: the Prophylaxis With Oral Penicillin in Children With Sickle Cell Anemia (PROPS) study showing that penicillin prophylaxis reduces morbidity and mortality from invasive pneumococcal disease at least until the age of 5 years;[5] the Multicenter Study of Hydroxyurea (MSH) showing the reduction of painful episodes and acute chest syndrome by hydroxyurea in adults;[6] and the Stroke Prevention Trial in Sickle Cell Anemia (STOP) showing evidence for primary stroke prevention using transcranial Doppler measurements and long-term blood transfusion.[7] Further studies have demonstrated extended benefits of hydroxyurea, including in primary stroke prevention,[8] and most importantly have shown its effectiveness in sub-Saharan Africa.[9] It is now widely accepted that specialist care should include neonatal screening, prophylaxis against infection, primary stroke prevention, and widespread use of hydroxyurea. However, even with these interventions, median life expectancy is still reduced by 20 or 30 years in SCA,[10] and this standard of care in only available in high-income countries. This improvement in life expectancy has mostly been achieved through the application of basic supportive medical care and has had little impact in African countries where the disease predominates and the majority of patients still die in childhood.[11] However, the situation seems to be improving, with specific treatments for SCD beginning to emerge and many clinical trials including patients in Africa.

Emerging Therapeutic Approaches

Reducing the Damage Caused by HbS Polymerization

Although almost every measurable parameter is abnormal in SCD, all pathology arises from a single point mutation in the β-globin gene, which is only expressed in red cells, and the tendency of deoxygenated sickle hemoglobin (HbS) to polymerize. Inhibition of HbS polymerization has proved remarkably difficult, but other therapeutic options are starting to emerge, particularly targeting downstream consequences of polymerization.

Allogeneic Hematopoietic Stem Cell Transplantation

Allogeneic hematopoietic stem cell transplantation (HSCT) is the only curative treatment currently available for SCD. It was first performed successfully for SCA in the early 1980s in a girl who also had acute myeloid leukemia[12] and subsequently has been extended as a treatment for SCD itself. It is still performed relatively rarely. For example, in Europe, approximately 200 HSCTs for SCD were performed in 2017,[13] compared to a birth rate of about 3000 patients per year.[14] Several factors limit the use of HSCT in SCD at the moment: toxicity, availability of donors, cost, availability of expertise, and facilities. Although outcomes using human leukocyte antigen (HLA)-matched sibling donors in children are good and improving, with mortality of about 5%, the outcomes using medical treatment are also good and improving, and only 10% to 20% patients have suitable sibling donors. One of the main developments emerging in this area is the expansion of the potential pool of donors by using unrelated matched donors or haploidentical relatives. To date, the results from these transplantations are significantly worse than those using HLA-identical siblings and are only justified in clinical trials and for the most severely affected patients.[15] As outcomes improve, this balance will change, although there is likely to be a parallel improvement in nontransplant outcomes. Progress in the development and deployment of HSCT strategies is presented in detail in Chapter 25.

Gene Correction and Addition

Gene therapy in its various forms for SCD is still in its infancy. Although there are now a large number of groups working in this area and many clinical trials, < 50 patients have currently undergone this treatment. Most clinical protocols to date involve gene addition,[16] with significant limitations in the efficiency of transfection; long-term outcomes are unknown, and it is unclear whether this will be a curative or ameliorative treatment. Protocols are starting to emerge involving gene editing with a view to directly correct the HbS mutation[17] or increase fetal hemoglobin (HbF) production, and it seems likely that these will become an increasing part of the therapeutic armamentarium in the next decades.[18] Use is currently limited by the toxicity of myeloablative chemotherapy, although developments such as in vivo gene correction may make this less of a problem. Progress in the development of gene therapy is detailed in Chapter 29.

Inhibition of HbS Polymerization

All of the complications of SCD stem from HbS polymerization, and complete inhibition of HbS polymerization would be curative. Over the years, many approaches have been tried to develop therapies based on this approach, with limited success. The most direct way of inhibiting polymerization is to develop small molecules to block contacts between the hemoglobin molecules at the points of polymerization. Few or no drugs with this mode of action have gotten close to clinical trials, which is perhaps surprising now that it is possible to design and engineer small molecules precisely. A particular problem with this approach is that there is up to 500 g of hemoglobin in adults, meaning that very large amounts of drug would need to be given and that toxicity would be likely unless the binding to HbS was specific, which is difficult to achieve. As design of small-molecule drugs progresses and dynamic protein structures are being modeled, it seems possible that such a small molecule will be developed and prove to be a highly effective treatment,[19] although currently, there are no trials of drugs with this mode of action.

Although specific small-molecule inhibitors of HbS polymerization are not available, an alternative strategy to inhibit polymerization has been successful: the induction of γ-globin synthesis, leading to increased erythrocyte HbF concentrations. This both dilutes the concentration of HbS in the cell and generates compound hemoglobin tetramers, containing both βs- and γ-globins, that terminate polymer formation. Hydroxyurea predominantly functions via this mechanism and is still the only widely used effective drug in SCD, with good evidence that it reduces the frequency and severity of acute complications and protects against progressive cerebrovascular disease.[8,20] Although hydroxyurea may have other pharmacologic effects, nearly all its therapeutic actions seem to come from HbF induction.[21] Several other drugs to promote HbF production are now in clinical trials, including decitabine, which modifies DNA methylation; pomalidomide, which reprograms transcription in hematopoietic stem cells[22]; metformin, which is a FOXO3 agonist[23]; and panobinostat, which is an histone deacetylase inhibitor.[24]

Another approach to inhibit HbS polymerization involves increasing the proportion of HbS in the R-state conformation, which does not polymerize. This necessitates increasing the oxygen affinity of HbS, either by chemically modifying the molecule or reducing concentrations of 2,3-diphosphoglycerate (2,3-DPG). Other molecules are known to increase the oxygen affinity of hemoglobin but have been difficult to use therapeutically because the drugs are either toxic or only weakly effective, such as vanillins. Recently, voxelotor has been specifically designed to have this effect, by covalently binding to the N-terminal of the α-globin chain. It seems to be well tolerated and to increase hemoglobin levels by 10 to 20 g/L, but it remains to be seen how this translates into clinical benefit.[25] Similarly, reducing the intraerythrocytic level of 2,3-DPG, which is increased in sickle erythrocytes, markedly reduces the rate of polymerization, although no current investigational agents target this directly. Potentially, drugs increasing pyruvate kinase activity may be beneficial in SCD for this reason.[26]

Reducing Red Blood Cell Dehydration and Hemolysis

Sickle erythrocytes are known to be leaky and, in particular, lose more potassium ions than they gain other cations, which causes a net water loss, increasing the concentration of HbS.[27,28] The delay between deoxygenation and the start of polymerization is dependent on the concentration of HbS raised to the power of 30, and therefore, a very small decrease in erythrocyte HbS concentration causes marked slowing of HbS polymerization.[29] Red blood cell hydration can be improved by either reducing plasma osmolarity or inhibiting cation loss through the membrane. Plasma hyponatremia, induced by intravenous 5% dextrose and desmopressin, causes some improvements in laboratory parameters but is difficult to maintain and causes symptoms of hyponatremia.[30] Senicapoc was used in a clinical trial to inhibit the Gardos channel and reduce cellular potassium loss and again caused significant improvements in red blood cell parameters, with reduced hemolysis but failed to reduce frequency of acute painful episodes.[31] In fact, in SCA patients, hemolysis improved but frequency of acute pain increased, possibly related to the increased hematocrit. A partially similar phenotypic effect is seen when SCA is coinherited with α thalassemia trait.[32,33] Inhibition of erythrocyte cation loss continues to be an interesting therapeutic candidate mechanism, although few agents are being actively developed in this area at the moment.

Various interventions, such as those inhibiting HbS polymerization or improving red blood cell hydration, also inevitably lead to a reduction in hemolysis. Hemolysis is harmful in itself, with the release of hemoglobin and other red blood cell constituents into the plasma.[34] Many association studies suggest that reducing hemolysis offers some benefits, although it remains to be shown directly whether reducing hemolysis is beneficial per se, independent of reduced vaso-occlusion and anemia.

Treatment of Vascular Endothelial Dysfunction

A lot of the pathology of SCD results from vascular endothelial dysfunction, particularly chronic complications such as pulmonary hypertension, cerebrovascular disease, and leg ulcers.[35] The origin of this dysfunction is multifactorial, and hemolysis is an important part of the pathology.[36] So far, there are few or no treatments directly and specifically targeting vasculopathy, although treatments reducing vaso-occlusion, hemolysis, inflammation, and hypercoagulability are likely to reduce vascular endothelial damage. Early studies in sickle cell mice suggest that infusions of haptoglobin, to chaperone free hemoglobin molecules, may have some beneficial effects.[37]

Anticoagulation, Antiplatelet Agents, and Antiadhesion Molecules

Laboratory and clinical data support the idea that one of the downstream consequences of HbS polymerization is an increased tendency for abnormal blood clotting in both arteries and veins, as shown by increased incidence of venous thrombosis, and abnormalities in platelet functions, coagulation factors, and the abnormal expression of adhesion molecules, both on vascular endothelium and blood corpuscles[38] (see Chapter 22 on thrombophilia in SCD). There is a fairly long history of clinical trials of anticoagulants and antiplatelet drugs, which so far have not shown convincing benefit, although ongoing trials include a heparin derivative, factor Xa inhibitors, and an oral inhibitor of adenosine monophosphate (ADP)-mediated platelet activation.[39] Interestingly, a recent clinical trial of a P-selectin blocker, crizanlizumab, showed a significant reduction in vaso-occlusive complications.[40] Crizanlizumab has recently been licensed for use in the United States and is undergoing further trials in children in Europe. However, clinical trials of other drugs with a predominantly antiadhesion mode of action have failed to show benefit, including poloxamer,[39] rivipansel,[41] and sevuparin.[42]

Blood Transfusion

Blood transfusion is useful in SCD principally to correct anemia or to reduce the number of circulating erythrocytes able to sickle, cause vaso-occlusion, and hemolyze. The use of blood transfusion is well established in SCD, although few clinical trials have assessed benefit, other than in primary stroke prevention and to a lesser extent prevention of perioperative complications. Blood can be given as a simple top-up transfusion or as an exchange transfusion, depending on the starting hemoglobin and the targets for postexchange levels of hemoglobin and percent HbS. Advances in blood transfusion seem likely to involve the increased use of extended genotypic blood grouping, the reduction of complications with hemolytic transfusion reactions,[43] and in the more distant future, the use of cultured blood units that are negative for all potentially immunogenic antigens.[44] More clinical trials may also better define the role of blood transfusion in different clinical situations, including pregnancy, progressive liver disease, and priapism.

Reducing Oxidative Stress and Reperfusion Injury

Oxidative stress is a slightly vague term applying to conditions in which there is evidence of abnormal oxidation of molecules, such as the generation of methemoglobin. Biomarker studies suggest that this is one of the many downstream problems in SCD. Oxidative stress seems to arise from 2 main sources: intravascular hemolysis releasing free hemoglobin and heme into the circulation and tissue infarction releasing other cellular contents. Tissue ischemia also results in further damage, when vaso-occlusion is relieved and reperfusion of the damaged tissue occurs.[21] Many different drugs with antioxidant activity are available, and >10 different trials of antioxidants in SCD have been undertaken. Most notably, a randomized controlled trial of L-glutamine in SCA showed a significant decrease in the number of painful episodes per year, from a median of 4 to 3 episodes.[45] It is still unclear how useful this moderate decrease in pain will be in clinical practice, although the drug is now licensed for use in the United States and more evidence should start to emerge.

Anti-inflammatory Drugs

In SCD, acute and chronic inflammation occurs as a result of tissue infarction, ischemia, and high levels of free heme.[46] Inflammation seems to be an important part of many pathologies, including acute chest syndrome, leg ulcers, vasculopathy, and splenic infarction. Nonsteroidal anti-inflammatory drugs are perhaps the most commonly prescribed drugs in SCD to control acute pain and, to a lesser extent, chronic pain. Many drugs with anti-inflammatory actions are currently being assessed in SCD, including selectin antagonists (crizanlizumab, rivipansel), statins, interleukin-1β blockers, omega-3 fatty acids, and intravenous immunoglobulins.[39] Many of these drugs have multiple actions apart from being anti-inflammatories, and it remains to be seen whether any of these will make it into routine clinical practice.

Treatment of Acute Complications

The best-known burden of SCD is the vaso-occlusive crisis (VOC). VOCs are acute, excruciatingly painful events and are the leading cause of hospital and emergency department (ED) utilization.[47] Although SCD is considered a rare disease in the United States, the burden of ED care and subsequent hospitalization is high. In 2006, total charges for all sickle cell ED visits in the United States was estimated to be $356 million.[48] In 2011, there were 317,557 ED visits for people with SCD, and 82% of these visits were by people aged 18 years and older. In addition, 30-day readmission rates for this patient population are the highest of any recorded diagnosis, at 31.9%.[49] These estimates suggest that SCD confers a significant burden on the patient, with a parallel excessive impact on the health care system.

Although VOC is the most common complication of SCD, there have been no randomized controlled trials evaluating best practices for managing these events. Using an expert panel, Wang et al[50] developed a set of quality measures for the treatment of children with SCD. This group identified 41 measures that could be used to assess health systems quality of care for children with SCD. Two of these measures were for the management of acute pain. The first measure was that children who present with an acute pain episode should receive a parenteral analgesic within 60 minutes of registration or 30 minutes of triage. The second measure was that there should be a reassessment of pain level repeated within 30 minutes of the first dose of analgesic. These metrics are now being used in guidelines to assist in improving outcomes for patients, but the evidence on which they are based is quite limited. The current standard of care for the management of acute painful events has remained unchanged for the past 40 years and includes the use of intravenous hydration and parenteral pain medications. Which fluids and pain medications to use has never been rigorously investigated. Although there has been success in developing novel therapies to prevent VOC, therapies to treat acute VOC have not been successful. Studies using inhaled nitric oxide, rivipansel, poloxamer-188, and sevuparin have all failed to meet their primary end points. The concern with developing therapies for acute management is the end point of resolution of VOC, which is subjective, making these studies enormously challenging to design and complete. Improving the ability to prevent and treat painful events will be a tremendous advance for those living with SCD.

Another important aspect of the management of acute painful events is consideration of where that management occurs. A number of studies have demonstrated that dedicated acute care facilities such as "day hospitals" or "infusion clinics" that provide care exclusively to people with SCD provide improved outcomes over standard ED care.[51,52] In addition, studies have shown that the use of patient-specific treatment plans can improve care in the ED.[53] Regardless of where care is provided, it is clear that improving access to high-quality care in the acute setting is an essential component to improving outcomes.

Multidisciplinary Care

Access to high-quality care entails having a broad range of providers available to provide care. In addition to identifying nephrologists, pulmonologists, orthopedic surgeons, retinal specialists, and others with expertise in managing patients with sickle cell complications that fall within their specialty, there is a need to have additional team members who can help with the day-to-day management of complex physical, mental, and social issues that arise in the care of people with SCD.

A key member of any comprehensive team is someone versed in the management of chronic pain. The Pain in Sickle Cell Epidemiologic Study was the first to show the burden of chronic pain in people living with SCD, with 30% of subjects reporting pain in >95% of collected diary days.[54] Other studies show that almost 70% of adults report having chronic pain.[55] Only recently has the sickle community defined chronic pain in SCD in order to aid in research and clinical care around this prevalent complication of the disease.[56] Treatment of chronic pain has long centered on the use of opioid therapy, of which the benefits have been called into question.[57] Although there may be limitations to the use of chronic opioid therapy, there has been very little research done on alternatives. The lack of evidence to drive care necessitates having someone on the sickle care team with expertise in chronic pain management.

The intertwining of pain and psychological comorbidities among those with SCD necessitates easy access to psychological services in comprehensive sickle cell care. The prevalence of depression is significantly higher in individuals with SCD than in the general African American population, and individuals with depression have more pain.[58] Anxiety and depression have also been found to predict pain intensity and pain interference.[59] In addition to psychiatric comorbidities, the effect of stroke and silent cerebral infarcts on patients' ability to adhere to therapy, complete educational goals, and maintain employment needs to be addressed. Studies have demonstrated lower IQ scores and executive dysfunction in children and adults with SCD.[60-62] Access to comprehensive sickle care includes the ability to obtain formal neuropsychiatric testing and then provide access to therapy to assist patients with tools to overcome neurocognitive dysfunction.

There are limited data on the use of multidisciplinary models in the care of adults with SCD. These models have been shown to decrease acute care utilization in children in the United States and often consist of hematologists, pain management specialist, psychotherapists, nurses, and social workers.[63] These models have also been suggested as necessary to improve transition from pediatric to adult care, which remains an enormous challenge. Increased ED utilization and mortality have been seen and are of great concern for youth in the middle of transitioning to adult care.[64-66] Improvements in outcomes have been seen using multidisciplinary care models for children in other countries. In Italy, a multidisciplinary clinic including pediatric hematologists, residents, and nurses and, in India, a team including tribal nurses[67,68] have been able to improve outcomes by improving adherence to health care maintenance recommendations.

Multidrug Therapy

As more therapeutic options start to emerge, the possibility of combination therapy arises. Nearly all new drugs are assessed in combination with hydroxyurea, but it is appealing to attempt to block many of the downstream pathologic consequences of HbS polymerization and conceivable that such an approach may have significant, additive benefits. For example, the combination of a P-selectin blocker, an interleukin-1β blocker, a platelet inhibitor, a drug to reduce hemolysis, and an antioxidant might ameliorate many of the harmful consequences of HbS polymerization in a way that is analogous to the largely successful multidrug treatment of acute leukemia. However, many of these emerging drugs are expensive, making such combinations prohibitively costly, and the risk of side effects would be high. Equally, it seems unlikely that appropriate clinical trials will ever be performed to prove the efficacy of such approaches, and novel curative gene-editing approaches will start to predominate.

Conclusion

People living with SCD have had limited therapeutic options and significantly decreased life expectancy. The future, however, is looking bright, with a number of new therapies in late-phase development and many more in the pipeline. As new therapies become available, it will be imperative that people living with SCD have access to high-quality, multidisciplinary care that addresses both the physical and psychosocial aspects of the disease.

High-Yield Facts

- ◆ The range of treatment options in SCD is still very limited, despite recent advances and the development of several new drugs.
- ◆ It is encouraging that new drugs are emerging, although evidence of clinical efficacy is still very limited.
- ◆ These novel agents will be very expensive. The cost may be prohibitive in many high-income countries, and it is very difficult to see how they will help those in low-income countries, where the vast majority of patients live.
- ◆ There are still no treatments aimed at specifically treating the acute symptoms of SCD, such as pain and acute chest syndrome.

References

1. Chaplin H. *Lenabell. A Doctor's Memoir of a Remarkable Woman's Eighty Year Battle With Sickle Cell Disease.* Xlibris Corp; 2003.
2. Smith LA, Oyeku SO, Homer C, Zuckerman B. Sickle cell disease: a question of equity and quality. *Pediatrics.* 2006;117(5):1763-1770.
3. Grosse SD, Schechter MS, Kulkarni R, Lloyd-Puryear MA, Strickland B, Trevathan E. Models of comprehensive multidisciplinary care for individuals in the United States with genetic disorders. *Pediatrics.* 2009;123(1):407-412.
4. Office of Minority Health. Sickle cell disease: increasing access and improving care. US Department of Health and Human Services; 2011. https://minorityhealth.hhs.gov/assets/pdf/Checked/1/sickel_cell_anemia_factsheet.pdf. Accessed July 17, 2020.
5. Gaston MH, Verter JI, Woods G, et al. Prophylaxis with oral penicillin in children with sickle cell anemia. A randomized trial. *N Engl J Med.* 1986;314(25):1593-1599.
6. Charache S, Terrin ML, Moore RD, et al. Effect of hydroxyurea on the frequency of painful crises in sickle cell anemia. Investigators of the Multicenter Study of Hydroxyurea in Sickle Cell Anemia. *N Engl J Med.* 1995;332(20):1317-1322.
7. Adams RJ, McKie VC, Hsu L, et al. Prevention of a first stroke by transfusions in children with sickle cell anemia and abnormal results on transcranial Doppler ultrasonography. *N Engl J Med.* 1998;339(1):5-11.
8. Ware RE, Davis BR, Schultz WH, et al. Hydroxycarbamide versus chronic transfusion for maintenance of transcranial doppler flow velocities in children with sickle cell anaemia-TCD With Transfusions Changing to Hydroxyurea (TWiTCH): a multicentre, open-label, phase 3, non-inferiority trial. *Lancet.* 2016;387(10019):661-670.
9. Tshilolo L, Tomlinson G, Williams TN, et al. Hydroxyurea for children with sickle cell anemia in sub-Saharan Africa. *N Engl J Med.* 2019;380(2):121-131.
10. Gardner K, Douiri A, Drasar E, et al. Survival in adults with sickle cell disease in a high-income setting. *Blood.* 2016;128(10):1436-1438.
11. Makani J, Cox SE, Soka D, et al. Mortality in sickle cell anemia in Africa: a prospective cohort study in Tanzania. *PLoS One.* 2011;6(2):e14699.
12. Johnson FL, Look AT, Gockerman J, Ruggiero MR, Dalla-Pozza L, Billings FT 3rd. Bone-marrow transplantation in a patient with sickle-cell anemia. *N Engl J Med.* 1984;311(12):780-783.
13. Passweg JR, Baldomero H, Basak GW, et al. The EBMT activity survey report 2017: a focus on allogeneic HCT for nonmalignant indications and on the use of non-HCT cell therapies. *Bone Marrow Transplant.* 2019;54(10):1575-1585.

14. Piel FB, Patil AP, Howes RE, et al. Global epidemiology of sickle haemoglobin in neonates: a contemporary geostatistical model-based map and population estimates. *Lancet*. 2013;381(9861): 142-151.

15. de Montalembert M, Brousse V, Chakravorty S, et al. Are the risks of treatment to cure a child with severe sickle cell disease too high? *BMJ*. 2017;359:j5250.

16. Ribeil JA, Hacein-Bey-Abina S, Payen E, et al. Gene therapy in a patient with sickle cell disease. *N Engl J Med*. 2017;376(9):848-855.

17. Anzalone AV, Randolph PB, Davis JR, et al. Search-and-replace genome editing without double-strand breaks or donor DNA. *Nature*. 2019;576(7785):149-157.

18. Orkin SH, Bauer DE. Emerging genetic therapy for sickle cell disease. *Annu Rev Med*. 2019;70:257-271.

19. Eaton WA, Bunn HF. Treating sickle cell disease by targeting HbS polymerization. *Blood*. 2017;129(20):2719-2726.

20. Ware RE. How I use hydroxyurea to treat young patients with sickle cell anemia. *Blood*. 2010;115(26):5300-5311.

21. Ware RE, de Montalembert M, Tshilolo L, Abboud MR. Sickle cell disease. *Lancet*. 2017;390(10091):311-323.

22. Dulmovits BM, Appiah-Kubi AO, Papoin J, et al. Pomalidomide reverses gamma-globin silencing through the transcriptional reprogramming of adult hematopoietic progenitors. *Blood*. 2016; 127(11):1481-1492.

23. Zhang Y, Paikari A, Sumazin P, et al. Metformin induces FOXO3-dependent fetal hemoglobin production in human primary erythroid cells. *Blood*. 2018;132(3):321-333.

24. Bradner JE, Mak R, Tanguturi SK, et al. Chemical genetic strategy identifies histone deacetylase 1 (HDAC1) and HDAC2 as therapeutic targets in sickle cell disease. *Proc Natl Acad Sci U S A*. 2010; 107(28):12617-12622.

25. Vichinsky E, Hoppe CC, Ataga KI, et al. A phase 3 randomized trial of voxelotor in sickle cell disease. *N Engl J Med*. 2019;381(6): 509-519.

26. Yang H, Merica E, Chen Y, et al. Phase 1 single- and multiple-ascending-dose randomized studies of the safety, pharmacokinetics, and pharmacodynamics of AG-348, a first-in-class allosteric activator of pyruvate kinase R, in healthy volunteers. *Clin Pharmacol Drug Dev*. 2019;8(2):246-259.

27. Tosteson DC, Shea E, Darling RC. Potassium and sodium of red blood cells in sickle cell anemia. *J Clin Invest*. 1952;31(4):406-411.

28. Brugnara C. Sickle cell dehydration: pathophysiology and therapeutic applications. *Clin Hemorheol Microcirc*. 2018;68(2-3):187-204.

29. Hofrichter J, Ross PD, Eaton WA. Kinetics and mechanism of deoxyhemoglobin S gelation: a new approach to understanding sickle cell disease. *Proc Natl Acad Sci U S A*. 1974;71(12):4864-4868.

30. Rosa RM, Bierer BE, Thomas R, et al. A study of induced hyponatremia in the prevention and treatment of sickle-cell crisis. *N Engl J Med*. 1980;303(20):1138-1143.

31. Ataga KI, Reid M, Ballas SK, et al. Improvements in haemolysis and indicators of erythrocyte survival do not correlate with acute vaso-occlusive crises in patients with sickle cell disease: a phase III randomized, placebo-controlled, double-blind study of the Gardos channel blocker senicapoc (ICA-17043). *Br J Haematol*. 2011;153(1):92-104.

32. Higgs DR, Aldridge BE, Lamb J, et al. The interaction of alpha-thalassemia and homozygous sickle-cell disease. *N Engl J Med*. 1982;306(24):1441-1446.

33. Embury SH, Dozy AM, Miller J, et al. Concurrent sickle-cell anemia and alpha-thalassemia: effect on severity of anemia. *N Engl J Med*. 1982;306(5):270-274.

34. Reiter CD, Wang X, Tanus-Santos JE, et al. Cell-free hemoglobin limits nitric oxide bioavailability in sickle-cell disease. *Nat Med*. 2002;8(12):1383-1389.

35. Kato GJ, Steinberg MH, Gladwin MT. Intravascular hemolysis and the pathophysiology of sickle cell disease. *J Clin Invest*. 2017;127(3):750-760.

36. Kato GJ, Hebbel RP, Steinberg MH, Gladwin MT. Vasculopathy in sickle cell disease: Biology, pathophysiology, genetics, translational medicine, and new research directions. *Am J Hematol*. 2009;84(9):618-625.

37. Belcher JD, Chen C, Nguyen J, et al. Haptoglobin and hemopexin inhibit vaso-occlusion and inflammation in murine sickle cell disease: role of heme oxygenase-1 induction. *PLoS One*. 2018;13(4):e0196455.

38. Wun T, Brunson A. Sickle cell disease: an inherited thrombophilia. *Hematology Am Soc Hematol Educ Program*. 2016; 2016(1):640-647.

39. Telen MJ, Malik P, Vercellotti GM. Therapeutic strategies for sickle cell disease: towards a multi-agent approach. *Nat Rev Drug Discov*. 2019;18(2):139-158.

40. Ataga KI, Kutlar A, Kanter J, et al. Crizanlizumab for the prevention of pain crises in sickle cell disease. *N Engl J Med*. 2017;376(5): 429-439.

41. Pfizer. Pfizer announces phase 3 top-line results for rivipansel in patients with sickle cell disease experiencing a vaso-occlusive crisis. https://www.pfizer.com/news/press-release/press-release-detail/pfizer_announces_phase_3_top_line_results_for_rivipansel_in_patients_with_sickle_cell_disease_experiencing_a_vaso_occlusive_crisis. Accessed July 17, 2020.

42. Modus Therapeutics. Modus Therapeutics announces the results of its global, randomized, placebo-controlled phase 2 clinical trial evaluating sevuparin for the management of acute vaso-occlusive crisis (VOC) in patients with sickle cell disease (SCD). https://www.modustx.com/modus-therapeutics-announces-the-results-of-its-global-randomized-placebo-controlled-phase-2-clinical-trial/. Accessed July 17, 2020.

43. Chou ST, Westhoff CM. Application of genomics for transfusion therapy in sickle cell anemia. *Blood Cells Mol Dis*. 2017; 67():148-154.

44. Hawksworth J, Satchwell TJ, Meinders M, et al. Enhancement of red blood cell transfusion compatibility using CRISPR-mediated erythroblast gene editing. *EMBO Mol Med*. 2018;10(6):e8454.

45. Niihara Y, Miller ST, Kanter J, et al. A phase 3 trial of l-glutamine in sickle cell disease. *N Engl J Med*. 2018;379(3):226-235.

46. Mendonca R, Silveira AA, Conran N. Red cell DAMPs and inflammation. *Inflamm Res*. 2016;65(9):665-678.

47. Platt OS, Thorington BD, Brambilla DJ, et al. Pain in sickle cell disease. Rates and risk factors. *N Engl J Med*. 1991;325(1): 11-16.

48. Lanzkron S, Carroll CP, Haywood C Jr. The burden of emergency department use for sickle-cell disease: an analysis of the national emergency department sample database. *Am J Hematol*. 2010;85(10):797-799.

49. Elixhauser A, Steiner C. Readmissions to U.S. hospitals by diagnosis, 2010: Statistical Brief #153. 2006. http://www.ncbi.nlm.nih.gov/pubmed/24006550. Accessed July 17, 2020.

50. Wang CJ, Kavanagh PL, Little AA, Holliman JB, Sprinz PG. Quality-of-care indicators for children with sickle cell disease. *Pediatrics*. 2011;128(3):484-493.

51. Lanzkron S, Carroll CP, Hill P, David M, Paul N, Haywood C Jr. Impact of a dedicated infusion clinic for acute

management of adults with sickle cell pain crisis. *Am J Hematol.* 2015;90(5):376-380.

52. Benjamin LJ, Swinson GI, Nagel RL. Sickle cell anemia day hospital: an approach for the management of uncomplicated painful crises. *Blood.* 2000;95(4):1130-1136.

53. Tanabe P, Silva S, Bosworth HB, et al. A randomized controlled trial comparing two vaso-occlusive episode (VOE) protocols in sickle cell disease (SCD). *Am J Hematol.* 2018;93(2):159-168.

54. Smith WR, Penberthy LT, Bovbjerg VE, et al. Daily assessment of pain in adults with sickle cell disease. *Ann Intern Med.* 2008;148(2):94-101.

55. Lanzkron S, Little J, Field J, et al. Increased acute care utilization in a prospective cohort of adults with sickle cell disease. *Blood Adv.* 2018;2(18):2412-2417.

56. Field JJ, Ballas SK, Campbell CM, et al. Analgesic, anesthetic, and addiction clinical trial translations, innovations, opportunities, and networks-american pain society-american academy of pain medicine pain taxonomy diagnostic criteria for acute sickle cell disease pain. *J Pain.* 2019;20(7):746-759.

57. Carroll CP, Lanzkron S, Haywood C, et al. Chronic opioid therapy and central sensitization in sickle cell disease. *Am J Prev Med.* 2016;51(1 suppl 1):S69-S77.

58. Brandow AM, DeBaun MR. Key components of pain management for children and adults with sickle cell disease. *Hematol Oncol Clin North Am.* 2018;32(3):535-550.

59. Master S, Arnold C, Davis T, Shi R, Mansour RP. Anxiety, depression, pain intensity and interference in adult patients with sickle cell disease. *Blood.* 2016;128(22):1312.

60. Cichowitz C, Carroll CP, Strouse JJ, Haywood C Jr, Lanzkron S. Screening for neurocognitive dysfunction in an adult population with sickle cell disease. *Blood.* 2014;124(21):2717.

61. Hijmans CT, Fijnvandraat K, Grootenhuis MA, et al. Neurocognitive deficits in children with sickle cell disease: a comprehensive profile. *Pediatr Blood Cancer.* 2011;56(5):783-788.

62. Vichinsky EP, Neumayr LD, Gold JI, et al. Neuropsychological dysfunction and neuroimaging abnormalities in neurologically intact adults with sickle cell anemia. *JAMA.* 2010;303(18):1823-1831.

63. Brandow AM, Weisman SJ, Panepinto JA. The impact of a multidisciplinary pain management model on sickle cell disease pain hospitalizations. *Pediatr Blood Cancer.* 2011;56(5):789-793.

64. Crosby LE, Quinn CT, Kalinyak KA. A biopsychosocial model for the management of patients with sickle-cell disease transitioning to adult medical care. *Adv Ther.* 2015;32(4):293-305.

65. Blinder MA, Duh MS, Sasane M, Trahey A, Paley C, Vekeman F. Age-related emergency department reliance in patients with sickle cell disease. *J Emerg Med.* 2015;49(4):513-522.

66. McLaughlin JF, Ballas SK. High mortality among children with sickle cell anemia and overt stroke who discontinue blood transfusion after transition to an adult program. *Transfusion.* 2016;56(5):1014-1021.

67. Colombatti R, Montanaro M, Guasti F, et al. Comprehensive care for sickle cell disease immigrant patients: a reproducible model achieving high adherence to minimum standards of care. *Pediatr Blood Cancer.* 2012;59(7):1275-1279.

68. Nimgaonkar V, Krishnamurti L, Prabhakar H, Menon N. Comprehensive integrated care for patients with sickle cell disease in a remote aboriginal tribal population in southern India. *Pediatr Blood Cancer.* 2014;61(4):702-705.

Transfusion Therapy in Sickle Cell Disease

Authors: *Sally A. Campbell-Lee, Anoosha Habibi,*
Darrell J. Triulzi

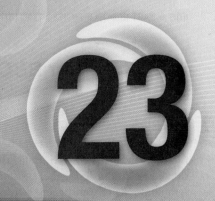

Chapter Outline

Overview

Red blood cell (RBC) transfusion has been shown to be beneficial as part of the treatment and management of sickle cell disease (SCD), whether as episodic treatment for an occurrence of acute anemia or as chronic transfusion for prevention of stroke recurrence. RBCs transfused to patients with SCD should, at minimum, be from donors negative for hemoglobin S (HbS), but patients may also benefit from leukoreduction of these blood components. As with any transfusion, RBC transfusion should only be used when the benefit to the patient outweighs the risks, which in this instance include transfusion-transmitted infectious diseases, transfusion reactions, RBC alloimmunization, and iron overload. However, because SCD patients have one of the highest incidences of RBC alloimmunization among transfused patients, strategies focused on prophylactic Rh and Kell antigen matching and the increased use of automated RBC exchange appear to mitigate the risks of RBC alloimmunization and transfusion-related iron overload, respectively. In the event of complex alloimmunization or hyperhemolysis, transfusion indications may be limited and transfusion may require preventative immunomodulatory therapies.

Indications for RBC Transfusion in SCD

Anemia

When the hemoglobin decreases below the patient's baseline value and symptoms occur, transfusion of RBCs can be considered by administering the fewest units necessary to alleviate symptoms. RBC transfusion increases hemoglobin, reduces the proportion of HbS in the circulation, and improves oxygen delivery. The underlying cause of the acute anemia, defined as a decrease in hemoglobin by ≥2 g/dL below the baseline value, should be investigated.[1] Acute anemia may be caused by aplastic crisis, splenic or hepatic sequestration, or delayed hemolytic transfusion reactions (if the patient has been transfused in the past 3-4 weeks), or it may be a harbinger of acute chest syndrome in a patient with a vaso-occlusive crisis (VOC).

Stroke and Stroke Prevention

Without preventative measures, 8% of children with SCD in high-income countries will have strokes by the age of 14 years.[2] In children with SCD, strokes are usually due to occlusion of the internal carotid or middle cerebral artery; however, adults may have hemorrhagic or ischemic strokes.[1] In sub-Saharan African countries and in India, before the age of 18 years, 50% of children with SCD will have either a stroke or a silent cerebral infarction.[3] Among the risk factors for cerebral ischemia in SCD are the existence of cerebral vasculopathy, anemia with a compensatory increase in cerebral blood flow and increased HbS percentage (HbS%) with decreasing cerebrovascular reserve, and a rapid increase in hemoglobin levels to >12 g/dL.[3] Thus, the primary goal of RBC transfusion in the treatment of acute stroke, prevention of primary stroke in those with abnormal transcranial Doppler ultrasound, and prevention of stroke recurrence is to reduce the HbS% to ≤30% and to maintain the hemoglobin close to 10 g/dL. In acute stroke, it is particularly important to rapidly reduce the HbS% to >30% and, where available, to perform automated RBC exchange (RBCX). When children who received a simple transfusion at the time of an acute stroke were compared to those who received RBCX, there was a 5-fold greater relative risk of a second stroke in simple transfusion recipients.[4] In a landmark randomized controlled trial of RBC transfusions every 3 to 6 weeks to maintain the HbS at <30% for prevention of primary stroke in children with elevated transcranial Dopplers, when compared to observation alone, there was a 92% relative risk reduction of primary stroke with transfusion.[5] Once patients have been started on chronic transfusion therapy for the prevention of repeat strokes, it has not been apparent that this therapy can be stopped without increasing the risk of recurrence.

In a continuation of their earlier study, Adams et al[6] evaluated the rate of stroke or reversion to an abnormal transcranial Doppler in children who had been on chronic transfusion therapy who were randomized to either cessation or continuation of transfusion. Within a mean of 4.5 months of stopping transfusion, 34% of patients reverted to elevated transcranial Doppler velocities and 5% developed stroke, whereas neither occurred in those who continued transfusion. Cessation of chronic transfusions when pediatric patients transition to adult sickle cell care has also been associated with poor outcomes. According to a retrospective review, 36% of patients who stopped chronic transfusion due to either refusal or noncompliance after transitioning to adult care died; causes of death included stroke and multiorgan failure.[7] However, transfusion may be switched to another therapy in certain patients. The TWiTCH (Transcranial Doppler With Transfusions Changing to Hydroxyurea) multicenter randomized trial showed that in 121 children who had abnormal Doppler studies, after 1 year of routine transfusion therapy and no demonstration of severe vasculopathy on magnetic resonance imaging (MRI) and angiography, patients could be safely switched to hydroxyurea therapy for stroke prevention.[8] Differences in the patient populations of these studies should be considered when interpreting these results. The TWiTCH study[8] enrolled children who had abnormal transcranial Doppler flow velocities (≥200 cm/s) but not severe vasculopathy or prior history of stroke, as did the studies from Adams et al.[5,6] However, in the study by McLaughlin and Ballas,[7] the subjects were adult patients who had strokes during childhood. As demonstrated in the TWiTCH study, hydroxyurea may be an option for primary stroke prevention instead of transfusion for some patients who are at risk but have not yet had a stroke.

Acute Chest Syndrome

Acute chest syndrome (ACS) has been defined as chest pain with a new pulmonary infiltrate, fever, tachypnea, wheezing, or cough. It is a leading cause of death in adults,[9] and its cause may be multifactorial, but most typically, it results from acute lung injury driven by infection, pulmonary vaso-occlusion, or fat embolism. The hemoglobin level may fall well below baseline values. ACS is treated with broad-spectrum antibiotics, oxygen, and transfusion of RBCs.

The apparent salutary effect of RBC transfusion in ACS has been reported since the 1980s. A retrospective review of 32 episodes of admission for ACS found that of the 23 patients who received simple transfusion within 24 hours of hospital admission, 100% had clinical and chest x-ray improvement. Five of the 9 patients who were not initially transfused had worsening of their condition but improvement with transfusion later in the course of their disease.[10] A later study by Emre et al[11] showed that children who received simple transfusion, partial exchange transfusion, or simple transfusion followed by whole blood exchange transfusion all had improvement in oxygenation after transfusion.

More recently, investigators have evaluated the manner of the provision of transfusion, simple or automated RBCX, in ACS. It has been postulated that with automated RBCX, in addition to removal of HbS RBCs and replacement with hemoglobin A (HbA) RBCs, inflammatory mediators such as secretory phospholipase A2 may be removed, which could lead to more rapid recovery. Secretory phospholipase A2 has been found to predict patients at risk for ACS, and a trial carried out by Styles et al[12] was designed to determine whether RBC transfusion can prevent ACS in patients with elevated phospholipase A2. In such patients, 5 of 8 patients randomized to no transfusion developed ACS, compared to none of the 7 patients who were transfused ($P = .026$).[12] The role therapeutic apheresis plays in the removal of other disease mediators in SCD is also supported by the demonstration of a decrease in heme concentration and increased haptoglobin and hemopexin with clinical improvement in SCD patients with acute multiorgan failure after therapeutic plasma exchange who were refractory to RBCX.[13] The mechanism for plasma exchange here is thought to be similar to its use in thrombotic thrombocytopenic purpura, where there is both removal of a disease-causing antibody (anti-ADAMTS13) by the apheresis machine and replacement of deficient antibody with normal donor plasma. However, currently for treatment of ACS, RBC transfusion, given either as simple transfusion or RBCX, is still predominately used.

In a comparison of 20 adult patients with SCD who received simple transfusion and 20 adult patients who received RBCX for treatment of ACS, the primary outcome was postprocedure length of stay. Both groups were otherwise similarly treated for their ACS. There was no significant difference in the postprocedure length of stay (5.6 days for RBCX vs 5.9 days for simple transfusion; $P = .82$) or the total length of stay (8.4 days for RBCX vs 8.0 days for simple transfusion; $P = .76$), but a larger number of RBC units were needed for the RBCX patients (10.3 units) compared to simple transfusion patients (2.4 units; $P < .001$).[14] Another comparison of children with ACS who received either simple transfusion or RBCX initially or simple transfusion followed by RBCX found no difference in the length of stay between any of the groups.[15] The group receiving RBCX initially had a higher clinical respiratory score than the other groups, but this score also improved significantly for both the initial simple transfusion and initial RBCX groups. The group that received initial simple transfusion followed by RBCX had worsening of the clinical respiratory score after simple transfusion. The authors concluded that the clinical respiratory score was useful to identify the most severely affected patients and that initial RBCX was safe and effective. However, both this study[15] and the one by Turner et al[14] concluded that additional study on the use of transfusion, either simple or RBCX, in ACS is needed. Until prospective studies of simple transfusion versus RBCX are available, an expert panel convened by the American Society for Apheresis[16] has recommended initial treatment with simple transfusion for patients with ACS who are anemic, followed by RBCX if there is no improvement. Patients presenting with ACS with a higher hemoglobin (≥9 g/dL) or who are more severely ill (oxygen saturation <90% on room air, progressive pulmonary infiltrates, and decreasing hemoglobin) are recommended to undergo RBCX, which mirrors the National Heart, Lung, and Blood Institute (NHLBI) guidelines.[1]

Pulmonary Hypertension

Pulmonary hypertension is defined as a mean pulmonary artery pressure ≥25 mm Hg at rest on right heart catherization. It is relatively common in SCD patients, with a minimum prevalence in adults of 6% to 10%, and is associated with a marked increase in mortality. Both precapillary and postcapillary forms are seen in SCD, with just over half of patients with precapillary pulmonary hypertension. In SCD, chronic intravascular hemolysis, abnormal nitric oxide signaling, thromboembolism, and hypoxia contribute to development of the precapillary form; chronic anemia and relative systemic hypertension leading to dilatation and concentric hypertrophy of the left ventricle are associated with the postcapillary form.[17] Because of the association of anemia and chronic hemolysis with pulmonary hypertension, RBC transfusion is a logical consideration for treatment.

A case report of 2 patients who received RBCX every 8 weeks, with a goal HbS after exchange of <10%, demonstrates the potential role of transfusion in the management of pulmonary hypertension in SCD. The first patient was also treated with sildenafil, diuretics, and iron chelation, whereas the second patient received sildenafil, diuretics, warfarin, and chelation. In the first patient, the tricuspid regurgitant velocity (TRV), a noninvasive estimate of pulmonary artery systolic pressure, was reversed from a maximum TRV of 3.6 m/s to undetectable after 7 RBCXs. In the second patient, the maximum TRV was reduced from 4.0 to 3.2 m/s after 4 RBCXs. These results suggest that pulmonary hypertension may be at least partly reversible if the HbS level is maintained at very low levels.[18] A prospective cross-sectional study of flow-mediated vasodilation and TRV in nontransfused and chronically transfused (both simple and RBCX) patients with SCD has also been performed. The most notable findings were the improvement in TRV and improved flow-mediated dilation in the transfused patients; in fact, a single transfusion in the chronically transfused cohort improved flow-mediated vasodilation.[19]

Turpin et al[20] retrospectively evaluated 13 patients with pulmonary hypertension who received chronic RBCX every 5 to 6 weeks over a median of 25 months. The RBCX targets were a postexchange hematocrit of ≥30% and a postexchange HbS% of <30%. After a median of 4 RBCXs, all 13 patients had improvement in right atrial pressure, brain natriuretic peptide, pulmonary vascular resistance, and New York Heart Association functional class. Although not recommended by the NHLBI expert panel guidelines,[1] chronic transfusion has been recommended for treatment of pulmonary hypertension in SCD, particularly for patients who do not tolerate or respond to hydroxyurea.[17] Larger prospective studies are necessary to further define the benefits versus the risks of this treatment in this clinical scenario. To that end, the SCD-CARRE randomized clinical trial will compare the current standard of care with monthly RBCX for adult patients with evidence of increased mortality risk (high TRV, moderately high TRV and elevated plasma N-terminal prohormone of brain natriuretic peptide, or presence of chronic kidney disease). This study will evaluate the impact of monthly RBCX on the number of emergency department or hospital visits for patients meeting enrollment criteria, as well as evidence of the impact on end-organ cardiac, lung, and kidney injury.[21]

Acute Multiorgan Failure

Acute multiorgan failure syndrome can occur following a severe vaso-occlusive pain crisis. It is defined as acute failure of 2 out of 3 organ systems: respiratory, hepatic, or renal. Fever, acute worsening of hemolysis and anemia, and the development of thrombocytopenia and nonfocal encephalopathy are also common in this syndrome. A case series of 17 episodes of multiorgan failure in 14 patients highlights the role of transfusion therapy.[22] Ten of the patients had HbSS disease and 4 had HbSC disease. Supportive care was provided, including intravenous fluids, parenteral pain medication, hemodialysis, and mechanical ventilation. In all 17 episodes, the patients received RBC transfusions. Eight episodes received simple transfusion, with a mean of 8 units per patient, and RBCX was used in 9 episodes, with a mean of 9 units per patient. After RBCX, the mean HbS% was 30%. Within 24 hours of initiation of transfusion, there was clinical improvement in all but 1 patient who died; pulmonary fat emboli were found on autopsy.[22] Although there are no published clinical trials of transfusion for this indication, the consensus of experts has been that in acute multiorgan failure in SCD, either simple or exchange transfusion should be instituted immediately.[1]

Preoperative Transfusion

SCD is associated with an increased risk of complications during surgery and anesthesia, in particular VOC and ACS. The Cooperative Study of Sickle Cell Disease included 717 patients who had surgical procedures. Patients receiving preoperative transfusion had a lower rate of SCD-related postoperative complications when undergoing low-risk procedures (12.9% without transfusion vs 4.8% with transfusion) such as inguinal hernia repair, myringotomy, or dilatation and curettage. Transfused and nontransfused patients undergoing moderate-risk surgeries (eg, tonsillectomy, cesarean section, cholecystectomy, hip replacement) had similar rates of SCD-related complications in the postoperative period (7.9% and 4.7%, respectively). All patients who had high-risk surgeries (eg, cardiac, intracranial, or thoracic) received preoperative transfusions; 16.7% had SCD-related complications.[23] A randomized controlled trial of an aggressive versus conservative preoperative transfusion regimen was published by Vichinsky et al[24] around the time of the Cooperative Study of Sickle Cell Disease. Patients were randomized to 2 groups: group 1 was transfused to a preoperative hemoglobin level of 10 g/dL and an HbS% <30%; group 2 was transfused to a hemoglobin level of 10 g/dL regardless of the HbS%. Ten patients in both group 1 (31 patients) and group 2 (35 patients) developed ACS in the postoperative period; however, there were only half as many transfusion-related complications (predominantly new alloantibodies and delayed hemolytic transfusion reactions) in group 2 compared to group 1 (7% vs 14%).[24]

The Transfusion Alternatives Preoperatively in Sickle Cell Disease (TAPS) study was a recent randomized controlled multicenter trial comparing nontransfused to transfused patients who had low- and medium-risk surgeries.[25] The transfusion goal was a hemoglobin level of 10 g/dL with an HbS% <60% obtained by simple transfusion or partial RBCX. Thirty-nine percent of the nontransfused patients had postoperative complications, and 27% developed ACS. Of the transfused patients, only 15% had postoperative complications and 3% had ACS. Preoperative transfusion has become a standard recommendation for SCD patients who will receive regional or general anesthesia; usually, the transfusion goal is a hemoglobin level of 10 g/dL, but for patients who require high-risk surgery or who have a higher pretransfusion hemoglobin, RBCX may be needed preoperatively. Most of the patients in the previously described studies had HbSS disease; for example, in patients in the Cooperative Study of Sickle Cell Disease study, 77% had HbSS, 14% had HbSC, 5.7% had HbS-β^0 thalassemia, and 3% had HbS-β^{0+} thalassemia.[23] Additional evaluation of patients with SCD types other than HbSS who have surgery requiring regional or general anesthesia is warranted, as is identification of conditions for which it is best to use simple versus exchange transfusion.

Transfusion Method: Simple Versus Exchange

Simple Transfusion

The traditional method of RBC transfusion for almost all patients regardless of the diagnosis has been administration of 1 unit at a time by either gravity infusion or through an infusion pump. For both gravity infusion and infusion pump administration, standard blood administration tubing with a 170- to 260-μm macroaggregate filter should be used. Use of an infusion pump can provide a controlled rate of delivery over a specified amount of time, which can be beneficial in patients with SCD and severe anemia who have expanded plasma volumes and who may require slower than normal infusion rates to avoid circulatory overload. The infusion pump manufacturer's instructions should be consulted to evaluate whether the pump can be used for blood transfusion and, in particular, to determine whether cellular components such as RBCs may be damaged by the pump.[26]

Simple transfusion can be used for patients with SCD when there is a need to increase oxygen-carrying capacity without a need to acutely lower the amount of sickle hemoglobin. The usual clinical situations when simple transfusion is used are those arising from degrees of anemia that are much lower than usual, such as in aplastic crisis and splenic sequestration. Each RBC unit infused should be from a donor who is negative for sickle trait (HbAA rather than HbAS). Transfusion of 1 RBC unit will increase the hemoglobin by 1 g/dL and the hematocrit by 3%. Offsetting this improvement in oxygen-carrying ability due to the increase in the hematocrit is an increase in blood viscosity, which subsequently reduces tissue perfusion. Blood containing sickle hemoglobin is known to have increased viscosity compared to HbAA blood at the same hematocrit levels; in SCD patients, the effect of HbS on viscosity is counterbalanced by the lower baseline hematocrit levels.[27] An in vivo study of mixtures of HbSS and HbAA RBCs where oxygen tension and shear rate were measured showed that viscosity increases more steeply with increasing hematocrit when a larger proportion of RBCs are HbSS.[28]

Based on these earlier studies, it has been concluded that simple transfusion when the HbS% is >60% will lead to a significant increase in viscosity, as opposed to when the HbS% is <40%, which will result in minimal impact on viscosity. Transfusion guidelines also state that in SCD it is best to avoid transfusing patients to total hematocrits >30% to avoid substantial increases in viscosity and subsequent reduction in oxygen-delivering capacity.[29] However, more recent in vivo studies[30] using mixtures of autologous HbSS and donor HbAA RBCs suspended in plasma from patients with SCD, as opposed to being suspended in buffer as performed in previous studies,[28] provide testing under conditions that account for plasma-mediated RBC interactions. Under these experimental conditions, Alexy et al[30] confirmed that the viscosity increased as the hematocrit and proportion of HbS RBCs increased but found that this was also dependent on shear flow rates and oxygenation levels. Simulating simple transfusion conditions, when the total hematocrit of the suspension of HbSS and HbAA RBCs in patient plasma was increased from 25% to 35% and enough donor HbAA RBCs were added to the suspension of RBCs in SCD patient plasma to decrease the HbS% from 100% to 50%, there was an increase in oxygen transport effectiveness at the higher hematocrit at a high shear flow rate (300/s); however, at a lower shear flow rate (5/s), there was a decrease in oxygen transport effectiveness. The authors concluded that the optimal hematocrit may depend on not just the HbS%, but also the shear flow rates in relevant tissue (lung vs brain vs bone marrow) and the patient's clinical status.[30]

There are several reports in the literature of adverse outcomes in patients given simple transfusions either of too great a volume or at rates that were too fast. A case of a 25-year-old woman with HbSS whose usual hemoglobin level was between 5 and 7 g/dL was chronicled.[31] The patient presented with a hemoglobin of 3.8 g/dL at a routine outpatient visit. She was admitted to a hospital and received 6 units of RBCs within a 24-hour period. Although her hematocrit had increased to 31%, her systolic and diastolic blood pressures increased by 30 mm Hg, she developed headaches within 9 hours of the last transfusion, and she died of cerebral hemorrhage within 72 hours. Other similar cases have also been reported in the literature.[32,33] Often referred to as hyperviscosity syndrome, this iatrogenic complication can be avoided by transfusion of the minimum number of units needed for stabilization, close monitoring of patients during transfusion, and appropriate posttransfusion hemoglobin goals. For most situations, this means not transfusing to a hemoglobin >10 g/dL.

RBCX Transfusion

RBCX transfusion is a procedure performed by removal of a portion of the patient's whole blood and replacement with donor RBCs mixed with other fluids such as saline, albumin, or plasma. RBCX results in rapidly lowered percentages of total HbS. When used chronically, RBCX reduces the rate of iron accumulation because iron is removed with whole blood during the procedure. Indications for chronic RBCX include prevention of stroke recurrence, reduction in frequency of ACS episodes, and prevention of complications related to pregnancy.[34] RBCX is also used acutely and, most commonly, is indicated for acute stroke or ACS to rapidly reduce the HbS% to ≤30%. Other indications for acute RBCX include multiorgan failure, intrahepatic cholestasis, and preoperatively prior to general anesthesia.

RBCX can be performed manually or by automated methods (also called erythrocytapheresis). Manual RBCXs are more commonly performed in small children, usually weighing <25 kg. After obtaining vascular access, whole blood is removed by phlebotomy, and equivalent volumes of RBCs and additional fluids are infused (isovolemic exchange). This procedure requires close medical supervision during and immediately after completion but is an option in resource-limited areas where equipment for automated RBCX is not available or when a patient cannot tolerate automated exchange transfusion. In a demonstration of the efficiency of manual RBCX in a chronic transfusion program for SCD, Koehl et al[35] showed that the mean HbS decrease was 18.8% for manually exchanged patients versus 21.5% for those on automated exchange. Although the amount of donor RBCs used in manually exchanged patients was slightly higher than in patients on automated exchange, ferritin levels between the 2 groups of exchange patients were comparable. Koehl et al[35] also provide a useful video demonstration of their isovolemic exchange technique (which can be accessed at https://www.jove.com/video/55172/), which includes supplementation with oral calcium to prevent citrate toxicity due to the citrate anticoagulant in the RBC component. This may be useful for smaller children (weight <45 kg) or adults who may be sensitive to the citrate. Table 23-1 details volumes for removal and transfusion in manual RBCX in adults.[36]

Use of automated RBCX requires large-bore peripheral or central vascular access, blood cell separator apheresis machines, trained operators, and large amounts of compatible RBCs. Table 23-2 details the guidelines for central venous access for RBCX based on patient size.[37] There are 2 types of apheresis machines available in the United States that perform automated RBCX. Both operate in the same manner: whole blood is removed by vascular access from the patient and enters a centrifuge through a plastic disposable tubing kit after being mixed with citrate anticoagulant. The blood components are separated in the centrifuge. Based on patient height, weight, starting hematocrit, and goal hematocrit, as well as the desired proportion of HbS to be removed, referred to as the fraction of cells remaining (FCR), the machine calculates the volume of the patient's RBCs that need to be removed to meet procedure goals. RBCs that are removed are collected into a waste bag and are replaced with donor RBCs, which are mixed with the patient's residual blood components and returned to the patient in a return vascular access line. The blood draw, centrifugation, and return occur as continuous flow during the procedure.

TABLE 23-1 Manual RBC exchange method

1. Calculate exchange volume as 1.5 × patient RBC volumes:

    a. Patient's RBC volume = Hematocrit × total blood volume

    b. Standard RBC volume per unit is approximately 180 mL (unit hematocrit 60% × 300 mL[a])

    c. Number of units = 1.5 × RBC volume/180

Example: Patient hematocrit = 25, total blood volume = 5000 mL

Patient RBC volume = 0.25 × 5000 = 1250 mL

1.5 × 1250 mL/180 = 6.9, or 7 units of RBCs

2. Perform manual exchange in adult:

    a. Bleed 500 mL and then infuse 500 mL of 0.9% saline or 5% albumin.

    b. Bleed 500 mL and then infuse 2 RBC units.

    c. Repeat steps a and b until volume of RBC units administered is equal to planned exchange volume.

[a]Most RBC units in the United States are stored in additive solution and have a volume of approximately 300 mL and hematocrit of 60%. Occasionally, RBC units stored in anticoagulant preservative solution are available (commonly citrate, phosphate, dextrose, adenine [CPDA]), and these units will have a volume of approximately 250 mL and hematocrit of 78%.

Abbreviation: RBC, red blood cell.

Adapted, with permission, from Shaz B. Red cell exchange and other therapeutic alterations of red cell mass. In McLeod BC, Weinstein R, Winters JL, Szczepiorkowski ZM, eds. *Apheresis: Principles and Practice*. 3rd ed. AABB Press; 2010:393.

One machine available in the United States is the Amicus Separator System, manufactured by Fresenius-Kabi, Inc.[38] The software operating the machine includes algorithms for fluid pumps, which adjust removal and replacement volumes to achieve the targeted FCR and goal hematocrit in response to patient parameters entered by the operator. The extracorporeal volume of the disposable tubing kit, 160 mL, is somewhat smaller than that of the other platform available, which can be beneficial for smaller patients. The other system is the Spectra

TABLE 23-2 Central venous access catheter size guide for red blood cell exchange

Weight (kg)	Apheresis/dialysis catheter size
10-20	Dual-lumen 7F
21-30	Dual-lumen 8F
31-40	Dual-lumen 8F or 9F
41-50	Dual-lumen 10F or 11.5F
>50	Dual-lumen >11.5F

Adapted, with permission, from Kim HC. Red cell exchange: special focus on sickle cell disease. *ASH Educ Book*. 2014;2014(1):450-456.

Optia Blood Cell Separator, manufactured by Terumo BCT (Lakewood, CO),[39] which replaced the older COBE-Spectra system. The Spectra Optia uses continuous flow and centrifugation to separate whole blood into its components and also requires citrate anticoagulant to prevent clotting within the disposable plastic tubing. Software controls the pumps and calculates volumes based on patient parameters entered by the operator as well. The extracorporeal volume of the Spectra Optia is 185 mL. Patients for whom this represents 15% or more of their total blood volume require priming of the disposable tubing with RBC to avoid abrupt worsening of anemia at the start of the procedure. Both machines are also capable of performing depletion and exchange procedures in addition to RBCX. A depletion/exchange procedure is different from an exchange in that the patient's RBCs are removed isovolemically and are replaced with albumin or saline until a calculated nadir hematocrit is reached. The machine then transitions to an exchange procedure to complete the goals for HbS removal and final hematocrit. The benefit of a depletion/exchange procedure is that a smaller volume of replacement RBCs is needed. In an evaluation of the safety of the Spectra Optia for RBCX, patients who underwent depletion/exchange used a mean of 1.5 L of replacement RBCs versus 2 L for exchange procedures.[40]

Vascular Access

Peripheral access is preferred because it has the lowest complication rate of all access procedures; the most common complications are bruising and hematoma formation. Access requires a 16- to 18-gauge needle, with a 19- to 20-gauge needle for the return line; each needle is usually placed in one of the antecubital veins.[41] If used for chronic exchange, the antecubital veins must be preserved and should not be used for blood draws or other procedures. As patients with SCD age, their peripheral vascular access typically becomes exhausted. This poses a barrier to exchange transfusion[34] because it requires a steady blood flow via a catheter that tolerates high negative pressure without collapse. Alternative forms of access are required for such patients.

Central vascular access is often considered the next option for patients without good peripheral access. Central access should be rigid, have at least two lumens, and be of the same type that can be used for dialysis. The placement site depends on the length of time the access is needed (ie, acute, short term, or chronic). The femoral vein is the least preferred site due to its high risk of infection but is often used for acute access needs because it can be placed at the bedside in an emergency. Subclavian and internal jugular vein placements have higher risks of complications such as pneumothorax and hemothorax, but their risk has been reduced by the use of ultrasound-guided placement. The right internal jugular vein is preferred over the left for anatomic reasons. Central vascular access placed in the subclavian vein has a lower risk of infection, but with long-term use, there is a risk of subclavian vein stenosis. For either the subclavian or internal jugular vein location, confirmation of placement by chest x-ray prior to use is necessary.[41] When short-term emergent access is needed, central vascular catheters are a good option. However, for long-term or chronic access, these are usually not acceptable for most patients secondary to the increased risk of infection and limitations on activities such as bathing. For chronic use of central vascular access, tunneled placement, where a portion of the catheter is passed under the skin, is recommended to circumvent these restrictions.

Another option for access during chronic RBCX is placement of an implantable port. Surgically placed, usually beneath the clavicle, the ports are made of a metal reservoir covered with a membrane. The reservoir is connected to a central line placed in the subclavian or internal jugular vein. The port is accessed using noncoring needles. Anticoagulation with instilled heparin or sodium citrate is required when not in use. There are several ports available for use in RBCX: the dual-lumen Vortex port (AngioDynamics, Latham, NY), Bard Powerport Duo MRI (Bard Access Systems, Salt Lake City, UT), and the Powerflow Implantable Apheresis IV port (Bard Peripheral Vascular, Tempe, AZ). A retrospective cohort study of adults with SCD requiring chronic RBCX compared the complications of peripheral, temporary central vascular catheters with those of implantable ports (dual-lumen Vortex ports).[42] In 20 patients with implantable ports, 6 ports were removed for infection and 1 for malfunction after a mean of 171 days (±120 days). Procedures performed with implanted ports had an increased rate of access alarms requiring nurse intervention, longer procedure times, and a lower inlet flow rate. The authors attributed these differences to the longer length and smaller internal radius of the central catheters in the implantable ports. Lawicki et al[43] compared procedures performed in 5 patients with Vortex ports and 4 patients with the Bard Powerport Duo MRI. Procedures using the Bard port had a lower mean inlet flow rate (42.1 mL/min) versus the Vortex port (45.2 mL/min). The differences seen in this study were attributed to the smaller diameter of the Bard port (9.5F) compared to the Vortex port (11.4F). However, each of these ports has been used successfully in patients with SCD requiring long-term vascular access

Thrombus formation associated with central catheters or ports is decreased with prophylactic heparin instillation but can still occur. The thrombus may develop gradually, eventually occluding the lumens of the port. When resistant flow is noted during aspiration of a port lumen, alteplase or urokinase can be used to release the blockage.[41] Patients with long-term vascular access should be closely monitored for the development of device-related thrombosis because this can lead to partial or complete occlusion of vessel, postthrombotic syndrome, pulmonary embolism, and, of particular concern for a patient who needs chronic RBCX, loss of vascular access. Risk factors for catheter-associated thrombus formation include insertion site (femoral > jugular > subclavian), catheter tip placement, and patient-related factors such as age, body mass index, and presence of thrombophilia,[44] although much of the data used to derive therapy recommendations are from oncology or other patients and case series often do not include SCD patients. Superior vena cava syndrome should be recognized

when facial edema and swelling above the neck are seen in a patient who has longer-term vascular access. Recombinant tissue plasminogen activator was used with success in a patient with SCD and superior vena cava syndrome who was receiving a bone marrow transplant.[45]

Arteriovenous fistulas are not a common option for vascular access in SCD due to the high rate of complications. In a study of 23 patients with SCD who had arteriovenous fistulas placed for chronic RBCX, 19 patients (73%) had a complication, with 17 patients experiencing thrombosis and 14 developing stenosis. The mean life span of the fistulas was 51 months.[46] However, in patients with renal failure who require dialysis, an arteriovenous fistula is a more appropriate choice for vascular access.

Future Directions

RBC transfusion is a cornerstone of therapy in SCD, both for emergent and chronic indications. However, information on the optimal utilization of transfusion therapy in several common complications of SCD is lacking. This includes the most common complication, VOC. Management of VOC focuses on the use of parenteral opioids for severe pain management and incentive spirometry to reduce the risk of ACS. Current guidelines for transfusion in SCD state that for uncomplicated VOC, transfusion is not indicated.[47] This recommendation was of moderate strength from the expert panel, but the evidence was admittedly of low quality. Sobota et al[48] demonstrated a correlation between receipt of transfusion and decreased readmission rate in children admitted for VOC. A larger, more recent study by Nouraie and Gourdeuk[49] showed that simple transfusion during admission for VOC is common and may have some benefit for certain patients. This study included >39,000 hospital admissions of 4348 adult Medicaid beneficiaries admitted with VOC between 2007 and 2012. There was a reduced odds of mortality and of readmission within 30 days for the 32% of admissions during which a simple transfusion was administered. A reduced length of stay was also seen for a subset of patients with chronic kidney disease. Hemolytic reactions and transfusion-related acute lung injury were seen in 0.1% of admissions when transfusions were given. Further studies examining the potential role of transfusion in the management of VOC are needed.

Another horizon for future developments in transfusion therapy for SCD is in blood component modification or adjunctive therapy after transfusion. During storage of RBCs, hemolysis and accumulation of toxins, such as iron, hemoglobin, and hemin, occur, which lead to tissue injury. Acute and chronic transfusion leads to saturation of transferrin, decreased plasma hemopexin and haptoglobin, and accumulation of hemin. Supplemental treatment with transferrin, hemopexin, and haptoglobin after transfusion has been proposed as potential treatment and is being explored in entities with intravascular and extravascular hemolysis.[50]

Because of blood's relatively short shelf life, requirement for refrigerated storage, risk of transfusion-transmitted infectious disease, and alloimmunization, there continues to be interest in the development of blood substitutes to use in place of or as an adjunct to allogeneic blood products. Due to improvements in blood safety related to transfusion-transmitted infectious disease, any version of a blood substitute eventually approved for use in the United States will have to show superior outcomes compared to the current blood components.[51] The most likely application of blood substitutes for patients with SCD would be for critical clinical situations where patients were so highly alloimmunized that finding compatible RBCs is nearly impossible. Although there has been some progress on this front since efforts began shortly after the end of World War II, currently there are still no US Food and Drug Administration (FDA)-approved blood substitutes available in the United States. Hemoglobin-based oxygen carriers were initially produced by lysis of RBC and isolating hemoglobin; however, upon infusion, hypertension, renal failure, and cardiac complications occurred due to the toxicity of free hemoglobin and nitric oxide scavenging.[52] Subsequently, other chemical forms of hemoglobin-based oxygen carriers were developed. The most successful has been polymerized cross-linked hemoglobin, which includes Hemopure (Biopure, Cambridge, MA) and Polyheme (Northfield Labs, Evanston, IL). Hemopure is produced from bovine blood, whereas Polyheme is manufactured from human RBCs. Although clinical trials of both products have taken place and both forms have been anecdotally used in patients with SCD,[53,54] neither has been approved by the FDA, and only one, Hemopure, is currently available for compassionate use in the United States.[52]

Adverse Events of Transfusion in SCD

Iron Overload

Transfusion indications have increased in recent years in children and adults with SCD, and it is not uncommon for a patient on monthly RBC transfusions to have received >200 units over the span of several years. Each unit of RBCs contains 200 to 250 mg of iron,[26] and in the absence of losses, the iron will be deposited in the body, resulting in end-organ damage to the liver, heart, or endocrine glands.[55,56]

Repeated RBC transfusions increase the saturation of transferrin, which carries iron in the plasma, and when saturated beyond 85%, free iron appears in the plasma as non–transferrin-bound iron (NTBI). As NTBI circulates, it produces oxidative damage and also enters the liver through unregulated pathways including zinc or calcium transporters or endocytosis. Labile plasma iron (LPI) is a toxic, highly reactive form of NTBI, capable of unregulated penetration into target organs such as the liver, heart, and endocrine glands. LPI accumulates in tissues and is capable of forming free radicals, leading to tissue damage such as cirrhosis.[57]

Observational studies have been informative on how best to monitor patients with SCD for the development of transfusion-related iron overload as well as which therapies to use. Information on the extent of iron overload was gathered from patients treated at the Northern California Comprehensive Sickle Center on chronic transfusion therapy.[58] The study included 20 patients with HbSS disease who had been on chronic transfusion for a mean of 57 months (range, 12-146 months). Even though 19 patients were receiving deferoxamine during the study, there was a positive correlation between the quantity of iron and the amount of time on chronic transfusion therapy. Liver biopsies showed mild to moderate inflammation or fibrosis, despite the high ferritin levels (average serum ferritin level at biopsy was 2686 ng/nL), with 64% of iron staining found within hepatocytes. There was no correlation between the average serum ferritin and quantitative iron on liver biopsy or length of time on transfusion therapy.

Patients on chronic transfusion therapy should be monitored closely for iron overload; however, those who receive frequent episodic transfusions should also be monitored but are often missed.[56] A serum ferritin level >1000 ng/mL is considered evidence of iron overload[1] but is unreliable for evaluating iron status independently. Liver iron best correlates with total-body iron concentrations; thus, liver biopsy has been the standard for diagnosis of iron overload. However, because liver biopsy is an invasive procedure, it has been replaced by MRI assessment of liver iron stores, which exploits the disturbance of the magnetic field by iron, resulting in predictable rates of image darkening (referred to as R2 and R2*), which correlates with a liver iron concentration (LIC).[57] A normal LIC is between 0.8 and 1.5 mg/g dry weight of liver; significant liver iron loading is said to occur at an LIC >20 mg/g dry weight.[56]

Treatment of Iron Overload

Iron overload in SCD is treated with phlebotomy, chelation therapy, and utilization of automated RBCX. Phlebotomy can be considered in patients with SCD who have reasonably high hemoglobin levels on hydroxyurea. Automated RBCX maintains iron balance with approximately equal replacement of HbS RBC with HbA donor RBC. RBCX is not a treatment for iron overload per se but can help manage it by reducing the rate of iron accumulation compared to simple transfusion. Driss et al[59] demonstrated in 43 patients receiving chronic automated RBCX that 32 patients did not develop evidence of iron overload. For the 11 patients with iron overload, the mean initial serum ferritin decreased from 2480 to 1058 μg/mL; 7 of the 11 patients did not require chelation.[59]

In the United States, guidelines for evidence-based management of SCD recommend a comprehensive program to monitor and treat iron overload in sickle cell patients. They propose the introduction of chelation therapy when an increase in liver iron stores of 7 mg/g dry weight is recorded, when the cumulative transfusion count reaches 120 mL/kg RBCs, or when serum ferritin levels at steady state are ≥1000 μg/mL.[1] Other experts state that chelation therapy should begin after 10 transfusions when the serum ferritin is >1000 μg/L or the LIC is >3 mg/d dry weight liver. In the United States and Europe, 3 drugs are available for iron chelation therapy: deferoxamine (parenteral), deferiprone (oral table or solution), and deferasirox (oral tablet)

TABLE 23-3 Iron chelators

	Deferoxamine	Deferiprone	Deferasirox
First available in United States	1968	1999	2005
Method of administration	Parenteral	Oral	Oral 2 forms: dispersible tablet (ExJade) and film-coated tablet (Jadenu)
Plasma half-life	30 minutes	3 hours	8-16 hours
Usual dose	40-50 mg/kg/d, administered over 10-24 hours[a]	75-100 mg/kg/d administered every 8 hours	20-40 mg/kg/d once daily (ExJade) 14-28 mg/kg/d once daily (Jadenu)
Excretion	Urine; fecal at higher dose	Urine	Fecal
Use in decreased renal function	Can be used; dialysable	Can be used; dialysable	Nephrotoxic; should not be used unless totally dialysis dependent
Removal of cardiac iron	Effective, especially by continuous infusion	Most effective at removal of cardiac iron	Effective over long periods
Advantages	Long experience; can be given intravenously	Most effective for cardiomyopathy	Can be given once per day
Toxicity	Local reactions, allergic reactions, retinal damage, hearing loss, osteoporosis, growth failure	Gastrointestinal, arthralgias, transient transaminitis, rare idiosyncratic agranulocytosis	Glomerular filtration rate increases in 30%, proteinuria, rare renal failure, moderate gastrointestinal toxicity, rare gastrointestinal bleeding

[a]Should be given as continuous infusion over 24 hours in cardiac failure.
Adapted from Coates TD, Wood JC. How we manage iron overload in sickle cell patients. *Br J Haematol*. 2017;177(5):703-716.

(Table 23-3). Deferiprone is preferred for the treatment of cardiac iron overload in SCD, and in severe cases, a combination of chelation therapies may be required. The selection of a drug for chelation therapy must also consider which regimen a patient is most likely to adhere to (parenteral vs oral) and side effects such as nephrotoxicity.[56]

RBC Alloimmunization

Historical Considerations

RBC transfusion has been a proven cornerstone of treatment for SCD for decades. One of the recognized and sometimes therapy-limiting complications of RBC transfusion is alloimmunization to transfused RBC antigens. Clinical consequences of RBC alloimmunization include increased complexity of compatibility testing, difficulty finding units, delays in transfusion, and an increased risk of delayed hemolytic reactions. Reports of the frequency of alloimmunization have varied widely. Almost 30 years ago, Rosse et al[60] in the Cooperative Study of Sickle Cell Disease reported the first large epidemiologic study of this complication in >1800 patients with SCD. The reported overall RBC alloimmunization rate was 18.6% and was clearly related to the number of transfusions, usually occurring within the first 15 transfusions. Of those patients who made an antibody, 45% made only 1 antibody, whereas 17% made ≥4 distinct antibodies. Importantly, this study defined the most common specificities of the alloantibodies made, including D, E, C, K, and the Lewis antigens. Antibodies to the Lewis antigens are generally not clinically significant. The same year, Vichinsky et al[61] published a smaller study of 107 transfused African American patients with SCD, reporting an alloimmunization rate of 30% and also showing E, C, and K as the most common RBC antibody specificities followed by Jk[b]. This study examined the role of racial differences between donors (90% White) and patients with SCD and found significant differences in antigen frequency that likely accounted for the high rate of RBC alloimmunization.

It is likely that variability in reported rates of alloimmunization among studies is primarily related to differences in the donor-patient racial demographics. For instance, a study of 245 transfused patients with SCD in Detroit reported an alloimmunization rate of 7.8%.[62] Other factors that could have affected the reported rate of alloimmunization are the sensitivity of the methods for antibody detection, mixtures of patients populations (SC disease and/or sickle β thalassemia) and differences in the numbers of transfusions in the study population. These early observational studies showing which antibody specificities are most likely to be encountered and the role of racial disparity between donors and patients with SCD would be confirmed by others and serve as the basis for subsequent studies of prophylactic antigen-matching transfusions to reduce RBC alloimmunization.

Prophylactic Antigen Matching

Single-center studies of prophylactic antigen matching have shown a major reduction in alloimmunization rates.[63,64] Ambruso et al[63] matched for Rh, Kell, Kidd, and Duffy blood group antigens, so-called extended phenotype matching, and reported a 90% reduction in the per-unit risk of alloimmunization. Tahhan et al[64] provided blood matched for Rh, Kell, Duffy, and S to 40 patients and reported a 0% alloimmunization rate compared to 34.8% in 46 matched controls. A multicenter observational study of SCD patients with ACS transfused with Rh- and Kell-matched units reported a 1% alloimmunization rate[65] versus a 7% rate of new alloimmunization in a multicenter randomized controlled trial of aggressive versus conservative transfusions for perioperative management of patients with SCD transfused without matching.[24] A multicenter randomized controlled trial of transfusion using Rh and Kell matching versus standard of care treatment for stroke prevention in SCD reported an alloimmunization rate of 8.0% (5 of 63 patients).[66] Four of the 5 patients developed single antibodies to E or Kell, and in these cases, alloimmunization could have likely been prevented by strict adherence to the matching protocol.[66] A follow-up study examining whether Rh- and Kell-matched transfusions could be discontinued for these patients confirmed the low rate of 2% alloimmunization in the transfused cohort.[6] These data suggest that strict adherence to transfusion of Rh- and Kell-matched units will reduce the rate of RBC alloimmunization to 0% to 7% of patients.

One question regarding prophylactic antigen matching is whether doing more extensive matching beyond Rh and Kell to include Duffy, Kidd, and Ss antigens and potentially other antigens is efficacious and feasible. This was studied by Castro et al[67] in 351 transfused patients with SCD who had an overall alloimmunization rate of 39%. They showed that if Rh and Kell matching had been done, it would have prevented 53.3% of the patients from becoming alloimmunized versus 70.8% if the matching had been extended to include Duffy, Kidd, and Ss antigens. However, 13.6% of White donors would be expected to be matched for the Rh and Kell antigens versus only 0.6% for the extended phenotype matching. A single-center study of 99 patients with SCD who were managed with extended phenotype units matched for Rh, Kell, Duffy, Kidd, Lewis, and MNSs reported an alloimmunization rate of 7%.[68] Only 34% of units were fully matched, however, which likely accounted for an alloimmunization rate similar to that observed with Rh and Kell matching alone. The conclusion is that although there is some incremental added benefit from extended phenotype matching, it is impractical in regions with a high proportion of White donors. Routine blood group testing of donors using molecular methods may make extended antigen matching more feasible, particularly in regions with a larger proportion of minority donors.

Historical data have repeatedly shown that RBC alloimmunization is dose related to the number of transfusions. For this reason, physicians have considered chronic RBCX as

associated with a greater risk of alloimmunization compared to simple transfusion. When RBC antigen-matching strategies are used, there are data to question this assumption.[20,68] In a study of 99 patients with SCD who were managed with extended matched transfusion, half of the patients received RBCX transfusions, and only 7 (7%) of 99 patients became alloimmunized, 1 each to Le[a] and Kp[a], 2 to M, and 3 to RhD in patients who were RhD variants. A more recent small study of 13 patients who received Rh- and Kell-matched transfusions for RBCX every 5 to 6 weeks for a median of 27 months reported only 1 patient (7%) who developed a new RBC antibody 3 years after starting RBCX.[20] These preliminary data suggest that in the era of prophylactic matching there may not be a materially increased risk of RBC alloimmunization associated with chronic RBCX compared with simple transfusion.

National guidelines and recommendations have been published regarding prevention and management of RBC alloimmunization in patients with SCD.[1,69,70] In 2014, the National Institutes of Health published an expert panel report titled "Evidence-Based Management of Sickle Cell Disease," which made the following recommendation: "RBC units that are to be transfused to individuals with SCD should include matching for C, E and K antigens (moderate recommendation, low-quality evidence)."[1] RhD antigen matching was considered a given. Similar recommendations have been proposed by other groups,[69] including the International Collaboration for Transfusion Medicine Guidelines, although the evidence supporting their recommendation was judged as being of very low quality using GRADE (Grading of Recommendations Assessment, Development and Evaluation) methodology.[69] Thus, the current recommended strategy for preventing and managing RBC alloimmunization in patients with SCD is as follows:

1. Patients with SCD should have a complete RBC phenotype performed by serology or genotyping of RBC blood groups by molecular methods, preferably before transfusion support is required.[69]

2. In nonalloimmunized patients, transfusions should be prophylactically matched for Rh (C, c, E, e) and Kell antigens.[1,69,70]

3. In patients who become alloimmunized with a clinically significant RBC alloantibody, extended phenotype/genotyped-matched units (Duffy, Kidd, Ss) should be provided to the extent feasible.[69,70] Consultation with the transfusion medicine physician is advisable for RBC alloimmunized patients to tailor the optimal transfusion management strategy.

Molecular Phenotyping of Recipients and Donors

The genomic approach to blood groups has been shown to have many advantages in the context of SCD. Serology may not be cost-effective and may not provide sufficiently precise information to match the RBCs delivered according to the antibodies produced by the recipient. Patient genotyping is necessary in the following situations:

- Recent transfusion episodes precluding blood group phenotyping. This technique can be used to determine the phenotype of patients who have recently undergone transfusion. In such cases, molecular biology techniques are much more reliable than the usual serologic tests.

- Typing for blood group systems or antigens for which there are no commercially available reagents (Dombrock). In some cases, molecular biology approaches are the only viable alternative.

- Detection of molecular variants involved in mismatched situations, especially for the RH blood group system. This technique is suitable for patients with antibodies against antigens that are present, suggesting the presence of a variant (eg, in situations in which serologic testing detects an anti-C antibody and the patient is known to be C antigen positive).

- Detection of rare blood groups (U negative, RH:−18, RH:−34, RH:−46).

- A positive direct antiglobulin test.

In situations in which serologic tests are not routinely performed on the donor, genotyping can help to select donor units with more extensive antigen matching to the recipients than just ABO/RhD. The screening of rare blood groups useful for patients is also possible by genotyping, together with the determination of low-frequency antigen expression in donors that might lead to immunization in patients. However, molecular biology laboratories with accreditation, specialization, and expertise in this field are rare, limiting the large-scale adoption of molecular phenotyping in SCD.

International Considerations: Observational Studies and Prophylactic Antigen-Matching Protocols Outside of the United States

The regulatory level of transfusion safety in each country is different, and there are limited resources that affect transfusion availability in some areas. The high incidence of alloimmunization in Western countries results from significant differences in the antigens present in donors and recipients. The incidence of alloimmunization is much lower in the absence of such differences.

In Africa, a large continent faced with multiple infectious risks, transfusion policy differs between countries. Most African countries currently have no access to phenotyped units or to units depleted of leukocytes. According to World Health Organization reports, intrafamily donations are common, particularly in low-resource countries, whereas in others, blood donation is remunerated. In India, patients generally receive RBC units crossmatched for ABO and RhD antigens. In Western India, Kell antigen matching is not recommended, but partial Rh (C, c, E, e) and MNS matching is recommended and has reduced the risk of alloimmunization by 75%.[71] In France and elsewhere in Europe, SCD patients receive crossmatch-compatible RBCs phenotyped for the ABO, Rh, and KEL systems. Extended matching for Duffy, Kidd, and MNS is proposed for patients considered to be high responders or with known alloimmunization.

Risk Factors for RBC Alloimmunization

RBC alloimmunization is an important complication of transfusion. Identification of risk factors for alloimmunization related to blood component or recipient characteristics could lead to therapies or blood component modifications that could reduce alloimmunization risk.

Blood Component Factors

Longer-stored RBCs have been associated with adverse outcomes related to transfusion in observational studies,[72] but the association has not been maintained in prospective studies.[73] In a murine model of RBC alloimmunization, longer-stored RBCs showed increased immunogenicity compared with fresher RBCs.[74] In a retrospective study of 166 patients with SCD transfused between 2005 and 2012, 11% of patients had made alloantibodies, and the median age of RBCs transfused was 20 days. There was an association with alloimmunization after transfusion of longer-stored RBCs, with significantly increased risk after transfusion of RBCs stored for 35 days.[75] The current body of data is insufficient to recommend preferential use of fresh units. The priority remains finding units matched for ABO, Rh, and Kell antigens.

An additional area to examine would be leukoreduction. Donor white blood cells release interleukin-6, tumor necrosis factor-α, and interleukin-1β and likely contribute to much of the storage lesion of RBCs.[76] Murine models have also shown that leukoreduction can affect RBC alloimmunization.[77] Campbell-Lee et al[78] demonstrated in their retrospective study of 476 transfused SCD patients that alloimmunized patients were more likely to have received non-leukoreduced RBCs prior to alloimmunization. Prospective studies would be necessary to further examine the role of storage age and leukoreduction of RBCs in alloimmunization.

Recipient Factors

Rh blood group alloantibodies are the most common alloantibodies made by transfused patients with SCD. Rh variants, which are altered antigens caused by amino acid substitutions in the Rh proteins, are very common in persons of African descent, including those with SCD. In one study, 182 patients with SCD who received Rh- and Kell-matched transfusions from African American donors were examined; 146 antibodies among 71 chronic and 9 episodically transfused patients were found. Ninety-one antibodies were unexplained antibodies, 56 were seen in patients who were serologically positive for the antigen they had become immunized against, and 35 were seen in antigen-negative recipients who had received antigen-negative RBCs. Eighty-seven percent of individuals who were RH genotyped had variant alleles.[79] Thus, commonly used strategies for Rh antigen matching leave patients exposed to risk for alloimmunization either due to their Rh variants or potential variants from African American donors, who would most likely express their needed RBC phenotype. The Rh variants associated with alloimmunization need to be further defined because matching for Rh variants is not feasible for most

TABLE 23-4 Single nucleotide polymorphisms associated with red blood cell alloimmunization in sickle cell disease

Study	Single nucleotide polymorphism	Increase or decrease in alloimmunization	Comment
Meinderts et al[85]	FCGR2C.nc-ORF	3-fold lower risk	Strongest association for antigens other than Rh or Kell
Oliveira et al[83]	−318C/T of *CTLA4*	Heterozygosity associated with increased risk	
Sippert et al[84]	TNFA-308 G/A (rs 1800629) DRB1*15	Increased risk Overrepresented in Rh alloimmunization	
Tatari-Calderone et al[86]	HLA-DQ2, DQ3, DQ5 HLA-DQB1	Increased frequency in nonalloimmunized Decreased alloimmunization	
Williams et al[82]	ADRA1B LINC01847	Increased risk	

blood centers. Recently, next-generation sequencing testing using whole-exome sequencing has been shown to be of use in detecting relevant Rh variants in this population.[80]

Recipient inflammatory state at the time of transfusion has been linked to RBC alloimmunization in SCD patients. Fasano et al[81] evaluated 52 alloimmunized patients with SCD who had been transfused during various clinical scenarios that have been deemed inflammatory. Transfusions given during inflammatory clinical events were associated with alloimmunization, with the strongest association seen for transfusions given during VOC or ACS. Other studies in which clinical status during transfusion for nonalloimmunized and alloimmunized patients was evaluated have not found similar associations.[78]

More than one gene regulates the immune response to transfusion, but investigators have been attempting to identify which polymorphisms are most important in alloimmunization related to SCD. Recently, several single nucleotide polymorphisms have been identified in SCD patients that are associated with increased risk of alloimmunization,[82-84] as well as protection from alloimmunization.[85,86] These single nucleotide polymorphisms are further detailed in Table 23-4.

Recognition and Diagnosis of Delayed Serologic Transfusion Reaction, Delayed Hemolytic Transfusion Reaction, and Hyperhemolysis

Definition

Delayed serologic transfusion reactions (DSTRs) are defined as the development of new antibodies against transfused RBCs without clinical hemolysis. The posttransfusion sample demonstrates a positive direct antiglobulin test (DAT) due to immunoglobulin G (IgG) sensitization of RBCs, and a new RBC alloantibody is identified by immunohematologic testing.[87]

However, delayed hemolytic transfusion reactions (DHTRs) are a clinical and biologic complication of transfusion. Hemolysis occurs with a decline in hemoglobin to the pretransfusion value or even lower than the pretransfusion value. There is an increase in markers of hemolysis, including lactate dehydrogenase (LDH) and hemoglobinuria. It occurs between 24 hours and 28 days after transfusion.[70,88] Clinical evidence of hemolysis includes an inadequate posttransfusion hemoglobin increment, increased reticulocyte count, and decreased haptoglobin. There is also an elevation of LDH and indirect bilirubin levels, which decline in the following days. Hemolysis seen in DHTR is usually extravascular due to clearance of IgG-sensitized RBCs through phagocytosis. This leads to inflammatory cytokine production, albeit at a lower level than in an acute hemolytic transfusion reaction. Due to this inflammatory response and lack of complement activation, patients often only present with fever, malaise, and symptoms of worsening anemia.[89] This is in further contrast to hyperhemolysis syndrome. Very serious cases of DHTR are called hyperhemolysis syndrome. The distinction between DHTR and hyperhemolysis syndrome is somewhat blurred. Some teams consider hyperhemolysis syndrome to be a severe form of DHTR as opposed to a separate entity. We will refer to the classical form of DHTR as *DHTR without hyperhemolysis* and will refer to hyperhemolysis syndrome as *DHTR with hyperhemolysis*. DHTR with hyperhemolysis is defined as follows[90]:

1. Severe anemia after transfusion with posttransfusion hemoglobin value lower than pretransfusion hemoglobin. Reticulocytopenia may develop.

2. Evidence of hemolysis (at least 1 of the following: increased LDH, hemoglobinemia, hemoglobinuria, or hyperbilirubinemia).

3. Rapid decrease in HbA% compared to the posttransfusion HbA%, which can allow for a rapid diagnosis of DHTR (http://www.reamondor.aphp.fr/nomogram-2/). This approach requires laboratory data for hemoglobin levels and HbA% obtained within 48 hours of transfusion. French guidelines recommend the determination of hemoglobin and HbA% after transfusion in patients with SCD.[91]

The most common presenting symptom is dark urine after transfusion. Most patients also have symptoms consistent with VOC, and about half develop a secondary ACS. Patients may develop pulmonary hypertension and end-organ damage during the episode. DHTR-related mortality was 6% in SCD patients, but DHTR was not even mentioned in some previous mortality studies.[92]

No relationship has yet been established between the presence or absence of antibodies and the severity of this syndrome.[92,93] The initial presentation may be of a DHTR without hyperhemolysis, with a positive DAT and detectable new alloantibody. However, many cases present without detectable new alloantibody, either a completely negative antibody screen and DAT or a positive DAT with only autoantibody and no alloantibody. In the series from Habibi et al,[92] in 62% (61/99) of their cases, newly formed antibodies were identified after transfusion. In 38% (38/99) if cases, no new antibodies were detected, and in 61% (23/38) of these cases, no antibodies were ever detected in the pre- or posttransfusion period. SCD patients produce more autoantibodies than the general population,[68,94-97] suggesting that SCD patients have a genetic predisposition to develop autoantibodies, reflecting a general dysfunction of the immune system.[98] DHTR with hyperhemolysis can progress rapidly to become fatal.[99,100] It is important to recognize this syndrome because giving additional RBC transfusions during these episodes exacerbates the anemia; treatment centers on transfusion avoidance with close monitoring and administration of intravenous immunoglobulin with or without high-dose steroids.[101,102] There have also been reports regarding the use of rituximab and eculizumab.[102] Details regarding treatment of this syndrome will be covered elsewhere.

Incidence

There are no published series detailing the incidence of delayed serologic transfusion reactions among only patients with SCD. One series that did not focus exclusively on SCD found an overall incidence of 0.66%.[87] The incidence of DHTR without hyperhemolysis has mostly been evaluated in retrospective studies. At a time when patients were matched only for ABO and RhD, high incidence rates (11.5%-16%) were reported, but with more extensive matching, more recent studies have reported much lower rates (4%-7%).[103] In all retrospective studies, the authors stressed the high probability of missed diagnoses, particularly if the clinical signs were mild. Because of the more recent recognition of DHTR with hyperhemolysis and likelihood of missed diagnoses due to its nature, there is little information on its overall incidence. In a national study from France, 99 cases of DHTR with hyperhemolysis were identified in 69 patients over a 12-year period.[92]

Pathophysiology

Previous Delayed Serologic Transfusion Reaction and Activation of Complement and the Membrane Attack Complex in DHTR

The mechanism involved in DHTR without hyperhemolysis is the destruction of transfused antigen-positive RBCs by an antibody recognizing that antigen. The titers of RBC alloantibodies produced after primary alloimmunization frequently fall and become less detectable over time (evanescence) and may remain undetected in the serum in the pretransfusion antibody screening test. The most commonly evanescent clinically significant antibodies in SCD patients are anti-Js[a], Fy[b], S, Jk[b], Fy[a], C, E, and Kell.[104] However, antibodies that are not classically clinically significant, such as anti-M or anti-HI antibodies, may also been involved.[98,105] Some antibodies against variant RH blood group antigens have also been implicated in DHTR without hyperhemolysis, as have antibodies associated with rare blood groups (U antigen of MNS blood group). Two factors impacting the ability of the blood bank laboratory to detect antibodies over time are (1) the antibody detection test method (tube testing is less sensitive than gel or solid phase methods)[106] and (2) the fact that posttransfusion evaluation for RBC alloimmunization within the time frame of increased likelihood of detection of new alloantibodies (ie, within 4-21 days) is not routinely performed (ie, a posttransfusion antibody screen).[107] During the primary immune response, immunoglobulin M (IgM) antibody is produced first, which then switches to IgG antibody. This immunoglobulin class switching is driven by cytokines from activated T cells, which also drive the development of memory B cells. In an anamnestic response seen in a DHTR without hyperhemolysis, upon reexposure of the foreign RBC antigen to T cells, there is an increase in the level of IgG antibody within several days. Because prior clonal expansion of B cells has already occurred, there will be an increased amount of IgG produced compared to the primary immune response. IgG antibody specific for the foreign RBC antigen binds to the antigen sites on the RBC membrane. This leads to extravascular hemolysis by phagocytes in the reticuloendothelial system. IgG antibodies are usually not efficient at complete activation of complement. Activation of complement usually occurs in intravascular hemolysis but can also occasionally be seen in DHTR without hyperhemolysis. This feature is blood group specific, with antibodies of the Kidd and Duffy blood groups more commonly activating complement compared to other non-ABO blood group antibodies.[26]

DHTR With Hyperhemolysis

The pathophysiology of DHTR with hyperhemolysis has not been defined, but there have been 3 postulated mechanisms:

(1) destruction of autologous RBC through "bystander hemolysis," (2) suppression of erythropoiesis, and (3) macrophage activation.

Destruction of Autologous RBCs Through "Bystander Hemolysis"

Petz[108] and Garratty[109] first described bystander hemolysis as immune hemolysis of cells that are negative for the antigen against which the relevant antibody is directed. The recipient's autologous RBCs may be destroyed along with transfused allogeneic RBCs. The studies performed by Ness et al[87] show that posttransfusion autoantibody production or sensitization of antigen-negative autologous RBCs was not uncommon even in DHTR without hyperhemolysis. Because patients with SCD are transfused with HbA RBCs, the fractions of HbS and HbA after transfusion are useful markers to evaluate this notion. In the series from King et al,[100] in all 5 patients described, there was substantial loss of HbA RBCs; in 2 of these patients, there was also loss of HbS RBCs, marking potential destruction of autologous RBCs. In addition, Win et al[110] demonstrated increases in both HbA and HbS in urine by high-performance liquid chromatography urinalysis over days 2 through 4 after a DHTR with hyperhemolysis. Some authors have suggested that in the absence of posttransfusion hemoglobin fraction determinations, DHTR with hyperhemolysis can be diagnosed as a significant decrease in hemoglobin levels of >25% between 4 and 21 days after transfusion. This decrease in hemoglobin levels is correlated with a larger increase in LDH levels than during a crisis, hemoglobinuria, and the rapid disappearance of HbA over several days.[92,111] In the series by Habibi et al[92] of 99 DHTR cases, the median decrease in hemoglobin levels was 4.6 g/dL (range, 3.1-5.3 g/dL), and the median value of maximum LDH was 1335 IU/L (range, 798-2086 IU/L). Changes of this magnitude are rarely observed during a simple VOC. Figure 23-1 details how use of a nomogram can aid in diagnosis of DHTR.

Suppression of Erythropoiesis

Suppression of erythropoiesis after destruction of allogenic RBCs was felt to be a mechanism for the severe anemia seen by Petz et al[99] in their series of 5 patients. The authors argue that because transfusion also suppresses erythropoiesis and the survival of autologous RBCs in patients with SCD is shortened, when there is additional destruction of allogeneic RBCs, it should be expected that severe anemia can result.

Macrophage Activation

HbS RBCs adhere to macrophages more avidly than HbA RBCs, and HbS reticulocytes adhere to vascular endothelium by vascular cell adhesion molecule 1 (VCAM1), which is also on macrophages.[90] Fluctuations of some plasma factors during inflammation, for example, could alter the RBC membrane

To use the nomogram, fill the yellow boxes with appropriate values.

	First assessment (AFTER the index transfusion)	Second assessment (at DHTR suspicion)
Date	12/06/2016 (day/month/year)	20/06/2016 (day/month/year)
Total Hb, g/dL	8.0	6.0
HbA percentage, %	25.0	10.0

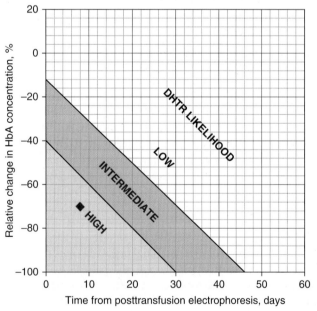

FIGURE 23-1 **This nomogram is proposed to estimate the likelihood of delayed hemolytic transfusion reaction (DHTR) in sickle cell disease patients.** To use the nomogram, the relative change in a patient's hemoglobin A (HbA) concentration and the time interval since posttransfusion electrophoresis are plotted. If the resulting point is above and to the right of the upper limit line, DHTR likelihood is low. If the point is below and to the left of the lower limit line, DHTR likelihood is high. If the point is between the 2 lines, DHTR likelihood is intermediate. Patients without a posttransfusion hemoglobin electrophoresis cannot be evaluated with the use of the nomogram. The relative change in HbA concentration is calculated as 100 × (HbA concentration at DHTR suspicion − posttransfusion HbA concentration)/posttransfusion HbA concentration, with HbA concentration expressed in g/dL (percent HbA × total hemoglobin in g/dL). Nomogram adapted from Mekontso Dessap A, Pirenne F, Razazi K, et al. A diagnostic nomogram for delayed hemolytic transfusion reaction in sickle cell disease. *Am J Hematol.* 2016;91(12):1181-1184.

and expose phosphatidyl serine (PS). An increase in PS expression on the RBC membrane is a marker of the "suicide" of RBCs, with accelerated aging leading to eryptosis. However, the plasma factors inducing an increase in PS expression on transfused RBCs remain unknown. Excessive PS exposure can also increase RBC binding to complement and the destruction of these cells by macrophages. This mechanism could potentially explain the occurrence of DHTR with hyperhemolysis in the absence of antibodies.[104] Inflammatory clinical conditions in SCD can promote alloimmunization, as has already been demonstrated.[81] However, the inflammatory context is not sufficient in itself to reduce the life span of the transfused RBCs. Mekontso et al[91] showed that transfusion outcomes were similar in intensive care patients with severe complications and significant inflammatory syndromes when compared to patients on long-term transfusion treatment. The trigger factor for the cascade of events resulting in hyperhemolysis thus remains unknown.

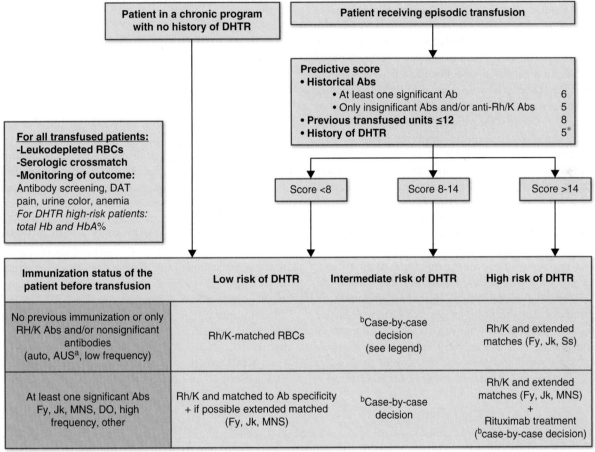

*This risk score is underestimated in this document and should be modified to 8-14.

FIGURE 23-2 Recommended transfusion guidelines for patients with sickle cell disease (SCD). All transfused patients with SCD should receive serologically crossmatch-compatible leukodepleted red blood cells (RBCs) and be monitored carefully by performing regular antibody (Ab) screening tests including direct antiglobulin test (DAT) and checking for pain, urine color, and signs of anemia. Total hemoglobin (Hb) and hemoglobin A percentage (HbA%) measurements are recommended for patients at high risk of delayed hemolytic transfusion reaction (DHTR). Patients on a chronic transfusion protocol are considered at low risk for DHTR. For patients receiving episodic transfusions, 3 criteria, assigned different point values based on statistical analysis, are considered DHTR risk factors: (1) History of RBC immunization. A point value of 6 is given if the patient has a history of at least 1 clinically significant antibody (other than anti-Rh or anti-K) classically known to be involved in transfusion reactions, such as anti-Jk[b], Fy[a], S, or HrS. A point value of 5 is given if the patient has a history of only anti-Rh/-K and/or antibodies considered not clinically significant (eg, autoantibodies or nonspecific antibodies). Thus, a patient who has an anti-Rh plus an anti-Jk[b] is given a point value of 6 (and not 6 + 5). (2) Cumulative transfusions of ≤12 units. (3) A previous DHTR. By adding the point values, a DHTR risk score is calculated and transfusion is tailored accordingly. Patients with a score of <8 are considered low risk. Patients transfused episodically who have a low risk of DHTR are transfused with Rh- (D, C, E, c, e) and K-matched RBCs, which is extended to Fy, Jk, and Ss only if the patient has developed antibodies against any of these antigens. [a]AUS, antibody with unknown specificity. [b]Patients who score between 8 and 14 have an intermediate risk. For such patients, the extent of matching should be based on their DHTR history and number of previous transfusions; those with no history of DHTR who have been transfused only a few times are considered at a lower risk similar to low-risk patients, but they should still be monitored closely. However, for patients with intermediate DHTR risk who have a history of DHTRs and few transfusions in the past (≤12 transfusions), we generally consider them high risk, and they receive extended matched RBCs (Fy, Jk, Ss). Patients with a score of >14 are considered at high DHTR risk. Episodically transfused patients with a high risk of DHTR (based on the predictive score) always receive extended matched RBCs (Fy, Jk, Ss). Prophylactic rituximab use should be considered for patients with a history of alloantibodies and severe DHTR.

Transfusion Precautions for Preventing DHTR

SCD patients with known RBC alloantibodies should receive RBCs that lack the clinically significant antigens to which they have become sensitized. Reducing the risk of DHTR without hyperhemolysis due to an anamnestic antibody response requires screening for antibodies after each transfusion to ensure identification of antibodies that may become undetectable before the next transfusion. This is not routine practice but should be considered for SCD patients due to their higher than usual risk of RBC alloimmunization. All adverse events related to transfusion should be clearly noted in the patient's transfusion records and communicated to the clinician to guide decisions concerning subsequent transfusion events. Patients should also be made aware of their alloimmunization status. Many institutions provide a wallet card that includes the name and phone number of the hospital blood bank that identified the antibodies. Alternatively, patients have worn medical alert identification bracelets. Either way, it is important for RBC alloimmunization information to be shared if the patient is seeking care at an institution other than where their care is usually received.

In patients with a history of DHTR with hyperhemolysis, the indications for transfusion are restricted to life-threatening situations. In such cases, if transfusion is considered essential, preventive immunomodulatory treatment may be required if the patient is already immunized. Preventive treatment should be discussed by the SCD reference center and the blood center on a case-by-case basis. In all cases, the known antibodies should be taken into account, and immunized patients should be provided with RBCs that have been matched for the patient's extended RBC phenotype. The most immunogenic blood groups should be taken into account in transfusion decisions, even if the patient has not yet developed antibodies against them. Patients can be prepared by erythropoietin and hydroxyurea treatments before surgery or during a pregnancy to prevent or decrease the need for transfusion.[112]

Narbey and al[113] performed a prospective study in which they calculated a risk score for DHTR with hyperhemolysis. They found that patients frequently undergoing transfusion did not develop DHTR with hyperhemolysis, whereas individuals with RBC alloimmunization or a history of DHTR were at high risk of developing DHTR. Their findings suggest that patients who have undergone a large number of transfusions with no history of DHTR with hyperhemolysis are not at risk, whereas the response status of patients who have undergone only a few transfusions remains unknown. Figure 23-2 demonstrates guidelines for stratification of transfusion decisions based on whether or not a patient has a high or low predictive score of DHTR.[70] Further studies are required to refine the definitions of high- and low-risk status, to guide transfusion decisions, and to minimize the risk of DHTR with hyperhemolysis.

Conclusion

Red blood cell transfusion, delivered by simple or exchange transfusion methods, is a therapeutic cornerstone in the management of patients with sickle cell disease. This therapy is used in primary prevention for cerebral vasculopathy or secondary prevention in severe organ damage or acute complications. The beneficial effects of transfusion therapy observed in recent clinical studies, and the lack of effective treatments for this population, have led to increased transfusions. Although red blood cell transfusions can save lives, red blood cell alloimmunization, a major complication of transfusion, has a much higher incidence in patients with sickle cell disease than in other patient groups. Hemolytic transfusion reactions, which occur frequently in alloimmunized patients, are often under-diagnosed, particularly because the symptoms and the biomarkers of the hemolysis mimic those of acute vaso-occlusive crisis. Transfusion indications in SCD patients should be decided on a case-by-case basis, taking into account each individual history of transfusion.

Case Study

A 26-year-old woman with SCD (homozygous hemoglobin S) received a transfusion of 3 units of RBCs during hip replacement surgery. The patient had a history of osteonecrosis of the hip, thrombosis, and 4 episodes of ACS requiring admission to intensive care. She was not taking hydroxyurea. The patient was blood group AB and RhD positive and had been transfused a total of 19 units of RBCs in her lifetime. She had become alloimmunized to Le^a, C^w, and HI. Her RBC phenotype was: C− E+ c+ e+ K− Fy^a− Fy^b− Jk^a+ Jk^b+ M− N+ S+ s+ Le^a− Le^b− P1+.

At steady state, her hemoglobin was approximately 8 g/dL. On postoperative day 6, she developed ACS, dark urine, and worsening anemia with relative reticulocytopenia and an increase in LDH to 1600 IU/L. The patient was transferred to the intensive care unit for close monitoring. Her hemoglobin dropped to a nadir of 3.5 g/dL. The diagnosis of DHTR with hyperhemolysis was quickly confirmed by nomogram (Figure 23-3B; see Mekontso et al[91]), and treatment was started. Further transfusion was avoided.

The patient received infusions of immunoglobulin, erythropoietin, and intravenous iron. The presence of relative reticulocytopenia motivated the use of high doses of erythropoietin to stimulate the production of RBCs.

A new type and screen was sent to the blood bank, and immunohematologic investigation revealed no new RBC alloantibodies. Extended phenotyped RBCs were available in case the patient developed organ failure. The graph in Figure 23-3A details the decrease in hemoglobin and hemoglobin A percentage after the transfusion during surgery.

Case Study: Continued

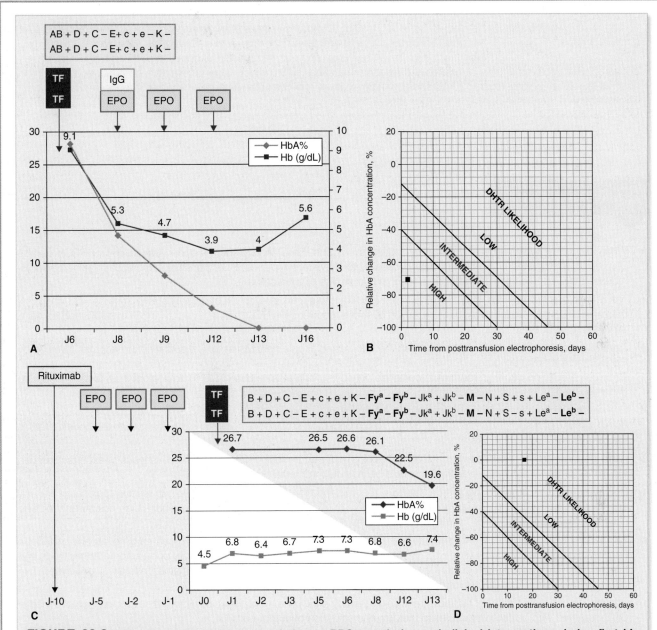

FIGURE 23-3 Clinical laboratory values in relation to RBC transfusion and clinical interventions during first hip replacement (A), normogram showing likelihood of DHTR during first hip replacement (B), and clinical laboratory values in relation to RBC transfusion and clinical treatment during severe ACS episode 2 years after second surgery (C). DHTR, delayed hemolytic transfusion reaction; EPO, erythropoietin; Hb, hemoglobin; HbA, hemoglobin A; IgG, immunoglobulin G; TF, transfusion.

The same patient was rehospitalized for a second hip replacement surgery a few years later. At that point, recommendations for the management of osteonecrosis had evolved. The patient received treatment with hydroxycarbamide a few weeks in advance combined with erythropoietin to reduce the likelihood of postoperative anemia. The target hemoglobin was 10 g/dL, taking into account that, on average, patients lose 4 g of hemoglobin after a hip replacement. Extensively phenotype-matched RBCs were reserved for her (matching not just Rh and Kell, but also prophylactic matching for Duffy, Kidd, and MNS blood groups), taking into account all the antibodies found. Treatment with rituximab at 1 month before surgery and corticosteroids 15 days before the procedure was started. The patient received her surgery and did not require transfusion in the postoperative period.

Case Study: Continued

The patient was hospitalized 2 years after her second surgery for very severe ACS requiring intensive care. Her hemoglobin level dropped drastically to 4.5 g/dL. This time, the patient received rituximab and erythropoietin. However, this time, the decision was made to transfuse because despite the erythropoietin, the hemoglobin did not rise and signs of organ failure appeared. She received 2 units of extended phenotype-matched RBCs, which were crossmatch compatible, taking into account her alloantibodies. Figures 23-3C and 23-3D detail the phenotype of the units given and her response to transfusion. This time, transfusion was effective despite the clinical context.

High-Yield Facts

◆ When the hemoglobin decreases below the patient's baseline value and symptoms occur, transfusion of RBCs can be considered, administering the fewest units necessary to alleviate symptoms. RBC transfusion increases the hemoglobin, reduces the proportion of HbS in the circulation, and improves oxygen delivery.

◆ The primary goal of RBC transfusion in the treatment of acute stroke, prevention of primary stroke in those with abnormal transcranial Doppler ultrasounds, and prevention of stroke recurrence in SCD is to reduce the HbS% to ≤30% and to maintain or increase the hemoglobin close to 10 g/dL.

◆ Transfusion of patients with ACS should initially be done using simple transfusion for patients who are anemic, followed by RBCX if there is no improvement. Patients presenting with ACS with a higher hemoglobin (≥9 g/dL) or who are more severely ill (oxygen saturation <90% on room air, progressive pulmonary infiltrates, and decreasing hemoglobin) are recommended to undergo RBCX.

◆ Chronic transfusion has been recommended for treatment of pulmonary hypertension in SCD, particularly for patients who do not tolerate or respond to hydroxyurea,[15] but larger prospective studies are necessary to further define the benefits versus the risks of this treatment in this clinical scenario.

◆ Although there are no published clinical trials of transfusion for acute multiorgan failure, the consensus of experts has been that either simple or exchange transfusion should be instituted immediately.[1]

◆ Preoperative transfusion has become a standard recommendation for SCD patients who will receive regional or general anesthesia; usually, the transfusion goal is a hemoglobin of 10 g/dL, but for patients who require high-risk surgery or who have a higher pretransfusion hemoglobin, RBCX may be needed preoperatively.

◆ Simple transfusion can be used for patients with SCD when there is a need to increase oxygen-carrying capacity without a need to acutely lower the amount of HbS. Exchange transfusion can be performed manually or by automated methods and is used when there is a need to rapidly lower the HbS%. Use of exchange transfusion, whether manual or automated, can be limited by vascular access, which can be complicated by thrombosis and infection.

◆ Patients on chronic or frequent episodic transfusion therapy should be monitored closely for iron overload. Iron overload in SCD is treated with phlebotomy, chelation therapy, and utilization of automated RBCX.

◆ Approximately 30% of transfused SCD patients produce alloantibodies to foreign RBC antigens, most commonly against Rh antigens. Prophylactic antigen matching of donor RBCs for Rh C and E antigens, as well as the K1 antigen, reduces the prevalence of alloimmunization to 7%.

◆ Patients with SCD should have a complete RBC phenotype performed by serology or genotyping of RBC blood groups by molecular methods, preferably before transfusion support is required.[58] Consultation with a transfusion medicine physician for alloimmunized patients is advised before beginning chronic transfusion therapy.

◆ Transfusion recipient risk factors for RBC alloimmunization include number of units transfused and the degree of antigen disparity between recipient and donor. There are several single nucleotide polymorphisms that have been identified in SCD patients that are associated with increased risk of alloimmunization[69-71] and protection from alloimmunization.[72,73]

◆ DHTR without hyperhemolysis can occur when there is an anamnestic response to previous RBC alloimmunization. These reactions can be prevented by closely monitoring transfused SCD patients for new RBC alloantibodies and ensuring patient alloimmunization and transfusion history is available.

◆ DHTR with hyperhemolysis is a life-threatening reaction resulting in severe anemia, below pretransfusion levels, that can occur even after transfusion of compatible RBCs that are phenotype matched.

References

1. National Institutes of Health. Evidence-based management of sickle cell disease: expert panel report. Published September 2014. https://www.nhlbi.nih.gov/health-topics/evidence-based-management-sickle-cell-disease. Accessed July 15, 2020.

2. Hirtz D, Kirkham FJ. Sickle cell disease and stroke. *Pediatr Neurol.* 2019;95:34-41.

3. DeBaun MR, Kirkham FJ. Central nervous system complications and management in sickle cell disease. *Blood.* 2016;127(7):829-838.

4. Hulbert ML, Scothorn DJ, Panepinto JA, et al. Exchange blood transfusion compared with simple transfusion for first overt stroke is associated with a lower risk of subsequent stroke: a retrospective cohort study of 137 children with sickle cell anemia. *Pediatrics.* 2006;149(5):710-712.

5. Adams RJ, McKie VC, Hsu LL, et al. Prevention of a first stroke by transfusions in children with sickle cell anemia and abnormal results on transcranial Doppler ultrasonography. *N Engl J Med.* 1998;339(1):5-11.

6. Adams RJ, Brambilla D, Optimizing Primary Stroke Prevention in Sickle Cell Anemia (STOP 2) Trial Investigators. Discontinuing prophylactic transfusions used to prevent stroke in sickle cell disease. *N Engl J Med.* 2005;353(26):2769-2778.

7. McLaughlin JF, Ballas SK. High mortality among children with sickle cell anemia and overt stroke who discontinue blood transfusion after transition to an adult program. *Transfusion.* 2016;56(5):1014-1021.

8. Ware RE, Davis BR, Schultz WH, et al. Hydroxycarbamide versus chronic transfusion for maintenance of transcranial doppler flow velocities in children with sickle cell anemia–TCD with Transfusions Changing to Hydroxyurea (TwiTCH): a multicentre, open label, phase 3, non-inferiority trial. *Lancet.* 2016;387(10019):661-670.

9. Ware RE, de Montalembert M, Tshilolo L, Abboud M. Sickle cell disease. *Lancet.* 2017;390:311-323.

10. Mallouh AA, Asha M. Beneficial effect of blood transfusion in children with sickle cell chest syndrome. *Am J Dis Child.* 1988;142(2):178-182.

11. Emre U, Miller ST, Gutierez M, et al. Effect of transfusion in acute chest syndrome of sickle cell disease. *J Pediatr.* 1995;127(6):901-904.

12. Styles LA, Abboud M, Larkin S, et al. Transfusion prevents acute chest syndrome predicted by elevated secretory phospholipase A2. *Br J Haematol.* 2007;136(2):343-344.

13. Louie JE, Anderson CJ, Fomani KFM, et al. Case series supporting heme detoxification via therapeutic plasma exchange in acute multiorgan failure syndrome resistant to red blood cell exchange in sickle cell disease. *Transfusion.* 2018;58(2):470-479.

14. Turner JM, Kaplan JB, Cohen HW, Billett HH. Exchange versus simple transfusion for acute chest syndrome in sickle cell anemia adults. *Transfusion.* 2009;49:863-868.

15. Saylors RL, Watkins B, Saccente S, Tang X. Comparison of automated red cell exchange transfusion and simple transfusion for the treatment of children with sickle cell disease acute chest syndrome. *Pediatr Blood Cancer.* 2013;60:1952-1956.

16. Sarode R, Ballas SK, Garcia A, et al. Red blood cell exchange: 2015 American Society for Apheresis consensus conference on the management of patients with sickle cell disease. *J Clin Apher.* 2017;32(5):342-367.

17. Gordeuk VR, Castro OL, Machado RF. Pathophysiology and treatment of pulmonary hypertension in sickle cell disease. *Blood.* 2016;127(7):820-828.

18. Tsitsikas DA, Seligman H, Sirigireddy B, et al. Regular automated red cell exchange transfusion in the management of pulmonary hypertension in sickle cell disease. *Br J Haematol.* 2014;167(5):707-710.

19. Detterich JA, Kato RM, Rabai M, et al. Chronic transfusion therapy improves but does not normalize systemic and pulmonary vasculopathy in sickle cell disease. *Blood.* 2015;126(6):703-710.

20. Turpin M, Chantalat-Auger C, Parent F, et al. Chronic blood exchange transfusions in the management of pre-capillary pulmonary hypertension complicating sickle cell disease. *Eur Respir J.* 2018;52:1800272.

21. ClinicalTrials.gov. Sickle Cell Disease and CardiovAscular Risk - Red Cell Exchange Trial (SCD-CARRE). https://www.clinical-trials.gov/ct2/show/NCT04084080. Accessed July 15, 2020.

22. Hassell KL, Eckman JR, Lane PA. Acute multiorgan failure syndrome: a potentially catastrophic complication of severe sickle cell pain episodes. *Am J Med.* 1994;96:155-162.

23. Koshy M, Weiner SJ, Miller ST, et al. Surgery and anesthesia in sickle cell disease. *Blood.* 1995;86(10):3676-3684.

24. Vichinsky EP, Haberkern CM, Neumayr L, et al. A comparison of conservative and aggressive transfusion regimens in the perioperative management of sickle cell disease. *N Engl J Med.* 1995;333:206-213.

25. Howard J, Malfroy M, Llewelyn C, et al. The transfusion alternatives preoperatively in sickle cell disease (TAPS) study: a randomised, controlled, multicentre clinical trial. *Lancet.* 2013;381:930-938.

26. Jorgenson M. *AABB Technical Manual.* In: Fung MK, eds. American Association of Blood Banks; 2017.

27. Chien S, Usami S, Bertles JF. Abnormal rheology of oxygenated blood in sickle cell anemia. *J Clin Invest.* 1970;49(4):623-634.

28. Schmalzer EA, Lee JO, Brown AK, Usami S, Chien S. Viscosity of mixtures of sickle and normal red cells at varying hematocrit levels: implications for transfusion. *Transfusion.* 1987;27:228-233.

29. Josephson CD, Su LL, Hillyer KL, Hillyer CD. Transfusion in the patient with sickle cell disease: a critical review of the literature and transfusion guidelines. *Transfus Med Rev.* 2007;21(2):118-133.

30. Alexy T, Pais E, Armstrong JK, et al. Rheologic behavior of sickle and normal red blood cell mixtures in sickle plasma: implications for transfusion therapy. *Transfusion.* 2006;46:912-918.

31. Serjeant G. Blood transfusion in sickle cell disease: a cautionary tale. *Lancet.* 2003;361:1659-1660.

32. Warth JA. Hypertension and a seizure following transfusion in an adult with sickle cell anemia. *Arch Intern Med.* 1984;144(3):607-608.

33. Royal JE, Seeler RA. Hypertension, convulsions, and cerebral haemorrhage in sickle-cell anaemia patients after blood-transfusions. *Lancet.* 1978;312:1207.

34. Kelly S, Quirolo K, Marsh A, et al. Erythrocytapheresis for chronic transfusion therapy in sickle cell disease: survey of current practices. *Transfusion.* 2016;56:2877-2888.

35. Koehl B, Missud F, Holvoet L, et al. Continuous manual exchange transfusion for patients with sickle cell disease: an efficient method to avoid iron overload. *J Vis Exp.* 2017;14:55172.

36. Shaz B. Red cell exchange and other therapeutic alterations of red cell mass. In McLeod BC, Weinstein R, Winters JL,

Szczepiorkowski ZM, eds. *Apheresis: Principles and Practice.* 3rd ed. AABB Press; 2010:393.

37. Kim HC. Red cell exchange: special focus on sickle cell disease. *ASH Educ Book.* 2014;2014(1):450-456.

38. Center for Biologics Evaluation and Research. 510k premarket notification: AMICUS Separator System. US Food and Drug Administration. December 4, 2018. https://www.accessdata.fda.gov/cdrh_docs/pdf18/K180615.pdf. Accessed February 12, 2019.

39. Center for Biologics Evaluation and Research. 510k premarket notification: Spectra Optia Apheresis System. US Food and Drug Administration. March 2, 2018. https://www.accessdata.fda.gov/scripts/cdrh/cfdocs/cfPMN/pmn.cfm?ID=K172590. Accessed July 6, 2019.

40. Quirolo K, Bertolone S, Hassell K, et al. The evaluation of a new apheresis device for automated red blood cell exchange procedures in patients with sickle cell disease. *Transfusion.* 2015;55:775-781.

41. Otrock ZK, Thibodeaux SR, Jackups R. Vascular access for red blood cell exchange. *Transfusion.* 2018;58:569-579.

42. Shrestha A, Jawa Z, Koch KL, et al. Use of a dual lumen port for automated red cell exchange in adults with sickle cell disease. *J Clin Apher.* 2015;30:353-358.

43. Lawicki S, Craig-Owens L, Bream PR, Eichbaum Q. Indwelling ports for prophylactic RBCXs in sickle cell patients: comparison of bard and vortex ports. *J Clin Apher.* 2018;33:666-670.

44. Rajasekhar A, Streiff MD. How I treat central venous access device-related upper extremity deep vein thrombosis. *Blood.* 2017;129:2727-2736.

45. Ramdas J, Haymon M, Ward K, et al. Treatment of superior vena cava syndrome with recombinant tissue plasminogen activator in a sickle cell patient undergoing bone marrow transplantation. *Pediatr Hematol Oncol.* 2001;18(1):71-77.

46. Delville M, Manceau S, Abdalla NA, et al. Arteriovenous fistula for automated red blood cell exchange in patients with sickle cell disease: complications and outcomes. *Am J Hematol.* 2017;92(2):136-140.

47. Yawn BP, Buchanan GR, Afenyi-Annan AN, et al. Management of sickle cell disease: summary of the 2014 evidence-based report by expert panel members. *JAMA.* 2014;312(10):1033-1048.

48. Sobota A, Graham DA, Neufeld EJ, et al. 30 day readmission rates following hospitalization for pediatric sickle cell crisis at freestanding Children's hospitals: risk factors and hospital variation. *Pediatr Blood Cancer.* 2012;58:61-65.

49. Nouraie M, Gordeuk V. Blood transfusion and 30 day readmission rate in adult patients hospitalized with sickle cell disease crisis. *Transfusion.* 2015;55:2331-2338.

50. Buehler PN, Karnaukhova E. When might transferrin, hemopexin or haptoglobin administration be of benefit following the transfusion of red blood cells? *Curr Opin Hematol.* 2018;25:452-458.

51. Quirolo K. Hemoglobin based oxygen carriers: a long road from bench to bedside. *Pediatr Hematol Oncol.* 2007;24(6):461-463.

52. Bialis C, Moser C, Sims CA. Artificial oxygen carriers and red blood cell substitutes: a historic overview and recent developments toward military and clinical relevance. *J Trauma Acute Care Surg.* 2019;87(1S suppl 1):S48-S58.

53. Janssen van Doorn K, Diltoer M, Servotte S, et al. Transfusion of polymerized bovine haemoglobin in a patient with sickle cell anaemia and severe allo-immunization: a case report. *Acta Clin Belg.* 2001;56:191-194.

54. Raff JP, Dobson CE, Tsai HM. Transfusion of polymerised human haemoglobin in a patient with severe sickle-cell anaemia. *Lancet.* 2002;360:464-465.

55. de Montalembert M, Ribeil JA, Brousse V, et al. Cardiac iron overload in chronically transfused patients with thalassemia, sickle cell anemia, or myelodysplastic syndrome. *PLoS One.* 2017;12(3):e0172147.

56. Coates TD, Wood JC. How we manage iron overload in sickle cell patients. *Br J Haematol.* 2017;177(5):703-716.

57. Wood JC. The use of MRI to monitor iron overload in SCD. *Blood Cells Mol Dis.* 2017;67:120-125.

58. Harmatz P, Butensky E, Quirolo K, et al. Severity of iron overload in patients with sickle cell disease receiving chronic red blood cell transfusion therapy. *Blood.* 2000;96:76-79.

59. Driss F, Moh-Klaren J, Pela AM, Tertian G. Regular automated erythrocytapheresis in sickle cell patients. *Br J Haematol.* 2011;154:656-659.

60. Rosse WF, Gallagher D, Kinney TR, et al. Transfusion and alloimmunization in sickle cell disease. *Blood.* 1990;76:1431-1437.

61. Vichinsky EP, Earles A, Johnson RA, et al. Alloimmunization in sickle cell anemia and transfusion of racially unmatched blood. *N Engl J Med.* 1990;322:1617-1621.

62. Sarnaik S, Schornack J, Lusher JM. The incidence of development of irregular red cell antibodies in patients with sickle cell anemia. *Transfusion.* 1986;26:249-252.

63. Ambruso DR, Githens JH, Alcorn R, et al. Experience with donors matched for minor blood group antigens in patients with sickle cell anemia who are receiving chronic transfusion therapy. *Transfusion.* 1987;27:94-98.

64. Tahhan HR, Holbrook CT, Braddy LR, et al. Antigen-matched donor blood in the transfusion management of patients with sickle cell disease. *Transfusion.* 1994;34:562-569.

65. Vichinsky EP, Neumayr LD, Earles AN, et al. Causes and outcomes of the acute chest syndrome in sickle cell disease *N Engl J Med.* 2000;342:1855-1865.

66. Vichinsky EP, Luban NLC, Wright E, et al. Prospective RBC phenotype matching in a stroke-prevention trial in sickle cell anemia: a multicenter transfusion trial. *Transfusion.* 2001;41:1086-1092.

67. Castro O, Sandler SG, Houston-Yu P, et al. Predicting the effect of transfusion only phenotype-matched RBCs to patients with sickle cell disease: theoretical and practical implications. *Transfusion.* 2002;42:684-690.

68. LaSalle-Williams M, Nuss R, Le T, et al. Extended red blood cell antigen matching for transfusions in sickle cell disease: a review of a 14-year experience from a single center. *Transfusion.* 2011;51:1732-1739.

69. Compernolle V, Chou ST, Tanael S, et al. Red blood cell specifications for patients with hemoglobinopathies: a systematic review and guideline. *Transfusion.* 2018;58:1555-1566.

70. Pirenne F, Yazdanbakhsh K. How I safely transfuse patients with sickle-cell disease and manage delayed hemolytic transfusion reactions. *Blood.* 2018;131(25):2773-2781.

71. Gogri H, Kulkarni S, Vasantha K, et al. Partial matching of blood group antigens to reduce alloimmunization in Western India. *Transfus Apher Sci.* 2016;54:390-395.

72. Pettila V, Westbrook AJ, Nichol AD, et al. Age of red blood cells and mortality in the critically ill. *Crit Care.* 2011;15(2):R116.

73. Cooper DJ, McQuilten ZK, Nichol A, et al. Age of red cells for transfusion and outcomes in critically ill adults. *N Engl J Med.* 2017;377(19):1858-1867.

74. Hendrickson JE, Hod EA, Spitalnik SL, et al. Immunohematology: storage of murine red blood cells enhances alloantibody responses to an erythroid-specific model antigen. *Transfusion.* 2010;50:642-648.

75. Desai PC, Deal AM, Pfaff ER, et al. Alloimmunization is associated with older age of transfused red blood cells in sickle cell disease. *Am J Hematol.* 2015;90(8):691-695.

76. Lannan KL, Sahler J, Spinelli SL, et al. Transfusion immunomodulation: the case for leukoreduced and (perhaps) washed transfusions. *Blood Cells Mol Dis.* 2013;50(1):61-68.

77. Ryder AB, Zimring JC, Hendrickson JE. Factors influencing RBC alloimmunization: lessons learned from murine models. *Transfus Med Hemother.* 2014;41:406-419.

78. Campbell-Lee SA, Gvozdjan K, Choi KM, et al. Red blood cell alloimmunization in sickle cell disease: assessment of transfusion protocols during two time periods. *Transfusion.* 2018;58:1588-1596.

79. Chou ST, Jackson T, Vege S, et al. High prevalence of red blood cell alloimmunization in sickle cell disease despite transfusion from Rh-matched minority donors. *Blood.* 2013;122(6):1062-1071.

80. Chou ST, Flanagan JM, Vege S, et al. Whole-exome sequencing for RH genotyping and alloimmunization risk in children with sickle cell anemia. *Blood Adv.* 2017;1(18):1414-1422.

81. Fasano RM, Booth GS, Miles M, et al. Red blood cell alloimmunization is influenced by recipient inflammatory state at time of transfusion in patients with sickle cell disease. *Br J Haematol.* 2014; 168:291-300.

82. Williams LM, Qi Z, Batai K, et al. A locus on chromosome 5 shows African ancestry-limited association with alloimmunization in sickle cell disease. *Blood Adv.* 2018;2:3637-3647.

83. Oliveira VB, Dezan MR, Gomes FCA. -318C/T polymorphism of the CTLA-4 gene is an independent risk factor for RBC alloimmunization among sickle cell disease patients. *Int J Immunogenet.* 2017;44:219-224.

84. Sippert EA, Visentainer JEL, Alves HV, et al. Red blood cell alloimmunization in patients with sickle cell disease: correlation with HLA and cytokine gene polymorphisms. *Transfusion.* 2017;57:379-389.

85. Meinderts SM, Sins JWR, Fijnvandraat K, et al. Nonclassical FCGR2C haplotype is associated with protection from red blood cell alloimmunization in sickle cell disease. *Blood.* 2017;130(19): 2121-2130.

86. Tatari-Calderone Z, Gordish-Dressman H, Fasano R, et al. Protective effect of HLA-DQB1 alleles against alloimmunization in sickle cell disease. *Hum Immunol.* 2016;77:35-40.

87. Ness PM, Shirey RS, Thoman SK, Buck SA. The differentiation of delayed serologic and delayed hemolytic transfusion reactions: incidence, long-term serologic findings, and clinical significance. *Transfusion.* 1990;30(8):688-693.

88. US Centers for Disease Control and Prevention. National Healthcare Safety Network Biovigilance Component Hemovigilance Module Surveillance Protocol. Version 2.2 January 2016. www.cdc.gov/nhsn. Accessed July 15, 2020.

89. Davenport RD, Burdick M, Moore SA, Kunkel SL. Cytokine production in IgG-mediated red cell incompatibility. *Transfusion.* 1993;33:19-24.

90. Win N. Hyperhemolysis syndrome in sickle cell disease. *Exp Rev Hematol.* 2009;2(2):111-115.

91. Mekontso Dessap A, Pirenne F, Razazi K, et al. A diagnostic nomogram for delayed hemolytic transfusion reaction in sickle cell disease. *Am J Hematol.* 2016;91(12):1181-1184.

92. Habibi A, Mekontso-Dessap A, Guillaud C, et al. Delayed hemolytic transfusion reaction in adult sickle-cell disease: presentations, outcomes, and treatments of 99 referral center episodes. *Am J Hematol.* 2016;91(10):989–994.

93. Yazdanbakhsh K, Ware RE, Noizat-Pirenne F. Red blood cell alloimmunization in sickle cell disease: pathophysiology, risk factors, and transfusion management. *Blood.* 2012;120(3): 528–537.

94. Castellino SM, Combs MR, Zimmerman SA, et al. Erythrocyte autoantibodies in paediatric patients with sickle cell disease receiving transfusion therapy: frequency, characteristics and significance. *Br J Haematol.* 1999;104(1):189-194.

95. Aygun B, Padmanabhan S, Paley C, Chandrasekaran V. Clinical significance of RBC alloantibodies and autoantibodies in sickle cell patients who received transfusions. *Transfusion.* 2002;42(1):37-43.

96. Garratty G. Autoantibodies induced by blood transfusion. *Transfusion.* 2004;44(1):5-9.

97. Young PP, Uzieblo A, Trulock E, Lublin DM, Goodnough LT. Autoantibody formation after alloimmunization: are blood transfusions a risk factor for autoimmune hemolytic anemia? *Transfusion.* 2004;44(1):67-72.

98. Ibanez C, Habibi A, Mekontso-Dessap A, et al. Anti-HI can cause a severe delayed hemolytic transfusion reaction with hyperhemolysis in sickle cell disease patients. *Transfusion.* 2016;56(7):1828-1833.

99. Petz LD, Calhoun L, Shulman IA, Johnson C, Herron RM. The sickle cell hemolytic transfusion reaction syndrome. *Transfusion.* 1997;37(4):382-392.

100. King KE, Shirey RS, Lankiewicz MW, et al. Delayed hemolytic transfusion reactions in sickle cell disease: simultaneous destruction of recipient's red cells. *Transfusion.* 1997;37:376-381

101. Win N, Sinha S, Lee E, Mills W. Treatment with intravenous immunoglobulin and steroids may correct severe anemia in hyperhemolytic transfusion reactions: case report and literature review. *Transfus Med Rev.* 2010;24:64-67.

102. Pirenne F, Bartolucci P, Habibi A. Management of delayed hemolytic transfusion reaction in sickle cell disease: prevention, diagnosis, treatment. *Transfus Clin Biol J Soc Francaise Transfus Sang.* 2017;24(3):227–231.

103. Pineda AA, Vamvakas EC, Gorden LD, Winters JL, Moore SB. Trends in the incidence of delayed hemolytic and delayed serologic transfusion reactions. *Transfusion.* 1999;39(10): 1097-1103

104. Siddon AJ, Kenney BC, Hendrickson JE, Tormey CA. Delayed haemolytic and serologic transfusion reactions: pathophysiology, treatment and prevention. *Curr Opin Hematol.* 2018;25: 459-467.

105. Vidler JB, Gardner K, Amenyah K, Mijovic A, Thein SL. Delayed haemolytic transfusion reaction in adults with sickle cell disease: a 5-year experience. *Br J Haematol.* 2015;169(5):746–753.

106. Winters JL, Richa EM, Bryant SC, et al. Polyethylene glycol antiglobulin tube versus gel microcolumn: influence on the incidence of delayed hemolytic transfusion reactions and delayed serologic transfusion reactions. *Transfusion.* 2010;50: 1444-1452.

107. Schonewille H, van de Watering LM, Loomans DS, Brand A. Red blood cell alloantibodies after transfusion: factors influencing incidence and specificity. *Transfusion.* 2006;46(2):250-256.

108. Petz LD. Bystander immune cytolysis. *Transfus Med Rev.* 2006;20(2):110-140.

109. Garratty G. The James Blundell Award Lecture 2007: do we really understand immune red cell destruction? *Transfus Med.* 2008;18(6):321-334.

110. Win N, Doughty H, Telfer P, et al. Hyperhemolytic transfusion reaction in sickle cell disease. *Transfusion.* 2001;41:323-328.

111. Noizat-Pirenne F. Transfusion and sickle cell disease: axes of transfusion safety optimization. *Transfus Clin Biol.* 2014;21;77-84.

112. Gardner K, Hoppe C, Mijovic A, Thein SL. How we treat delayed haemolytic transfusion reactions in patients with sickle cell disease. *Br J Haematol.* 2015;170(6):745–756.

113. Narbey D, Habibi A, Chadebech P, et al. Incidence and predictive score for delayed hemolytic transfusion reaction in adult patients with sickle cell disease. *Am J Hematol.* 2017;92(12):1340-1348.

Clinical Trials: State of the Art and Lessons Learned

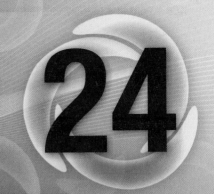

Authors: *Laura M. De Castro, Ramasubramanian Kalpatthi, Marilyn J. Telen*

Chapter Outline

Overview

In 1973, patients with sickle cell disease (SCD) due to homozygosity for hemoglobin S (HbSS) were estimated to have a median life expectancy of slightly more than 14 years,[1] and thus, the disease was essentially a disease of childhood. However, in the observational Cooperative Study of Sickle Cell Disease (CSSCD), data collected between 1977 and 1988 showed that approximately 85% of children with HbSS lived to adulthood.[2] Furthermore, in the CSSCD, child mortality peaked early, occurring among children aged 1 to 3 years, and was due predominantly to infections such as *Streptococcus pneumoniae* sepsis. Since the CSSCD natural history study, hallmark interventional clinical trials have significantly impacted the disease's natural history by establishing standards of care, helping prevent serious complications, and improving quality of life and survival in SCD. In this chapter, we first review those clinical trials that have had major impact on clinical practice and patient survival (Figure 24-1 and Table 24-1). We also summarize the major observational studies that have substantially affected clinical practice in the care of patients with SCD in Table 24-2. Subsequent sections in this chapter address the key achievements and challenges of clinical trials in SCD.

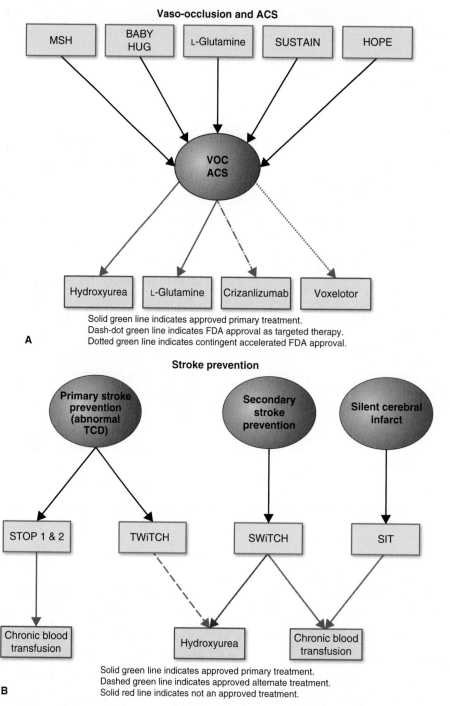

FIGURE 24-1 Major clinical trials in sickle cell disease (SCD). Many contemporary efforts endeavor to find and validate new therapeutic targets, often one or more of the many abnormalities observed in red blood cells containing predominantly hemoglobin S. Others, however, focus on downstream effects on various organs or physiologic pathways, attempting to prevent or slow organ damage. ACS, acute chest syndrome; Hb, hemoglobin; HbS, sickle hemoglobin; HSCT, hematopoietic stem cell transplantation; SCI, silent cerebral infarction; TCD, transcranial Doppler; VOC, vaso-occlusive crisis.

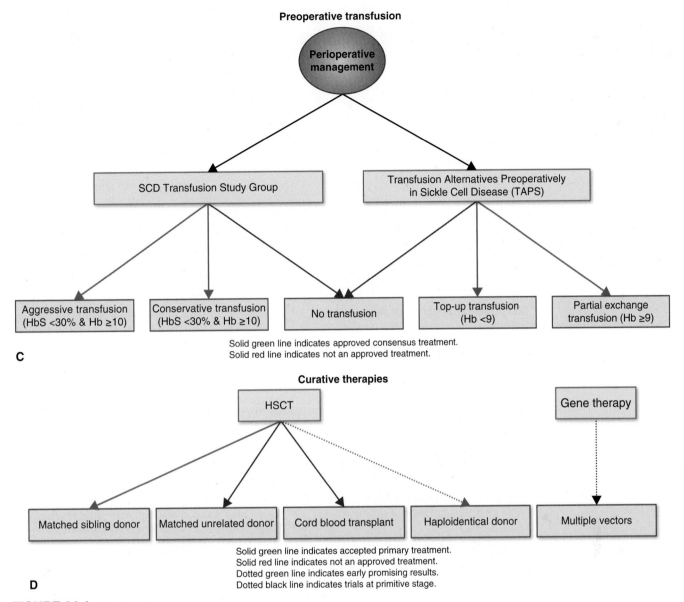

FIGURE 24-1 (*Continued*)

Infection Prevention

In the first landmark clinical trial in SCD, Prophylaxis With Oral Penicillin in Children With Sickle Cell Anemia (PROPS), Gaston et al[3] demonstrated the unequivocal benefit of penicillin prophylaxis on the morbidity and mortality of pneumococcal sepsis in children with SCD. In this trial, children with SCD aged 3 to 36 months were randomized to penicillin V (n = 105) or placebo (n = 110). This trial was terminated early because the interim analysis showed an 84% relative risk reduction, with 2 and 13 episodes of pneumococcal sepsis in the penicillin and placebo group, respectively. In addition, 3 deaths occurred in the placebo group due to invasive pneumococcal disease (IPD), whereas there were no deaths in the placebo group. This led to the practice of initiating penicillin prophylaxis shortly after birth and continuing until at least 5 years of age for children with SCD in developed countries.[4] However, there remained a

challenge regarding how to identify these young children with SCD at birth to initiate early penicillin prophylaxis. This issue was addressed by a seminal study of initiation of newborn screening for SCD, which set the standard of care for all children born with SCD.[5] Vichinsky et al[5] introduced newborn screening for SCD in California, along with comprehensive care that included early diagnosis and notification, education about how to palpate the spleen, and instructions about when to seek medical attention for prompt fever management and early treatment of splenic sequestration. Subsequently, all states in the United States started newborn screening, early comprehensive care, and penicillin prophylaxis, thus leading to a new standard of care for children with SCD. Implementation of routine administration of 23-valent pneumococcal polysaccharide vaccine and conjugated pneumococcal vaccines (PCV7 and PCV13) has since further reduced the incidence of IPD and its associated mortality in children with SCD.[6-8]

TABLE 24-1 Landmark clinical trials with major clinical practice impact in SCD

Trial and reference	Major findings	Lessons learned
Prophylaxis With Oral Penicillin in Children With Sickle Cell Anemia (PROPS)[3]	Oral penicillin prophylaxis significantly decreased morbidity (84% relative risk reduction) and mortality due to IPD in children with HbSS disease or HbS-β^0 thalassemia; 2 episodes of IPD occurred in the penicillin group (n = 105) vs 13 episodes of IPD in the placebo group (n = 110).	The study led to the recommendation of instituting universal newborn screening for SCD to permit early penicillin prophylaxis. However, this trial did not include patients with other SCD genotypes such as HbSC and HbS-β^+ thalassemia that are at risk of developing delayed, severe IPD due to functional asplenia.
Prophylaxis With Oral Penicillin in Children With Sickle Cell Anemia II (PROPS II)[4]	The study found no significant difference in the incidence of IPD between continuing penicillin prophylaxis (2 episodes [1%]) vs placebo (4 episodes [2%]) in 400 children with HbSS disease or HbS-β^0 thalassemia aged ≥5 years with mean follow-up of 3.2 years. There was no mortality due to IPD in either group.	The study concluded that penicillin prophylaxis can be safely discontinued in children with SCD aged ≥5 years who have not had a prior IPD or splenectomy, have received 2 doses of PCV23 vaccine, and are receiving comprehensive care. Like PROPS, other SCD genotypes were not included. Vaccine efficacy and splenic function were not assessed in this trial.
Multicenter Study of Hydroxyurea (MSH)[9]	Compared to placebo, hydroxyurea significantly reduced pain crises (median, 4.5 vs 2.5 per year; P <.001), ACS (51 vs 25 patients; P <.001), and transfusion requirement (73 vs 48 patients; P = .001) in adults with HbSS disease.	The MSH trial led to the FDA approval of hydroxyurea as the first drug to treat patients with SCD. MSH did not include other SCD genotypes, particularly HbS-β^0 thalassemia, which is severe. Patients who consumed higher doses of opioids were also excluded, possibly preventing patients with severe or chronic pain from entering study.
Stroke Prevention Trial in Sickle Cell Anemia (STOP)[14]	Prospective screening with TCD and randomization of children with HbSS disease or HbS-β^0 thalassemia (ICA or MCA velocities ≥200 cm/s) to CBT (n = 63) or standard of care (n = 67) resulted in early termination of trial (median follow-up, 1.75 years), with 1 stroke in CBT cohort vs 11 strokes in standard-of-care group, respectively.	Because there was a 92% stroke risk reduction in the CBT group, the STOP trial established the standard of practice of using TCD as an effective screening tool to identify SCD children who are at risk of stroke. The STOP trial did not include other SCD genotypes, and TCD velocities in both groups at study termination were not published. Baseline MRI was not obtained routinely; thus, the potential confounding influence of SCI on the development of stroke is unknown.
Stroke Prevention Trial in Sickle Cell Anemia 2 (STOP 2)[17]	Children with HbSS disease or HbS-β^0 thalassemia with abnormal TCD velocities who received CBT for >30 months with normalization of TCD were randomized to continuation of CBT (n = 38) or discontinuation of CBT (n = 41). The trial was terminated early because 2 children developed stroke and 14 had reversion of TCD to higher-risk range in the CBT discontinuation group, whereas none of these events occurred in the CBT continuation group.	This trial led to the recommendation to continue CBT indefinitely in children with SCD who have abnormal TCD velocities. Although the 2 strokes in the CBT discontinuation group were preceded by reversion to abnormal TCD velocities, not all patients with recurrence of high-risk TCD velocities would have been likely to develop stroke, as described in the STOP study. Age, an important factor of developing stroke with elevated TCD as demonstrated in the STOP study, was not factored into the conclusion of the STOP 2 results. Eight patients (20%) in the CBT discontinuation group neither developed stroke nor reverted to high-risk TCD velocities.
BABY HUG[11]	Prospective, double-blind randomization of young children with HbSS disease or HbS-β^0 thalassemia aged 9-18 months to receive hydroxyurea (n = 96) or placebo (n = 97) failed to show differences in primary end points (preservation of spleen and renal function). However, as in the MSH trial, there was significantly decreased incidence of VOC, dactylitis, ACS, and transfusion requirements in the hydroxyurea group.	Hydroxyurea showed major clinical and laboratory benefits. Fixed dose of hydroxyurea (20 mg/kg/d), shorter duration (2 years with 3 months of clinical hold of hydroxyurea), and suboptimal end point measurements were felt to be responsible for the failure to demonstrate the primary end point differences. Nonetheless, hydroxyurea was well tolerated, without major side effects. Neutropenia was the only major toxicity, but it was only mild to moderate, without any increased risk of serious infections. BABY HUG follow-up studies are just completed, and results are pending at this time.

(continued)

TABLE 24-1 Landmark clinical trials with major clinical practice impact in SCD (Continued)

Trial and reference	Major findings	Lessons learned
Stroke With Transfusions Changing to Hydroxyurea (SWiTCH)[20]	This prospective, randomized, noninferiority trial comparing transfusion/chelation to hydroxyurea/phlebotomy for secondary stroke prevention was terminated early due to futility of not achieving the composite primary outcome (liver iron concentration and stroke recurrence)	Although within the noninferiority margin, there was a trend for increased stroke risk in the hydroxyurea/phlebotomy group compared to the transfusion/chelation group (7 strokes in 67 patients vs 0 strokes in 66 patients, respectively). There were more subjects with previous recurrent strokes and baseline severe cerebral vasculopathy in the hydroxyurea/phlebotomy group, but the difference was not significant. Thus, transfusion remains the standard of care for children with SCA and previous history of stroke.
Transcranial Doppler With Transfusions Changing to Hydroxyurea (TWiTCH)[21]	This prospective, randomized, noninferiority trial comparing hydroxyurea/phlebotomy (n = 60) to transfusion/chelation (n = 61) for primary stroke prevention in children with elevated TCD velocities ≥200 cm/s was terminated early. Hydroxyurea was noninferior in maintaining TCD velocities and associated with significant decrease in iron overload in liver as measured by FerriScan R2-MRI ($P = .001$). There were no strokes or conversion to abnormal TCD in either arm. There were 3 TIAs in both arms during the study period.	Hydroxyurea is noninferior to blood transfusion in maintaining TCD velocities and can be safely offered for primary prevention of stroke in children with HbSS with elevated TCD velocities provided they have received blood transfusion for some period of time and do not have a history of stroke, TIA, or baseline severe cerebral vasculopathy. The optimal duration of transfusion before switching to hydroxyurea was not addressed but averaged 4 years in the study.
Silent Infarct Transfusion Trial (SIT)[29]	In this prospective, single-blind trial, children with SCD (age 5-15 years) with ≥1 SCI detected on MRI with normal TCD velocities were randomized to receive either CBT (n = 99) or standard of care (n = 97). With a median follow-up of 3 years, there were 6 events in the CBT group (1 stroke and 5 new or enlarged SCIs) and 14 events in the standard-of-care group (7 strokes and 7 new or enlarged SCIs).	Compared to standard of care, CBT showed a 58% relative risk reduction for overt strokes or new or enlarged SCIs. However, wide implementation of MRI screening is yet to be adopted in clinical practice. There were 9 new alloantibodies in 4 subjects in the CBT group (alloimmunization rate of 0.278 per 10 units of red blood cells). The burden of iron overload due to CBT was not addressed in this trial.
L-Glutamine[34]	Prospective, double-blind, phase III trial of oral L-glutamine supplementation (n = 152) or placebo (n = 78) in children and adults (age 5-58 years) with HbSS disease or HbS-β⁰ thalassemia showed that L-glutamine supplementation resulted in a 25% reduction in pain crises ($P = .005$) and fewer hospitalizations over 48 weeks.	This study led to the FDA approval of L-glutamine (Endari) for the prevention of acute sickle cell complications such as VOC and ACS. Biologic markers of oxidative stress or endothelial adhesion were not analyzed in this study.

Abbreviations: ACS, acute chest syndrome; CBT, chronic blood transfusion; FDA, US Food and Drug Administration; ICA, internal carotid artery; IPD, invasive pneumococcal disease; MCA, middle cerebral artery; MRI, magnetic resonance imaging; SCA, sickle cell anemia (HbSS); SCD, sickle cell disease; SCI, silent cerebral infarct; TIA, transient ischemic attack; TCD, transcranial Doppler; VOC, vaso-occlusive pain crisis.

Hydroxyurea Therapy as a Disease-Modifying Agent

In the randomized, double-blind, placebo-controlled Multicenter Study of Hydroxyurea (MSH), Charache et al[9] found that hydroxyurea significantly reduced the number of vaso-occlusive pain crises (VOCs), the incidence of acute chest syndrome (ACS), and transfusion requirements in 299 adults with HbSS and severe SCD. In addition, patients who responded to hydroxyurea treatment had improved quality of life.[10] This led to the US Food and Drug Administration's (FDA) approval of hydroxyurea as the first disease-modifying drug therapy for adults with SCD in 1998. Because organ damage was not evaluated in the MSH trial and organ damage can occur very early in life, the BABY HUG trial was then designed to address the efficacy of hydroxyurea in preventing organ damage in very young children

TABLE 24-2 Pivotal observational studies in SCD

Reference	Study information	Major findings	Implications for clinical practice
Falletta et al,[4] 1995	Discontinuing penicillin prophylaxis in children with SCA (PROPS II)	6 children had IPD, 2 (1%) in the penicillin group and 4 (2%) in the placebo group (relative risk, 0.5), in 400 children with SCA with a mean follow-up of 3.2 years.	Penicillin prophylaxis can be safely discontinued at age 5 in children with SCA if there is no previous history of IPD or splenectomy.
Gaston et al,[154] 1987	Cooperative Study of Sickle Cell Disease (CSSCD)	Multi-institutional study that followed 3800 patients with SCD from birth to adulthood (1977-1988).	The study helped understand the natural history of SCD and provided important information about disease severity and survival.
Vichinsky et al,[155] 2000	National Acute Chest Syndrome Study Group	Fat embolism and infection (atypical bacteria) were the most common causes (38%) of ACS episodes with identifiable causes in 538 patients with 671 episodes of ACS.	The addition of macrolide antibiotic to treat ACS became the standard of care.
Vichinsky et al,[156] 2001	RBC phenotype matching in SCD	Reduced alloimmunization rate and hemolytic transfusion reactions in 61 patients who received RBCs that were phenotypically matched for C, E, and Kell antigens in the STOP trial.	Matching for C, E, and Kell antigens in SCD patients receiving RBC transfusion (especially chronic blood transfusion) has become a standard practice.
Smith et al,[157] 2005	Pain in Sickle Cell Epidemiologic Study (PiSCES)	Prospective longitudinal etiologic and methodologic study of pain in 232 young adults and adults with SCD aged 16-64 years.	The study led to the introduction of the pain diary concept in SCD and helped elucidate the prevalence of daily and chronic pain and the impact of pain on health outcomes.
Gladwin et al,[158] 2004	Pulmonary hypertension in SCD	Of 195 patients who had Doppler echocardiograms, 32% of patients had pulmonary hypertension (tricuspid regurgitant jet velocity ≥2.5 m/s), which was strongly associated with increased mortality.	The study showed the importance of echocardiography as a noninvasive screening tool for pulmonary hypertension in SCD.

Abbreviations: ACS, acute chest syndrome; IPD, invasive pneumococcal disease; RBC, red blood cell; SCA, sickle cell anemia; SCD, sickle cell disease.

with SCD. BABY HUG trial was a phase III, multicenter, randomized, double-blind clinical trial in which 193 infants with SCD aged 9 to 18 months were enrolled to receive either hydroxyurea (fixed dose of 20 mg/kg/d) or placebo.[11] The primary outcomes (preservation of spleen and renal function) were not different between the groups. However, like the MSH study, there were significant reductions in VOC, ACS, dactylitis, and transfusion requirements in the hydroxyurea group. Moreover, hydroxyurea was well tolerated, and the toxicity was limited to only mild and moderate neutropenia without increased risk of bacteremia or serious infections.[12] Building on the results of BABY HUG, the FDA granted approval for hydroxyurea for children with SCD older than 2 years of age in 2017 based on the additional safety and efficacy data from the European Sickle Cell Disease Cohort study (ESCORT HU, NCT02516579).

Stroke Prevention

Primary Stroke Prevention

Stroke is one of the most devastating complications of SCD, with approximately 11% of children with HbSS developing stroke by age 20 years before the implementation of transcranial Doppler

(TCD) screening.[13] One of the most impressive advancements in SCD history is the advent of primary stroke prevention by TCD screening in children with SCD who are at high risk for stroke. The landmark Stroke Prevention Trial in Sickle Cell Anemia (STOP) demonstrated that prophylactic blood transfusions resulted in a 92% relative risk reduction of overt stroke in children with SCD who had abnormal cerebral blood flow velocity (≥200 cm/s) identified by TCD.[14] Subsequently, routine TCD screening at least annually in children with SCD starting at age 2 years, along with preventive chronic blood transfusion (CBT) for those who have abnormal TCD velocities, has become the new standard of care. As a result, the rate of strokes and stroke-related hospitalizations has dramatically decreased, and overt stroke in children with SCD is a rarity nowadays.[15,16] The subsequent Optimizing Primary Stroke Prevention in Sickle Cell Anemia (STOP 2) trial was conducted to determine the appropriate duration of the preventive blood transfusion therapy to decrease primary stroke. The results of this study showed that preventive blood transfusion therapy for primary stroke prevention might be needed indefinitely. Patients randomized to discontinue CBT had a higher frequency of either overt stroke or reversal to abnormal TCD velocities, which are associated with higher stroke risk.[17]

Secondary Stroke Prevention

The recurrent risk of secondary stroke is approximately 70% in individuals who have suffered a clinically apparent first stroke. Importantly, this risk is reduced to 13% with CBT.[18,19] However, indefinite CBT for both primary and secondary stroke prevention is associated with iron overload requiring chelation; alloimmunization; requirement of central venous line placement and its associated complications, such as infections and thrombosis; and a high health care burden for patients and parents as a result of monthly clinic visits. Due to these drawbacks of chronic transfusion, as well as the several recognized clinical benefits of hydroxyurea, the National Heart, Lung, and Blood Institute (NHLBI) sponsored the Stroke With Transfusions Changing to Hydroxyurea (SWiTCH) trial. SWiTCH was a noninferiority trial in which children with SCD and a prior history of iron overload were randomized to receive either standard treatment (transfusions with chelation, n = 66) or alternate treatment (hydroxyurea with phlebotomy, n = 67). Its primary end point was defined as a composite of recurrent stroke and liver iron concentration.[20] There were 7 recurrent strokes in the alternate treatment group but no recurrent strokes in the standard treatment group. Although recurrent stroke in the alternate treatment group was within the noninferiority margin, the trial was terminated early because there was no difference in liver iron concentration between these 2 treatment groups. Thus, continuation of the trial was considered to be futile in reaching the composite primary outcome. The authors noted that there were more subjects with previous recurrent strokes and baseline severe cerebral vasculopathy in the hydroxyurea/phlebotomy group compared to the transfusion/chelation group, although this difference was not statistically significant. Thus, CBT remains the standard of care for secondary stroke prevention in children and adolescents with SCD. Moreover, due to lack of data in older patients, this practice is often continued into adulthood.

Hydroxyurea as an Alternative for Primary Stroke Prevention

Despite hydroxyurea being deemed ineffective for secondary stroke prevention, the NHLBI also sponsored a clinical trial to investigate its efficacy in primary stroke prevention. The Transcranial Doppler With Transfusions Changing to Hydroxyurea (TWiTCH) was another noninferiority trial that studied children with SCD and abnormal TCD velocities. The children studied had had no previous strokes and no baseline severe cerebral vasculopathy; they had also received at least 1 year of CBT. Study participants were randomized to receive either continued CBT or hydroxyurea and phlebotomy.[21] In contrast to SWiTCH, the rationale for the TWiTCH study was supported by previous studies that clearly demonstrated decreasing TCD velocities with hydroxyurea treatment.[22-24] This trial was also terminated early because noninferiority (maximum TCD velocity with a noninferiority margin of 15 cm/s) was shown in the interim analysis to support the efficacy of hydroxyurea in maintaining low TCD velocities. The final model-based TCD velocities were 143 ± 1.6 and 138 ± 1.6 cm/s in children who received standard transfusion versus hydroxyurea, respectively (noninferiority, $P = 8.82 \times 10^{-16}$; post hoc superiority, $P = .023$). The investigators concluded that hydroxyurea can be a safe alternative to CBT for primary prevention of stroke in children with sickle cell anemia who have received at least 1 year of blood transfusions and have no magnetic resonance angiography–defined severe vasculopathy.

Silent Cerebral Infarct

Silent cerebral infarct (SCI) is the most common neurologic injury, occurring in 30% of children with SCD.[25] The presence of SCI is associated with an increased risk of overt stroke, poor academic achievement, and lower IQ scores.[26-28] The Silent Infarct Transfusion Trial was a single-blind clinical trial that randomized children aged 5 to 15 years who had ≥1 SCI detected on magnetic resonance imaging (MRI) to receiving either CBT (n = 99) or standard of care (n = 97). CBT showed a 58% relative risk reduction in overt strokes or new or enlarged SCIs compared to standard of care (2 vs 4.8 events per 100 patient-years, respectively; $P = .04$).[29] However, implementation of routine screening for SCI has not yet been widely accepted because the detection of SCI requires a brain MRI, which often necessitates sedation and/or general anesthesia, especially in young children.

Hematopoietic Stem Cell Transplantation

Hematopoietic stem cell transplantation (HSCT) has been recommended as a treatment option for children who have either a history of stroke or abnormal TCD velocities in the context of SCD. However, there is limited information available on the efficacy of HSCT in either primary or secondary stroke prevention. Nonetheless, in a recent multicenter, nonrandomized, controlled intervention trial of matched sibling donor HSCT (DREPAGREFFE), Bernaudin et al[30] reported that matched sibling donor HSCT significantly reduced TCD velocities at 1 year compared to standard treatment (transfusions with option to switch to hydroxyurea) (129 cm/s vs 170 cm/s, respectively; $P < .001$). These results were sustained at 3 years of follow-up. In addition, no strokes, sickle cell symptoms, or chronic graft-versus-host disease (GVHD) occurred in the transplant group.

Prevention of Acute Sickle Cell Complications

VOC and ACS are the most common causes of hospitalizations in children and adults with SCD. Until recently, hydroxyurea was the only drug available for prevention of these acute sickle cell complications. Oxidative stress has been postulated as one of the major contributors to the complex pathophysiology of SCD. Sickle red blood cells (RBCs) have a lower redox ratio (NADPH/NAD), and this phenomenon has been associated with a higher hemolytic rate and pulmonary arterial hypertension.[31] Oral supplementation of L-glutamine raises this redox ratio in sickle RBCs and is associated with decreased endothelial adhesion.[32,33] In a multicenter, double-blind, placebo-controlled, phase III clinical trial involving 230 children and adults with SCD, oral supplementation of L-glutamine (Endari) significantly decreased pain crises (median, 3 vs 4 crises; P = .005), ACS (17.2% vs 46.3%; P = .003), and the number of hospitalizations for sickle cell pain–related events (median 2 vs 3 hospitalizations; P = .005) compared to placebo.[34] These improvements, which appeared in patients both taking and not taking hydroxyurea, led to FDA approval in 2017 of L-glutamine (Endari) for the prevention of acute complications of SCD such as VOC and ACS.

Increased cellular adhesion has also been identified as a critical component of vaso-occlusion in SCD and involves adhesion of both RBCs[35-38] and leukocytes,[39,40] as well as activation of platelets and endothelial cells (reviewed in Telen et al[41]) Not surprisingly, therefore, several studies have attempted to demonstrate the utility of antiadhesive therapies in SCD. A phase II, double-blind, randomized, placebo-controlled clinical trial of crizanlizumab (Adakveo, formerly SEG101), a humanized monoclonal antibody that binds to P-selectin and blocks its interaction with P-selectin glycoprotein ligand 1 (PSGL-1), has recently been completed,[42] and crizanlizumab was approved by the FDA as a therapeutic option for prevention of vaso-occlusive episodes for all SCD types in November 2019.

Although vaso-occlusion clearly occurs in animal models due to cell adhesion in the absence of red cell sickling, polymerization of sickle hemoglobin (HbS) is a pathophysiologic hallmark of SCD and contributes to both mechanical small-vessel occlusion as well as hemolysis and the downstream inflammatory sequelae of that process (reviewed in Telen et al[41]). In a multicenter, phase III, double-blind, randomized, placebo-controlled trial (HOPE), daily administration of an oral anti-sickling agent, voxelotor (Oxbryta, formerly GBT440) was associated with significantly increased hemoglobin levels and reduced markers of hemolysis, but a not significantly different annualized incidence rate of VOC, compared to placebo in patients with SCD aged 12 to 64 years.[43] Voxelotor was also approved by the FDA in November 2019, although for the indication of improvement of anemia rather than reduction of vaso-occlusive episodes. Thus, it remains to be seen to what extent either of these drugs will produce major changes in clinical practice and patient outcomes.

Perioperative Management

Individuals with SCD undergoing elective or emergency surgical procedures are at risk for excess morbidity (VOC and ACS) and mortality, underscoring the importance of optimal perioperative management in these patients.[44] Preoperative blood transfusions have long been used as one of the strategies to minimize this risk, but there has been little consensus about the best transfusion management (eg, exchange transfusion to reduce the percent HbS or conservative "top up" simple transfusion). In a multicenter study, Vichinsky et al[45] randomized 551 patients with SCD who underwent 604 surgeries to receive either exchange transfusion to reduce HbS to ≤30%, with total

hemoglobin ≥10 g/dL (n = 278 patients with 303 procedures), or conservative transfusion to achieve a hemoglobin ≥10 g/dL (n = 273 patients with 301 procedures). In that study, both groups had a similar incidence of serious complications (31% in the exchange transfusion group and 35% in the conservative transfusion group) with a 10% risk of ACS in both. However, the risk of transfusion-related complications was higher with exchange transfusion compared to simple transfusion (14% vs 7%, respectively; odds ratio, 2.15 [95% confidence interval, 1.23-3.77]). The vast majority of subjects in the study were young and were undergoing relatively low-risk procedures, such as tonsillectomy and cholecystectomy; therefore, the optimal transfusion regimen for older patients with more comorbidities or undergoing higher-risk surgeries remains to be defined. In the Transfusion Alternatives Preoperatively in Sickle Cell Disease (TAPS) trial, Howard et al[46] randomized children and adults with SCD who were scheduled for low- or medium-risk surgeries to 1 of 2 groups: preoperative transfusion (n = 36) or no transfusion (n = 34). This trial was halted early because there were more clinically important complications (ACS being the most common) in the no transfusion group compared to those who received preoperative transfusion (39% vs 15%; P = .023). Based on these studies, the 2014 SCD expert panel report recommends preoperative blood transfusion to bring the hemoglobin level to 10 g/dL in children and adults with SCD prior to any surgical procedure that involves general anesthesia.[47] There is no published evidence regarding preoperative transfusions for individuals with HbSC and other SCD genotypes with high baseline hemoglobin. However, the decision for preoperative transfusion for patients with SCD, either simple or exchange, should be individualized based on the level of risk associated with surgical procedures and, more importantly, the patients' clinical status and comorbidities.

Curative Therapies

HSCT is the only curative treatment currently available for individuals with SCD. Since the first bone marrow transplantation in 1984, approximately 2000 individuals with SCD have received allogeneic HSCT.[48,49] Excellent outcomes have been reported in an international survey of 1000 SCD patients who received human leukocyte antigen (HLA)-matched sibling donor (MSD) HSCT (1986-2013), with event-free and overall survival rates of 91.4% and 92.9%, respectively, accompanied by a 7% mortality rate.[48] The majority of the patients included in that report, however, were <16 years old (85%), and 87% received myeloablative conditioning regimens. In contrast, adults with SCD often have comorbidities such as pulmonary hypertension and chronic kidney disease that increase the risk of toxicities associated with myeloablative regimens. To overcome this, nonmyeloablative regimens have been studied in adults receiving HSCT for SCD. Hsieh et al[50] reported a 97% overall survival rate in 30 adults who underwent MSD HSCT with a nonmyeloablative conditioning regimen (low-dose total-body irradiation and alemtuzumab) and sirolimus for GVHD prophylaxis. There was no acute or chronic GVHD in these patients. However, most SCD patients do not have an HLA-MSD. Thus, the Blood and Marrow Transplant Clinical Trials Network conducted the Sickle Cell Unrelated Donor Transplant (SCURT) trial using a reduced conditioning regimen in children and adolescents with SCD. The cord blood arm was prematurely stopped due to a high transplant rejection rate (5 of 8 children), and the bone marrow transplantation arm had a high frequency of extensive chronic GVHD (38%), rendering these strategies unsafe.[51] HSCT from related haploidentical donors is another option to increase the donor pool and cure rate. The number of these transplants has been low, although early results have been encouraging. Research accomplishments and future research are described in more detail in Chapter 25.

Several gene therapy trials in SCD have been ongoing since the first reported successful gene therapy attempt using a lentiviral vector in a child with HbSS.[52] These approaches, along with the American Society of Hematology's (ASH) Sickle Cell Disease Initiative, including its ASH Research Collaborative SCD Clinical Trials Network, and the NHLBI's Cure Sickle Cell Initiative, both of which commenced existence in 2018, are expected to improve the clinical outcomes and raise the chance of cure of this debilitating disease. Gene therapy research is covered more thoroughly in Chapter 29.

Study Design and Performance

The simple single nucleotide change in the gene encoding the β chain of hemoglobin A belies the complicated pathophysiology resulting from it. Despite the restriction of hemoglobin expression to red cells and their precursors, the presence of HbS—alone or in combination with other hemoglobin variants that participate in deoxygenated hemoglobin polymer formation—gives rise to a broad range of RBC abnormalities as well as adverse effects on essentially all the major organs of the body. Thus, many contemporary efforts endeavor to find and validate new therapeutic targets, often one of the many abnormalities observed in RBCs containing predominantly HbS. Other efforts, however, focus on downstream processes affecting various organs or pathophysiologic pathways in attempt to prevent or slow organ damage. Thus, when contemplating the discovery and validation of new therapeutics for SCD, many challenges must be overcome.

First, a decision must be made as to the therapeutic target. One could clearly target the abnormal gene by replacing or correcting it. Or, one could use other therapies, such as hydroxyurea, to target normal regulation of hemoglobin genes, especially the "switching" mechanism that turns off normal fetal γ hemoglobin (required by fetal hemoglobin [HbF]) while activating the adult β globin. Alternatively, one could target the abnormal function of HbS and attempt to forestall polymerization of HbS, for example, through manipulation of its oxygen affinity.

Challenges can arise from the fact that SCD is a relatively rare disease, especially in resource-rich countries with the means to conduct clinical trials. SCD is also quite variable, necessitating that relatively large populations be studied in order to identify statistically significant and clinically meaningful effects. Of course, clinical trials most often follow and often build on evidence obtained through studies in animal models. That natural sequence of events, however, is only useful when the animal models fairly accurately represent the pathophysiology of the human disease.

Discovering, testing, and improving therapies for SCD has thus proven quite challenging indeed. In other diseases, both common and rare, these challenges are often met with the use of biomarkers of disease activity and algorithms for risk stratification in order to make clinical studies as efficient as possible. Although many biomarkers have been studied, they have thus far proven of quite limited utility. Attempts at risk stratification have also met with only a small degree of success because the data about natural history of SCD are also inadequate. Furthermore, enrollment in clinical trials, in the face of small patient populations, constrained resources, and a degree of mistrust between patients and providers, has also remained problematic. As a result, development of drugs for SCD has been slow. As mentioned earlier, hydroxyurea gained its first FDA approval for adults with SCD in 1998 and was approved for children almost 20 years later, in 2017. However, recent FDA approval of three new drugs, L-Glutamine (2017), crizanlizumab (2019) and voxelotor (2019) for SCD is encouraging.

Identifying Therapeutic Targets

Some of the many pathophysiologic processes that occur as part of SCD, along with classes of compounds that could address them, are illustrated in Figure 24-2. Hemolysis and consequent anemia are the hallmarks of SCD. However, the effects of hemolysis extend beyond anemia; the usually robust erythropoietic response results in reticulocytosis, as well as release of hemoglobin and microparticles into the plasma. Toxic levels of heme also contribute to the downstream processes of membrane damage, decreased nitric oxide bioavailability, procoagulant hemostatic abnormalities, production and release of vasoactive and proinflammatory compounds, blood cell adhesion and activation, and endothelial activation and injury. These developments then play a role in causing inflammation, vaso-occlusion, and ischemia-reperfusion injury.[53]

To date, a number of pathophysiologic processes have been targeted by new potential pharmacotherapeutics over the past several decades, using many different strategies.

The hyperactivated coagulation system of SCD was targeted early in the history of therapeutics for SCD, using antiplatelet and anticoagulant drugs. However, although it was recognized early that markers of activation of coagulation were elevated in SCD,[54,55] a fuller understanding of the many pathways of coagulation activation present in SCD has continued to grow. Among the mechanisms now known to contribute to coagulation activation are increased expression of tissue factor by monocytes and endothelial cells,[56-58] expression of phosphatidylserine by both sickle RBCs and microparticles,[59] and release

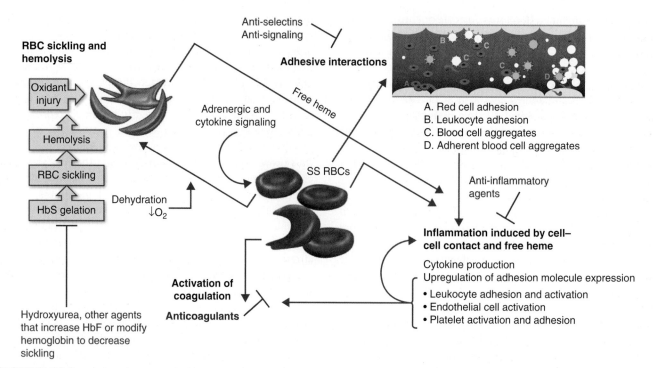

RBC sickling and hemolysis

Oxidant injury

Hemolysis

RBC sickling

HbS gelation

Dehydration ↓O₂

Hydroxyurea, other agents that increase HbF or modify hemoglobin to decrease sickling

Adrenergic and cytokine signaling

SS RBCs

Activation of coagulation

Anticoagulants

Anti-selectins Anti-signaling

Adhesive interactions

Free heme

A. Red cell adhesion
B. Leukocyte adhesion
C. Blood cell aggregates
D. Adherent blood cell aggregates

Anti-inflammatory agents

Inflammation induced by cell–cell contact and free heme

Cytokine production
Upregulation of adhesion molecule expression
• Leukocyte adhesion and activation
• Endothelial cell activation
• Platelet activation and adhesion

FIGURE 24-2 **The complex and highly interactive pathophysiology of sickle cell disease.** Sickle cell disease pathophysiology stems from the presence of abnormal hemoglobin in the red blood cells (RBCs) but sets in motion a complex series of interactive pathologic processes involving hemolysis, cell adhesion, cell activation, coagulation, and inflammation. Of note, many of these feed into each other, so that together they produce a vicious cycle of interrelated processes that tend to exacerbate each other. Potential therapeutic targets abound among many different physiologic pathways. HbF, fetal hemoglobin; HbS, sickle hemoglobin.

of free heme from hemolysis itself.[60,61] The combined effects of multiple prothrombotic pathways, involving multiple components of the coagulation cascade, are increased thrombin generation and platelet activation. Thus, many approaches to decreasing activation of coagulation have been studied.

Among antiplatelet agents, trials have studied the effects of prasugrel, ticlopidine, aspirin, piroxicam, and eptifibatide. However, as early as the 1980s, 4 trials of aspirin showed no consistent effect on frequency of VOCs.[62-65] More recently, prasugrel was studied in the pediatric age group. However, after animal studies and phase II results suggested potential for a clinical effect,[66,67] a large, multicenter, randomized, placebo-controlled trial showed no significant effect on vaso-occlusion or other clinical end points, despite a modest platelet inhibitory effect.[68]

Likewise, anticoagulants were also studied early in the history of clinical trials for SCD. However, these studies were small and inconclusive. Studies of warfarin exhibited little or no benefit measured by the frequency of VOCs while being associated with significant bleeding, despite being effective in lowering the otherwise high levels of detectable D-dimer in plasma.[69,70] Heparin and low-molecular-weight heparin, due to the requirement for intravenous or subcutaneous administration, have mostly been studied only in the setting of acute VOC, although one study of low-dose unfractionated heparin prophylaxis in 4 patients, spanning several years, did show an approximately 70% decrease in days requiring hospitalization for pain, as well as in emergency department visits.[71]

Low-molecular-weight heparins, however, remain of uncertain value for the treatment of acute VOC.[72,73]

Recent and current late-stage clinical trials at this time have focused on numerous other critical pathophysiologic processes, including oxidative damage; hemoglobin polymerization, cell sickling, and hemolysis; and cell adhesion. L-Glutamine, explored due to its potential to improve antioxidant capacity, was approved by the FDA for use in SCD based primarily on a phase III study of 230 pediatric and adult patients,[34] as discussed earlier in this chapter.

Hemoglobin polymerization and cell sickling have been explored as therapeutic targets in trials of the drug voxelotor (GBT-440). Voxelotor directly inhibits the polymerization of HbS by binding to hemoglobin and shifting the oxygen dissociation curve so that hemoglobin does not release oxygen as easily. When voxelotor is administered to people, a concentration-dependent left shift of the oxygen equilibrium curves is observed.[74] In phase III human studies, voxelotor significantly increased hemoglobin levels and reduced markers of hemolysis, even in the approximately two-thirds of patients taking hydroxyurea, although it did not have a significant effect on frequency of vaso-occlusive episodes.[43] This is perhaps similar to the previously demonstrated effect of senicapoc (ICA-17043), another compound investigated for its ability to decrease sickling and hemolysis by a different mechanism. Senicapoc is a Gardos channel inhibitor that blocks cell dehydration; by improving cell hydration, it lowers the cellular concentration of hemoglobin and thereby decreases the rate of hemoglobin polymerization, which is concentration dependent.[75] However, although it significantly raised hemoglobin levels in a phase III study, it also failed to lessen the rate of VOC.[76]

Thus far, efforts to target cell adhesion with novel pharmacologic agents have been somewhat more successful, despite the plethora of potentially targetable adhesion receptor-ligand interactions that can be shown to be active in vitro and in sickle mice (reviewed in Telen[77]). In one instance, crizanlizumab, a humanized monoclonal antibody against P-selectin, was tested for its ability to reduce the frequency of VOC. In a successful phase II, randomized, placebo-controlled study of 198 subjects who received crizanlizumab or placebo every 4 weeks, high-dose crizanlizumab (5 mg/kg) was associated with a 45.3% lower median rate of pain crises (1.63 vs 2.98; $P = .01$) compared to placebo.[42] Phase III studies of crizanlizumab were ongoing at the time of this writing.

A second antiadhesive drug, rivipansel (originally GMI-1070), has also been studied, although in this case for the indication of acute vaso-occlusive pain because rivipansel has a relatively short half-life, unlike an antibody. Rivipansel is a small carbohydrate molecule that inhibits selectin-mediated adhesion, with highest affinity for E-selectin. In mice, rivipansel improved blood flow in small vessels, reduced RBC-leukocyte interactions, and improved survival of sickle cell mice from tumor necrosis factor (TNF)-induced VOC, with mortality reduced from 100% to 50%.[78] After a successful phase I study,[79] a small randomized, placebo-controlled phase II study showed significant reduction in opioid requirements with rivipansel and a large, but not statistically significant, reduction in mean length of hospitalization required for treatment of VOC.[80] A phase III trial was subsequently undertaken and enrollment was completed; however, announcement of initial results, as yet unpublished, indicated that the trial failed to achieve its primary and secondary end points.

Thus, both historical and current investigations of potential therapeutics for SCD have targeted multiple pathophysiologic targets. Given the "vicious cycle" of pathophysiology shown in Figure 24-2, it remains undetermined whether intervention at one point rather than another would be most efficacious in forestalling vaso-occlusion, inflammation, and end-organ damage.

Choosing Therapeutic End Points

As is easily understood from the previous brief synopses of selected recent clinical studies of novel therapeutic agents, not only must investigators choose a therapeutic target, but they must also choose a suitable clinical end point. Those used in studies thus far include anemia, hemolysis, and frequency or length of VOC episodes (with concomitant reduction of need for opioid medication), frequency of ACS and prevention of primary or secondary stroke.

Several factors contribute to making specific end points particularly suitable to clinical trials. In clinical studies, the end point that indicates a favorable response to a treatment may be a laboratory value (eg, improvement in baseline anemia, 6-minute walk test result), a clinical measurement (eg, days requiring hospitalization, physical exam findings such as presence, absence, or size of leg ulcers), or a subjective measurement or patient-reported outcome (eg, pain score). Lab measurements are not affected by the subjective interpretation of the health care provider but may have their own limitations (eg, the unreliability of hemoglobin A1c in a patient with shortened RBC life span) and may not be a good reflection of overall health and subjective well-being. Clinical measures may be provider and site dependent. Subjective measures, such as pain scores and quality of life measures, may depend on the interviewer and the patient, and pain scores are notoriously difficult to compare between individuals. Overall, there is also the philosophical and practical question of whether changes that do not translate into clearly documentable improved survival, relief of suffering, or substantially enhanced patient perceptions of well-being are meaningful enough to warrant approval of a new therapeutic agent.

Considering Effect Size

When choosing an end point, the investigators also must be able to estimate the effect size they hope or expect to achieve because the likelihood that a study will be able to detect an association between a predictor variable (ie, drug or placebo) and an outcome variable (end point) depends on the actual magnitude of the association—the effect size. Ordinarily, statisticians perform power calculations to estimate how many subjects will be needed to demonstrate a statistically significant effect as a result of the treatment to be tested. In addition, the investigators need to decide what minimum effect size would be considered clinically significant and whether the needed study population size is achievable. However, the true effect size is usually not known until after the study is completed.

Therefore, investigators often define their study population according to the characteristics they expect will lead to the largest effect size in the shortest amount of time. Thus, a study of a drug chosen because of its potential to decrease hemolysis would be best performed in patients with higher degrees of hemolysis, although a particular drug may not be effective in extremely high hemolytic rates. Similarly, most studies designed to prevent VOC require a minimum baseline frequency because patients who experience 0 to 1 event per year would have to be treated and followed for a very long time before a difference could be observed, whereas patients who experience ≥3 VOCs per year would need to be followed for a much shorter time in order to observe significant reductions in VOC rate, as was observed in the MSH trial.[81]

Effect size and the clinical significance of the effect size observed are also important. In some large studies, for example, a dietary change reduced blood pressure by 2 to 3 mm Hg (high to medium sodium intake) or more substantially by 7 to 11 mm Hg (high to low sodium intake).[82] Although there might be statistical significance, due to the large size of the population studied, few clinicians would think that adding a new drug to a patient's antihypertensive regimen would be worth the potential cost and side effects if the blood pressure decrement was likely to be 2 to 3 mm Hg, whereas a 10-mm Hg reduction might be viewed as clinically meaningful. Similarly, if the average patient with VOC is hospitalized for 5 days, a 2-day decrease in length of stay would be considered clinically significant by most physicians,[80] whereas a 1- to 2-hour decrease would likely not be considered as meriting the medication in question.[83]

Subject Enrollment

SCD is a rare disease, with most likely no more than 100,000 individuals of all ages with the disease in the United States. Furthermore, as many as half of patients lack reliable health insurance coverage, and financial resources to allow them to travel to clinical trial sites, and access to centers that conduct clinical trials in SCD. Not surprisingly, therefore, trials in SCD have often struggled to meet their target enrollments and have required much longer enrollment periods than initially hoped for. Nonetheless, due to dedicated physicians and research personnel, pharma-sponsored clinical drug trials have recently been meeting their expected enrollment numbers. However, this achievement has also proven to be expensive, because it has required long enrollment times using many participating sites, and subjects have often required financial support to participate. In the future, therefore, efforts should be directed toward creating a clinical trial infrastructure and conducting clinical trials in areas of high SCD prevalence, namely Africa and India. This effort has now begun, with the support of the National Institutes of Health (NIH), other foundations, and national programs located in Africa and India, and this effort is discussed further later in this chapter. Consequently, successes are now starting to accrue. For instance, a recent study documenting the feasibility and safety of using hydroxyurea in children in sub-Saharan Africa showed that hydroxyurea treatment was feasible and safe in children in that population[84]; >600 children received hydroxyurea for at least 3 years and experienced a reduced incidence of VOC, infections, malaria, transfusions, and death without an undue rate of drug-related adverse events. Hopefully, therefore, the participation of centers with large patient populations outside of resource-rich countries in the Americas and Europe will accelerate clinical trial development and drug discovery for SCD.

Patient Selection and Risk Stratification

As discussed earlier, present and future clinical trials in SCD are likely to involve drugs that potentially act through a wide variety of mechanisms, and the study end points can similarly be expected to be varied. In addition, SCD, even when defined as homozygosity for HbS, is clinically quite variable. Although more than three-quarters of patients are likely to experience ACS at least once in their lifetime,[85] many other sequelae—such as stroke, sickle cell nephropathy (SCN), priapism in males, and pulmonary arterial hypertension (PAH)—only occur in a minority of patients.[86,87] It has been assumed that some

of these differences in disease expression among individuals with the same hemoglobin diagnosis arise from genetic polymorphisms, but these have been definitively demonstrated in only a very few cases. Perhaps the best documented effect of a genetic variant outside the hemoglobin genes and their regulators are the *ApoL1* polymorphisms associated with SCN.[88-91] In addition, the phenotype varies when HbS is co-inherited with other hemoglobin mutations, such as a β thalassemia allele, or hemoglobins C, D, E, or O. Compound heterozygosity for HbS and other mutations has its own typical natural history and most frequent sequelae, usually with considerable overlap with HbSS but also with significant differences.

One of the most frequently used end points for SCD clinical trials is a meaningful decrease in frequency of VOC. However, although painful VOC comprises the paradigmatic presentation of SCD, the frequency of VOC varies widely among patients, as well as during the lifetime of individuals. Furthermore, there is no gold standard for diagnosis of VOC. Pain is a subjective, patient-reported symptom, and there is no objective measure for degree of pain. Although various pain scales have been tested and employed, they remain most useful when tracking the course of pain in an individual patient. Such scales have yielded widely discrepant results when patients are compared to one another. Moreover, for many adult patients with both chronic pain and avascular necrosis of 1 or more joints or leg ulcers, it can be hard to differentiate between an acute VOC episode and exacerbation of chronic pain. Thus, if frequency of VOC is to be the primary end point of a clinical study of a drug with prophylactic potential, the study must be designed to clearly define VOC. Lack of universally accepted guidelines to define VOC has led to inconsistent approaches among studies.

The definition of VOC in most trials has included (1) a painful episode with no other apparent cause (eg, trauma, infection in the painful area[s]) and (2) requirement for medical attention to treat pain. However, beyond those elements, different studies have used a variety of defining characteristics. In the MSH trial,[92] VOC was defined as an episode of pain requiring a visit to a medical facility and having no other apparent cause other than SCD. Furthermore, the visit had to last at least 4 hours and require treatment with either parenteral opioids or nonsteroidal anti-inflammatory drugs, although oral or transdermal opioids qualified in institutions where parenteral opioids were not available. In addition, discrete episodes of ACS, hepatic sequestration, and priapism were considered VOC. In the phase II trial of crizanlizumab, a somewhat similar definition was used. However, there was no time of treatment requirement, and treatment with both oral and parenteral opioids was qualifying; both hepatic and splenic sequestration, as well as priapism and ACS, were considered qualifying events. Finally, an independent blinded crisis review committee adjudicated what qualified as VOC.[42]

Somewhat different definitions have been used for studying drugs considered as potential treatments for acute VOC, in which the primary end point is a measure of time to resolution of VOC, such as time to hospital discharge or time to report of resolution of VOC symptoms. In a study of poloxamer 188, study entry required hospitalization for VOC and requirement for parenteral opioids.[83] In addition, the study included not only patients with HbSS and HbS-β⁰ thalassemia, but also patients with HbSC and HbS-β⁺ thalassemia, whereas the MSH trial did not include subjects with HbSC and HbS-β⁺ thalassemia. The poloxamer study also enrolled both children and adults, whereas the initial MSH study only enrolled adults. Finally, the poloxamer study mandated administration of study drug within 12 hours of presentation, in an attempt to ensure that treatment was provided during the most acute phase of the episode. Another recent study of treatment for acute VOC, the phase II study of rivipansel, also required hospital admission and administration of parenteral opioids but included only HbSS and HbS-β⁰ thalassemia genotypes; however, it allowed up to 24 hours from patient presentation to study drug administration.[80] It further limited enrollment to patients who had had ≤5 episodes of VOC in the past 6 months in an attempt to exclude patients being admitted for treatment of exacerbation of chronic pain.

End-Organ Damage

When seeking to design a clinical study of an intervention aimed at preventing or treating end-organ–related outcomes, an ability to identify patients at highest risk for a specific adverse outcome, such as progression of chronic kidney disease, is likely to result in a trial demonstrating a larger effect size with a smaller number of subjects. Studies of life expectancy in SCD clearly demonstrate an association of survival with specific types of end-organ damage, including stroke, SCN, and PAH, with the latter often used loosely to include anyone with an elevated tricuspid regurgitant jet velocity (TRV).[86,87] Other types of organ damage, such as priapism, skin ulcers, and avascular necrosis of bone, are also extremely distressing to patients, even when not life threatening. Therefore, many clinical studies have focused and continue to focus on preventing and treating these sequelae of SCD.

When exploring ways to improve or prevent the deterioration of kidney function, for example, we can consider the signs of kidney dysfunction we generally use in clinical medicine, such as presence or absence of proteinuria or hematuria and measurement of estimated or measured glomerular filtration rate (eGFR or mGFR). However, in the case of SCN, these are relatively insensitive measures, in that proteinuria does not appear until there is substantial kidney injury and eGFR remains normal or above normal in many SCD patients due to the hyperfiltration usually present in older children and young adults. Thus, for a trial of a drug candidate for the prevention of SCN, none of these measures would identify individuals at high risk of developing SCN, although they would identify people who were already developing the disorder. Likewise, for a drug designed to retard the deterioration of renal function, being able to predict who is likely to suffer rapid renal functional decline would make a clinical study more powerful.[93]

In the case of PAH, it is clear that individuals with SCD who have TRVs ≥2.5 m/s have markedly worse survival, with a mortality rate 6- to 10-fold higher than other patients with SCD,[86,87,94-96] despite the fact that they do not all have right heart catheterization–documentable PAH as usually defined in patients without SCD. However, requirements to prevent pulmonary hypertension, which occurs in about 20% to 30% of adults with SCD, may be different from those needed to treat it. Thus, it again becomes problematic to identify the study population needed to answer the study question. For a potential preventative therapy, one would like to be able to identify patients at high risk for developing PAH but who do not yet have it. For those with PAH, one might want to identify those at highest risk of early mortality, again to focus the therapeutic trial on the patients at risk.

These types of conundrums clearly arose in the STOP trial. Although the investigators were able to demonstrate that regular transfusion prevented stroke in almost all children at high risk, as identified by TCD measurements, they may have transfused a large number of patients who would never have suffered strokes.[14] Unfortunately, when MRI data were combined with TCD results, they did not significantly improve the investigators' ability to predict which subjects were at highest risk of stroke.[14]

Biomarkers

A biomarker is a quantifiable indicator of a biologic condition, often used in the study of both normal and pathologic biologic processes, as well as to study pharmacologic responses to a therapeutic intervention. The term *biomarker* is sometimes used to include a variety of clinical measures. Thus, molecular, histologic, radiographic, and physiologic characteristics can be considered types of biomarkers. In SCD, measures such as TCD, the 6-minute walk test and TRV might fall into this category. Other biomarker measures might include quantitation of proteins, metabolites, and gene expression.

Role of Biomarkers in Clinical Trials and Pitfalls of Using Biomarkers

Biomarkers have been used in many disciplines to identify individuals who are susceptible to or at risk for developing a specific disease or condition. Such biomarkers are especially useful when attempting prophylactic studies, such as of vaccinations. They can also serve to select at-risk populations for long-term longitudinal studies aimed at understanding or preventing a specific disease consequence. By doing so, biomarkers allow clinical studies to be more time and cost efficient. Biomarkers can also be used in the diagnosis of a condition; for example, proteinuria can be considered a biomarker for SCN. In that case, however, patients with the condition, rather than at risk for it, are identified. Further along the continuum, biomarkers may enable monitoring of disease progression or identification of prognosis, that is, which individuals with the condition are most likely to do poorly, experiencing either more rapid advancement of their condition or even accelerated mortality from it. For example, several biomarkers have been shown to be strongly linked to mortality in SCD. These include soluble vascular cell adhesion molecule 1 (sVCAM1), soluble intercellular adhesion molecule 1 (sICAM1), and pro-brain natriuretic peptide (pro-BNP)[86,94,97]; in each case, the higher the value, the shorter is the expected survival. However, biomarkers do not always perform as expected. One study, for example, found that sICAM1 levels were significantly decreased in HbSC patients with retinopathy compared to those without ocular disease.[98] Biomarkers are also used in the context of clinical studies to monitor response to therapy (eg, changes in cellular function) and to demonstrate that an intervention has indeed caused a biologic response. Biomarkers can also be used to monitor safety of an intervention by measuring the presence or extent of toxicity related to an intervention. And finally, biomarkers are sometimes used as surrogate end points as a substitute for direct measures of how a patient feels, functions, or survives. Unlike most primary end points in clinical trials, a surrogate end point does not directly measure the effect of an intervention but is expected to predict clinical benefit (or harm) based on the scientific evidence demonstrating a strong linkage between the biomarker and the clinical end point of interest.

Irrespective of the purpose for which a biomarker is used, both the biomarker and the technology to measure it must be validated. The analytical assay to be used must be well characterized with respect to its sensitivity, specificity, reliability, and reproducibility. The quality of the biomarker for its purpose must be supported with high-quality evidence of association between the biomarker and the disease state or therapeutic response that it is meant to represent. Furthermore, the measure must be strongly correlated to a meaningful clinical outcome. Ideally, the correlation between a biomarker and the disease state with which it correlates should have a clear mechanism of association, although these are not often clearly demonstrated.

Peptide and Protein Biomarkers

Historically, many or even most biomarkers studied in the context of SCD have been proteins or peptides because these are more readily measured by standard and relatively inexpensive technologies. Overall, many protein and peptide biomarkers are elevated in SCD patients as compared to those without SCD. Further, many of these biomarkers, as well as others, are comparatively elevated during VOC compared to steady state. In general, such biomarkers may be classified as representative of classes of pathophysiologic processes, as shown in Table 24-3.

Genomics and Other Omics

Clinical, environmental, genetic, and proteomic factors all contribute to risk for specific sequelae in SCD. Thus, identifying these risk factors may provide an opportunity to identify at-risk patients early in the process of end-organ damage in order to most beneficially pursue therapeutic approaches. However, many markers of end-organ damage reflect relatively late-stage disease processes. Consequently, it is difficult

to identify at-risk SCD patients prior to end-organ damage. Nonetheless, markers for early detection of organ dysfunction, including genetic modifiers and metabolomic and proteomic markers, are essential to the design of efficient clinical trials targeting prevention of end-organ damage in order to combat these outcomes in a rare disease population such as patients with SCD.

To date, most investigations have considered simple risk models for organ-specific phenotypes, primarily examining a single genetic or biologic marker at a time, without gaining increased statistical power from identifying multiomic predictors of both disease-specific and multiple correlated outcomes. However, one single nucleotide polymorphism (SNP) is unlikely to exert a large effect on risk, whereas the combination of multiple independent SNPs may exert a stronger influence, especially in the context of other clinical or demographic factors. Complex genetic models have been used to predict risk of stroke[99] and HbF[100] in small SCD cohorts, and a risk scoring system for rapid eGFR decline has recently been described.[93] However, as available SCD data sets grow, along with the depth of phenotypic and genotypic information they contain, it is reasonable to anticipate greatly enhancing our power to design and improve predictive models of SCD-related organ dysfunction and functional decline, thus making targeted clinical trials more practical and enrollment more achievable.

Almost 2 decades of research have led to the identification of genetic variants that may contribute to various clinical outcomes. The genetic alteration most firmly associated with a specific clinical outcome is alteration of the *APOL1* gene, which contributes to SCN,[88-91] as well as to kidney disease in other settings. Association of variants in *APOL1* with proteinuria in SCD was first described in the Outcome Modifying Genes in Sickle Cell Disease (OMG-SCD) cohort,[89] and this finding was subsequently replicated in several other SCD cohorts.[101-103] However, variation at the *APOL1* locus explains only a portion of overall SCN risk, as the frequency of proteinuria associated with risk genotypes ranged from 35% to 50%, suggesting additional genetic factors may also contribute to risk for renal dysfunction in SCD. Others have reported association of SCN with genetic variants identified by candidate gene studies or exome sequencing studies,[101,104-106] although for the most part, these associations have not been replicated. The pathophysiology of SCN may indeed also be distinct from other forms of kidney disease and thus be most influenced by different genetic factors. The trajectory of renal decline in SCD patients is also steeper than renal decline in African Americans without SCD.[93] Thus, genetic modifiers influencing renal function in patients with SCD remain to be fully elucidated.

Stroke is another outcome that produces major morbidity and mortality in SCD. Using TCD studies in children, investigators found that children at high risk can be identified and that most strokes can be prevented by CBT.[14] However, 20 years on, screening with TCD remains the only clinical prognostic tool available, and CBT remains the treatment recommended for children at high risk of stroke. Because only a minority of high-risk children experienced an overt stroke

TABLE 24-3 Selected biomarkers reflecting pathophysiologic processes in sickle cell disease

Erythrocyte biology	Inflammation	Coagulation (including platelet activation)	Neutrophil and monocyte activation	Endothelium: activation and adhesion	Hemolysis, heme and heme catabolism, and oxidant stress
Adhesion[159,160]	IL-1β[161]	Thrombin generation assay[162]	Soluble L-selectin (sL-SEL)[163]	Soluble P-selectin (sP-SEL)[97]	Haptoglobin[164]
Deformability (EI) c/s deoxygenation[165]	IL-10[166-168]	TAT[169]	IL-8[167,168,170-172]	Soluble E-selectin (sE-SEL)[97]	Hemopexin[173]
Phosphatidylserine (PS) exposure[174-178]	IL-2[166,179]	D-dimer[54,55]	IL-6[167,168,170,180]	sVCAM1[87,97]	Lactate dehydrogenase (LDH)[181]
Reactive oxygen species (ROS)[182]	IL-3[183]	Soluble tissue factor[184]	PMN degranulation[185]	sICAM1[97]	ROS[182]
Oxidative damage to membrane proteins	Plasma HMGB1[186]	Soluble CD40 ligand (sCD40L)[187]	NETs[188]		
Cellular GSH content[189]	NF-κB[190]		Tumor necrosis factor-α[161,167,168,170,180]		
PIGF[191-194]			hsCRP[164,184]		
ERK phosphorylation[37,195-197]			MIP-1α[167]		
Cellular cAMP content[198]					
Cellular ATP content[199]					

Abbreviations: ATP, adenosine triphosphate; cAMP, cyclic adenosine monophosphate; EI, elongation index; GSH, glutathione; HMGB1, high mobility group box 1; hsCRP, high-sensitivity C-reactive protein; IL, interleukin; MIP-1α, macrophage inflammatory protein-1α; NETs, neutrophil extracellular traps; NF-κB, nuclear factor-κB; PIGF, placental growth factor; PMN, polymorphonuclear leukocyte; sICAM1, soluble intercellular adhesion molecule 1; sVCAM1, soluble vascular cell adhesion molecule 1; TAT, thrombin-antithrombin.

during approximately 18 months of follow-up (10% per year) without transfusion,[14] the relatively poor positive predictive value of TCD as a screening test means that many children are transfused to prevent overt stroke in a few. Thus far, the search for other factors, such as genetic variants that might contribute to risk, has produced no validated and accepted answers.[107] However, one study has suggested that plasma protein markers may eventually be useful for this purpose. Tewari et al[108] have shown that children with silent strokes have alterations in proteins in the coagulation and atherosclerosis pathways, although there were no genetic polymorphisms associated with these changes.

Epigenetic factors, such as DNA methylation and histone modification, have been a major focus of recent efforts to ameliorate SCD through upregulation of HbF production, and these efforts are now also moving into the realm of gene therapy. These issues are discussed elsewhere in this book.

However, epigenetic factors may also have effects outside of hemoglobin switching and globin gene expression. MicroRNAs (miRNAs) are well recognized to affect gene expression and are a focus of intense research interest.[109] *KLF, Bcl11A,* and *Sox6,* all of which in turn affect HbF expression.[110] In a study of epigenetic changes associated with hydroxyurea treatment, the investigators found that the degree of methylation of the (G)γ-globin promoter was inversely correlated to baseline HbF levels but was only slightly minimally changed by hydroxyurea treatment. However, hydroxyurea treatment was associated with significantly altered miRNA expression, and expression of both miR-26b and miR-151-3p was associated with HbF levels at steady state after hydroxyurea treatment.[109] However, miRNA expression is altered in SCD even without hydroxyurea treatment and may affect other disease-modifying processes, such as oxidative stress defense mechanisms,[111,112] which in turn can affect hemolytic rate and degree of anemia.

Likewise, metabolomic analysis can offer potentially useful insights because it analyzes the summary results of genomic, transcriptomic, and proteomic events occurring together, thus providing a functional readout of cellular, tissue, and organism biochemistry.[113] The metabolome comprises the small molecules produced by cells, and it is possible to examine metabolomes of different tissues in an organism. In SCD, metabolomic analysis has been performed on RBCs, plasma, and urine. In each instance, such analysis offers an unbiased look at how the biochemical status of the contributing cells or tissues relates to cell, tissue, and even organism phenotype. Metabolomic examination of erythrocytes, for example, has shown that there are detectable differences in numerous pathways between normal and sickle RBCs, including in glycolysis, in glutathione and ascorbate metabolism, and in metabolites associated with membrane turnover, among other findings.[114] Nonetheless, glycolysis end-products such as pyruvate and lactate were shown to be present in normal amounts in sickle compared to normal RBCs in one study, suggesting that glycolysis occurs fairly normally in sickle RBCs.[115] However, the same study found reduced glutathione, which reflects reduced antioxidant capacity. Sickle RBCs also contain increased amounts of 2,3-diphosphoglycerate, which increases off-loading of oxygen from hemoglobin and thus potentiates sickling as oxygen tension decreases. Metabolomic analysis of whole blood from sickle mice confirmed that adenosine is increased in comparison with normal mouse blood and further showed that inhibition of the adenosine signaling cascade reduced sickling and improved inflammation and disease progression in sickle mice.[116]

Metabolomic analysis may also help distinguish between patients with a high or low risk of specific SCD complications. Indeed, 2 groups have now used metabolomics, as well as other biomarkers and clinical parameters, to study SCN and progression of renal dysfunction. Elsherif et al[117] performed an exploratory study of plasma metabolomics in patients with SCD with and without proteinuria. This study found that several measured metabolites, including dimethylamine, betaine, proline, glutamate, and lysine, were substantially altered in patients with proteinuria, a sign of SCN. in addition, a longitudinal study of progression of SCN found that asymmetric dimethylarginine and quinolinic acid were associated with rapid renal function decline.[93]

Ultimately, longitudinal studies of integrated biomarkers derived from proteomics, transcriptomics, metabolomics, and other analysis platforms are needed to determine their relationships to SCD severity, as measured by such events as frequency of VOC and occurrence of end-organ damage.[118]

Applicability of In Vitro and Animal Models in Preclinical Studies

SCD has not been identified to occur spontaneously in mice, necessitating the need to create a sickle hemoglobinopathy in mice using molecular genetic techniques. Two steps were

required for success: removal, or "knock out," of native murine hemoglobin genes and insertion of functional human globin genes leading to synthesis of human hemoglobin containing 2 α and 2 β chains. Currently, there are 2 murine models of SCD that meet the key criteria of eliminating expression of murine globins while enabling expression of human α- and β-globins.[119,120] These models, unlike earlier ones, also enable expression of human HbF during fetal development, reducing but not eliminating in utero and early postnatal mortality in homozygous HbS mice. Surviving mice do closely mimic the human disease in many respects. They are anemic with high levels of hemolysis and robust reticulocytosis, have easily inducible in vivo sickling and vaso-occlusion (in response to stimuli such as hypoxia, free heme, and inflammatory cytokines such as TNF-α), and suffer damage to a variety of important organ systems, including the brain and kidney.

So-called sickle mice, however, only incompletely imitate human SCD. Although they suffer many of the same types of end-organ damage as do human SCD patients, there are distinct differences. For example, both types of mice have enlarged rather than infarcted, shrunken, and nonfunctional spleens, as seen in adult humans. In addition, in studies of cell-cell interactions, the mouse models also show their differences. On the cellular-biochemical level, murine RBCs do not express BCAM/Lu or CD44, 2 adhesion receptors that are expressed by human RBCs and contribute to cell-cell interactions. BCAM/Lu mediates adhesion to both endothelial laminin and leukocyte α4β1 integrin, whereas CD44 also mediates RBC–white blood cell interactions with extracellular matrix and integral membrane proteins. Thus, for reasons that have yet to be fully understood, several trials in humans have failed to duplicate the robust "clinical" responses seen in sickle mice. For example, the platelet inhibitor prasugrel attenuated both basal and agonist-stimulated platelet activation in the Berkeley murine model of SCD.[67] However, a prospective randomized trial of prasugrel to prevent VOC in children and adolescents with SCD showed that prasugrel did not significantly reduce the rate of VOC compared to placebo.[121] Likewise, the pan-selectin blocker rivipansel showed pronounced activity in preventing and ameliorating VOC in sickle cell mice,[78] as well as reduced opioid need during VOC during a phase II study.[80] Nonetheless, a recent phase III study showed that the same compound failed to shorten vaso-occlusive episodes in patients with SCD.[122] Likewise, the heparinoid sevuparin showed robust antiadhesive activity in a mouse model, including prevention of vaso-occlusion,[38] but failed to show a meaningful clinical benefit by shortening VOC events in patients with SCD (NCT02515838).[123]

Therapeutic Pitfalls and Unexpected Sequelae

Potential therapeutic interventions may be aimed at ameliorating or preventing one or more of the many sequelae of SCD, including anemia, pain due to vessel occlusion and consequent tissue hypoxia, and end-organ damage. Likewise, interventions may also exacerbate aspects of SCD, such as anemia, pain frequency, or organ health. For example, senicapoc, a Gardos channel inhibitor, had been shown in a preclinical study and a phase II study in SCD patients to limit solute and water loss, resulting in preservation of sickle RBC hydration.[75,124] Because polymerization of deoxygenated HbS is in part dependent on intracellular hemoglobin concentration, it was theorized that senicapoc could improve sickle RBC survival. Senicapoc was studied in a phase III trial to determine whether it could decrease the frequency of VOC in the presence or absence of hydroxyurea.[76] In the latter study, senicapoc was again shown to significantly increase hemoglobin levels and result in decreased numbers of dense cells associated with sickling. However, the study was terminated early due to a lack of efficacy in lessening the frequency of VOC compared to placebo. Nonetheless, some evidence derived from the phase II study suggests that raising hemoglobin levels may have meaningful beneficial effects. In the 35 subjects who received the study drug and experienced a hemoglobin increase of at least 0.5 g/dL in the phase II study, significant decreases were observed in N-terminal prohormone of brain natriuretic peptide (NT-proBNP), a marker of heart failure, pulmonary hypertension, and shortened life expectancy.[125]

In another example, studies of sildenafil were undertaken as a treatment for SCD-associated PAH, a condition that impairs quality of life and significantly shortens survival.[126] PAH is a frequent complication of SCD that is associated with hemolysis and impaired nitric oxide bioavailability in hemolytic diseases generally. In an early study, therapy with sildenafil appeared safe and seemed to improve both the degree of PAH as well as exercise capacity.[127] However, in a larger phase III study, the NIH stopped the trial (known as Walk-PHaSST) nearly 1 year earlier than anticipated due to safety concerns, when data from the first 33 subjects receiving the drug showed that they experienced significantly more medical problems than those who had received placebo. Pain episodes severe enough to require hospitalization were the most common of these problems.

Thus, as we see in these studies, the complex pathophysiology of SCD may result in some pharmacologic agents resulting in a benefit in one parameter usually considered in SCD, while at the same time giving rise to adverse outcomes in other parameters.

Challenges From the Patient Perspective

The challenges facing clinical investigators are multifactorial and can be considered from different perspectives, as discussed earlier. From the patients' and study participants' point of view, trust is frequently cited as a main roadblock, but lack of awareness about trials, socioeconomic factors, and communication issues, such as fear that trial involvement would have a negative effect on the patient's relationship with their physician, are also all very relevant. Racial and cultural differences between the patients and the study team; complexity and stringency of

the protocol; presence of a placebo or no-treatment group; and target recruitment, enrollment, and completion of study visits are the most frequent areas in which challenges to performance of clinical trials have been observed.[128-132]

Historical Perspectives

Mistrust in clinical trials in general and specifically by the African American community appears to have strong roots in the historic events surrounding the unethical and immoral, racially based malpractice of the US Public Health Service. The Tuskegee Study of Untreated Syphilis in the Negro Male, which was carried out in Macon County, Alabama, from 1932 to 1972,[133,134] documented the natural history of untreated syphilis and continued despite the availability of medical treatment. In response to the Tuskegee study's ethical missteps, regulations were created to manage human participant research, including the creation of the National Commission for the Protection of Human Subjects of Biomedical and Behavioral Research in 1974 and establishment of regulatory systems ranging from individual informed consent and supervision by local institutional review boards to federally set standards, including the Common Rule (45 CFR 46).[135] Nonetheless, mistrust by participants of the systems meant to protect research participants continues to make many individuals cautious about participation in clinical trials, especially among minorities, women, and other underrepresented populations.[136-138]

Patient-Centered Considerations

SCD is more prevalent in the following ethnic groups: people of African descent, including African Americans; Hispanics from the Caribbean and Central and South America; and people of Middle Eastern, Asian, Indian, and Mediterranean ancestry,[139,140] most of which are considered ethnic minority groups in the United States. There is a lack of data detailing the current percentage of patients with SCD who identify themselves as African American or belonging to other minority race or ethnicity groups, such as Hispanics, due to lack of sufficiently large sample sizes in surveys, incomplete diagnostic work or testing inadequacies, and missing or misleading ethnicity data.[141] Demographics of 336 children enrolled in Michigan Medicaid in 2014 and classified by hemoglobin status included 78% African Americans, 2% Whites, 0% Asians, and 19% unknown; 1 child was identified as Hispanic.[142] More than 95% of the patients with SCD participating in hallmark clinical trials in the United States have defined themselves racially as Black or African American, including 96% in BABY HUG trial (NCT00006400)[143] and 95% in the phase III trial of L-glutamine (NCT01179217).[34] Individuals with SCD, mainly due to their race and socioeconomic status, are considered to belong to "special populations," defined as age (minors <18 years of age or adults >65 years), historically underrepresented ethnic or racial groups, and people who live in rural areas.[144] The term *special populations* has been used interchangeably with *vulnerable populations* and *diverse populations*, and the inconsistent terminology may complicate comparisons across studies.[145]

Several SCD clinical trials of significant relevance have been terminated early and/or did not achieve their enrollment goals due to low enrollment.[130,146] A recent study by Suarez et al[147] attempted to characterize SCD pain phenotypes in adults with SCD and controlled for African ancestry. The study report highlighted the recruitment and completion challenges; for example, 49% of study visits were cancelled, often due to patients experiencing pain, and there was only an 80% study participant retention rate. They concluded that patients' struggles with illness, chronic pain, and their life situations resulted in many challenges both for recruitment and completion of study visits. Their data also—and critically—showed that a key factor in overcoming those challenges was gaining the trust of patients with SCD and establishing a participant-centered approach.[134,147]

Future of Clinical Research in SCD

Challenges in Enrollment

Two publications derived from the BABY HUG study—the landmark clinical trial on the use of hydroxyurea in young children with SCD—provide insight into the challenges of designing and executing such a fundamental study in SCD from the patient, patient's parent/guardian, and research team perspectives. In this study, reasons for declining participation and concerns during participation included frequency of clinic visits and lab tests (cited by 25% as reasons for declining participation), fear or avoidance of research, lack of transportation, excessive distance from home to the clinical center, increased costs or effects on health insurance, lack of family support, fear of research-associated loss of control of decision making, and mistrust of research or medical providers.[142,148]

Challenges Presented by SCD

An unequivocal challenge of exceptional importance for planning, but also for enrollment and completion, is posed by issues intrinsic to SCD itself. Estimates calculate the number of individuals affected with SCD in Africa to be between 12 and 15 million, whereas there are 70,000 to 100,000 cases in the United States,[149] where most of the clinical trials on SCD have been developed and implemented. The relatively low disease prevalence in the United States and the lack of a nationwide or global SCD patient registry present a major challenge for the design and conduct of clinical trials.

In addition, patients experiencing pain, a hallmark of SCD, frequently encounter difficulties presenting to scheduled appointments, including routine clinic appointments or clinical trial study visits. This translates to low enrollment, frequent failure to document study end points, and loss of participant follow-up. Other disease-related challenges are associated with the significant site-to-site variability of patient care protocols, such as dissimilarity in clinical practice for dosing and administering oral and parental opioid analgesics at different clinical sites. A combined effect of these challenges is the difficulty in establishing generalizable study end points, as well as the standardization of clinical trial study schedules and protocols.[130,148]

Protocol-Related Challenges

Protocol-related concerns, highlighted by the BABY HUG study, include the complexity of the trial, opposition to randomization and the use of a placebo, the potential for negative side effects, burdensome testing, and recruitment of potentially vulnerable subjects. Other elements in the design of clinical trials—such as definition of end points, unanticipated severe toxicity, and monitoring requirements—were addressed early in the study implementation phase, mainly by the initiation of a Feasibility and Safety Pilot Study, which was designed to ensure intensive monitoring of the first 40 BABY HUG study randomized subjects. These approaches, designed to monitor for a variety of adverse occurrences and address challenges early, contributed to the successful completion of the study.[143,150]

Another SCD clinical trial experience also provided significant insight regarding the challenges and barriers of performing studies in the SCD population. The IMPROVE trial, a randomized controlled trial of patient-controlled analgesia for sickle cell painful episodes, was designed as a multicenter, acute intervention randomized clinical trial of 2 methods of patient-controlled analgesia for acute painful episodes. The study was designed and executed by the NHLBI-sponsored Sickle Cell Disease Clinical Research Network but was terminated early due to inadequate enrollment (NCT00999245).[130,148] Obstacles to patient accrual identified at the end of the study included inability of most of the sites (17 of 31 sites) to enroll patients and the short duration of the available enrollment period for those 14 sites that were able to enroll study participants. Protocol design components also contributing to difficulty in accrual included both the complex dosing schedule and the study eligibility criteria. Local site-specific barriers were also identified as associated with site and study team performances, including poor communication with the research team about potentially eligible patients in the emergency department, where study enrollment began; involvement of multiple departments; the requirement for staff availability during weekends and after hours; protocol acceptance by staff and providers; competing protocols; and other overarching staff limitations. The investigators concluded that each of these study-related difficulties needs to be systematically addressed to guarantee the success of future studies in SCD. Notably, most of the challenges and barriers preventing successful clinical trial execution are not exclusive to SCD and may be encountered in studies conducted in other populations.[136,137,151]

Collaborations: National and International

Interest in and participation of patients with SCD and their relatives in research in general, and specifically in clinical trials, remain challenging but have also evolved over the years, in part due to efforts by federal agencies, private institutions, and other professional and lay organizations. These efforts are multilevel and range from improving patients' awareness of and education about both SCD and clinical trials to involving patients and their advocates in the design and implementation of clinical trials. Efforts have included emphasizing study aims, outcomes, and methodology that matter to the patients, as well as the creation of clinical trials networks to improve standardization of study design methodology and clinical trial conduct.

Partnering With Pharma and Federal Agencies and Professional Society Initiatives

In the past 10 years, the interest of not-for-profit institutions, such as the Patient-Centered Outcomes Research Institute (PCORI) and the American Society of Hematology (ASH) Research Collaborative, in enhancing patient engagement and participation in decisions involving research and clinical trial planning appears to have positively impacted the SCD patient community's knowledge of and interest in participating in clinical trials.

PCORI is a nonprofit organization authorized by Congress to fund comparative clinical effectiveness research. Its mission is to help people make informed health care decisions and improve health care delivery and outcomes by producing and promoting high-integrity, evidence-based information that comes from research guided by patients and their caregivers, among others.

In 2018, as part of a comprehensive and long-term initiative, ASH's Research Priorities for Sickle Cell Disease, ASH created the ASH Research Collaborative and its first SCD Clinical Trials Network (CTN), with the aim of accelerating the development of new therapies for patients with SCD. One of the SCD CTN key subcommittees is the Patient Engagement and Education Subcommittee, underscoring the role that patients

with SCD should have in steering future clinical research in this area.

An example of an innovative international partnership of investigators and clinical institutions, formed with support from an established pharmaceutical partner, was the recently concluded REACH trial. This clinical trial involved collaboration between investigators in North America and Africa, with donation of the study drug, hydroxyurea, by the pharmaceutical industry. This study demonstrated both that rigorous clinical trials could be performed in Africa, a relatively resource-poor setting, and that hydroxyurea could be safely and beneficially used in that setting. In addition, this study highlighted use of a consensus-based therapeutic research protocol (NCT01966731).[152,153]

Conclusion

In summary, the long-term and transformative involvement of traditional funding sources, such as the NIH and especially the NHLBI, the National Institute of Diabetes and Digestive and Kidney Diseases, PCORI, and the Doris Duke Charitable Foundation, remains a strong force of support for current and future clinical trials in SCD. In addition, the interest of biopharma startup companies, together with the involvement of established pharmaceutical companies, appears to be at unprecedented heights. Not only are they investing in the development of new therapeutics and sponsoring clinical trials, but perhaps as importantly, they are also supporting SCD community- and patient-based initiatives, including grassroots efforts to provide education and advocacy for SCD (eg, oneSCDvoice [https://www.onescdvoice.com/], Novartis's STEP [Solutions to Empower Patients] Program). Thus, the prospects for new and innovative clinical research on the many aspects of SCD (eg, clinical outcomes, psychosocial issues, curative interventions) is brighter than ever.

High-Yield Facts

◆ Historically, clinical trials for sickle cell disease have been characterized by difficulty in reaching enrollment goals and ill-defined endpoints, although more recent trials have improved subject participation.

◆ New and innovative clinical studies of many aspects of SCD, for example, clinical outcomes, psychosocial issues, curative interventions, etc., are currently stronger and better positioned for success than before, in large part due to

- Availability of federal, pharma, professional societies, and private foundations support;
- Better definition of study aims and biomarkers;
- Emphasis on patient-reported outcomes research; and
- Active participation by patients and their advocates in study design, planning, and enrollment.

◆ The recent FDA approval of three new SCD-modifying drugs represents a significant advance in the availability of multidrug therapy to address key SCD complications, although it remains to be seen to what extent these new drugs will produce major changes in clinical practice and patient outcomes.

References

1. Diggs LM. Anatomic lesions in sickle cell disease. In: Abramson H, Bertles JF, Wethers DL, eds. *Sickle Cell Disease: Diagnosis, Management, Education, and Research.* C.V. Mosby; 1973.

2. Leikin SL, Gallagher D, Kinney TR, Sloane D, Klug P, Rida W. Mortality in children and adolescents with sickle cell disease. Cooperative Study of Sickle Cell Disease. *Pediatrics.* 1989;84(3):500-508.

3. Gaston MH, Verter JI, Woods G, et al. Prophylaxis with oral penicillin in children with sickle cell anemia. A randomized trial. *N Engl J Med.* 1986;314(25):1593-1599.

4. Falletta JM, Woods GM, Verter JI, et al. Discontinuing penicillin prophylaxis in children with sickle cell anemia. Prophylactic Penicillin Study II. *J Pediatr.* 1995;127(5):685-690.

5. Vichinsky E, Hurst D, Earles A, Kleman K, Lubin B. Newborn screening for sickle cell disease: effect on mortality. *Pediatrics.* 1988;81(6):749-755.

6. Adamkiewicz TV, Sarnaik S, Buchanan GR, et al. Invasive pneumococcal infections in children with sickle cell disease in the era of penicillin prophylaxis, antibiotic resistance, and 23-valent pneumococcal polysaccharide vaccination. *J Pediatr.* 2003;143(4):438-444.

7. Halasa NB, Shankar SM, Talbot TR, et al. Incidence of invasive pneumococcal disease among individuals with sickle cell disease before and after the introduction of the pneumococcal conjugate vaccine. *Clin Infect Dis.* 2007;44(11):1428-1433.

8. Oligbu G, Collins S, Sheppard C, et al. Risk of invasive pneumococcal disease in children with sickle cell disease in England: a national observational cohort study, 2010-2015. *Arch Dis Child.* 2018;103(7):643-647.

9. Charache S, Terrin ML, Moore RD, et al. Effect of hydroxyurea on the frequency of painful crises in sickle cell anemia. Investigators of the Multicenter Study of Hydroxyurea in Sickle Cell Anemia. *N Engl J Med.* 1995;332(20):1317-1322.

10. Ballas SK, Barton FB, Waclawiw MA, et al. Hydroxyurea and sickle cell anemia: effect on quality of life. *Health Qual Life Outcomes.* 2006;4:59.

11. Wang WC, Ware RE, Miller ST, et al. Hydroxycarbamide in very young children with sickle-cell anaemia: a multicentre, randomised, controlled trial (BABY HUG). *Lancet.* 2011;377(9778):1663-1672.

12. Thornburg CD, Files BA, Luo Z, et al. Impact of hydroxyurea on clinical events in the BABY HUG trial. *Blood.* 2012;120(22):4304-4310; quiz 4448.

13. Ohene-Frempong K, Weiner SJ, Sleeper LA, et al. Cerebrovascular accidents in sickle cell disease: rates and risk factors. *Blood.* 1998;91(1):288-294.

14. Adams RJ, McKie VC, Hsu L, et al. Prevention of a first stroke by transfusions in children with sickle cell anemia and abnormal results on transcranial doppler ultrasonography. *N Engl J Med.* 1998;339(1):5-11.

15. Enninful-Eghan H, Moore RH, Ichord R, Smith-Whitley K, Kwiatkowski JL. Transcranial Doppler ultrasonography and prophylactic transfusion program is effective in preventing overt stroke in children with sickle cell disease. *J Pediatr.* 2010;157(3):479-484.

16. McCavit TL, Xuan L, Zhang S, Flores G, Quinn CT. National trends in incidence rates of hospitalization for stroke in children with sickle cell disease. *Pediatr Blood Cancer.* 2013;60(5):823-827.

17. Adams RJ, Brambilla D, Optimizing Primary Stroke Prevention in Sickle Cell Anemia Trial Investigators. Discontinuing prophylactic transfusions used to prevent stroke in sickle cell disease. *N Engl J Med.* 2005;353(26):2769-2778.

18. Pegelow CH, Adams RJ, McKie V, et al. Risk of recurrent stroke in patients with sickle cell disease treated with erythrocyte transfusions. *J Pediatr.* 1995;126(6):896-899.

19. Powars D, Wilson B, Imbus C, Pegelow C, Allen J. The natural history of stroke in sickle cell disease. *Am J Med.* 1978;65(3):461-471.

20. Ware RE, Helms RW, SWiTCH Investigators. Stroke With Transfusions Changing to Hydroxyurea (SWiTCH). *Blood.* 2012;119(17):3925-3932.

21. Ware RE, Davis BR, Schultz WH, et al. Hydroxycarbamide versus chronic transfusion for maintenance of transcranial doppler flow velocities in children with sickle cell anaemia: TCD With Transfusions Changing to Hydroxyurea (TWiTCH): a multicentre, open-label, phase 3, non-inferiority trial. *Lancet.* 2016;387(10019):661-670.

22. Kratovil T, Bulas D, Driscoll MC, Speller-Brown B, McCarter R, Minniti CP. Hydroxyurea therapy lowers TCD velocities in children with sickle cell disease. *Pediatr Blood Cancer.* 2006;47(7):894-900.

23. Lagunju I, Brown BJ, Sodeinde O. Hydroxyurea lowers transcranial Doppler flow velocities in children with sickle cell anaemia in a Nigerian cohort. *Pediatr Blood Cancer.* 2015;62(9):1587-1591.

24. Zimmerman SA, Schultz WH, Burgett S, Mortier NA, Ware RE. Hydroxyurea therapy lowers transcranial Doppler flow velocities in children with sickle cell anemia. *Blood.* 2007;110(3):1043-1047.

25. Bernaudin F, Verlhac S, Arnaud C, et al. Impact of early transcranial Doppler screening and intensive therapy on cerebral vasculopathy outcome in a newborn sickle cell anemia cohort. *Blood.* 2011;117(4):1130-1140; quiz 1436.

26. Bernaudin F, Verlhac S, Freard F, et al. Multicenter prospective study of children with sickle cell disease: radiographic and psychometric correlation. *J Child Neurol.* 2000;15(5):333-343.

27. Pegelow CH, Macklin EA, Moser FG, et al. Longitudinal changes in brain magnetic resonance imaging findings in children with sickle cell disease. *Blood.* 2002;99(8):3014-3018.

28. Schatz J, Brown RT, Pascual JM, Hsu L, DeBaun MR. Poor school and cognitive functioning with silent cerebral infarcts and sickle cell disease. *Neurology.* 2001;56(8):1109-1111.

29. DeBaun MR, Gordon M, McKinstry RC, et al. Controlled trial of transfusions for silent cerebral infarcts in sickle cell anemia. *N Engl J Med.* 2014;371(8):699-710.

30. Bernaudin F, Verlhac S, Peffault de Latour R, et al. Association of matched sibling donor hematopoietic stem cell transplantation with transcranial Doppler velocities in children with sickle cell anemia. *JAMA.* 2019;321(3):266-276.

31. Morris CR, Suh JH, Hagar W, et al. Erythrocyte glutamine depletion, altered redox environment, and pulmonary hypertension in sickle cell disease. *Blood.* 2008;111(1):402-410.

32. Niihara Y, Matsui NM, Shen YM, et al. L-glutamine therapy reduces endothelial adhesion of sickle red blood cells to human umbilical vein endothelial cells. *BMC Blood Disord.* 2005;5:4.

33. Niihara Y, Zerez CR, Akiyama DS, Tanaka KR. Oral L-glutamine therapy for sickle cell anemia: I. Subjective clinical improvement and favorable change in red cell NAD redox potential. *Am J Hematol.* 1998;58(2):117-121.

34. Niihara Y, Miller ST, Kanter J, et al. A phase 3 trial of L-glutamine in sickle cell disease. *N Engl J Med.* 2018;379(3):226-235.

35. Udani M, Zen Q, Cottman M, et al. Basal cell adhesion molecule/lutheran protein. The receptor critical for sickle cell adhesion to laminin. *J Clin Invest.* 1998;101(11):2550-2558.

36. Zennadi R, Moeller BJ, Whalen EJ, et al. Epinephrine-induced activation of LW-mediated sickle cell adhesion and vaso-occlusion in vivo. *Blood.* 2007;110(7):2708-2717.

37. Zennadi R, Whalen EJ, Soderblom EJ, et al. Erythrocyte plasma membrane-bound ERK1/2 activation promotes ICAM-4-mediated sickle red cell adhesion to endothelium. *Blood.* 2012; 119(5):1217-1227.

38. Telen MJ, Batchvarova M, Shan S, et al. Sevuparin binds to multiple adhesive ligands and reduces sickle red blood cell-induced vaso-occlusion. *Br J Haematol.* 2016;175(5):935-948.

39. Turhan A, Weiss LA, Mohandas N, Coller BS, Frenette PS. Primary role for adherent leukocytes in sickle cell vascular occlusion: a new paradigm. *Proc Natl Acad Sci U S A.* 2002;99(5):3047-3051.

40. Zennadi R, Chien A, Xu K, Batchvarova M, Telen MJ. Sickle red cells induce adhesion of lymphocytes and monocytes to endothelium. *Blood.* 2008;112(8):3474-3483.

41. Telen MJ, Malik P, Vercellotti GM. Therapeutic strategies for sickle cell disease: towards a multi-agent approach. *Nat Rev Drug Discov.* 2019;18(2):139-158.

42. Ataga KI, Kutlar A, Kanter J, et al. Crizanlizumab for the prevention of pain crises in sickle cell disease. *N Engl J Med.* 2017;376(5):429-439.

43. Vichinsky E, Hoppe CC, Ataga KI, et al. A phase 3 randomized trial of voxelotor in sickle cell disease. *N Engl J Med.* 2019;381(6):509-519.

44. Koshy M, Weiner SJ, Miller ST, et al. Surgery and anesthesia in sickle cell disease. Cooperative Study of Sickle Cell Diseases. *Blood.* 1995;86(10):3676-3684.

45. Vichinsky EP, Haberkern CM, Neumayr L, et al. A comparison of conservative and aggressive transfusion regimens in the perioperative management of sickle cell disease. The Preoperative Transfusion in Sickle Cell Disease Study Group. *N Engl J Med.* 1995;333(4):206-213.

46. Howard J, Malfroy M, Llewelyn C, et al. The Transfusion Alternatives Preoperatively in Sickle Cell Disease (TAPS) study: a randomised, controlled, multicentre clinical trial. *Lancet.* 2013;381(9870):930-938.

47. Yawn BP, Buchanan GR, Afenyi-Annan AN, et al. Management of sickle cell disease: summary of the 2014 evidence-based report by expert panel members. *JAMA.* 2014;312(10):1033-1048.

48. Gluckman E, Cappelli B, Bernaudin F, et al. Sickle cell disease: an international survey of results of HLA-identical sibling hematopoietic stem cell transplantation. *Blood.* 2017;129(11):1548-1556.

49. Johnson FL, Look AT, Gockerman J, Ruggiero MR, Dalla-Pozza L, Billings FT 3rd. Bone-marrow transplantation in a patient with sickle-cell anemia. *N Engl J Med.* 1984;311(12):780-783.

50. Hsieh MM, Fitzhugh CD, Weitzel RP, et al. Nonmyeloablative HLA-matched sibling allogeneic hematopoietic stem cell transplantation for severe sickle cell phenotype. *JAMA.* 2014;312(1):48-56.

51. Shenoy S, Eapen M, Panepinto JA, et al. A trial of unrelated donor marrow transplantation for children with severe sickle cell disease. *Blood.* 2016;128(21):2561-2567.

52. Ribeil JA, Hacein-Bey-Abina S, Payen E, et al. Gene therapy in a patient with sickle cell disease. *N Engl J Med.* 2017;376(9):848-855.

53. Hebbel RP, Osarogiagbon R, Kaul D. The endothelial biology of sickle cell disease: inflammation and a chronic vasculopathy. *Microcirculation.* 2004;11(2):129-151.

54. Devine DV, Kinney TR, Thomas PF, Rosse WF, Greenberg CS. Fragment D-dimer levels: an objective marker of vaso-occlusive crisis and other complications of sickle cell disease. *Blood.* 1986;68(1):317-319.

55. Francis RB Jr. Elevated fibrin D-dimer fragment in sickle cell anemia: evidence for activation of coagulation during the steady state as well as in painful crisis. *Haemostasis.* 1989;19(2):105-111.

56. Shet AS, Aras O, Gupta K, et al. Sickle blood contains tissue factor-positive microparticles derived from endothelial cells and monocytes. *Blood.* 2003;102(7):2678-2683.

57. Chantrathammachart P, Mackman N, Sparkenbaugh E, et al. Tissue factor promotes activation of coagulation and inflammation in a mouse model of sickle cell disease. *Blood.* 2012;120(3): 636-646.

58. Setty BN, Key NS, Rao AK, et al. Tissue factor-positive monocytes in children with sickle cell disease: correlation with biomarkers of haemolysis. *Br J Haematol.* 2012;157(3):370-380.

59. Setty BN, Rao AK, Stuart MJ. Thrombophilia in sickle cell disease: the red cell connection. *Blood.* 2001;98(12):3228-3233.

60. Sparkenbaugh EM, Chantrathammachart P, Wang S, et al. Excess of heme induces tissue factor-dependent activation of coagulation in mice. *Haematologica.* 2015;100(3):308-314.

61. Shah N, Welsby IJ, Fielder MA, Jacobsen WK, Nielsen VG. Sickle cell disease is associated with iron mediated hypercoagulability. *J Thromb Thrombolysis.* 2015;40(2):182-185.

62. Greenberg J, Ohene-Frempong K, Halus J, Way C, Schwartz E. Trial of low doses of aspirin as prophylaxis in sickle cell disease. *J Pediatr.* 1983;102(5):781-784.

63. Osamo NO, Photiades DP, Famodu AA. Therapeutic effect of aspirin in sickle cell anaemia. *Acta Haematol.* 1981;66(2):102-107.

64. Ozsoylu S. Aspirin in sickle-cell anaemia. *Acta Haematol.* 1982;68(4):347.

65. Zago MA, Costa FF, Ismael SJ, Tone LG, Bottura C. Treatment of sickle cell diseases with aspirin. *Acta Haematol.* 1984;72(1):61-64.

66. Wun T, Soulieres D, Frelinger AL, et al. A double-blind, randomized, multicenter phase 2 study of prasugrel versus placebo in adult patients with sickle cell disease. *J Hematol Oncol.* 2013;6:17.

67. Ohno K, Tanaka H, Samata N, et al. Platelet activation biomarkers in Berkeley sickle cell mice and the response to prasugrel. *Thromb Res.* 2014;134(4):889-894.

68. Heeney MM, Hoppe CC, Rees DC. Prasugrel for sickle cell vaso-occlusive events. *N Engl J Med.* 2016;375(2):185-186.

69. Ahmed S, Siddiqui AK, Iqbal U, et al. Effect of low-dose warfarin on D-dimer levels during sickle cell vaso-occlusive crisis: a brief report. *Eur J Haematol.* 2004;72(3):213-216.

70. Salvaggio JE, Arnold CA, Banov CH. Long-term anti-coagulation in sickle-cell disease. A clinical study. *N Engl J Med.* 1963;269:182-186.

71. Chaplin H Jr, Monroe MC, Malecek AC, Morgan LK, Michael J, Murphy WA. Preliminary trial of minidose heparin prophylaxis for painful sickle cell crises. *East Afr Med J.* 1989;66(9): 574-584.

72. Qari MH, Aljaouni SK, Alardawi MS, et al. Reduction of painful vaso-occlusive crisis of sickle cell anaemia by tinzaparin in a double-blind randomized trial. *Thromb Haemost.* 2007;98(2):392-396.

73. van Zuuren EJ, Fedorowicz Z. Low-molecular-weight heparins for managing vaso-occlusive crises in people with sickle cell disease. *Cochrane Database Syst Rev.* 2015;12:CD010155.

74. Hutchaleelaha A, Patel M, Washington C, et al. Pharmacokinetics and pharmacodynamics of voxelotor (GBT440) in healthy adults and patients with sickle cell disease. *Br J Clin Pharmacol.* 2019;85(6):1290-1302.

75. Stocker JW, De Franceschi L, McNaughton-Smith GA, Corrocher R, Beuzard Y, Brugnara C. ICA-17043, a novel Gardos channel blocker, prevents sickled red blood cell dehydration in vitro and in vivo in SAD mice. *Blood.* 2003;101(6):2412-2418.

76. Ataga KI, Reid M, Ballas SK, et al. Improvements in haemolysis and indicators of erythrocyte survival do not correlate with acute vaso-occlusive crises in patients with sickle cell disease: a phase III randomized, placebo-controlled, double-blind study of the Gardos channel blocker senicapoc (ICA-17043). *Br J Haematol.* 2011;153(1):92-104.

77. Telen MJ. Beyond hydroxyurea: new and old drugs in the pipeline for sickle cell disease. *Blood.* 2016;127(7):810-819.

78. Chang J, Patton JT, Sarkar A, Ernst B, Magnani JL, Frenette PS. GMI-1070, a novel pan-selectin antagonist, reverses acute vascular occlusions in sickle cell mice. *Blood.* 2010;116(10):1779-1786.

79. Wun T, Styles L, DeCastro L, et al. Phase 1 study of the E-selectin inhibitor GMI 1070 in patients with sickle cell anemia. *PloS One.* 2014;9(7):e101301.

80. Telen MJ, Wun T, McCavit TL, et al. Randomized phase 2 study of GMI-1070 in SCD: reduction in time to resolution of vaso-occlusive events and decreased opioid use. *Blood.* 2015;125(17):2656-2664.

81. Charache S, Barton FB, Moore RD, et al. Hydroxyurea and sickle cell anemia. Clinical utility of a myelosuppressive "switching" agent. The Multicenter Study of Hydroxyurea in Sickle Cell Anemia. *Medicine.* 1996;75(6):300-326.

82. Sacks FM, Svetkey LP, Vollmer WM, et al. Effects on blood pressure of reduced dietary sodium and the Dietary Approaches to Stop Hypertension (DASH) diet. *N Engl J Med.* 2001;344(1):3-10.

83. Orringer EP, Casella JF, Ataga KI, et al. Purified poloxamer 188 for treatment of acute vaso-occlusive crisis of sickle cell disease: a randomized controlled trial. *JAMA.* 2001;286(17):2099-2106.

84. Tshilolo L, Tomlinson G, Williams TN, et al. Hydroxyurea for children with sickle cell anemia in sub-Saharan Africa. *N Engl J Med.* 2019;380(2):121-131.

85. Afenyi-Annan A, Kail M, Combs MR, Orringer EP, Ashley-Koch A, Telen MJ. Lack of Duffy antigen expression is associated with organ damage in patients with sickle cell disease. *Transfusion.* 2008;48(5):917-924.

86. De Castro LM, Jonassaint JC, Graham FL, Ashley-Koch A, Telen MJ. Pulmonary hypertension associated with sickle cell disease: clinical and laboratory endpoints and disease outcomes. *Am J Hematol.* 2008;83(1):19-25.

87. Elmariah H, Garrett ME, De Castro LM, et al. Factors associated with survival in a contemporary adult sickle cell disease cohort. *Am J Hematol.* 2014;89(5):530-535.

88. Anderson BR, Howell DN, Soldano K, et al. In vivo modeling implicates APOL1 in nephropathy: evidence for dominant negative effects and epistasis under anemic stress. *PLoS Genet.* 2015;11(7):e1005349.

89. Ashley-Koch AE, Okocha EC, Garrett ME, et al. MYH9 and APOL1 are both associated with sickle cell disease nephropathy. *Br J Haematol.* 2011;155(3):386-394.

90. Kormann R, Jannot AS, Narjoz C, et al. Roles of APOL1 G1 and G2 variants in sickle cell disease patients: kidney is the main target. *Br J Haematol.* 2017;179(2):323-335.

91. Saraf SL, Shah BN, Zhang X, et al. APOL1, alpha-thalassemia, and BCL11A variants as a genetic risk profile for progression of chronic kidney disease in sickle cell anemia. *Haematologica.* 2017;102(1):e1-e6.

92. Charache S, Terrin ML, Moore RD, et al. Design of the multicenter study of hydroxyurea in sickle cell anemia. *Cont Clin Trials.* 1995;16(6):432-446.

93. Xu JZ, Garrett ME, Soldano KL, et al. Clinical and metabolomic risk factors associated with rapid renal function decline in sickle cell disease. *Am J Hematol.* 2018;93(12):1451-1460.

94. Gladwin MT, Barst RJ, Gibbs JS, et al. Risk factors for death in 632 patients with sickle cell disease in the United States and United Kingdom. *PloS One.* 2014;9(7):e99489.

95. Klings ES, Machado RF, Barst RJ, et al. An official American Thoracic Society clinical practice guideline: diagnosis, risk stratification, and management of pulmonary hypertension of sickle cell disease. *Am J Respir Crit Care Med.* 2014;189(6):727-740.

96. Sachdev V, Kato GJ, Gibbs JS, et al. Echocardiographic markers of elevated pulmonary pressure and left ventricular diastolic dysfunction are associated with exercise intolerance in adults and adolescents with homozygous sickle cell anemia in the United States and United Kingdom. *Circulation.* 2011;124(13):1452-1460.

97. Kato GJ, Martyr S, Blackwelder WC, et al. Levels of soluble endothelium-derived adhesion molecules in patients with sickle cell disease are associated with pulmonary hypertension, organ dysfunction, and mortality. *Br J Haematol.* 2005;130(6):943-953.

98. Cruz PR, Lira RP, Pereira Filho SA, et al. Increased circulating PEDF and low sICAM-1 are associated with sickle cell retinopathy. *Blood Cells Mol Dis.* 2015;54(1):33-37.

99. Sebastiani P, Ramoni MF, Nolan V, Baldwin CT, Steinberg MH. Genetic dissection and prognostic modeling of overt stroke in sickle cell anemia. *Nat Genet.* 2005;37(4):435-440.

100. Milton JN, Gordeuk VR, Taylor JG, Gladwin MT, Steinberg MH, Sebastiani P. Prediction of fetal hemoglobin in sickle cell anemia using an ensemble of genetic risk prediction models. *Circ Cardiovasc Genet.* 2014;7(2):110-115.

101. Geard A, Pule GD, Chetcha Chemegni B, et al. Clinical and genetic predictors of renal dysfunctions in sickle cell anaemia in Cameroon. *Br J Haematol.* 2017;178(4):629-639.

102. Saraf SL, Zhang X, Shah B, et al. Genetic variants and cell-free hemoglobin processing in sickle cell nephropathy. *Haematologica.* 2015;100(10):1275-1284.

103. Schaefer BA, Flanagan JM, Alvarez OA, et al. Genetic modifiers of white blood cell count, albuminuria and glomerular filtration rate in children with sickle cell anemia. *PLoS One.* 2016;11(10):e0164364.

104. Saraf SL, Viner M, Rischall A, et al. HMOX1 and acute kidney injury in sickle cell anemia. *Blood.* 2018;132(15):1621-1625.

105. Liu CT, Garnaas MK, Tin A, et al. Genetic association for renal traits among participants of African ancestry reveals new loci for renal function. *PLoS Genet.* 2011;7(9):e1002264.

106. Morris AP, Le TH, Wu H, et al. Trans-ethnic kidney function association study reveals putative causal genes and effects on kidney-specific disease aetiologies. *Nat Commun.* 2019;10(1):29.

107. Belisario AR, Silva CM, Velloso-Rodrigues C, Viana MB. Genetic, laboratory and clinical risk factors in the development of overt ischemic stroke in children with sickle cell disease. *Hematol Transfus Cell Ther.* 2018;40(2):166-181.

108. Tewari S, Renney G, Brewin J, et al. Proteomic analysis of plasma from children with sickle cell anemia and silent cerebral infarction. *Haematologica.* 2018;103(7):1136-1142.

109. Walker AL, Steward S, Howard TA, et al. Epigenetic and molecular profiles of erythroid cells after hydroxyurea treatment in sickle cell anemia. *Blood.* 2011;118(20):5664-5670.

110. Costa D, Capuano M, Sommese L, Napoli C. Impact of epigenetic mechanisms on therapeutic approaches of hemoglobinopathies. *Blood Cells Mol Dis.* 2015;55(2):95-100.

111. Chen SY, Wang Y, Telen MJ, Chi JT. The genomic analysis of erythrocyte microRNA expression in sickle cell diseases. *PloS One.* 2008;3(6):e2360.

112. Sangokoya C, Telen MJ, Chi JT. microRNA miR-144 modulates oxidative stress tolerance and associates with anemia severity in sickle cell disease. *Blood.* 2010;116(20):4338-4348.

113. Patti GJ, Yanes O, Siuzdak G. Innovation: metabolomics: the apogee of the omics trilogy. *Nat Rev Mol Cell Biol.* 2012;13(4):263-269.

114. Darghouth D, Koehl B, Junot C, Romeo PH. Metabolomic analysis of normal and sickle cell erythrocytes. *Transfus Clin Biol.* 2010;17(3):148-150.

115. Darghouth D, Koehl B, Madalinski G, et al. Pathophysiology of sickle cell disease is mirrored by the red blood cell metabolome. *Blood.* 2011;117(6):e57-e66.

116. Adebiyi MG, Manalo JM, Xia Y. Metabolomic and molecular insights into sickle cell disease and innovative therapies. *Blood Adv.* 2019;3(8):1347-1355.

117. Elsherif L, Pathmasiri W, McRitchie S, Archer DR, Ataga KI. Plasma metabolomics analysis in sickle cell disease patients with albuminuria: an exploratory study. *Br J Haematol.* 2019;185(3):620-623.

118. Goodman SR, Pace BS, Hansen KC, et al. Minireview: multiomic candidate biomarkers for clinical manifestations of sickle cell severity: early steps to precision medicine. *Exp Biol Med (Maywood).* 2016;241(7):772-781.

119. Paszty C, Brion CM, Manci E, et al. Transgenic knockout mice with exclusively human sickle hemoglobin and sickle cell disease. *Science.* 1997;278(5339):876-878.

120. Ryan TM, Ciavatta DJ, Townes TM. Knockout-transgenic mouse model of sickle cell disease. *Science.* 1997;278(5339):873-876.

121. Heeney MM, Hoppe CC, Abboud MR, et al. A multinational trial of prasugrel for sickle cell vaso-occlusive events. *N Engl J Med.* 2016;374(7):625-635.

122. Pfizer. Pfizer announces phase 3 top-line results for rivipansel in patients with sickle cell disease experiencing a vaso-occlusive crisis. https://www.pfizer.com/news/press-release/press-release-detail/pfizer_announces_phase_3_top_line_results_for_rivipansel_in_patients_with_sickle_cell_disease_experiencing_a_vaso_occlusive_crisis. Accessed July 18, 2020.

123. BioSpace. Modus therapeutics announces the results of its global, randomized, placebo-controlled phase 2 clinical trial evaluating sevuparin for the management of acute vaso-occlusive crisis (VOC) in patients with sickle cell disease (SCD). https://www.biospace.com/article/-modus-therapeutics-announces-the-results-of-its-global-randomized-placebo-controlled-phase-2-clinical-trial-evaluating-sevuparin-for-the-management-of-acute-vaso-occlusive-crisis-voc-in-patients-with-sickle-cell-disease-scd-/. Accessed July 18, 2020.

124. Ataga KI, Smith WR, De Castro LM, et al. Efficacy and safety of the Gardos channel blocker, senicapoc (ICA-17043), in patients with sickle cell anemia. *Blood.* 2008;111(8):3991-3997.

125. Minniti CP, Wilson J, Mendelsohn L, et al. Anti-haemolytic effect of senicapoc and decrease in NT-proBNP in adults with sickle cell anaemia. *Br J Haematol.* 2011;155(5):634-636.

126. Castro O, Hoque M, Brown BD. Pulmonary hypertension in sickle cell disease: cardiac catheterization results and survival. *Blood.* 2003;101(4):1257-1261.

127. Machado RF, Martyr S, Kato GJ, et al. Sildenafil therapy in patients with sickle cell disease and pulmonary hypertension. *Br J Haematol.* 2005;130(3):445-453.

128. Mills EJ, Seely D, Rachlis B, et al. Barriers to participation in clinical trials of cancer: a meta-analysis and systematic review of patient-reported factors. *Lancet Oncol.* 2006;7(2):141-148.

129. Outlaw FH, Bourjolly JN, Barg FK. A study on recruitment of black Americans into clinical trials through a cultural competence lens. *Cancer Nurs.* 2000;23(6):444-451; quiz 451-442.

130. Peters-Lawrence MH, Bell MC, Hsu LL, et al. Clinical trial implementation and recruitment: lessons learned from the early closure of a randomized clinical trial. *Contemp Clin Trials.* 2012;33(2):291-297.

131. Scharff DP, Mathews KJ, Jackson P, Hoffsuemmer J, Martin E, Edwards D. More than Tuskegee: understanding mistrust about research participation. *J Health Care Poor Underserved.* 2010;21(3):879-897.

132. Shavers-Hornaday VL, Lynch CF, Burmeister LF, Torner JC. Why are African Americans under-represented in medical research studies? Impediments to participation. *Ethn Health.* 1997;2(1-2):31-45.

133. Caplan AL. Twenty years after. The legacy of the Tuskegee Syphilis Study. When evil intrudes. *Hastings Cent Rep.* 1992;22(6):29-32.

134. Harris Y, Gorelick PB, Samuels P, Bempong I. Why African Americans may not be participating in clinical trials. *J Natl Med Assoc.* 1996;88(10):630-634.

135. Wood A, Grady C, Emanuel EJ. The crisis in human participants research: identifying the problems and proposing solutions. Paper presented at the President's Council on Bioethics, Bethesda, MD, 2002.

136. Advani AS, Atkeson B, Brown CL, et al. Barriers to the participation of African-American patients with cancer in clinical trials: a pilot study. *Cancer.* 2003;97(6):1499-1506.

137. Ford JG, Howerton MW, Lai GY, et al. Barriers to recruiting underrepresented populations to cancer clinical trials: a systematic review. *Cancer.* 2008;112(2):228-242.

138. Swanson GM, Ward AJ. Recruiting minorities into clinical trials: toward a participant-friendly system. *J Natl Cancer Inst.* 1995;87(23):1747-1759.

139. Alsaeed ES, Farhat GN, Assiri AM, et al. Distribution of hemoglobinopathy disorders in Saudi Arabia based on data from the premarital screening and genetic counseling program, 2011-2015. *J Epidemiol Glob Health.* 2018;7(suppl 1):S41-S47.

140. Lippi G, Mattiuzzi C. Updated worldwide epidemiology of inherited erythrocyte disorders. *Acta Haematol.* 2020;143(3):196-203.

141. Lorey FW, Arnopp J, Cunningham GC. Distribution of hemoglobinopathy variants by ethnicity in a multiethnic state. *Genet Epidemiol.* 1996;13(5):501-512.

142. Reeves SL, Jary HK, Gondhi JP, Kleyn M, Dombkowski KJ. Health outcomes and services in children with sickle cell trait, sickle cell anemia, and normal hemoglobin. *Blood Adv.* 2019;3(10):1574-1580.

143. Wynn L, Miller S, Faughnan L, et al. Recruitment of infants with sickle cell anemia to a phase III trial: data from the BABY HUG study. *Contemp Clin Trials.* 2010;31(6):558-563.

144. Winter SS, Page-Reeves JM, Page KA, et al. Inclusion of special populations in clinical research: important considerations and guidelines. *J Clin Transl Res.* 2018;4(1):56-69.

145. Yancey AK, Ortega AN, Kumanyika SK. Effective recruitment and retention of minority research participants. *Annu Rev Public Health.* 2006;27:1-28.

146. Haywood C Jr, Lanzkron S, Diener-West M, et al. Attitudes toward clinical trials among patients with sickle cell disease. *Clin Trials.* 2014;11(3):275-283.

147. Suarez ML, Schlaeger JM, Angulo V, et al. Keys to recruiting and retaining seriously ill African Americans with sickle cell disease in longitudinal studies: respectful engagement and persistence. *Am J Hosp Palliat Care.* 2020;37(2):123-128.

148. Dampier CD, Smith WR, Wager CG, et al. IMPROVE trial: a randomized controlled trial of patient-controlled analgesia for sickle cell painful episodes: rationale, design challenges, initial experience, and recommendations for future studies. *Clin Trials.* 2013;10(2):319-331.

149. Hassell KL. Population estimates of sickle cell disease in the U.S. *Am J Prev Med.* 2010;38(4 suppl):S512-S521.

150. Thompson BW, Miller ST, Rogers ZR, et al. The pediatric hydroxyurea phase III clinical trial (BABY HUG): challenges of study design. *Pediatr Blood Cancer.* 2010;54(2):250-255.

151. Branson RD, Davis K Jr, Butler KL. African Americans' participation in clinical research: importance, barriers, and solutions. *Am J Surg.* 2007;193(1):32-39; discussion 40.

152. McGann PT, Williams TN, Olupot-Olupot P, et al. Realizing effectiveness across continents with hydroxyurea: enrollment and baseline characteristics of the multicenter REACH study in Sub-Saharan Africa. *Am J Hematol.* 2018;93(4):537-545.

153. Quinn CT. Extending the global reach of hydroxyurea. *Hematologist.* 2015;12(6):15.

154. Gaston M, Smith J, Gallagher D, et al. Recruitment in the Cooperative Study of Sickle Cell Disease (CSSCD). *Control Clin Trials.* 1987;8(4 suppl):131S-140S.

155. Vichinsky EP, Neumayr LD, Earles AN, et al. Causes and outcomes of the acute chest syndrome in sickle cell disease. National Acute Chest Syndrome Study Group. *N Engl J Med.* 2000;342(25):1855-1865.

156. Vichinsky EP, Luban NL, Wright E, et al. Prospective RBC phenotype matching in a stroke-prevention trial in sickle cell anemia: a multicenter transfusion trial. *Transfusion.* 2001;41(9):1086-1092.

157. Smith WR, Bovbjerg VE, Penberthy LT, et al. Understanding pain and improving management of sickle cell disease: the PiSCES study. *J Natl Med Assoc.* 2005;97(2):183-193.

158. Gladwin MT, Sachdev V, Jison ML, et al. Pulmonary hypertension as a risk factor for death in patients with sickle cell disease. *N Engl J Med.* 2004;350(9):886-895.

159. Hebbel RP, Boogaerts MA, Eaton JW, Steinberg MH. Erythrocyte adherence to endothelium in sickle-cell anemia. A possible determinant of disease severity. *N Engl J Med.* 1980;302(18):992-995.

160. Hebbel RP, Eaton JW, Steinberg MH, White JG. Erythrocyte/endothelial interactions and the vasocclusive severity of sickle cell disease. *Prog Clin Biol Res.* 1981;55:145-162.

161. Francis RB Jr, Haywood LJ. Elevated immunoreactive tumor necrosis factor and interleukin-1 in sickle cell disease. *J Natl Med Assoc.* 1992;84(7):611-615.

162. Shah N, Thornburg C, Telen MJ, Ortel TL. Characterization of the hypercoagulable state in patients with sickle cell disease. *Thromb Res.* 2012;130(5):e241-e245.

163. Benkerrou M, Delarche C, Brahimi L, et al. Hydroxyurea corrects the dysregulated L-selectin expression and increased H(2)O(2) production of polymorphonuclear neutrophils from patients with sickle cell anemia. *Blood.* 2002;99(7):2297-2303.

164. Bourantas KL, Dalekos GN, Makis A, Chaidos A, Tsiara S, Mavridis A. Acute phase proteins and interleukins in steady state sickle cell disease. *Eur J Haematol.* 1998;61(1):49-54.

165. Rab MAE, van Oirschot BA, Bos J, et al. Rapid and reproducible characterization of sickling during automated deoxygenation in sickle cell disease patients. *Am J Hematol.* 2019;94(5):575-584.

166. Musa BOP, Onyemelukwe GC, Hambolu JO, Mamman AI, Isa AH. Pattern of serum cytokine expression and T-cell subsets in sickle cell disease patients in vaso-occlusive crisis. *Clin Vaccine Immunol.* 2010;17(4):602-608.

167. Qari MH, Dier U, Mousa SA. Biomarkers of inflammation, growth factor, and coagulation activation in patients with sickle cell disease. *Clin Appl Thromb Hemost.* 2012;18(2):195-200.

168. Graido-Gonzalez E, Doherty JC, Bergreen EW, Organ G, Telfer M, McMillen MA. Plasma endothelin-1, cytokine, and prostaglandin E2 levels in sickle cell disease and acute vaso-occlusive sickle crisis. *Blood.* 1998;92(7):2551-2555.

169. Kurantsin-Mills J, Ofosu FA, Safa TK, Siegel RS, Lessin LS. Plasma factor VII and thrombin-antithrombin III levels indicate increased tissue factor activity in sickle cell patients. *Br J Haematol.* 1992;81(4):539-544.

170. Pathare A, Al Kindi S, Alnaqdy AA, Daar S, Knox-Macaulay H, Dennison D. Cytokine profile of sickle cell disease in Oman. *Am J Hematol.* 2004;77(4):323-328.

171. Lanaro C, Franco-Penteado CF, Albuqueque DM, Saad ST, Conran N, Costa FF. Altered levels of cytokines and inflammatory mediators in plasma and leukocytes of sickle cell anemia patients and effects of hydroxyurea therapy. *J Leukocyte Biol.* 2009;85(2):235-242.

172. Michaels LA, Ohene-Frempong K, Zhao H, Douglas SD. Serum levels of substance P are elevated in patients with sickle cell disease and increase further during vaso-occlusive crisis. *Blood.* 1998;92(9):3148-3151.

173. Vendrame F, Olops L, Saad STO, Costa FF, Fertrin KY. Differences in heme and hemopexin content in lipoproteins from patients with sickle cell disease. *J Clin Lipidol.* 2018;12(6):1532-1538.

174. Al Balushi H, Hannemann A, Rees D, Brewin J, Gibson JS. The effect of antioxidants on the properties of red blood cells from patients with sickle cell anemia. *Front Physiol.* 2019;10:976.

175. Barber LA, Palascak MB, Qi X, Joiner CH, Franco RS. Activation of protein kinase C by phorbol ester increases red blood cell scramblase activity and external phosphatidylserine. *Eur J Haematol.* 2015;95(5):405-410.

176. Sabina RL, Wandersee NJ, Hillery CA. Ca2+-CaM activation of AMP deaminase contributes to adenine nucleotide dysregulation and phosphatidylserine externalization in human sickle erythrocytes. *Br J Haematol.* 2009;144(3):434-445.

177. Wautier MP, Heron E, Picot J, Colin Y, Hermine O, Wautier JL. Red blood cell phosphatidylserine exposure is responsible for increased erythrocyte adhesion to endothelium in central retinal vein occlusion. *J Thromb Haemost.* 2011;9(5):1049-1055.

178. Weiss E, Rees DC, Gibson JS. Role of calcium in phosphatidylserine externalisation in red blood cells from sickle cell patients. *Anemia.* 2011;2011:379894.

179. Setty BN, Kulkarni S, Rao AK, Stuart MJ. Fetal hemoglobin in sickle cell disease: relationship to erythrocyte phosphatidylserine exposure and coagulation activation. *Blood.* 2000;96(3): 1119-1124.

180. Hibbert JM, Hsu LL, Bhathena SJ, et al. Proinflammatory cytokines and the hypermetabolism of children with sickle cell disease. *Exp Biol Med (Maywood).* 2005;230(1):68-74.

181. Kato GJ, McGowan V, Machado RF, et al. Lactate dehydrogenase as a biomarker of hemolysis-associated nitric oxide resistance, priapism, leg ulceration, pulmonary hypertension, and death in patients with sickle cell disease. *Blood.* 2006;107(6): 2279-2285.

182. Antwi-Boasiako C, Dankwah GB, Aryee R, Hayfron-Benjamin C, Donkor ES, Campbell AD. Oxidative profile of patients with sickle cell disease. *Med Sci (Basel).* 2019;7(2):17.

183. Rodrigues L, Costa FF, Saad ST, Grotto HZ. High levels of neopterin and interleukin-3 in sickle cell disease patients. *J Clin Lab Anal.* 2006;20(3):75-79.

184. Mohan JS, Lip GY, Wright J, Bareford D, Blann AD. Plasma levels of tissue factor and soluble E-selectin in sickle cell disease: relationship to genotype and to inflammation. *Blood Coagul Fibrinolysis.* 2005;16(3):209-214.

185. de Franceschi L, Malpeli G, Scarpa A, et al. Protective effects of S-nitrosoalbumin on lung injury induced by hypoxia-reoxygenation in mouse model of sickle cell disease. *Am J Physiol Lung Cell Mol Physiol.* 2006;291(3):L457-L465.

186. Xu H, Wandersee NJ, Guo Y, et al. Sickle cell disease increases high mobility group box 1: a novel mechanism of inflammation. *Blood.* 2014;124(26):3978-3981.

187. Lee SP, Ataga KI, Orringer EP, Phillips DR, Parise LV. Biologically active CD40 ligand is elevated in sickle cell anemia: potential role for platelet-mediated inflammation. *Arterioscler Thromb Vasc Biol.* 2006;26(7):1626-1631.

188. Chen G, Zhang D, Fuchs TA, Manwani D, Wagner DD, Frenette PS. Heme-induced neutrophil extracellular traps contribute to the pathogenesis of sickle cell disease. *Blood.* 2014;123(24): 3818-3827.

189. Detterich JA, Liu H, Suriany S, et al. Erythrocyte and plasma oxidative stress appears to be compensated in patients with sickle cell disease during a period of relative health, despite the presence of known oxidative agents. *Free Radic Biol Med.* 2019;141:408-415.

190. Loomis Z, Eigenberger P, Redinius K, et al. Hemoglobin induced cell trauma indirectly influences endothelial TLR9 activity resulting in pulmonary vascular smooth muscle cell activation. *PloS One.* 2017;12(2):e0171219.

191. Brittain JE, Hulkower B, Jones SK, et al. Placenta growth factor in sickle cell disease: association with hemolysis and inflammation. *Blood.* 2010;115(10):2014-2020.

192. Hagag AA, Elmashad G, Abd El-Lateef AE. Clinical significance of assessment of thrombospondin and placenta growth factor levels in patients with sickle cell anemia: two centers egyptian studies. *Med J Hematol Infect Dis.* 2014;6(1):e2014044.

193. Perelman N, Selvaraj SK, Batra S, et al. Placenta growth factor activates monocytes and correlates with sickle cell disease severity. *Blood.* 2003;102(4):1506-1514.

194. Sundaram N, Tailor A, Mendelsohn L, et al. High levels of placenta growth factor in sickle cell disease promote pulmonary hypertension. *Blood.* 2010;116(1):109-112.

195. Soderblom EJ, Thompson JW, Schwartz EA, et al. Proteomic analysis of ERK1/2-mediated human sickle red blood cell membrane protein phosphorylation. *Clin Proteomics.* 2013;10(1):1.

196. Zennadi R. MEK inhibitors, novel anti-adhesive molecules, reduce sickle red blood cell adhesion in vitro and in vivo, and vasoocclusion in vivo. *PloS One.* 2014;9(10):e110306.

197. Zhao Y, Schwartz EA, Palmer GM, Zennadi R. MEK1/2 inhibitors reverse acute vascular occlusion in mouse models of sickle cell disease. *FASEB J.* 2016;30(3):1171-1186.

198. Ugurel E, Connes P, Yavas G, et al. Differential effects of adenylyl cyclase-protein kinase A cascade on shear-induced changes of sickle cell deformability. *Clin Hemorheol Microcirc.* 2019;73(4): 531-543.

199. Hoffman JF. Erythrocyte ATP, a possible therapeutic approach for sickle cell disease. *Am J Hematol.* 2019;94(5):E117.

Hematopoietic Stem Cell Transplantation in Sickle Cell Disease

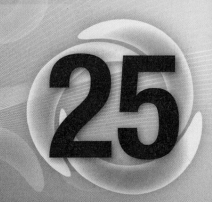

25

Authors: Alexis Leonard, John F. Tisdale, Lakshmanan Krishnamurti, Mark C. Walters

Chapter Outline

Overview

Sickle cell disease (SCD) is the most common inherited hemoglobinopathy worldwide and is associated with substantial morbidity, high health care utilization, and premature mortality. Although hydroxyurea (HU), chronic blood transfusions, and L-glutamine decrease SCD-associated complications, they do not eliminate them and thus need to be continued indefinitely. Allogeneic hematopoietic stem cell transplantation (HSCT) is the only currently available curative option for patients with SCD. Disease-free survival (DFS) in children and young adults with SCD is >95% after a myeloablative regimen using a human leukocyte antigen (HLA)-matched sibling donor. Mixed donor chimerism with ≥20% donor myeloid cells is associated with predominant donor-derived erythropoiesis due to normal donor red blood cell (RBC) survival compared to the ineffective erythropoiesis of SCD. Thus, reduced-intensity conditioning (RIC) and nonmyeloablative conditioning appear efficacious and safe for adults with an HLA-identical sibling donor who may otherwise be unable to tolerate myeloablative conditioning. HSCT is still largely underused in part due to the lack of available matched donors for patients with SCD and concerns about morbidity and mortality from transplantation conditioning, graft-versus-host disease (GVHD), and graft rejection. Approaches to improve the safety, efficacy, and applicability of HSCT for SCD that are currently being tested in clinical trials include novel low-intensity conditioning, novel graft manipulation techniques to reduce the risk of GVHD, novel strategies for GVHD prophylaxis, and the use of alternate sources of hematopoietic progenitor cells including HLA-haploidentical donors (matched at 50% of HLA alleles), umbilical cord blood (UCB), and matched unrelated donors. Simultaneously, significant advances in gene therapy suggest that a universal cure(s) for SCD might soon be available that eliminates major limitations of allogeneic transplantation, and this is being investigated in multiple clinical trials.

Introduction

SCD encompasses a group of disorders caused by the homozygous inheritance of sickle hemoglobin (HbS) or the inheritance of HbS in a variety of double heterozygous states with other β-globin gene variants. Although there are various clinical phenotypes, the hallmarks of SCD include chronic anemia, chronic inflammation, recurrent vaso-occlusive crises, acute and chronic pain, stroke, organ damage and risk of failure, and early mortality.[1]

SCD is a global health problem with a need for cure. Approximately 5% of the world's population carries trait genes for hemoglobin disorders, mainly SCD and thalassemia.[2] Approximately 300,000 babies with severe hemoglobin disorders are born each year, although by 2050, this is estimated to increase to >400,000.[3] In well-resourced countries, >94% of children with SCD now survive until age 18 years because of significant reductions in excess early childhood mortality though newborn screening, penicillin prophylaxis, and vaccinations.[4,5] Thus, disease management has shifted to a chronic disease model that addresses long-term complications, reduced quality of life, and early mortality faced in adulthood.[6] In the United States, SCD is a public health concern with high health care costs,[7] affecting approximately 100,000 Americans who have fewer US Food and Drug Administration (FDA)-approved treatment options and less access to comprehensive care teams than people with other genetic disorders.[8-10] HU,

which was approved by the FDA for use in adults in 1998 and children in 2017, has been proven to be efficacious in reducing SCD-related complications and improving survival in clinical trials and in clinical practice.[11-14] The efficacy and safety of HU have resulted in the routine consideration of its introduction for the treatment of children as early as 9 months of age before the occurrence of any SCD-related complications. However, HU must be continued indefinitely with close monitoring, all of which may contribute to the low uptake and adherence with this drug. L-Glutamine was approved for use in SCD by the FDA in 2018, and Voxeletor and Crizanlizumab were approved by the FDA in 2019. As such, the role of these drug in the management of patients with SCD remains unclear. In addition, the cost of these new drugs may be prohibitive in their widespread use in amelioration of the severity of SCD. Chronic blood transfusion therapy requires patients' time and commitment and does not fully eliminate the consequences of the disease. Cure after allogeneic HSCT may reduce disease burden and improve outcomes and quality of life for patients with SCD and potentially reduce health care costs over the long term.[15-18] Barriers remain however to the acceptability and broad applicability of HSCT for SCD.

Since the first HSCT in 1984 in a pediatric patient with SCD and acute myelogenous leukemia (AML), thousands of patients have successfully undergone HSCT with an HLA-identical sibling donor, with >90% of all patients cured of SCD.[19] HSCT is an established therapeutic option when a patient has a clinical indication and an HLA-identical sibling donor. Unfortunately, only approximately 14% of patients with SCD in the United States have a matched sibling donor and only 19% have a well-matched unrelated donor in the donor registry.[20,21] Matched unrelated donor transplantation, umbilical cord blood transplantation (UCBT), and haploidentical transplantation may improve access to HSCT, but complications, risks, and severity after alternate donor HSCT currently limit the broad use of these therapies.

As the outcomes and options improve for allogenic HSCT in SCD, parallel progress in autologous gene therapy for the cure of SCD is occurring. Whereas allogeneic transplantation is limited by donor availability, the potential for morbidity and mortality from transplant conditioning, GVHD, and graft rejection, gene therapy, either by gene addition or gene editing targeting autologous hematopoietic stem cells (HSCs), is currently being investigated in multiple clinical trials and is discussed in more detail elsewhere in this book.

Historical Perspective

In 1984, an 8-year-old girl with AML and known HbSS disease underwent a curative bone marrow (BM) HSCT in the setting of her malignancy.[22] The patient was treated according to the St. Jude AML-80 therapy protocol, where patients who had a suitably matched HLA donor were treated with HSCT. The patient's 4-year-old brother, who carried the sickle cell trait (HbAS), was ABO compatible and HLA identical. After myeloablative conditioning with total-body irradiation (TBI) and cyclophosphamide (CY), the patient was engrafted; she was cured of her AML, her SCD complications stopped, and she demonstrated the hemoglobin electrophoresis pattern of her brother. This case served as proof of principle that SCD could be successfully treated by HSCT and that an HbAS donor was acceptable.

Within the next decade, the first cohort of children and young adults were treated by HSCT for SCD in Brussels, Belgium.[23] A group of 12 asymptomatic patients with mild phenotypes (median age, 2 years) were transplanted prior to returning to Africa, where mortality rates can exceed 50% for children under age 5 depending on access to care. After myeloablative conditioning with oral busulfan (BU), CY, and 750 cGy of thoracoabdominal radiation for recipients older than age 12 years, 11 patients were cured of their SCD. One patient who sustained secondary graft failure was successfully rescued with a second HSCT.

A larger, expanded cohort in France and Belgium subsequently demonstrated sustained donor HSC engraftment in 36 of 42 patients; all those with sustained engraftment were free of ongoing crises due to SCD, 1 patient died, and 2 of the 5 patients with initial graft rejection successfully underwent secondary HSCT.[24] The summarized Belgian experience of 50 patients demonstrated overall survival (OS), event-free survival (EFS), and DFS rates of 93%, 82%, and 85%, respectively, with the subgroup with milder phenotype who were returning to Africa fairing somewhat better.[25] Simultaneously, in the United States, the first multicenter trial investigating HSCT in pediatric patients with SCD reported similarly encouraging OS and EFS rates of 93% and 84%, respectively, with important lessons learned from patients treated early on this trial.[26] These results led to the era of multicenter clinical trials for matched sibling donor HSCT for SCD from the late 1980s to the present.

Over the past several decades, clinical studies investigating HSCT for SCD have tackled the problems of graft rejection and regimen-related toxicity and have expanded the donor options. Factors such as BM stress erythropoiesis, alloimmunization from frequent blood transfusions, and an immunocompetent host all contribute to increased graft rejection and disease recurrence, whereas years of chronic organ damage in patients with SCD can complicate the HSCT process and make preparative regimens excessively toxic. Unlike HSCT for a hematologic malignancy, stable mixed chimerism with the natural enrichment of donor RBCs in the blood can elicit a curative outcome; therefore, nonmyeloablative preparative regimens may be feasible and important for this patient population. Additionally, because there is no benefit of GVHD in nonmalignant disorders, minimizing GVHD risk is imperative. Where there are limitations in donor availability and conditioning regimens and occurrences of graft rejection or life-threatening GVHD, investigations into nonmyeloablative conditioning regimens, expanded donor sources, and improved post-HSCT supportive care are ongoing.

Indications for HSCT

Despite being a monogenic disorder, the clinical phenotypes of SCD are extremely variable. There are few reliable predictors of disease severity that would easily elucidate patients whose risk of disease sequelae clearly outweighs the risk of potential morbidity and mortality from HSCT. Given its investigational nature, the first large multicenter trial in the United States investigating HSCT for SCD selected patients who appeared to have a high risk of severe morbidity and early death as defined by 9 disease-based criteria.[26] Of these 9 criteria, clinical stroke, recurrent vaso-occlusive pain, and recurrent acute chest syndrome (ACS) defined HSCT indications among all 22 enrolled patients. Exclusionary criteria included older patients (>15 years old) and those with significant end-organ damage (lung, liver, or renal insufficiency) or low performance scores (Lansky score <70). Despite reporting high OS and EFS rates at 4 years of 91% and 73%, respectively, the authors acknowledged that the "optimal timing of marrow transplantation in the course of sickle cell anemia remains uncertain, in part because of the unpredictable nature of the disease."[26]

Over the past 2 decades, there have been significant improvements in preparative regimens, supportive care, and management of complications. The risk-benefit ratio of HSCT based on these improved outcomes and a better understanding of disease progression have expanded eligibility considerations, for example, to include patients with end-organ complications[27] or those with lower performance scores (Lansky score >40).[28] In 2014, an expert panel published consensus-based recommendations on the indications for HSCT and transplant management.[29] The panel recommended that "young patients with symptomatic SCD who have an HLA-matched sibling donor should be transplanted as early as possible."[29] For those who do not meet these criteria, "HSCT from unrelated BM or CB donors should only be considered in the presence of at least one of the indications suggested by Walters et al[26] and should be performed only in the context of controlled trials in experienced centers."[29]

Symptomatic SCD is not clearly defined, and thus, there are no universal, widely adopted indications for HSCT. The presence of central nervous system (CNS) disease, however, is generally acceptable as an indication for HSCT; 20% of children with previous strokes and cerebral vasculopathy may experience second overt strokes within 5 years, and up to 45% may experience progressive cerebral infarcts despite adequate transfusion therapy.[30,31] Thus, currently, therapy for CNS vasculopathy is palliative in nature and does not prevent progression of CNS lesions. Recurrent vaso-occlusive crisis despite HU, recurrent ACS, osteonecrosis, sickle nephropathy, RBC alloimmunization, pulmonary hypertension, and recurrent splenic sequestration encompass other "severe" disease complications that should be considered indications for HSCT[32]. Exclusionary criteria for studies are narrowing as treatment options and supportive care expand, but generally, they include a Karnofsky or Lansky functional performance score <70, acute hepatitis or evidence of moderate or severe bridging fibrosis or cirrhosis on biopsy, severe renal impairment, severe cardiac disease, stage III or IV sickle lung disease, demonstrated lack of compliance with medical care, seropositivity for HIV, and uncontrolled infections.

Although HLA-identical HSCT should be considered in those with symptomatic SCD and an HLA-matched sibling donor, this option is underutilized. Over 20% of patients are likely to meet disease severity criteria for consideration of HSCT and they have a 10% to 15% likelihood of having an HLA-identical donor. If the majority of eligible patients with available donors were to undergo HSCT, it is anticipated that there should be roughly 10,000 patients in the United States who might pursue HSCT. However, only 1200 patients with HSCT were reported in the Center for International Blood and Marrow Transplant Research (CIBMTR) registry as of 2014[33]. This is surprising because several studies have reported patient and parent willingness to consider HSCT.[34,35] Whereas HSCT has the best outcome when performed before irreversible organ damage has occurred, the inability to predict disease severity prior to overt clinical symptoms or organ damage and concern for patient autonomy in the pediatric setting have limited patient referral and provider comfort with offering or recommending curative therapy. The importance of a shared decision-making model among providers, patients, and their families is imperative to ensure acceptable considerations are addressed regarding the various potential risks and benefits of choosing to either decline or undergo HSCT.[36] Although there may be consensus to offer HSCT to those who have experienced an overt stroke and a consensus not to offer HSCT to patients with milder disease such as hereditary persistence of fetal hemoglobin or HbS-β[+] disease, other disease criteria are less straightforward, and therefore, any determination of an acceptable risk-benefit trade-off can only be made by an individual patient or the patient's parents after thoughtful and informed discussion. Such discussions should center around the inability to precisely predict SCD severity, the cumulative organ damage from SCD, and harm that may occur by not electively performing early HSCT. Although outcomes worsen with age, these discussions must compare options to the low-risk, but major complications from HSCT, including death or significant organ toxicity, such as endocrine dysfunction and infertility, secondary malignancy, and the substitution of one chronic morbidity (SCD) for another (GVHD). Whereas pediatric mortality has declined significantly since the 1970s, allowing more patients to survive into adulthood, mortality rates for adults have increased during the same period, and thus, therapeutic options that improve median survival are needed.[6]

HLA-Identical Sibling Allogeneic HSCT

Early experience after myeloablative HSCT for SCD suggested stable donor-host hematopoietic chimerism is sufficient for phenotypic cure; therefore, nonmyeloablative conditioning and RIC were investigated. Initially, these studies showed inferior results compared with myeloablative conditioning due to a high rate of graft rejection that typically occurred after postgrafting immunosuppression was withdrawn.[37,38] More recently, the use of sirolimus for postgrafting immunosuppression and donor regulatory T-cell expansion has improved the results of nonmyeloablative HSCT for SCD,

which show an acceptable OS and EFS with very little morbidity or GVHD.[27,39] Between 1986 and 2013, >1000 patients have received an HLA-identical sibling HSCT with either myeloablative conditioning or RIC, with 5-year EFS and OS rates of 91.4% and 92.9%, respectively[19] (Figure 25-1). Regardless of conditioning regimen, EFS in HLA-identical sibling HSCT is overall lower with increasing age at transplantation and higher for transplantations performed after 2006 given improvements in supportive care and prevention and management of complications.

Myeloablative Conditioning

Initial trials in HSCT for SCD used myeloablative conditioning regimens with BM from HLA-identical siblings as the HSC source (Table 25-1).[23-26,40,41] The Multicenter Investigation of Bone Marrow Transplantation was a collaboration between HSCT centers in Europe and North and South America that generated essential data over several publications detailing outcomes after myeloablative HSCT in children and adolescents with SCD.[26,42,43] In an initial report, 22 pediatric patients with symptomatic SCD were treated with myeloablative doses of BU in combination with highly immunosuppressive doses of CY (similar to European studies[40,41]) and T-cell depletion with antithymocyte globulin (ATG) or alemtuzumab. Combinations of methotrexate and cyclosporine (CsA) or CsA and prednisone were used for GVHD prophylaxis. EFS and OS rates at 4 years were 73% and 91%, respectively, with most of the failures from graft rejection or disease recurrence. Follow-up results in 59 patients at a median of 42 months addressed the prevention of neurologic complications (goals for blood pressure, hemoglobin and platelet count, and magnesium level).[42,43] EFS and OS rates were improved to 93% and 84%, respectively, with 7% treatment-related mortality (TRM), 19% acute and chronic GVHD, and donor chimerism between 11% and 100%. None of the 50 patients with donor engraftment experienced SCD-related crises, including pain, stroke, or ACS, after engraftment, and those with a prior history of stroke had stable or improved cerebral imaging.

Subsequent studies with larger cohorts using similar preparative regimens (± fludarabine,[44] ± HU,[45] substitution of treosulfan for BU[46]) published EFS rates ranging from 82% to 100% and OS ranging from 91% to 100% (Table 25-1).[25,26,42-50] EFS was improved further with the addition of ATG,[43,51] showing an improvement in the 5-year EFS from 86% to 95% in patients treated after 2000 with the addition of ATG. An updated cohort of 215 patients who received no ATG, ATG at a dose of 10 to 15 mg/kg, or ATG at dose of 20 mg/kg reported a similar DFS of 95% with ATG and demonstrated that the high ATG dose (20 mg/kg) significantly reduced chronic GVHD without enhancing viral infections.[52] EFS was also noted to be higher in patients who received HU before HSCT, with an EFS at 8 years of 97.1%, which was significantly higher than the EFS in those who did not receive HU prior to HSCT ($P <.001$).[45,53] The overall rates of acute and chronic GVHD using a CsA-based immunosuppressive

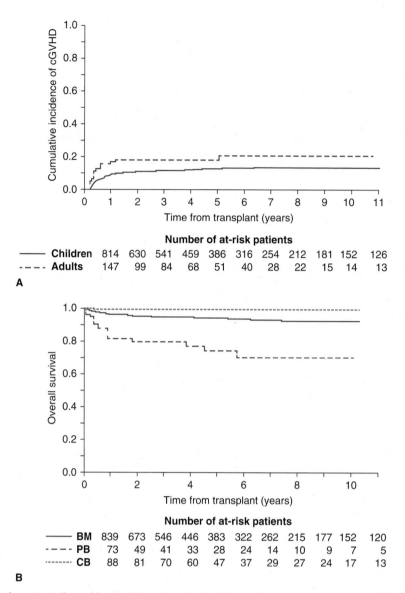

FIGURE 25-1 **Human leukocyte antigen–identical hematopoietic stem cell transplantation for sickle cell disease between 1986 and 2013: influence of age and stem cell source on outcomes. A.** Cumulative incidence of chronic graft-versus-host disease (cGVHD) in adults and children. **B.** Overall survival according to stem cell source. BM, bone marrow; CB, cord blood; PB, peripheral blood. Reproduced, with permission, from Gluckman E, Cappelli B, Bernaudin F, et al. Sickle cell disease: an international survey of results of HLA-identical sibling hematopoietic stem cell transplantation. *Blood*. 2017;129(11):1548-1556.

regimen ranged between 10% and 22%, although GVHD was a main cause of TRM in several studies.[43,44,47,49] A Belgian cohort determined treatment options based on access to optimal care; group 1 was composed of permanent residents of a European country who satisfied the traditional inclusion criteria as previously defined in SCD,[26] and group 2 consisted of asymptomatic patients (median age, 2 years).[25] Differences in outcome included higher OS (88% in group 1 vs 100% in group 2), EFS (76% vs 93% in group 2), and DFS (80% vs 93% in group 2), lower rejection (25% vs 7% in group 2; *P* <.001), and lower GVHD (none in group 2) in group 2. Although this was not a randomized comparison, the benefit of performing HSCT before SCD progression occurs was illustrated.

Important lessons were learned over the course of these initial studies. First, the addition of ATG appears to decrease the risk of graft rejection from 22.6% to 3%, improving the EFS, and should be considered in HSCT myeloablative preparative regimens[45,47] (Figure 25-2). Second, there is an increased incidence of neurologic complications including seizures and fatal intracranial hemorrhage (ICH) in this patient population, for which anticonvulsant prophylaxis during BU and throughout the duration of CsA administration is warranted, in addition to maintaining platelets (>50,000/μL), hemoglobin (9-10 g/dL), and blood pressure and repleting magnesium levels.[54] Third, stable mixed chimerism with a reduction rather than an elimination of residual host hematopoiesis is sufficient for a strong

TABLE 25-1 Myeloablative HSCT in patients with SCD with HLA-identical sibling donors

Study	Walters et al, 1996/2000/2001[26,42,43]	Vermylen et al, 1998[25]	Bernaudin et al, 2007[47]	Panepinto et al, 2007[50]	McPherson et al, 2011[49]	Lucarelli et al, 2014[44]	Bhatia et al, 2014[48]	Dedeken et al, 2014[45]	Strocchio et al, 2015[46]	Krishnamurti et al, 2019[64]
Location	United States (multicenter)	Belgium	France	CIBMTR	United States (Atlanta)	Rome	United States (New York)	Belgium	Italy	USA (multicenter STRIDE)
Date	1991-2000	1986-1997	1988-2004	1989-2002	1993-2007	2004-2013	NR	1988-2013	2007-2014	2012-2015
No. of patients	59	50	87	67	27	40	18	50	30	17
Age range (years)	3-15	9 months-23	2-22	2-27	3-17	2-17	2-20	1-15	1-18	17-36[a]
Source (BM/CB)	59/0	48/2	74[a]/10	54/4	27/0	40/0	15/3	39/3	22/4[b]	22/0[a]
Preparative regimen	BU 14 mg/kg, CY 200 mg/kg, ATG/alemtuzumab	BU 16 mg/kg, CY 200 mg/kg, ± TLI or ATG	BU 16 mg/kg, CY 200 mg/kg, ± ATG	BU 16 mg/kg, CY 200 mg/kg	BU 14 mg/kg, CY 200 mg/kg, ATG	BU 14 mg/kg, CY 200 mg/kg, ATG, ± Flu 30 mg/m²	BU 13-16 mg/kg, Flu 180 mg/m², alemtuzumab	BU 13-18 mg/kg, CY 200 mg/kg, ± ATG, ± HU	BU 16 mg/kg or treosulfan 14 g/m², Flu 40 mg/m², TT 10 mg/kg, ± ATG	BU 13.2 mg/kg, Flu 175 mg/m², ATG
GVHD prophylaxis	CsA ± MTX ± Pred	CsA ± MTX	CsA ± MTX	CsA, MTX	CsA, MTX	CsA, MTX, Pred	Tacrolimus, MMF	CsA, MTX	CsA, MTX	CsA or tacrolimus + MTX
OS	93%	93%	93%	97%	96%	91%	100%	94%	100%	94%
EFS	84%	82%	86%	85%	96%	91%	100%	86%	93%	94%
Rejection	8%	10%	7%	13%	0	0	0	8%	7%	6% (n = 1)
TRM	7% (n = 4)	2% (n = 1)	7% (n = 6)	4% (n = 3)	4% (n = 1)	9% (n = 3)	0	4%	0	6% (n = 1)
GVHD (acute/chronic)[c]	19% (acute + chronic)	20%/20%	20%/13%	10%/22%	12%/4%	18%/5%	17%/11%	22%/20%	7%/7%	18%/29%
% Donor chimerism	11%-100%; 26% stable mixed chimerism	<10%-100%	5%-95%; 25%-40% with mixed chimerism	9 had mixed red cell chimerism (HbS >50%)	62%-100%	25%-100%	86%-93%	15%-100%	70%-100%	>97% whole blood

(continued)

TABLE 25-1 Myeloablative HSCT in patients with SCD with HLA-identical sibling donors (Continued)

Study	Walters et al, 1996/2000/2001[26,42,43]	Vermylen et al, 1998[25]	Bernaudin et al, 2007[47]	Panepinto et al, 2007[50]	McPherson et al, 2011[49]	Lucarelli et al, 2014[44]	Bhatia et al, 2014[48]	Dedeken et al, 2014[45]	Strocchio et al, 2015[46]	Krishnamurti et al, 2019[64]
Complications	Seizures 48%; GVHD was the main cause of TRM (n = 3)	Seizures 36%	Seizures 16%; GVHD was the main cause of TRM (n = 4)	Seizures 20%	Seizures 16%; GVHD was the main cause of TRM (n = 1)	Seizures 23%; GVHD was the main cause of TRM (n = 3)	NR	Seizures 22%	NR	NR
End-organ changes	No post-transplant pain, stroke, or ACS after engraftment; those with a prior history of stroke had stable or improved cerebral imaging	Recovery of spleen function present in 7/10; gonadal dysfunction present in those (6 boys, 8 girls) transplanted around puberty	No new ischemic lesions were detected after engraftment, and cerebral velocities were significantly reduced	NR	NR	No post-transplant pain, stroke, or ACS	Neurologic, pulmonary, and cardio-vascular function were stable or improved at 2 years	All patients with elevated arterial cerebral velocities before HSCT had conditional or normal values afterward	No SCD-related adverse events after engraftment	1 death from PRES; patients had improvement in physical function, reduction in pain, and stable brain imaging
Notes	In response to neurologic complications, anticonvulsant therapy was added, and parameters were set for BP, Hb, Plt count, and Mg level	Group of 14 asymptomatic patients (median age, 2 years) transplanted before returning to Africa had lower rejection and GVHD	Rejection rate dropped from 22.6% to 3% and EFS increased to 95% when ATG was added; CB transplant recipients did not develop GVHD; no TRM after the 40th transplant or with CB	Half of those who rejected received more than 10 blood transfusions prior to HSCT	Lower busulfan AUC was seen with partial donor chimerism versus full donor chimerism (P = .022)	No deaths in non-Black African patients	Reduced toxicity, myeloablative conditioning regimen; all episodes of GVHD resolved	EFS at 8 years (97.4%) was significantly higher than EFS in those who did not receive HU prior to HSCT (58.3%; P <.001)	Treosulfan-based regimen provides sufficient immunosuppression to achieve high rate of engraftment	NR

[a]Four patients had 1 HLA mismatch.

[b]Four patients received CB, 3 received BM plus CB, and 1 received peripheral mobilized stem cells.

[c]GVHD grades 2–4.

Abbreviations: ACS, acute chest syndrome; ATG, antithymocyte globulin; AUC, area under the curve; BM, bone marrow; BP, blood pressure; BU, busulfan; CB, cord blood; CIBMTR, Center for International Blood and Marrow Transplant Research; CsA, cyclosporine; CY, cyclophosphamide; EFS, event-free survival; Flu, fludarabine; GVHD, graft-versus-host disease; Hb, hemoglobin; HbS, hemoglobin S; HLA, human leukocyte antigen; HSCT, hematopoietic stem cell transplantation; HU, hydroxyurea; Mg, magnesium; MMF, mycophenolate mofetil; MTX, methotrexate; NR, not reported; Plt, platelet; Pred, prednisone; OS, overall survival; SCD, sickle cell disease; TLI, total lymphoid irradiation; TRM, treatment-related mortality; TT, thiotepa.

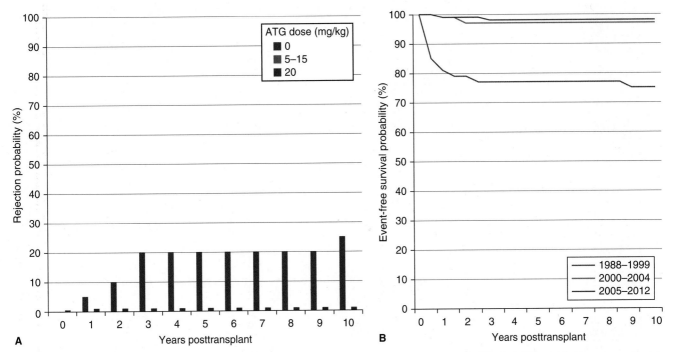

FIGURE 25-2 **Impact of antithymocyte globulin (ATG) and transplant year on outcome. A.** Effect of ATG and its dose on graft rejection incidence. **B.** Event-free survival depicted according to the interval when the transplant was performed.

clinical benefit. This occurs when there is a minority of donor cells contributing to erythropoiesis with a survival advantage compared with short-lived sickle RBCs.

Nonmyeloablative Conditioning

Less toxic, nonmyeloablative conditioning was tested as an efficacious and safer option to myeloablation. Myeloablative therapy is limited by the short- and long-term toxicities of BU/CY, including infertility and gonadal failure, secondary malignancy, and severe organ toxicity in older patients who have impaired organ function or consequences of chronic RBC transfusions before HSCT. By using reduced toxicity with immunomodulatory conditioning, engraftment may still be achieved and allow older adults who have accumulated end-organ damage, those refractory to HU, or those who have developed severe alloimmunization precluding RBC transfusion to be eligible for curative therapy.

Early trials with nonmyeloablative conditioning were notable for high rates of graft failure and disease recurrence (Table 25-2).[37,38,55] The CsA-based immunosuppressive regimen continued to demonstrate GVHD, and after CsA was stopped, patients often rejected their grafts.[38] Based on concerns regarding calcineurin-induced neurologic complications and worsening of renal function and on a novel mechanism for inducing immunologic tolerance, Hsieh et al[27,39] substituted CsA with sirolimus (formerly known as rapamycin) in a regimen using low-dose TBI and alemtuzumab and demonstrated

minimal rejection and no acute or chronic GVHD. Unlike calcineurin inhibitors that inhibit the activation and secretion of interleukin (IL)-2, sirolimus inhibits the secondary IL-2 receptor–dependent signal transduction required for T-cell proliferation. Thus, activated T cells cannot proliferate and become anergic, promoting T-cell tolerance and thus minimizing the risk of GVHD.[56] Furthermore, the novel preparative regimen of TBI at 300 cGy with alemtuzumab for T-cell depletion was chosen for several reasons: the elimination of BU/CY made veno-occlusive disease unlikely, low-dose radiation was sufficient for engraftment,[57] and alemtuzumab had improved infusional tolerance and superior prophylaxis against GVHD over ATG in patients with SCD.[58,59] In addition, alemtuzumab remains detectable for several weeks after infusion and deletes alloreactive T cells during subsequent donor engraftment and initial immune reconstitution. Older patients (n = 30) were successfully transplanted with granulocyte colony-stimulating factor–mobilized peripheral blood stem cells (PBSCs) with EFS and OS rates of 87% and 97%, respectively; a 13% rejection rate; no TRM; and no acute or chronic GVHD. In addition, 15 engrafted patients discontinued immunosuppression medication with continued stable donor chimerism and no GVHD. These results have been confirmed at 2 other centers in 13 adults and 16 children. OS and EFS were 100% and 93%, respectively, in adults and 100% (OS and EFS) in children, and there was no TRM or acute or chronic GVHD in either cohort.[60,61] One patient in

TABLE 25-2 Nonmyeloablative HSCT for patients with SCD

Study	Horan et al, 2005[37]	Iannone et al, 2003[38]	Jacobsohn et al, 2004[55]	Krishnamurti et al, 2008[62]	Matthes-Martin et al, 2013[63]	King et al, 2015[28]	Hsieh et al, 2014[27]	Saraf et al, 2016[61]	Guilcher et al, 2019[60]
Location	USA (Rochester)	USA (multicenter)	USA (Chicago)	USA (multicenter)	Austria	USA (multicenter)	USA (NIH)	USA (Chicago)	Canada
Date	2001-2002	1999-2001	2000-2004	NR	2004-2011	2003-2014	2004-2013	2011-2014	2013-2017
No. of patients	3	6	3	7	8	43	30	13	16
Age range (years)	9-30	3-20	4-22	6-18	3-24	0-20	16-65	17-40	3-18
Source (BM/CB)	3/0	6/0	0/0[b]	7/0	7/1	51/1[c]	0/0[b]	0/0[b]	0/0[b]
Preparative regimen	Flu 125 mg/m², TBI 200 cGy, ATG	Flu 150 mg/m², TBI 200 cGy, ± ATG	BU 6.4 mg/kg, Flu 180 mg/m², ATG	BU 6.4 mg/kg IV or 8 mg/kg PO, Flu 175 mg/kg, TLI 500 cGy, ATG	Flu 160 mg/m², melphalan 140 mg/m², ± TLI 200 cGy, ± TT 10 mg/kg, ± ATG	Flu 140-150 mg/m², melphalan 140 mg/m², alemtuzumab	TBI 300 cGy, alemtuzumab	TBI 300 cGy, alemtuzumab	TBI 300 cGy, alemtuzumab
GVHD prophylaxis	MMF, CsA	MMF, CsA, or tacrolimus	CsA, MMF	CsA, MMF	CsA, MMF	CsA or tacrolimus ± MTX, MMF, Pred	Sirolimus	Sirolimus	Sirolimus
OS	100%	100%	67%	100%	100%	93%	97%	100%	100%
EFS	33%	0	0	86%	100%	91%	87%	93%	100%
Rejection	67% (n = 2)	100% (n = 6)	67% (n = 2)	14% (n = 1)	0	2% (n = 1)[c]	13% (n = 4)	7% (n = 1)	0
TRM	0	0	33% (n = 1)	0	0	7%	0	0	0
GVHD (acute/chronic)[d]	0/0	17%/0	0/100%	7%/7%	0/0	23%/13%[d]	0/0	0/0	0/0
% Donor chimerism	0%-100% (n = 1)	25%-85%	9%-100%	50%-90%	20%-97%; 100% donor erythropoiesis	16%->90%	34%-62% lymphoid; 70%-100% myeloid	Median 81% (31%-98%)	>20% myeloid

Complications, end-organ changes, notes	Pure red cell aplasia in engrafted patient due to major ABO incompatibility; 1 patient had a stroke during period of low engraftment; no SCD-related complications occurred and pulmonary function improved; rejection occurred in all but 1 patient after immunosuppression was weaned	During the period of mixed chimerism, none experienced pain, ACS, or stroke; all patients rejected their grafts once immune suppression was weaned	Death due to extensive chronic GVHD	All patients had stable head imaging and lung function as measured by pulmonary function testing; normal renal function was regained in all patients; 5 patients had splenic regeneration	Renal volume and structure normalized in 4 of 5 patients with nephropathy; all patients showed normal growth; 3 of 4 female postpubertal patients had regular gonadal hormone levels	All deaths were related to GVHD and occurred in patients aged 17-18; all patients who engrafted were transfusion independent; no strokes or pulmonary complications of SCD were noted, and pain symptoms subsided within 6 months posttransplant	Serious adverse events (n = 38) were related to pain, infection, abdominal events, and sirolimus-related toxic effects; however, no acute SCD-related complications, hepatic sinusoidal obstructive syndrome, or cerebral complications from immunosuppression; 15 engrafted patients discontinued immunosuppression with stable donor chimerism and no GVHD	Patient with secondary graft failure was not compliant with sirolimus; patients had normalized hemoglobin and improved cardiopulmonary and QoL parameters including bodily pain, general health, and vitality	No sickling crises after HSCT have been observed; 12 of 16 patients discontinued sirolimus (3 have not yet reached 1 year after HSCT)

[a] Entire cohort (n = 22) included 17 patients who received marrow from an HLA-identical sibling donor and 5 patients who received marrow from an 8/8 HLA-allele matched unrelated donor.

[b] All donor sources were granulocyte colony-stimulating factor CD34+-mobilized peripheral blood stem cells.

[c] Patient who rejected received an umbilical CB graft and subsequently underwent a successful BM transplant.

[d] GVHD grades 2-4.

[e] Includes 9 patients with other nonmalignant diseases.

Abbreviations: ACS, acute chest syndrome; ATG, antithymocyte globulin; BM, bone marrow; BU, busulfan; CB, cord blood; CsA, cyclosporine; CY, cyclophosphamide; EFS, event-free survival; Flu, fludarabine; GVHD, graft-versus-host disease; HLA, human leukocyte antigen; HSCT, hematopoietic stem cell transplantation; IV, intravenous; MTX, methotrexate; NIH, National Institutes of Health; NR, not reported; OS, overall survival; PO, oral; Pred, Prednisone; PRES, posterior reversible encephalopathy syndrome; QoL, quality of life; SCD, sickle cell disease; TBI, total-body irradiation; TLI, total lymphoid irradiation; TRM, treatment-related mortality; TT, thiotepa; URD, unrelated donor; USA, United States of America.

501

the adult cohort had secondary graft failure due to sirolimus noncompliance.

In other series, patients have received various conditioning regimens including fludarabine, low-dose BU, varying doses of TBI, melphalan, and/or ATG/alemtuzumab (Table 25-2).[28,62-64] Fludarabine is an antimetabolite drug with immunosuppressive properties that can potentiate the effects of alkylating agents such as BU/CY, allowing for reduced doses of alkylating agents.[65] Two studies (n = 43, n = 17) demonstrated EFS and OS rates of 91% to 94% and 93% to 94%, respectively, with acute and chronic GVHD rates of 18% to 23% and 13% to 29%, respectively, using a calcineurin-based immunosuppressive regimen.[28,64] Smaller series (n = 7-8) have shown an OS rate of 100%, with minimal graft rejection and minimal to no acute or chronic GVHD.

Transplant Considerations: Age, Graft Source, Conditioning, and Transplant Period

The largest international survey of results of HLA-identical sibling HSCT identified several key factors associated with survival after transplantation: age, graft type, and transplant period.[19] One thousand patients aged 0 to 54 years received an HLA-identical sibling transplant for SCD with either myeloablative conditioning (n = 873) or RIC (n = 125) from donor BM (n = 839), peripheral blood (PB; n = 73), or cord blood (CB; n = 88) stem cell sources between 1986 and 2013 at 106 centers in 23 countries worldwide. The authors concluded that HLA-identical sibling transplantation for SCD offers excellent long term survival (OS, 93%), there is no difference in EFS or OS based on preparative regimen (myeloablative vs nonmyeloablative), and EFS is improved in patients transplanted after 2006.

When an indication for transplantation is identified, data support early referral for patients with an HLA-matched sibling given a 5-year OS (95% vs 81%; *P* <.001), EFS (93% vs 81%; *P* <.001), and GVHD-free survival (86% vs 77%; *P* <.001) advantage for patients <16 years old compared to those ≥16 years old.[19] In multivariate analysis, for every 1-year increment in age, there was a 4% increase in the hazard ratio (HR) for acute GVHD, a 2% increase for chronic GVHD, a 9% increase in HR for treatment failure (graft failure or death), and a 10% increase for death. Similar reports in single-institution or multi-institutional studies of non–HLA-matched sibling transplantation have demonstrated higher rates of mortality in patients ≥16 years old[66] or less GVHD and GVHD-related mortality in younger patients.[67]

The balance of potential benefits of long-term survival after curative transplantation, however, is individualized in the context of patient age, disease status, donor match, and other unmeasurable, sometimes personal factors. Whereas the 5-year OS of 95% in patients <16 years old after an HLA-identical transplantation compares favorably to the Dallas Newborn Cohort,[68] a direct comparison of transplantation versus standard of care (ie, nontransplant therapies) is needed. Sickle Cell Transplantation to Prevent Disease Exacerbation is a multicenter study comparing myeloablative HSCT with HLA-matched related or unrelated donors with standard of care in patients with severe SCD (BMT CTN 1503, NCT02766465), with results anticipated by 2021.

Donor Stem Cell Source

HSCT can be accomplished by cells harvested from BM or UCB or mobilized from the PB and collected by apheresis (Figure 25-3). Within the CIBMTR, European Group for

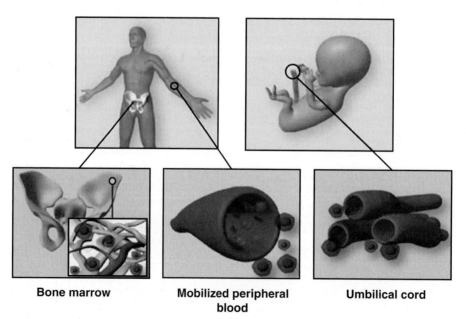

Bone marrow   **Mobilized peripheral blood**   **Umbilical cord**

FIGURE 25-3 The sources of hematopoietic cells for transplantation are depicted: bone marrow, mobilized peripheral blood, and umbilical cord blood. Modified with permission from Spinger Nature. Ratajczak MZ et al. Pivotal role of paracrine effects in stem cell therapies in regenerative medicine: can we translate stem cell-secreted paracrine factors and microvesicles into better therapeutic strategies? *Leukemia*. 2012;26(6):1166-73. Copyright 2012.

Blood and Marrow Transplantation (EBMT), and EUROCORD data set, BM was the predominant stem cell source (87%), compared to PB (7%) or CB (9%).[21] Of note, the median age of transplantation for recipients of BM, PB, and CB was 9.4, 18.7, and 6.1 years, respectively ($P <.001$), and most recipients of BM (88%; 742 of 838 recipients) and CB (95%; 84 of 88 recipients) transplantation received myeloablative regimens, compared with only 65% of patients (47 of 72 patients) who received PB transplantation. Median times to granulocyte and platelet recovery were shorter after transplantation with BM (18 and 25 days, respectively) and PB (15 and 18 days, respectively) compared with CB cells (27 and 37 days, respectively; $P <.001$). Multivariate analysis demonstrated lower OS for PB transplantation recipients compared to BM recipients (HR, 2.6; $P = .019$), with age considered a continuous variable in the adjusted Cox regression analysis.

More recently, many studies have used PBSCs as the donor stem cell source as the best available method to obtain high cell numbers, with many haploidentical protocols using this method for ease of CD34+ isolation. When 2 donors are otherwise equally HLA matched, donor selection may consider ABO match, the presence of alloantibodies directed toward donor RBC antigens, donor-specific HLA antibodies, and matching donor/recipient cytomegalovirus (CMV) serostatus.

Unrelated Donor Sources

Access to an alternative donor source of hematopoietic cells is critical for expanding HSCT. Matched and mismatched unrelated BM and UCB expand the donor pool and have successfully been used in pediatric malignant and nonmalignant hereditary and acquired hematologic and immunologic disorders.[69] Unrelated BM or UCB HSCT for patients with SCD remains limited, however, due in part to less common, more diverse haplotypes in African populations and an underrepresentation of ethnic minorities in the donor registries worldwide.[70,71] The probability of identifying a suitable donor in the unrelated BM registry increases from 19% to 76% for African Americans if 7/8 HLA matches are considered acceptable.[20] Similarly, 90% of children <43 months old may have an adequate single cord, as defined by a total nucleated cell count >5 × 10^7/kg and matched at 5/6 to 6/6 of the major histocompatibility loci (HLA-A, HLA-B, HLA-DRB1), which increases to >97% if smaller cell dose (allowing for the use of double cords or in vitro expansion) or 4/6 HLA matching is allowed.[72] Relaxing the stringency of HLA matching, however, is likely to increase the rates of rejection and/or GVHD. Therefore, according to the expert panel, "due to the lack of matched donors in the registries there are no firm data on outcome of HSCT from unrelated donors for SCD, and, therefore, the advantages and disadvantages of this option cannot be adequately addressed."[29] HSCT from unrelated BM or CB is thus recommended to be considered for severe disease and only in a clinical trial at experienced centers.

UCBT

Lower rates of GVHD and TRM were noted in several studies investigating myeloablative conditioning for HLA-identical sibling HSCT patients who used CB as the donor source.[47,73] UCB is a rich source of hematopoietic stem and progenitor cells with extensive proliferative capacity that has the advantage of lowered risk of GVHD compared to marrow transplantation.[74] This lowered risk of GVHD may allow for a greater degree of mismatch but is balanced by a higher rate of graft rejection, poor immune reconstitution, and a prolonged period of hematologic recovery where there is a high risk for infection.[75] Many trials using primarily unrelated UCB as the donor source are limited by the small numbers of patients treated and show high rates of graft rejection and infection (Table 25-3).[67,73,76-79] The sickle cell unrelated donor transplant trial of the Blood and Marrow Transplant Clinical Trials Network (BMT CTN 0601) was a phase II study of the toxicity and efficacy of unrelated donor HSCT in children with severe SCD using an RIC regimen (NCT00745420). The UCB arm of this trial was suspended due to a high incidence of graft rejection (63%) with a DFS of 37.5% noted at 1 year.[77]

Efforts to improve upon existing outcomes include changes to preparative regimens, the use of cellular therapy such as antiviral specific cytotoxic T lymphocytes to reduce infectious complications, and expansion of CB products to reduce the period of neutropenia and enhance engraftment.[80,81] A study investigating mesenchymal stromal cells to support expansion of HSCT and encourage engraftment of UCB showed that mesenchymal stromal cells were ineffective, and the study was terminated early due to lack of engraftment and excessive mortality from opportunistic infections, GVHD, and ICH.[82] The RIC regimen that failed to provide engraftment in BMT CTN 0601 was modified to include HU and thiotepa (TT), and results suggested improved outcomes with a median follow-up of 2-years.[83] The DFS and OS rates in 9 patients were 78% and 100%, respectively. Eight patients had bacterial infections, viral infections, or reactivations; 1 patient had graft rejection after CMV reactivation; and GVHD occurred in 33% of the patients (n = 3).

The UCBT transplant experience after related, HLA-identical sibling CB transplantation is identical to BM HSCT, confirming the importance of an HLA-matched sibling for success regardless of donor cell source. The most recent update comparing HLA-identical sibling BM versus UCB transplant outcomes for 485 recipient cases with thalassemia major or SCD was published from the CIBMTR and EBMT registry data from US and European transplant centers.[67] One hundred sixty patients with SCD who underwent HSCT were included in this analysis, of whom 30 patients received CB as their donor source. Compared to those who received BM, those who received CB had delayed neutrophil recovery (BM, 19 days, range, 8-56 days; vs CB, 23 days; range, 9-60 days; $P = .002$) but less acute and chronic GVHD (acute GVHD: 21% with BM vs 11% with CB; $P = .04$; chronic GVHD, 12% with BM vs 7% with CB; $P = .12$). None of the patients who received CB developed extensive

TABLE 25-3 Umbilical cord blood hematopoietic stem cell transplantation in patients with sickle cell disease

Study	Locatelli et al, 2003[67]	Adamkiewicz et al, 2007[76]	Radhakrishnan et al, 2013[78]	Ruggeri et al, 2011[79]	Kamani et al, 2012[77]	Locatelli et al, 2013[73]	Abraham et al, 2017[83]
Location	EUROCORD	USA (multicenter)	USA (New York)	Retrospective review	USA (multi-center SCURT trial)	EUROCORD, Oakland	USA (multicenter)
Date	1994-2001	NR	2004-2010	1996-2009	2008-2012	1994-2005	2009-NR
No. of patients	11	7	8	16	8	160	9
Age range (years)	1-12	1-12	1-10	3-17	7-16	1-24	3-10
Source (BM/CB)	CB	CB	CB	CB	CB	130/30	CB
Relationship	Related	Unrelated	Unrelated	Unrelated	Unrelated	Related	Unrelated
HLA match	6/6 (n = 41); 5/6 (n = 3)[a]	5/6 (n = 2); 4/6 (n = 5)	NR	6/6 (n = 2); 5/6 (n = 4); 4/6 (n = 10)	5/6 (n = 8)	HLA-identical	5/6 (n = 7); 6/6 (n = 2)
TNC dose (range)	4.0×10^7/kg $(1.2\text{-}10 \times 10^7$/kg)[a]	5.7×10^7/kg $(1.5\text{-}9.3 \times 10^7$/kg)	NR	4.9×10^7/kg $(1.1\text{-}9 \times 10^7$/kg)	6.4×10^7/kg $(3.1\text{-}7.6 \times 10^7$/kg)	3.9×10^7/kg (NR)	5.9×10^7/kg $(3.9\text{-}8.5 \times 10^7$/kg)
Median CD34+ cell dose (range)	NR	2.3×10^5/kg $(0.5\text{-}6 \times 10^5$/kg)	NR	NR	1.5×10^5/kg $(0.2\text{-}2.3 \times 10^5$/kg)	NR	2.4×10^5/kg $(1.2\text{-}8.0 \times 10^5$/kg)
Preparative regimen	BU, CY, ATG/ alemtuzumab, ± TT, Flu	BU 3.5 mg/kg-40 mg/m², CY 50-60 mg/kg, Flu 25-35 mg/m², ATG ± TLI 200-750 cGy	BU 3.2-4 mg/kg, Flu 30 mg/m², alemtuzumab	Combinations of BU, CY, ATG, Flu, melphalan, alemtuzumab, TLI/ TBI	Flu 30 mg/ m², melphalan 140mg/m², alemtuzumab	BU 16 mg/kg, CY 200 mg/kg, ± treosulfan, ± Flu ± ATG	HU, TT 4 mg/kg, Flu 30 mg/m², melphalan 140 mg/m², alemtuzumab
GVHD prophylaxis	CsA ± MTX ± tacrolimus ± Pred	CsA, methylprednisolone ± MMF ± tacrolimus	MMF, tacrolimus	CsA or tacrolimus or Pred or MMF or MTX	CsA or tacrolimus + MMF	CSA ± MTX	CsA or tacrolimus + MMF
OS	100%	43%	63%	94%	88%	95%/97%[b]	100%
EFS	90%	43%[c]	50%	50%	38%	92%/90%[d]	78%
Rejection	9%	43%	38%	44%	63%	7%/10%[b]	22% (n = 2)
TRM	0	14% (n = 1)	38% (n = 3)	6% (n = 1)	13% (n = 1)	5% (n = 18)/3% (n = 3)[b]	0

GVHD (acute/chronic)[e]	11%/6%[a]	57%/14%	50%/13%	23%/16%[f]	25%/13%	21%/11%(acute)[b]; 12%/7%(chronic)	33%/33%
% Donor chimerism	45%-100%	75%-76%	NR	9 with complete donor chimerism	3 with complete donor chimerism	NR	>90%
Complications and notes	Use of MTX for GVHD prophylaxis was associated with a greater risk of treatment failure	57% (n = 4) developed significant viral infections	3 deaths were due to infection in patients with primary graft failure	1 death from chronic GVHD; in multivariate analysis, DFS was higher with CB units containing TNC dose >5 × 10^7/kg	19 infections in 6 patients; 2 serious neurologic complications (ICH, PRES); 1 death from chronic GVHD; CB arm of this trial was suspended due to high incidence of graft rejection	GVHD was the most frequent cause of death in patients after BM transplantation, whereas no CB recipient died of GVHD; cell dose did not influence outcomes	Viral and bacterial infection developed in 8 patients; in the 2 patients who rejected grafts, both were HLA-mismatched and 1 rejection occurred after an early CMV infection; of 5 patients with preexisting cerebral vasculopathy, 1 had improvement, 3 were stable, and 1 was pending

[a]Includes 33 patients with thalassemia and 11 patients with SCD in the cohort; HLA typing specifically for SCD not reported.

[b]Includes 325 patients with thalassemia and 160 patients with SCD in the cohort.

[c]Patient rejected graft 8 months after first failed umbilical CB transplant but developed sustained engraftment after a second umbilical CB transplant with an immunosuppressive but not myeloablative regimen.

[d]DFS for sickle cell cohort only, BM/umbilical CB.

[e]GVHD grades 2-4.

[f]Includes 35 patients with thalassemia and 16 patients with SCD in the cohort.

Abbreviations: ATG, antithymocyte globulin; BM, bone marrow; BU, busulfan; CB, cord blood; CMV, cytomegalovirus; CsA, cyclosporine; CY, cyclophosphamide; DFS, disease-free survival; EFS, event-free survival; Flu, fludarabine; GVHD, graft versus host disease; HLA, human leukocyte antigen; HU, hydroxyurea; ICH, intracranial hemorrhage; MMF, mycophenolate mofetil; MTX, methotrexate; NR, not reported; OS, overall survival; Pred, prednisone; PRES, posterior reversible encephalopathy syndrome; SCD, sickle cell disease; SCURT, Sickle Cell Unrelated Donor Transplant; TBI, total-body irradiation; TLI, total lymphoid irradiation; TNC, total nucleated cell; TRM, treatment-related mortality; TT, thiotepa; USA, United States of America.

chronic GVHD or died of GVHD-related complications. It must be noted, however, that those who received CB were younger than those who received BM (combined thalassemia and SCD median age, 5.9 years for CB vs 8.1 years for BM; P = .02), and therefore, it cannot be excluded that the younger age of CBT recipients could have contributed to their lower incidence and severity of GVHD in comparison with BM recipients. The 6-year OS rates for all patients were 95% and 97% for BM and CB HSCT, respectively (P = .92), and the 6-year DFS rates for patients with SCD were 92% and 90%, respectively. Two patients who received CB had primary graft failure and were successfully retransplanted from the same donor. Six patients had secondary graft failure at a median time of 151 days (range, 51-202 days). In this study, the cell dose infused did not influence the outcome of patients given CB, and there was no difference in the cumulative incidence of primary graft failure.

HLA-Matched Unrelated Donor

The current experience of unrelated donor HSCT with marrow for SCD is limited. Small studies have demonstrated mixed results from unrelated HLA-matched HSCT (Table 25-4): 97% chimerism with no GVHD (n = 1),[84] graft rejection of 17% without any acute or chronic GVHD (n = 6),[46] or no graft rejection (1 patient received a second HSCT with success after rejecting the first graft) with 50% chronic GVHD (n = 2).[85] The largest group (n = 29) reported EFS and OS rates of 69% and 79%, respectively.[66] TRM rate was 28% and GVHD was the cause of 7 deaths. The rate of chronic GVHD was 62%. Of note, all deaths except 1 occurred in recipients ≥16 years old. The authors concluded that although the 1-year EFS met the prespecified target of ≥75%, this regimen could not be considered sufficiently safe for widespread adoption without modifications to achieve more effective GVHD prevention. Therefore, investigators are currently exploring the tolerability of the costimulation blocking agent abatacept (CTLA4-Ig) when added to standard GVHD prophylaxis (NCT02867800). This preparative regimen will include RIC conditioning with fludarabine, melphalan, and alemtuzumab, with TT to promote engraftment.

Results of a pilot study of BM transplantation in young adults with severe SCD after 1 year show outcomes similar to previous trials using RIC.[27,64,86] The authors reported 1-year EFS and OS rates of 86.4% and 90.9%, respectively, in all patients (matched related donor, n = 17; matched unrelated donor, n = 5), a single graft rejection after unrelated donor HSCT, minimal GVHD, and 2 deaths from ICH related to posterior reversible encephalopathy syndrome and chronic GVHD. This regimen is now being tested in a comparative trial of HSCT and standard of care based on the availability of a suitable HLA-matched related or unrelated donor (BMT CTN 1503, NCT01565616).

Mismatched Unrelated Donor Transplantation

By pursuing alternate unrelated donors matched at 7/8 HLA loci by high-resolution typing, it might be possible to expand HSCT as in malignant disorders; however, in nonmalignant

disorders, a higher risk of chronic GVHD is unacceptable. Methods for success must therefore reduce the GVHD risk. Methods include T-cell depletion (in vivo or in vitro), CD34 selection, or $\alpha\beta$CD3$^+$ T-cell depletion. One patient who received a T-cell receptor $\alpha\beta^+$CD19$^+$-depleted PBSC graft from an 8/12 HLA-mismatched unrelated donor had 61% donor chimerism and survives event free.[87] Posttransplantation complications included Epstein-Barr virus (EBV) reactivation treated with rituximab and grade 2 acute GVHD, which responded to treatment. Another patient with a follow-up of 50 months received a CD34$^+$-selected PBSC graft from a 9/10 unrelated donor, had 92% chimerism, and had no acute or chronic GVHD.[84] The course was complicated by posttransplantation lymphoproliferative disorder, which was successfully treated with low-dose radiation, rituximab, a very-low-dose donor lymphocyte infusion, and EBV-specific cytotoxic T lymphocytes.

In summary, the role of unrelated BM or CB transplantation in patients with SCD is uncertain, in part due to small numbers of patients treated. Successful outcomes have been reported, but indications and an optimal treatment regimen have not been established. Optimized conditioning regimens (eg, the addition of TT), improved and refined donor/recipient HLA matching, higher cell dose for CB, identification of anti-HLA antibodies, and improved effectiveness of GVHD prophylaxis will be needed to extend unrelated donor HSCT for SCD.

Haploidentical Transplantation

Haploidentical transplantation promises an expanded donor pool of biologic parents, biologic children, full or half siblings, or even extended family donors to patients with SCD who otherwise satisfy eligibility requirements for HSCT but lack a suitable matched related or unrelated donor. An HLA-haploidentical donor shares exactly 1 HLA haplotype with the recipient but is mismatched for a variable number of HLA genes on the unshared haplotype. The major challenge of HLA-haploidentical HSCT is therefore the bidirectional alloreactivity, leading to high incidences of graft rejection and GVHD. Unlike patients with hematologic malignancies who are pretreated with chemotherapy and irradiation, patients with SCD may have a higher risk of graft rejection due to an intact, activated immune system, a lifetime of anemia and chronic inflammation, and alloimmunization with donor sensitization related to pre-HSCT transfusion exposures. To broaden the availability of transplantation to more patients, engraftment without GVHD is a lofty goal.

Novel strategies in T-cell depletion are highlighted by ongoing studies of haploidentical HSCT for SCD. These include in vivo posttransplantation CY (PTCy) and ex vivo infusion of CD34 positively selected donor grafts. In contrast to nonselective in vivo T-cell depletion with ATG or alemtuzumab, which have long half-lives,[88,89] high-dose PTCy targets short-acting depletion of alloreactive T cells without adversely affecting immune reconstitution and passive transfer of immunity (Figure 25-4). Ex vivo T-cell depletion avoids CY-induced toxicity. Promoting engraftment and/or enriching antiviral immunity are theoretically possible in ex vivo models, for example, by enriching or expanding

TABLE 25-4 Unrelated donor HSCT in patients with SCD

Study	Mynarek et al, 2013[85]	Strocchio et al, 2015[46]	Gilman et al, 2017[84]	Shenoy et al, 2016[66]	Krishnamurti et al, 2019[64]
Location	Germany	Italy	USA (North Carolina)	USA (multicenter SCURT trial)	USA (multicenter STRIDE trial)
Date	2000-20009	2007-2014	2009-2015	2008-2014	2012-2015
No. of patients	2	6	2	29	5
Age range (years)	6-8	27-48	5-13	6-19	17-36[a]
Source (BM/PBSC)	2/0	5/1	0/2	29/0	22/0[a]
Relationship	Unrelated	Unrelated	Unrelated	Unrelated	Unrelated
HLA match	10/10	12/12	9/10 (n = 1); 10/10 (n = 1)	8/8 (n = 29)	8/8
Preparative regimen	BU 3.8 mg/kg, Flu 30 mg/m², ATG	Flu 40 mg/m², TT 10 mg/kg, treosulfan 14 g/m², ATG	Flu 40 mg/m², TT 5 mg/kg, melphalan 140 mg/m², ATG	Flu 30 mg/m², melphalan 140 mg/m², alemtuzumab	BU 13.2 mg/kg, Flu 150 mg/m², ATG
GVHD prophylaxis	Tacrolimus or CsA and MTX	CsA, MTX	DLI, MTX	CsA or tacrolimus, MTX, methylprednisolone	CsA or tacrolimus, MTX
OS	100%	100%	100%	79%	80%
EFS	100%	83%	100%	69%	60%
Rejection	50%	17%	0	10%	20%
TRM	0	0	0	28% (n = 8)	20% (n = 1)
GVHD (acute/chronic)[b]	0/50%	0/0	0/0	28%/62%	20%/20%
% Donor chimerism	>89%	70%-100%	92%-97%	>90%	>97% whole blood
Complications and notes	1 patient developed graft failure and received a successful second unrelated 10/10 BM HSCT; this patient developed chronic extensive GVHD after the second HSCT	No SCD-related adverse events after engraftment	PTLD developed in 1 patient successfully treated with low-dose radiation, rituximab, a very low dose DLI, and EBV-specific cytotoxic T lymphocytes	GVHD was the main cause of TRM (n = 7); a 34% incidence of PRES was noted; although the 1-year EFS met the target (≥75%), this regimen is not sufficiently safe for widespread use without modifications for more effective GVHD prophylaxis	1 death due to severe, chronic GVHD; 1 patient had secondary graft failure followed by a successful second URD BM transplantation

[a]Entire cohort (n = 22) included 17 patients who received marrow from an HLA-identical sibling donor and 5 patients who received marrow from an 8/8 HLA-allele matched unrelated donor.
[b]GVHD grades 2-4.
Abbreviations: ATG, antithymocyte globulin; BM, bone marrow; BU, busulfan; CsA, cyclosporine; CY, cyclophosphamide; DLI, donor lymphocyte infusion; EBV, Epstein-Barr virus; EFS, event-free survival; Flu, fludarabine; GVHD, graft-versus-host disease; HLA, human leukocyte antigen; HSCT, hematopoietic stem cell transplantation; ICH, intracranial hemorrhage; MTX, methotrexate; OS, overall survival; PBSC, peripheral blood stem cell; PRES, posterior reversible encephalopathy syndrome; PTLD, posttransplantation lymphoproliferative disorder; SCD, sickle cell disease; SCURT, Sickle Cell Unrelated Donor Transplant; STRIDE, Bone Marrow Transplant in Young Adults With Severe Sickle Cell Disease; TRM, treatment-related mortality; TT, thiotepa; URD, unrelated donor; USA, United States of America.

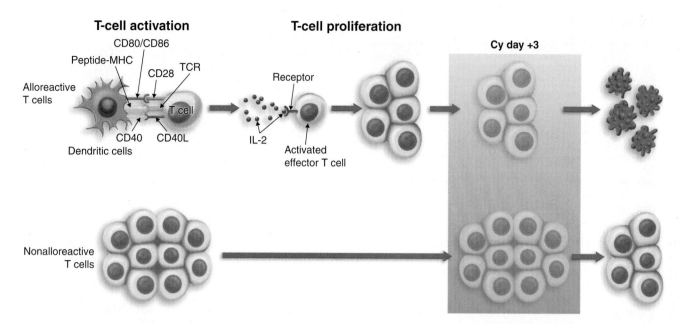

FIGURE 25-4 **Depiction of T-cell activation and T-cell proliferation with cytokine secretion that follows antigen recognition and presentation by the host dendritic cell.** The process is abrogated by high-dose cyclophosphamide (Cy) administered 3 days after transplant, which elicits T-cell depletion in vivo. In contrast, nonalloreactive T cells that are not activated after transplant are spared. IL-2, interleukin-2; MHC, major histocompatibility complex; TCR, T-cell receptor. Reproduced with permission from Springer Nature. Luznik L and Fuchs EJ. High-dose, post-transplantation cyclophosphamide to promote graft-host tolerance after allogeneic hematopoietic stem cell transplantation. *Immunol Res.* 2010;47(1-3):65-77.) Copyright 2010.

the graft to allow for larger doses of HSCs while maintaining a fixed T-cell dose or adding back virus-specific T cells. Extensive ex vivo T-cell depletion, however, can cause delayed immune reconstitution and promote viral reactivation and infection.

PTCy

In vivo, high-dose CY administered on days 3 and 4 after HSCT targets donor and recipient proliferating, alloreactive T cells,[90] but high-level, cell nonautonomous secretion of aldehyde dehydrogenase protects quiescent HSCs from CY.[91] An RIC regimen consisting of fludarabine, low-dose TBI, and pretransplantation CY was used in initial studies in high-risk malignancies. In SCD, ATG was added to the regimen to promote engraftment of donor cells.[47] The initial phase I trial in high-risk malignancies gave a single dose of PTCy (50 mg/kg) on day +3. This dosing was associated with a high incidence of graft rejection and severe GVHD (60% with 1 death).[92] Subsequent studies comparing single-dose administration versus 2-dose administration (50 mg/kg per dose) on days +3 and +4 showed no difference in acute GVHD but a trend ($P = .05$) toward less extensive chronic GVHD in the 2-dose group.[93] In general, postgrafting immunosuppression with mycophenolate mofetil and tacrolimus or sirolimus (and the administration of corticosteroids in the conditioning regimen) was commenced after PTCy to avoid inhibition of activated, proliferating donor-derived alloreactive T cells.[94]

The first series of SCD patients treated by HLA-haploidentical transplantation showed a low rate of GVHD (Table 25-5).[95] No patient developed either acute or chronic GVHD, PTCy caused limited serious toxicities, and all patients were alive a median of 711 days after HSCT. However, graft rejection

occurred in 42.8% of the recipients. To reduce graft rejection, the TBI dose was increased from 200 cGy to 400cGy. Rejection was 6% (n = 1) in 17 patients (12 patients with SCD and 5 with β thalassemia).[96] EFS and OS rates were 100% and 94%, respectively; most patients achieved full donor chimerism; and all patients were alive at a median of 705 days after HSCT. Rates of acute and chronic GVHD were 29% and 18%, respectively, with resolution of GVHD in all patients at most recent follow-up and 88% of patients off immunosuppression. In another study, 23 patients with severe disease (21 patients with SCD and 2 patients with β thalassemia) were treated with nonmyeloablative conditioning including 400 cGy of TBI and escalating doses of PTCy (cohort 1: 0 doses; cohort 2: 1 dose; cohort 3: 2 doses).[97] A mean HSCT-specific comorbidity index of 6 reflected patients with cirrhosis, heart failure, and end-stage renal disease. The engraftment rate improved from 1 (33%) of 3 patients in cohort 1 to 5 (63%) of 8 patients in cohort 2 and 10 (83%) of 12 patients in cohort 3. Percentage of donor myeloid and CD3 chimerism also improved with subsequent cohorts. There was no TRM, OS was 87%, and there was no grade 2 to 4 acute or extensive chronic GVHD. At a median follow-up of 3.17 years (range, 0.67-6.16 years), 0% of patients in cohort 1, 25% in cohort 2, and 50% in cohort 3 remained free of their disease. An additional protocol is ongoing for patients with high risk of graft rejection that uses pentostatin and oral CY before transplant to further deplete recipient lymphocytes in an attempt to decrease the rate of graft rejection (NCT02105766).

The addition of TT to the conditioning regimen might also improve donor engraftment with an acceptable toxicity profile. A multidisciplinary haploidentical BM transplantation

TABLE 25-5 Haploidentical transplantation with posttransplantation cyclophosphamide in patients with SCD

Study	Bolaños-Meade et al, 2012[95]	Dhedin et al, 2016[99]	Fitzhugh et al, 2017[97]	Wiebking et al, 2017[10]	Frangoul et al, 2018[100]	Pawlowska et al, 2018[101]	de al Fuente et al, 2019[98]	Bolaños-Meade et al, 2019[96]
Location	USA (Johns Hopkins)	France, UK, USA	USA (NIH)	Germany	USA (Tennessee)	USA (California)	France, UK, USA	USA (Johns Hopkins)
Date	2006-2011	NR	2009-2016	NR	2014-2016	2016-2017	NR	2014-2017
No. of patients	14	22	23[a]	3	4	4	15[b]	17[c]
Age range (years)	15-42	3-18	20-56	5-20	12-23	13-23	12-26	6-31
HLA match	NR	NR	5/10 (n = 5); 6/10 (n = 5); 7/10 (n = 8); 8/10 (n = 5)	5/10 (n = 5); 6/10 (n = 1)	NR	NR	NR	NR
Median CD34+ cell dose (range)	5.24 × 10^6/kg (4.4-8.7 × 10^6/kg)	3.63 × 10^6/kg (NR)	12.2 × 10^6/kg (7.0-29.7 × 10^6/kg)	7.5 × 10^6/kg (3.5-8.3 × 10^6/kg)	NR	1.86-5 × 10^6/kg	3 × 10^6/kg (2.35-4.80 × 10^6/kg)	4 × 10^6/kg (2.71-6.14 × 10^6/kg)
Median CD3+ cell count (range)	3.61 × 10^7/kg (3.29-6.59 × 10^7/kg)	NR	3.8 × 10^8/kg (1.86-8.1 × 10^8/kg)	60 × 10^6/kg (54-251 × 10^6/kg)	NR	NR	NR	4.5 × 10^7/kg (2.9-7.1 × 10^7/kg)
Preparative regimen	Flu 30 mg/m^2, CY 14.5 mg/kg, TBI 200 cGy, ATG	Azathioprine + HU followed by Flu 150 mg/m^2, CY 29 mg/kg, TT 10 mg/kg, ATG, TBI 200 cGy	TBI 400 cGY, alemtuzumab	Flu 30 mg/m^2, CY 14.5 mg/kg, TT 5 mg/kg, treosulfan 14 g/m^2, alemtuzumab	ATG, Flu 30 mg/m^2, CY 14.5 mg/kg, TT 10 mg/kg, TBI 200 cGy	Flu 40 mg/m^2 + dexamethasone 25 mg/m^2 followed by BU 120 mg/m^2, Flu 35 mg/m^2, ATG	Flu 30 mg/m^2, CY 14.5 mg/kg, TT 10 mg/kg, TBI 200 cGY, ATG	Flu 30 mg/m^2, CY 14.5 mg/kg, TBI 400 cGy, ATG
GVHD prophylaxis	CY 50 mg/kg × 2, tacrolimus or sirolimus, MMF	CY 50 mg/kg × 2, sirolimus, MMF	Sirolimus, CY 0 mg/kg (cohort 1), 50 mg/kg (cohort 2), or 100 mg/kg (cohort 3)	CY 50 mg/kg × 2, MMF, tacrolimus	CY 50 mg/kg × 2, MMF, sirolimus	CY 50 mg/kg × 2, tacrolimus or sirolimus, MMF	CY 50 mg/kg × 2, sirolimus, MMF	CY 50 mg/kg × 2, sirolimus or MMF
OS	100%	82%	87%	100%	100%	100%	100%	100%
EFS	50%	86%	0 cohort 1; 25% (n = 2) cohort 2; 50% (n = 6) cohort 3	100%	100%	100%	93%	94%
Rejection	42.3% (n = 6)[d]	NR	65%	0	0	0	6% (n = 1)	6% (n = 1)
TRM	0	14% (n = 3)	0	0	0	0	0	0

(continued)

509

TABLE 25-5 Haploidentical transplantation with posttransplantation cyclophosphamide in patients with SCD (Continued)

Study	Bolaños-Meade et al, 2012[95]	Dhedin et al, 2016[99]	Fitzhugh et al, 2017[97]	Wiebking et al, 2017[10]	Frangoul et al, 2018[100]	Pawlowska et al, 2018[101]	de al Fuente et al, 2019[98]	Bolaños-Meade et al, 2019[96]
GVHD (acute/chronic)[e]	0/0	18% (acute + chronic)	0/0	0/0	100%/0	0/75%	20%/6%	29%/18%
% Donor chimerism	11%-100%	NR	33%-79%	100%	100%	99%-100%	99%-100%	11%-100%
Complications, endorgan changes, and notes	PRES was not encountered in the patients who received sirolimus instead of tacrolimus (incidence 21% for patients on tacrolimus) No new cerebrovascular events, ACS, or priapism Pain medicines eventually tapered in 10 of the 11 patients with engraftment; rejection rate reported at 43%; however, an additional patient had 5% chimerism and return of SCD	Mortality was mainly from infectious complications and macrophage activation syndrome; 2 patients had secondary graft failure (9.1%) Preliminary evidence indicates that there is no benefit for the 2-drug preconditioning regimen with azathioprine (HU plus TT) when compared to addition of TT alone	15 patients developed bacteremia; 1 developed PTLD; 2 developed high-grade myelodysplastic syndrome with fibrosis with 1 death; 7 severe adverse events occurred possibly or definitely as a result of sirolimus NR Increased incidence of viral reactivation seen in cohort 3; therefore, likely related to 2 doses of posttransplantation CY; high sirolimus levels used peritransplant likely led to complications; all other complications resolved when the sirolimus level was reduced	Asymptomatic CMV reactivation was seen in 2 patients; all patients are off immune suppression	Grade 2 acute GVHD developed in all 4 patients and all responded to corticosteroid therapy; 1 episode of VOD; 3 patients had CMV reactivation No SCD-related complications following transplant; follow-up evaluation at 1 year after transplant showed no change in the brain MRI and no change in baseline organ function compared to pretransplant evaluation	2 patients had high titers of anti-HLA antibodies No pain episodes or other SCD-related complications after transplantation; 1 patient continues with chronic pain requiring ongoing opioids Preference was given to healthy, younger male donors with a lower number of mismatches on the non-shared haplotype, to the donors with non-inherited maternal haplotype mismatch, and to ABO-compatible donors and donors with the same CMV status (for those CMV negative)	60% developed viral reactivation (n = 9) No new cerebrovascular events, ACS, or priapism 3 of 9 patients who were opioid-dependent before transplant had persistent chronic pain after transplantation requiring daily opioid use	SCD pain crisis after ATG treatment was seen in all 12 patients with SCD; 1 of the 16 engrafted patients remained transfusion dependent, and 14 (88%) discontinued immunosuppression; GVHD was resolved in all patients, and no patients were receiving systemic GVHD therapy

[a]Cohort included a total of 21 patients with SCD and 2 with β thalassemia.

[b]Cohort who received thiotepa (n = 15) after the stopping rule was met when 2 of 3 patients had engraftment failure without thiotepa (n = 3) in the first cohort.

[c]Cohort included a total of 12 patients with SCD and 5 with β thalassemia.

[d]One patient had 11% chimerism but no symptoms of SCD at follow-up >700 days.

[e]GVHD grades 2-4.

Abbreviations: ACS, acute chest syndrome; ATG, antithymocyte globulin; BU, busulfan; CMV, cytomegalovirus; CY, cyclophosphamide; EFS, event-free survival; Flu, fludarabine; GVHD, graft-versus-host disease; HLA, human leukocyte antigen; HU, hydroxyurea; MMF, mycophenolate mofetil; MRI, magnetic resonance imaging; NIH, National Institutes of Health; NR, not reported; OS, overall survival; PRES, posterior reversible encephalopathy syndrome; PTLD, posttransplantation lymphoproliferative disorder; SCD, sickle cell disease; TBI, total-body irradiation; TRM, treatment-related mortality; TT, thiotepa; UK, United Kingdom; USA, United States of America; VOD, vaso-occlusive disease.

consortium is investigating the addition of TT to the CY, fludarabine, TBI, and ATG backbone (NCT03240731).[98,99] At a median follow-up of 13 months, rejection decreased from 60% (3 of 5 patients) to 6% (1 of 15 patients) after the addition of TT, with 100% OS and low rates of acute and chronic GVHD (20% and 6%, respectively).[98] A second cohort in this study included 22 pediatric patients with TT and preconditioning with 3 months of azathioprine and HU.[99] OS was 86%, with 9% graft rejection, 14% TRM, and 18% acute and chronic GVHD. Mortality was mainly from infectious complications and macrophage activation syndrome. Other smaller studies that include TT conditioning reported 100% OS and EFS, no TRM, and either no GVHD or mild GVHD that responded to treatment.[100-102]

The results of HLA-haploidentical transplantation with PTCy show an acceptable toxicity profile with excellent OS and very little acute and chronic GVHD. The addition of TT or TBI 400 cGy to the preparative regimen appears to improve engraftment and is being evaluated in an ongoing multicenter trial of HLA-haploidentical BM transplantation in adults with severe disease and in children with silent and overt stroke (BMT CTN 1507, NCT03263559).

Ex Vivo T-Cell–Depleted Approach

The ex vivo model of CD3[+]-depleted, CD34[+]-selected grafts is a labor-intensive process with a track record of poor immune reconstitution after depletion of natural killer cells and mature γδ T cells. Approximately 2×10^6/kg CD34[+] cells are adequate for recovery of hematopoiesis in the HLA-matched allogeneic setting[103]; however, higher doses will be needed after HLA-mismatched haploidentical transplantation where rejection is a concern. Ex vivo T-cell depletion by CD34[+] enrichment can increase total cell numbers and accomplish targeted CD3[+] depletion, αβ-T-cell depletion, or CD45RA depletion to promote passive immunity and immune reconstitution.[104-106] Early trials of high-dose CD34[+]-selected HSCT incompletely depleted alloreactive T cells. Therefore, ongoing trials in SCD are adapting ex vivo strategies that optimize and target T-cell depletion and use an intense preparative regimen (Table 25-6).[84,87,107,108] Reports to date are limited by small numbers of patients.

A single center reported results after haploidentical HSCT in 8 patients who received grafts with CD3[+] depletion and CD34[+] selection.[107] There were high rates of acute and chronic GVHD (40% and 75%, respectively), and 2 patients died of

TABLE 25-6 Haploidentical transplantation with ex vivo T-cell depletion in patients with SCD

Study	Dallas et al, 2013[107]	Gilman et al, 2017[84]	Marzollo et al, 2017[87]	Gaziev et al, 2018[111]	Foell et al, 2019[110]
Location	USA (St. Jude)	USA (North Carolina)	Italy	Italy	Germany
Date	NR	2009-2015	2010-2015	2012-2017	NR
No. of patients	8	8	2	14[a] (n = 3 SCD)	20
Age range (years)	4-17	8-23	13-16	3-15	3-31
HLA match	3/6 (n = 6); 4/6 (n = 2)	5/10 (n = 3); 6/10 (n = 3); 7/10 (n = 1); 9/10 (n = 1)	NR	5/10 (n = 10); 6/10 (n = 3); 7/10 (n = 1)	5/10 (n = 12); 6/10 (n = 4); 7/10 (n = 3); 8/10 (n = 1)
Ex-vivo T-cell depletion method	CD34[+] selection	CD34[+] selection	TCRαβ, CD19[+] depletion	TCRαβ, CD19[+] depletion	CD3[+]/CD19[+] depleted (n = 15); TCRαβ, CD19[+] depletion (n = 5)
Median CD34[+] cell dose (range)	25.4×10^6/kg (6-57×10^6/kg)	18×10^6/kg (9-25×10^6/kg)	14.3×10^6/kg	15.7×10^6/kg	13×10^6/kg (8-78×10^6/kg)
Median CD3[+] cell count (range)	0.07×10^6/kg (0.006-0.168×10^6/kg)	$<1 \times 10^3$/kg	NR	NR	14×10^3/kg (4-706×10^3/kg)
Preparative regimen	BU 900 ng/mL, Flu 150-200 mg/m^2, TT 10 mg/kg, ATG, muromonab-CD3 (n = 3) or HU + azathioprine followed by BU 900 ng/mL, TT 10 mg/kg, CY 200 mg/kg, muromonab-CD3 (n = 5)	Flu 40 mg/m^2, TT 5 mg/kg, melphalan 140 mg/m^2, ATG	Flu 40 mg/m^2, TT 8-10 mg/kg, treosulfan 14 g/m^2, ATG	Preconditioning with Flu 150 mg/m^2, HU, azathioprine; BU 14 mg/kg, TT 10 mg/kg, CY 200 mg/kg, ATG	Flu 40 mg/m^2, TT 5 mg/kg, treosulfan 14 g/m^2, ATG

(continued)

TABLE 25-6 Haploidentical transplantation with ex vivo T-cell depletion in patients with SCD (Continued)

Study	Dallas et al, 2013[107]	Gilman et al, 2017[84]	Marzollo et al, 2017[87]	Gaziev et al, 2018[111]	Foell et al, 2019[110]
GVHD prophylaxis	MMF	DLI, MTX	None	CsA, MMF or CsA, methylprednisolone	MMF, CsA or tacrolimus
OS	75%	88%	100%	84%	90%
EFS	38%	88%[a]	100%	64%	90%
Rejection	38%	13% (n = 1)	0	14%	NR
TRM	25% (n = 2)	13% (n = 1)	0	14%	10%
GVHD (acute/chronic)[b]	40%/75%	25%/13%	50%/0	28%/21%	35% (grade 1-2)/20%
% Donor chimerism	100%	>94%	88%-100%	NR	100%
Complications, end-organ changes, and notes	GVHD was the main cause of TRM (n = 2) No stroke, pulmonary hypertension, ACS, proteinuria, or hematuria observed in patients after successful HSCT; however, the patients who underwent myeloablative matched related donor HSCT demonstrated progressive declines in renal, pulmonary, and cardiac function over time that have not been reported previously[c] Of the 2 patients who died, 1 had received the highest CD3+ dose in the graft, and the other developed severe chronic lung GVHD after receiving a DLI	PTLD developed in 2 patients No sickle-related complications after transplant; 2 patients with elevated tricuspid regurgitant jet velocity had a decrease; no progression of cerebrovascular disease; no pulmonary changes	No sickle-related complications Resolution (n = 1) or improvement (n = 1) of cerebral vascular stenosis; height, weight, and thyroid function normalized after HSCT; 1 patient had normal pubertal development while the other had secondary gonadal failure No viral reactivation seen	Viral reactivation was common; incidence of PTLD was 23%	In the T-haplo-HSCT group, 2 patients died from CMV pneumonitis and a macrophage activation syndrome; 1 patient in the T-haplo-HSCT group requires renal replacement therapy because of BK virus nephritis; high rates of viral reactivation/ infection were noted

[a]One patient rejected initial graft but engrafted after second haploidentical transplant.
[b]GVHD grades 2-4.
[c]Study also reported on 14 patients who underwent matched related donor HSCT.
Abbreviations: ACS, acute chest syndrome; ATG, antithymocyte globulin; BU, busulfan; CMV, cytomegalovirus; CsA, cyclosporine; CY, cyclophosphamide; DLI, donor lymphocyte infusion; EFS, event-free survival; Flu, fludarabine; GVHD, graft-versus-host disease; HSCT, hematopoietic stem cell transplantation; HU, hydroxyurea; MMF, mycophenolate mofetil; MTX, methotrexate; NR, not reported; OS, overall survival; PTLD, posttransplantation lymphoproliferative disorder; SCD, sickle cell disease; TCR, T-cell receptor; TRM, treatment-related mortality; TT, thiotepa; USA, United States of America.

GVHD. Patients who received a high dose of CD3+ T cells or donor lymphocyte infusion had a high risk of mortality. Other approaches using CD34+-selected PBSC grafts show rapid engraftment and a low incidence of GVHD,[84] with one larger multicenter study including T-cell add back reporting a 1-year OS of 88% in 17 patients, with acute and chronic GVHD rates of 7% and 20%, respectively.[109] Two patients died due to complications from GVHD and 1 died of vaso-occlusive disease, whereas the remainder are alive and free of SCD symptoms with a median follow-up of 711 days.

A cohort of 20 patients in Germany received either CD3$^+$/CD19$^+$ (n = 15) or T-cell receptor αβ (TCRαβ) (n = 5) depletion, with EFS and OS rates of 90%, TRM rate of 10% (n = 2), and acute and chronic GVHD rates of 35% and 20%, respectively.[110] All patients had full donor chimerism, although high rates of viral reactivation or infection were noted, including 1 death from uncontrolled CMV pneumonitis. In a smaller series, 14 patients with thalassemia (n = 11) or SCD (n = 3) received grafts with TCRαβ and CD19$^+$ depletion and reported EFS and OS rates of 84% and 64%, respectively.[111] Graft failure occurred in 2 thalassemia patients (14%), with acute and chronic GVHD rates of 28% and 21%, respectively. One patient died of chronic GVHD. Viral reactivation was common, including a 23% incidence of EBV-related posttransplantation lymphoproliferative disorder. Compared to a historical group of patients who received CD34$^+$-selected grafts (n = 32) or CD34$^+$-selected and CD3$^+$/CD19$^+$-depleted grafts (n = 8), TCRαβ/CD19$^+$-depleted grafts were associated with a reduced incidence of graft failure (54% vs 14%; P = .048); however, delayed immune reconstitution and associated morbidity and mortality were similarly problematic between groups.

The addition of various T-cell depletion methods after CD34 selection over the past several years has shown significant improvement in minimizing rejection and GVHD after HLA-haploidentical transplantation. Current and future work to optimize the haploidentical HSCT results includes trials investigating pretransplantation immunosuppressive therapy (NCT03279094, NCT02757885); use of a nonmyeloablative regimen (NCT02678143, NCT01850108, NCT03240731, NCT03263559) with a CD34$^+$-selected graft (NCT02165007, NCT01461837), a CD4$^+$ T-cell–depleted graft (NCT03249831), a CD3/CD19-depleted graft with CD45$^+$RA$^+$ depletion (NCT03653338); or use of PBSCs after nonmyeloablative conditioning (NCT03077542). Other active and recruiting trials for HSCT in patients with SCD, as listed on ClinicalTrials.gov as of February 2019, are listed in Table 25-7.

Long-Term Effects After Transplantation

A consensus summary reviewing long-term follow-up results and identifying research priorities in late effects after HSCT in children with SCD and thalassemia[112] has now been followed up with comprehensive late effects screening guidelines.[113] In general, patients with stable donor engraftment after HSCT do not experience sickle-related complications after HSCT, with stabilization or even improvement in end-organ pathology. This is balanced by a significant risk of infertility, which remains a significant concern for patients and their families.[26,27,39,45,47,114] A recent analysis of the long-term effects of 59 children with SCD who underwent HSCT between 1991 and 2000 strongly suggests that, in addition to a lack of painful or other clinical events related to SCD in patients with durable engraftment of donor cells, most individuals are also protected from subclinical progression of end-organ damage and CNS dysfunction that is associated with sickle-related pathophysiology.[114]

Neurologic Outcomes

Children with stroke and successful engraftment are generally protected from a second stroke or further silent ischemic lesions after HSCT, including those with progressive cerebrovascular disease.[47,114] Patients with elevated arterial cerebral velocities before HSCT have conditional or normal values afterward, and often the brain magnetic resonance imaging (MRI) scans demonstrate stable or improved appearance after HSCT.[27,39,42,45,47,87,114-116] In those with more severe baseline MRI findings, however, there may be clinically silent parenchymal and vascular changes on MRI after HSCT despite 100% donor chimerism and normal erythropoiesis.[107,117] In a prospective study of 9 children over a period of 7 months to 6.5 years after HSCT, none of the patients had new overt strokes, although 5 patients had new, persistent changes including leukoencephalopathy or increased size of a preexisting lesions.[117] None of 2 patients lacking pre-HSCT CNS lacunae or infarction had MRI changes after transplantation; however, parenchymal changes occurred in all 7 patients with evidence of lacunae or infarction before HSCT (P = .0278). Despite these MRI changes, cognitive function remained stable >3 years after HSCT. It is unlikely that cognitive deficits will be reversed after HSCT, although this possibility has not been systematically evaluated. It is important to note, however, that any neurologic complications that occur during the course of HSCT such as posterior reversible encephalopathy syndrome or ICH may contribute additional cognitive effects, including complications from chronic GVHD.[118] Overall, post-HSCT MRI findings tend to show that a majority of patients have stable CNS disease, with improvement in some patients and potential worsening in a small proportion of patients.[119] However, it is not yet clear if the incidence of new CNS injury after HSCT is less frequent than occurs during supportive care with regular RBC transfusions in high-risk individuals.

Gonadal Function and Fertility

Two important long-term complications after myeloablative HSCT are gonadal failure and the risk of infertility. The risk of these complications is influenced by pretransplantation HU use, transfusion-associated iron overload, and recurrent priapism. Posttransplantation infertility is caused by myeloablative and gonadotoxic chemotherapeutic agents and radiation and is affected by the stage of pubertal development at HSCT.[114,120,121] Females have a finite number of ovarian follicles, which are particularly sensitive to gonadotoxic chemotherapy, with high rates of ovarian failure (65%-84%) after HSCT.[122,123] In males, chemotherapy-only regimens may be safer than regimens containing TBI,[124] although azoospermia or oligospermia is common given spermatogonial germ cell sensitivity to gonadotoxic therapy.[122] RIC regimens, particularly those that omit gonadotoxic alkylating agents such as BU and CY, have the potential to be less toxic on gonadal function.[125]

The multicenter study of BM transplantation for SCD reported gonadal function after myeloablative HSCT[114]; low testosterone and abnormal luteinizing hormone and follicle-stimulating hormone levels were reported in 77% and 30% of

TABLE 25-7 Clinical trials for HSCT in SCD in 2019

ClinicalTrials.gov Identifier	Title	Status	Regimen	Donor source	Age (yr)	No. of pts	Start date	Study objective	Location
NCT03279094	Haploidentical Transplantation With Pre-Transplant Immunosuppressive Therapy for Patients With SCD	Recruiting	Myeloablative	Haploidentical	1-30	15	October 2017	To evaluate safety and toxicity of 2 cycles of pretransplantation immunosuppressive therapy followed by myeloablative preparative regimen and allogeneic HSCT from a haploidentical donor	USA, California City of Hope Medical Center
NCT03121001	Study of HLA-SCT to Treat Clinically Aggressive SCD	Recruiting	Reduced intensity	Haploidentical	16-60	50	April 28, 2017	To determine engraftment at day +60 following HLA-haploidentical HSCT protocol using immunosuppressive agents and low-dose TBI for conditioning and posttransplantation cyclophosphamide	USA, Illinois University of Illinois at Chicago
NCT03077542	Nonmyeloablative Haploidentical PB Mobilized HPCT for SCD	Recruiting	Nonmyeloablative	Haploidentical	2-80	84	April 6, 2017	To evaluate safety, efficacy, and tolerance of a nonmyeloablative haploidentical PB mobilized HPCT for SCD	USA, Maryland National Institutes of Health
NCT03249831	Nonmyeloablative Conditioning Regimen With Haploidentical T-Cell–Depleted PB Transplant for Patients With Severe SCD	Recruiting	Nonmyeloablative	Haploidentical	18-45	6	November 2017	To evaluate safety and feasibility of nonmyeloablative conditioning and CD4+ T-cell–depleted grafts for haploidentical HSCT	USA, California City of Hope Medical Center
NCT03240731	HLA Haploidentical Bone Marrow Transplant in Patients With Severe SCD (DREPHAPLO)	Recruiting	Reduced intensity	Haploidentical	15-40	15	August 10, 2017	To evaluate haploidentical BMT after RIC, with prevention of GVHD based on posttransplantation cyclophosphamide	France, multicenter

NCT Number	Title	Status	Conditioning	Donor	Age	N	Start Date	Objective	Location
NCT03263559	Haploidentical Bone Marrow Transplantation in Sickle Cell Patients (BMT CTN 1507)	Recruiting	Reduced intensity	Haploidentical	5-45	80	October 3, 2017	To estimate the efficacy and toxicity of haploidentical BMT in patients with SCD stratified into 2 groups: (1) children with SCD with strokes; and (2) adults with severe SCD	USA, multicenter
NCT01461837	Haploidentical T-Cell–Depleted Transplantation in High-Risk SCD (HaploSCD)	Recruiting	Myeloablative	Haploidentical	2-20	20	January 2012	To investigate myeloablative conditioning followed by familial haploidentical T-cell–depleted allogeneic HSCT in patients with high-risk SCD	USA, multicenter
NCT03653338	T-Cell–Depleted Alternative Donor Bone Marrow Transplant for SCD and Thalassemia (SCD)	Recruiting	Reduced intensity	Haploidentical	5-40	5	August 2, 2018	To evaluate RIC and ex vivo T-cell depletion methods in the setting of mismatched donor transplantation	USA, Pennsylvania Children's Hospital of Pittsburgh of UPMC
NCT03367546	Haploidentical Allogeneic HSCT (HaploHCT) Following RIC for Selected High-Risk Nonmalignant Diseases	Recruiting	Reduced intensity	Haploidentical	≤25	20	July 2, 2018	To evaluate T-cell–replete RIC haploidentical donor allogeneic HSCT	USA, Minnesota Masonic Caner Center at University of Minnesota
NCT02165007	Haploidentical HSCT	Recruiting	Reduced intensity	Haploidentical, CD34+-selected graft	Up to age 22	15	January 2015	To assess safety and toxicity of RIC haploidentical HSCT using CD34+-selected graft	USA, Washington, DC Children's National Medical Center

(continued)

TABLE 25-7 Clinical trials for HSCT in SCD in 2019 (Continued)

ClinicalTrials .gov Identifier	Title	Status	Regimen	Donor source	Age (yr)	No. of pts	Start date	Study objective	Location
NCT02678143	A Pilot Study of Nonmyeloablative Conditioning for Mismatched HSCT for Severe SCD	Recruiting	Nonmyeloablative	Haploidentical, mismatched unrelated	>19	20	April 26, 2016	To evaluate safety and feasibility of nonmyeloablative conditioning in haploidentical or 1 antigen mismatch unrelated HSCT for adult patients with severe SCD	USA, Missouri Washington University
NCT02105766	Nonmyeloablative PB Mobilized HPCT for SCD and Beta Thalassemia in People With Higher Risk of Transplant Failure	Recruiting	Nonmyeloablative	HLA-matched	16-80	162	April 1, 2014	To see if low-dose radiation (300 rads), oral cyclophosphamide, pentostatin, and sirolimus help a body to better accept donor stem cells	USA, Maryland National Institutes of Health
NCT02038478	Allograft for SCD and Thalassemia	Recruiting	Nonmyeloablative	HLA-matched	18-45	50	January 2014	To determine safety and therapeutic potential of a nonmyeloablative PB-mobilized HPCT	USA, Texas University of Texas Southwestern Medical Center
NCT00061568	Improving the Results of Bone Marrow Transplantation for Patients With Severe Congenital Anemias	Recruiting	Nonmyeloablative	HLA-matched	2-80	150	May 23, 2003	To evaluate nonmyeloablative conditioning in adults with severe SCD	USA, Maryland National Institutes of Health
NCT03421756	Stem Cell Transplant in Patients With Severe SCD	Recruiting	Nonmyeloablative	HLA-matched related donor	18-40	12	March 29, 2018	To evaluate matched-related donor allogeneic stem cell transplantation in adults with severe SCD using a matched-sibling PBSC graft with a nonmyeloablative conditioning regimen (alemtuzumab)	USA, Pennsylvania UPMC Hillman Cancer Center

NCT Number	Title	Status	Conditioning	Donor	Age	Enrollment	Start Date	Objective	Location
NCT03587272	Minimizing Toxicity in HLA-Identical Related Donor Transplantation for Children With SCD (SUN)	Recruiting	Nonmyeloablative	HLA-matched related donor	2–21	30	April 17, 2018	To determine if HLA-identical sibling donor transplantation using alemtuzumab, low-dose TBI, and sirolimus (Sickle Transplant Using a Nonmyeloablative Approach, "SUN") can decrease the toxicity of transplant while achieving a high cure rate for children with SCD	USA, Washington, DC Children's National Medical Center
NCT03214354	Nonmyeloablative Stem Cell Transplant in Children With SCD and a Major ABO-Incompatible Matched Sibling Donor (Sickle-MAID)	Recruiting	Nonmyeloablative	HLA-matched related donor	1–19	12	July 5, 2017	To evaluate the safety and efficacy of a nonmyeloablative conditioning regimen for allogeneic HSCT in pediatric patients with SCD who have a matched related major ABO-incompatible donor	Canada, Alberta Alberta Children's Hospital
NCT01962415	RIC for Nonmalignant Disorders Undergoing UCBT, BMT, or PBSCT (HSCT+RIC)	Recruiting	Reduced intensity	HLA-matched related or unrelated UCB 4/6, 5/6, or 6/6 or HLA-matched unrelated donor BM or PB progenitor graft 8/8 or 7/8	2 months–35	30	February 4, 2014	To evaluate efficacy of using an RIC regimen with UCBT, double-cord UCBT, matched unrelated donor, BM transplant, or PBSC transplant in patients with nonmalignant disorders	USA, Pennsylvania Children's Hospital of Pittsburgh of UPMC

(continued)

TABLE 25-7 Clinical trials for HSCT in SCD in 2019 (Continued)

ClinicalTrials .gov Identifier	Title	Status	Regimen	Donor source	Age (yr)	No. of pts	Start date	Study objective	Location
NCT01850108	Nonmyeloablative Conditioning and BMT	Recruiting	Nonmyeloablative	HLA-matched related donor or haploidentical	2-70	25	May 2013	To evaluate efficacy of a nonmyeloablative regimen for partially HLA-mismatched and HLA-matched BM	USA, Tennessee Vanderbilt-Ingram Cancer Center
NCT02766465	BMT vs Standard of Care in Patients With Severe SCD (BMT CTN 1503) (STRIDE2)	Recruiting	Myeloablative	HLA-matched related or unrelated donor	15-40	200	November 2016	To compare BMT to standard care	USA, multicenter
NCT00408447	Stem Cell Transplant in SCD and Thalassemia	Recruiting	Nonmyeloablative	HLA-matched related or unrelated donor	1 month-30	60	September 2004	To evaluate nonmyeloablative conditioning	USA, New York Morgan Stanley Children's Hospital, New York-Presbyterian
NCT02776202	HLA-Identical Sibling Donor Bone Marrow Transplantation for Individuals With Severe SCD Using a RIC Regimen	Recruiting	Reduced intensity	HLA-matched sibling donor	3-18	15	May 2016	To investigate HSCT with an RIC conditioning regimen	Saudi Arabia, King Abdul Aziz Medical City for National Guard
NCT03128996	Reduced Intensity Conditioning and Familial HLA-Mismatched BMT for Nonmalignant Disorders	Recruiting	Reduced intensity	HLA-mismatched donor	≤21	29	March 20, 2017	To evaluate an RIC regimen consisting of hydroxyurea, alemtuzumab, fludarabine, thiotepa, and melphalan in a familial HLA-mismatched BMT	USA, Missouri Washington University

NCT Number	Title	Status	Conditioning	Donor	Age	N	Start Date	Objective	Location
NCT03214354	Nonmyeloablative SCT in Children With SCD and a Major ABO-Incompatible Matched Sibling Donor (Sickle-MAID)	Recruiting	Nonmyeloablative	Matched related	1-19	12	July 5, 2017	To evaluate safety and efficacy of nonmyeloablative conditioning for allogeneic HSCT in pediatric patients with SCD who have a matched related major ABO-incompatible donor	Canada, Alberta Alberta Children's Hospital
NCT01499888	Phase I/II Study of Allogeneic SCT for Clinically Aggressive SCD	Recruiting	Nonmyeloablative	Matched related	16-60	15	November 11, 2011	To determine engraftment and transplant-related morbidity and mortality after nonmyeloablative allogeneic HSCT using immunesuppressive agents and low-dose TBI without standard chemotherapy in patients with aggressive SCD	USA, Illinois University of Illinois at Chicago
NCT02757885	Transplantation Using Reduced-Intensity Approach for Patients with SCD From Mismatched Family Donors of Bone Marrow (TRANSFORM)	Recruiting	Reduced intensity	Mismatched family donor BM	15-40	15	April 2016	To learn if it is possible and safe to treat persons with severe SCD by HSCT from HLA half-matched related donors	USA, Georgia Children's Healthcare of Atlanta
NCT02867800	Abatacept for GVHD Prophylaxis After HSCT for Pediatric SCD	Recruiting	Reduced intensity	Unrelated	3-20	10	July 2016	To assess tolerability of the co-stimulation blocking agent abatacept (CTLA4-Ig) when added to standard GVHD prophylaxis	USA and Canada, multicenter

Abbreviations: BM, bone marrow; BMT, bone marrow transplantation; GVHD, graft-versus-host disease; HLA, human leukocyte antigen; HPCT, hematopoietic precursor cell transplantation; HSCT, hematopoietic stem cell transplantation; PB, peripheral blood; PBSC, peripheral blood stem cells; PBST, peripheral blood stem cell transplantation; RIC, reduced-intensity conditioning; SCD, sickle cell disease; SCT, stem cell transplantation; TBI, total-body irradiation; UCB, umbilical cord blood; UCBT, umbilical cord blood transplant; UPMC, University of Pittsburgh Medical Center; USA, United States of America.

men, respectively, with 57% of females developing ovarian failure. Ovarian failure after HSCT is more common in postpubertal females,[47,120] whereas prepubertal therapy may be a risk factor in males.[120] Many prepubertal females also develop primary amenorrhea after HSCT and receive hormone replacement therapy to promote the development of secondary sexual characteristics.[43,107] However, spontaneous puberty and successful pregnancies have been reported.[45,47,87,126]

Discussions about the risks of gonadal dysfunction and infertility should be individualized, and pre-HSCT sperm and ovarian cryopreservation should be offered[127] with the knowledge that some methods are only available on research protocols and not covered by health insurance policies. Other options include embryo cryopreservation, hormonal suppression, and gonadal shielding during TBI, whereas experimental options for prepubertal children include oocyte and testicular and ovarian tissue cryopreservation. Periprocedural SCD-related complications after fertility preservation treatment have been reported.[128] Successful oocyte preservation has been reported in a woman who underwent a matched sibling donor HSCT,[129] whereas successful ovarian tissue cryopreservation and reimplantation after HSCT resulted in a live birth to a mother with SCD who underwent myeloablative HSCT at the age of 14 years.[130] In general, patients with SCD have rarely conceived children naturally after both myeloablative and nonmyeloablative conditioning regimens.[27,39,45] Patients have delivered healthy babies, although fertility data are less promising than in patients with thalassemia who have undergone HSCT.[125,131,132] As has been shown in patients with thalassemia, fertility may be better preserved when HSCT is performed in young, prepubertal children, where the risk of gonadal damage may be attenuated by reduced-toxicity regimens, although when not possible, hormonal therapy may be of benefit.[125,131-133]

End-Organ Changes

For those with recurrent ACS or pulmonary hypertension, pulmonary function tests are often stable or improved,[42,84,114] although this is not seen in all patients.[107] In adults transplanted with a nonmyeloablative regimen, mean tricuspid regurgitant velocity improved from 2.84 m/s (95% confidence interval [CI], 2.71-2.99 m/s) before HSCT to 2.33 m/s (95% CI, 2.14-2.51 m/s) 3 years after HSCT ($P = .01$ for tricuspid regurgitant velocity 2.6-2.9 m/s, and $P <.001$ for tricuspid regurgitant velocity ≥3 m/s, mixed-model regression),[27] and this effect is similarly seen in the pediatric population.[84] Although mild tricuspid regurgitation has been reported after HSCT, jet velocities are normal with no clinical impact on cardiac function.[107] As for other measurable outcomes, linear growth is generally unchanged, whereas weight growth velocity does improve.[44,47,87] Splenic reticuloendothelial dysfunction appears to improve in young patients after HSCT,[47,61,134,135] and penicillin prophylaxis can be stopped in the absence of GVHD or splenectomy.[25] Normal fatty replacement of bone occurs in patients with a history of osteonecrosis,[47] although others report no radiographic improvement.[25] In patients with sickle cell nephropathy and proteinuria, renal function is stable after transplantation,[27,39] and in some patients, there is improved renal function.[63]

Pain, Hospitalization, and Health-Related Quality of Life

Most importantly, patients and parents report a markedly improved quality of life after successful HSCT.[17,61,83] In the majority of cases, it is possible to discontinue immunosuppressive medication 6 to 12 months after HSCT with a return to normal school and work life. Mean annual hospitalization rate declined from 3.23 (95% CI, 1.83-4.63) the year before HSCT to 0.11 (95% CI, 0.04-0.19) the third year after transplant, and a majority of patients were able to successfully wean from narcotics.[27] Successful HSCT leads to resolution of pain in the large majority of SCD patients; however, there is a subgroup of patients who continue to receive opioids for chronic pain after HSCT. Although there is a significant reduction in the prescription of both short- and long-acting opioids after HSCT (91% to 40% for short-acting and 40% to 15% for long-acting opioids), 40% of patients report persistent pain treated by opioids, with pain outcomes after HSCT potentially influenced by pre-HSCT pain characteristics including higher pain burden (higher pain admissions and higher pain intensity ratings), more symptoms of anxiety, and more probable use of long-acting opioids before HSCT.[136] Despite continued use of opioids in these patients, however, there is a significant improvement in pain intensity, pain impact, satisfaction with social role, and physical function after HSCT.

Coverage and Cost Considerations

SCD is a chronic disease with cumulative organ damage where management becomes more costly in older compared with younger patients. Total lifetime charges to age 50 exceed $8 million, with patient fees of $200,000 from ages 0 to 5 that increase to >$7 million in patients age 17 to 50 years.[16] SCD in the United States accounts for an estimated $1.6 billion per year in health care costs[137] and ranks fifth among the top 10 diagnoses of hospital stays among Medicaid superusers.[138] Although maximizing HU therapy, optimizing management of sickle cell pain, and discovering new therapeutic targets are essential, a greater focus on curative approaches for this disease might also represent a suitable strategy to reduce personal lifetime health care costs and improve quality of life.

Although the up-front costs of HSCT and gene therapy are significant, quality-adjusted life-years (QALYs) gained and the potential to reduce overall lifetime health care costs may render curative therapy cost-effective. Median HSCT cost per patient is estimated at $467,747 (range, $344,029-$799,219),[15] although this may be nearly 50% lower in patients who receive a nonmyeloablative regimen.[18] Costs for gene therapy are less certain; however, many aspects will go into the cost model, including a need to shift from fee-for-service to value-based payment systems.

There are significant issues around how to finance immediate costs for deferred benefits, and evaluation of the economic and QALY impacts of curative therapies for the treatment of severe SCD is needed. Current data suggest that health care utilization after HSCT is significantly reduced[15,27] and quality of life is improved,[17,61] although optimal therapy, particularly in the pediatric setting, is not well defined. A previous hypothetical model suggested that HSCT does not have a significant QALY advantage over chronic transfusions in patients with an elevated cerebral blood flow velocity by transcranial Doppler; however, outcomes after HSCT have improved since this study, which highlights the need for nonhypothetical research.[139] An active study is directly comparing standard therapy to HSCT in young adult patients with severe SCD (BMT CTN 1503, NCT02766465). When addressing health care costs, however, hidden costs are often not factored into health care estimates, including loss of wages due to frequent health care visits and unemployment among patients and parents. Furthermore, there are no dedicated data on improvement in mental health conditions such as depression after curative therapy that similarly affects health care expenditures. Mental health conditions such as depression are 5 times higher in patients with SCD, and total health care costs for adult SCD patients with depression are more than double those of SCD patients without depression.[140] Improved quality of life may mitigate depression, and less health care utilization may translate into improved job stability and sustained access to health care coverage. These improvements directly benefit patients and their families and potentially reduce health care expenditures.

Conclusion

Allogeneic HSCT has curative potential in SCD yet is underused due to a lack of suitable donors and concerns over long term effects of HSCT. Although risks must be weighed against the benefits of any medical intervention, the ability to cure patients, a lack of overt SCD manifestations in most patients after allogeneic HSCT, and stabilization or improvement of subclinical SCD pathology supports the view that conventional BM transplantation offers a favorable risk-benefit balance for patients with severe SCD who are living with a life-limiting disease with limited therapeutic options to reduce disease severity. When there are limitations in donor availability or conditioning regimens, graft rejection, or life-threatening GVHD, studies into nonmyeloablative conditioning regimens, expanded donor sources, and improved post-HSCT supportive care are promising. Given the scarcity of available treatments for SCD, each of these contributions is significant and aims to reduce disease burden and improve outcomes and quality of life for patients with SCD, and ultimately, they may reduce health care costs over the long term.

Case Studies

Patient 1

A 27-year-old man had HbSS complicated by frequent vaso-occlusive pain crises, 3 episodes of ACS associated with a moderate diffusion defect on pulmonary function testing, frequent transfusions with subsequent iron overload and RBC alloimmunization, proteinuria, and arteriovenous malformations proved by brain imaging. The pain events increased in number and intensity during late adolescence and early adulthood, causing more frequent and longer hospitalizations, which were managed by chronic opioid administration.

Pretransplantation Medications

Pretransplantation medications included HU, deferasirox, lisinopril, and hydromorphone (Dilaudid) as needed.

Transplantation Course

This patient received a nonmyeloablative HLA-identical sibling allogeneic HSCT at age 22 after preparation with alemtuzumab and 400 cGy of TBI. He received sirolimus for posttransplantation immunosuppression. He had an uncomplicated transplant course and was discharged home 19 days after transplantation.

Long-Term Follow-Up

The patient is currently 5 years post-HSCT, and he has stable mixed chimerism (99% donor myeloid, 83% donor CD3 chimerism) and no GVHD. There is a donor hemoglobin electrophoresis pattern (F <1.0%; A2 3.6%; A 67.7%; S 28.3%), and the hemoglobin is normal (14.4 g/dL). He has normal renal and hepatic function. There is no proteinuria and no hypertension. He has a normal ferritin, cortisol, follicle-stimulating hormone, luteinizing hormone, insulin, and progesterone levels. The brain magnetic resonance angiography and pulmonary function tests are stable; the echocardiogram and 6-minute walk distance also are normal. He has had no emergency department visits or hospitalizations for pain in the past 5 years and is not receiving any medications.

Patient 2

A 21-year-old woman had HbSS complicated by stroke requiring chronic RBC transfusions with subsequent iron overload, frequent vaso-occlusive pain treated with chronic opioid analgesics, history of central venous catheter infections with removal, ACS treated in the intensive care unit, and depression.

Case Studies: Continued

Pretransplantation Medications
Pretransplantation medications included oxycodone, duloxetine, folate, vitamin B_{12}, vitamin D, ondansetron, and diphenhydramine (Benadryl) as needed.

Transplantation Course
This patient underwent a nonmyeloablative HLA-haploidentical sibling allogeneic BM transplant at age 19. The conditioning regimen consisted of BU, fludarabine, and rabbit ATG. She received a combination of tacrolimus and methotrexate to prevent GVHD. Oocyte retrieval and cryopreservation were pursued before transplantation. Her inpatient transplantation course was complicated by culture-negative neutropenic fever and diarrhea positive for adenovirus. Neutrophil and platelet recovery occurred 23 and 28 days after transplantation, respectively. She was discharged home 31 days after transplantation.

Long-Term Follow-Up
Two years after transplantation, this patient had full donor chimerism (100% donor T cells) and was transfusion independent. There was no GVHD. Posttransplantation chronic pain was managed with a combination of oral and parenteral opioid analgesics, but these were tapered and stopped 7 months after transplantation. The brain MRI showed no new white matter lesions. Although urinalysis was negative for protein, there was persistent hypertension. The echocardiogram and pulmonary function tests were normal. She commenced a program of regular phlebotomy for posttransplantation management of iron overload.

Patient 3
A 14-year-old girl had HbSS complicated by chronic pain and repeated acute vaso-occlusive pain episodes requiring >15 hospitalizations over the past 3 years.

Pretransplantation Medications
HU was the only pretransplantation medication the patient was taking.

Transplantation Course
This patient underwent a nonmyeloablative HLA-haploidentical allogeneic BM transplant at age 13 years. The conditioning regimen consisted of fludarabine, CY, TT, 200 cGy of TBI, and rabbit ATG followed by 2 doses of posttransplantation CY. She received sirolimus for posttransplantation immunosuppression. Oocyte retrieval and cryopreservation were pursued before transplantation. Her inpatient transplantation course was complicated by EBV reactivation. She had neutrophil and platelet recovery 28 and 34 days after transplantation, respectively. She was discharged home 40 days after transplantation.

Long-Term Follow-Up
This patient is 18 months posttransplantation and has full donor chimerism (100% donor T cells), is off immunosuppression, and is transfusion independent. There is no GVHD. The patient has had no SCD-related complications following transplant. Her chronic pain was managed by a multidisciplinary team and resolved gradually over the 12 months following BM transplantation. Follow-up evaluation at 1 year after transplantation showed stable brain MRI and no change in baseline organ function compared to pretransplantation evaluation. Her weight has increased from the 10th to the 25th percentile.

High-Yield Facts

◆ HSCT with BM, UCB, or PBSCs is an established therapeutic option for patients with symptomatic SCD and an HLA-matched sibling donor with OS and EFS rates of >90%.

◆ Stable mixed chimerism with a reduction rather than an elimination of hemoglobin S is sufficient to overcome the pathogenic phenotype. Nonmyeloablative but immunosuppressive conditioning regimens reduce toxicity and, therefore, may extend more patients the ability to undergo HSCT who would otherwise be limited by myeloablative conditioning. A large review of myeloablative versus nonmyeloablative conditioning in >1000 patients showed no difference in OS and EFS based on the preparative regimen but did demonstrate OS benefit in younger transplant recipients.

◆ When an HLA-identical sibling does not exist, alternative donor sources should be pursued for symptomatic patients with SCD and done only on a clinical trial. Results for BM and CB transplantation from unrelated donors are limited by small patient numbers, with high rates of graft rejection, GVHD, and TRM. Haploidentical transplantation provides an expanded donor pool with current goals aimed at improving engraftment while lowering the risk of GVHD by employing in vivo and ex vivo T-cell depletion methods.

High-Yield Facts (Cont.)

◆ In general, patients with stable donor engraftment after HSCT do not experience sickle-related complications after HSCT, with stabilization or even improvement in end-organ pathology. This is balanced by a significant risk of infertility, which remains an important concern for patients and their families.

◆ SCD is a chronic disease with numerous costly complications and uncertainties that worsen throughout a patient's life. There are significant issues regarding how to finance immediate costs for curative therapies, and evaluation of the economic and quality of life impacts of curative therapies is needed.

References

1. Paulukonis ST, Eckman JR, Snyder AB, et al. Defining sickle cell disease mortality using a population-based surveillance system, 2004 through 2008. *Public Health Rep.* 2016;131(2):367-375.

2. Modell B, Darlison M. Global epidemiology of haemoglobin disorders and derived service indicators. *Bull World Health Org.* 2008;86(6):480-487.

3. Piel FB, Hay SI, Gupta S, et al. Global burden of sickle cell anaemia in children under five, 2010-2050: modelling based on demographics, excess mortality, and interventions. *PLoS Med.* 2013;10(7):e1001484.

4. Grosse SD, Odame I, Atrash HK, et al. Sickle cell disease in Africa: a neglected cause of early childhood mortality. *Am J Prev Med.* 2011;41(6 suppl 4):S398-S405.

5. Quinn CT, Rogers ZR, McCavit TL, Buchanan GR. Improved survival of children and adolescents with sickle cell disease. *Blood.* 2010;115(17):3447-3452.

6. Lanzkron S, Carroll CP, Haywood C Jr. Mortality rates and age at death from sickle cell disease: U.S., 1979-2005. *Public Health Rep.* 2013;128(2):110-116.

7. Ashley-Koch A, Yang Q, Olney RS. Sickle hemoglobin (HbS) allele and sickle cell disease: a HuGE review. *Am J Epidemiol.* 2000;151(9):839-845.

8. Grosse SD, Schechter MS, Kulkarni R, et al. Models of comprehensive multidisciplinary care for individuals in the United States with genetic disorders. *Pediatrics.* 2009;123(1):407-412.

9. Strouse JJ, Lobner K, Lanzkron S, et al. NIH and national foundation expenditures for sickle cell disease and cystic fibrosis are associated with pubmed publications and FDA approvals. *Blood.* 2013;122(21):1739.

10. Smith LA, Oyeku SO, Homer C, et al. Sickle cell disease: a question of equity and quality. *Pediatrics.* 2006;117(5):1763-1770.

11. Steinberg MH, Barton F, Castro O, et al. Effect of hydroxyurea on mortality and morbidity in adult sickle cell anemia: risks and benefits up to 9 years of treatment. *JAMA.* 2003;289(13):1645-1651.

12. Wang WC, Ware RE, Miller ST, et al. Hydroxycarbamide in very young children with sickle-cell anaemia: a multicentre, randomised, controlled trial (BABY HUG). *Lancet.* 2011;377(9778):1663-1672.

13. Ware RE. How I use hydroxyurea to treat young patients with sickle cell anemia. *Blood.* 2010;115(26):5300-5311.

14. Zimmerman SA, Schultz WH, Burgett S, et al. Hydroxyurea therapy lowers transcranial Doppler flow velocities in children with sickle cell anemia. *Blood.* 2007;110(3):1043-1047.

15. Arnold SD, Brazauskas R, He N, et al. Clinical risks and healthcare utilization of hematopoietic cell transplantation for sickle cell disease in the USA using merged databases. *Haematologica.* 2017;102(11):1823-1832.

16. Ballas SK. The cost of health care for patients with sickle cell disease. *Am J Hematol.* 2009;84(6):320-322.

17. Bhatia M, Kolva E, Cimini L, et al. Health-related quality of life after allogeneic hematopoietic stem cell transplantation for sickle cell disease. *Biol Blood Marrow Transplant.* 2015;21(4):666-672.

18. Saenz C, Tisdale JF. Assessing costs, benefits, and risks in chronic disease: taking the long view. *Biol Blood Marrow Transplant.* 2015;21(7):1149-1150.

19. Gluckman E, Cappelli B, Bernaudin F, et al. Sickle cell disease: an international survey of results of HLA-identical sibling hematopoietic stem cell transplantation. *Blood.* 2017;129(11):1548-1556.

20. Gragert L, Eapen M, Williams E, et al. HLA match likelihoods for hematopoietic stem-cell grafts in the U.S. registry. *N Engl J Med.* 2014;371(4):339-348.

21. Walters MC, Patience M, Leisenring W, et al. Barriers to bone marrow transplantation for sickle cell anemia. *Biol Blood Marrow Transplant.* 1996;2(2):100-104.

22. Johnson FL, Look AT, Gockerman J, et al. Bone-marrow transplantation in a patient with sickle-cell anemia. *N Engl J Med.* 1984;311(12):780-783.

23. Vermylen C, Cornu G, Philippe M, et al. Bone marrow transplantation in sickle cell anaemia. *Arch Dis Child.* 1991;66(10):1195-1198.

24. Vermylen C, Cornu G. Bone marrow transplantation for sickle cell disease. The European experience. *Am J Pediatr Hematol Oncol.* 1994;16(1):18-21.

25. Vermylen C, Cornu G, Ferster A, et al. Haematopoietic stem cell transplantation for sickle cell anaemia: the first 50 patients transplanted in Belgium. *Bone Marrow Transplant.* 1998;22(1):1-6.

26. Walters MC, Patience M, Leisenring W, et al. Bone marrow transplantation for sickle cell disease. *N Engl J Med.* 1996;335(6):369-376.

27. Hsieh MM, Fitzhugh CD, Weitzel RP, et al. Nonmyeloablative HLA-matched sibling allogeneic hematopoietic stem cell transplantation for severe sickle cell phenotype. *JAMA.* 2014;312(1):48-56.

28. King AA, Kamani N, Bunin N, et al. Successful matched sibling donor marrow transplantation following reduced intensity conditioning in children with hemoglobinopathies. *Am J Hematol.* 2015;90(12):1093-1098.

29. Angelucci E, Matthes-Martin S, Baronciani D, et al. Hematopoietic stem cell transplantation in thalassemia major and sickle cell disease: indications and management recommendations from an international expert panel. *Haematologica.* 2014;99(5):811-820.

30. Hulbert ML, McKinstry RC, Lacey JL, et al. Silent cerebral infarcts occur despite regular blood transfusion therapy after first strokes in children with sickle cell disease. *Blood.* 2011;117(3):772-779.

31. Scothorn DJ, Price C, Schwartz D, et al. Risk of recurrent stroke in children with sickle cell disease receiving blood transfusion therapy for at least five years after initial stroke. *J Pediatr.* 2002;140(3):348-354.

32. Kassim AA, Sharma D. Hematopoietic stem cell transplantation for sickle cell disease: the changing landscape. *Hematol Oncol Stem Cell Ther.* 2017;10(4):259-266.

33. Bhatia M, Sheth S. Hematopoietic stem cell transplantation in sickle cell disease: patient selection and special considerations. *J Blood Med.* 2015;6:229-238.

34. Chakrabarti S, Bareford D. A survey on patient perception of reduced-intensity transplantation in adults with sickle cell disease. *Bone Marrow Transplant.* 2007;39(8):447-451.

35. Meier ER, Dioguardi JV, Kamani N. Current attitudes of parents and patients toward hematopoietic stem cell transplantation for sickle cell anemia. *Pediatr Blood Cancer.* 2015;62(7):1277-1284.

36. Nickel RS, Kamani NR. Ethical challenges in hematopoietic cell transplantation for sickle cell disease. *Biol Blood Marrow Transplant.* 2018;24(2):219-227.

37. Horan JT, Liesveld JL, Fenton P, et al. Hematopoietic stem cell transplantation for multiply transfused patients with sickle cell disease and thalassemia after low-dose total body irradiation, fludarabine, and rabbit anti-thymocyte globulin. *Bone Marrow Transplant.* 2005;35(2):171-177.

38. Iannone R, Casella JF, Fuchs EJ, et al. Results of minimally toxic nonmyeloablative transplantation in patients with sickle cell anemia and beta-thalassemia. *Biol Blood Marrow Transplant.* 2003;9(8):519-528.

39. Hsieh MM, Kang EM, Fitzhugh CD, et al. Allogeneic hematopoietic stem-cell transplantation for sickle cell disease. *N Engl J Med.* 2009;361(24):2309-2317.

40. Bernaudin F, Souillet G, Vannier JP, et al. Bone marrow transplantation (BMT) in 14 children with severe sickle cell disease (SCD): the French experience. GEGMO. *Bone Marrow Transplant.* 1993;12(suppl 1):118-121.

41. Vermylen C, Cornu G, Ferster A, et al. Bone marrow transplantation in sickle cell disease: the Belgian experience. *Bone Marrow Transplant.* 1993;12(suppl 1):116-117.

42. Walters MC, Patience M, Leisenring W, et al. Stable mixed hematopoietic chimerism after bone marrow transplantation for sickle cell anemia. *Biol Blood Marrow Transplant.* 2001;7(12):665-673.

43. Walters MC, Storb R, Patience M, et al. Impact of bone marrow transplantation for symptomatic sickle cell disease: an interim report. Multicenter Investigation of Bone Marrow Transplantation for Sickle Cell Disease. *Blood.* 2000;95(6):1918-1924.

44. Lucarelli G, Isgrò A, Sodani P, et al. Hematopoietic SCT for the Black African and non-Black African variants of sickle cell anemia. *Bone Marrow Transplant.* 2014;49(11):1376-1381.

45. Dedeken L, Lê PQ, Azzi N, et al. Haematopoietic stem cell transplantation for severe sickle cell disease in childhood: a single centre experience of 50 patients. *Br J Haematol.* 2014;165(3):402-408.

46. Strocchio L, Zecca M, Comoli P, et al. Treosulfan-based conditioning regimen for allogeneic haematopoietic stem cell transplantation in children with sickle cell disease. *Br J Haematol.* 2015;169(5):726-736.

47. Bernaudin F, Socie G, Kuentz M, et al. Long-term results of related myeloablative stem-cell transplantation to cure sickle cell disease. *Blood.* 2007;110(7):2749-2756.

48. Bhatia M, Jin Z, Baker C, et al. Reduced toxicity, myeloablative conditioning with BU, fludarabine, alemtuzumab and SCT from sibling donors in children with sickle cell disease. *Bone Marrow Transplant.* 2014;49(7):913-920.

49. McPherson ME, Hutcherson D, Olson E, et al. Safety and efficacy of targeted busulfan therapy in children undergoing myeloablative matched sibling donor BMT for sickle cell disease. *Bone Marrow Transplant.* 2011;46(1):27-33.

50. Panepinto JA, Walters MC, Carreras J, et al. Matched-related donor transplantation for sickle cell disease: report from the Center for International Blood and Transplant Research. *Br J Haematol.* 2007;137(5):479-485.

51. Bernaudin F, Socie G, Kuentz M, et al. Related myeloablative stem cell transplantation (SCT) to cure sickle cell anemia (SCA): update of French results. *Blood.* 2010;116(21):3518.

52. Bories D, Bories D, Dalle JH, et al. Sickle cell anemia and HSCT: relation between ATG, chimerism, GVHD and outcome in myeloablative genoidentical transplants for the SFGM-TC. *Blood.* 2013;122(21):971.

53. Brachet C, Azzi N, Demulder A, et al. Hydroxyurea treatment for sickle cell disease: impact on haematopoietic stem cell transplantation's outcome. *Bone Marrow Transplant.* 2004;33(8):799-803.

54. Walters MC, Sullivan KM, Bernaudin F, et al. Neurologic complications after allogeneic marrow transplantation for sickle cell anemia. *Blood.* 1995;85(4):879-884.

55. Jacobsohn DA, Duerst R, Tse W, Kletzel M. Reduced intensity haemopoietic stem-cell transplantation for treatment of non-malignant diseases in children. *Lancet.* 2004;364(9429):156-162.

56. Powell JD, Lerner CG, Schwartz RH. Inhibition of cell cycle progression by rapamycin induces T cell clonal anergy even in the presence of costimulation. *J Immunol.* 1999;162(5):2775-2784.

57. Powell JD, Fitzhugh C, Kang EM, et al. Low-dose radiation plus rapamycin promotes long-term bone marrow chimerism. *Transplantation.* 2005;80(11):1541-1545.

58. Chakraverty R, Peggs K, Chopra R, et al. Limiting transplantation-related mortality following unrelated donor stem cell transplantation by using a nonmyeloablative conditioning regimen. *Blood.* 2002;99(3):1071-1078.

59. Kottaridis PD, Milligan DW, Chopra R, et al. In vivo CAMPATH-1H prevents graft-versus-host disease following nonmyeloablative stem cell transplantation. *Blood.* 2000;96(7):2419-2425.

60. Guilcher GMT, Monagel DA, Nettel-Aguirre A, et al. Nonmyeloablative matched sibling donor hematopoietic cell transplantation in children and adolescents with sickle cell disease. *Biol Blood Marrow Transplant.* 2019;25(6):1179-1186.

61. Saraf SL, Oh AL, Patel PR, et al. Nonmyeloablative stem cell transplantation with alemtuzumab/low-dose irradiation to cure and improve the quality of life of adults with sickle cell disease. *Biol Blood Marrow Transplant.* 2016;22(3):441-448.

62. Krishnamurti L, Kharbanda S, Biernacki MA, et al. Stable long-term donor engraftment following reduced-intensity hematopoietic cell transplantation for sickle cell disease. *Biol Blood Marrow Transplant.* 2008;14(11):1270-1278.

63. Matthes-Martin S, Lawitschka A, Fritsch G, et al. Stem cell transplantation after reduced-intensity conditioning for sickle cell disease. *Eur J Haematol.* 2013;90(4):308-312.

64. Krishnamurti L, Neuberg DS, Sullivan KM, et al. Bone marrow transplantation for adolescents and young adults with sickle cell disease: results of a prospective multicenter pilot study. *Am J Hematol.* 2019;94(4):446-454.

65. Horan JT, Haight A, Lagerlof Dioguardi J, et al. Using fludarabine to reduce exposure to alkylating agents in children with sickle cell disease receiving busulfan, cyclophosphamide, and antithymocyte globulin transplant conditioning: results of a dose de-escalation trial. *Biol Blood Marrow Transplant.* 2015;21(5):900-905.

66. Shenoy S, Eapen M, Panepinto JA, et al. A trial of unrelated donor marrow transplantation for children with severe sickle cell disease. *Blood.* 2016;128(21):2561-2567.

67. Locatelli F, Rocha V, Reed W, et al. Related umbilical cord blood transplantation in patients with thalassemia and sickle cell disease. *Blood.* 2003;101(6):2137-2143.

68. Quinn CT, Lee NJ, Shull EP, et al. Prediction of adverse outcomes in children with sickle cell anemia: a study of the Dallas Newborn Cohort. *Blood.* 2008;111(2):544-548.

69. Cairo MS, Rocha V, Gluckman E, et al. Alternative allogeneic donor sources for transplantation for childhood diseases: unrelated cord blood and haploidentical family donors. *Biol Blood Marrow Transplant.* 2008;14(1 suppl 1):44-53.

70. Krishnamurti L, Abel S, Maiers M, Flesch S. Availability of unrelated donors for hematopoietic stem cell transplantation for hemoglobinopathies. *Bone Marrow Transplant.* 2003;31(7):547-550.

71. Switzer GE, Bruce JG, Myaskovsky L, et al. Race and ethnicity in decisions about unrelated hematopoietic stem cell donation. *Blood.* 2013;121(8):1469-1476.

72. Justus D, Perez-Albuerne E, Dioguardi J, et al. Allogeneic donor availability for hematopoietic stem cell transplantation in children with sickle cell disease. *Pediatr Blood Cancer.* 2015;62(7):1285-1287.

73. Locatelli F, Kabbara N, Ruggeri A, et al. Outcome of patients with hemoglobinopathies given either cord blood or bone marrow transplantation from an HLA-identical sibling. *Blood.* 2013;122(6):1072-1078.

74. Broxmeyer HE, Douglas GW, Hangoc G, et al. Human umbilical cord blood as a potential source of transplantable hematopoietic stem/progenitor cells. *Proc Natl Acad Sci U S A.* 1989;86(10):3828-3832.

75. Ballen KK, Gluckman E, Broxmeyer HE. Umbilical cord blood transplantation: the first 25 years and beyond. *Blood.* 2013;122(4):491-498.

76. Adamkiewicz TV, Szabolcs P, Haight A, et al. Unrelated cord blood transplantation in children with sickle cell disease: review of four-center experience. *Pediatr Transplant.* 2007;11(6):641-644.

77. Kamani NR, Walters MC, Carter S, et al. Unrelated donor cord blood transplantation for children with severe sickle cell disease: results of one cohort from the phase II study from the Blood and Marrow Transplant Clinical Trials Network (BMT CTN). *Biol Blood Marrow Transplant.* 2012;18(8):1265-1272.

78. Radhakrishnan K, Bhatia M, Geyer MB, et al. Busulfan, fludarabine, and alemtuzumab conditioning and unrelated cord blood transplantation in children with sickle cell disease. *Biol Blood Marrow Transplant.* 2013;19(4):676-677.

79. Ruggeri A, Eapen M, Scaravadou A, et al. Umbilical cord blood transplantation for children with thalassemia and sickle cell disease. *Biol Blood Marrow Transplant.* 2011;17(9):1375-1382.

80. Horwitz ME, Chao NJ, Rizzieri DA, et al. Umbilical cord blood expansion with nicotinamide provides long-term multilineage engraftment. *J Clin Invest.* 2014;124(7):3121-3128.

81. Parikh S, Brochstein JA, Wease S, et al. A novel therapy for sickle cell disease (SCD): co-transplantation of Nicord [ex vivo expanded umbilical cord blood (UCB) progenitor cells with nicotinamide] and an unmanipulated unrelated UCB graft leads to successful engraftment and cure of severe SCD. *Biol Blood Marrow Transplant.* 2018;24(3):S191-S192.

82. Kharbanda S, Smith AR, Hutchinson SK, et al. Unrelated donor allogeneic hematopoietic stem cell transplantation for patients with hemoglobinopathies using a reduced-intensity conditioning regimen and third-party mesenchymal stromal cells. *Biol Blood Marrow Transplant.* 2014;20(4):581-586.

83. Abraham A, Cluster A, Jacobsohn D, et al. Unrelated umbilical cord blood transplantation for sickle cell disease following reduced-intensity conditioning: results of a phase I trial. *Biol Blood Marrow Transplant.* 2017;23(9):1587-1592.

84. Gilman AL, Eckrich MJ, Epstein S, et al. Alternative donor hematopoietic stem cell transplantation for sickle cell disease. *Blood Adv.* 2017;1(16):1215-1223.

85. Mynarek M, Bettoni da Cunha Riehm C, Brinkmann F, et al. Normalized transcranial Doppler velocities, stroke prevention and improved pulmonary function after stem cell transplantation in children with sickle cell anemia. *Klin Padiatr.* 2013;225(3):127-132.

86. Shenoy S, Grossman WJ, DiPersio J, et al. A novel reduced-intensity stem cell transplant regimen for nonmalignant disorders. *Bone Marrow Transplant.* 2005;35(4):345-352.

87. Marzollo A, Calore E, Tumino M, et al. Treosulfan-based conditioning regimen in sibling and alternative donor hematopoietic stem cell transplantation for children with sickle cell disease. *Mediterr J Hematol Infect Dis.* 2017;9(1):e2017014.

88. Bunn D, Lea CK, Bevan DJ, et al. The pharmacokinetics of antithymocyte globulin (ATG) following intravenous infusion in man. *Clin Nephrol.* 1996;45(1):29-32.

89. Morris EC, Rebello P, Thomson KJ, et al. Pharmacokinetics of alemtuzumab used for in vivo and in vitro T-cell depletion in allogeneic transplantations: relevance for early adoptive immunotherapy and infectious complications. *Blood.* 2003;102(1):404-406.

90. Luznik L, Jones RJ, Fuchs EJ. High-dose cyclophosphamide for graft-versus-host disease prevention. *Curr Opin Hematol.* 2010;17(6):493-499.

91. Emadi A, Jones RJ, Brodsky RA. Cyclophosphamide and cancer: golden anniversary. *Nat Rev Clin Oncol.* 2009;6(11):638-647.

92. O'Donnell PV, Luznik L, Jones RJ, et al. Nonmyeloablative bone marrow transplantation from partially HLA-mismatched related donors using posttransplantation cyclophosphamide. *Biol Blood Marrow Transplant.* 2002;8(7):377-386.

93. Luznik L, O'Donnell PV, Symons HJ, et al. HLA-haploidentical bone marrow transplantation for hematologic malignancies using nonmyeloablative conditioning and high-dose, posttransplantation cyclophosphamide. *Biol Blood Marrow Transplant.* 2008;14(6):641-650.

94. Nomoto K, Eto M, Yanaga K, et al. Interference with cyclophosphamide-induced skin allograft tolerance by cyclosporin A. *J Immunol.* 1992;149(8):2668-2674.

95. Bolaños-Meade J, Fuchs EJ, Luznik L, et al. HLA-haploidentical bone marrow transplantation with posttransplant cyclophosphamide expands the donor pool for patients with sickle cell disease. *Blood.* 2012;120(22):4285-4291.

96. Bolaños-Meade J, Cooke KR, Gamper CJ, et al. Effect of increased dose of total body irradiation on graft failure associated with HLA-haploidentical transplantation in patients with severe haemoglobinopathies: a prospective clinical trial. *Lancet Haematol.* 2019;6(4):e183-e193.

97. Fitzhugh CD, Hsieh MM, Taylor T, et al. Cyclophosphamide improves engraftment in patients with SCD and severe organ damage who undergo haploidentical PBSCT. *Blood Adv.* 2017;1(11):652-661.

98. de la Fuente J, Dhedin N, Koyama T, et al. Haploidentical bone marrow transplantation with post-transplantation cyclophosphamide plus thiotepa improves donor engraftment in patients with sickle cell anemia: results of an international learning collaborative. *Biol Blood Marrow Transplant.* 2019;25(6):1197-1209.

99. Dhedin N, de la Fuente J, Bernaudin F, et al. Haploidentical bone marrow transplant with post-transplant cytoxan plus thiotepa improves donor engraftment in patients with sickle cell anemia: results of an international multicenter learning collaborative. *Blood.* 2016;128(22):1233.

100. Frangoul H, Evans M, Isbell J, et al. Haploidentical hematopoietic stem cell transplant for patients with sickle cell disease using thiotepa, fludarabine, thymoglobulin, low dose cyclophosphamide, 200 cGy tbi and post transplant cyclophosphamide. *Bone Marrow Transplant.* 2018;53(5):647-650.

101. Pawlowska AB, Cheng JC, Karras NA, et al. HLA haploidentical stem cell transplant with pretransplant immunosuppression for patients with sickle cell disease. *Biol Blood Marrow Transplant.* 2018;24(1):185-189.

102. Wiebking V, Hütker S, Schmid I, et al. Reduced toxicity, myeloablative HLA-haploidentical hematopoietic stem cell transplantation with post-transplantation cyclophosphamide for sickle cell disease. *Ann Hematol.* 2017;96(8):1373-1377.

103. Villalon L, Odriozola J, Laraña JG, et al. Autologous peripheral blood progenitor cell transplantation with <2 × 10(6) CD34(+)/kg: an analysis of variables concerning mobilisation and engraftment. *Hematol J.* 2000;1(6):374-381.

104. Airoldi I, Bertaina A, Prigione I, et al. Gammadelta T-cell reconstitution after HLA-haploidentical hematopoietic transplantation depleted of TCR-alphabeta+/CD19+ lymphocytes. *Blood.* 2015;125(15):2349-2358.

105. Diaz MA, Pérez-Martínez A, Herrero B, et al. Prognostic factors and outcomes for pediatric patients receiving an haploidentical relative allogeneic transplant using CD3/CD19-depleted grafts. *Bone Marrow Transplant.* 2016;51(9):1211-1216.

106. Triplett BM, Shook DR, Eldridge P, et al. Rapid memory T-cell reconstitution recapitulating CD45RA-depleted haploidentical transplant graft content in patients with hematologic malignancies. *Bone Marrow Transplant.* 2015;50(7):968-977.

107. Dallas MH, Triplett B, Shook DR, et al. Long-term outcome and evaluation of organ function in pediatric patients undergoing haploidentical and matched related hematopoietic cell transplantation for sickle cell disease. *Biol Blood Marrow Transplant.* 2013;19(5):820-830.

108. Foell J, Pfirstinger B, Rehe K, et al. Haploidentical stem cell transplantation with CD3(+)-/CD19(+)- depleted peripheral stem cells for patients with advanced stage sickle cell disease and no alternative donor: results of a pilot study. *Bone Marrow Transplant.* 2017;52(6):938-940.

109. Talano J-A, Moore TB, Keever-Taylor CA, et al. Promising results at 1 year follow-up following familial haploidentical (FHI) T-cell depleted (TCD) with CD34 enrichment and T-cell (CD3) addback allogeneic stem cell transplantation in patients with high-risk sickle cell disease (SCD) (IND 14359). *Blood.* 2017;130(suppl 1):4602.

110. Foell J, Schulte JH, Pfirstinger B, et al. Haploidentical CD3 or alpha/beta T-cell depleted HSCT in advanced stage sickle cell disease. *Bone Marrow Transplant.* 2019;54(11):1859-1867.

111. Gaziev J, Isgrò A, Sodani P, et al. Haploidentical HSCT for hemoglobinopathies: improved outcomes with TCRalphabeta(+)/CD19(+)-depleted grafts. *Blood Adv.* 2018;2(3):263-270.

112. Shenoy S, Angelucci E, Arnold SD, et al. Current results and future research priorities in late effects after hematopoietic stem cell transplantation for children with sickle cell disease and thalassemia: a consensus statement from the Second Pediatric Blood and Marrow Transplant Consortium International Conference on Late Effects after Pediatric Hematopoietic Stem Cell Transplantation. *Biol Blood Marrow Transplant.* 2017;23(4):552-561.

113. Shenoy S, Gaziev J, Angelucci E, et al. Late effects screening guidelines after hematopoietic cell transplantation (HCT) for hemoglobinopathy: consensus statement from the Second Pediatric Blood and Marrow Transplant Consortium International Conference on Late Effects after Pediatric HCT. *Biol Blood Marrow Transplant.* 2018;24(7):1313-1321.

114. Walters MC, Hardy K, Edwards S, et al. Pulmonary, gonadal, and central nervous system status after bone marrow transplantation for sickle cell disease. *Biol Blood Marrow Transplant.* 2010;16(2):263-272.

115. Bernaudin F, Verlhac S, Peffault de Latour R, et al. Association of matched sibling donor hematopoietic stem cell transplantation with transcranial Doppler velocities in children with sickle cell anemia. *JAMA.* 2019;321(3):266-276.

116. King AA, McKinstry RC, Wu J, et al. Functional and radiologic assessment of the brain after reduced-intensity unrelated donor transplantation for severe sickle cell disease: Blood and Marrow Transplant Clinical Trials Network Study 0601. *Biol Blood Marrow Transplant.* 2019;25(5):e174-e178.

117. Woodard P, Helton KJ, Khan RB, et al. Brain parenchymal damage after haematopoietic stem cell transplantation for severe sickle cell disease. *Br J Haematol.* 2005;129(4):550-552.

118. Padovan CS, Yousry TA, Schleuning M, et al. Neurological and neuroradiological findings in long-term survivors of allogeneic bone marrow transplantation. *Ann Neurol.* 1998;43(5):627-633.

119. Bodas P, Rotz S. Cerebral vascular abnormalities in pediatric patients with sickle cell disease after hematopoietic cell transplant. *J Pediatr Hematol Oncol.* 2014;36(3):190-193.

120. Borgmann-Staudt A, Rendtorff R, Reinmuth S, et al. Fertility after allogeneic haematopoietic stem cell transplantation in childhood and adolescence. *Bone Marrow Transplant.* 2012;47(2):271-276.

121. Smith-Whitley K. Reproductive issues in sickle cell disease. *Hematology Am Soc Hematol Educ Program.* 2014;2014(1):418-424.

122. Joshi S, Savani BN, Chow EJ, et al. Clinical guide to fertility preservation in hematopoietic cell transplant recipients. *Bone Marrow Transplant.* 2014;49(4):477-484.

123. Loren AW, Chow E, Jacobsohn DA, et al. Pregnancy after hematopoietic cell transplantation: a report from the late effects working committee of the Center for International Blood and Marrow Transplant Research (CIBMTR). *Biol Blood Marrow Transplant.* 2011;17(2):157-166.

124. Anserini P, Chiodi S, Spinelli S, et al. Semen analysis following allogeneic bone marrow transplantation. Additional data for evidence-based counselling. *Bone Marrow Transplant.* 2002; 30(7):447-451.

125. Madden LM, Hayashi RJ, Chan KW, et al. Long-term follow-up after reduced-intensity conditioning and stem cell transplantation for childhood nonmalignant disorders. *Biol Blood Marrow Transplant.* 2016;22(8):1467-1472.

126. Brachet C, Heinrichs C, Tenoutasse S, et al. Children with sickle cell disease: growth and gonadal function after hematopoietic stem cell transplantation. *J Pediatr Hematol Oncol.* 2007;29(7):445-450.

127. Practice Committee of American Society for Reproductive Medicine. Fertility preservation in patients undergoing gonadotoxic therapy or gonadectomy: a committee opinion. *Fertil Steril.* 2013;100(5):1214-1223.

128. Pecker LH, Maher JY, Law JY, et al. Risks associated with fertility preservation for women with sickle cell anemia. *Fertil Steril.* 2018;110(4):720-731.

129. Dovey S, Krishnamurti L, Sanfilippo J, et al. Oocyte cryopreservation in a patient with sickle cell disease prior to hematopoietic stem cell transplantation: first report. *J Assist Reprod Genet.* 2012;29(3):265-269.

130. Demeestere I, Simon P, Dedeken L, et al. Live birth after autograft of ovarian tissue cryopreserved during childhood. *Hum Reprod.* 2015;30(9):2107-2109.

131. Rahal I, Galambrun C, Bertrand Y, et al. Late effects after hematopoietic stem cell transplantation for beta-thalassemia major: the French national experience. *Haematologica.* 2018;103(7): 1143-1149.

132. Santarone S, Natale A, Olioso P, et al. Pregnancy outcome following hematopoietic cell transplantation for thalassemia major. *Bone Marrow Transplant.* 2017;52(3):388-393.

133. Gharwan H, Neary NM, Link M, et al. Successful fertility restoration after allogeneic hematopoietic stem cell transplantation. *Endocr Pract.* 2014;20(9):e157-e161.

134. Ferster A, Bujan W, Corazza F, et al. Bone marrow transplantation corrects the splenic reticuloendothelial dysfunction in sickle cell anemia. *Blood.* 1993;81(4):1102-1105.

135. Nickel RS, Seashore E, Lane PA, et al. Improved splenic function after hematopoietic stem cell transplant for sickle cell disease. *Pediatr Blood Cancer.* 2016;63(5):908-913.

136. Darbari DS, Liljencrantz J, Ikechi A, et al. Pain and opioid use after reversal of sickle cell disease following HLA-matched sibling haematopoietic stem cell transplant. *Br J Haematol.* 2019;184(4):690-693.

137. Kauf TL, Coates TD, Huazhi L, et al. The cost of health care for children and adults with sickle cell disease. *Am J Hematol.* 2009;84(6):323-327.

138. Jiang HJ, Weiss AJ, Barrett ML, et al. *Characteristics of Hospital Stays for Super-Utilizers by Payer, 2012: Statistical Brief #190, in Healthcare Cost and Utilization Project (HCUP) Statistical Briefs.* Agency for Healthcare Research and Quality; 2006.

139. Nietert PJ, Abboud MR, Silverstein MD, et al. Bone marrow transplantation versus periodic prophylactic blood transfusion in sickle cell patients at high risk of ischemic stroke: a decision analysis. *Blood.* 2000;95(10):3057-3064.

140. Adam SS, Flahiff CM, Kamble S, et al. Depression, quality of life, and medical resource utilization in sickle cell disease. *Blood Adv.* 2017;1(23):1983-1992.

Emergent Clinical Complications of Sickle Cell Disease

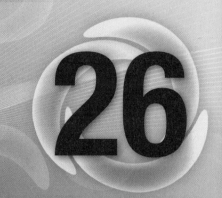

Authors: *Marcus Carden, Jeffrey Glassberg,*
Claudia R. Morris

Chapter Outline

Overview

Sickle cell disease (SCD) comprises a group of recessively inherited hemoglobinopathies that impact approximately 100,000 adults and children of various ethnicities and backgrounds in the United States and millions more worldwide.[1,2] Although the clinical features of SCD vary from patient to patient, common clinical complaints in the emergency department (ED) result from a persistent hemolytic anemia and vasculopathy within the microcirculation, which leads to repeated episodes of vaso-occlusion and ischemia-reperfusion that can result in acute and chronic end-organ damage of every organ system.[3,4] Patients with SCD have a shortened life expectancy compared to the general population due to these complications; however, most children with SCD in the United States can now expect to live to adulthood thanks to modern medical advances, including mandatory neonatal hemoglobinopathy screening, disease-specific immunization practices, early initiation of penicillin prophylaxis, hydroxyurea therapy, transfusion protocols, and parent education.[5]

Patients with SCD spend a great deal of time in an ED, yet care in the ED is a neglected area of sickle cell research. The negative attitudes toward SCD patients with pain have been compounded by racial stereotypes, the effects of the disease in limiting educational and employment opportunities, suboptimal medical coverage, and the large doses of opioids often required to obtain pain relief.[6] Ethnic disparities in ED care have been reported,[7-9] and adults with SCD experience longer delays in the initiation of analgesics compared to other patients with pain.[10] Barriers to rapid care in the ED are common across the country, including overcrowding, low nurse-to-patient ratios, insufficient staff coverage, inadequate funding, and slow flow of patients to the wards, in addition to high patient acuity of other patients in a busy ED.

The term *sickler* is often used by medical practitioners to refer to children and adults with SCD. Although using a label is common practice in the ED to rapidly refer to a specific patient (*CF'er* is used for a patient with cystic fibrosis and *asthmatic* for a patient with asthma) and often not meant to be derogatory, many patients with SCD find the term offensive.[11] In fact, the term *sickler* is pervasively used across the United States, and studies have found that emergency medicine physician use of the term *sickler* is associated with negative attitudes toward people with SCD.[11,12] Ultimately, this is a term that should be avoided in practice.

The total financial costs of SCD admissions from the ED are nearly $2 billion per year in the United States.[13] The transition from pediatric to adult care is an especially vulnerable time for these patients, during which ED utilization dramatically increases, likely due to both biologic and social causes.[14-16] Some literature suggests that admissions may be avoided by reducing stigmatization and improving care delivered in the ED, which is cited as a top priority area in great need of improvement by the SCD community and experts who provide ongoing care for patients with SCD.[11,17] As such, early consultation with a hematologist or other provider with SCD expertise may provide guidance for management and disposition when pediatric or adult patients present to the ED with complex issues. This is especially important in EDs with a low volume of patients with SCD, where physicians may be unfamiliar with treatments for this rare disease.

Variable Clinical Manifestations of SCD: Children Versus Adults

The frequency and presenting symptoms of complications in SCD will vary by age. In the infant, functional asplenia develops, although the exact age is variable.[18] As a result, however, all children with SCD should be considered immunocompromised due to abnormal splenic function. With age, progressive renal, pulmonary, liver, neurologic, and cardiac damage occurs. Both large and small vessels are affected in SCD, and both acute and chronic, and often asymptomatic, organ damage may occur.[19,20]

Despite an improvement in life expectancy over the past 50 years from approximately 10 years to approximately 45 years,[21] death in infancy and childhood is still a significant risk, with approximately 6% mortality in patients with homozygous sickle hemoglobin (HbS) prior to 18 years of age[5] and death historically peaking between 1 and 3 years of age.[22] The statistics are even more unfavorable in areas where access to care is limited, particularly in low-income countries. Sepsis is the primary cause of death, most commonly associated with *Streptococcus pneumoniae*. Acute anemic complications, acute chest syndrome (ACS), and stroke are also significant causes of mortality and morbidity in children. After age 10 years, cerebrovascular accidents and traumatic events surpass sepsis as the major causes of death.[21,23] By adulthood, ACS, pulmonary hypertension, chronic kidney disease, and sudden death account for the majority of mortality.

Sickle cell anemia is a chronic disease with acute and often life-threatening complications that frequently bring patients to the ED. Early recognition of complications and aggressive treatment initiated in the ED can dramatically improve patient survival.[24-26] Rehydration, oxygen, antibiotics, attention to respiratory status, and transfusion for precipitous decreases in hemoglobin can be critical lifesaving interventions.[25,27] This chapter summarizes emergency management approaches to common complications encountered in children and adults with SCD.

Emergent Complications of SCD

Complications of SCD affect every organ system and are often infectious, vaso-occlusive, and/or hyperhemolytic in nature.[28] Symptoms of SCD can develop as early as 4 to 6 months of age but more typically manifest between the ages of 1 and 2 years.[19,20,29] The etiology, clinical presentation, differential diagnosis, evaluation, and management of common complications are summarized in the following sections. Obtaining vital signs and performing a thorough history and physical exam are a crucial part of the evaluation regardless of the presenting complaint. Early consultation with a hematology specialist should always be considered when evaluating a patient with SCD in the ED.

Vaso-occlusive Pain Episodes

Acute pain is the hallmark of SCD and the most challenging aspect of sickle cell care in the ED.[30] Nationally, 78% of the nearly 200,000 annual ED visits for SCD are for a complaint of pain.[31] However, many studies find that ED physicians misunderstand SCD pain.[32,33] Studies indicate that 53% of ED physicians believe that >20% of SCD patients are addicted to opioids, whereas 22% of ED physicians believe that >50% of SCD patients are addicted to opioids.[34] Improved ED physician education is essential to improve negative attitudes commonly perceived by families dealing with SCD when seeking emergency care.

Pain may result from inflammatory, nociceptive, and neuropathic pathways.[35,36] Vaso-occlusive pain episodes (VOE) are the most common complication of SCD and are thought to result from small-vessel obstruction and resultant local tissue ischemia and damage.[35,37] Sickle-related pain is often referred to as a *pain crisis*,[38] which, similar to the term *sickler*, may carry a derogatory connotation for the individual with SCD and is not an ideal term. The preferred descriptor for sickle-related pain is vaso-occlusive pain *episode*, rather than *crisis*.

Patients with VOEs are optimally cared for in a day-hospital setting staffed by clinicians dedicated to SCD pain management because these facilities have been shown to reduce hospital admission rates. However, resources are often not available to establish them at all institutions.[39,40] As such, VOEs are the primary reason patients with SCD seek ED care and are hospitalized in the United States.[41,42] The pain can be unpredictable, often without a known or identifiable trigger, but some patients can pinpoint a certain cause, such as change in weather, dehydration, or stress. VOEs can start as early as 6 months of age in children, soon after fetal hemoglobin (HbF) begins to wane. The pain can be excruciating and debilitating and should be treated as a true medical emergency. Many pediatric and adult

patients treat their pain at home long before presenting to an ED and seek emergency care only after the pain becomes unbearable.[43,44] Adolescence and transition from pediatric to adult care are periods of exceptional reliance on ED care for VOE in SCD.[15]

Pain may be due to uncomplicated VOEs; however, it may also be the harbinger of more serious, life-threatening complications in SCD, including ACS, multisystem organ failure, or delayed hemolytic transfusion reaction. Thus, in addition to pain assessment with a validated, age-appropriate tool such as the Wong-Baker FACES Pain Rating Scale for children over age 3 and adults (Figure 26-1)[45] or the Numeric Pain Rating Scale, which is an 11-point scale of 0 (no pain) to 10 (worst possible pain) for patient self-reporting of pain in adults and children ≥10 years old,[46] obtaining an accurate history from the patient and/or family members is crucial to appropriate management. It should not only address the acute pain complaint, but also characterize the severity of the patient's disease and the patient's other comorbidities and complaints, as well as review the patient's medical record if available, with attention to baseline hemoglobin level and platelet count. Determining whether the specific pain a patient is experiencing resembles the patient's typical sickle-related pain is an important step in evaluating the etiology of pain. Atypical pain can be a red flag warranting additional clinical workup.

Children may present with excessive crying and may be developmentally unable to communicate the specifics of their pain. Dactylitis, also referred to as hand-foot syndrome (Figure 26-2), is a unique complication of SCD in infants and young children, manifesting as swelling of the hands and feet due to bone infarctions in red marrow. Prior to, or in the absence of, newborn screening, dactylitis or splenomegaly (with or without signs of sequestration) often revealed the diagnosis of SCD. Adult patients commonly present with pain in the chest, abdomen, and long bones, without any additional clinical exam findings.[47] Therefore, a broad differential diagnosis should be considered in patients with a complaint of pain to ensure the pain is not perniciously masquerading as an uncomplicated VOE (Table 26-1).

Laboratory studies are indicated for all patients (unless a specific multidisciplinary care plan dictates otherwise) who present to the ED for VOE and should include at minimum a

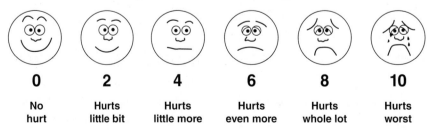

Wong-Baker FACES® Pain Rating Scale

0	2	4	6	8	10
No hurt	Hurts little bit	Hurts little more	Hurts even more	Hurts whole lot	Hurts worst

FIGURE 26-1 **Wong-Baker FACES Pain Rating Scale.** Vaso-occlusive pain assessment in the emergency department should be performed using a validated, age-appropriate tool such as the Wong-Baker FACES Pain Rating Scale for children over age 3 and in adults. Wong-Baker FACES Foundation (2020). Wong-Baker FACES® Pain Rating Scale. Retrieved 10/26/2020 with permission from http://www.WongBakerFACES.org. Originally published in *Whaley & Wong's Nursing Care of Infants and Children*. © Elsevier Inc.

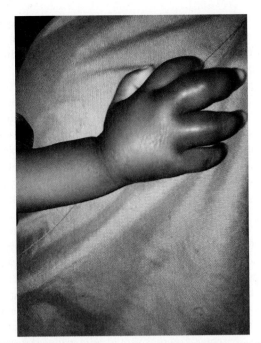

FIGURE 26-2 Dactylitis in a child with sickle cell disease (SCD). Also referred to as hand-foot syndrome, dactylitis is a unique complication of SCD in infants and young children, manifesting as swelling of the hands and feet due to bone infarctions in red marrow. Prior to or in the absence of newborn screening, dactylitis often revealed the diagnosis of SCD. Photograph provided with permission by Dr. U.A. Shehu (Department of Pediatrics, Bayero University, Aminu Kano Teaching Hospital, Kano, Nigeria) and Dr. H. Bello-Manga (Department of Hematology, Kaduna State University, Barau Dikko Teaching Hospital, Kaduna, Nigeria).

TABLE 26-1 Differential diagnosis by location of pain masquerading as an uncomplicated vaso-occlusive episode

Location	Differential diagnosis[a]
Head/skull	Stroke, meningitis
Ribs/chest	Acute chest syndrome/pneumonia, asthma, pulmonary embolism, fat embolus, costochondritis, gastroesophageal reflux, acute coronary syndrome, rib infarction
Abdomen	Acute chest syndrome/pneumonia, cholelithiasis/cholecystitis, appendicitis, pregnancy, ovarian torsion, menstrual pain, pelvic inflammatory disease, renal calculi, renal infarction, urinary tract infection, acute splenic sequestration
Bones/joints/ extremities	Dactylitis, osteomyelitis, septic arthritis, osteonecrosis/avascular necrosis of hip or shoulder

[a]Differential diagnoses presented are not meant to be comprehensive. Other etiologies should be considered based on clinician judgment.

complete blood count (CBC) with differential and reticulocyte count. Standard evaluation of liver and kidney function studies varies by institution but is recommended for symptoms that include abdominal pain or for patients known to have renal dysfunction. Elevated baseline white blood cell (WBC) counts have been associated with increased ED utilization and early death in patients with SCD and may be related to the complexity of SCD pathophysiology.[21,48] A WBC count above baseline, and certainly >20,000/μL, may indicate a potential infection or other complication. It should also be noted that hemoglobin levels often are near baseline or elevated during VOE, and if the patient has a significant decrease of 1 to 2 g/dL, the clinician should be alerted to other potential anemic complications or early ACS. Under the appropriate circumstances, blood culture, urinalysis and urine culture, urine pregnancy test, evaluation for pelvic inflammatory disease, and chest radiograph should be considered if clinically indicated. Abdominal imaging should be considered if the patient has abdominal pain, if there is jaundice or scleral icterus worse than baseline on physical exam, or if there is concern for hepatosplenomegaly or complications from cholelithiasis that may results from chronic hemolysis. Additional imaging studies, including contrasted studies or magnetic resonance imaging (MRI) of the brain in case of severe headache, should be considered in the appropriate clinical circumstances and with consultation of a hematologist. Blood typing and screening, hemoglobin electrophoresis (to quantify pretransfusion HbS), and a direct Coombs test (direct antiglobulin test) may also be considered if there is concern the patient may need a transfusion and/or there is suspicion the patient is having a delayed hemolytic transfusion reaction. We encourage early blood typing for all admitted adult patients to identify individuals for whom it will be difficult to find blood, before there is an emergent need for transfusion.

Pain reported by the patient and/or family members is the gold standard for VOE assessment because there are no labs or clinical findings that can adequately and accurately quantify the severity of pain.[49] Appropriate and timely treatment of SCD-related pain is the standard of care, and choice of therapy should be based on severity of symptoms. Analgesics, including opioids and nonsteroidal anti-inflammatory drugs (NSAIDs), and gentle hydration are mainstays of therapy for treating sickle cell–related VOE. Unfortunately, disparities in pain management of patients with SCD compared to others with chronic pain have been reported and are in part due to negative attitudes toward patients with SCD, language bias, and certain racial sterotypes.[12,30,50,51] Recent studies have confirmed that racial bias impacts how some medical providers think about pain in Black versus White people, which may also play a role in undertreatment recommendations for patients with SCD in the ED.[52] In addition, although some ED providers are worried about addiction among patients with SCD receiving opioids for pain, studies suggest <10% of patients with SCD likely have a true opioid addiction.[51,53-55] Therefore, opioids should not be consciously withheld from patients reporting pain due to perceptions of drug-seeking behavior.

The Centers for Disease Control and Prevention (CDC) guidelines for limiting opioid use specifically excluded patients with SCD.[56] If there is a concern that an individual may have addiction or opioid misuse disorder, a comprehensive psychosocial assessment obtained by the primary clinicians managing the patient is indicated to formulate a plan that may or may not include opioids for acute pain. This should be done after the acute event that generated concern and not during an acute, ongoing VOE. In addition, because of tolerance, patients with SCD often require substantial amounts of opioids for pain control, and therefore, appropriate amounts should be administered. As with anyone who receives opioids in the ED, SCD patients should be monitored closely for symptoms of respiratory depression. If prescriptions for outpatient management of pain are given at the time of ED discharge, patients (adults and children) should not be given >3 days of opioids in accordance with the CDC recommendations, and they should be encouraged to follow up with their primary sickle cell provider if more prolonged opiate regimens are needed.[56]

2014 National Heart, Lung, and Blood Institute Pain Guidelines

All patients with SCD and a complaint of pain should be triaged as an Emergency Severity Index (ESI) level 2 and moved into the ED immediately.[55] According to the 2014 National Heart, Lung, and Blood Institute (NHLBI) guidelines, patients with VOE presenting to the ED should be treated with an analgesic within 30 minutes of triage or 60 minutes of arrival[49] (Figure 26-3). Although oral medications can be trialed, intravenous (IV) access should be attempted as soon as possible in preparation to administer parenteral medications for patients experiencing moderate to severe pain, typically defined by a numeric pain score of ≥6. Alternatives include subcutaneous or intranasal (IN) medications as a bridge while waiting for IV placement.[57] Studies have shown that administration of IN fentanyl as the first parenteral medication improves adherence to NHLBI guidelines by decreasing time to administration of first parenteral opioid. IN fentanyl rapidly reduces pain and may improve discharge rates of pediatric patients from the ED.[57-59] Adequate dosing of IN fentanyl by weight is limited by the volume that can be delivered intranasally. IN fentanyl may therefore be a more ideal option for younger children compared to larger adolescents and adults. There is also a lack of high-quality evidence regarding the use of IN fentanyl in adult patients with VOE; however, some EDs have used it with success.

IN fentanyl dosing is as follows: 1.5 µg/kg IN per dose; administer second dose 5 minutes later (maximum dose, 100 µg). The dose should be divided equally between each nare (not to exceed 1 mL per nare); IN fentanyl is contraindicated if the patient has a current upper respiratory infection or nasal infection/obstruction or if there is concern for stroke, altered level of consciousness, or any form of head injury.[57,58]

The cornerstone of VOE management is parenteral analgesia with IV opiates. Personal treatment plans are ideal for patients with VOE. Individualized pain plans (IPPs) have been shown to be beneficial for both pediatric and adult patients in the ED.[60,61] IPPs may improve pain control, reduce time to second opioid, and reduce admission rates, while also improving patient experience in the ED. Optimally, these plans are built in collaboration with hematologists and ED providers.

For patients without treatment plans or those with frequent ED utilization, type and dosing of IV opioids should be based on previous visits. IV opioids, such as morphine or hydromorphone, should be administered within 60 minutes of presentation, and the patient's pain should be reassessed every 15 to 30 minutes, with additional IV opioids provided for persistent moderate to severe pain.

Many patients with SCD have had years of exposure to opioids, and such exposure leads to experience of care, ideas of what has worked and what has not, and tolerance to lower doses of opioids. Studies also have shown that patients with SCD may have altered neural pathways and hyperalgesia that may impact their response to opioid therapies.[36,62,63] Therefore, if initial analgesic therapy does not provide prompt relief despite appropriate titration, alternative therapies may need to be considered. Patients with uncontrolled pain despite 2 to 3 doses of parenteral opioids should be considered for admission to the hospital. Utilization of patient-controlled analgesia is ideal when available.[64]

Meperidine should be avoided in SCD. Its metabolite, normeperidine, is a renally cleared central nervous system (CNS) irritant. As such, it may accumulate in the blood in the setting of underlying kidney dysfunction, leading to seizures or other CNS complications.

Adjunctive Pain Therapies

Nonopiate therapies are also often used during VOEs. NSAIDs, including IV ketorolac, have been used for synergism and opioid-sparing effects, although reports of benefits on VOE course are mixed.[65-69] Clinicians should exercise caution when using this class of drugs in patients with renal dysfunction. Reports of NSAID use inducing acute kidney injury during VOE have been described in the literature.[70-72]

Oral antihistamines, such as diphenhydramine, may be needed if patients experience opioid-induced histamine release and pruritus. Use of IV diphenhydramine is discouraged during VOE treatment outside of cases of allergic reaction or anaphylaxis because it can cause a euphoric effect and respiratory depression in some cases.

Ondansetron should be considered for nausea and vomiting. Supplemental oxygen is unnecessary during uncomplicated VOE but should be administered to keep oxygen levels >92%. In cases of decreased oxygen saturation, harm from hypoxemia outweighs concerns about suppressed reticulocytosis reported in a small, uncontrolled case series.[73]

Investigational Therapies

There are a growing number of investigational therapies for acute VOE. Ketamine, an activator of the N-methyl-D-aspartate receptor, has been anecdotally used to treat VOE in the ED and inpatient units. Small, uncontrolled studies and case reports in adults and children suggest it may be safe and effective and

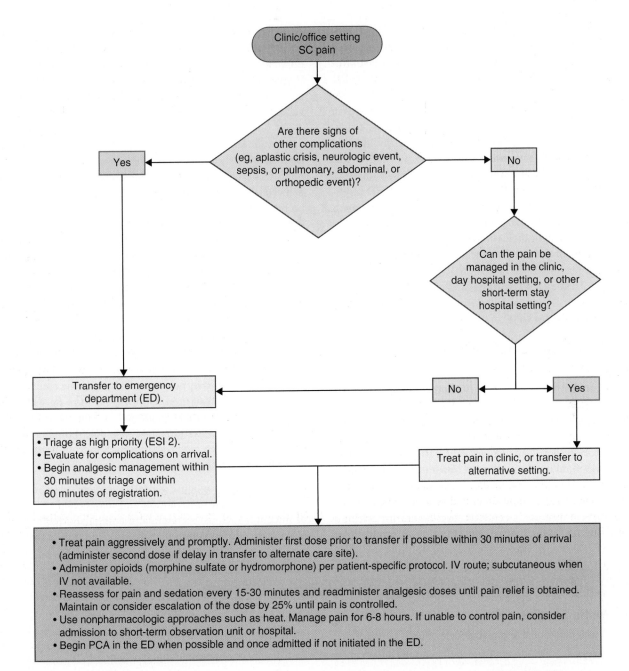

FIGURE 26-3 2014 National Heart, Lung, and Blood Institute guidelines for management of acute vaso-occlusive pain. Adapted from National Heart, Lung, and Blood Institute. Evidence-based management of sickle cell disease. https://www.nhlbi.nih.gov/health-topics/evidence-based-management-sickle-cell-disease. Accessed July 23, 2020.

may reduce need for opioid administration.[74-76] However, controlled trials are needed before routine use can be justified.[77] A recent randomized controlled noninferiority trial of ketamine (1 mg/kg) compared to IV morphine for children with SCD and pain demonstrated comparable analgesic effectiveness, but ketamine was associated with an 11-fold increased risk of transient, non–life-threatening side effects.[78] Low-dose ketamine protocols for VOE should be used in consultation with pain management experts.

Nitric oxide gas inhalation,[79] IV magnesium,[80,81] regadenoson (adenosine A2a receptor agonist),[82] and vepoloxamer (MST-188)[83,84] failed to demonstrate benefits in large randomized controlled trials. IV arginine therapy significantly reduced total parenteral opioid use by 54% (1.9 ± 2.0 mg/kg vs 4.1 ± 4.1 mg/kg; $P = .02$) and lowered pain scores at discharge compared to placebo in a small clinical trial.[85,86] Although rivipansel (GMI-1070) had demonstrated opioid-sparing efficacy in a phase II randomized trial,[87] the phase III trial failed to achieve efficacy end points.[88] IV immunoglobulins (IVIGs) are also being trialed.[89,90]

As SCD has gained interest among researchers and the pharmaceutical industry in search of novel treatments for pain, many patients who come to the ED for pain management may be on studies assessing the effectiveness of drugs to prevent or treat VOE. Providers should be aware of whether patients are on investigational studies and must specifically ask about this. Descriptions of specific trials are beyond the scope of this chapter, but they are described elsewhere in this book and in various reviews.[86,91-93]

There is growing interest from both patients and clinicians in the use of integrative adjunctive therapies to treat acute sickle-related pain that warrant further investigation,[62] including acupuncture,[62,94-96] yoga,[97] hypnosis,[98] music therapy,[99] and virtual reality.[100] In one study of 63 caregivers of children with SCD, >70% used complementary therapies to treat pain.[89] ED physicians should inquire about the use of both investigational medications and complementary therapies, including nutritional supplements, as part of their routine evaluation for VOE. Recommendations for the approach to the patient with SCD and acute pain are summarized in Box 26-1; opioid and nonopioid strategies for treating pain in the ED are found in Box 26-2.

Use of IV Fluids for VOE

Due to insensible losses, hyposthenuria, and reduced oral fluid intake, some patients with SCD and VOE may be dehydrated upon presentation to the ED. Although oral hydration in the ED is preferred, hydration with IV fluids is common, inexpensive, and anecdotally considered by many hematologists and ED physicians as an integral part of VOE management. Use of IV fluids is a common pharmacologic intervention for VOE in the ED. However, evidence regarding the ideal type and tonicity of IV fluid to administer and how IV fluids impact red blood cell (RBC) adhesiveness during the vaso-occlusive process is lacking.[101] In vitro and in vivo studies have shown that lowering serum osmolality (by hydrating the erythrocyte and thus diluting and reducing the concentration of intracellular

HbS) can reduce erythrocyte sickling, improve deformability, and reduce adhesion to endothelium.[102-105] The 2014 NHLBI guidelines on SCD management suggest IV fluids be used when euvolemic patients cannot maintain oral hydration.[49] However, excess IV fluids should be avoided, given their association with potential fluid overload and risk for atelectasis and ACS.[106] Bolusing crystalloid fluids should be avoided unless the patient shows clinical signs of severe hypovolemia or dehydration. Caution should be used when using a normal saline (NS) bolus in particular, because it has been associated with worse pain control in children with SCD and VOE.[107-109] This may be related to its excessive tonicity, low pH, and risk of causing hyperchloremic metabolic acidosis (ie, high tonicity can theoretically dehydrate erythrocytes and increase HbS concentration, and the low pH can facilitate HbS deoxygenation). Hydration with hypotonic fluids (dextrose 5% [D5] plus ½ NS or D5 plus ¼ NS) at 1 to 1.5 times maintenance rate should be used in patients who cannot tolerate oral fluids; however, there is a paucity of data to guide recommendations.[109]

Note that from a mechanistic standpoint, HbS polymerization is proportional to the concentration of HbS in the erythrocyte to the 34th power (small changes in concentration can have major changes in polymerization) and the extent of HbS deoxygenation. Thus, interventions that increase RBC dehydration (ie, hypertonic IV solutions) or right shift the hemoglobin-oxygen dissociation curve (low pH) should be avoided.

Fever and Infections

Infection is a leading cause of death in patients with SCD. Fever is a very common presentation and may herald the presence of infection such as bacteremia, meningitis, osteomyelitis, or other sources of infection that are also common in the general

---

| **Box 26-1** | **Approach to the Patient With SCD and Acute Pain** |

Diagnostic Studies

1. CBC with differential and reticulocyte count
2. Electrolytes to include renal function in adults and in children with a history of abnormal renal function
3. Urinalysis, urine culture (for abdominal pain or dysuria)
4. Pulse oximetry
5. Chest x-ray when clinically indicated (fever, chest pain, respiratory symptoms, abdominal/back pain)

Caveat: Normally a patient's hemoglobin should be at baseline during a VOE; therefore, a decrease in hemoglobin below baseline should alert the evaluating physician to a possible acute anemic complication or early acute chest syndrome. Any additional diagnostic workup is dictated by individual symptoms and specific areas of pain:

◆ Symptoms of dehydration: Serum electrolytes.

◆ Fever: Diagnostic studies for fever. Aggressively evaluate for infection.

◆ Chest pain: Evaluate for ACS and asthma; electrocardiogram (ECG) in adult.

◆ Bone pain: Consider osteomyelitis if clinically indicated.

◆ Joint pain (hip, shoulder): Consider radiographic study or more advanced imaging to evaluate for avascular necrosis or acute septic arthritis.

(continued)

Box 26-1	Approach to the Patient With SCD and Acute Pain (Continued)

◆ Abdominal pain: Consider complete metabolic panel to include liver function tests. Most SCD patients with abdominal pain require no diagnostic imaging. However, localized tenderness or peritoneal signs (especially with fever) warrant surgical consultation and/or diagnostic imaging (abdominal ultrasound or computed tomography [CT]). Caution is warranted when obtaining a CT with contrast, particularly in a patient with reduced renal function.[110] Contrast studies should be obtained in consultation with a hematologist. Additional studies for abdominal pain may include a urinalysis and culture, urine pregnancy test, evaluation for possible pelvic inflammatory disease in females >13 years old (urine screen for gonorrhea/chlamydia polymerase chain reaction), abdominal films, liver function tests (for right upper quadrant pain or jaundice), ultrasound to evaluate for appendicitis (and ovarian torsion in females), splenic sequestration (if HbSC or HbS-β+ thalassemia), or gallstones/gallbladder disease

◆ Severe headache: Consider evaluation for stroke, intracranial hemorrhage, and other dangerous causes of headache if not improving. Headache can be the only clinical manifestation of a stroke early on in SCD.

Management

1. See Figure 26-3. Follow the 2014 NHLBI guidelines.

   • Triage at ESI level 2.

   • Treat pain adequately and timely with parenteral opioids initiated within 60 minutes of ED arrival.

   • Reassess pain every 15 to 30 minutes, with readministration of IV opioids for persistent moderate to severe pain.

   • Analgesic therapy should be titrated to provide prompt relief. Therapy choice is based on pain severity. Continuous IV infusion of opioid using patient-controlled analgesia devices is ideal, but should only be used in institutions familiar with its use.

   • Opioids are currently the drug of choice for pain management in the ED. Dosing should be individualized for each patient, and frequent reassessment of the patient is critical.

   • Avoid the pain pendulum by giving opioids at fixed intervals rather than waiting for pain to recur after relief.

   • Monitor for signs of oversedation and decreased respiratory drive.

   • Monitor patients receiving opioids with pulse oximetry.

   • Use adjunctive therapies as appropriate: IV ketorolac, oral diphenhydramine, and warm packs to painful areas.

   • Evaluate for other causes of pain.

   • Consider hydration with hypotonic saline at maintenance rate.

   • Avoid NS bolus for euvolemic patients with SCD presenting for acute pain management (but appropriately treat dehydration with 20 mL/kg of crystalloid fluid bolus).

   • Consider admission if no better after 2 to 3 rounds of parenteral opioids.

Admission Criteria for VOE

◆ Pain not controlled in ED

◆ Persistent tachycardia

◆ Hypotension

◆ Fever >101°F (38.3°C)

◆ Signs of significant infection

◆ Aplastic or hyperhemolytic event

◆ Acute decrease in hemoglobin >1 g/dL

◆ Pregnancy

◆ Hepatic syndrome

◆ New infiltrate on chest x-ray

◆ Prolonged priapism

◆ New CNS finding

◆ Acute abdomen

◆ Hypoxemia

◆ Acidosis

| Box 26-2 | Opioid and Nonopioid Strategies for Treating Pain in the ED |

1. IN fentanyl: 1.5 µg/kg IN per dose; administer second dose 5 minutes later (maximum dose, 100 µg). Divide dose equally between each nare (not to exceed 1 mL per nare).

2. Morphine (0.1-0.15 mg/kg IV dose every 1-3 hours; maximum, 10 mg/dose).

3. Hydromorphone (0.01-0.015 mg/kg IV dose; maximum, 2 mg/dose).

4. Ketorolac (0.5 mg/kg IV dose; maximum, 30 mg). Avoid in patients with abnormal renal function.

5. NSAIDs (in patients with normal renal function) or acetaminophen (in patients with normal liver function) may be used for mild to\ moderate uncomplicated pain.

6. Diphenhydramine (1-2 mg/kg given orally; maximum, 50 mg) may be needed due to opioid-induced histamine release. IV administration may have euphoric effects and should be avoided, unless the patient has signs of severe reaction.

7. Consider ondansetron (0.15 mg/kg IV single dose), for nausea or vomiting.

8. Low-dose ketamine protocols for pain management should be used in consultation with pain management experts.

population. VOE itself can also sometimes be associated with hyperpyrexia. The definition of a fever has not been rigorously studied, and although the NHLBI guidelines suggest using 38.5°C (101.5°F) as a cutoff for fever, some institutions use 38.0°C (100.4°F)[111] or 38.3°C (101°F).[49] Infants and young children are at particularly high risk for serious bacterial infection due to an immunocompromised state from early onset of splenic autoinfarction and dysfunction, resulting in an inability to properly clear bacterial organisms from the bloodstream. SCD is also associated with defects in the alternate complement pathway and low nitric oxide bioavailability. Preventative measures, including penicillin prophylaxis and immunization against encapsulated organisms including *Haemophilus influenzae* and *S pneumoniae*, have significantly reduced the incidence of sepsis and mortality among children.[5] Guidelines for managing adults and children with fever in the ED are based mainly on expert opinion because substantial evidence-based prospective studies are lacking.[112]

Patients with SCD and fever at home should seek medical attention immediately. The ED evaluation of fever includes a careful physical exam and investigation for infectious etiologies. According to the NHLBI guidelines, all patients should have a CBC with differential, reticulocyte count, blood culture (peripherally and/or from central venous catheter, if present), and urinalysis with urine culture if there is suspicion of urinary source. Lumbar puncture should be considered in patients with signs of meningitis. Stool cultures or gastrointestinal polymerase chain reaction panels should be obtained if prolonged or bloody diarrhea is present. In patients with localized or multifocal bone tenderness, skeletal films should be obtained to evaluate for osteomyelitis and consideration given to an orthopedics consult. Chest radiographs (CXRs) should be ordered on any patient with fever or respiratory symptoms (eg, shortness of breath, tachypnea, chest pain, cough, abnormal lung exam/rales, hypoxemia)[111,113] or a past history of ACS.[113]

Fever may be the only symptom of ACS in children (see section on pulmonary complications and ACS).[111] ACS is defined as a new infiltrate on CXR (lobar consolidation, excluding atelectasis) in a patient with SCD and at least 1 of the following: fever, cough, sputum production, tachypnea, dyspnea, or new hypoxia. As a lung injury syndrome, ACS can present with different manifestations, including pneumonia, acute respiratory distress syndrome, and pulmonary infarction. Manifestations of ACS (which include pneumonia in an SCD patient, although etiology from infectious causes versus infarct is not always apparent) can vary from mild with very few symptoms to severe. Symptoms include fever, rapid breathing, shortness of breath, chest pain, and cough.[114] Pneumonia in children with SCD may present with abdominal pain and/or no complaints beyond fever, particularly in children <10 years of age. The second most common clinical finding in children with ACS is a normal lung exam.[111,114,115] The lone finding of fever without additional respiratory symptoms in a child with a past history of ACS may also be indicative of recurrent ACS.[113] Thus, consideration should be given to a 2-view CXR (anterior-posterior and lateral) on any pediatric patient presenting with fever and a low threshold to obtain a CXR in adults with SCD and fever.

An ultrasound should be considered in patients with abdominal pain and fever to evaluate for signs of cholecystitis, appendicitis, or splenic sequestration. Antibiotics should be administered promptly, preferably within 60 minutes of ED presentation, and should cover *S pneumoniae* and gram-negative enteric organisms (eg, ceftriaxone).[116] Although potentially fatal cases of acute ceftriaxone-induced immune hemolytic anemia[117-119] or splenic sequestration[120] have been reported, they are rare, and use of ceftriaxone remains the gold standard treatment for fever in patients with SCD. However, awareness of this complication is important among ED providers because early diagnosis and proper treatment of hemolytic anemia is essential to improve patient outcome. IVIG plus supportive measures have been reported to be beneficial in a case of life-threatening ceftriaxone-induced hemolytic anemia in a previously healthy 3-year-old girl.[120] Ceftriaxone should be avoided in any patient with SCD who has a history of ceftriaxone-induced hemolysis.

Patients with SCD and fever who are not ill appearing may be discharged after a dose of ceftriaxone and close follow-up. ED discharge criteria for fever in a child with SCD are summarized later in this chapter.[55,121] Infants ≤6 months old with SCD and fever should be admitted for IV antibiotics, monitoring, and supportive care. Viral infections, including influenza, may cause greater morbidity in patients with SCD and can be an etiology of ACS. Therefore, if a patient presents with fever during influenza season, the patient should be screened for influenza infection and started preemptively on oseltamivir while awaiting the results of the influenza swab. See Box 26-3 for the approach to fever in SCD.

Acute Anemia

Sickle erythrocytes have an average life span of 5 to 20 days[122] due to a chronic hemolytic anemia with hemoglobin values ranging from 6 to 9 g/dL. Patients also have high reticulocyte

---

Box 26-3	Approach to Fever in SCD

Diagnostic Studies

1. Complete history and physical exam and vitals, including pulse oximetry
2. CBC with differential and reticulocyte count
3. Blood culture
4. CXR (anterior-posterior and lateral)
5. Influenza swab (during flu season)
6. Urinalysis and urine culture (for dysuria, abdominal pain, infants/toddlers)
7. Stool culture (if diarrhea is present)
8. Lumbar puncture in any patient with symptoms of meningitis (strongly consider in patients <1 year old with slightest CNS indication)
9. Evaluation for osteomyelitis; if high fever and localized bone pain, consider bone scan, skeletal films; early orthopedic consultation
10. Type and screen/crossmatch for extreme pallor, respiratory or neurologic symptoms, or acute splenic enlargement (see section on transfusion for specific blood bank orders)

Management

1. Prompt IV or intramuscular dose of ceftriaxone (75 mg/kg; maximum, 2 g) while awaiting lab results (consider vancomycin, 20 mg/kg IV [maximum dose, 1250 mg] for severe illness/sepsis)
2. Add oral erythromycin or azithromycin for ACS/pneumonia; admission for ACS
3. Oseltamivir during flu season while awaiting influenza test results.
4. See following Admission Criteria indications
5. For known/suspected cephalosporin allergy: consider levofloxacin (10 mg/kg IV; maximum dose, 750 mg) if no concern for CNS infection; consider meropenem (40 mg/kg IV; maximum dose, 2 g) plus vancomycin for CNS infection

Admission Criteria: Fever

◆ Clinical signs or suspicion of serious bacterial infection or systemic toxicity
◆ All infants aged 0 to 6 months
◆ Patients with temperature ≥40°C (≥104°F)
◆ Central line present
◆ WBC >30,000/μL or <5000/μL
◆ Platelet count <100,000/μL
◆ Hemoglobin <5 g/dL
◆ Hemoglobin decrease ≥2 g/dL
◆ Evidence of additional acute complications: severe pain, aplastic crisis, splenic sequestration, ACS, stroke, priapism
◆ Endemic *S pneumoniae* in community is *not* sensitive to the antibiotic provided
◆ Immunizations *not* up to date
◆ Patient has a past history of sepsis
◆ Persistent tachycardia, hypotension, or hypoperfusion
◆ Evidence of dehydration
◆ Concerns about compliance
◆ Twenty-four-hour follow-up phone-call contact at minimum is available; may need repeat dose of ceftriaxone in ED or at next-day clinic visit

counts, often accounting for 5% to 20% of the total erythrocyte mass in circulation. As such, any further insult to the circulating sickle RBCs or RBC production itself can lead to sudden, severe, and life-threatening anemia as the bone marrow is unable to adequately compensate. Common symptoms of acute anemia include worsening fatigue, shortness of breath, scleral icterus, dark urine, or multisystem organ failure from reduced end-organ perfusion. In addition to causes of acute anemia in the general population, the following etiologies need to be considered in patients with SCD. Box 26-4 summarizes the approach to the SCD patient with acute anemia.

Parvovirus Infection/Transient RBC Aplasia

Transient RBC aplasia is most commonly caused by an acute infection with parvovirus B19, which results in transient suppression of RBC production (5-7 days) via a direct cytotoxic effect on erythroid precursors via the P antigen.[123] The incidence of parvovirus infection is higher in children compared to adults with SCD. With approximately 11.3 events per 100 patient-years, 62% of these infections result in transient RBC aplasia.[124] Previously referred to as an *aplastic crisis*, infection with parvovirus B19 leads to severe anemia, with hemoglobin well below the baseline. Patients may be lethargic or tachycardic and, in some cases, may even present with syncope or signs of heart failure. The reticulocyte count is extremely low or even zero in patients with transient RBC aplasia. Other cytopenias, including reduced leukocyte and platelet count, may also be seen. Patients often need emergent blood transfusion support and should be admitted for close observation. Adequate follow-up is important because bone marrow recovery may take several days.

Splenic Sequestration

Splenic sequestration manifests with a sudden enlargement of the spleen and a life-threatening decrease in hemoglobin, typically by at least 2 g/dL below baseline value. More common in children <5 years old, splenic sequestration can be associated with high rates of mortality. Infants may present with hypovolemic shock.[125] However, it may present later in life among adolescents or adults with hemoglobin SC or HbS-β⁺ thalassemia who have persistent splenic tissue. On exam, the spleen can be palpated in the left upper quadrant and sometimes even down to the umbilicus. Thrombocytopenia is often present, but unlike in transient RBC aplasia, the reticulocyte count is variable. According to the NHLBI guidelines, patients with hypovolemia and sequestration should be quickly resuscitated with IV fluids. In consultation with a hematologist, patients should also be cautiously transfused to raise hemoglobin to a stable level while avoiding overtransfusion or giving blood too quickly, which can trigger complications such as pain, stroke, and ACS.[49] Although typically not initiated in the ED, exchange transfusion may be considered in consultation with a hematologist and/or transfusion medicine expert. All patients with acute splenic sequestration should be admitted; hemoglobin and neurologic examinations should

---

Box 26-4 | **Approach to the Sickle Cell Patient With Anemia**

Diagnostic Studies

1. CBC with differential and reticulocyte count
2. Type and screen/crossmatch blood for possible emergent packed RBC transfusion

Management

Acute Splenic Sequestration Crisis

1. Simple transfusion to hemoglobin of 9 to 10 g/dL with monitoring for reverse sequestration.
2. Exchange transfusion (typically in intensive care unit) for signs of cardiopulmonary distress (hypoxemia, respiratory distress, clinical evidence of shock): remove 75% blood volume and replace with packed RBCs/NS(50/50); simple transfusion is indicated while preparing for exchange transfusion if there is going to be a significant delay because this is a life-threatening complication.
3. Admit to hospital.
4. Consider giving 2 separate small aliquot transfusions over 3 hours with furosemide in between to prevent respiratory compromise due to fluid overload (post-ED management).
5. Consider splenectomy if patient is >2 years old or if patient is <2 years old and has no evidence of splenic function (post-ED management).
6. Chronic transfusion program until age 2 years; maintain HbS <30% if patient is <2 years old and splenic function is intact (post-ED management).

Aplastic Crisis

1. Treatment is symptomatic; typically resolves in 1-2 weeks.
2. Close follow-up in asymptomatic patients.
3. Transfuse packed RBCs for severe anemia (hemoglobin <5 g/dL) or for associated cardiopulmonary compromise.
4. Admit to hospital.

Hyperhemolysis (Without Concern for Delayed Hemolytic Transfusion Reaction)

1. Evaluate for and treat underlying cause or trigger (including infection, VOE, ACS).
2. Transfuse packed RBCs for severe anemia (10 mL/kg over 3-4 hours).
3. Reduction of HbS to <30% of total circulating RBCs will effectively prevent further sickling; exchange transfusion may be needed based on severity of crisis.
4. Admit to hospital (may require intensive care).

---

be monitored frequently because of the potential for neurologic complications due to hyperviscosity as blood remobilizes from the spleen when the condition resolves, a condition also known as autotransfusion.

Delayed Hemolytic Transfusion Reaction

Delayed hemolytic transfusion reaction is the result of hemolysis of donor erythrocytes that occurs between 1 and 28 days after a blood transfusion due to alloimmunization and can occur despite adequate phenotype matching of donor RBCs.[126-128] Patients may present with VOE-like symptoms, and due to the potential for life-threatening delayed hemolytic transfusion reaction, clinicians should always ask patients with SCD and VOE complaints when they received their last transfusion. Patients with a previous life-threatening episode of delayed hemolytic transfusion reaction are at increased risk for delayed hemolytic transfusion reaction in the future.[129] If a patient presents with a lower hemoglobin level just after recent transfusions and with no source of blood loss, an urgent hematology consultation is warranted. Hemoglobin electrophoresis will show a lower than expected hemoglobin A (HbA) percentage. Hyperhemolysis can be seen in patients with delayed hemolytic transfusion reaction, and this life-threatening clinical scenario is heralded by the destruction of both the transfused RBCs and also the patient's own RBCs, so-called *bystander hemolysis*.[130-133] Patients may present with clinical and laboratory findings consistent with excessive hemolysis, along with reticulocytopenia and multisystem organ failure. Transfusions may paradoxically worsen hemolysis.[129] Patients should be comanaged with hematology and transfusion medicine specialists and will often require hospital admission and potentially intensive care for close monitoring and hemodynamic support.

Bone Marrow Suppression From Hydroxyurea

In patients who take hydroxyurea, fluctuations in adherence, renal function, and other factors may lead to excessive myelosuppression and iatrogenic acute anemia. Typically, patients manifest leukopenia with their anemia, and thrombocytopenia is also common. If myelosuppression from hydroxyurea is suspected, the drug should be temporarily suspended until counts improve; the patient's hematologist may consider restarting hydroxyurea at a lower dose.

Pulmonary Complications

Patients with SCD will often present to the ED with pulmonary complaints. Acute and chronic pulmonary complications will compromise oxygenation and contribute to a relentless cycle of RBC vaso-occlusion. ACS/pneumonia, asthma, pulmonary hypertension, and thromboembolic disease are common.[134] Oxygen should always be used for low pulse oximetry measurements to maintain oxygen saturations >92%, despite anecdotal reports against oxygen use in a small case series that demonstrated an adverse impact of extended use of high levels of oxygen supplement on reticulocytosis.[73] However, routine oxygen use is not indicated without signs of hypoxemia or respiratory distress.

Acute pulmonary disease is estimated to be hundreds of times more frequent for SCD patients than for the general population (overall incidence, 10.5 cases per 100 patient-years).[135] Abnormal pulmonary function has been identified in >80% of adults and children with SCD[136,137] and is characterized by airway obstruction, restrictive lung disease, abnormal diffusing capacity, and hypoxemia. Poor baseline lung function may contribute to acute events. Pulmonary symptoms in the ED will vary by age and carry a fairly large differential diagnosis, which includes ACS/pneumonia; asthma; pulmonary hypertension; pulmonary embolus; aspiration pneumonia; atelectasis; chest trauma; VOE of the abdomen, ribs, sternum, or back; sepsis; splenic sequestration and infarction; stroke or acute anemic crisis with cardiopulmonary compromise; congestive heart failure; and acute myocardial infarction in adult patients. The most common pulmonary complications are discussed in detail in other chapters of this book; however, emergency management of the most frequent pulmonary complications is summarized in the following sections. The approach to the patient with SCD and pulmonary complaints is summarized in Box 26-5.

Box 26-5 Approach to the Sickle Cell Patient With Pulmonary Complaints

Diagnostic Studies

1. A good history and review of systems; evaluate for asthma symptoms
2. Pulse oximetry
3. CXR (anterior-posterior and lateral)
4. CBC with differential and reticulocyte count
5. Blood culture if fever is present or suspect ACS
6. Type and screen/crossmatch in patients with moderate to severe respiratory distress, if ACS is suspected, or if a pneumonia is identified on CXR even without respiratory symptoms, because hemoglobin can drop precipitously during ACS
7. Ventilation/perfusion scan or chest CT when significant chest symptoms exist with normal CXR
8. ECG (prolonged QTc has been reported in children and adults with SCD[197-199])
9. Doppler echocardiography if pulmonary hypertension or congestive heart failure is suspected
10. *Caveat:* Indications for arterial blood gas on room air should be considered similar to the general population

(continued)

| Box 26-5 | Approach to the Sickle Cell Patient With Pulmonary Complaints (Continued) |

Management

1. Ascertain rapidity of onset and other historical factors such as asthma, severe limb pain, or a past history of thromboembolism or pulmonary hypertension.

2. Ascertain temperature and severity of hypoxia. Attempt to correct low pulse oximetry by deep breathing, thereby showing low tidal volumes secondary to splinting from pain. Provide adequate analgesia to allow deep inspiration.

3. Examine lungs for signs of consolidation, air trapping, wheezing, and pleural changes. Egophony and rales may be present before radiographic changes.

4. CXR is indicated with any severe chest symptoms, hypoxemia, or fever. Cardiac hypertrophy may be present at baseline, but compare to prior films for acute changes. Any new infiltrate and a fever should be considered ACS and warrant admission. See ACS section and Chapter 12.

5. Because half of patients with ACS present with pain and a normal CXR that becomes positive with time and hydration (usually within 72 hours), an additional CXR may be needed after admission if there continues to be a suspicion for ACS.

6. If ACS is suspected, ensure hydration and oxygenation. Empiric antibiotics, including a macrolide or quinolone in addition to a parenteral broad-spectrum antibiotic appropriate to local microbial susceptibilities, are routinely started. Oseltamivir should be given preemptively during flu season. If symptoms are severe, then consider steroids and early transfusion. If the hemoglobin is too high for simple transfusion, consult hematology for urgent erythrocytapheresis.

7. In the presence of wheezing, institute treatments directed at bronchospasm and asthma.

8. If the history and physical examination suggest a pulmonary embolism, then Doppler evaluation and CT angiogram should be obtained. SCD is not a contraindication to IV contrast. However, renal dysfunction is common in adults with SCD and poses the same relative risks as in other patients. D-dimer levels are elevated at baseline and further in VOE and, therefore, cannot be used to screen for pulmonary embolism.

9. For severe dyspnea or chest pain without a clear cause, Doppler echocardiography is indicated to screen for pulmonary hypertension. If increased pulmonary pressure is suspected (over about 35 mm Hg), then admission is warranted for further evaluation. Brain natriuretic peptide (BNP) may be helpful because most patients with significant pulmonary hypertension have a BNP >500 pg/mL.[200]

10. Any acute lung compromise warrants admission for further observation and treatment.

ACS

ACS is the second most common complication of SCD, is one of the most frequent conditions at time of death, and carries a 3% mortality rate.[115] It is a complex condition of bone marrow emboli, infection, and vascular shunting. Physician recognition of ACS is suboptimal, given that few respiratory symptoms may be present early on.[111,113,114]

ACS is defined as a new infiltrate on CXR (lobar consolidation, excluding atelectasis) in a patient with SCD and at least 1 of the following: fever, cough, tachypnea, dyspnea, or new hypoxemia.[138] Children tend to present to the ED with fever and cough and often have a normal lung exam,[111,114] whereas adults tend to present with chest or extremity pain[114] (Figure 26-4). See earlier section on fever and infections for more details. Patients who present to the ED with symptoms of cough, chest pain, tachypnea, abnormal lung exam, or a past history of ACS are at higher risk of ACS when presenting with fever[113]; however, clinical assessment alone is not reliable in identifying ACS (Figure 26-5).[113] Studies have shown that >60% of children will present with a normal lung exam early on,[111,113] requiring high clinical suspicion.[114] The incidence of ACS in febrile children with SCD has decreased from approximately 27% to 17% over the past 20 years,[139] but presenting symptoms in the ED remain similar.[113]

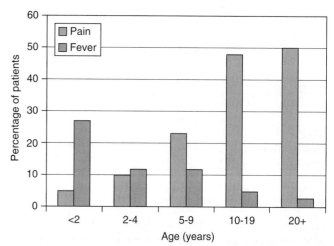

FIGURE 26-4 Age-specific events preceding acute chest syndrome (ACS). Children with sickle cell disease tend to present to the emergency department with fever as a primary symptom of ACS, with children <2 years old at highest risk, whereas adolescents and adults more frequently present with chest or extremity pain, with overlapping symptoms of vaso-occlusive pain. Reproduced with permission Vichinsky EP, Styles LA, Colangelo LH, Wright EC, Castro O, Nickerson B. Acute chest syndrome in sickle cell disease: clinical presentation and course. Cooperative Study of Sickle Cell Disease. *Blood.* 1997;89(5):1787-1792.

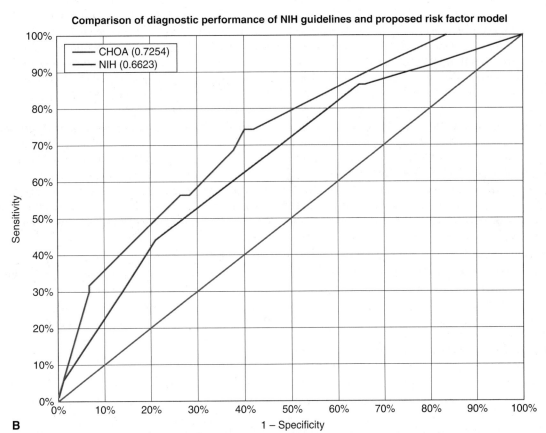

Adjusted point estimates and 95% CI for odds ratios

Model	Odds ratio (95% CI)	P	AUC
CHOA			
History of ACS, yes vs no	2.91 (1.59–5.34)	<0.01	
Chest pain, yes vs no	2.55 (1.16–5.62)	0.02	0.7254
Cough, yes vs no	3.36 (1.59–7.10)	<0.01	
Abnormal lung physical exam, yes vs no	2.35 (1.26–4.36)	<0.01	
NIH guidelines			
Shortness of breath, yes vs no	3.08 (0.85–11.24)	0.09	
Cough, yes vs no	3.35 (1.61–6.95)	<0.01	0.6623
Abnormal breathing (rales), yes vs no	6.26 (0.29–135.60)	0.24	
Tachypnea, yes vs no	1.78 (1.02–3.10)	0.04	

A

Comparison of diagnostic performance of NIH guidelines and proposed risk factor model

B

FIGURE 26-5 Risk factors for acute chest syndrome (ACS). A. Adjusted point estimates and 95% confidence intervals (CIs) for odds ratios comparing risk stratification models recommended by National Heart, Lung, and Blood Institute (NHLBI) of the National Institutes of Health (NIH) compared to Lazarus and colleagues at Children's Healthcare of Atlanta (CHOA). **B.** Comparison of diagnostic performance of NIH guidelines for obtaining a chest radiograph (CXR) in febrile patients with sickle cell disease (SCD) versus proposed CHOA risk factor model. Clinical assessment alone is a poor predictor of ACS. The majority of patients with ACS will have a normal lung exam. In children, a past history of ACS alone is a significant risk factor for repeat ACS presenting with fever. Based on risk stratification by Lazarus and colleagues, any symptom of chest pain, cough, abnormal lung exam, or a past history of ACS is an independent risk factor for ACS, with an area under the curve (AUC) of 0.7254. This is superior to the current NHLBI recommendations for obtaining a CXR with an AUC of 0.6623 (*P* = .04). However, an AUC <0.80 is still insufficient to accurately identify all ACS, and neither are ideal prediction models. Given the mortality and morbidity associated with ACS, emergency department physicians should consider obtaining a CXR for all patients with SCD and fever. Reproduced with permission Lazarus SG, Kelleman M, Adisa O, et al. Are we missing the mark? Fever, respiratory symptoms, chest radiographs, and acute chest syndrome in sickle cell disease. *Am J Hematol.* 2016;91(8):E332-E333.

A routine CXR should be obtained as a standard aspect of a fever workup in SCD, regardless of age, given the high mortality and morbidity.[111,113] Progression to hypoxia, decreasing hemoglobin, increasing lactate dehydrogenase or other biomarkers of increased hemolysis, decreasing platelets, and multilobar pneumonia is a common scenario for ACS, particularly in adults. An acute worsening of obstructive disease and an "asthma-like" syndrome develop in many children with ACS[140] and respond to bronchodilators.[114] It may be difficult to differentiate between symptoms of an asthma exacerbation versus those of ACS. Thus, clinicians should consider treating for both.[141] Almost half of those diagnosed with ACS in the Cooperative Study of Sickle Cell Disease were initially admitted to the hospital for another reason, commonly pain, with a mean hospital stay of 2.5 days before diagnosis of ACS. ACS may also manifest as abdominal pain or back pain. Duration of illness can be prolonged, often 10 to 12 days, and mechanical ventilation is required in 13% of patients. Symptoms of ACS are different in adults and children (Figure 26-4). In addition, the etiology of ACS is varied and includes both viral and bacterial infections, fat embolism from bone marrow ischemia,[142] hypoventilation due to thoracic bone infarction or opiate administration, and thromboembolic events. Infection is a more common trigger in children, whereas pain and pulmonary fat emboli are more common in adults. Pleural effusions are less common in children compared to adults. ACS is often accompanied by a decreasing hemoglobin and platelet count and a significant increase in WBC count, laboratory findings that should alert the evaluating physician to an increased risk of ACS. Complications of ACS are common and include respiratory failure, neurologic events (11% of hospitalizations), altered mental status, seizures, and death.[114] One study examined 84 consecutive hospitalized patients with ACS and found that 13% had clinical manifestations of right heart failure, placing them at the highest risk for mechanical ventilation and death.[143] These data suggest that acute pulmonary hypertension and right heart dysfunction represent major comorbidities during ACS.

Approximately 50% of ACS cases initially present as a VOE with a normal CXR, and one risk factor is preceding limb pain, likely secondary to marrow infarct, which may encourage marrow emboli.[144] Any new CXR infiltrate accompanied by a fever in a person with SCD should be treated as ACS. Management involves rapid delivery of antibiotics to include a cephalosporin (eg, ceftriaxone; see section on fever for more details) and a macrolide to cover the high percentage of atypical bacteria noted in bronchoscopy studies of SCD.[144] If a patient with pneumonia continues to clinically deteriorate, transfusion should be initiated. Early transfusions anecdotally appear to abort or lessen the severity of ACS.[145] Secretory phospholipase A2 (sPLA2) in plasma is an inflammatory mediator felt to be, in part, responsible for the acute lung injury of fat embolism syndrome and may be a unique biomarker of ACS and correlated with clinical severity.[146] Early transfusion was shown to prevent the development of ACS predicted by elevated sPLA2 levels,[145] but the shortcomings of the PROACTIVE feasibility study suggest that more investigation is needed to determine the potential clinical role of sPLA2.[147] Procalcitonin also may be used[148] but requires further investigation.

Some studies have shown that corticosteroids may attenuate the course of ACS in the short term, but rebound pain and increased length of stay with a risk of readmission after discharge have been noted.[149,150] Keeping the oxygenation >92% by nasal cannula is important to decrease the risk of deoxy-HbS polymerization. Incentive spirometry has also shown marked improvement in outcomes.[151] Bilevel positive airway pressure has been used with success as noninvasive ventilation

to support patients with ACS in some institutions[152] and should be considered for clinical deterioration because it might avoid need for intubation. In addition, pain from pleurisy from lung infarction may lead to hypoventilation and atelectasis, a known risk factor of ACS. NS bolus should be avoided unless the patient is showing signs of hypotension or severe dehydration, and maintenance fluids should be restricted given risks of excess fluid overload to contribute to or worsen ACS.[106] Point-of-care lung ultrasound has a reported 95% sensitivity and specificity to identify community-acquired pneumonia in children.[153] Preliminary studies suggest a potential role of lung ultrasound to identify ACS,[154,155] requiring further investigation given the potential to minimize radiation exposure.

Distinguishing ACS from pulmonary embolism in the ED can be challenging in adult patients. Hypoxia and chest pain, elevated D-dimer levels, ventilation/perfusion mismatches, and abnormal CT angiogram findings are common to both conditions. In particular, both ACS and pulmonary thrombosis share findings of pulmonary infarct, and pulmonary thrombosis is present in up to 17% of patients with ACS.[156,157] Patients with SCD are often in a hypercoagulable state,[158] with increased markers of activation of the coagulation system and decreased levels of antithrombotic factors such as protein C and protein S.[159] If a pulmonary embolism is suspected, it should be treated as in a person without SCD. There is no strong evidence to support the use of therapeutic anticoagulation in ACS, although hemostatic activation could contribute to its pathogenesis and pulmonary thrombosis may complicate its course. ACS in SCD is discussed further in Chapter 12.

By adulthood, baseline pulmonary function is abnormal in approximately 90% of patients with SCD.[136] Regardless of the cause, severe pulmonary symptoms require admission and inpatient follow-up and evaluation.

Wheezing and Asthma

Asthma is discussed in more details in Chapter 11. However, asthma is a common comorbid factor in SCD,[160-167] and patients with SCD may present to the ED with wheezing. The incidence of asthma in SCD is much higher than expected compared to rates in the general population, particularly in children.[165] The estimated prevalence of obstructive lung disease in SCD children ranges from 8% to 57%,[168-172] independent of an asthma diagnosis, whereas a restrictive pattern and diffusion defects are more commonly seen in older children and adults.[136,173] Hypoxemia induced by bronchoconstriction and inflammation associated with asthma exacerbations will contribute to HbS polymerization and subsequent complications of SCD, which may further exacerbate hypoxemia in a vicious cycle. Wheezing, intercostal and supraclavicular retractions, cough (worse at night), shortness of breath, and exercise intolerance should alert the ED physician to a possible asthma exacerbation. Triggers are those typical for asthma in non-SCD children: viral upper respiratory infections, cigarette smoke, air pollution, cold temperatures, allergies, pets, and exercise.

Asthma predisposes to complications of SCD, such as pain episodes,[174-178] ACS,[179,180] and stroke,[180] and is associated with increased mortality.[181,182] A randomized controlled trial of inhaled steroids in nonasthmatic patients with SCD demonstrated reduced pain[183] and inflammatory markers,[183,184] highlighting the need for further study. Early recognition and aggressive standard-of-care management of asthma may prevent serious pulmonary complications and reduce mortality. However, data regarding the identification and management of asthma in SCD are limited; adherence to NHLBI guidelines for the treatment of asthma in the general population is recommended.[185-187] It is difficult to clinically differentiate an asthma exacerbation from ACS in children. If unclear, treat for both.[141]

Treatment with aerosolized β-agonists often results in substantial clinical improvement. Maximizing lung oxygenation by treating the bronchoreactive component of the disease may decrease the sickling process and prevent further progression. Concern for rebound symptoms has affected clinical utilization of corticosteroids for wheezing and asthma among many practitioners. However, steroids should not be withheld for asthma when clinically indicated. Patients requiring corticosteroids should be admitted for monitoring and supportive care. A slow taper of corticosteroids over 2 weeks may be necessary and should be done in consultation with a pulmonary specialist familiar with SCD. Many experts use shorter courses (1-2 days) of systemic glucocorticoids to treat asthma exacerbation in patients with SCD because this is thought to reduce the rates of rebound VOE. More details on reactive airway disease in SCD are provided in Chapter 11.

Pulmonary Hypertension

Pulmonary hypertension is an increasingly recognized complication of chronic hemolytic anemias, including SCD, with a prevalence of 6% to 11% (based on mean pressure of ≥25 mm Hg, although the World Health Organization now suggests pulmonary hypertension be defined by pressure ≥20 mm Hg).[188-190] Pulmonary hypertension is associated with 10-fold increased risk of mortality in adults and is linked with increasing age.[191] Clinical implications for children are unknown at this time but under investigation.[182,192-194] An acute increase in pulmonary artery pressures occurs during VOE, ACS, and exercise[43,195] that may be clinically relevant during acute events. Guidelines for the evaluation and treatment of pulmonary hypertension in SCD have recently been developed by a committee commissioned by the American Thoracic Society.[196] For more discussion of pulmonary hypertension, see Chapter 14.

Cardiovascular Complications: Chest Pain, Arrhythmias, and Sudden Death

In the prehydroxyurea era, when life expectancy was much shorter than it is today, atherosclerosis and myocardial infarction were rare among patients with sickle cell anemia.[201] However, as the sickle cell population ages and survives longer, heart abnormalities are becoming more prevalent.[202,203] A complete differential diagnosis for chest pain in the ED is beyond the scope of this chapter but involves prioritization of various diagnoses based on the patient's age and the potential of a missed diagnosis to cause morbidity and mortality.

This general approach to ED chest pain should be modified to accommodate diagnoses that are more likely in SCD such as pulmonary embolism and ACS (discussed earlier in section on pulmonary complications). Cardiac complications, including acute coronary syndromes and acute complications of valvular heart disease, are discussed here. The approach to the SCD patient with chest pain is summarized in Box 26-6.

Acute Coronary Syndromes

Acute focal myocardial ischemia, caused by atherosclerotic heart disease, is rare in SCD, and few publications are available to estimate prevalence or incidence rates. Analysis of national inpatient sample data found a concurrent diagnosis of SCD in 0.02% of admissions for acute myocardial infarction (defined by International Classification of Diseases, 10th Edition codes).[204] Abnormalities in myocardial perfusion, especially during VOE, are common[205-207] in children with SCD, and subclinical myocardial ischemia is thought to contribute to structural heart disease later in life; however, the etiology is not focal atherosclerotic coronary artery occlusion. Cardiac enzyme elevations are not seen in this type of ischemia because it results in myocardial apoptosis in contrast to classic myocardial infarction, which causes necrosis and cell rupture.[208] This type of ischemia, which would manifest as changes in ECG and new focal wall motion abnormality on echocardiogram without cardiac enzyme elevation, should be treated with therapy to reduce sickling (ie, blood transfusion), rather than typical percutaneous coronary interventions. For traditional atherosclerotic acute coronary syndromes, current-generation cardiac troponin testing works well in SCD.[209] Elevated cardiac enzymes should prompt consideration of traditional cardiac interventions such as stenting or balloon angioplasty. We recommend testing for acute coronary syndromes according to guidelines for the general population, including ECG, cardiac enzymes, and further testing guided by the presenting symptoms, age, and risk factors for coronary artery disease.

Structural Heart Disease and Systolic and Diastolic Dysfunction

Anemia lowers the oxygen-carrying capacity of blood, so patients with SCD maintain higher cardiac output but have limited functional reserve to increase output to the heart in conditions of acute stress.[210] Chronically, this leads to cardiomegaly and systolic (left greater than right) dysfunction. Patients with cardiac iron overload may also develop diastolic dysfunction and restrictive cardiomyopathy.[208] In the ED, patients may present acutely with fluid overload from right- or left-sided heart failure. Patients are also at increased risk of iatrogenic fluid overload from blood transfusions or IV fluids; diuretics may be indicated to restore fluid balance. For this reason, BNP (and N-terminal proBNP [NT-proBNP]) levels are useful in the evaluation of chest pain and shortness of breath in the ED.

Sudden Death and Arrhythmia

Up to 41% of patients with SCD die suddenly.[211,212] The etiology of sudden death in SCD is multifactorial, but it is important

Box 26-6	Approach to the Sickle Cell Patient With Chest Pain

Diagnostic Studies

1. A good history and review of systems; evaluate for symptoms suggestive of pulmonary embolism, myocardial ischemia, or pneumonia
2. Pulse oximetry
3. ECG (to evaluate for signs of active ischemia and QTc interval prolongation)
4. CXR (anterior-posterior and lateral)
5. For unstable patients, immediate bedside echocardiography to identify emergent reversible causes (cardiac tamponade, right heart strain, aortic dissection flap)
6. CBC with differential and reticulocyte count
7. Electrolytes and renal function studies
8. Hemolysis labs (lactate dehydrogenase, bilirubin)
9. Troponin
10. BNP or NT-proBNP if available and congestive heart failure is suspected
11. D-dimer may be useful if suspicion for pulmonary embolism is high enough that CT angiography or ventilation/perfusion scan is planned because this may be useful for trending
12. Blood culture if fever is present or there is suspicion for ACS
13. Type and screen/crossmatch in patients with moderate/severe respiratory distress, if ACS is suspected, or if a pneumonia is identified on CXR even without respiratory symptoms because hemoglobin can drop precipitously during ACS
14. Ventilation/perfusion scan or chest CT when significant chest symptoms exist with normal CXR
15. Doppler echocardiography if pulmonary hypertension or congestive heart failure is suspected

Management

1. Obtain IV access and cardiac monitor with pulse oximetry; provide supplemental oxygen if saturation is <92%.
2. Provide aggressive analgesia for VOE, but evaluate frequently for worsening hypoxia and respiratory depression after opioid administration.
3. For patients with pulmonary embolism and myocardial ischemia, admit for further cardiac monitoring and risk stratification (may need intensive care unit).
4. For patients with *confirmed* pulmonary embolism, initiate anticoagulation with unfractionated or low-molecular-weight heparin.
5. For patients with persistent tachycardia, hypoxia, hypotension, or echocardiographic evidence of right heart strain, consult critical care and strongly consider thrombolytics.
6. For patients with renal dysfunction and suspected pulmonary embolism, if vital signs are stable, admission and delayed ventilation/perfusion scan are preferred over emergent CT angiography for pulmonary embolism.
7. For active myocardial ischemia, emergent cardiology consultation is indicated. Unless there is clear evidence of coronary artery occlusion, management should focus on treatment of SCD (ie, transfusion) rather than interventional revascularization.

for the ED physician to consider potentially preventable causes such as ventricular arrhythmias. QTc prolongation is common in SCD and can be caused by pulmonary hypertension and medications. Providers should ensure that a recent QTc measurement (within the past 6 months, or sooner if medications have changed) is on file before administering QT-prolonging medications such as ondansetron, methadone, macrolides, and albuterol, to name a few drugs commonly administered to patients with SCD. Although several factors are known to increase the risk of sudden death in SCD, no studies have evaluated the possible benefits of more intense cardiac monitoring during admission. When placing orders for admission, patients with a prior history of high tricuspid regurgitant jet velocity, ACS, or long QTc interval should be considered for telemetry monitoring.[212]

Neurologic Complications

As a vasculopathy, the CNS of patients with SCD is often affected. Recognition and acute symptom management of certain high-risk complications are important in the ED setting. Neurologic complications in SCD include stroke, headache and migraines, silent cerebral infarcts, meningitis, cerebral venous sinus thrombosis, transient ischemic attacks, posterior reversible encephalopathy, and seizures.[213]

Stroke

Stroke is one of the most devastating complications of SCD and can affect children and adults. Approximately 11% of patients with homozygous SCD (HbSS disease, sickle cell anemia) experienced a stroke by 19 years of age and 24% by 45 years of age in the prescreening era.[214] With transcranial Doppler screening and chronic transfusion protocols, the prevalence has decreased to 1% by late adolescence.[215] Although stroke risk is not increased in African American patients with sickle cell trait,[216] SCD-related ischemic infarcts are the number one reason for stroke in pediatrics and more common in children <10 years old. Hemorrhagic strokes are more common in older patients with SCD, although they may be seen in children with hypertension, aneurysms, and recent blood transfusions or treatment with corticosteroids.[217] Sequelae of recurrent CNS insults may impact patients' cognition and memory, which should be considered in the management of patients with SCD in the ED.[218] Stroke should be considered in the differential diagnosis in any child with SCD who was fully ambulatory and has developed an abnormal gait or refuses to bear weight. Children may also be more likely to present with altered mental status compared to adults.

Many factors are thought to contribute to the risk of stroke in SCD, including vascular pathology such as large-vessel stenosis and moyamoya, abnormal sickle RBC adhesion, endothelial cell dysfunction, and impaired oxygenation in the setting of anemia. Adults may also be at particularly increased risk due to conventional comorbid risk factors such as diabetes, hypertension, and atrial fibrillation.[213] If stroke is suspected in a patient with SCD, immediate neuroimaging is imperative in the workup. Due to time constraints, CT scan should be considered initially, although MRI is preferred when available. If a head CT scan is negative and pretest probability is high for ischemic stroke, MRI should be obtained. Magnetic resonance with arteriography or venography should be considered in the appropriate setting (ie, if there is concern for significant large-vessel vasculopathy or cerebral venous sinus thrombosis, respectively). If there is substantial delay in obtaining neuroimaging and the suspicion for stroke is high, initiation of transfusion therapy (simple vs exchange) should be considered in the ED.

Initial evaluation for neurologic symptoms should include baseline laboratory studies that include point-of-care testing for hypoglycemia, electrolytes, CBC, type and crossmatch (see transfusion section for specific blood orders for transfusion), and determination of the percentage of HbS hemoglobin in the peripheral blood.[215] Treatment of stroke includes neurology consultation, blood pressure control, and airway management. Rapid consultations with hematology and the blood bank is imperative because the mainstay of therapy for ischemic stroke in SCD is exchange transfusion. The goal is to substantially reduce HbS and improve oxygenation to the CNS.[219] Simple transfusion should be considered when an exchange is not emergently feasible, taking care not to increase the patient's hemoglobin to >10 g/dL because this can lead to hyperviscosity and further neurologic injury.[215] Data on the use of thrombolytics in the setting of ischemic stroke in SCD are limited.[220] The risk of symptomatic hemorrhagic transformation is theoretical and not substantiated by a retrospective analysis.[221] Because the use of thrombolytics, such as tissue plasminogen activator, has not been prospectively studied in patients with SCD and ischemic stroke, its use should be in accordance with institutional guidelines and in consultation with a neurologist

---

Box 26-7 | Approach to the Sickle Cell Patient With Possible Stroke

Diagnostic Studies

1. Emergent head CT (without contrast)
2. Head MRI if available
3. Lumbar puncture if meningitis is suspected
4. Arteriography in follow-up for stroke to more fully evaluate cerebral infarction

Management

1. Start parenteral hydration immediately.
2. Initiate emergent exchange transfusion, with goal to lower HbS level to 30%.
3. Simple transfusion is not recommended due to concerns of hyperviscosity.
4. Initiate seizure control as clinically warranted.
5. Pharmacologic agents to decrease cerebral edema should be considered if the patient becomes somnolent or if edema is confirmed on imaging.
6. Provide neurosurgical and neurologic consultation early on.
7. Long-term chronic transfusions are necessary for secondary prevention, particularly in children.
8. Thromboembolic agents for ischemic stroke have not been evaluated in SCD.

---

and hematologist. The approach to the SCD patient with a possible stroke is summarized in Box 26-7.

Ocular Complications

Several ocular conditions related to SCD may be seen in the ED setting. Traumatic hyphema, or grossly visible blood in the anterior chamber of the eye, is typically the result of trauma or surgery and can result in permanent vision loss. The risk of complications increases in patients with a large amount of blood in the anterior chamber, which is an ocular emergency in patients with SCD as well as those with sickle cell trait[222] (Figure 26-6). Low partial pressure of oxygen (Po_2) and low pH in the aqueous humor can trigger acute vaso-occlusion of RBCs, even in a patient with sickle trait, which can subsequently block the flow of aqueous humor, leading to sharp increases in intraocular pressure. Permanent ischemic damage to the optic nerve may occur within 24 hours. Given the high risk of morbidity, a rapid hemoglobin solubility blood test (Sickledex; Streck Labs) should be checked in all patients with a hyphema, even those without known SCD, because many individuals are unaware of their sickle trait status. Some children's hospitals have access to patients' newborn screening test results, which is an alternative to performing a Sickledex test if newborn screening is negative for SCD or sickle trait.

Due to abnormal rheologic properties and hypercoagulability often encountered in patients with SCD, hyphemas may be

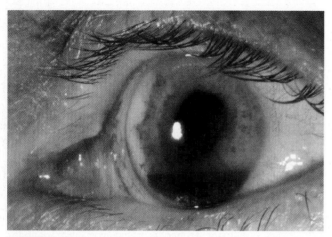

FIGURE 26-6 **Hyphema.** Blood in the anterior chamber of the eye, usually caused by trauma, is an ophthalmologic emergency in patients with sickle cell disease or sickle trait. Photograph provided and used with permission by Sean Grout, OCT-C (The Kittner Eye Center, University of North Carolina School of Medicine, Chapel Hill, NC).

associated with development of acute narrow-angle glaucoma, rebleeding into the hyphema, and complications such as optic nerve atrophy and central retinal artery occlusion. All patients with eye trauma and SCD should have a detailed history obtained, as well as visual acuity and visual field testing, slit-lamp examination, intraocular pressure measurements, and consideration for emergent ophthalmologic consultation. An open-globe injury must be excluded before any examination or procedure that might create pressure to the eyeball, including tonometry, is performed. It should be noted, however, that increased intraocular pressures may be seen in the presence of trauma even without a hyphema.[223] The majority of hyphemas will resolve with medical management alone; however, approximately 5% of traumatic hyphemas will require surgery.[224-226]

Other ophthalmologic emergencies in SCD result from ischemia and perfusion injuries to the eye and include vitreous hemorrhage as a consequence of neovascularization of the retina, ophthalmic artery or vein occlusion, and ischemic optic neuropathy.[227-229] The treatment of these maladies often includes improving oxygenation and reducing HbS, which can be accomplished with simple blood transfusion or erythrocytapheresis in consultation with hematologists and transfusion experts. Additional treatments for traumatic hyphema and other ocular emergencies should be considered in consultation with an ophthalmologist and may include the following[225,230]: placement of the patient in supine position with the head of the bed elevated 30 to 45 degrees and an eye shield placed to prevent further trauma; treatment of acute angle closure glaucoma if intraocular pressure is ≥24 mm Hg with timolol (other agents such as pilocarpine, brimonidine, apraclonidine, or dorzolamide should be considered as second or third agents); and strong consideration for admission for close monitoring and serial intraocular pressure measurements. Although not specifically trialed in the setting of SCD, the antifibrinolytic agent ε-aminocaproic acid may be associated with decreased incidence of secondary hemorrhage.[225] Ophthalmic complications of SCD are covered in detail in Chapter 20. The approach to the SCD patient with hyphema is summarized in Box 26-8.

| **Box 26-8** | **Approach to the Sickle Cell Patient With Hyphema** |

Management

1. Place patient in supine position, with head elevated 30 to 45 degrees, and use an eye shield to prevent further trauma.

2. Provide topical analgesia with a drop of proparacaine or tetracaine eye drops in patients without a globe rupture.

3. Treat nausea and/or vomiting with antiemetics (ondansetron) to minimize increased intraocular pressure.

4. Treat for acute angle closure glaucoma for intraocular pressure ≥24 mm Hg with timolol 0.5% ophthalmic twice a day. Pilocarpine 2% (1 drop every 15 minutes) should also be used. Management for persistent elevation of intraocular pressure should be determined in consultation with ophthalmologist.

5. Avoid NSAIDS because they may increase risk of rebleeding.

6. Provide emergent ophthalmologic consultation.

7. Admit to the hospital.

Abdominal Complications

Abdominal Pain

Abdominal pain in SCD may be the manifestation of uncomplicated VOE, but other causes include constipation, which occurs frequently in patients on chronic opioids, splenic sequestration in the pediatric patient, splenic or renal infarction, or sequelae of sickle hepatopathy. Also considered in the differential diagnosis should be other common causes of abdominal pain in the non-SCD patient, including appendicitis, urinary tract infection, acute gastroenteritis, pancreatitis, pelvic inflammatory disease or pregnancy in fertile females, kidney stones, gastroesophageal reflux, and gastritis, among others. The ED workup should be directed accordingly. Vomiting and/or diarrhea may be associated with abdominal pain and may help guide the differential diagnosis. However, nausea and vomiting may also be side effects of opioids given to treat the pain. Ondansetron (if QTc on ECG is normal) should be considered to treat nausea/vomiting while an etiology of the symptoms is sought. Patients who are vomiting should be assessed for dehydration and should receive an IV fluid bolus when dehydration or significant fluid losses through vomiting, diarrhea, or poor oral intake of fluids are noted. Heart rate is not an ideal measure of dehydration because tachycardia may not always be present early on; urine output and capillary refill are more helpful. The ideal IV fluid to use in SCD is currently unknown,[109] but 20 mL/kg of NS or lactated Ringer's solution is commonly used for children who are hypovolemic, whereas no more than 1 L of fluid should be given to an adult patient unless managing hypotension and/or sepsis.

Hepatobiliary Dysfunction

Sickle hepatopathy may include cholelithiasis/cholecystitis in the setting of pigment stone formation from chronic hemolysis, acute (on chronic) hepatitis in the setting of blood transfusions and secondary hemochromatosis, hepatic sequestration or infarction, or other common diagnoses seen in patients without SCD.[231-233]

Sickle hepatopathy includes both acute and chronic hepatobiliary complications and can present differently in adult and pediatric patients.[234-236] Acute hepatic sequestration is a clinical emergency and may present with sudden liver enlargement and a ≥2 g/dL decrease in hemoglobin from baseline.[237] Patients with acute liver or cholestatic pathology such as acute intrahepatic cholestasis may have sudden right upper quadrant pain, jaundice or scleral icterus out of proportion to baseline, light-colored stools, mild or markedly elevated liver function tests with extreme hyperbilirubinemia, and thrombocytopenia or coagulation abnormalities.[238]

Imaging studies, such as ultrasound, abdominal CT, or MRI, should be performed in all patients with significant abdominal pain and worrisome findings on liver function tests. Choosing studies that minimize radiation exposure should be considered as part of the medical decision-making process, although this may not always be feasible. Acute cholecystitis should be treated with antibiotics and surgical consultation. Per the NHLBI guidelines, if surgery is needed, consultation with a hematologist should be obtained for possible preoperative blood transfusions to prevent postoperative complications.[49] Patients with acute hepatic sequestration or acute intrahepatic cholestasis may also benefit from exchange transfusion.

Genitourinary Complications

It should be noted that patients with SCD often have a urine-concentrating defect that begins early in childhood. They also tend to have relatively low serum creatinine and blood urea nitrogen levels, likely due to a high glomerular filtration rate along with a high rate of creatinine secretion in the distal tubules.[239] Therefore, a mildly elevated creatinine level >1.0 mg/dL is not normal and warrants further evaluation, especially if it is higher than previous values. NSAIDs should be used with caution in such patients, and in consultation with hematology, considering risks versus benefits.

Hematuria

The kidney can be a harsh environment for sickle RBCs, whereby abrupt changes in osmolarity and pH can lead to repeated VOEs in the renal vasculature and result in renal infarcts.[70,240] When severe, such infarcts in the renal medulla or papillary structures can lead to flank pain mimicking pyelonephritis and result in microscopic or gross hematuria that can sometimes lead to significant anemia. When suspected, patients should be treated with hypotonic IV fluids at maintenance and analgesics, avoiding the use of NSAIDs. Imaging should be performed in adults to rule out renal medullary carcinoma, an aggressive kidney malignancy primarily found in patients with sickle cell trait or SCD.[241] The differential diagnosis of gross hematuria also includes urinary tract infection, a common cause of hematuria in non-SCD patients; urethritis; trauma; glomerulonephritis; and renal calculi. Although it occurs more frequently in adults, hematuria is an uncommon problem in children with SCD and

should be evaluated acutely when present, including consultation with hematology and nephrology.

Proteinuria

Macro- and microalbuminuria are also common in adults with SCD and may be associated with hypertension. Proteinuria may be noted on urinalysis but is typically not an acute problem requiring attention in the ED setting. There is a high prevalence of chronic kidney disease in patients with SCD, which is associated with intravascular hemolysis[242] and will be discussed in detail in Chapter 16.

Priapism

Priapism is an undesirable and often painful erection experienced by approximately 35% to 40% of men and adolescent boys with SCD.[243] Repeated episodes of priapism can lead to permanent damage and erectile dysfunction. Priapism in SCD can be separated into 2 subtypes: low-flow and high-flow. High-flow, nonischemic priapism is rare in patients with SCD, typically results from trauma and disruption in arterial blood flow to the corpora cavernosa, and often self-resolves without a visit to the ED. Low-flow, veno-occlusive priapism accounts for the majority of episodes in SCD and results from venous outflow obstruction in the corpora cavernosa, leading to a reduction in blood flow within the penile arteries and subsequent tissue ischemia and intense pain.[244]

The mechanism of SCD-related priapism is likely multifactorial but includes hemolysis-mediated dysregulation of the arginine–nitric oxide signaling pathway, downregulated phosphodiesterase 5 protein expression, and dysregulation of adenosine-mediated vasodilation in the penis.[245-251] Depletion of nitric oxide through chronic hemolysis with cell-free hemoglobin scavenging and increased intravascular arginase is thought to play a role.[247,252] Triggers of priapism are often unknown but may be associated with VOE, dehydration, or sexual intercourse. Most instances of ischemic priapism are brief, recurrent episodes (stuttering priapism) that are self-limited and last from several minutes to hours. However, males with SCD are often educated by their sickle cell providers to seek emergency medical attention once the painful priapism episode lasts ≥4 hours given the increased risk of penile compartment syndrome associated with irreversible damage and permanent erectile dysfunction when episodes last >6 hours.[244]

Hematologists will often counsel male patients to try oral pseudoephedrine at home based on anecdotal experiences.[253] However, urology experts believe it is unlikely that oral phenylephrine will be successful in the emergent treatment of priapism and may add to the effect of injected phenylephrine and theoretically increase the possibility of hypertension if both were used. Although pseudoephedrine was not recommended by the 2003 consensus of the American Urological Society recommendation,[254] it is not contraindicated and may be considered in the ED if not already taken prior to arrival. Treatment options for priapism in SCD are limited and not evidence based, including hydration, alkalization, analgesia, oxygen supplementation, and exchange transfusion.[246,255-257] A 2017 Cochrane Database analysis found a lack of evidence for the benefits or risks of treatment options, including stilbestrol, sildenafil, and ephedrine, compared to placebo.[255] Because treatment is influenced by observational studies and case reports, NHLBI guideline recommendations are based on low-quality evidence and expert opinion.[49] Episodes lasting >4 hours should be considered a urologic emergency, and patients should be immediately triaged in the ED and treated conservatively with oral or IV analgesics and hydration, similar to treatment for VOE. Anxiolytics may be helpful to reduce stress from anticipated pain. Penile aspiration and α-agonist injection may be considered, but further treatment should truly be guided by urology consultation if conservative management does not significantly improve the priapism.

Case reports have described a therapeutic benefit from oral α-adrenergic agonists such as pseudoephedrine, phosphodiesterase 5 inhibitors such as sildenafil,[247,248,258] IV arginine,[249] and IV ketamine,[259] but controlled trials are lacking. A recent pediatric case series suggests inhaled nitrous oxide gas may represent a novel treatment option for priapism in the ED.[253] Nitrous oxide gas is an inhalational medication that has anxiolytic, amnestic, potent venodilatory, and mild to moderate analgesic properties and is frequently used in the ED setting.[260,261] It also has a rapid onset of action (<5 minutes) and recovery (<5 minutes) and can help facilitate IV placement. Of interest, it has been used in France for patients with SCD and VOE not initially responding to IV opioids.[262]

If priapism persists despite initial conservative measures, a urologist may need to perform needle aspiration and corporal irrigation with an α-adrenergic agent such as epinephrine. RBC transfusions are not helpful for acute priapism episodes. However, if surgical intervention (ie, shunting) is needed, a hematologist should be consulted for potential perioperative simple or exchange transfusion management recommendations. Priapism is presented in more detail in Chapter 19.

Pregnancy

Women with SCD have a 6-fold increased risk of maternal death compared to those without SCD, as well as increased risk for other obstetric complications including preterm births, preeclampsia, stillbirths, and infants who are small for gestational age.[263,264] These complications may be related to placental infarcts. Other complications, including a higher incidence of VOE, thromboembolic events, and postoperative complications after cesarean section, may also occur.[265] Because patients with SCD may have proteinuria, elevated liver enzymes, and hypertension at baseline, surveillance for many pregnancy-related complications can be challenging. Pain from SCD may worsen during pregnancy for some women. Opioids are not contraindicated in pregnancy, but NSAIDs should be avoided. Any complex presentation of a pregnant woman with SCD mandates experienced obstetrics consultation with or without hematology involvement.

Skin Complaints: Leg Ulcers

Leg ulcers are a chronic symptom for some patients with SCD.[266] Although the mainstay treatment for leg ulcers is prevention, patients with SCD may present to the ED due to severe pain or signs of superimposed infection at the site of ulceration. Due to evidence of venostasis in the ulcer bed and with SCD being a vasculopathy, concomitant venous thromboembolism should also be considered in the appropriate setting.[267] After a thorough exam and history (including evaluating for trauma and complaints of changes in pain, smell, or swelling), imaging may be necessary to rule out osteomyelitis. Other comorbidities that may predispose to ulceration, such as diabetes, should be considered. Cultures of the ulcer are of variable utility and may just reveal skin colonization. A therapeutic trial of antibiotics covering common skin flora may reduce ulcers, but if this has been unsuccessful, evaluation for *Pseudomonas* or methicillin-resistant *Staphylococcus aureus* should be undertaken. Patients with symptoms of bacteremia should be admitted, and consultations to infectious disease and wound specialists may be warranted if specialists are available. Although there are no reports of acute efficacy, benefits have been reported with topical sodium nitrite paste[268,269] and arginine therapy,[270-273] whereas peripheral blood stem cell transplantation was associated with healing in a pilot study.[274,275] Leg ulcers are covered extensively in Chapter 4.

Transfusions

Due to the heterogeneity of SCD, clinical manifestations that may vary with age, and other comorbid underlying chronic disease states, patients will have variable baseline hemoglobin levels. The use of RBC transfusions in the ED for acute complications related to SCD is rarely indicated, but when it is, patients should be matched for C, E, and Kell antigens if at all possible. Recommended specific requirements for ordering blood for transfusion are summarized in Boxes 26-9 and 26-10. Furthermore,

---

Box 26-9 | Approach to the Patient With SCD Needing Transfusion

Management

1. Ascertain transfusion history and frequency, amounts of blood transfused, and history of transfusion reactions.

2. Calculate the number of milliliters needed to obtain a posttransfusion hemoglobin of 8 to 9 mg/dL without exceeding 11.5 mg/dL. Round to the nearest number of units (approximately 250-300 mL of RBCs/unit).

3. If a patient with a high hemoglobin needs transfusion for a nonanemia indication, then exchange transfusion is needed, and hematologic consultation is required.

4. Order leukoreduced, HbS-negative RBCs matched for Kell, C, and E antigens. If these units are not available, hematologic consultation is needed to find the most compatible units

5. Premedication before transfusions is not standardized, but often oral acetaminophen 650 mg and diphenhydramine 50 mg are common. Loratadine 10 mg orally can also be given as premedication for pruritus. With adults, furosemide 20 mg IV is often given if the number of units exceeds 2 or if vascular congestion, dyspnea, or high blood pressure develops during transfusions.

Box 26-10	Summary of Recommendations for Transfusion Therapy for Patients With SCD in the ED	
Blood bank order specifications for SCD		**Indications for acute therapeutic transfusion**
◆ Order type and screen/crossmatch (ie, indirect Coombs)		◆ Stroke
◆ Order crossmatch units that are:		◆ Splenic sequestration
• ABO/Rh(D) compatible		◆ Aplastic crisis
• Rh (C/c, E/e) and K antigen matched		◆ Acute chest syndrome
• Leukoreduced		◆ Multisystem organ failure
• HbS negative		◆ Hepatopathy
• Extended antigen match (eg, Kidd, Duffy) if patient has history of alloantibodies		◆ Emergent preoperative state
◆ Order direct Coombs (direct antiglobulin test) for all patients if there is concern for delayed hemolytic transfusion reaction		◆ Severe symptomatic anemia
		◆ Severe hemolysis (ie, delayed hemolytic transfusion reaction)
		◆ Severe bleeding

Note. Some centers also routinely irradiate blood units because eligibility for stem cell transplantation for SCD is expanding.

although the decision to provide an emergent transfusion for severely ill patients should be left to clinical judgement, the use of RBC transfusions in nonill patients should be done in consultation with the blood bank and/or hematologist. The dangers of unnecessary and inappropriately matched transfusion include infection, alloimmunization, iron overload, and delayed hemolytic transfusion reaction. In addition, raising the hematocrit unnecessarily in patients with SCD can increase the risk of hyperviscosity, reduced cerebral blood flow, and stroke.[276-278] Transfusion medicine topics are discussed further in Chapter 23.

Conclusion

For decades, the care of patients with SCD has focused on early diagnosis and prevention of complications through prophylactic antibiotics, transfusions, and US Food and Drug Administration–approved drugs such as hydroxyurea. More recently, significant progress has been made toward a cure through advances in bone marrow transplant and gene therapy research. However, the acute treatment of SCD complications in the ED has remained suboptimal[279] and a neglected area of research. In recognition of the need to improve the care offered to patients with SCD in the ED, the American College of Emergency Physicians, in collaboration with multiple public, private, and professional partners, has recently created the Emergency Department Sickle Cell Care Coalition (EDSC[3]). Its purpose is to provide a national forum dedicated to the improvement of the emergency care of patients with SCD in the United States. The primary objective of the EDSC[3] is to promote evidence-based emergency care and optimize provider-patient-family communication in the delivery of the emergency care for patients with SCD. Its focus includes dissemination of research findings locally and nationally, education of ED providers and patients regarding appropriate management of SCD-related pain and other complications, advocacy, community outreach, and health care performance in order to develop appropriate metrics to improve emergency care. A strong partnership between emergency medicine physicians and hematologists will lead to the best outcomes for patients with SCD requiring emergency care and will ultimately move the field forward.

Case Study

A 3-year-old boy with hemoglobin SS disease presented to the ED after 3 days of limping and difficulty bearing weight on his right leg. There was no history of trauma. On exam, he was afebrile and had no pain with manipulation of the right leg. Past medical history included normal transcranial Doppler studies at 2- and 3-year check-ups with his sickle cell provider. A CBC showed a hemoglobin of 8.0 g/dL (baseline) with an absolute reticulocyte count of 13%, whereas the WBC and platelet counts were within normal range. An x-ray of the right hip and leg demonstrated no evidence of fracture or arthritis. CT of the head was unremarkable. A sedated MRI/magnetic resonance angiography of the brain demonstrated numerous T2-hyperintense lesions in the left-sided cerebral white matter with narrowing of the supraclinoid internal carotid artery on the left side. In consultation with transfusion medicine and the hematology team, he was type and crossmatched and started on a simple transfusion with 10 mL/kg of packed RBCs matched for Rh D, C, and E and Kell while being admitted to the pediatric intensive care unit for an exchange transfusion with a goal HbS of <30%. Always consider stroke in your differential diagnosis when evaluating a patient with SCD.

> ## High-Yield Facts
>
> ### Children Are Not Small Adults[a]
>
> ◆ Fever is a more common presentation of ACS in children; pain is more common in adults.
>
> ◆ Splenic sequestration is a life-threatening cause of acute anemia in young children prior to spleen autoinfarction, which typically occurs by age 5 years. Sequestration can also occur in adults with milder SCD phenotypes (eg, HbSC and HbS-β⁺ thalassemia).
>
> ◆ Young infants and children ≤5 years old are at high risk for sepsis, pneumonia, meningitis, and osteomyelitis due to functional asplenia.
>
> ◆ Children between 2 and 10 years of age are at highest risk for stroke: headaches and neurologic symptoms should trigger a careful evaluation for stroke.
>
> ◆ Dactylitis is one of the earliest manifestations of SCD; it is typically seen in infants <6 months but can occur through age 4.
>
> ◆ Pain should be managed aggressively regardless of age; children may not verbalize pain as well as adults.
>
> ◆ Asthma is very common in children with SCD; loss of reversibility and restrictive lung disease develop in adulthood.
>
> ---
>
> [a]*Reproduced with permission, from Morris CR. Sickle cell emergencies. In: Wang NE, ed.* Manual of Pediatric Emergency Medicine. *Cambridge University Press; 2011:360-369.*

> ## High-Yield Facts
>
> ### Symptoms Warranting Emergent Medical Attention[a]
>
> ◆ Signs of infection: fever >101°F, cough, tachypnea, respiratory difficulty, irritability, feeding difficulties
>
> ◆ Signs of severe anemia: pallor, scleral icterus or jaundice (more than baseline), lethargy, weakness
>
> ◆ Signs indicating possible dehydration: vomiting, diarrhea, oliguria/fewer wet diapers
>
> ◆ Signs of stroke: headache, altered level of consciousness, focal deficits, abnormal neurologic exam
>
> ◆ Moderate/severe pain
>
> ◆ Other signs: abdominal pain or organomegaly, dactylitis, screams when touched (infants/children)
>
> ---
>
> [a]*Reproduced with permission, from Morris CR. Sickle cell emergencies. In: Wang NE, ed.* Manual of Pediatric Emergency Medicine. *Cambridge University Press; 2011:360-369.*

References

1. Hassell KL. Population estimates of sickle cell disease in the U.S. *Am J Prev Med.* 2010;38(4 suppl):S512-S521.
2. Piel FB, Patil AP, Howes RE, et al. Global epidemiology of sickle haemoglobin in neonates: a contemporary geostatistical model-based map and population estimates. *Lancet.* 2013;381(9861):142-151.
3. Kato GJ, Piel FB, Reid CD, et al. Sickle cell disease. *Nat Rev Dis Primers.* 2018;4:18010.
4. Piel FB, Steinberg MH, Rees DC. Sickle cell disease. *N Engl J Med.* 2017;377(3):305.
5. Quinn CT, Rogers ZR, McCavit TL, Buchanan GR. Improved survival of children and adolescents with sickle cell disease. *Blood.* 2010;115(17):3447-3452.
6. Ballas SK. New era dawns on sickle cell pain. *Blood.* 2010;116(3):311-312.
7. Tamayo-Sarver JH, Hinze SW, Cydulka RK, Baker DW. Racial and ethnic disparities in emergency department analgesic prescription. *Am J Public Health.* 2003;93(12):2067-2073.
8. Richardson LD, Babcock Irvin C, Tamayo-Sarver JH. Racial and ethnic disparities in the clinical practice of emergency medicine. *Acad Emerg Med.* 2003;10(11):1184-1188.
9. Fiscella K, Franks P, Gold MR, Clancy CM. Inequality in quality: addressing socioeconomic, racial, and ethnic disparities in health care. *JAMA.* 2000;283(19):2579-2584.
10. Lazio MP, Costello HH, Courtney DM, et al. A comparison of analgesic management for emergency department patients with sickle cell disease and renal colic. *Clin J Pain.* 2010;26(3):199-205.

11. Glassberg J, Tanabe P, Richardson L, Debaun M. Among emergency physicians, use of the term "sickler" is associated with negative attitudes toward people with sickle cell disease. *Am J Hematol.* 2013;88(6):532-533.

12. Glassberg JA, Tanabe P, Chow A, et al. Emergency provider analgesic practices and attitudes toward patients with sickle cell disease. *Ann Emerg Med.* 2013;62(4):293-302.e210.

13. Lanzkron S, Carroll CP, Haywood C Jr. The burden of emergency department use for sickle-cell disease: an analysis of the national emergency department sample database. *Am J Hematol.* 2010;85(10):797-799.

14. Brousseau DC, Owens PL, Mosso AL, Panepinto JA, Steiner CA. Acute care utilization and rehospitalizations for sickle cell disease. *JAMA.* 2010;303(13):1288-1294.

15. Paulukonis ST, Harris WT, Coates TD, et al. Population based surveillance in sickle cell disease: methods, findings and implications from the California registry and surveillance system in hemoglobinopathies project (RuSH). *Pediatr Blood Cancer.* 2014;61(12):2271-2276.

16. Blinder MA, Duh MS, Sasane M, Trahey A, Paley C, Vekeman F. Age-related emergency department reliance in patients with sickle cell disease. *J Emerg Med.* 2015;49(4):513-522.e511.

17. Glassberg JA. Improving emergency department-based care of sickle cell pain. *Hematology Am Soc Hematol Educ Program.* 2017;2017(1):412-417.

18. Pearson HA, Gallagher D, Chilcote R, et al. Developmental pattern of splenic dysfunction in sickle cell disorders. *Pediatrics.* 1985;76(3):392-397.

19. Bunn HF. Pathogenesis and treatment of sickle cell disease. *N Engl J Med.* 1997;337(11):762-769.

20. Stuart MJ, Nagel RL. Sickle-cell disease. *Lancet.* 2004;364(9442):1343-1360.

21. Platt OS, Brambilla DJ, Rosse WF, et al. Mortality in sickle cell disease. Life expectancy and risk factors for early death. *N Engl J Med.* 1994;330(23):1639-1644.

22. Leikin SL, Gallagher D, Kinney TR, Sloane D, Klug P, Rida W. Mortality in children and adolescents with sickle cell disease. Cooperative Study of Sickle Cell Disease. *Pediatrics.* 1989;84(3):500-508.

23. Sebastiani P, Nolan VG, Baldwin CT, et al. A network model to predict the risk of death in sickle cell disease. *Blood.* 2007;110(7):2727-2735.

24. Vichinsky E, Lubin BH. Suggested guidelines for the treatment of children with sickle cell anemia. *Hematol Oncol Clin North Am.* 1987;1(3):483-501.

25. Vichinsky EP. Sickle cell disease. In: Schwartz GR, ed. *Principles and Practice of Emergency Medicine.* Lea & Febiger; 1992:2019-2025.

26. Freeman L. Sickle cell disease and other hemoglobinopathies: approaches to emergency diagnosis and treatment. *Emerg Med Pract.* 2001;3:1-24.

27. Vichinsky E. Comprehensive care in sickle cell disease: its impact on morbidity and mortality. *Semin Hematol.* 1991;28:220.

28. Hoppe C, Styles L, Vichinsky E. The natural history of sickle cell disease. *Curr Opin Pediatr.* 1998;10(1):49-52.

29. Gill FM, Sleeper LA, Weiner SJ, et al. Clinical events in the first decade in a cohort of infants with sickle cell disease. *Blood.* 1995;86(2):776-783.

30. Tanabe P, Artz N, Mark Courtney D, et al. Adult emergency department patients with sickle cell pain crisis: a learning collaborative model to improve analgesic management. *Acad Emerg Med.* 2010;17(4):399-407.

31. Yusuf HR, Atrash HK, Grosse SD, Parker CS, Grant AM. Emergency department visits made by patients with sickle cell disease: a descriptive study, 1999-2007. *Am J Prev Med.* 2010;38(4 suppl):S536-S541.

32. Haywood C Jr, Lanzkron S, Ratanawongsa N, et al. The association of provider communication with trust among adults with sickle cell disease. *J Gen Intern Med.* 2010;25(6):543-548.

33. Zempsky WT. Treatment of sickle cell pain: fostering trust and justice. *JAMA.* 2009;302(22):2479-2480.

34. Shapiro BS, Benjamin LJ, Payne R, Heidrich G. Sickle cell-related pain: perceptions of medical practitioners. *J Pain Symptom Manage.* 1997;14(3):168-174.

35. Ballas SK, Gupta K, Adams-Graves P. Sickle cell pain: a critical reappraisal. *Blood.* 2012;120(18):3647-3656.

36. Tran H, Gupta M, Gupta K. Targeting novel mechanisms of pain in sickle cell disease. *Blood.* 2017;130(22):2377-2385.

37. Embury SH. The not-so-simple process of sickle cell vasoocclusion. *Microcirculation.* 2004;11(2):101-113.

38. Savitt TL, Smith WR, Haywood C, Creary MS. Use of the word "crisis" in sickle cell disease: the language of sickle cell. *J Natl Med Assoc.* 2014;106(1):23-30.

39. Benjamin LJ, Swinson GI, Nagel RL. Sickle cell anemia day hospital: an approach for the management of uncomplicated painful crises. *Blood.* 2000;95(4):1130-1136.

40. Wright J, Bareford D, Wright C, et al. Day case management of sickle pain: 3 years experience in a UK sickle cell unit. *Br J Haematol.* 2004;126(6):878-880.

41. Tanabe P, Myers R, Zosel A, et al. Emergency department management of acute pain episodes in sickle cell disease. *Acad Emerg Med.* 2007;14(5):419-425.

42. Platt OS, Thorington BD, Brambilla DJ, et al. Pain in sickle cell disease. Rates and risk factors. *N Engl J Med.* 1991;325(1):11-16.

43. Dampier C, Ely E, Eggleston B, Brodecki D, O'Neal P. Physical and cognitive-behavioral activities used in the home management of sickle pain: a daily diary study in children and adolescents. *Pediatr Blood Cancer.* 2004;43(6):674-678.

44. Smith WR, Penberthy LT, Bovbjerg VE, et al. Daily assessment of pain in adults with sickle cell disease. *Ann Intern Med.* 2008;148(2):94-101.

45. Hockenberry MJ, Wilson D. *Wong's Essentials of Pediatric Nursing.* 8th ed. Mosby; 2009.

46. Breivik EK, Bjornsson GA, Skovlund E. A comparison of pain rating scales by sampling from clinical trial data. *Clin J Pain.* 2000;16(1):22-28.

47. McClish DK, Smith WR, Dahman BA, et al. Pain site frequency and location in sickle cell disease: the PiSCES project. *Pain.* 2009;145(1-2):246-251.

48. Curtis SA, Danda N, Etzion Z, Cohen HW, Billett HH. Elevated steady state WBC and platelet counts are associated with frequent emergency room use in adults with sickle cell anemia. *PloS One.* 2015;10(8):e0133116.

49. Yawn BP, Buchanan GR, Afenyi-Annan AN, et al. Management of sickle cell disease: summary of the 2014 evidence-based report by expert panel members. *JAMA.* 2014;312(10):1033-1048.

50. P Goddu A, O'Conor KJ, Lanzkron S, et al. Do words matter? Stigmatizing language and the transmission of bias in the medical record. *J Gen Intern Med.* 2018;33(5):685-691.

51. Haywood C Jr, Lanzkron S, Hughes MT, et al. A video-intervention to improve clinician attitudes toward patients with sickle cell disease: the results of a randomized experiment. *J Gen Intern Med.* 2011;26(5):518-523.

52. Hoffman KM, Trawalter S, Axt JR, Oliver MN. Racial bias in pain assessment and treatment recommendations, and false beliefs about biological differences between blacks and whites. *Proc Natl Acad Sci U S A.* 2016;113(16):4296-4301.

53. Solomon LR. Treatment and prevention of pain due to vaso-occlusive crises in adults with sickle cell disease: an educational void. *Blood.* 2008;111(3):997-1003.

54. Elander J, Lusher J, Bevan D, Telfer P. Pain management and symptoms of substance dependence among patients with sickle cell disease. *Soc Sci Med.* 2003;57(9):1683-1696.

55. Glassberg J. Evidence-based management of sickle cell disease in the emergency department. *Emerg Med Pract.* 2011;13(8):1-20; quiz 20.

56. Dowell D, Haegerich TM, Chou R. CDC guideline for prescribing opioids for chronic pain–United States, 2016. *MMWR Recomm Rep.* 2016;65(1):1-49.

57. Akinsola B, Hagbom R, Zmitrovich A, et al. Impact of intranasal fentanyl in nurse initiated protocols for sickle cell vaso-occlusive pain episodes in a pediatric emergency department. *Am J Hematol.* 2018; doi: 10.1002/ajh.25144.

58. Kavanagh PL, Sprinz PG, Wolfgang TL, et al. Improving the management of vaso-occlusive episodes in the pediatric emergency department. *Pediatrics.* 2015;136(4):e1016-e1025.

59. Fein DM, Avner JR, Scharbach K, Manwani D, Khine H. Intranasal fentanyl for initial treatment of vaso-occlusive crisis in sickle cell disease. *Pediatr Blood Cancer.* 2017;64:6.

60. Tanabe P, Silva S, Bosworth HB, et al. A randomized controlled trial comparing two vaso-occlusive episode (VOE) protocols in sickle cell disease (SCD). *Am J Hematol.* 2018;93(2):159-168.

61. Schefft MR, Swaffar C, Newlin J, Noda C, Sisler I. A novel approach to reducing admissions for children with sickle cell disease in pain crisis through individualization and standardization in the emergency department. *Pediatr Blood Cancer.* 2018;65(10):e27274.

62. Aich A, Jones MK, Gupta K. Pain and sickle cell disease. *Curr Opin Hematol.* 2019;26(3):131-138.

63. Tran H, Sagi V, Leonce Song-Naba W, et al. Effect of chronic opioid therapy on pain and survival in a humanized mouse model of sickle cell disease. *Blood Adv.* 2019;3(6):869-873.

64. Averbukh Y, Porrovecchio A, Southern WN. Patient controlled analgesia for vaso-occlusive crisis: a cohort study. *Clin J Pain.* 2019;35(8):686-690.

65. Goodman E. Use of ketorolac in sickle-cell disease and vaso-occlusive crisis. *Lancet.* 1991;338(8767):641-642.

66. Wright SW, Norris RL, Mitchell TR. Ketorolac for sickle cell vaso-occlusive crisis pain in the emergency department: lack of a narcotic-sparing effect. *Ann Emerg Med.* 1992;21(8):925-928.

67. Perlin E, Finke H, Castro O, et al. Enhancement of pain control with ketorolac tromethamine in patients with sickle cell vaso-occlusive crisis. *Am J Hematol.* 1994;46(1):43-47.

68. Hardwick WE Jr, Givens TG, Monroe KW, King WD, Lawley D. Effect of ketorolac in pediatric sickle cell vaso-occlusive pain crisis. *Pediatr Emerg Care.* 1999;15(3):179-182.

69. Beiter JL Jr, Simon HK, Chambliss CR, Adamkiewicz T, Sullivan K. Intravenous ketorolac in the emergency department management of sickle cell pain and predictors of its effectiveness. *Arch Pediatr Adolesc Med.* 2001;155(4):496-500.

70. Nath KA, Hebbel RP. Sickle cell disease: renal manifestations and mechanisms. *Nat Rev Nephrol.* 2015;11(3):161-171.

71. Baddam S, Aban I, Hilliard L, Howard T, Askenazi D, Lebensburger JD. Acute kidney injury during a pediatric sickle cell vaso-occlusive pain crisis. *Pediatr Nephrol.* 2017;32(8):1451-1456.

72. Simckes AM, Chen SS, Osorio AV, Garola RE, Woods GM. Ketorolac-induced irreversible renal failure in sickle cell disease: a case report. *Pediatr Nephrol.* 1999;13(1):63-67.

73. Embury SH, Garcia JF, Mohandas N, Pennathur-Das R, Clark MR. Effects of oxygen inhalation on endogenous erythropoietin kinetics, erythropoiesis, and properties of blood cells in sickle-cell anemia. *N Engl J Med.* 1984;311(5):291-295.

74. Young JR, Sawe HR, Mfinanga JA, et al. Subdissociative intranasal ketamine plus standard pain therapy versus standard pain therapy in the treatment of paediatric sickle cell disease vaso-occlusive crises in resource-limited settings: study protocol for a randomised controlled trial. *BMJ Open.* 2017;7(7):e017190.

75. Palm N, Floroff C, Hassig TB, Boylan A, Kanter J. Low-dose ketamine infusion for adjunct management during vaso-occlusive episodes in adults with sickle cell disease: a case series. *J Pain Palliat Care Pharmacother.* 2018;32(1):20-26.

76. Nobrega R, Sheehy KA, Lippold C, Rice AL, Finkel JC, Quezado ZMN. Patient characteristics affect the response to ketamine and opioids during the treatment of vaso-occlusive episode-related pain in sickle cell disease. *Pediatr Res.* 2018;83(2):445-454.

77. Alshahrani MS, Asonto LP, El Tahan MM, et al. Study protocol for a randomized, blinded, controlled trial of ketamine for acute painful crisis of sickle cell disease. *Trials.* 2019;20(1):286.

78. Lubega FA, DeSilva MS, Munube D, et al. Low dose ketamine versus morphine for acute severe vaso occlusive pain in children: a randomized controlled trial. *Scand J Pain.* 2018;18(1):19-27.

79. Gladwin MT, Kato GJ, Weiner D, et al. Nitric oxide for inhalation in the acute treatment of sickle cell pain crisis: a randomized controlled trial. *JAMA.* 2011;305(9):893-902.

80. Brousseau DC, Scott JP, Hillery CA, Panepinto JA. The effect of magnesium on length of stay for pediatric sickle cell pain crisis. *Acad Emerg Med.* 2004;11(9):968-972.

81. Brousseau DC, Scott JP, Badaki-Makun O, et al. A multicenter randomized controlled trial of intravenous magnesium for sickle cell pain crisis in children. *Blood.* 2015;126(14):1651-1657.

82. Field JJ, Majerus E, Gordeuk VR, et al. Randomized phase 2 trial of regadenoson for treatment of acute vaso-occlusive crises in sickle cell disease. *Blood Adv.* 2017;1(20):1645-1649.

83. Orringer EP, Casella JF, Ataga KI, et al. Purified poloxamer 188 for treatment of acute vaso-occlusive crisis of sickle cell disease: a randomized controlled trial. *JAMA.* 2001;286(17):2099-2106.

84. Gibbs WJ, Hagemann TM. Purified poloxamer 188 for sickle cell vaso-occlusive crisis. *Ann Pharmacother.* 2004;38(2):320-324.

85. Morris CR, Kuypers FA, Lavrisha L, et al. A randomized, placebo-controlled trial of arginine therapy for the treatment of children with sickle cell disease hospitalized with vaso-occlusive pain episodes. *Haematologica.* 2013;98(9):1375-1382.

86. Morris CR, Hamilton-Reeves J, Martindale RG, Sarav M, Ochoa Gautier JB. Acquired amino acid deficiencies: a focus on arginine and glutamine. *Nutr Clin Pract.* 2017;32(suppl 1):30S-47S.

87. Telen MJ, Wun T, McCavit TL, et al. Randomized phase 2 study of GMI-1070 in SCD: reduction in time to resolution of vaso-occlusive events and decreased opioid use. *Blood.* 2015;125(17):2656-2664.

88. Genetic Engineering & Biotechnology News. Pfizer, GlycoMimetics phase III drug fails phase III trial for sickle cell

complication [press release]. 2019. https://www.genengnews.com/news/pfizer-glycomimetics-phase-iii-drug-fails-phase-iii-trial-for-sickle-cell-complication/. Accessed July 23, 2020.

89. Yoon SL, Black S. Comprehensive, integrative management of pain for patients with sickle-cell disease. *J Altern Complement Med.* 2006;12(10):995-1001.

90. Manwani D, Chen G, Carullo V, et al. Single-dose intravenous gammaglobulin can stabilize neutrophil Mac-1 activation in sickle cell pain crisis. *Am J Hematol.* 2015;90(5):381-385.

91. Telen MJ. Beyond hydroxyurea: new and old drugs in the pipeline for sickle cell disease. *Blood.* 2016;127(7):810-819.

92. Moerdler S, Manwani D. New insights into the pathophysiology and development of novel therapies for sickle cell disease. *Hematology Am Soc Hematol Educ Program.* 2018;2018(1):493-506.

93. Kapoor S, Little JA, Pecker LH. Advances in the treatment of sickle cell disease. *Mayo Clin Proc.* 2018;93(12):1810-1824.

94. Lu K, Cheng MC, Ge X, et al. A retrospective review of acupuncture use for the treatment of pain in sickle cell disease patients: descriptive analysis from a single institution. *Clin J Pain.* 2014;30(9):825-830.

95. Tsai SL, Niemtzow RC, Brown M, et al. Acupuncture and integrative medicine in pediatrics. *Med Acupunct.* 2018;30(2):61-67.

96. Tsai SL, Reynoso E, Shin DW, Tsung JW. Acupuncture as a nonpharmacologic treatment for pain in a pediatric emergency department. *Pediatr Emerg Care.* 2018; doi: 10.1097/PEC.0000000000001619.

97. Moody K, Abrahams B, Baker R, et al. A randomized trial of yoga for children hospitalized with sickle cell vaso-occlusive crisis. *J Pain Symptom Manage.* 2017;53(6):1026-1034.

98. Bhatt RR, Martin SR, Evans S, et al. The effect of hypnosis on pain and peripheral blood flow in sickle-cell disease: a pilot study. *J Pain Res.* 2017;10:1635-1644.

99. Rodgers-Melnick SN, Matthie N, Jenerette C, et al. The effects of a single electronic music improvisation session on the pain of adults with sickle cell disease: a mixed methods pilot study. *J Music Ther.* 2018;55(2):156-185.

100. Agrawal AK, Robertson S, Litwin L, et al. Virtual reality as complementary pain therapy in hospitalized patients with sickle cell disease. *Pediatr Blood Cancer.* 2019;66(2):e27525.

101. Okomo U, Meremikwu MM. Fluid replacement therapy for acute episodes of pain in people with sickle cell disease. *Cochrane Database Syst Rev.* 2017;7:CD005406.

102. Guy RB, Gavrilis PK, Rothenberg SP. In vitro and in vivo effect of hypotonic saline on the sickling phenomenon. *Am J Med Sci.* 1973;266(4):267-277.

103. Rosa RM, Bierer BE, Thomas R, et al. A study of induced hyponatremia in the prevention and treatment of sickle-cell crisis. *N Engl J Med.* 1980;303(20):1138-1143.

104. Carden MA, Fay M, Sakurai Y, et al. Normal saline is associated with increased sickle red cell stiffness and prolonged transit times in a microfluidic model of the capillary system. *Microcirculation.* 2017;24(5). doi: 10.1111/micc.12353.

105. Carden MA, Fay ME, Lu X, et al. Extracellular fluid tonicity impacts sickle red blood cell deformability and adhesion. *Blood.* 2017;130(24):2654-2663.

106. Howard J, Hart N, Roberts-Harewood M, et al. Guideline on the management of acute chest syndrome in sickle cell disease. *Br J Haematol.* 2015;169(4):492-505.

107. Carden MA, Patil P, Ahmad ME, Lam WA, Joiner CH, Morris CR. Variations in pediatric emergency medicine physician practices for intravenous fluid management in children with sickle

cell disease and vaso-occlusive pain: a single institution experience. *Pediatr Blood Cancer.* 2018;65(1). doi: 10.1002/pbc.26742.

108. Self WH, Semler MW, Wanderer JP, et al. Balanced crystalloids versus saline in noncritically ill adults. *N Engl J Med.* 2018;378(9):819-828.

109. Carden MA, Brousseau DC, Ahmad FA, et al. Normal saline bolus use in pediatric emergency departments is associated with poorer pain control in children with sickle cell anemia and vaso-occlusive pain. *Am J Hematol.* 2019;94(6):689-696.

110. Losco P, Nash G, Sone P, Ventre J. Comparison of the effects of radiographic contrast media on dehydration and filterability of red blood cells from donors homozygous for hemoglobin A or hemoglobin S. *Am J Hematol.* 2001;68:149-158.

111. Morris C, Vichinsky E, Styles L. Clinician assessment for acute chest syndrome in febrile patients with sickle cell disease: is it accurate enough? *Ann Emerg Med.* 1999;34(1):64-69.

112. Savage WJ, Buchanan GR, Yawn BP, et al. Evidence gaps in the management of sickle cell disease: a summary of needed research. *Am J Hematol.* 2015;90(4):273-275.

113. Lazarus SG, Kelleman M, Adisa O, et al. Are we missing the mark? Fever, respiratory symptoms, chest radiographs, and acute chest syndrome in sickle cell disease. *Am J Hematol.* 2016;91(8):E332-E333.

114. Vichinsky EP, Styles LA, Colangelo LH, Wright EC, Castro O, Nickerson B. Acute chest syndrome in sickle cell disease: clinical presentation and course. Cooperative Study of Sickle Cell Disease. *Blood.* 1997;89(5):1787-1792.

115. Vichinsky E, Neumayr L, Earles A, et al. Causes and outcomes of the acute chest syndrome in sickle cell disease. National Acute Chest Syndrome Study Group. *N Engl J Med.* 2000;342:1855-1865.

116. Wang CJ, Kavanagh PL, Little AA, Holliman JB, Sprinz PG. Quality-of-care indicators for children with sickle cell disease. *Pediatrics.* 2011;128(3):484-493.

117. Arndt PA, Leger RM, Garratty G. Serologic characteristics of ceftriaxone antibodies in 25 patients with drug-induced immune hemolytic anemia. *Transfusion.* 2012;52(3):602-612.

118. Bernini JC, Mustafa MM, Sutor LJ, Buchanan GR. Fatal hemolysis induced by ceftriaxone in a child with sickle cell anemia. *J Pediatr.* 1995;126(5 Pt 1):813-815.

119. Neuman G, Boodhan S, Wurman I, et al. Ceftriaxone-induced immune hemolytic anemia. *Ann Pharmacother.* 2014;48(12):1594-1604.

120. Van Buren NL, Gorlin JB, Reed RC, Gottschall JL, Nelson SC. Ceftriaxone-induced drug reaction mimicking acute splenic sequestration crisis in a child with hemoglobin SC disease. *Transfusion.* 2018;58(4):879-883.

121. Wilimas JA, Flynn PM, Harris S, et al. A randomized study of outpatient treatment with ceftriaxone for selected febrile children with sickle cell disease. *N Engl J Med.* 1993;329(7):472-476.

122. Franco RS. The measurement and importance of red cell survival. *Am J Hematol.* 2009;84(2):109-114.

123. Brown KE, Anderson SM, Young NS. Erythrocyte P antigen: cellular receptor for B19 parvovirus. *Science (New York, NY).* 1993;262(5130):114-117.

124. Smith-Whitley K, Zhao H, Hodinka RL, et al. Epidemiology of human parvovirus B19 in children with sickle cell disease. *Blood.* 2004;103(2):422-427.

125. Emond AM, Collis R, Darvill D, Higgs DR, Maude GH, Serjeant GR. Acute splenic sequestration in homozygous

sickle cell disease: natural history and management. *J Pediatr.* 1985;107(2):201-206.

126. Gardner K, Hoppe C, Mijovic A, Thein SL. How we treat delayed haemolytic transfusion reactions in patients with sickle cell disease. *Br J Haematol.* 2015;170(6):745-756.

127. Dean CL, Maier CL, Chonat S, et al. Challenges in the treatment and prevention of delayed hemolytic transfusion reactions with hyperhemolysis in sickle cell disease patients. *Transfusion.* 2019;59(5):1698-1705.

128. de Montalembert M, Dumont MD, Heilbronner C, et al. Delayed hemolytic transfusion reaction in children with sickle cell disease. *Haematologica.* 2011;96(6):801-807.

129. Pirenne F, Yazdanbakhsh K. How I safely transfuse patients with sickle-cell disease and manage delayed hemolytic transfusion reactions. *Blood.* 2018;131(25):2773-2781.

130. Petz LD, Calhoun L, Shulman IA, Johnson C, Herron RM. The sickle cell hemolytic transfusion reaction syndrome. *Transfusion.* 1997;37(4):382-392.

131. Win N, New H, Lee E, de la Fuente J. Hyperhemolysis syndrome in sickle cell disease: case report (recurrent episode) and literature review. *Transfusion.* 2008;48(6):1231-1238.

132. Win N. Hyperhemolysis syndrome in sickle cell disease. *Expert Rev Hematol.* 2009;2(2):111-115.

133. Talano JA, Hillery CA, Gottschall JL, Baylerian DM, Scott JP. Delayed hemolytic transfusion reaction/hyperhemolysis syndrome in children with sickle cell disease. *Pediatrics.* 2003;111 (6 Pt 1):e661-e665.

134. Minter K, Gladwin M. Pulmonary complications of sickle cell anemia. A need for increased recognition, treatment, and research. *Am J Respir Crit Care Med.* 2001;164:2016-2019.

135. Vichinsky E, Styles L. Pulmonary complications. *Hematol Oncol Clin North Am.* 1996;10(6):1275-1287.

136. Klings ES, Wyszynski DF, Nolan VG, Steinberg MH. Abnormal pulmonary function in adults with sickle cell anemia. *Am J Respir Crit Care Med.* 2006;173(11):1264-1269.

137. Hagar W, Michlitsch J, Gardner J, Vichinsky EP, Morris CR. Clinical differences between children and adults with pulmonary hypertension and sickle cell disease. *Br J Haematol.* 2008; 140(1):104-112.

138. Vichinsky EP, Styles LA, Colangelo LH, et al. Acute chest syndrome in sickle cell disease: clinical presentation and course. *Blood.* 1997;89(5):1787-1792.

139. Chang TP, Kriengsoontorkij W, Chan LS, Wang VJ. Clinical factors and incidence of acute chest syndrome or pneumonia among children with sickle cell disease presenting with a fever: a 17-year review. *Pediatr Emerg Care.* 2013;29(7): 781-786.

140. Neumayr L, Morris CR, Wen A, et al. Reversible loss of pulmonary function induced by acute chest syndrome in sickle cell disease. *Blood.* 2005;106(abstr 315):96a.

141. Morris CR. Asthma management: re-inventing the wheel in sickle cell disease. *Am J Hematol.* 2009;84(4):234-241.

142. Vichinsky EP, Williams R, Das M, et al. Pulmonary fat embolism: a distinct cause of severe acute chest syndrome in sickle cell anemia. *Blood.* 1994;83(11):3107-3112.

143. Mekontso Dessap A, Leon R, Habibi A, et al. Pulmonary hypertension and cor pulmonale during severe acute chest syndrome in sickle cell disease. *Am J Respir Crit Care Med.* 2008;177(6):646-653.

144. Vichinsky EP, Neumayr LD, Earles AN, et al. Causes and outcomes of the acute chest syndrome in sickle cell disease.

National Acute Chest Syndrome Study Group. *N Engl J Med.* 2000;342(25):1855-1865.

145. Styles LA, Abboud M, Larkin S, Lo M, Kuypers FA. Transfusion prevents acute chest syndrome predicted by elevated secretory phospholipase A2. *Br J Haematol.* 2007;136(2):343-344.

146. Styles LA, de Jong K, Vichinsky E, Lubin B, Adams R, Kuypers F. Increased RBC phosphatidylserine exposure in sickle cell disease patients at risk for stroke by transcranial doppler ultrasound. *Blood.* 1997;90(10):604a.

147. Styles L, Wager CG, Labotka RJ, et al. Refining the value of secretory phospholipase A2 as a predictor of acute chest syndrome in sickle cell disease: results of a feasibility study (PROACTIVE). *Br J Haematol.* 2012;157(5):627-636.

148. Alsayed S, Marzouk S, Mousa E. Serum procalcitonin as a predicting value in severity and prognosis of CAP in sickle cell-patients. *J Egypt Soc Parasitol.* 2013;43(3):657-668.

149. Sobota A, Graham DA, Heeney MM, Neufeld EJ. Corticosteroids for acute chest syndrome in children with sickle cell disease: variation in use and association with length of stay and readmission. *Am J Hematol.* 2010;85(1):24-28.

150. Kumar R, Qureshi S, Mohanty P, Rao SP, Miller ST. A short course of prednisone in the management of acute chest syndrome of sickle cell disease. *J Pediatr Hematol Oncol.* 2010;32(3):e91-e94.

151. Bellet PS, Kalinyak KA, Shukla R, Gelfand M, Rucknagel DL. Incentive spirometry to prevent acute pulmonary complications in sickle cell diseases. *N Engl J Med.* 1995;333:699-703.

152. Adisa O, Bhutta A, Taylor N, Gee B, Buchanan I, Morris C. Use of BiPAP in the management of acute chest syndrome (ACS) in children with sickle cell disease. Paper presented at the Pediatric Academy Society Annual Meeting, Baltimore, MD, 2016.

153. Balk DS, Lee C, Schafer J, et al. Lung ultrasound compared to chest X-ray for diagnosis of pediatric pneumonia: a meta-analysis. *Pediatr Pulmonol.* 2018;53(8):1130-1139.

154. Cohen S, Malik Z, Hagbom R, et al. Lung ultrasound for evaluating acute chest syndrome in pediatric patients with sickle cell disease: so easy even a medical student can do it. Paper presented at the American Institute of Ultrasound Medicine, New York, New York, 2016.

155. Daswani DD, Shah VP, Avner JR, Manwani DG, Kurian J, Rabiner JE. Accuracy of point-of-care lung ultrasonography for diagnosis of acute chest syndrome in pediatric patients with sickle cell disease and fever. *Acad Emerg Med.* 2016;23(8):932-940.

156. Mekontso Dessap A, Deux JF, Habibi A, et al. Lung imaging during acute chest syndrome in sickle cell disease: computed tomography patterns and diagnostic accuracy of bedside chest radiograph. *Thorax.* 2014;69(2):144-151.

157. Mekontso Dessap A, Deux JF, Abidi N, et al. Pulmonary artery thrombosis during acute chest syndrome in sickle cell disease. *Am J Respir Crit Care Med.* 2011;184(9):1022-1029.

158. Singer ST, Ataga KI. Hypercoagulability in sickle cell disease and beta-thalassemia. *Curr Mol Med.* 2008;8(7):639-645.

159. Schnog JB, Mac Gillavry MR, van Zanten AP, et al. Protein C and S and inflammation in sickle cell disease. *Am J Hematol.* 2004;76(1):26-32.

160. Morris CR. Asthma management: reinventing the wheel in sickle cell disease. *Am J Hematol.* 2009;84(4):234-241.

161. Newaskar M, Hardy KA, Morris CR. Asthma in sickle cell disease. *ScientificWorldJournal.* 2011;11:1138-1152.

162. Palma-Carlos AG, Palma-Carlos ML, Costa AC. "Minor" hemoglobinopathies: a risk factor for asthma. *Allerg Immunol (Paris).* 2005;37(5):177-182.

163. Strunk RC, Brown MS, Boyd JH, Bates P, Field JJ, DeBaun MR. Methacholine challenge in children with sickle cell disease: a case series. *Pediatr Pulmonol.* 2008;43(9):924-929.

164. Field JJ, DeBaun MR. Asthma and sickle cell disease: two distinct diseases or part of the same process? *Hematology Am Soc Hematol Educ Program.* 2009;2009:45-53.

165. Shilo NR, Lands LC. Asthma and chronic sickle cell lung disease: a dynamic relationship. *Paediatr Respir Rev.* 2011;12(1):78-82.

166. Field JJ, Stocks J, Kirkham FJ, et al. Airway hyperresponsiveness in children with sickle cell anemia. *Chest.* 2011;139(3):563-568.

167. Koumbourlis AC, Zar HJ, Hurlet-Jensen A, Goldberg MR. Prevalence and reversibility of lower airway obstruction in children with sickle cell disease. *J Pediatr.* 2001;138(2):188-192.

168. Boyd JH, DeBaun MR, Morgan WJ, Mao J, Strunk RC. Lower airway obstruction is associated with increased morbidity in children with sickle cell disease. *Pediatr Pulmonol.* 2009;44(3):290-296.

169. Leong MA, Dampier C, Varlotta L, Allen JL. Airway hyperreactivity in children with sickle cell disease. *J Pediatr.* 1997;131:278-283.

170. Koumbourlis A, Zar H, Hurlet-Jensen A, Goldberg M. Prevalence and reversibility of lower airway obstruction in children with sickle cell disease. *J Pediatr.* 2001;138:188-192.

171. Santoli F, Zerah F, Vasile N, Bachir D, Galacteros F, Atlan G. Pulmonary function in sickle cell disease with or without acute chest syndrome. *Eur Respir J.* 1998;12:1124-1129.

172. Arteta M, Campbell A, Nouraie M, et al. Abnormal pulmonary function and associated risk factors in children and adolescents with sickle cell anemia. *J Pediatr Hematol Oncol.* 2014;36(3):185-189.

173. Sen N, Kozanoglu I, Karatasli M, Ermis H, Boga C, Eyuboglu FO. Pulmonary function and airway hyperresponsiveness in adults with sickle cell disease. *Lung.* 2009;187(3):195-200.

174. Boyd JH, Macklin EA, Strunk RC, Debaun MR. Asthma is associated with acute chest syndrome and pain in children with sickle cell anemia. *Blood.* 2006;108(9):2923-2927.

175. Glassberg J, Spivey JF, Strunk R, Boslaugh S, DeBaun MR. Painful episodes in children with sickle cell disease and asthma are temporally associated with respiratory symptoms. *J Pediatr Hematol Oncol.* 2006;28(8):481-485.

176. Field JJ, Macklin EA, Yan Y, Strunk RC, DeBaun MR. Sibling history of asthma is a risk factor for pain in children with sickle cell anemia. *Am J Hematol.* 2008;83(11):855-857.

177. Knight-Perry JE, Field JJ, Debaun MR, Stocks J, Kirkby J, Strunk RC. Hospital admission for acute painful episode following methacholine challenge in an adolescent with sickle cell disease. *Pediatr Pulmonol.* 2009;44(7):728-730.

178. Paul R, Minniti CP, Nouraie M, et al. Clinical correlates of acute pulmonary events in children and adolescents with sickle cell disease. *Eur J Haematol.* 2013;91(1):62-68.

179. Boyd JH, Moinuddin A, Strunk RC, DeBaun MR. Asthma and acute chest in sickle-cell disease. *Pediatr Pulmonol.* 2004;38(3):229-232.

180. Nordness ME, Lynn J, Zacharisen MC, Scott PJ, Kelly KJ. Asthma is a risk factor for acute chest syndrome and cerebral vascular accidents in children with sickle cell disease. *Clin Mol Allergy.* 2005;3(1):2.

181. Boyd JH, Macklin EA, Strunk RC, Debaun MR. Asthma is associated with increased mortality in patients with sickle cell anemia. *Haematologica.* 2007;92:1115-1118.

182. Nouraie M, Rana S, Castro O, et al. Predictors of mortality in children and adolescents with sickle cell disease: the PUSH study. *Blood.* 2011;118:abst 515.

183. Glassberg J, Minnitti C, Cromwell C, et al. Inhaled steroids reduce pain and sVCAM levels in individuals with sickle cell disease: a triple-blind, randomized trial. *Am J Hematol.* 2017;92(7):622-631.

184. Langer AL, Leader A, Kim-Schulze S, Ginzburg Y, Merad M, Glassberg J. Inhaled steroids associated with decreased macrophage markers in nonasthmatic individuals with sickle cell disease in a randomized trial. *Ann Hematol.* 2019;98(4):841-849.

185. National Heart, Lung, and Blood Institute. New NHLBI guidelines for the diagnosis and management of asthma. *Lippincott Health Promot Lett.* 1997;2(7):1, 8-9.

186. Corrarino J. New guidelines for diagnosis and management of asthma. *MCN Am J Matern Child Nurs.* 2008;33(2):136.

187. Moore WC. Update in asthma 2007. *Am J Respir Crit Care Med.* 2008;177(10):1068-1073.

188. Gladwin MT. Prevalence, risk factors and mortality of pulmonary hypertension defined by right heart catheterization in patients with sickle cell disease. *Exp Rev Hematol.* 2011;4(6):593-596.

189. Gladwin MT, Vichinsky E. Pulmonary complications of sickle cell disease. *N Engl J Med.* 2008;359(21):2254-2265.

190. Parent F, Bachir D, Inamo J, et al. A hemodynamic study of pulmonary hypertension in sickle cell disease. *N Engl J Med.* 2011;365(1):44-53.

191. Gladwin M, Sachdev V, Jison M, et al. Pulmonary hypertension as a risk factor for death in patients with sickle cell disease. *N Engl J Med.* 2004;350:22-31.

192. Minniti CP, Sable C, Campbell A, et al. Elevated tricuspid regurgitant jet velocity in children and adolescents with sickle cell disease: association with hemolysis and hemoglobin oxygen desaturation. *Haematologica.* 2009;94(3):340-347.

193. Kato GJ, Onyekwere OC, Gladwin MT. Pulmonary hypertension in sickle cell disease: relevance to children. *Pediatr Hematol Oncol.* 2007;24(3):159-170.

194. Morris CR. Vascular risk assessment in patients with sickle cell disease. *Haematologica.* 2011;96(1):1-5.

195. Machado RF, Kyle Mack A, Martyr S, et al. Severity of pulmonary hypertension during vaso-occlusive pain crisis and exercise in patients with sickle cell disease. *Br J Haematol.* 2007;136(2):319-325.

196. Klings ES, Machado RF, Barst RJ, et al. An official American Thoracic Society clinical practice guideline: diagnosis, risk stratification, and management of pulmonary hypertension of sickle cell disease. *Am J Respir Crit Care Med.* 2014;189(6):727-740.

197. Mueller BU, Martin KJ, Dreyer W, Bezold LI, Mahoney DH. Prolonged QT interval in pediatric sickle cell disease. *Pediatr Blood Cancer.* 2006;47(6):831-833.

198. Boga C, Kozanoglu I, Yeral M, Bakar C. Assessment of corrected QT interval in sickle-cell disease patients who undergo erythroapheresis. *Transfus Med.* 2007;17(6):466-472.

199. Akgul F, Seyfeli E, Melek I, et al. Increased QT dispersion in sickle cell disease: effect of pulmonary hypertension. *Acta Haematol.* 2007;118(1):1-6.

200. Machado RF, Anthi A, Steinberg MH, et al. N-terminal pro-brain natriuretic peptide levels and risk of death in sickle cell disease. *JAMA.* 2006;296(3):310-318.

201. Barrett O Jr, Saunders DE Jr, McFarland DE, Humphries JO. Myocardial infarction in sickle cell anemia. *Am J Hematol.* 1984;16(2):139-147.

202. Pannu R, Zhang J, Andraws R, Armani A, Patel P, Mancusi-Ungaro P. Acute myocardial infarction in sickle cell disease: a systematic review. *Crit Pathw Cardiol.* 2008;7(2):133-138.

203. Gladwin MT, Sachdev V. Cardiovascular abnormalities in sickle cell disease. *J Am Coll Cardiol.* 2012;59(13):1123-1133.

204. Ogunbayo GO, Misumida N, Olorunfemi O, et al. Comparison of outcomes in patients having acute myocardial infarction with versus without sickle-cell anemia. *Am J Cardiol.* 2017;120(10): 1768-1771.

205. de Montalembert M, Maunoury C, Acar P, Brousse V, Sidi D, Lenoir G. Myocardial ischaemia in children with sickle cell disease. *Arch Dis Child.* 2004;89(4):359-362.

206. Acar P, Maunoury C, de Montalembert M, Dulac Y. [Abnormalities of myocardial perfusion in sickle cell disease in childhood: a study of myocardial scintigraphy]. *Arch Mal Coeur Vaiss.* 2003;96(5):507-510.

207. Maunoury C, Acar P, de Montalembert M, Sidi D. Myocardial perfusion in children with sickle cell disease. *Am J Cardiol.* 2003;91(3):374-376.

208. Voskaridou E, Christoulas D, Terpos E. Sickle-cell disease and the heart: review of the current literature. *Br J Haematol.* 2012;157(6):664-673.

209. Aslam AK, Rodriguez C, Aslam AF, Vasavada BC, Khan IA. Cardiac troponin I in sickle cell crisis. *Int J Cardiol.* 2009;133(1): 138-139.

210. Alpert BS, Gilman PA, Strong WB, et al. Hemodynamic and ECG responses to exercise in children with sickle cell anemia. *Am J Dis Child.* 1981;135(4):362-366.

211. Manci EA, Culberson DE, Yang YM, et al. Causes of death in sickle cell disease: an autopsy study. *Br J Haematol.* 2003;123(2):359-365.

212. Gladwin MT. Cardiovascular complications and risk of death in sickle-cell disease. *Lancet.* 2016;387(10037):2565-2574.

213. DeBaun MR, Kirkham FJ. Central nervous system complications and management in sickle cell disease. *Blood.* 2016;127(7):829-838.

214. Ohene-Frempong K, Weiner SJ, Sleeper LA, et al. Cerebrovascular accidents in sickle cell disease: rates and risk factors. *Blood.* 1998;91(1):288-294.

215. Kassim AA, Galadanci NA, Pruthi S, DeBaun MR. How I treat and manage strokes in sickle cell disease. *Blood.* 2015;125(22):3401-3410.

216. Hyacinth HI, Carty CL, Seals SR, et al. Association of sickle cell trait with ischemic stroke among African Americans: a meta-analysis. *JAMA Neurol.* 2018;75(7):802-807.

217. Strouse JJ, Hulbert ML, DeBaun MR, Jordan LC, Casella JF. Primary hemorrhagic stroke in children with sickle cell disease is associated with recent transfusion and use of corticosteroids. *Pediatrics.* 2006;118(5):1916-1924.

218. Vichinsky EP, Neumayr LD, Gold JI, et al. Neuropsychological dysfunction and neuroimaging abnormalities in neurologically intact adults with sickle cell anemia. *JAMA.* 2010;303(18):1823-1831.

219. Hulbert ML, Scothorn DJ, Panepinto JA, et al. Exchange blood transfusion compared with simple transfusion for first overt stroke is associated with a lower risk of subsequent stroke: a retrospective cohort study of 137 children with sickle cell anemia. *J Pediatr.* 2006;149(5):710-712.

220. Strouse JJ, Lanzkron S, Urrutia V. The epidemiology, evaluation and treatment of stroke in adults with sickle cell disease. *Expert Rev Hematol.* 2011;4(6):597-606.

221. Adams RJ, Cox M, Ozark SD, et al. Coexistent sickle cell disease has no impact on the safety or outcome of lytic therapy in acute ischemic stroke: findings from Get With the Guidelines-Stroke. *Stroke.* 2017;48(3):686-691.

222. Mowatt L, Chambers C. Ocular morbidity of traumatic hyphema in a Jamaican hospital. *Eur J Ophthalmol.* 2010;20(3):584-589.

223. Coats DK, Paysse EA, Kong J. Unrecognized microscopic hyphema masquerading as a closed head injury. *Pediatrics.* 1998;102(3 Pt 1):652-654.

224. Andreoli C, Gardiner M. Traumatic hyphema: clinical features and diagnosis. UpToDate Published 2018.

225. Gharaibeh A, Savage HI, Scherer RW, Goldberg MF, Lindsley K. Medical interventions for traumatic hyphema. *Cochrane Database Syst Rev.* 2011;1:CD005431.

226. Liebmann JM. Management of sickle cell disease and hyphema. *J Glaucoma.* 1996;5(4):271-275.

227. Saidkasimova S, Shalchi Z, Mahroo OA, et al. Risk factors for visual impairment in patients with sickle cell disease in London. *Eur J Ophthalmol.* 2016;26(5):431-435.

228. Do BK, Rodger DC. Sickle cell disease and the eye. *Curr Opin Ophthalmol.* 2017;28(6):623-628.

229. Perlman JI, Forman S, Gonzalez ER. Retrobulbar ischemic optic neuropathy associated with sickle cell disease. *J Neuroophthalmol.* 1994;14(1):45-48.

230. Walton W, Von Hagen S, Grigorian R, Zarbin M. Management of traumatic hyphema. *Surv Ophthalmol.* 2002;47(4): 297-334.

231. Ebert EC, Nagar M, Hagspiel KD. Gastrointestinal and hepatic complications of sickle cell disease. *Clin Gastroenterol Hepatol.* 2010;8(6):483-489; quiz e470.

232. Yohannan MD, Arif M, Ramia S. Aetiology of icteric hepatitis and fulminant hepatic failure in children and the possible predisposition to hepatic failure by sickle cell disease. *Acta Paediatr Scand.* 1990;79(2):201-205.

233. DeVault KR, Friedman LS, Westerberg S, Martin P, Hosein B, Ballas SK. Hepatitis C in sickle cell anemia. *J Clin Gastroenterol.* 1994;18(3):206-209.

234. Gardner K, Suddle A, Kane P, et al. How we treat sickle hepatopathy and liver transplantation in adults. *Blood.* 2014; 123(15):2302-2307.

235. Ahn H, Li CS, Wang W. Sickle cell hepatopathy: clinical presentation, treatment, and outcome in pediatric and adult patients. *Pediatr Blood Cancer.* 2005;45(2):184-190.

236. Pecker LH, Patel N, Creary S, et al. Diverse manifestations of acute sickle cell hepatopathy in pediatric patients with sickle cell disease: a case series. *Pediatr Blood Cancer.* 2018;65(8): e27060.

237. Hatton CS, Bunch C, Weatherall DJ. Hepatic sequestration in sickle cell anaemia. *Br Med J (Clin Res Ed).* 1985;290(6470): 744-745.

238. Haydek JP, Taborda C, Shah R, et al. Extreme hyperbilirubinemia: an indicator of morbidity and mortality in sickle cell disease. *World J Hepatol.* 2019;11(3):287-293.

239. Airy M, Eknoyan G. The kidney in sickle hemoglobinopathies. *Clin Nephrol.* 2017;87(2):55-68.

240. Naik RP, Derebail VK. The spectrum of sickle hemoglobin-related nephropathy: from sickle cell disease to sickle trait. *Expert Rev Hematol.* 2017;10(12):1087-1094.

241. Alvarez OA. Renal medullary carcinoma: the kidney cancer that affects individuals with sickle cell trait and disease. *J Oncol Pract.* 2017;13(7):424-425.

242. Kato GJ, Steinberg MH, Gladwin MT. Intravascular hemolysis and the pathophysiology of sickle cell disease. *J Clin Invest.* 2017;127(3):750-760.

243. Rogers ZR. Priapism in sickle cell disease. *Hematol Oncol Clin North Am.* 2005;19(5):917-928, viii.

244. Anele UA, Le BV, Resar LM, Burnett AL. How I treat priapism. *Blood.* 2015;125(23):3551-3558.

245. Anele UA, Burnett AL. Erectile dysfunction after sickle cell disease-associated recurrent ischemic priapism: profile and risk factors. *J Sex Med.* 2015;12(3):713-719.

246. Broderick GA. Priapism and sickle-cell anemia: diagnosis and nonsurgical therapy. *J Sex Med.* 2012;9(1):88-103.

247. Kato GJ. Priapism in sickle-cell disease: a hematologist's perspective. *J Sex Med.* 2012;9(1):70-78.

248. Bivalacqua TJ, Musicki B, Hsu LL, Berkowitz DE, Champion HC, Burnett AL. Sildenafil citrate-restored eNOS and PDE5 regulation in sickle cell mouse penis prevents priapism via control of oxidative/nitrosative stress. *PloS One.* 2013;8(7):e68028.

249. Morris CR. Alterations of the arginine metabolome in sickle cell disease: a growing rationale for arginine therapy. *Hematol Oncol Clin North Am.* 2014;28(2):301-321.

250. Sopko NA, Matsui H, Hannan JL, et al. Subacute hemolysis in sickle cell mice causes priapism secondary to NO imbalance and PDE5 dysregulation. *J Sex Med.* 2015;12(9):1878-1885.

251. Claudino MA, Franco-Penteado CF, Corat MA, et al. Increased cavernosal relaxations in sickle cell mice priapism are associated with alterations in the NO-cGMP signaling pathway. *J Sex Med.* 2009;6(8):2187-2196.

252. Kato GJ, McGowan V, Machado RF, et al. Lactate dehydrogenase as a biomarker of hemolysis-associated nitric oxide resistance, priapism, leg ulceration, pulmonary hypertension, and death in patients with sickle cell disease. *Blood.* 2006;107(6):2279-2285.

253. Greenwald M, Gutman, CK, Morris CR. Resolution of acute priapism in two children with sickle cell disease who received nitrous oxide gas. *Acad Emerg Med.* 2019 Sep;26(9):1102-1105.

254. Montague DK, Jarow J, Broderick GA, et al. American Urological Association guideline on the management of priapism. *J Urol.* 2003;170(4 Pt 1):1318-1324.

255. Chinegwundoh FI, Smith S, Anie KA. Treatments for priapism in boys and men with sickle cell disease. *Cochrane Database Syst Rev.* 2017;9:CD004198.

256. Olujohungbe A, Burnett AL. How I manage priapism due to sickle cell disease. *Br J Haematol.* 2013;160(6):754-765.

257. Ballas SK, Lyon D. Safety and efficacy of blood exchange transfusion for priapism complicating sickle cell disease. *J Clin Apheresis.* 2016;31(1):5-10.

258. Bialecki ES, Bridges KR. Sildenafil relieves priapism in patients with sickle cell disease. *Am J Med.* 2002;113(3):252.

259. Zipper R, Younger A, Tipton T, et al. Ischemic priapism in pediatric patients: Spontaneous detumescence with ketamine sedation. *J Pediatr Urol.* 2018;14(5):465-466.

260. Tobias JD. Applications of nitrous oxide for procedural sedation in the pediatric population. *Pediatr Emerg Care.* 2013;29(2):245-265.

261. Babl FE, Oakley E, Seaman C, Barnett P, Sharwood LN. High-concentration nitrous oxide for procedural sedation in children: adverse events and depth of sedation. *Pediatrics.* 2008;121(3):e528-532.

262. Galeotti C, Courtois E, Carbajal R. How French paediatric emergency departments manage painful vaso-occlusive episodes in sickle cell disease patients. *Acta Paediatr.* 2014;103(12):e548-e554.

263. Oteng-Ntim E, Meeks D, Seed PT, et al. Adverse maternal and perinatal outcomes in pregnant women with sickle cell disease: systematic review and meta-analysis. *Blood.* 2015;125(21):3316-3325.

264. de Montalembert M, Deneux-Tharaux C. Pregnancy in sickle cell disease is at very high risk. *Blood.* 2015;125(21):3216-3217.

265. Howard J, Oteng-Ntim E. The obstetric management of sickle cell disease. *Best Pract Res Clin Obstet Gynaecol.* 2012;26(1):25-36.

266. Minniti CP, Eckman J, Sebastiani P, Steinberg MH, Ballas SK. Leg ulcers in sickle cell disease. *Am J Hematol.* 2010;85(10):831-833.

267. Minniti CP, Delaney KM, Gorbach AM, et al. Vasculopathy, inflammation, and blood flow in leg ulcers of patients with sickle cell anemia. *Am J Hematol.* 2014;89(1):1-6.

268. Connor JL Jr, Sclafani JA, Kato GJ, Hsieh MM, Minniti CP. Brief topical sodium nitrite and its impact on the quality of life in patients with sickle leg ulcers. *Medicine (Baltimore).* 2018;97(46):e12614.

269. Minniti CP, Gorbach AM, Xu D, et al. Topical sodium nitrite for chronic leg ulcers in patients with sickle cell anaemia: a phase 1 dose-finding safety and tolerability trial. *Lancet Haematol.* 2014;1(3):e95-e103.

270. Novelli E, Delaney K, Axelrod K, Morris C, Minniti C. Arginine therapy in a patient with Hb-SS disease and refractory leg ulcers. Paper presented at the Sickle Cell Disease Association of America Annual Convention, Baltimore, MD, 2012.

271. Koshy M, Askin M, McMahon L, et al. Arginine butyrate in sickle cell leg ulcers: interim findings of a phase II trial. Paper presented at the 24th Annual Meeting of the National Sickle Cell Disease Program, Philadelphia, PA, 2000.

272. McMahon L, Tamary H, Askin M, et al. A randomized phase II trial of arginine butyrate with standard local therapy in refractory sickle cell leg ulcers. *Br J Haematol.* 2010;151(5):516-524.

273. Morris CR, Morris SM Jr, Hagar W, et al. Arginine therapy: a new treatment for pulmonary hypertension in sickle cell disease? *Am J Respir Crit Care Med.* 2003;168:63-69.

274. Connor JL Jr, Minniti CP, Tisdale JF, Hsieh MM. Sickle cell anemia and comorbid leg ulcer treated with curative peripheral blood stem cell transplantation. *Int J Low Extrem Wounds.* 2017;16(1):56-59.

275. Meneses JV, Fortuna V, de Souza ES, et al. Autologous stem cell-based therapy for sickle cell leg ulcer: a pilot study. *Br J Haematol.* 2016;175(5):949-955.

276. Jan K, Usami S, Smith JA. Effects of transfusion on rheological properties of blood in sickle cell anemia. *Transfusion.* 1982;22(1):17-20.

277. Schmalzer EA, Lee JO, Brown AK, Usami S, Chien S. Viscosity of mixtures of sickle and normal red cells at varying hematocrit levels. Implications for transfusion. *Transfusion.* 1987;27(3):228-233.

278. Hurlet-Jensen AM, Prohovnik I, Pavlakis SG, Piomelli S. Effects of total hemoglobin and hemoglobin S concentration on cerebral blood flow during transfusion therapy to prevent stroke in sickle cell disease. *Stroke.* 1994;25(8):1688-1692.

279. Morris CR, Ahmad F, Bennett J, et al. Pediatric emergency department adherence to the 2014 National Heart, Lung, and Blood Institute guidelines targeting analgesic therapy in the management of vaso-occlusive pain episodes in children with sickle cell disease: a multicenter perspective. *Blood* 2016;128:1016.

Psychosocial Burden in Sickle Cell Disease

Authors: *Allison A. King, Sherif M. Badawy, Julie Panepinto, Kofi Anie, Charles Jonassaint, Marsha Treadwell*

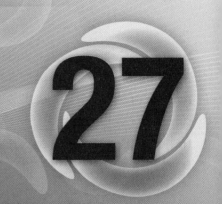

Chapter Outline

Overview

Sickle cell disease (SCD) has been described in Africa for centuries. Characteristics of the disease have become incorporated into local languages, impacting cultural understanding of the course and symptomology of SCD. For example, the prominence of sickle cell pain is the basis upon which SCD has been named in certain Ghanaian cultures. These names—*chwechweechwe* ("gnawing"; Ga), *nuidudui* ("biting"; Ewe), and *ahotutuo* ("body pinching"; Twi)—reflect the lived experiences of individuals affected by the disease.[1] Other names—*onye kye ba* ("s/he is not one who would live"; Twi)—capture the expectation of early mortality. Still others—*ogbanje* ("child who comes and goes"; Igbo) and *sika be sa* ("money will finish"; Twi)—reflect the emotional and financial impact on the family.[2]

SCD was first named in Western medicine following the 1910 description of "peculiar-shaped red blood cells" in a West Indian dental student experiencing anemia, pain, respiratory problems, and leg ulcers.[3] The inheritance pattern, clinical course, and pathophysiologic features of this "new" disease were delineated over the next 40 years, as was the basis of the disease in an abnormality in the hemoglobin molecule.[4] The field of molecular biology owes much to SCD as "the first molecular disease" that generated new scientific strategies and discoveries.[5] However, the disease remained largely invisible clinically and in public awareness through the late 1940s, resulting in preventable morbidities and mortality.[6,7]

After World War II, medical breakthroughs illuminated the clinical burdens of SCD (eg, pain, risk of early mortality) and approaches to clinical management, such as infection prevention.[8] At the same time, the disease's origin was firmly linked to the African continent, and clinical research and public awareness of SCD became fraught with racism and stigmatization.[9] Public health efforts to prevent the disease resulted in many African Americans feeling forced to undergo sickle cell trait testing and subsequently facing discrimination in employment and in receiving health insurance.[10] To activists such as the Black Panthers, the invisibility and pain experienced by individuals with SCD became an embodiment of the African American experience and a reflection of the community's sociopolitical oppression.[11] The Black Panther party championed health as a human right and emphasized the inadequate funding designated for SCD care and research. Reports on funding disparities from SCD advocates, such as hematologist Robert Scott, MD, prompted the US Congress to provide funding for sickle cell trait screening and counseling, public awareness campaigns, research, and comprehensive SCD health care.[8]

During the early 1970s, the National Sickle Cell Disease Program launched at the National Heart, Lung, and Blood Institute (NHLBI), heralding major advancements in SCD care and research.[12] These advancements included the development of a newborn screen for SCD and the ultimate implementation of universal screening in every US state; providing SCD-positive infants with daily prophylactic penicillin to prevent fatal infections; educating parents about the signs of medical emergencies; and preventing strokes through screening and regular blood transfusions. In 1998, hydroxyurea became the first US Food and Drug Administration (FDA)-approved agent for preventing severe sickle cell pain episodes, reducing the number of acute health care visits, and reducing the frequency of acute chest syndrome. Despite these advances in care, funding for the 10 comprehensive sickle cell centers financed under the National Sickle Cell Disease Control Act was abruptly discontinued in 2007, and in some instances, the centers have disbanded.

Recent approval of glutamine and active clinical trials evaluating P-selectin inhibition[13] and antipolymerization small molecules[14] are encouraging. More recent research advancements include stem cell transplantation, gene therapy, and the identification of genetic modifiers associated with SCD severity. Despite such breakthroughs in SCD research, individuals with SCD and their families have largely experienced no increases in their quality of life.[8] SCD remains characterized by stunning levels of infant mortality in low-resource settings[15] and by disparities in health outcomes and health resources, even in developed countries.[16-18] As we examine the relationship between social determinants of health and health outcomes in SCD, we recognize that racism and stigma remain critical facets of sickle cell care, policy, and research.

SCD-Related Racism, Discrimination, and Stigmatization

A recent meta-analysis of 293 studies published between 1983 and 2013 synthesized data on racism as a determinant of health.[19] Discrimination based on race, ethnicity, and/or nationality was associated with poor mental, physical, and general health. African Americans who reported repeated experiences of racial discrimination were found to exhibit impaired physical and mental health functioning (specifically increased pain), lower adherence to provider recommendations, and delays in seeking medical care.

Findings within sickle cell populations mirror these results. In one study, 71 adults with SCD provided reports of their experiences with discrimination in healthcare settings and completed measures of laboratory pain sensitivity (heat and pressure).[20] Ratings on the Interpersonal Processes of Care discrimination subscale were positively associated with reports of clinical pain severity and heightened sensitivity to laboratory-induced pain. Higher ratings of discrimination were also associated with reported symptoms of depression, higher stress levels, and poor sleep quality.

Individuals with SCD, their family members, and their health care providers believe that race affects the quality of SCD health care.[21] In the Improving Patient Outcomes With Respect and Trust (IMPORT) study of 273 adolescents and adults with SCD, patients reporting experiences of discrimination in the health care system were 53% more likely to report nonadherence with provider recommendations.[22] Trust in medical professionals mediated the relationship between discrimination and nonadherence; trust also contributes to disparities in health outcomes. Other research suggests that providers make negative judgments about patients with SCD and that providers consistently overestimate the risk of opioid addiction in patients with SCD compared to patients with other pain syndromes, which may incite cycles of undertreatment, bias, and mistrust.[23,24] Experiences of discrimination can affect coping; in a study of 51 adults with SCD reporting on pain-coping strategies, pain experiences, and health care injustice, those who reported experiences of health care injustice also reported more problematic pain-coping strategies, including catastrophizing (ruminating on the pain experience and feeling helpless about it) and isolation, compared with patients who did not report health care injustice.[25]

Although individuals with SCD and their families report a burden of race-based discrimination from health care providers, they also report disease-based discrimination. This includes more reports of discrimination with aging-out of pediatric care and discrimination associated with being misbelieved when in pain.[22] Adults with SCD who use emergency departments more frequently and who experience greater frequency and severity of pain reported more disease-based discrimination.

Disparities in health care provision result from discrimination, which is a type of stigma, although it is not expressed explicitly. Stigma is a Greek word that was conceptualized as a shaming attribute or a social identity that reduces an individual "from a whole and usual person to a tainted, discounted one."[26] Therefore, stigmatization occurs when a person possesses (or is believed to possess) "some attribute or characteristic that conveys a social identity that is devalued in a particular social context."[27]

A review of stigma in SCD studies identified 4 interactive domains, namely: (1) the social consequences of stigma; (2) the effect of stigma on psychological well-being; (3) the effect of stigma on physiologic well-being; and (4) the impact of stigma on patient-provider relationships and care-seeking behaviors.[28] Health-related stigma is prominent and may appear to result from racial prejudice.[29]

Linus Pauling, who was famously awarded 2 undivided Nobel Prizes and first described SCD as a molecular disease, was accused of racism when he suggested that carriers of genetic diseases including SCD should not procreate. Specifically, he stated, "I have suggested that the time might come in the future when information about heterozygosity in such serious genes as the sickle cell anemia gene would be tattooed on the forehead of the carriers, so that young men and women would at once be warned not to fall in love with each other."[30] This is consistent with the Greek description of stigma, which refers to a type of marking or tattoo that was cut or burnt into the skin of criminals, slaves, or traitors in order to visibly identify them as blemished or morally tainted people who were avoided or shunned, particularly in public places.[26]

President Nixon's subsequent press statement assumed Linus Pauling meant young African American persons, affirming that SCD "strikes only blacks and no one else." This seems to have resulted in early stigmatization that has persisted until today. Unfortunately, stigmatization and discrimination did not end with the passage of the National Sickle Cell Anemia Control Act in 1972.[31] Legislation from several states that was enacted to mandate screening for SCD among African Americans (ie, targeted screening) was construed by their communities to be discriminatory and stigmatizing because this led to denial of education, employment opportunities, and insurance for those with sickle cell trait. However, given that SCD was perceived to predominantly affect African Americans, implementation of newborn screening programs was quite slow in adoption, despite federal government funding.[32]

Since 2006, all 50 states in the United States screen for SCD with newborn screening.[32] Universal screening allows for early protection from infection and education for parents regarding risks of SCD-related complications. Newborns with sickle cell trait can also be identified through newborn screening, but follow-up with families regarding the results vary from state to state. Some controversy exists with screening for sickle cell trait among the military and college athletes. Sudden death is rare but feared. Within the military, reports of rhabdomyolysis or heat stroke among African American troops raised concern. However, further analysis demonstrated that these events occurred at a rate similar to all recruits.[33,34] Currently, universal precautions to prevent overheating and exertion are implemented in the military, protecting all military personnel independent of trait status. In the National Collegiate Athletic Association (NCAA), an analysis of 2 million athlete-years found an elevated risk for exertional death among individuals with sickle cell trait (5 times that those without sickle cell trait) but low overall risk (0.02%) in general.[35] Counseling those with trait and disease with recommendations to avoid exertion and dehydration appears to be the most prudent approach to offer both opportunity and protection to all. Adequate research on sickle cell trait and its implications remains lacking.

Research Participation

Racism, discrimination, and stigmatization can contribute to limited engagement by ethnic minority populations in research designed to test various treatment options, including curative therapies.[36] The issue is complex, with one study showing over-representation of African Americans in phase I safety studies but significant underrepresentation in phase III trials.[36] Issues that contribute to challenges to research participation for populations with SCD include mistrust of the health care system due to abuse and exploitation, as previously cited, as well as mistrust of research.[37-39] In separate focus group studies, parents of children with SCD expressed cultural mistrust (ie, suspicion of the broader society due to the history of racism and unfair treatment in the United States) and mistrust in medical professionals as barriers to research participation.[37,38]

In a cross-sectional survey of 154 parents/caregivers of children with SCD and 88 adolescents or young adults (AYAs) with SCD, factors contributing to mistrust as well as benefits and barriers to research participation were examined.[39] For caregivers, mistrust correlated with religious beliefs countering medical science and instrumental support provided by the researchers (eg, incentives, concrete support such as transportation). Higher perceived stress and lack of previous experience with research contributed to mistrust for caregivers. Male AYAs expressed the most mistrust, and for AYAs generally, lower instrumental support correlated with lower mistrust.

In a qualitative study of perceived benefits and barriers to clinical trial participation, children and AYAs with SCD (aged 10-29 years) and parents wanted the potential benefits of the research to outweigh potential harm and unmanageable study demands.[40] This and other studies highlight the importance of social determinants of health and practical considerations as contributing to research participation, including time required and other demands based on the study design.[41] In a large (N = 542), transregional survey study of parents and adults with SCD from throughout the United States, less than half of participants were interested in studies that required blood draws and hospital admission. Male gender, younger age, and depressive symptoms were predictive of interest in the least invasive studies. For parents, lower health literacy in fact predicted interest in studies requiring hospital admissions. Patient literacy about research participation can be dependent on access to knowledgeable health care providers who can educate patients about clinical trials and who have positive views of their patients and of clinical trials themselves.[42]

In an effort to improve the future care and clinical trial participation of people with SCD, we need a better understanding of the social determinants that significantly impact the population's daily lives and care. Social determinants may specifically influence the impact of the diagnosis and the experience of disease complications, particularly pain. Figure 27-1 depicts our conceptual model of the complex cycle of complications that can begin with external stressors triggering or

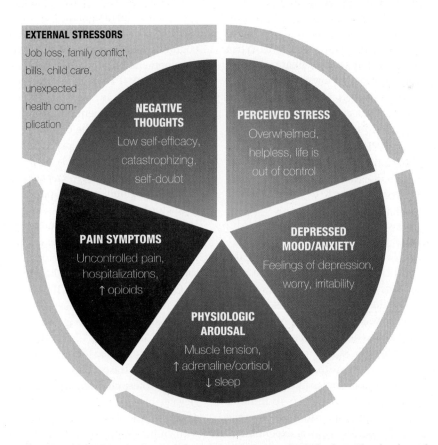

FIGURE 27-1 **A conceptualization of the biopsychosocial model adapted to show the hypothesized mechanisms linking behavioral and social factors to physiological pain and complication in sickle cell disease.**

exacerbating mood. A physiologic response to stress is well known, and the changes worsen pain. In the following sections, we summarize some of the most common external stressors that impact the lives of individuals with SCD.

The Economics of SCD in the United States

Within the United States, there are approximately 100,000 people with SCD, and >90% are African American.[43] Based on studies using claims data[44] and the Silent Cerebral Infarct Multi-Center Clinical Trial (SIT),[45] we estimate that 60% to 70% of children with SCD receive health coverage through Medicaid. One of the primary criteria for Medicaid eligibility is a family's low income, so this means that the majority of these families are living at or near poverty. Based on US Census data, 20% of children in the United States live in poverty.[46] In the screening phase of SIT, the primary caregivers of 536 school-aged children reported the family's income per capita. Well over 50% of these families were living with incomes per capita that were below the poverty level.[45]

African American families are more likely to live in poverty than White non-Hispanic families in the United States. However, the prevalence of poverty is even greater among families with SCD. Possibly, the demands of being available to care for a child with both acute and chronic needs make full-time employment a challenge.[47] In qualitative studies, parents of children report that these factors are significant and present barriers to holding a job.[48] At the child's birth, however, most of the families are already living at or near poverty level. When children are born into poverty, the family's financial status rarely improves enough to move out of low-income status.[49] For example, between 1979 and 2008, families who represented the bottom three-fifths of the average after-tax income brackets gained 40% in income, whereas the top 20% gained 65% in income over the same period. Most striking was that the top 1% of the tax brackets gained 275% in income over the 29-year period.[50]

Adults with SCD are also less likely to hold full-time employment. In 1985, the Cooperative Study of Sickle Cell Disease (CSSCD), a prospective cohort study funded by NHLBI, reported the unemployment status of 340 adults with SCD. The highest rate of unemployment was 56% among males who were not the head of their household. Among the men and women who were the heads of their households, 35% were unemployed. For comparison, the unemployment rate of non-patient controls was 13% to 16%. Fifteen to 26% of the adult patients were disabled compared to only 4% of controls.[51]

The cost of care for people with SCD is significant. The total lifetime health costs of a patient with SCD is almost a million dollars, and the yearly health care costs are >$10,000 for children and >$30,000 for adults with SCD.[52] To think of this in another way, a report of statewide insurance coverage found that children with SCD incurred medical expenditures that were 6 to 11 times higher than those of children without

SCD.[53] With the advent of new medications approved by the FDA for SCD, these costs are expected to continue to increase. Even after Medicaid expansion, gaps in insurance coverage remain for adults with SCD.[54]

For patients who are trying to work and support a household in addition to covering chronic medical needs, these financial burdens are significant barriers. One significant advance in US history that protects people with SCD is the Americans With Disabilities Act. In 1990, the US Congress passed this act, which protects qualified individuals with SCD from discrimination in employment.[55] For adults who are well enough to work, this type of protection was a noteworthy step forward.

Education

Chronic diseases are a critical component in the relationship between health and education, impacting both academic attainment and achievement. In the United States, 1 in 4 adolescents has a chronic disease.[56] Chronic illnesses among children increases the risk for academic failure.[57,58] Youth with chronic health conditions miss more school, are less connected to the school environment, and experience higher dropout rates.[59,60] Studies of children with SCD are consistent with these findings.

Early Childhood Development

Cognitive disparities are evident as early as infancy in children with SCD. One of the early investigations was a single-center study at Duke University. A total of 89 children between 6 and 36 months of age and their parents were evaluated. The Bayley Scales of infant Development-II was used to measure cognitive and neuromotor functioning. On both the mental developmental index (MDI) and the psychomotor developmental index (PDI), the percentage of children who scored in an at-risk range increased over time. In fact, the percentage of children with mental developmental concerns increased from 1.5% at 6 months of age (n = 66) to 46% at 36 months of age (n = 26). From a psychomotor standpoint, the proportion increased from 15.1% to 28% among the same sample. Regression models were created to predict the MDI and the PDI. Hemoglobin phenotype was a statistically significant predictor in both models, and a parent's attributional style of learned helplessness contributed an equal amount to the MDI. Daily stress, the child's phenotype, decreased knowledge of child development, and decreased efficacy all contributed to the prediction of parental distress.[61]

Over the next few years, the literature evolved to suggest that biologic variables may play a larger role in development than previously suspected. A group in London studied 28 infants with SCD at 3, 9, and 12 months of age using the Bayley Infant Neurodevelopmental Screener.[62] Transcranial Doppler (TCD), which is an ultrasound of the middle cerebral artery, was measured for these children. This measure was completed because elevated blood flow velocity in children between 2 and 16 years of age with hemoglobin SS and Sβ^0 thalassemia is associated with an increased risk of stroke.[63] The children also had pulse oximetry performed to measure the oxygen saturation of the blood because desaturation was identified as a risk factor for stroke as well.[64] Among 14 infants with SCD and 14 ethnically matched controls, the children with SCD were more likely to score in a range indicating greater risk for developmental delay as compared with the controls. At the age of 9 months, the raw scores from the Bayley Infant Neurodevelopmental Screener negatively correlated with TCD velocity and positively correlated with levels of hemoglobin. In total, the proportion of infants with SCD who scored in the moderate- to high-risk range for developmental delay rose from 14.3% at 3 months to 58.3% at 12 months.[62]

Developmental delay was associated with disease-related variables in another single-center cohort. The group included 50 children between the ages of 12 and 42 months. Parents were interviewed to complete the Vineland Adaptive Behavior Scale communication and motor domains.[65] The children were administered the Denver II[66] to assess their development. A total of 30% of the children had suspect scores, and 18% of the children were considered suspect in the language domain. The children with suspect scores were more likely to have lower language scores on the Vineland Adaptive Behavior Scale, lower hematocrit levels, and higher velocities on the TCD.[67]

In other groups of toddlers, disease-related variables did not significantly affect the children's development.[68,69] In a cohort of 88 3-year-old children with SCD, 50% had scores below the normal cutoff for their age on the Brigance Early Childhood Developmental Inventory.[70] When comparing the pass group with the fail group, the group that failed the screening test were more likely to have parents who did not graduate high school, and no biologic factors were associated with the failing scores.[68] The other cohort of toddlers included 26 children with SCD with a mean age of 51.7 months.[69] Only 7 children had TCD or magnetic resonance imaging (MRI) results, and all were unremarkable. The hemoglobin level had no association with the children's IQ score as measured by the Wechsler Preschool and Primary Scale Intelligence, Third Edition.[71] The mean IQ was 89.0 (range, 74-104). The family's income and the parental level of education were positively correlated with the children's language, memory/attention, and visual/spatial scores.[69] Within a single-center cohort of 43 infants and toddlers with SCD, >50% of children scored significantly below average on cognition and expressive language subscales on the Bayley Scales of Infant and Toddler Development (BSID-III).[72] SCD severity was not associated with patient scores. Socioeconomic status determined by the Diez-Roux method[73] positively correlated ($r = 0.401$, $P < .01$) with the home environment. Scores from the Home Observation Measurement of the Environment (HOME) correlated ($r = 0.360$, $P < .05$) with the cognitive subscale on the BSID-III. Other studies have identified similar trends.[68,69] On the basis of the result of these last few studies, it appears that environmental and family factors have more of an impact on early childhood development in this population than does the disease.

One early intervention for parents of young children with SCD proved feasibility of a home visitation program. In a single-arm, prospective cohort of 35 children with SCD between the ages of 3 and 36 months, their caregivers received monthly home visitation to encourage positive parent-child interactions. The mean scores within all 5 subtests of the BSID-III improved between enrollment and exit, with significant changes within cognitive ($P = .016$) and expressive language domains ($P = .002$). The home environment was a significant predictor of cognitive development.[74] These results support the concept that the home environment is modifiable by teaching caregivers ways to enrich the child's early experiences.

High School Graduation

Nearly 20% of children with SCD experience grade retention at least once, and >60% of children with SCD and silent cerebral infarcts have either failed a grade or received special education services.[45,75] Children who experience grade retention are at higher risk for high school dropout[76] and higher emergency department utilization as adults.[77]

The earliest description of the high school graduation rate of students with SCD came from the CSSCD. At that time in the early 1980s, 71% of the adults in that cohort graduated from high school. This rate was 4% lower than the Black US population during the same period.[51] In 2012, the graduation rate of 108 teenage students with SCD in St. Louis, Missouri, was 10% to 20% below the state average for those who lived in the county and city.[78]

In the US general population, adults without a high school diploma are likely to die 9 years earlier than college graduates.[79] For adolescents with SCD, patterns of school absence are often established early in life, creating lost learning opportunities, limiting motivation, compromising student relationships with teachers and peers, and impacting later academic attainment and achievement.[59,60,80-84] Improving the high school graduation rate for students with SCD may help improve both their health and earning potential.

Higher Education

Few studies have measured the rates of college education among adults with SCD. Again, the CSSCD is one of the earliest and largest descriptions. Only 8% of the patients had a 4-year college education, compared to 13% of African Americans in the United States in the same time period.[51] Male patients had the lowest rate of college graduation at 6%.[51] In a more recent cohort of 50 adults with SCD, 20% of the patients earned at least a 4-year degree.[85] These patients with a higher level of education also had a higher IQ and a higher rate of employment.

Mental Health

SCD is associated with a myriad of physical complications that require significant medical management; however, many patients living with SCD also suffer from psychological complications and mental health issues that frequently go unrecognized and untreated.[86-90] The need for mental health screening and treatment is often underappreciated. Several psychosocial stressors and behavioral challenges may put individuals with SCD at risk for developing major depression or other mental disorders. Mental health disorders and maladaptive stress coping responses are well-known risk factors for chronic pain and poor health outcomes in the general population. In turn, chronic pain and poor health outcomes can also precede the development of mental health disorders.

Depression

Symptoms related to depression, including social isolation, irritability, feelings of helplessness, depressed mood, and suicidality, are often seen among both children and adults with SCD.[89,91-94] Chronic pain and opioids can exacerbate other depressive symptoms, such as fatigue, poor appetite or weight loss, and sleep disturbance. It is not surprising, therefore, that children and adults with SCD are at an elevated risk of developing depression. Point prevalence estimates for major depressive disorders in people with SCD have varied widely between studies, from about 20% to 57%.[86,95-97] These rates are significantly higher than the rates typically seen in the general population.[98,99] When comparing African American adults with and without SCD, adults with SCD reported an 11% higher prevalence of depression compared to their healthy counterparts.[100]

The true prevalence of clinically significant depression in SCD remains unclear. Most studies regarding patients with SCD only report data from mental health screening tests or are underpowered to provide population estimates. Given the limitations of self-report depressive symptoms scales in detecting major depression based on *Diagnostic and Statistical Manual of Mental Disorders, Fifth Edition* (DSM) criteria, particularly in African American populations, the available studies do not provide an accurate estimate of the prevalence of major depression in SCD. One study[95] employed a validated structured clinical interview to assess depression and found that 26% of patients met criteria when interviewed; however, about 40% of patients met criteria for depression based on their self-reported symptoms on the Center for Epidemiologic Studies Depression Scale (CES-D) scale.[95] In a study of children with SCD who underwent a structured clinical interview, 12.5% met criteria for major depression.[92] Similarly, another study using a clinical interview to diagnose DSM disorders in children and adolescents found that 13% of patients with SCD met criteria for major depression, a prevalence that was not significantly different from other patients visiting a pediatric outpatient facility.[101]

Although limited, these data on prevalence of major depressive disorders in adults and children with SCD may suggest that either depression screening provides an overestimate of the actual diagnosis of major depression in this population or that patients are less forthcoming during a clinical interview than on a self-report scale. We were unable to find any other studies assessing major depression in adult patients with SCD using structured clinical interviews, and the current studies in both adult and pediatric populations have small sample sizes. Further, only one study has compared a clinical interview to

a validated depressive symptoms screening tool.[95] Given the current state of the literature, the true prevalence of major depression among adults with SCD remains unclear, as does the accuracy of depression screening tools and the suggested clinical cut points.

Almost all SCD studies are based on clinical samples because it is difficult to identify patients in the community who may or may not visit outpatient clinics. Not only has this been a limitation for studies of mental health in SCD, but it may also negatively skew our understanding of SCD as a whole. In addition, the prevalence of depression and other psychological complications might appear artificially high because current studies only include data from the patients with the most severe disease course who are attending a clinic.

Cultural Differences in Presentation

Because the majority of patients with SCD in the United States are ethnic/racial minorities, we must consider cultural differences in the presentation of depressive symptoms. African Americans are much less likely to seek treatment for depression, but they are more likely to experience chronic depression and rate their condition as severe or disabling.[102,103] Therefore, a less severe but more chronic form of depression, called dysthymic disorder, may be more prevalent in individuals with SCD. Indeed, a retrospective study of children with SCD found dysthymic disorder present 9 times more frequently than major depressive disorder.[104]

In addition, given the perceived stigma associated with mental health disorders in the African American community, it is also likely that typical symptoms of depression are not often endorsed by American Americans with SCD. Among African American men, depression may be considered a sign of personal weakness, and many members of the community believe that mental illness should be addressed within the family unit or religious organizations.[105] Many African American patients with SCD may be reluctant to express symptoms of depression, such as depressed mood and feelings of hopelessness, directly to their providers. Instead, they will more likely report culturally acceptable symptoms such as irritability, fatigue, stress, and pain.

Diagnosis of Depression

Although a large proportion of patients with SCD are at risk for mental health disorders, depression is rarely diagnosed (and even more rarely adequately treated) with routine SCD care. Unfortunately, the issue of underdiagnosed depression is not unique to the SCD community. Patients in need of mental health services typically receive care from their primary care providers, not from psychologists or psychiatrists, and primary care providers only diagnose depression in about half of all patients who meet the diagnostic criteria for the disorder. Symptoms of depression that may manifest as behavioral dysfunction are often attributed to physiologic illness; thus, physicians develop treatment plans that target the assumed physiologic illness without treating the underlying mental disorder. As a result, neither the patient's behavioral nor physiologic outcomes improve. A lack of essential mental health treatment may exacerbate the challenges associated with treating SCD, especially in patients who are considered "problematic" due to frequent or inappropriate health care utilization. Depression is a known risk factor for emergency department visits[106] and hospital admissions and readmissions.[107] Therefore, health care providers must appropriately screen for and treat depression in patients with SCD to effectively treat and manage SCD as a whole.

Anxiety

Compared to the relatively high rate of depression in patients with SCD, anxiety symptoms are reported much less frequently. Anxiety is highly correlated with depression in the general population.[108] In a large epidemiologic study of adults with SCD, only 6.5% presented with clinically significant symptoms of anxiety.[93] When anxiety was assessed during routine clinic visits, only 29% of adults reported anxiety.[94] Anxiety symptoms among children and adolescents may be even lower.[108] In other chronic pain syndromes, symptoms of depression and anxiety may be masked by use of substances.[109] Data from the Pain in Sickle Cell Epidemiology Study (PiSCES) indicated that approximately one-third of adults with SCD surveyed met criteria for alcohol abuse and one-third met criteria for depression/anxiety.[110] Interestingly, individuals who abused alcohol reported greater pain relief from opioids compared to those who did not use alcohol.

Sleep-Wake Disorders

Patients with SCD regularly experience abnormal sleep, characterized by frequent arousals and reduced total sleep time. In an animal study comparing mice with sickle cell phenotype versus mice with sickle cell trait, the phenotype mice exhibited significantly decreased total non–rapid eye movement sleep time but no change in total rapid eye movement sleep time. The phenotype mice also took longer to resume sleep after a wake period compared to the trait mice (3.2 ± 0.3 minutes v 1.9 ± 0.2 minutes; P <.05). The disrupted sleep patterns observed in the phenotype mice were not better accounted for by obstructive sleep apnea.[111] This animal study suggests that not only do behavioral factors, such as sleep hygiene, pain symptoms, and chronic opioid use, negatively affect sleep, but biologic factors may also play a role in disrupting sleep patterns as well. In a cohort of 328 adults with SCD, 70% had sleep disturbances.[86] More research is needed to understand the factors driving these disturbances.

Posttraumatic Stress Disorder

Posttraumatic stress disorder (PTSD) is an exaggerated fear or anxiety response to a traumatic event where the person was exposed to death, threatened death, or violence. The main symptoms of PTSD are persistent reexperiencing of the traumatic event, avoidance of trauma-related stimuli, negative thoughts and mood, and hyperarousal or hypervigilance. This disorder has been relatively ignored in the SCD literature and clinical care. Although children and adults with SCD may often report or exhibit symptoms consistent with PTSD in response to a traumatizing hospitalization for severe pain, the reported stressor (eg, severe pain episode requiring medical attention) does not meet DSM criteria for a traumatic event. Recent debates in mental health literature question the definition of a "traumatic event," and some experts suggest that whether someone experiences a DSM-congruent or DSM-incongruent stressor makes little difference in whether the event results in PTSD symptoms.[112,113] One study evaluated PTSD in SCD by semistructured interview using hospitalization for a severe pain episode as the traumatic event and found that 27% (3 of 11) of children and 40% (4 of 11) of their parents met diagnostic criteria.[114] Apart from this study, no other data have systematically examined the prevalence of PTSD in patients with SCD. However, there is a recognized need to consider PTSD secondary to severe pain episodes in SCD, particularly in the context of depression and anxiety that may increase risk of posttrauma symptoms.[115] For individuals with SCD who perceive the onset of a pain episode and subsequent hospital stay as a traumatic, life-threatening experience, expanding the definition of a traumatic event may enable them to access a wider array of mental health services.

Factors Increasing Risk for Mental Health Disorders in SCD

Stress and the Effects of Chronic Illness

The unpredictable and chronic nature of the disease can be a source of significant psychological and socioeconomic stress to both patients and their family members.

Low Socioeconomic Status

The SCD population is subject to high rates of poverty, low educational attainment, and a lack of environmental resources, which are already independent risk factors for depression in SCD.[100] These psychosocial stressors are exacerbated by a patient's belief that society holds a negative attitude toward SCD and those affected.

Negative Social Interactions and Perceived Discrimination

As noted earlier, when individuals with SCD seek medical treatment, they often report poor interactions with medical providers and express a general distrust of the health care system. These negative interactions, perceived lack of support, and discrimination can contribute to increased stress and mental health symptoms.[116]

Effects of Anemia on the Brain

Chronic anemia can have negative acute and chronic effects on brain health.[117] Data from non-SCD older adults suggest that even mild anemia can increase risk for depressive symptoms and lower quality of life. There are no direct data showing an effect of anemia on mental health in SCD; however, it is likely that the same mechanisms linking anemia to poorer cognitive functioning in SCD may also contribute to increased risk for mental health disorders in this population. Taken together, the multiple sources of biologic, psychological, and social stress put individuals with SCD, especially those with the most severe disease, at heightened risk for depression and other mental health complications.[118]

Mental Health and Pain Outcomes

Although studies exploring depression and SCD are limited, evidence suggests that depressive symptoms may increase the risk for poor disease outcomes, particularly pain.[119] Patterns of depressed moods and negative thoughts can make it more difficult for people with SCD to cope with pain,[120] and patients with more depressive symptoms experience more frequent and severe acute vaso-occlusive pain events.[86,93] Psychological stress and the negative stress response are also associated with poor pain outcomes and disability.[121-123] Gil et al[123] found that among adults with SCD, daily stress and negative mood were positively associated with fluctuations in same-day SCD pain. Increased stress levels also predicted pain increase during the following 2 days. Similarly, in a group of adolescents with SCD, daily increases in stress and negative mood were associated with increased pain, increased health care utilization, and reduced school and social activity on the same day as the increased stress levels and negative mood.[124]

A reciprocal relationship exists between pain and depression. Negative thoughts and low mood may elevate perceived stress and pain, which in turn can increase negative affect.[120,125] In patients with SCD, unpredictable acute pain and unrelenting chronic pain can lead to deleterious negative thoughts and low self-efficacy, causing patients to feel overwhelmed and helpless. This perceived stress increases depression and anxiety, as well as physiologic arousal and vaso-occlusion, which can directly trigger a pain crisis.[126]

Mental Health and Health Care Utilization

The relationship between mental health and health care utilization may be heterogeneous depending on patient disease severity and risk for health care utilization.[127] Several studies have found no association between mental health and health care utilization, whereas others have reported significant associations. In their 2011 study, Carroll et al[106] showed a strong association between depression and frequency of emergency department visits. These data make a convincing case for mental health as a risk factor for increased health care utilization. However, compared to other studies that did not show an association, Carroll et al[106] restricted their data to include only adults with a medically documented mental health disorder, and they used a more stringent definition of high utilization (ie, ≥4 encounters in 1 year). Thus, they performed analyses on an extreme group with respect to disease severity and health care use.

The association between depression and health care utilization may be much stronger for individuals with SCD who have severe disease and frequent pain episodes or complications. In contrast, for those who do not present with severe disease, depressive symptoms may not exacerbate their outcomes. Thus, screening for depression may be important for all patients with SCD, but identifying symptoms indicative of major depression is particularly important for patients with frequent complications and a severe disease presentation.

Depression is not the only factor linked to health care utilization and poor health outcomes in patients with SCD. Other negative psychological factors related to depression have also been associated with health care utilization and may account for the observed depression-utilization association. Daily stress and negative mood have been associated with increased self-reported health care use in both adolescents and adults.[123,125,128] In a group of children and adolescents, emotional suppression and somatization were associated with parent-reported number of hospitalizations over the past 12 months, even after controlling for SCD type and pain.[129] In pediatrics, some evidence suggests that poorer psychological adjustment of the caregivers can lead to increased health care utilization among children with SCD.[130,131] Also, more frequent health care visits can negatively impact both physical and mental quality of life.[132,133] Therefore, several other potential causal factors may confound the association between depression and health care utilization.

Mental Health Screening Tests

A variety of mental health screening tests have been used to assess mental health in SCD, all of which have been validated in other primary care or chronic disease populations.[108] It is unclear, however, what screening tests are valid for use in SCD and how they can be used most effectively. To our knowledge, only one study has attempted to determine the validity of cut-off scores used in the SCD population. Grant et al[95] found that using traditional cutoff scores for the CES-D led to 25% of the patients being falsely identified as having depression when compared to the diagnosis determined by a clinical interview. However, when more stringent cutoff scores are used, 10% to 14% of patients can be misidentified as not having depression when they actually do. Fatigue and other somatic symptoms could potentially lead to high false-positive rates for depression and other mental health disorders in patients with SCD when self-reporting is used. There is also the likelihood that individuals with SCD (especially African Americans) will underreport mental health symptoms due to perceived stigma, fear of having pain treatments withheld, and a lack of general education about mental health symptoms. Given the link between mental health, somatic symptoms, and health care utilization,[108] adequate health care should err toward treatment of false-positive mental health diagnoses, particularly where a low-risk, behavioral assessment can serve as the first line of treatment.

Treatment of Mental Health Issues in SCD

Few psychological intervention studies address behavioral or mental health issues in patients with SCD, and even fewer have attempted to specifically address depression. Further, due to methodologic limitations of the existing body of evidence, it is difficult to determine whether there are interventions that will be effective for treating depression in SCD. A systematic review found 11 studies testing psychological interventions in patients with SCD,[134] but only one of these studies examined depression as an outcome, finding that a psychoeducational intervention did not decrease depressive symptoms in pediatric patients with SCD.[135] Four studies tested the efficacy of cognitive-behavioral therapy on pain, coping, and health care utilization. The findings were mixed, and because of the poor quality of these studies (eg, small sample size, no control group, unclear intervention protocol), the impact of cognitive-behavioral therapy, or any other evidence-based mental health treatment, on behavioral outcomes in SCD is unclear.[134] One study offered 6 manual-assisted individual cognitive-behavioral therapy sessions to 35 adults with SCD and found no significant differences in pain or health care utilization after the intervention. Patients also reported a reduced level of anxiety, but not depression, after the cognitive-behavioral therapy; however, the lack of efficacy may have been due to high dropout (14 of 35). Patient engagement and retention may be as important, or more important, than the intervention itself. Despite the significant psychosocial burden and mental health issues in this population, there are still no high-quality studies testing the effectiveness of an evidence-based treatment for mental health disorders in patients with SCD. More recently, there have been attempts to implement electronic therapy in SCD care. These studies are covered later in this chapter.

Patient-Reported Outcomes in SCD

A patient-reported outcome (PRO) has been defined as "an outcome reported directly by patients themselves and not interpreted by an observer."[136] PROs include patients' report of social or physical functioning, pain or other symptoms,

treatment satisfaction, stigma, medication adherence, sleep quality, and health-related quality of life (HRQOL).[136] HRQOL is a PRO that is defined as "a multidimensional concept that usually includes self-report of the way in which physical, emotional, social, or other domains of well-being are affected by a disease or its treatment."[136] A proxy-reported outcome has also commonly been used to evaluate PROs and/or HRQOL among pediatric populations (ie, parent-proxy) and has been defined as "a measurement based on a report by someone other than the patient reporting as if he or she is the patient."[137] Major international health policy and regulatory authorities, as well as patients, have recognized the value of PRO assessment in clinical trials to inform clinical decision making, pharmaceutical labeling claims, and product reimbursement and to influence health care policy.[137-139] The inclusion of PROs in clinical trial protocols should be planned and reported according to the SPIRIT-PRO guidelines.[140] In addition, the routine assessment of PROs in clinical settings has shown several benefits, such as enhancing patient-provider communication, improving patients' satisfaction, assisting in shared decision-making process, monitoring improvement or deterioration of health, and creating a patient-centered environment.[141] Importantly, assessing PROs in clinical settings has not increased the duration of the visit.[142]

SCD is characterized by frequent, recurrent, unexpected, and debilitating pain episodes; increased risk for silent and overt strokes; and several comorbidities, such as renal and cardiopulmonary disease.[143] These complications, particularly pain episodes, lead to significant impairment in PROs among individuals with SCD in different domains across their life span. Physical and psychosocial impairments are especially salient and are comparable to or worse than those of other chronic illnesses.[144-147] Our conceptual framework (Figure 27-2) summarizes key patient- and SCD-related factors that contribute to PROs in SCD and their relationship to SCD complications and health care utilization in this population. Earlier studies showed better PROs in children and adults with SCD who received hydroxyurea, compared to those who

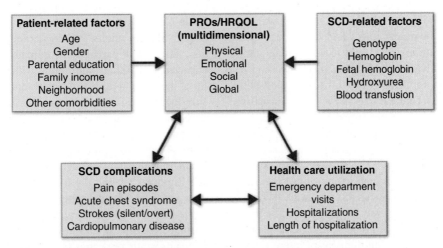

FIGURE 27-2 Key patient- and sickle cell disease (SCD)-related factors that contribute to patient-reported outcomes (PROs) in SCD and their relationship to SCD. HRQOL, heath-related quality of life.

did not.[148,149] Patients with higher hydroxyurea adherence rates also showed better PROs.[150] In contrast, more frequent SCD-related hospitalizations and emergency department visits and/or longer length of stay during hospitalizations were found to be associated with worse PRO scores, particularly for pain, fatigue, physical function mobility, depression, and social isolation.[145-147,150-155] Previous studies showed an association between worse PRO scores and female sex, older age,[147,153,156-160] low family income, poor neighborhood, low parental education, and associated comorbidities.[153,161,162] Further, Dampier et al[147] reported worse PRO scores in patients with hemoglobin SS and SB⁰ thalassemia, compared to other genotypes, which was not seen in other published studies.[153,156,163] Other reported factors associated with worse PRO scores include neurobehavioral comorbidities (eg, developmental delay or attention deficit disorder) and laboratory markers (eg, low hemoglobin and low fetal hemoglobin).[145,149] Evaluating PROs among children and/or adults with SCD is key to better understand their individual functioning and well-being. PRO research has also been informative to individuals with SCD, their families, and health care professionals because it provides an opportunity to measure the impact of treatment, uniquely focusing on the perspective of the patient, and provides information necessary to tailor therapies.

A number of factors should be considered when evaluating PROs in patients with SCD, such as participants' age, generic versus disease-specific approach, and psychometric properties of the available measures. For adults with SCD, a self-report PRO measure would suffice, whereas in children, having both self-report and parent-proxy versions of the measure would be preferred, especially if it includes a wide age range (infants up to 18 years). Prior work has shown that proxy-report of PROs is complementary to patient self-report of PROs.[164] For example, Seid et al[164] have shown that parent proxy-report of PROs may be used to predict outcomes such as health care costs in children. Using PRO measures that have been tested in patients with SCD and demonstrated strong psychometric properties (eg, reliability, validity, and responsiveness) should be a key consideration when determining which measures to use to assess well-being in this vulnerable population.[165] Moreover, there has been an ongoing debate regarding the use of generic versus disease-specific PRO measures, and each approach has its own advantages and disadvantages.[166] Generic measures provide an opportunity to better understand SCD burden on an individual's well-being in comparison to healthy individuals and populations with other chronic health conditions.[146,147,167-169] In contrast, disease-specific measures have high specificity and are better suited to examine differences within patients with SCD in response to treatment or interventions and across various patient groups (eg, SCD genotypes and treatment vs controls).[170-172] Therefore, most experts in the field recommend using a combination of both generic and disease-specific measures to assess PROs in SCD.[144,145,166,173] Finally, participant burden (ie, survey fatigue) should be minimized, and the administration of PROs should be as brief as possible and focused on the relevant domains of interest, particularly when used in clinical settings.

TABLE 27-1 Commonly used patient-reported outcome measures in sickle cell disease (SCD)

Pediatric SCD	Adult SCD
SCD specific	SCD specific
PedsQL SCD module	ASCQ-Me
Generic	Generic
PedsQL generic core scales	SF-36
Pediatric PROMIS measures	Adult PROMIS measures
Child Health Questionnaire	WHOQOL-BREF

Abbreviations: ASCQ-Me, Adult Sickle Cell Quality of Life Measurement Information System; PedsQL, Pediatric Quality of Life; PROMIS, Patient Reported Outcomes Measurement Information System; SF-36, Medical Outcomes Study Questionnaire Short Form 36; WHOQOL-BREF, World Health Organization Quality of Life-BREF.

Over the past few decades, several PRO measures have been used and evaluated in SCD (Table 27-1), whereas only a few have been developed and validated specifically for this population. The most commonly used generic HRQOL measures for children with SCD are the PedsQL generic core scales and the Child Health Questionnaire. The Medical Outcomes Study Questionnaire Short Form 36 (SF-36) and the World Health Organization Quality of Life-BREF (WHOQOL-BREF) are widely used for adults.[144,145,174] The National Institutes of Health (NIH)-endorsed Patient Reported Outcomes Measurement Information System (PROMIS) has been evaluated recently among pediatric and adult patients with SCD, using both short forms and computerized adaptive testing (CAT).[156,163,173,175-179] There have been a number of validation studies that evaluated the psychometric properties of these measures in patients with SCD and supported the use of these measures in this population.[167-169,180-183] More recently, SCD-specific PRO measures became available, including the PedsQL SCD module for children and the NIH-endorsed Adult Sickle Cell Quality of Life Measurement Information System (ASCQ-Me) for adults.[170-173] In particular, pain, physical function, fatigue, and psychosocial domains have been consistently impacted in children and adults with SCD (Table 27-2).[144,145] All of these age-appropriate generic and SCD-specific measures were found to have sound psychometric properties and would be recommended for use to evaluate PROs in patients with SCD. However, in SCD, the clinically important differences in PRO scores is only known for the PedsQL Generic Core Scales, Multidimensional Fatigue Scale, and the disease-specific PedsQL SCD module.[183] Clinically important differences have not yet been established for the other measures. Ongoing work as part of the Pediatric Patient Reported Outcomes for Children with Chronic Diseases Consortium (PEPR Consortium, https://www.peprconsortium.org) aims to establish the clinically important differences for pediatric PROMIS domains.

TABLE 27-2 Commonly affected PRO domains and suggested age-appropriate PRO measures

	Generic PROs	SCD-specific PROs
Pediatric measures	**PROMIS**	**PedsQL SCD**
Age	Self-report (8-17 years old) Proxy-report (5-17 years old)	Self-report (5-18 years old) Proxy-report (2-18 years old)
Domains		
Pain	Pain interference Pain intensity Pain behavior Pain quality–sensory Pain quality–affective	Pain and hurt Pain impact Pain management and control
Physical	Physical function–mobility Physical activity Physical stress experiences Strength impact	Physical health
Fatigue	Fatigue	Fatigue module
Psychosocial	Depressive symptoms Anxiety Peer relationships Psychological stress experiences	Worry I Worry II Emotions
Adult measures	**PROMIS**	**ASCQ-Me**
Age	≥18 years old	≥18 years old
Domains		
Pain	Pain behavior Pain intensity Pain quality–neuropathic Pain quality–nocioceptive	Pain episodes Pain impact
Physical	Physical function Physical function–mobility Physical function–upper extremity	Stiffness impact
Fatigue	Fatigue	
Psychosocial	Depression Anxiety Social isolation Satisfaction with social roles	Emotional impact Social functioning impact

Abbreviations: ASCQ-Me, Adult Sickle Cell Quality of Life Measurement Information System; PRO, patient-reported outcome; PROMIS, Patient Reported Outcomes Measurement Information System; SCD, sickle cell disease.

The mode of PRO assessment is another important consideration. PRO measures can be administered either using paper and pencil or electronically (e-PROs). The use of e-PROs has several advantages: (1) provides more accurate, complete, high-quality, and timely data; (2) improves compliance to study protocol (eg, reminders and real-time monitoring); (3) minimizes recall bias and secondary data entry errors; (4) allows for CAT approach; (5) allows easier implementation of skip patterns; (6) results in less administrative burden; (7) allows for potential cost savings with less paper printing;

and (8) provides a patient-friendly approach with high acceptance rates.[184-186] In addition, regulators (eg, FDA), the Professional Society for Health Economics and Outcomes Research (ISPOR), the International Society for Quality of Life Research (ISOQOL), and the ePRO Consortium encourage the use of e-PROs.[140,185,187]

Mobile Health Behavioral Interventions in SCD

Self-management has been defined as the individual's ability to manage the symptoms, treatment, physical and psychological consequences, and lifestyle changes inherent to living with a chronic illness.[188] Self-management is a critical skill for individuals with SCD as they encounter frequent challenges related to pain management, adequate hydration, balanced nutrition, clinic attendance, and adherence to medication regimens, especially during the transition from pediatric to adult care settings. In particular, medication adherence is a key component of patients' self-management skills. Individuals with SCD with more adherence barriers, as well as negative perceptions of hydroxyurea or SCD, reported lower adherence rates, had worse PRO scores, and had more frequent SCD-related complications and increased health care utilization.[175,176,189] Earlier data suggest that SCD complications have led to >230,000 emergency department visits per year with an annual health expenditure of $1.5 billion.[190,191] Novel interventions in SCD, such as the integration of personal technology tools, have the potential to improve health outcomes and self-management for individuals with SCD.

Adolescents and adults with SCD have ubiquitous access to personal technologies, including smartphones, tablets, laptops, and desktops.[41,192-194] Individuals with SCD have reported interest in using these personal devices to manage their SCD.[41,192-194] These technologic solutions are well integrated with the way health care is delivered currently because more and more people use technology to obtain and maintain information about a chronic illness, such as SCD, or to track a healthy lifestyle.[195,196] In addition, previous studies showed a relationship between improved health outcomes and shared decision making, enhanced patient activation, and engagement in medical care,[197-199] all of which can be facilitated by mobile health (mHealth) interventions.[200-204] mHealth is defined as "an emerging field in the intersection of medical informatics, public health and business, referring to health services and information delivered or enhanced through the Internet and related technologies."[205] mHealth interventions have gained momentum and have become more widely acceptable and, therefore, should be leveraged to enhance self-management skills among individuals with SCD to optimize their health outcomes.

There is growing evidence that the use of technologic interventions contributes to improved self-care skills for individuals.[206-208] In addition, data support the overall feasibility, acceptability, and efficacy of mHealth interventions in improving health outcomes,[209-214] including for those with SCD,[215] although the cost-effectiveness of these interventions remains unclear.[216] A recent systematic review evaluated the evidence for mHealth interventions to support self-management in children and adults with SCD.[215] All mHealth studies were conducted in the United States, and most were for children or adolescents (69%) and had a sample size of ≤50 participants (75%).[215] These mHealth interventions were focused on improving medication adherence, self-management, pain/symptom monitoring, coping skills training, cognitive training, education, guided relaxation, or cognitive-behavioral therapy.[215] Various technologic tools were used in these studies, including text messaging, native mobile or web-based applications (apps), mobile directly observed therapy, internet-delivered cognitive-behavioral therapy, electronic pill bottles, or interactive gamification.[215] Almost all mHealth studies showed evidence to support the preliminary efficacy of these interventions.[215] The majority of studies reported high satisfaction and acceptability of the interventions among study participants of various age groups.[215] These findings are further supported by 2 recent studies that provided promising evidence for the efficacy of mHealth interventions to improve medication adherence and disease knowledge[217] as well as mental health using cognitive-behavioral therapy.[218] A number of mHealth intervention studies in SCD are ongoing.[219-221] Despite the current evidence, future mHealth studies using rigorous methodology and theoretical frameworks with clearly defined clinical outcomes are still warranted to examine the efficacy, effectiveness, and cost-effectiveness of these interventions in children and adults with SCD.

Conclusion

Experiences and exposures influence physical and emotional health, no less for individuals with SCD compared with the general population. Although risk factors can be reduced and protective factors enhanced to improve health and well-being, individuals with SCD are at particular risk for psychological, social, and cognitive challenges due to higher prevalence of poverty, lower educational attainment, stigmatization, health care disparities, and disease processes. There are a small number of trials to date evaluating interventions that target enhanced coping and self-management, some using novel modes of delivery such as mHealth. Family education and cognitive-behavioral therapy are most promising but do not yet meet criteria for well-established interventions in SCD due to heterogeneity of methods and measurement and small sample sizes that preclude definitive statements about efficacy. The field is ripe to rigorously test diverse interventions that promote positive coping, and the number of active trials (many multisite) of psychological, social, and cognitive interventions registered on ClinicalTrials.gov has burgeoned in recent years.

Future directions for research within this field include evaluation of targeted, problem-focused treatments to reduce symptoms and prevent ongoing or escalating distress; evaluation of sensitive periods when interventions should be delivered, if needed; community collaborations to address the range of social determinants of health; and consortia, including shared measurement, that focus on enhancing resilience in SCD. The majority of individuals with SCD do indeed demonstrate resiliency in the face of multiple stressors. However, it is critical for health care providers and researchers to improve screening of potential challenges using PROs and other tools; to offer and evaluate best practices for supporting adults and children with SCD across the life span; and to recognize individual and institutional biases that must be addressed in order to ensure that health equity is attained and the long-standing and pervasive health disparities that have characterized SCD are eliminated.

Case Studies

Case 1. Shay is a 10-year-old with hemoglobin SS. He has a history of frequent headaches, attention deficit disorder, and frequent painful episodes. He had a relatively uncomplicated disease course until he was approximately 7 years old. His mother remained in the home to raise Shay until Shay went to school full time in first grade. His father worked as a public transit operator. Shay's parents developed marital discord, but both parents and Shay continued to live in the same household due to financial inability to maintain 2 households in a large urban city characterized by gentrification (ie, displacement of poor and working-class people of color). However, the situation became untenable, so Shay and his mother moved in with Shay's maternal grandmother. Shay's mother and grandmother also had a conflictual relationship. After some time, that living situation also became unsustainable, and Shay and his mother became homeless, floating between other relatives' homes. Shay's mother works as an Uber driver to maintain flexibility around Shay's frequent appointments and hospitalizations. Shay's family is receiving outpatient psychotherapy with the sickle cell team psychologist, but his pain episodes remain frequent and interfere significantly with Shay's ability to adequately function in school, at home, and with peers.

Case 2. Tiara is a 20-year-old African American female who is a student at a local community college, pursuing certification as a nursing assistant. She lives with her mother, stepfather, and half-sister not far from her maternal grandparents. Tiara was diagnosed on newborn screening with SCD, hemoglobin SS, and has been cared for at a comprehensive sickle cell center since infancy. Her maternal uncle also has hemoglobin SS and experiences severe symptoms including multiple episodes of acute chest syndrome and pain. At age 4, Tiara was identified as at risk for stroke on TCD and started a course of chronic transfusion therapy. She developed avascular necrosis of both hips and eventually had her right hip replaced. Other surgeries included a cholecystectomy and a tunneled venous port placement at age 15 as her venous access became increasingly difficult. Tiara complains of frequent headaches and has had progressive narrowing of her internal carotid artery despite monthly transfusions.

Tiara's maternal grandmother has provided primary support to Tiara and her mother since Tiara's diagnosis with SCD, as Tiara's mother was a single parent during her infancy and early childhood. However, the support of Tiara's grandmother has faded since Tiara's mother remarried 5 years ago. Although adherence with appointments, screenings, and preventive therapies including penicillin prophylaxis had been good, adherence with iron chelation therapy became challenging when Tiara's mother remarried. Although the stepfather is supportive, clinical staff had difficulty finding a clinic time to provide him with sickle cell education due to his work schedule. In addition, although Tiara graduated from high school, her clinical team became concerned that she was beginning to exhibit executive functioning difficulties (eg, appearing to have difficulty planning and tracking appointments). Impairments in executive functioning were confirmed on neuropsychological evaluation, but the family had transitioned responsibility for her appointment keeping and medication management to her in her late teens, based on her age. During this time, adherence with appointment keeping deteriorated, as did Tiara's adherence with iron chelation therapy, resulting in severe iron overload. Tiara's serum ferritin level is >10,000 ng/mL (goal is <2000 ng/mL), and on MRI, her current reading is 10,000 µg/g dry weight (goal is <7000 µg/g dry weight). The clinical team has held family meetings with Tiara, her mother, and her grandmother to encourage them to assist Tiara more with appointment keeping and adherence with iron chelation therapy. Unfortunately, there has been limited improvement.

Tiara reports depressed and anxious moods and increasing lack of motivation to be adherent with iron chelation therapy, as she has begun to struggle with managing her community college classes. Tiara's social worker used motivational interviewing to help understand barriers to adherence, and Tiara reported these were forgetting to take the medicine, not prioritizing iron chelation among her other responsibilities, and anxiety about needle insertion to administer the medication. Tiara reported that her emotions related to her disease included anger and sadness as she felt overwhelmed and burned out with the need to chelate daily but also reported having some challenges with accepting the need for chelation given that she did not feel "sick" as a result of her iron overload. An oral iron chelator was added to Tiara's medication regimen, but she complained of the taste and challenges with dissolving the formulation completely in water. Another family meeting was held, and Tiara's mother was convinced to become more involved with the iron chelation for a period of time.

High-Yield Facts

◆ Psychosocial stress triggers sympathetic arousal and a physiologic state (eg, increased catecholamines, inflammation, cellular adhesion, vasoconstriction, decreased oxygenation) that can cause a vaso-occlusive event for persons with SCD.

◆ Discrimination and stigmatization are common aspects of the lived experience of adults with SCD that can contribute to poor mental and physical health, as well as hinder engagement in medical care and clinical research.

◆ Lower socioeconomic status, neighborhood stressors, and limited access to social resources negatively impact some individuals' ability to successfully navigate life transitions and manage the complexities of their chronic condition.

◆ Across their life span, mental health disorders and impaired quality of life as measured by PROs are prevalent in patients with SCD and can be both a cause and consequence of disease complications, particularly pain episodes.

◆ Improving screening and treatment for mental health and stress-related disorders in SCD has the potential to improve outcomes and perceived quality of care.

References

1. Konotey-Ahulu FI. *The Sickle Cell Disease Patient.* Macmillan Press; 1991.

2. Dennis-Antwi JA, Culley L, Hiles DR, Dyson SM. "I can die today, I can die tomorrow": lay perceptions of sickle cell disease in Kumasi, Ghana at a point of transition. *Ethn Health.* 2011;16(4-5):465-481.

3. Savitt TL, Goldberg MF. Herrick's 1910 case report of sickle cell anemia: the rest of the story. *JAMA.* 1989;261(2):266-271.

4. Frenette PS, Atweh GF. Sickle cell disease: old discoveries, new concepts, and future promise. *J Clin Invest.* 2007;117(4):850-858.

5. Wailoo K. Sickle cell disease—a history of progress and peril. *N Engl J Med.* 2017;376(9):805-807.

6. Serjeant GR. The emerging understanding of sickle cell disease. *Br J Haematol.* 2001;112(1):3-18.

7. Savitt TL. The invisible malady: sickle cell anemia. *J Natl Med Assoc.* 1981;73(8):739.

8. Prabhakar H, Haywood C Jr, Molokie R. Sickle cell disease in the United States: looking back and forward at 100 years of progress in management and survival. *Am J Hematol.* 2010;85(5):346-353.

9. Tapper M. *In the Blood: Sickle Cell Anemia and the Politics of Race.* University of Pennsylvania Press; 1999.

10. Naik RP, Haywood C. Sickle cell trait diagnosis: clinical and social implications. *Hematology Am Soc Hematol Educ Program.* 2015;2015(1):160-167.

11. Nelson A. *Body and Soul: The Black Panther Party and the Fight Against Medical Discrimination.* University of Minnesota Press; 2011.

12. National Heart, Lung, and Blood Institute. *Sickle Cell Disease: Milestones in Research and Clinical Progress.* National Heart, Lung, and Blood Institute; 2018:10-7657.

13. Ataga KI, Kutlar A, Kanter J, et al. Crizanlizumab for the prevention of pain crises in sickle cell disease. *N Engl J Med.* 2016;376(5):429-439.

14. Vichinsky E, Hoppe CC, Ataga KI, et al. A phase 3 randomized trial of voxelotor in sickle cell disease. *N Engl J Med.* 2019;381(6):509-519.

15. Piel FB, Hay SI, Gupta S, Weatherall DJ, Williams TN. Global burden of sickle cell anaemia in children under five, 2010–2050: modelling based on demographics, excess mortality, and interventions. *PLoS Med.* 2013;10(7):e1001484.

16. Anand S, Theodore R, Mertens A, Lane PA, Krishnamurti L. Health disparity in hematopoietic cell transplantation for sickle cell disease: analyzing the association of insurance and socioeconomic status among children undergoing hematopoietic cell transplantation. *Blood.* 2017;130(suppl 1):4636.

17. Haywood C, Lanzkron S, Bediako S, et al. Perceived discrimination, patient trust, and adherence to medical recommendations among persons with sickle cell disease. *J Gen Intern Med.* 2014;29(12):1657-1662.

18. Elixhauser A, Steiner C. Readmissions to US hospitals by diagnosis, 2010. *Stat Brief.* 2006(153). https://pubmed.ncbi.nlm.nih.gov/24006550/. Accessed July 24, 2020.

19. Paradies Y, Ben J, Denson N, et al. Racism as a determinant of health: a systematic review and meta-analysis. *PloS One.* 2015; 10(9):e0138511.

20. Mathur VA, Kiley KB, Haywood Jr C, et al. Multiple levels of suffering: discrimination in health-care settings is associated with enhanced laboratory pain sensitivity in sickle cell disease. *Clin J Pain.* 2016;32(12):1076.

21. Nelson SC, Hackman HW. Race matters: perceptions of race and racism in a sickle cell center. *Pediatr Blood Cancer.* 2013; 60(3):451-454.

22. Haywood C, Diener-West M, Strouse J, et al. Perceived discrimination in health care is associated with a greater burden of pain in sickle cell disease. *J Pain Symptom Manage.* 2014;48(5):934-943.

23. Bediako SM, Moffitt KR. Race and social attitudes about sickle cell disease. *Ethn Health.* 2011;16(4-5):423-429.

24. Zempsky WT. Evaluation and treatment of sickle cell pain in the emergency department: paths to a better future. *Clin Pediatr Emerg Med.* 2010;11(4):265-273.

25. Ezenwa MO, Yao Y, Molokie RE, et al. Coping with pain in the face of healthcare injustice in patients with sickle cell disease. *J Immigr Minor Health.* 2017;19(6):1449-1456.

26. Goffman E. *Stigma: Notes on the Management of Spoiled Identity.* Touchstone; 1963.

27. Crocker J, Major B, Steele C. Social stigma. In: *Handbook of Social Psychology.* McGraw-Hill; 1998:504-553.

28. Bulgin D, Tanabe P, Jenerette C. Stigma of sickle cell disease: a systematic review. *Issues Mental Health Nurs.* 2018;39(8):675-686.

29. Royal CD, Jonassaint CR, Jonassaint JC, De Castro LM. Living with sickle cell disease: traversing 'race' and identity. *Ethn Health.* 2011;16(4-5):389-404.

30. Pauling L. Letter to S. Leonard Wadler. August 15, 1966. http://scarc .library.oregonstate.edu/coll/pauling/blood/people/pauling- linus.html. Accessed July 27, 2020.

31. US Government. The National Sickle Cell Anemia Control Act. Vol Public Law 92-294; US Government Printing Office; 1972:136-139.

32. Benson JM, Therrell BL Jr. History and current status of new- born screening for hemoglobinopathies. *Semin Perinatol.* 2010; 34(2):134-144.

33. Nelson DA, Deuster PA, Carter R 3rd, Hill OT, Wolcott VL, Kurina LM. Sickle cell trait, rhabdomyolysis, and mortality among U.S. Army soldiers. *N Engl J Med.* 2016;375(5):435-442.

34. Nelson DA, Deuster PA, O'Connor FG, Kurina LM. Sickle cell trait and heat injury among US Army soldiers. *Am J Epidemiol.* 2018;187(3):523-528.

35. Harmon KG, Drezner JA, Klossner D, Asif IM. Sickle cell trait associated with a RR of death of 37 times in National Colle- giate Athletic Association football athletes: a database with 2 million athlete-years as the denominator. *Br J Sports Med.* 2012;46(5):325-330.

36. Fisher JA, Kalbaugh CA. Challenging assumptions about minor- ity participation in US clinical research. *Am J Public Health.* 2011;101(12):2217-2222.

37. Omondi NA, Ferguson SES, Majhail NS, et al. Barriers to hematopoietic cell transplantation clinical trial participation of African-American and black youth with sickle cell disease and their parents. *J Pediatr Hematol Oncol.* 2013;35(4):289.

38. Lebensburger JD, Sidonio RF, DeBaun MR, Safford MM, Howard TH, Scarinci IC. Exploring barriers and facilitators to clinical trial enrollment in the context of sickle cell anemia and hydroxyurea. *Pediatr Blood Cancer.* 2013;60(8):1333-1337.

39. Stevens EM, Patterson CA, Li YB, Smith-Whitley K, Barakat LP. Mistrust of pediatric sickle cell disease clinical trials research. *Am J Prev Med.* 2016;51(1):S78-S86.

40. Patterson CA, Chavez V, Mondestin V, Deatrick J, Li Y, Barakat LP. Clinical trial decision making in pediatric sickle cell disease: a qualitative study of perceived benefits and barriers to partici- pation. *J Pediatr Hematol Oncol.* 2015;37(6):415-422.

41. Cronin RM, Hankins JS, Adams-Graves P, et al. Barriers and facilitators to research participation among adults, and parents of children with sickle cell disease: a trans-regional survey. *Am J Hematol.* 2016;91(10):E461-E462.

42. Haywood C, Lanzkron S, Diener-West M, et al. Attitudes toward clinical trials among patients with sickle cell disease. *Clin Trials.* 2014;11(3):275-283.

43. Hassell KL. Population estimates of sickle cell disease in the U.S. *Am J Prev Med.* 2010;38(4 suppl):S512-S521.

44. Panepinto J, Owens P, Mosso A, Steiner C, Brousseau D. Con- centration of hospital care for acute sickle cell disease-related visits. *Pediatr Blood Cancer.* 2012;59(4):685-689.

45. King AA, Rodeghier MJ, Panepinto JA, et al. Silent cerebral infarction, income, and grade retention among students with sickle cell anemia. *Am J Hematol.* 2014;89(10):E188-E192.

46. US Census Bureau. Fast facts. 2018. https://www.census.gov/ quickfacts/tn. Accessed July 27, 2020.

47. Kuhlthau KA, Perrin JM. Child health status and paren- tal employment. *Arch Pediatr Adolesc Med.* 2001;155(12): 1346-1350.

48. Burlew AK, Evans R, Oler C. The impact of a child with sickle cell disease on family dynamics. *Ann N Y Acad Sci.* 1989;565:161-171.

49. Osborne JW. Race and academic disidentification. *J Educ Psy- chol.* 1997;89(4):728-735.

50. Harris E, Sammartino F. Trends in the distribution of household income between 1979 and 2007. 2011. https://www.cbo.gov/ publication/42729. Accessed July 27, 2020.

51. Farber MD, Koshy M, Kinney TR. Cooperative Study of Sickle Cell Disease: demographic and socioeconomic characteristics of patients and families with sickle cell disease. *J Chronic Dis.* 1985;38(6):495-505.

52. Kauf TL, Coates TD, Huazhi L, Mody-Patel N, Hartzema AG. The cost of health care for children and adults with sickle cell disease. *Am J Hematol.* 2009;84(6):323-327.

53. Raphael JL, Dietrich CL, Whitmire D, Mahoney DH, Mueller BU, Giardino AP. Healthcare utilization and expenditures for low income children with sickle cell disease. *Pediatr Blood Can- cer.* 2009;52(2):263-267.

54. Kayle M, Valle J, Paulukonis S, et al. Impact of Medicaid expan- sion on access and healthcare among individuals with sickle cell disease. *Pediatr Blood Cancer.* 2020;67(5):e28152.

55. US Government. Americans With Disabilities Act of 1990, 328, 104(1990).

56. Centers for Disease Control and Prevention, National Center for Chronic Disease Prevention and Health Promotion, Depart- ment of Health. The right place for a healthy start. 2016. https:// www.cdc.gov/chronicdisease/resources/publications/aag/ healthy-schools.htm. Accessed May 28, 2019.

57. Krenitsky-Korn S. High school students with asthma: attitudes about school health, absenteeism, and its impact on academic achievement. *Pediatr Nurs.* 2011;37(2):61-68.

58. Boice MM. Chronic ilness in adolescence. *Adolescence.* 1998; 33:927-940.

59. Basch CE. Asthma and the achievement gap among urban minority youth. *J Sch Health.* 2011;81:606-613.

60. Basch CE. Healthier students are better learners: a missing link in school reforms to close the achievement gap. *J Sch Health.* 2011;81:593-598.

61. Thompson RJ Jr, Gustafson KE, Bonner MJ, Ware RE. Neuro- cognitive development of young children with sickle cell dis- ease through three years of age. *J Pediatr Psychol.* 2002;27(3): 235-244.

62. Hogan AM, Kirkham FJ, Prengler M, et al. An exploratory study of physiological correlates of neurodevelopmental delay in infants with sickle cell anaemia. *Br J Haematol.* 2006;132(1):99-107.

63. Adams R, McKie V, Nichols F, et al. The use of transcranial ultra- sonography to predict stroke in sickle cell disease. *N Engl J Med.* 1992;326:605-610.

64. Kirkham FJ, Hewes DK, Prengler M, Wade A, Lane R, Evans JP. Nocturnal hypoxaemia and central-nervous-system events in sickle-cell disease. *Lancet.* 2001;357(9269):1656-1659.

65. Sparrow S, Balla D, Cicchetti D. *Vineland Adaptive Behavior Scales.* American Guidance Service; 1984.

66. Frankenburger WK, Dodds J, Archer P, et al. *Denver II Training Manual.* Denver Developmental Materials; 1992.

67. Schatz J, McClellan CB, Puffer ES, Johnson K, Roberts CW. Neu- rodevelopmental screening in toddlers and early preschoolers with sickle cell disease. *J Child Neurol.* 2008;23(1):44-50.

68. Aygun B, Parker J, Freeman MB, et al. Neurocognitive screening with the Brigance Preschool Screen-II in 3-year-old children with sickle cell disease. *Pediatr Blood Cancer.* 2011;56(4):620-624.

69. Tarazi RA, Grant ML, Ely E, Barakat LP. Neuropsychological functioning in preschool-age children with sickle cell disease:

the role of illness-related and psychosocial factors. *Child Neuropsychol.* 2007;13(2):155-172.

70. Glascoe FP. *Inventory of Early Development II: Standardzation and Validation Manual.* Curriculum Associates; 2004.

71. Wechsler D. *Wechsler Preschool and Primary Scale of Intelligence™–Third Edition (WPPSI™–III).* The Psychological Corporation; 2002.

72. Drazen CH, Abel R, Gabir M, Farmer G, King AA. Prevalence of developmental delay and contributing factors among children with sickle cell disease. *Pediatr Blood Cancer.* 2016;63(3):504-510.

73. Diez Roux AV. Conceptual approaches to the study of health disparities. *Ann Rev Public Health.* 2012;33:41-58.

74. Fields ME, Hoyt-Drazen C, Abel R, et al. A pilot study of parent education intervention improves early childhood development among toddlers with sickle cell disease. *Pediatr Blood Cancer.* 2016;63(12):2131-2138.

75. Schatz J, Brown RT, Pascual JM, Hsu L, DeBaun MR. Poor school and cognitive functioning with silent cerebral infarcts and sickle cell disease. *Neurology.* 2001;56(8):1109-1111.

76. Roderick M. Grade retention and school dropout: investigating the association. *Am Educ Res J.* 1994;31(4):729-759.

77. Jonassaint CR, Beach MC, Haythornthwaite JA, et al. The association between educational attainment and patterns of emergency department utilization among adults with sickle cell disease. *Int J Behav Med.* 2016;23(3):300-309.

78. Harris KM, Dadekian JN, Abel RA, et al. Increasing educational attainment in adolescents with sickle cell disease. *Soc Work Public Health.* 2019;34(6):468-482.

79. National Center for Health Statistics. *Health, United States, 2011: With Special Feature on Socioeconomic Status and Health.* National Center for Health Statistics; 2012.

80. Krenitsky-Korn S. High school students with asthma: attitudes about school health, absenteeism, and its impact on academic achievement. *Pediatr Nurs.* 2011;37:61.

81. Mohai P, Kweon BS, Lee S, Ard K. Air pollution around schools is linked to poorer student health and academic performance. *Health Aff.* 2011;30:852-862.

82. Moonie S, Sterling DA, Figgs LW, Castro M. The relationship between school absence, academic performance, and asthma status. *J Sch Health.* 2008;78:140-148.

83. Moonie SA, Sterling DA, Figgs L, Castro M. Asthma status and severity affects missed school days. *J Sch Health.* 2006;76(1):18-24.

84. Taras H, Potts-Datema W. Childhood asthma and student performance at school. *J Sch Health.* 2005;75:296-312.

85. Sanger M, Jordan L, Pruthi S, et al. Cognitive deficits are associated with unemployment in adults with sickle cell anemia. *J Clin Exp Neuropsychol.* 2016;38(6):661-671.

86. Wallen GR, Minniti CP, Krumlauf M, et al. Sleep disturbance, depression and pain in adults with sickle cell disease. *BMC Psychiatry.* 2014;14:207.

87. Barrett DH, Wisotzek IE, Abel GG, et al. Assessment of psychosocial functioning of patients with sickle cell disease. *South Med J.* 1988;81(6):745-750.

88. Anie KA, Grocott H, White L, Dzingina M, Rogers G, Cho G. Patient self-assessment of hospital pain, mood and health-related quality of life in adults with sickle cell disease. *BMJ Open.* 2012;2(4):e001274.

89. Anie KA, Egunjobi FE, Akinyanju OO. Psychosocial impact of sickle cell disorder: perspectives from a Nigerian setting. *Glob Health.* 2010;6:2.

90. Thomas VJ, Taylor LM. The psychosocial experience of people with sickle cell disease and its impact on quality of life: qualitative findings from focus groups. *Br J Health Psychol.* 2002;7(part 3):345-363.

91. Lukoo RN, Ngiyulu RM, Mananga GL, et al. Depression in children suffering from sickle cell anemia. *J Pediatr Hematol Oncol.* 2015;37(1):20-24.

92. Benton TD, Boyd R, Ifeagwu J, Feldtmose E, Smith-Whitley K. Psychiatric diagnosis in adolescents with sickle cell disease: a preliminary report. *Curr Psychiatry Rep.* 2011;13(2):111-115.

93. Levenson JL, McClish DK, Dahman BA, et al. Depression and anxiety in adults with sickle cell disease: the PiSCES project. *Psychosom Med.* 2008;70(2):192-196.

94. Edwards CL, Green M, Wellington CC, et al. Depression, suicidal ideation, and attempts in black patients with sickle cell disease. *J Natl Med Assoc.* 2009;101(11):1090-1095.

95. Grant MM, Gil KM, Floyd MY, Abrams M. Depression and functioning in relation to health care use in sickle cell disease. *Ann Behav Med.* 2000;22(2):149-157.

96. Hasan SP, Hashmi S, Alhassen M, Lawson W, Castro O. Depression in sickle cell disease. *J Natl Med Assoc.* 2003;95(7):533-537.

97. Asnani MR, Fraser R, Lewis NA, Reid ME. Depression and loneliness in Jamaicans with sickle cell disease. *BMC Psychiatry.* 2010;10:40.

98. Narrow WE, Rae DS, Robins LN, Regier DA. Revised prevalence estimates of mental disorders in the United States: using a clinical significance criterion to reconcile 2 surveys' estimates. *Arch Gen Psychiatry.* 2002;59(2):115-123.

99. Kessler LG, Burns BJ, Shapiro S, et al. Psychiatric diagnoses of medical service users: evidence from the Epidemiologic Catchment Area Program. *Am J Public Health.* 1987;77(1):18-24.

100. Laurence B, George D, Woods D. Association between elevated depressive symptoms and clinical disease severity in African-American adults with sickle cell disease. *J Natl Med Assoc.* 2006;98(3):365-369.

101. Cepeda ML, Yang YM, Price CC, Shah A. Mental disorders in children and adolescents with sickle cell disease. *South Med J.* 1997;90(3):284-287.

102. Williams DR, Gonzalez HM, Neighbors H, et al. Prevalence and distribution of major depressive disorder in African Americans, Caribbean blacks, and non-Hispanic whites: results from the National Survey of American Life. *Arch Gen Psychiatry.* 2007;64(3):305-315.

103. Woodward AT, Taylor RJ, Abelson JM, Matusko N. Major depressive disorder among older African Americans, Caribbean blacks, and non-Hispanic whites: secondary analysis of the National Survey of American Life. *Depress Anxiety.* 2013;30(6):589-597.

104. Jerrell JM, Tripathi A, McIntyre RS. Prevalence and treatment of depression in children and adolescents with sickle cell disease: a retrospective cohort study. *Prim Care Companion CNS Disord.* 2011;13(2):PCC.10m01063.

105. Shim RS, Ye J, Baltrus P, Fry-Johnson Y, Daniels E, Rust G. Racial/ethnic disparities, social support, and depression: examining a social determinant of mental health. *Ethn Dis.* 2012;22(1):15-20.

106. Carroll CP, Haywood C Jr, Lanzkron S. Prediction of onset and course of high hospital utilization in sickle cell disease. *J Hosp Med.* 2011;6(5):248-255.

107. Cronin RM, Hankins JS, Byrd J, et al. Risk factors for hospitalizations and readmissions among individuals with sickle cell disease: results of a U.S. survey study. *Hematology.* 2019;24(1):189-198.

108. Toumi ML, Merzoug S, Boulassel MR. Does sickle cell disease have a psychosomatic component? A particular focus on anxiety and depression. *Life Sci.* 2018;210:96-105.

109. Zale EL, Maisto SA, Ditre JW. Interrelations between pain and alcohol: an integrative review. *Clin Psychol Rev.* 2015;37:57-71.

110. McClish DK, Smith WR, Levenson JL, et al. Comorbidity, pain, utilization, and psychosocial outcomes in older versus younger sickle cell adults: the PiSCES project. *Biomed Res Int.* 2017;2017:4070547.

111. O'Donnell BJ, Guo L, Ghosh S, et al. Sleep phenotype in the Townes mouse model of sickle cell disease. *Sleep Breath.* 2019; 23(1):333-339.

112. Franklin CL, Raines AM, Hurlocker MC. No trauma, no problem: symptoms of posttraumatic stress in the absence of a criterion a stressor. *J Psychopathol Behav Assess.* 2019;41(1):107-111.

113. Larsen SE, Pacella ML. Comparing the effect of DSM-congruent traumas vs. DSM-incongruent stressors on PTSD symptoms: a meta-analytic review. *J Anxiety Disord.* 2016;38:37-46.

114. Hofmann M, de Montalembert M, Beauquier-Maccotta B, de Villartay P, Golse B. Posttraumatic stress disorder in children affected by sickle-cell disease and their parents. *Am J Hematol.* 2007;82(2):171-172.

115. Alao AO, Soderberg M. Sickle cell disease and posttraumatic stress disorder. *Int J Psychiatr Med.* 2002;32(1):97-101.

116. Scott KD, Scott AA. Cultural therapeutic awareness and sickle cell anemia. *J Black Psychol.* 1999;25(3):316-335.

117. Vichinsky EP, Neumayr LD, Gold JI, et al. Neuropsychological dysfunction and neuroimaging abnormalities in neurologically intact adults with sickle cell anemia. *JAMA.* 2010;303(18): 1823-1831.

118. Anie KA. Psychological complications in sickle cell disease. *Br J Haematol.* 2005;129(6):723-729.

119. Reese FL, Smith WR. Psychosocial determinants of health care utilization in sickle cell disease patients. *Ann Behav Med.* 1997;19(2):171-178.

120. Edwards CL, Scales MT, Loughlin C, et al. A brief review of the pathophysiology, associated pain, and psychosocial issues in sickle cell disease. *Int J Behav Med.* 2005;12(3):171-179.

121. Tsao JC, Jacob E, Seidman LC, Lewis MA, Zeltzer LK. Psychological aspects and hospitalization for pain crises in youth with sickle-cell disease. *J Health Psychol.* 2014;19(3):407-416.

122. Porter LS, Gil KM, Sedway JA, Ready J, Workman E, Thompson RJ Jr. Pain and stress in sickle cell disease: an analysis of daily pain records. *Int J Behav Med.* 1998;5(3):185-203.

123. Gil KM, Carson JW, Porter LS, Scipio C, Bediako SM, Orringer E. Daily mood and stress predict pain, health care use, and work activity in African American adults with sickle-cell disease. *Health Psychol.* 2004;23(3):267-274.

124. Gil KM, Carson JW, Porter LS, et al. Daily stress and mood and their association with pain, health-care use, and school activity in adolescents with sickle cell disease. *J Pediatr Psychol.* 2003;28(5):363-373.

125. Wilson Schaeffer JJ, Gil KM, Burchinal M, et al. Depression, disease severity, and sickle cell disease. *J Behav Med.* 1999;22(2):115-126.

126. Shah P, Khaleel M, Thuptimdang W, et al. Mental stress causes vasoconstriction in sickle cell disease and normal controls. *Haematologica.* 2020;105(1):83-90.

127. Jonassaint CR, Jones VL, Leong S, Frierson GM. A systematic review of the association between depression and health care utilization in children and adults with sickle cell disease. *Br J Haematol.* 2016;174(1):136-147.

128. Porter EA. The role of stress and mood in sickle cell disease pain. *J Health Psychol.* 2000;5(1):53-63.

129. Tsao JCI, Jacob E, Seidman LC, Lewis MA, Zeltzer LK. Psychological aspects and hospitalization for pain crises in youth with sickle-cell disease. *J Health Psychol.* 2014;19(3):407-416.

130. Schlenz AM, Schatz J, Roberts CW. Caregiver psychological functioning in relation to pain and health care utilization in pediatric sickle cell disease. *Blood.* 2014;124(21):4844.

131. Brown RT, Connelly M, Rittle C, Clouse B. A longitudinal examination predicting emergency room use in children with sickle cell disease and their caregivers. *J Pediatr Psychol.* 2006;31(2):163-173.

132. Aisiku IP, Smith WR, McClish DK, et al. Comparisons of high versus low emergency department utilizers in sickle cell disease. *Ann Emerg Med.* 2009;53(5):587-593.

133. Treadwell MJ, Barreda F, Kaur K, Gildengorin G. Emotional distress, barriers to care, and health-related quality of life in sickle cell disease. *J Clin Outcomes Manage.* 2015;22(1):10-20.

134. Anie KA, Green J. Psychological therapies for sickle cell disease and pain. *Cochrane Database Syst Rev.* 2012;2:CD001916.

135. Kaslow NJ, Collins MH, Rashid FL, et al. The efficacy of a pilot family psychoeducational intervention for pediatric sickle cell disease (SCD). *Fam Syst Health.* 2000;18(4):381-404.

136. Calvert M, Blazeby J, Altman DG, et al. Reporting of patient-reported outcomes in randomized trials: the CONSORT PRO extension. *JAMA.* 2013;309(8):814-822.

137. US Department of Health and Human Services, Food and Drug Administration Center for Biologics Evaluation Research, Center for Devices and Radiological Health. Guidance for industry: patient-reported outcome measures: use in medical product development to support labeling claims: draft guidance. *Health Qual Life Outcomes.* 2006;4:79.

138. European Medicines Agency. Appendix 2 to the guideline on the evaluation of anticancer medicinal products in man: The use of patient-reported outcome (PRO) measures in oncology studies EMA/CHMP/292464/2014. https://www.ema.europa.eu/en/documents/other/appendix-2-guideline-evaluation-anticancer-medicinal-products-man_en.pdf. Accessed April 4, 2019.

139. Tunis SR, Stryer DB, Clancy CM. Practical clinical trials: increasing the value of clinical research for decision making in clinical and health policy. *JAMA.* 2003;290(12):1624-1632.

140. Calvert M, Kyte D, Mercieca-Bebber R, et al. Guidelines for inclusion of patient-reported outcomes in clinical trial protocols: the SPIRIT-PRO extension. *JAMA.* 2018;319(5): 483-494.

141. Dobrozsi S, Panepinto J. Patient-reported outcomes in clinical practice. *Hematology Am Soc Hematol Educ Program.* 2015; 2015(1):501-506.

142. Velikova G, Booth L, Smith AB, et al. Measuring quality of life in routine oncology practice improves communication and patient well-being: a randomized controlled trial. *J Clin Oncol.* 2004;22(4):714-724.

143. Piel FB, Steinberg MH, Rees DC. Sickle cell disease. *N Engl J Med.* 2017;376(16):1561-1573.

144. Panepinto JA. Health-related quality of life in patients with hemoglobinopathies. *Hematology Am Soc Hematol Educ Program.* 2012;2012:284-289.

145. Panepinto JA, Bonner M. Health-related quality of life in sickle cell disease: past, present, and future. *Pediatr Blood Cancer.* 2012; 59(2):377-385.

146. Dampier C, LeBeau P, Rhee S, et al. Health-related quality of life in adults with sickle cell disease (SCD): a report from the

comprehensive sickle cell centers clinical trial consortium. *Am J Hematol.* 2011;86(2):203-205.

147. Dampier C, Lieff S, LeBeau P, et al. Health-related quality of life in children with sickle cell disease: a report from the Comprehensive Sickle Cell Centers Clinical Trial Consortium. *Pediatr Blood Cancer.* 2010;55(3):485-494.

148. Thornburg CD, Calatroni A, Panepinto JA. Differences in health-related quality of life in children with sickle cell disease receiving hydroxyurea. *J Pediatr Hematol Oncol.* 2011;33(4):251-254.

149. Ballas SK, Barton FB, Waclawiw MA, et al. Hydroxyurea and sickle cell anemia: effect on quality of life. *Health Qual Life Outcomes.* 2006;4:59.

150. Badawy SM, Thompson AA, Lai JS, Penedo FJ, Rychlik K, Liem RI. Health-related quality of life and adherence to hydroxyurea in adolescents and young adults with sickle cell disease. *Pediatr Blood Cancer.* 2017;64(6):10.1002/pbc.26369.

151. Adeyemo TA, Ojewunmi OO, Diaku-Akinwumi IN, Ayinde OC, Akanmu AS. Health related quality of life and perception of stigmatisation in adolescents living with sickle cell disease in Nigeria: a cross sectional study. *Pediatr Blood Cancer.* 2015;62(7):1245-1251.

152. Ahmed AE, Alaskar AS, McClish DK, et al. Saudi SCD patients' symptoms and quality of life relative to the number of ED visits. *BMC Emerg Med.* 2016;16(1):30.

153. Amr MA, Amin TT, Al-Omair OA. Health related quality of life among adolescents with sickle cell disease in Saudi Arabia. *Pan Afr Med J.* 2011;8:10.

154. Jonassaint CR, Jones VL, Leong S, Frierson GM. A systematic review of the association between depression and health care utilization in children and adults with sickle cell disease. *Br J Haematol.* 2016;174(1):136-147.

155. Badawy SM, Thompson AA, Holl JL, Penedo FJ, Liem RI. Healthcare utilization and hydroxyurea adherence in youth with sickle cell disease. *Pediatr Hematol Oncol.* 2018;35(5-6):297-308.

156. Dampier C, Barry V, Gross HE, et al. Initial evaluation of the pediatric PROMIS(R) health domains in children and adolescents with sickle cell disease. *Pediatr Blood Cancer.* 2016;63(6):1031-1037.

157. Palermo TM, Schwartz L, Drotar D, McGowan K. Parental report of health-related quality of life in children with sickle cell disease. *J Behav Med.* 2002;25(3):269-283.

158. Dale JC, Cochran CJ, Roy L, Jernigan E, Buchanan GR. Health-related quality of life in children and adolescents with sickle cell disease. *J Pediatr Health Care.* 2011;25(4):208-215.

159. Jackson JL, Lemanek KL, Clough-Paabo E, Rhodes M. Predictors of health-related quality of life over time among adolescents and young adults with sickle cell disease. *J Clin Psychol Med Settings.* 2014;21(4):313-319.

160. Ingerski LM, Modi AC, Hood KK, et al. Health-related quality of life across pediatric chronic conditions. *J Pediatr.* 2010;156(4):639-644.

161. Palermo TM, Riley CA, Mitchell BA. Daily functioning and quality of life in children with sickle cell disease pain: relationship with family and neighborhood socioeconomic distress. *J Pain.* 2008;9(9):833-840.

162. Panepinto JA, Pajewski NM, Foerster LM, Sabnis S, Hoffmann RG. Impact of family income and sickle cell disease on the health-related quality of life of children. *Qual Life Res.* 2009;18(1):5-13.

163. Badawy SM, Barrera L, Cai S, Thompson AA. Association between participants' characteristics, patient-reported outcomes, and clinical outcomes in youth with sickle cell disease. *Biomed Res Int.* 2018;2018:8296139.

164. Seid M, Varni JW, Segall D, Kurtin PS. Health-related quality of life as a predictor of pediatric healthcare costs: a two-year prospective cohort analysis. *Health Qual Life Outcomes.* 2004;2:48.

165. Frost MH, Reeve BB, Liepa AM, Stauffer JW, Hays RD, Mayo/FDA Patient-Reported Outcomes Consensus Meeting Group. What is sufficient evidence for the reliability and validity of patient-reported outcome measures? *Value Health.* 2007;10(suppl 2):S94-S105.

166. Patrick DL, Deyo RA. Generic and disease-specific measures in assessing health status and quality of life. *Med Care.* 1989;27(3 suppl):S217-S232.

167. Asnani MR, Lipps GE, Reid ME. Validation of the SF-36 in Jamaicans with sickle-cell disease. *Psychol Health Med.* 2009;14(5):606-618.

168. Asnani MR, Lipps GE, Reid ME. Utility of WHOQOL-BREF in measuring quality of life in sickle cell disease. *Health Qual Life Outcomes.* 2009;7:75.

169. Panepinto JA, Pajewski NM, Foerster LM, Hoffmann RG. The performance of the PedsQL generic core scales in children with sickle cell disease. *J Pediatr Hematol Oncol.* 2008;30(9):666-673.

170. Keller SD, Yang M, Treadwell MJ, Werner EM, Hassell KL. Patient reports of health outcome for adults living with sickle cell disease: development and testing of the ASCQ-Me item banks. *Health Qual Life Outcomes.* 2014;12:125.

171. Panepinto JA, Torres S, Bendo CB, et al. PedsQL sickle cell disease module: feasibility, reliability, and validity. *Pediatr Blood Cancer.* 2013;60(8):1338-1344.

172. Panepinto JA, Torres S, Bendo CB, et al. PedsQL Multidimensional Fatigue Scale in sickle cell disease: feasibility, reliability, and validity. *Pediatr Blood Cancer.* 2014;61(1):171-177.

173. Keller S, Yang M, Treadwell MJ, Hassell KL. Sensitivity of alternative measures of functioning and wellbeing for adults with sickle cell disease: comparison of PROMIS(R) to ASCQ-Me. *Health Qual Life Outcomes.* 2017;15(1):117.

174. Sarri G, Bhor M, Abogunrin S, et al. Systematic literature review and assessment of patient-reported outcome instruments in sickle cell disease. *Health Qual Life Outcomes.* 2018;16(1):99.

175. Badawy SM, Thompson AA, Lai JS, Penedo FJ, Rychlik K, Liem RI. Adherence to hydroxyurea, health-related quality of life domains, and patients' perceptions of sickle cell disease and hydroxyurea: a cross-sectional study in adolescents and young adults. *Health Qual Life Outcomes.* 2017;15(1):136.

176. Badawy SM, Thompson AA, Liem RI. Beliefs about hydroxyurea in youth with sickle cell disease. *Hematol Oncol Stem Cell Ther.* 2018;11(3):142-148.

177. Dampier C, Jaeger B, Gross HE, et al. Responsiveness of PROMIS pediatric measures to hospitalizations for sickle pain and subsequent recovery. *Pediatr Blood Cancer.* 2016;63(6):1038-1045.

178. Bakshi N, Lukombo I, Belfer I, Krishnamurti L. Pain catastrophizing is associated with poorer health-related quality of life in pediatric patients with sickle cell disease. *J Pain Res.* 2018;11:947-953.

179. Bakshi N, Ross D, Krishnamurti L. Presence of pain on three or more days of the week is associated with worse patient reported outcomes in adults with sickle cell disease. *J Pain Res.* 2018;11:313-318.

180. Panepinto JA, O'Mahar KM, DeBaun MR, Loberiza FR, Scott JP. Health-related quality of life in children with sickle cell disease: child and parent perception. *Br J Haematol.* 2005;130(3):437-444.

181. DeWalt DA, Gross HE, Gipson DS, et al. PROMIS((R)) pediatric self-report scales distinguish subgroups of children within and across six common pediatric chronic health conditions. *Qual Life Res.* 2015;24(9):2195-2208.

182. Reeve BB, Edwards LJ, Jaeger BC, et al. Assessing responsiveness over time of the PROMIS((R)) pediatric symptom and function measures in cancer, nephrotic syndrome, and sickle cell disease. *Qual Life Res.* 2018;27(1):249-257.

183. Panepinto JA, Paul Scott J, Badaki-Makun O, et al. Determining the longitudinal validity and meaningful differences in HRQL of the PedsQL Sickle Cell Disease Module. *Health Qual Life Outcomes.* 2017;15(1):124.

184. Coons SJ, Eremenco S, Lundy JJ, O'Donohoe P, O'Gorman H, Malizia W. Capturing patient-reported outcome (PRO) data electronically: the past, present, and promise of ePRO measurement in clinical trials. *Patient.* 2015;8(4):301-309.

185. Coons SJ, Gwaltney CJ, Hays RD, et al. Recommendations on evidence needed to support measurement equivalence between electronic and paper-based patient-reported outcome (PRO) measures: ISPOR ePRO Good Research Practices Task Force report. *Value Health.* 2009;12(4):419-429.

186. Gwaltney CJ, Shields AL, Shiffman S. Equivalence of electronic and paper-and-pencil administration of patient-reported outcome measures: a meta-analytic review. *Value Health.* 2008;11(2):322-333.

187. US Food and Drug Administration. The voice of the patient: a series of reports from the U.S. Food and Drug Administration's (FDA's) Patient-Focused Drug Development Initiative. 2014. https://www.fda.gov/downloads/ForIndustry/UserFees/PrescriptionDrugUserFee/UCM418430.pdf. Accessed April 3, 2019.

188. Barlow J, Wright C, Sheasby J, Turner A, Hainsworth J. Self-management approaches for people with chronic conditions: a review. *Patient Educ Couns.* 2002;48(2):177-187.

189. Badawy SM, Thompson AA, Penedo FJ, Lai JS, Rychlik K, Liem RI. Barriers to hydroxyurea adherence and health-related quality of life in adolescents and young adults with sickle cell disease. *Eur J Haematol.* 2017;98(6):608-614.

190. Lanzkron S, Carroll CP, Haywood C Jr. The burden of emergency department use for sickle-cell disease: an analysis of the national emergency department sample database. *Am J Hematol.* 2010;85(10):797-799.

191. Centers for Disease Control and Prevention. Sickle cell disease: data & statistics. 2016. https://www.cdc.gov/ncbddd/sicklecell/data.html. Accessed April 4, 2018.

192. Badawy SM, Thompson AA, Liem RI. Technology access and smartphone app preferences for medication adherence in adolescents and young adults with sickle cell disease. *Pediatr Blood Cancer.* 2016;63(5):848-852.

193. Shah N, Jonassaint J, De Castro L. Patients welcome the Sickle Cell Disease Mobile Application to Record Symptoms via Technology (SMART). *Hemoglobin.* 2014;38(2):99-103.

194. Utrankar A, Mayo-Gamble TL, Allen W, et al. Technology use and preferences to support clinical practice guideline awareness and adherence in individuals with sickle cell disease. *J Am Med Inform Assoc.* 2018;25(8):976-988.

195. Fox S. Health information online. 2014. http://www.pewinternet.org/2014/02/13/health-information-online-2/. Accessed April 4, 2018.

196. Pew Research Internet. Mobile Fact Sheet. 2018. http://www.pewinternet.org/fact-sheet/mobile/. Accessed April 4, 2018.

197. Hibbard JH, Greene J. What the evidence shows about patient activation: better health outcomes and care experiences; fewer data on costs. *Health Aff (Millwood).* 2013;32(2):207-214.

198. Peters AE, Keeley EC. Patient engagement following acute myocardial infarction and its influence on outcomes. *Am J Cardiol.* 2017;120(9):1467-1471.

199. Sawesi S, Rashrash M, Phalakornkule K, Carpenter JS, Jones JF. The impact of information technology on patient engagement and health behavior change: a systematic review of the literature. *JMIR Med Inform.* 2016;4(1):e1.

200. Haas K, Martin A, Park KT. Text message intervention (TEACH) improves quality of life and patient activation in celiac disease: a randomized clinical trial. *J Pediatr.* 2017;185:62-67.e62.

201. John ME, Samson-Akpan PE, Etowa JB, Akpabio II, John EE. Enhancing self-care, adjustment and engagement through mobile phones in youth with HIV. *Int Nurs Rev.* 2016;63(4):555-561.

202. Knoerl R, Lee D, Yang J, et al. Examining the impact of a web-based intervention to promote patient activation in chemotherapy-induced peripheral neuropathy assessment and management. *J Cancer Educ.* 2018;33(5):1027-1035.

203. Milani RV, Lavie CJ, Bober RM, Milani AR, Ventura HO. Improving hypertension control and patient engagement using digital tools. *Am J Med.* 2017;130(1):14-20.

204. Solomon M, Wagner SL, Goes J. Effects of a Web-based intervention for adults with chronic conditions on patient activation: online randomized controlled trial. *J Med Internet Res.* 2012;14(1):e32.

205. Eysenbach G. What is e-health? *J Med Internet Res.* 2001;3(2):E20.

206. Al-Durra M, Torio MB, Cafazzo JA. The use of behavior change theory in Internet-based asthma self-management interventions: a systematic review. *J Med Internet Res.* 2015;17(4):e89.

207. de Jongh T, Gurol-Urganci I, Vodopivec-Jamsek V, Car J, Atun R. Mobile phone messaging for facilitating self-management of long-term illnesses. *Cochrane Database Syst Rev.* 2012;12:CD007459.

208. Holtz B, Lauckner C. Diabetes management via mobile phones: a systematic review. *Telemed J E Health.* 2012;18(3):175-184.

209. Thakkar J, Kurup R, Laba TL, et al. Mobile telephone text messaging for medication adherence in chronic disease: a meta-analysis. *JAMA Intern Med.* 2016;176(3):340-349.

210. Payne HE, Lister C, West JH, Bernhardt JM. Behavioral functionality of mobile apps in health interventions: a systematic review of the literature. *JMIR mHealth uHealth.* 2015;3(1):e20.

211. Majeed-Ariss R, Baildam E, Campbell M, et al. Apps and adolescents: a systematic review of adolescents' use of mobile phone and tablet apps that support personal management of their chronic or long-term physical conditions. *J Med Internet Res.* 2015;17(12):e287.

212. Badawy SM, Kuhns LM. Texting and mobile phone app interventions for improving adherence to preventive behavior in adolescents: a systematic review. *JMIR mHealth uHealth.* 2017;5(4):e50.

213. Badawy SM, Barrera L, Sinno MG, Kaviany S, O'Dwyer LC, Kuhns LM. Text messaging and mobile phone apps as interventions to improve adherence in adolescents with chronic health conditions: a systematic review. *JMIR mHealth uHealth.* 2017;5(5):e66.

214. Badawy SM, Thompson AA, Kuhns LM. Medication adherence and technology-based interventions for adolescents with chronic health conditions: a few key considerations. *JMIR mHealth uHealth.* 2017;5(12):e202.

215. Badawy SM, Cronin RM, Hankins J, et al. Patient-centered eHealth interventions for children, adolescents, and adults with sickle cell disease: systematic review. *J Med Internet Res.* 2018; 20(7):e10940.

216. Badawy SM, Kuhns LM. Economic evaluation of text-messaging and smartphone-based interventions to improve medication adherence in adolescents with chronic health conditions: a systematic review. *JMIR mHealth uHealth.* 2016;4(4):e121.

217. Anderson LM, Leonard S, Jonassaint J, Lunyera J, Bonner M, Shah N. Mobile health intervention for youth with sickle cell disease: Impact on adherence, disease knowledge, and quality of life. *Pediatr Blood Cancer.* 2018;65(8):e27081.

218. Jonassaint CR, Kang C, Prussien KV, et al. Feasibility of implementing mobile technology-delivered mental health treatment in routine adult sickle cell disease care. *Transl Behav Med.* 2020;10(1):58-67.

219. Creary S, Chisolm DJ, O'Brien SH. ENHANCE-(Electronic Hydroxyurea Adherence): a protocol to increase hydroxyurea adherence in patients with sickle cell disease. *JMIR Res Protoc.* 2016;5(4):e193.

220. Makubi A, Sasi P, Ngaeje M, et al. Rationale and design of mDOT-HuA study: a randomized trial to assess the effect of mobile-directly observed therapy on adherence to hydroxyurea in adults with sickle cell anemia in Tanzania. *BMC Med Res Methodol.* 2016;16(1):140.

221. Palermo TM, Zempsky WT, Dampier CD, et al. iCanCope with Sickle Cell Pain: design of a randomized controlled trial of a smartphone and web-based pain self-management program for youth with sickle cell disease. *Contemp Clin Trials.* 2018;74:88-96.

Therapeutic Options and Combination Therapy

Authors: Caterina P. Minniti, Jane S. Hankins

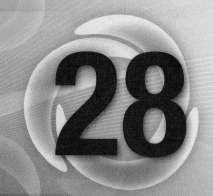

Chapter Outline

Overview

The therapeutic landscape for patients with sickle cell disease (SCD) has recently expanded, and health care practitioners now have several options of disease-modifying drugs that are sickle cell specific. As of 2020, in the United States, there are 4 Food and Drug Administration (FDA)-approved drugs for patients living with SCD: hydroxyurea, L-glutamine,[1] voxelotor,[2] and crizanlizumab.[3] Many more agents are currently being tested in phase II or III trials; therefore, we foresee that several new targeted therapies will be available by the end of the current decade. The treatment of individuals with SCD will become increasingly complex and, at the same time, mechanistically based, as a large number of these drugs are specifically being developed to affect and/or change the multifaceted pathophysiology of SCD.

Although hydroxyurea, also referred to as hydroxycarbamide, has been used by thousands of patients around the globe for >30 years[4] and clinicians can rely on decades of clinical and laboratory data to inform and guide its use,[5] fewer data exist for the 3 recently FDA-approved drugs—L-glutamine, voxelotor, and crizanlizumab. Therefore, many scientific and clinical questions remain about their mechanism of action, efficacy, effectiveness, and long-term safety profile. FDA-mandated postlicensing trials are planned or already under way to answer these remaining questions.

With increasing choices, clinicians who treat patients with SCD need to develop a systematic approach to evaluate and present different therapeutic options and, together with patients and their families, apply shared decision-making principles[6] to make final recommendations and decisions. Practitioners need to take into consideration both the clinical characteristics of each patient, such as their age and disease phenotype, and their values and preferences. Social circumstances (eg, home environment, occupation) and the drug's mechanism of action and route of administration should all be considered. Finally, insurance coverage and drug access need to be factored into the decision-making process. As with any disease, as newer drugs are developed, high costs may preclude drug access and become a substantial barrier, which creates and perpetuates inequity.

Although the new disease-modifying agents have not yet been compared to each other and have been given in combination with hydroxyurea in a very small subset of patients, some general guidance can be provided based on patients' clinical characteristics (eg, venous access, disease phenotype), age, and preferences. In this chapter, we provide recommendations on how to incorporate the new disease-modifying agents in clinical practice, given the newest evidence for their efficacy and mode of utilization.

Considering Sickle Cell Phenotype in the Choice of Therapy

When clinically evident, the patient's phenotype may be an important guide to therapy. Although on a spectrum and with substantial overlap, the phenotype in SCD can be divided into 2 main clinical subphenotypes: hemolytic and vaso-occlusive.[7] The FDA-approved labels of the disease-modifying agents provide guidance in the decision process in relation to the clinical SCD phenotype. Hydroxyurea is approved by the FDA for adults (aged ≥18 years) with SCD with ≥3 vaso-occlusive crisis (VOC) events in a 12-month period. In 2017, the FDA approved hydroxyurea for children aged ≥2 years with HbSS and HbS-β⁰ thalassemia and recurrent, moderate to severe VOC. In current practice, however, most hematologists will initiate hydroxyurea in children with HbSS and HbS-β⁰ thalassemia starting at 9 months of age and before complications occur, as recommended by the National Heart,

Lung, and Blood Institute guidelines.[8] This practice is likely to continue because the safety of hydroxyurea has been demonstrated by a large phase III trial and other prospective studies in pediatrics.[9,10] A new approach to personalize hydroxyurea dosing, informed by pharmacokinetics, appears promising and may predict the optimal dose of hydroxyurea in children.[11,12] If this approach is successfully validated and replicated, it may lead to better clinical response (higher fetal hemoglobin [HbF] level) with less toxicity.

Similarly to the Multicenter Study of Hydroxyurea (MSH) trial, the primary outcome measure of L-glutamine in its pivotal phase 3 trial, was reduction in the frequency of VOCs that lead to a visit to the emergency department or hospitalization.[13] Thus, L-glutamine use is recommended for patients who have VOC events, including pain or acute chest syndrome (ACS). In this study,[13] a subset of the participants was already exposed to stable hydroxyurea dosing. L-Glutamine can, therefore, be offered to individuals who either are or are not receiving hydroxyurea.

Approval of crizanlizumab was based on reduction of VOC events, and results in a more robust effect size than L-glutamine, as reported in its pivotal study.[3] Crizanlizumab at the 5mg/kg dosing provided approximately 45% reduction in VOC events, compared to the 33% reduction by L-glutamine.[3,14] The VOC decrease was accompanied by a reduction in hospitalization days and a delay in time to first and second VOC occurrence. Like L-glutamine, the crizanlizumab pivotal study included patients who were already exposed to hydroxyurea, and the reduction of pain was observed in both hydroxyurea-exposed and non–hydroxyurea-exposed individuals. Therefore, it is appropriate to offer crizanlizumab to patients with recurrent (>2 per year) VOC events in addition to hydroxyurea therapy.

Voxelotor, with its unique mechanism of action, targets the upstream key event in SCD, namely, polymerization of sickle hemoglobin (HbS). Voxelotor is a first-in-class agent that selectively and reversibly binds to the hemoglobin and keeps it in a high-oxygen-affinity conformation, reducing hemoglobin polymerization.[15,16] By preventing polymerization, hemolysis is reduced and hemoglobin concentration is increased. The FDA conditionally approved voxelotor based on a mean increase in hemoglobin concentration of 1 g/dL.[2] Its final approval is conditioned to phase IV studies that will test its efficacy in improving clinical outcomes in both adults and children (eg, VOC events, elevated transcranial Doppler velocities, skin ulcers). The hemoglobin threshold for initiating voxelotor is not yet defined and difficult to tease from available published data. Although the FDA did not require a hemoglobin threshold below which voxelotor would be indicated, we believe that the primary indication for this drug should be for patients with severe anemia due to hemolysis (elevated serum levels of lactate dehydrogenase, elevated reticulocytes, and elevated high indirect bilirubin). Recent promising, albeit limited, data on leg ulcer improvement seem to point toward a potential effect in decreasing end-organ damage with voxelotor[17]; however, studies should be conducted to test this hypothesis. Another logical target population for whom voxelotor could be beneficial are patients who are unable to receive red blood cell transfusions, either because of severe alloimmunization or a history of delayed hemolytic transfusion reaction, although clinical benefit has not yet been demonstrated in this clinical scenario.[18] Religious reasons precluding a red blood cell transfusion (eg, Jehovah's Witnesses) could also be a consideration for using voxelotor. Finally, voxelotor, like L-glutamine and crizanlizumab, was tested in patients concomitantly receiving hydroxyurea, and both hydroxyurea-treated and -untreated participants exhibited increases in the hemoglobin concentration.[2] Therefore, it is reasonable to offer voxelotor to individuals with SCD who are already treated with hydroxyurea.

Combination therapy of any of the 3 new agents (voxelotor, L-glutamine, or crizanlizumab) with hydroxyurea has not yet been formally investigated. There are data to suggest that these 3 new agents provide benefit in reducing VOC events (L-glutamine and crizanlizumab) and increasing hemoglobin concentration (voxelotor) despite current exposure to hydroxyurea. This means that hydroxyurea does not blunt the effect of these new agents, which does not equate to an additive or synergistic benefit when any of the new agents is combined with hydroxyurea (ie, synergistic effect of polytherapy). Importantly, none of the 3 pivotal studies of voxelotor, L-glutamine, and crizanlizumab suggested that using these agents in combination with hydroxyurea caused increased toxicity. Given the lack of data, however, the 2 following points should be emphasized when these drugs are discussed with patients prior to their initiation: (1) discontinuation of hydroxyurea when initiating any of the new agents is *not* advisable and should be discouraged since a direct comparison (hydroxyurea vs any of the new agents) has not been undertaken, and (2) it is unclear whether adding any of the new agents will enhance the effect of hydroxyurea, but there are data to suggest that it is safe to combine them.

Considering Sickle Cell Genotype in the Choice of Therapy

Most of the studies investigating the efficacy and effectiveness of disease-modifying therapies in SCD have been primarily performed in individuals with HbSS and HbS-β^0 thalassemia (also referred to as sickle cell anemia [SCA]). The level of evidence for hydroxyurea, for instance, in individuals with HbSC and HbS-β^+ thalassemia is insufficient, and the data on efficacy and safety are mostly inferred from studies in individuals with HbSS and HbS-β^0 thalassemia and come from small, observational, retrospective studies or underpowered prospective studies.[19-22] To date, no HbSC-specific therapy has been developed. Similarly, even though the co-inheritance of α thalassemia or hereditary persistence of HbF has been associated with a different spectrum of complications, their presence or absence has not been assessed in the drug registration trials. At this time, we are not able to personalize therapy based on the genotype or on known genetic modifiers

(eg, *BCL11A*). The phase II and III trials of crizanlizumab and voxelotor, respectively, included participants who did not have HbSS and/or HbS-β^0 thalassemia however, their numbers were small relative to HbSS and HbS-β^0 thalassemia participants, and the studies were not powered to detect clinical or laboratory differences according to the sickle genotype. As a group, all participants, regardless of the sickle genotype, benefited from these new agents; therefore, it is reasonable to offer crizanlizumab and voxelotor to individuals of any sickle genotype.

Considering Age in the Choice of Therapy

Age of the patients may be a strong influencer in choice of therapy. In the United States, the FDA has differentially approved disease-modifying therapy agents according to age: hydroxyurea for patients ≥2 years of age, L-glutamine for ≥5 years, voxelotor for ≥12 years, and crizanlizumab for ≥16 years. No upper age limit was specified in the prescribing label information. Pediatric prescribing of any of these agents below the age limit is considered off-label and should be monitored carefully. However, appropriate labeling for pediatric use of new (and old) drugs lags those of adults, and there might be an instance in which a child might benefit from one of the newer agents when no other options are available. The European Academy of Paediatrics and the European Society for Developmental Perinatal and Pediatric Pharmacology offer useful guidance on off-label use of new therapeutic agents in pediatrics.[23]

Considering Hydroxyurea Long-Term Effectiveness in the Choice of Therapy

Although there are insufficient data on the long-term (>15 or 20 years) effectiveness of hydroxyurea use, there are some data that suggest a decrease in maximum-tolerated dose and clinical effectiveness over time.[24] The progressive decline in hydroxyurea response and tolerated total daily dose is not well characterized or understood, but it is suggested to be due to progressive chronic kidney disease with declining secretion of erythropoietin and decreased bone marrow function (bone marrow reserve). Therefore, increase in hydroxyurea toxicities, such as myelosuppression, with a less robust increase in HbF limits the use of hydroxyurea in older patients. Although more research is necessary to investigate bone marrow reserve of emerging and older adults exposed or not to long-term hydroxyurea, it is a consideration when discussing the initiation of new disease-modifying agents.

As patients age, they often develop more sickle nephropathy and hepatopathy, and ammonia levels could increase after L-glutamine use.[25,26] It may be prudent to monitor changes in ammonia in patients with severe renal or hepatic disease and/or initiate it at a lower dose or frequency (ie, once a day) than currently recommended.

Considering the Route and Frequency of Administration in the Choice of Therapy

The route of administration is an important consideration in the selection of SCD therapeutic agents. Of the 4 FDA-approved SCD disease-modifying agents, crizanlizumab is the only nonoral agent. Crizanlizumab is given intravenously (IV) every 2 weeks for the first month, then monthly thereafter. Hydroxyurea and voxelotor are tablets given once daily, whereas L-glutamine is dosed orally twice daily and needs to be dissolved in a liquid of preference.

Many patients have poor venous access, especially as adults. Placement of a central line solely for the purpose of administering an IV medication will have to be weighed against the potential benefit to decrease VOC by approximately 50% with crizanlizumab.[3] Patients and parents may be unwilling to undergo an invasive procedure to have a central catheter placed and then to allocate extra time to attend a clinic or day hospital every 4 weeks indefinitely. Patients with a low total number of VOC episodes per year, such as those with <3 events per year, who compose the majority of patients, will have to weigh the inconvenience of coming to the hospital once a month (total of 12 visits over 1 year) to avoid an unplanned inpatient stay (typically 4-7 days in length depending on age). A discussion regarding the time commitment required to administer crizanlizumab in the hospital or clinic versus the convenience of using oral medications, such as L-glutamine, voxelotor, and hydroxyurea, to achieve a reduction in VOC events should take place.

Considering Medication Uptake in the Choice of Therapy

Recent data from administrative registries in the United States demonstrate that the uptake of hydroxyurea remains low (between 11% and 33%) in the SCD population, both among children and adults with SCD.[27,28] Worldwide, there is also suboptimal utilization of hydroxyurea despite intensive campaigns and educational initiatives promoting its use. In 2019, a large survey of patients (2145 patients, including children and adults) reported worldwide hydroxyurea use at 31%, with 42% of patients ever receiving a prescription for hydroxyurea.[29] The causes of this poor overall uptake of hydroxyurea are multiple and reflect providers' poor understanding or willingness to prescribe this medication, system barriers due to access (eg, lack of health coverage), and patients' low acceptance (eg, due to mistrust in the medication or lack of knowledge regarding its efficacy and toxicity) and low adherence to daily dosing (eg, due to forgetfulness, lack of motivation, fear of complications).[30-35]

Some of these uptake barriers can be addressed by allowing easier access to drug information, receipt of daily reminders, and development of habit-forming behaviors—all tasks supported by digital technology solutions, including mobile health (mHealth) applications. A few mHealth applications have been developed to foster greater patient medication adherence in SCD, including text message reminders and more complex multilevel interventions that involve education, 2-way communication with providers, direct feedback, and creation of a virtual social support network.[36-43] Future mHealth interventions should be flexible enough to incorporate multiple different medications, in addition to hydroxyurea, serving as a support tool for patients to increase their uptake of not one medication, but multiple medications.

The use of IV medication may be attractive to patients who prefer a single monthly dose, versus daily dosing, particularly those who face difficulties with daily medication adherence. However, oral medications may have overall better adherence over injectable formulations, as demonstrated by studies that compared adherence to the subcutaneous iron chelator deferoxamine versus the oral iron chelator deferasirox among patients with SCD and transfusional iron overload.[44,45] Further investigation regarding how the mode of administration impacts adherence should be undertaken.

A discussion regarding the added burden of polytherapy (ie, hydroxyurea in combination with other oral disease-modifying agents) should be incorporated in the decision-making process for initiating these new agents. For an average-size adult who takes 2000 mg/d of hydroxyurea and initiates voxelotor at 1500 mg/d, the total number of capsules per day will amount to 7. Although they can be ingested together, the increased number of capsules may pose a burden and negatively impact daily adherence. Furthermore, these patients are likely to be taking other drugs to control comorbidities and SCD complications such as hypertension, renal disease, iron overload, and chronic pain, further impacting their willingness to adhere do a daily treatment regimen.

The pace of the translation of discoveries into clinical practice has been slow in SCD. It took 17 years to translate into clinical practice the knowledge that blood transfusions prevented stroke among high-risk children who were screened with transcranial Doppler ultrasound.[46] The implementation and dissemination of new discoveries have been slow to reach the SCD population and promote public health benefits. The infrastructure for information dissemination and implementation of strategies needs to be enriched by implementation methods that can accelerate the pace of translation of evidence-based guidelines and knowledge into clinical practice.[47]

Considering the Patient's Preferences and Context in the Choice of Therapy

A shared decision model of selecting drugs needs to be used to increase patients' and their families' engagement in the decision process and subsequent ongoing treatment.[6] Understanding how SCD patients weigh risks and benefits for a treatment is essential for the clinician to prepare for the decision-making process dialog. Understanding the patients' lifestyle, their own perception of their health status, their level of knowledge of the therapy, and how they balance risks and benefits is important information that will inform how the clinician should frame the treatment discussion.[48-50]

Additionally, considering the health literacy level of patients is important. Health literacy is the degree to which individuals have the capacity to obtain, process, and understand basic health information and services needed to make appropriate health decisions (as defined by the Patient Protection and Affordable Care Act of 2010, Title V). Although few studies have formally measured the health literacy level of patients with SCD, all pointed to a low or very low health literacy level.[51,52] Decision tools that incorporate strategies to communicate new concepts accounting for low health literacy are needed. New decision tools have been developed and tested, and although decisional conflict has been reduced, they have been inconsistent in demonstrating improved patient knowledge and involvement in decision making.[53,54] Greater research should be devoted to developing decision tools that are effective in improving patient knowledge and can be translated to greater patient engagement with their treatment. Additionally, decision tools for health care providers within electronic medical records that use algorithms based on age and clinical phenotypes should be developed to automate the patient screening according to eligibility criteria and clinical indications for therapies. Table 28-1 summarizes the efficacy and safety data and can be used as a quick reference in preparation for treatment discussions.

TABLE 28-1 Comparison of characteristics of current FDA-approved disease-modifying therapies for sickle cell disease

	Hydroxyurea	L-Glutamine	Crizanlizumab	Voxelotor
Age (years)	≥2	≥5	≥16	≥12
Indication	↓ VOC, PRBC transfusion	↓ VOC	↓ VOC	↓ Hemoglobin
Mechanism of action	Decrease in HbS polymerization by improving HbF production	Increases NAD redox potential (antioxidant), decreases RBC adhesion	P-selectin inhibitor, reduces RBC and WBC vascular adherence	Decreases HbS polymerization by increasing Hb oxygen affinity
Genotypes[a]	HbSS and HbS-β^0 thalassemia[b]	Any	Any	Any
Initial daily dose	15 mg/kg (adults) 20 mg/kg (children)	<30 kg: 10 g 30-65 kg: 20 g >65 kg: 30 g	5 mg/kg	1500 mg
Dose escalation	Yes (to MTD)	No	No	No
Route	PO	PO	IV	PO
Frequency	Once daily	Twice daily	Monthly	Once daily
Monitoring	Yes[c]	None	None	None
Common toxicities	Myelosuppression,[d] nail discoloration, hair loss	Diarrhea[d]	Joint pain[d]	Headache, diarrhea[d]
Long-term toxicities	Possible infertility in males	Unknown	Unknown; possible development of antibodies against crizanlizumab	Unknown
Cost	$	$$$	$$$$$	$$$$$
Dose reductions	Renal function	None	None	Hepatic function

[a]Reflects genotypes in which the drug has been tested. The FDA label does not restrict to these genotypes.
[b]Hydroxyurea is used in patients with genotypes other than HbSS and HbS-β^0 thalassemia on an individual basis.
[c]Complete blood counts should be done at least once every 2 to 3 months if used at the doses outlined in the table.
[d]Reversible side effect.
Abbreviations: FDA, US Food and Drug Administration; Hb, hemoglobin; HbS, sickle hemoglobin; HbF, fetal hemoglobin; IV, intravenous; MTD, maximum-tolerated dose; NAD, nicotinamide adenine dinucleotide; PO, oral; PRBC, packed red blood cell; RBC, red blood cell; VOC, vaso-occlusive crisis.

A Potential Approach to SCD Therapy in 2021

In the absence of clinical guidelines for prescribing the new disease-modifying therapies L-glutamine, crizanlizumab, and voxelotor, we are proposing a rational and evidence-based approach. We present 5 common clinical scenarios that will illustrate how we recommend the use of these new agents. As a point of departure, because hydroxyurea is inexpensive and documented to reduce pain episodes and mortality, it will remain as the front-line therapy for treatment of individuals with SCD.

1. Average-risk HbSS and HbS-β⁰ thalassemia in child or adult with >1 VOC episode per year (pain or ACS)
   - We recommend initiating hydroxyurea (see Table 28-1 for dosing) and titrating to the maximum-tolerated dose (MTD; see Chapter 30 for details on how to dose escalate and monitor hydroxyurea).
   - If the patient is still symptomatic after 6 to 12 months of reasonably documented adherence to hydroxyurea therapy, add L-glutamine or crizanlizumab (see Table 28-1 for dosing), depending on patient's choice, availability of venous access, and age. We personally start with L-glutamine and would add or substitute crizanlizumab if approval is denied by insurance or there is lack of effectiveness after 6 months or documented side effects. If the patient displays important gastrointestinal side effects, we suggest lowering the dose (ie, 10 mg twice daily) and/or frequency (ie, once a day; expert opinion).
   - If the patient refuses hydroxyurea or has documented side effects from it, consider L-glutamine or crizanlizumab.
   - Monitor ammonia in patients with severe renal damage on L-glutamine, and start these patients at lower doses (expert opinion).

2. Highly hemolytic and anemic (ie, hemoglobin <7-8 g/dL, high bilirubin and reticulocyte count) HbSS and HbS-β⁰ thalassemia in child or adult with <1 acute pain episode per year
   - We recommend initiating hydroxyurea and titrating to MTD.
   - If the patient is still very anemic after 6 to 12 months of reasonably documented adherence to hydroxyurea therapy, add voxelotor 1500 mg/d.
   - If the patient refuses or cannot tolerate hydroxyurea, consider voxelotor as a single agent.
   - If the patient has >1 VOC per year and is >5 years old, add L-glutamine.
   - If the patient continues to have VOCs and/or has severe gastrointestinal symptoms, switch to crizanlizumab.

3. The patient with skin ulcers: A unique population is patients with leg ulcers and severe anemia. Often, hydroxyurea is either not initiated or stopped because of fears of aggravating ulcer status, despite no strong evidence of its toxicity. For these patients, it is reasonable to initiate voxelotor 1500 mg/d. If no improvement in ulcer status is observed

after 3 to 6 months, start (or resume) hydroxyurea 15 mg/day and titrate to MTD.

4. Patients who cannot be transfused because of severe alloimmunization, previous delayed hemolytic transfusion reactions, or refusal of transfusion based on religious beliefs
   - Start hydroxyurea (see Table 28-1 for dosing) and titrate to MTD.
   - If the patient is still very anemic after 6 to 12 months of reasonably documented adherence to hydroxyurea therapy, add voxelotor 1500 mg/d.
   - If the patient refuses or cannot tolerate hydroxyurea, consider single-agent voxelotor.

Clinicians should expect changes in high-performance liquid chromatography (HPLC) for patients on voxelotor. Voxelotor binding to alfa chain of hemoglobin results in shifts in the electrical charge of the hemoglobin molecule, which causes changes in the retention times on the cation exchange columns used in most HPLC instruments for hemoglobinopathies.[55] This phenomenon can be seen also on alkaline electrophoresis and chromatography electrophoresis instruments, although to different extents.

This interference is dose dependent, as is seen in Figure 28-1. In this case, the patient was tested before voxelotor was administered (Figure 28-1A), during open-label extension of voxelotor, 1500 mg/day (Figure 28-1B), and again, several weeks later. The interference shows a clear response to both the addition of the drug and its removal, showing that there is a quantifiable response to the treatment. It is important to be knowledgeable of this interference because it will be difficult to measure adequately HbS and HbF percentages in patients taking voxelotor. This could become an issue when the need for accuracy emerges, such as in patients who receive simple transfusions or exchange transfusions and are maintained at a certain HbS target level.

Finally, voxelotor therapy, changes in the hemoglobin concentration can be expected quickly (within 2 weeks), paralleling the changes in the appearance of peripheral blood (Figure 28-2).

5. Patients with frequent hospitalizations for pain and chronic pain syndromes
   - Start hydroxyurea (see Table 28-1 for dosing) and titrate to MTD.
   - If no improvement, consider adding crizanlizumab for at least 12 months.
   - Consider adding L-glutamine if pain control is not yet optimal or no IV access.

Conclusion

Patients and providers are cautious when initiating new treatments, regardless of the disease. The introduction of several new medications to the armamentarium of SCD treatment

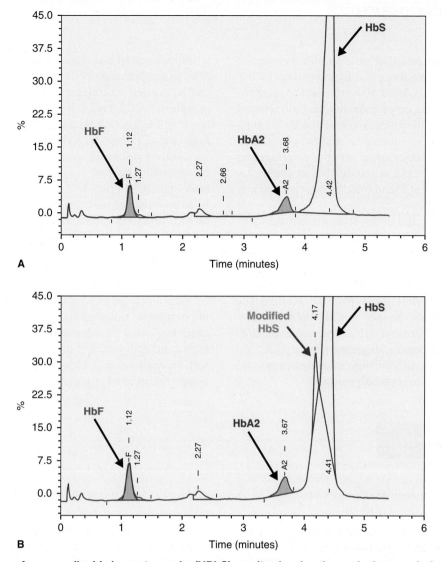

FIGURE 28-1 **High-performance liquid chromatography (HPLC) results showing the peak changes during voxelotor treatment.**
A. HPLC results before voxelotor treatment. There are three main peaks indicated by the black arrows: Fetal hemoglobin (HbF) on the left, Hb A2 in the middle and sickle hemoglobin (HbS) as the large peak on the right. No other major species are present. **B.** Same patient results after taking voxelotor for 4 weeks. Interferences on HbS peaks are clearly visible, as demonstrated by a second HbS peak to the left of the main HbS peak (red arrow), representing the voxelotor-modified HbS.

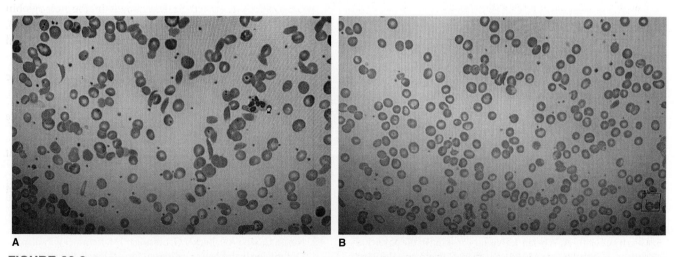

FIGURE 28-2 **Peripheral blood smears of a 49-year-old woman with HbSS, severe anemia and hemolysis, and recurrent leg ulcers who refused to take hydroxyurea because of lower extremity ulcers.** Baseline hemoglobin was 6 g/dL. After 2 weeks of voxelotor 1500 mg, hemoglobin increased to 7.4 g/dL, and bilirubin decreased from 3.2 to 1.7 mg/dL. **A.** Baseline peripheral smear. **B.** Two weeks after voxelotor initiation. Please note the significant decrease in sickled forms. Source: Dr. Caterina Minniti's clinical lab.

within a relatively short period of time stresses the need to develop guidelines for providers, patients, and parents as they consider the new options. Clinical research needs to incorporate end points that are not only measurable, but also relevant and directly beneficial to the patient and based on the patient's preferences and experiences. Patient-centered end points, such as improvement in appearance when jaundice decreases and improvement in fatigue, are not well studied but are commonly reported complications of SCD and could be incorporated into future clinical trials.

Newer and more powerful drugs alone are not sufficient to improve outcomes for SCD, and standardization and optimization of supportive and ancillary care are sorely needed. Improvement in supportive care is credited for a great portion of the improvement in survival in pediatric cancer therapies. As an example, we are just starting to explore the best fluid type and amount of hydration to be used during a VOC episode. Recent data suggest that the use of sodium-rich solutions, such as normal saline, is associated with greater risk for VOC and admissions.[56] Further research on supportive treatments will be key to continuing improving health outcomes.

As future directions, combination therapy should be formally investigated, including both new agents with hydroxyurea and cocktails of new agents (eg, crizanlizumab with voxelotor), with or without hydroxyurea. It is plausible that initiating a new therapy may lead to discontinuing hydroxyurea, which remains the main stay of therapy for individuals with SCD. Many patients do relatively well for decades and begin to have issues as they become older. How we weigh the use of new therapies in the emerging adults needs to be studied. Changing therapy may be as important as initiating it, as patient's age and their clinical picture evolves. Additionally, investigative tools that provide information accounting for patients' health literacy level will be paramount in ensuring patient participation in the decision-making process and their later engagement with their own care.

The outlook for patients with SCD and investigators is entering a new era in which more questions are being raised, but new hope is also increasing for our patients. Being able to candidly discuss the advantages and limitations of new treatments and systematically incorporate them into regular care will be challenging. Changes bring opportunities, and this decade brings more opportunities than ever.

High-Yield Facts

◆ The availability of disease-modifying therapies in SCD have been limited to hydroxyurea and transfusions for many decades.

◆ Since 2017, new disease-modifying therapy agents have been approved, but limited data regarding their efficacy and toxicity profiles are available.

◆ Although combination therapy is a goal in SCD, the lack of data regarding the combination of hydroxyurea and new disease-modifying therapy precludes clinician-informed decisions.

◆ The use of the new disease-modifying therapies should be guided by the existing body of literature, the patient's clinical status, and the patient's (and their family's) preferences, constituting the practice of shared decision making.

References

1. Anker MS, Haverkamp W, Anker SD. A phase 3 trial of l-glutamine in sickle cell disease. *N Engl J Med.* 2018;379(19):1879.

2. Vichinsky E, Hoppe CC, Ataga KI, et al. A phase 3 randomized trial of voxelotor in sickle cell disease. *N Engl J Med.* 2019; 381(6):509-519.

3. Ataga KI, Kutlar A, Kanter J, et al. Crizanlizumab for the prevention of pain crises in sickle cell disease. *N Engl J Med.* 2017; 376(5):429-439.

4. Platt OS, Orkin SH, Dover G, Beardsley GP, Miller B, Nathan DG. Hydroxyurea increases fetal hemoglobin production in sickle cell anemia. *Trans Assoc Am Physicians.* 1984;97:268-274.

5. McGann PT, Ware RE. Hydroxyurea therapy for sickle cell anemia. *Expert Opin Drug Saf.* 2015;14(11):1749-1758.

6. Charles C, Gafni A, Whelan T. Decision-making in the physician-patient encounter: revisiting the shared treatment decision-making model. *Soc Sci Med.* 1999;49(5):651-661.

7. Morris CR. Vascular risk assessment in patients with sickle cell disease. *Haematologica.* 2011;96(1):1-5.

8. Yawn BP, Buchanan GR, Afenyi-Annan AN, et al. Management of sickle cell disease: summary of the 2014 evidence-based report by expert panel members. *JAMA.* 2014;312(10):1033-1048.

9. Wang WC, Ware RE, Miller ST, et al. Hydroxycarbamide in very young children with sickle-cell anaemia: a multicentre, randomised, controlled trial (BABY HUG). *Lancet.* 2011;377(9778): 1663-1672.

10. Rigano P, De Franceschi L, Sainati L, et al. Real-life experience with hydroxyurea in sickle cell disease: a multicenter study in a cohort of patients with heterogeneous descent. *Blood Cells Mol Dis.* 2018;69:82-89.

11. McGann PT, Niss O, Dong M, et al. Robust clinical and laboratory response to hydroxyurea using pharmacokinetically guided dosing for young children with sickle cell anemia. *Am J Hematol.* 2019;94(8):871-879.

12. Nazon C, Sabo AN, Becker G, Lessinger JM, Kemmel V, Paillard C. Optimizing hydroxyurea treatment for sickle cell disease patients: the pharmacokinetic approach. *J Clin Med.* 2019;8(10):1701.

13. Niihara Y, Miller ST, Kanter J, et al. A phase 3 trial of l-glutamine in sickle cell disease. *N Engl J Med.* 2018;379(3):226-235.

14. Niihara Y, Matsui NM, Shen YM, et al. L-glutamine therapy reduces endothelial adhesion of sickle red blood cells to human umbilical vein endothelial cells. *BMC Blood Disord.* 2005;5:4.

15. Metcalf B, Chuang C, Dufu K, et al. Discovery of GBT440, an orally bioavailable r-state stabilizer of sickle cell hemoglobin. *ACS Med Chem Lett.* 2017;8(3):321-326.

16. Oksenberg D, Dufu K, Patel MP, et al. GBT440 increases haemoglobin oxygen affinity, reduces sickling and prolongs RBC half-life in a murine model of sickle cell disease. *Br J Haematol.* 2016;175(1):141-153.

17. Minniti CP, Knight-Madden J, Tonda M, Lehrer-Graiwer J, Biemond B. The impact of voxelotor treatment on leg ulcers in patients with SCD: analysis from the phase 3 HOPE study. Poster presented at the Annual Sickle Cell Disease and Thalassaemia Conference (ASCAT), London, England, October 23, 2019.

18. Shet AS, Mendelsohn L, Harper J, et al. Voxelotor treatment of a patient with sickle cell disease and very severe anemia. *Am J Hematol.* 2019;94(4):E88-E90.

19. Luchtman-Jones L, Pressel S, Hilliard L, et al. Effects of hydroxyurea treatment for patients with hemoglobin SC disease. *Am J Hematol.* 2016;91(2):238-242.

20. Wang W, Brugnara C, Snyder C, et al. The effects of hydroxycarbamide and magnesium on haemoglobin SC disease: results of the multi-centre CHAMPS trial. *Br J Haematol.* 2011;152(6):771-776.

21. Rezende PV, Santos MV, Campos GF, et al. Clinical and hematological profile in a newborn cohort with hemoglobin SC. *J Pediatr (Rio J).* 2018;94(6):666-672.

22. Yates AM, Dedeken L, Smeltzer MP, Lebensburger JD, Wang WC, Robitaille N. Hydroxyurea treatment of children with hemoglobin SC disease. *Pediatr Blood Cancer.* 2013;60(2):323-325.

23. Schrier L, Hadjipanayis A, Stiris T, et al. Off-label use of medicines in neonates, infants, children, and adolescents: a joint policy statement by the European Academy of Paediatrics and the European society for Developmental Perinatal and Pediatric Pharmacology. *Eur J Pediatr.* 2020;179(5):839-847.

24. Hankins JS, Aygun B, Nottage K, et al. From infancy to adolescence: fifteen years of continuous treatment with hydroxyurea in sickle cell anemia. *Medicine.* 2014;93(28):e215.

25. Heyland D, Muscedere J, Wischmeyer PE, et al. A randomized trial of glutamine and antioxidants in critically ill patients. *N Engl J Med.* 2013;368(16):1489-1497.

26. Kaiser S, Gerok W, Haussinger D. Ammonia and glutamine metabolism in human liver slices: new aspects on the pathogenesis of hyperammonaemia in chronic liver disease. *Eur J Clin Invest.* 1988;18(5):535-542.

27. Su ZT, Segal JB, Lanzkron S, Ogunsile FJ. National trends in hydroxyurea and opioid prescribing for sickle cell disease by office-based physicians in the United States, 1997-2017. *Pharmacoepidemiol Drug Saf.* 2019;28(9):1246-1250.

28. Brousseau DC, Richardson T, Hall M, et al. Hydroxyurea use for sickle cell disease among medicaid-enrolled children. *Pediatrics.* 2019;144(1):e20183285.

29. Osunkwo I, Andemariam B, Inusa B, et al. Impact of sickle cell disease symptoms on patients' daily lives: interim results from the international Sickle Cell World Assessment Survey (SWAY). Poster presented at American Society of Hematology Annual Meeting, Orlando, FL, December 8, 2019.

30. Badawy SM, Thompson AA, Lai JS, Penedo FJ, Rychlik K, Liem RI. Adherence to hydroxyurea, health-related quality of life domains, and patients' perceptions of sickle cell disease and hydroxyurea: a cross-sectional study in adolescents and young adults. *Health Qual Life Outcomes.* 2017;15(1):136.

31. Brandow AM, Jirovec DL, Panepinto JA. Hydroxyurea in children with sickle cell disease: practice patterns and barriers to utilization. *Am J Hematol.* 2010;85(8):611-613.

32. Haywood C Jr, Beach MC, Bediako S, et al. Examining the characteristics and beliefs of hydroxyurea users and nonusers among adults with sickle cell disease. *Am J Hematol.* 2011;86(1):85-87.

33. Lebensburger JD, Sidonio RF, Debaun MR, Safford MM, Howard TH, Scarinci IC. Exploring barriers and facilitators to clinical trial enrollment in the context of sickle cell anemia and hydroxyurea. *Pediatr Blood Cancer.* 2013;60(8):1333-1337.

34. Oyeku SO, Driscoll MC, Cohen HW, et al. Parental and other factors associated with hydroxyurea use for pediatric sickle cell disease. *Pediatr Blood Cancer.* 2013;60(4):653-658.

35. Strouse JJ, Heeney MM. Hydroxyurea for the treatment of sickle cell disease: efficacy, barriers, toxicity, and management in children. *Pediatr Blood Cancer.* 2012;59(2):365-371.

36. Alberts N, Badawy S, Hodges J, et al. Development of the mobile app "InCharge Health" to improve adherence to hydroxyurea in sickle cell disease: a user-centered design approach. *JMIR Mhealth Uhealth.* 2020;8(5):e14884.

37. Creary S, Chisolm D, Stanek J, Hankins J, O'Brien SH. A multidimensional electronic hydroxyurea adherence intervention for children with sickle cell disease: single-arm before-after study. *JMIR Mhealth Uhealth.* 2019;7(8):e13452.

38. Creary S, Chisolm DJ, O'Brien SH. ENHANCE-(Electronic Hydroxyurea Adherence): a protocol to increase hydroxyurea adherence in patients with sickle cell disease. *JMIR Res Protoc.* 2016;5(4):e193.

39. Creary SE, Gladwin MT, Byrne M, Hildesheim M, Krishnamurti L. A pilot study of electronic directly observed therapy to improve hydroxyurea adherence in pediatric patients with sickle-cell disease. *Pediatr Blood Cancer.* 2014;61(6):1068-1073.

40. Curtis K, Lebedev A, Aguirre E, Lobitz S. A medication adherence app for children with sickle cell disease: qualitative study. *JMIR Mhealth Uhealth.* 2019;7(6):e8130.

41. Leonard S, Anderson LM, Jonassaint J, Jonassaint C, Shah N. Utilizing a novel mobile health "selfie" application to improve compliance to iron chelation in pediatric patients receiving chronic transfusions. *J Pediatr Hematol Oncol.* 2017;39(3):223-229.

42. Anderson LM, Leonard S, Jonassaint J, Lunyera J, Bonner M, Shah N. Mobile health intervention for youth with sickle cell disease: impact on adherence, disease knowledge, and quality of life. *Pediatr Blood Cancer.* 2018;65(8):e27081.

43. Estepp JH, Winter B, Johnson M, Smeltzer MP, Howard SC, Hankins JS. Improved hydroxyurea effect with the use of text messaging in children with sickle cell anemia. *Pediatr Blood Cancer.* 2014;61(11):2031-2036.

44. Jordan LB, Vekeman F, Sengupta A, Corral M, Guo A, Duh MS. Persistence and compliance of deferoxamine versus deferasirox in Medicaid patients with sickle-cell disease. *J Clin Pharm Ther.* 2012;37(2):173-181.

45. Shah NR. Advances in iron chelation therapy: transitioning to a new oral formulation. *Drugs Context.* 2017;6:212502.

46. King AA, Baumann AA. Sickle cell disease and implementation science: a partnership to accelerate advances. *Pediatr Blood Cancer.* 2017;64(11):10.1002/pbc.26649.

47. DiMartino LD, Baumann AA, Hsu LL, et al. The sickle cell disease implementation consortium: translating evidence-based guidelines into practice for sickle cell disease. *Am J Hematol.* 2018;93(12):E391-E395.

48. Creary S, Zickmund S, Ross D, Krishnamurti L, Bogen DL. Hydroxyurea therapy for children with sickle cell disease: describing how caregivers make this decision. *BMC Res Notes.* 2015;8:372.

49. Hankins J, Hinds P, Day S, et al. Therapy preference and decision-making among patients with severe sickle cell anemia and their families. *Pediatr Blood Cancer.* 2007;48(7):705-710.

50. Jabour SM, Beachy S, Coburn S, Lanzkron S, Eakin MN. The role of patient-physician communication on the use of hydroxyurea in adult patients with sickle cell disease. *J Racial Ethn Health Disparities.* 2019;6(6):1233-1243.

51. Caldwell EP, Carter P, Becker H, Mackert M. The use of the newest vital sign health literacy instrument in adolescents with sickle cell disease. *J Pediatr Oncol Nurs.* 2018;35(5): 361-367.

52. Perry EL, Carter PA, Becker HA, Garcia AA, Mackert M, Johnson KE. Health literacy in adolescents with sickle cell disease. *J Pediatr Nursing.* 2017;36:191-196.

53. Crosby LE, Walton A, Shook LM, et al. Development of a hydroxyurea decision aid for parents of children with sickle cell anemia. *J Pediatr Hematol Oncol.* 2019;41(1):56-63.

54. Krishnamurti L, Ross D, Sinha C, et al. Comparative effectiveness of a web-based patient decision aid for therapeutic options for sickle cell disease: randomized controlled trial. *J Med Internet Res.* 2019;21(12):e14462.

55. Rutherford NJ, Thoren KL, Shajani-Yi Z, Colby JM. Voxelotor (GBT440) produces interference in measurements of hemoglobin S. *Clin Chim Acta.* 2018;482:57-59.

56. Carden MA, Brousseau DC, Ahmad FA, et al. Normal saline bolus use in pediatric emergency departments is associated with poorer pain control in children with sickle cell anemia and vaso-occlusive pain. *Am J Hematol.* 2019;94(6):689-696.

Gene Therapy for Sickle Cell Disease

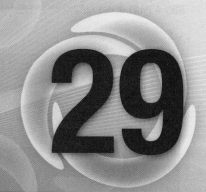

Authors: *Tim M. Townes, Marina Cavazzana*

Chapter Outline

Overview

The sickle mutation is a transversion from A to T in the sixth codon of the β-globin gene. The sixth codon is normally GAG, which encodes glutamic acid, but the transversion results in GTG, which encodes valine. Valine forms a hydrophobic projection on the surface of the hemoglobin tetramer ($\alpha_2\beta^S_2$; HbS), and when HbS releases oxygen, the valine fits into a natural hydrophobic pocket on a second tetramer in a nucleation event that stimulates the polymerization of thousands of HbS tetramers. The elongated polymers interact with each other to form a 14-stranded polymer, which is one of the most interesting and destructive polymers in nature. The HbS polymers convert normally pliable red blood cells (RBCs) into fragile, rigid rods and sickle-shaped structures that occlude small vessels and that lyse and release a host of products causing extensive tissue and organ damage.[1] Figure 29-1 is a magnetic resonance angiography of the brain of a young sickle cell patient who has suffered a massive stroke. Her left internal carotid artery is completely occluded and, therefore, invisible in the image. She has permanent right hemiplegia. Occlusions of smaller vessels in the brain in 53% of sickle patients result in "silent infarcts," which is a misnomer because they result in cognitive impairment.[2] Pathology caused by occlusions and by extensive oxidative stress in many other tissues and organs result in a severe disease that affects 100,000 patients in the United States and millions worldwide.

At present, the only curative approach for sickle cell disease (SCD) is allogeneic hematopoietic stem cell transplant (HSCT) with a full conditioning regimen and immunosuppression. The choice donor is represented by a human leukocyte antigen (HLA) genoidentical sibling even if some trials with matched unrelated donors or mismatched family donors are ongoing with significantly less satisfying results. The overall probability of survival for patients with SCD transplanted with an HLA-identical sibling graft ranges from 91% to 100%, with an event-free survival of 73% to 100%, and results are significantly better when the patients are transplanted early in life.[3]

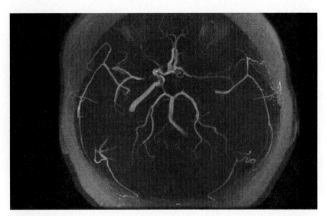

FIGURE 29-1 Magnetic resonance angiography of the brain of a young sickle patient who suffered a massive stoke. Her left internal carotid artery is completely occluded and, therefore, invisible in the image. She is permanently paralyzed on her right side. Occlusions of smaller vessels in the brain in 53% of sickle patients result in "silent infarcts," which are not at all "silent" because they result in cognitive impairment.

Gene Therapy by Gene Addition and Gene Editing

Modern molecular biology provides tools that can be used to develop an autologous, curative treatment for most if not all patients with SCD, and many dedicated scientists and clinicians are working diligently to bring a safe, efficacious, and cost-effective solution to individuals suffering from this debilitating disorder.

Gene Therapy by Gene Addition

Gene therapy by gene addition is characterized by the introduction into patients' derived hematopoietic stem and progenitor cells (HSPCs) of an extra copy of a functional β- or γ-globin gene; this functional transgene is expected to favorably compete against the production of the globin by the 2 sickle alleles. Despite the solid experience acquired in the field of genetically modified autologous transplantation, gene therapy for HbSS disease needs to address a number of issues such as:

- The source of HSPCs, which should enable administration of an adequate dose of transduced cells retaining stem cell properties and long-term engraftment capacity
- The choice of the bone marrow (BM) conditioning regimen tailored to create space for the gene corrected cells while reducing toxicity
- The dose of transduced HSPCs and the therapeutic level of transgene expression at the single progenitor level
- The presence of a favorable BM microenvironment to regenerate complete hematopoiesis initiated from corrected stem cells

Source of the HSPCs for the Ex Vivo Gene Addition

The accepted source of stem cells for gene addition therapy for HbSS patients was previously BM, harvested from the iliac crests. This precise recommendation followed the severe adverse events that occurred after several attempts to mobilize HSPCs into peripheral blood of sickle patients with granulocyte colony-stimulating factor (filgrastim). The temporal relationship between filgrastim administration, the rapid rise in the white blood cell count, and the severe adverse events were strongly suggestive of a causal link.[4-6]

The failure of HSPC procurement by a single BM harvest stimulated investigators to develop a reagent that safely and effectively mobilized HSPC into the peripheral blood. Plerixafor has led us and others to conceive new mobilization strategies under very precise circumstances in order to achieve a higher yield of CD34+ cells without side effects.[7-9]

Plerixafor (AMD3100; Mozobil) is a bicyclam molecule that selectively and reversibly antagonizes the binding of stromal cells derived factor-1 (SDF-1) to the chemokine CXC-receptor-4 (CXCR4) located on the surface of HSPCs, thus releasing stem cells from BM niches into the peripheral circulation. The mechanistic difference between plerixafor and filgrastim explains the small increase in the white blood cell count and the short time interval between plerixafor administration and HSPC mobilization. The use of plerixafor is currently approved by the US Food and Drug Administration and European Medicines Agency, in combination with filgrastim, in patients affected by lymphoma or multiple myeloma in whom cells mobilize poorly with filgrastim alone.[7-9]

Several clinical trials have demonstrated that plerixafor alone safely and rapidly mobilizes HSPCs in HbSS patients provided that the level of circulating HbS is maintained at <30% via erythrocyte exchanges and appropriate hydration with tight correction of electrolytes at all times during harvesting. Whether this procedure is safe in 100% of HbSS patients is still unknown, and only the enrollment of a significant number of patients can answer this important concern.

Comparative analysis of human HSPCs collected from BM or mobilized by filgrastim and/or plerixafor has highlighted differences and specific biologic properties among the different sources: immunophenotyping and global gene expression profiling have highlighted the superior characteristics of plerixafor-mobilized HSPCs, whereas competitive transplantation in NOD scid gamma (NSG) triple-knockout mice and in vivo imaging have allowed defining their homing capacity and their superior reconstitution potential. Although the overall yield of CD34+ cells is reduced by using plerixafor alone, this is counterbalanced by the superior stem cell characteristics of the harvest, which could support the elimination of filgrastim, provided that mobilization of an adequate cell dose can be achieved.

The Conditioning Regimen

The conditioning regimen is defined as the treatment necessary to assure the engraftment of gene-modified HSPCs that considers the pathophysiology of the disease and, in the case of autologous transplantation, the absence of a role for allogenic T cells to make space for transplanted cells.

The clinical history of gene therapy has indicated that in vivo selective advantage improves the efficacy of the treatment when the transplanted, genetically corrected hematopoietic stem cells (HSCs) are suboptimal, as shown for different severe combined immunodeficiency (SCID) forms.[10] In these cases, nonmyeloablative, minimally toxic conditioning regimens can be used successfully. In the case of HbSS disease, selective advantage has been well described for patients transplanted with an allogeneic graft, but unfortunately, different lines of evidence show that it is mostly limited to peripheral mature RBCs. One line of evidence comes from a multilineage analysis that we performed after HLA genoidentical allogeneic transplantation for SCD in patients who received a full conditioning regimen.[11] In this study, a median 2-fold increase between donor chimerism in peripheral RBCs versus BFU-E was observed; moreover, we showed that a minimal engraftment of 30% for an AA donor and 50% for an AS donor must be obtained to completely control the disease (ie, vaso-occlusive crisis and hemolytic anemia).

Lentiviral-based gene addition strategies and genome editing approaches (see later section on gene editing) at best generate a heterozygous phenotype in vitro; therapeutic hemoglobin accounts for at most 60% of the total hemoglobin types. For example, RBCs derived from HSPCs harboring multiple copies of a therapeutic lentiviral vector[12] generate an AS-like phenotype under optimal conditions. Our clinical data on SCD patients with mixed chimerism suggest that an HSPC genetic modification rate <30% would not be sufficient to cure the SCD phenotype. Altogether, these data allow us to recommend in sickle cell patients the use of genetically modified HSPCs with a vector copy number (VCN) >1 and myeloablative conditioning regimens to make sufficient space in the BM for transplanted cells.

The morbidity of myeloablative conditioning is reduced in gene therapy protocols compared to allogeneic HSCT, because immune suppression is not required in an autologous setting. Therefore, severe opportunistic infections and reactivation of endogenous viruses are avoided. Nevertheless, patients still face concerns related to infertility and sometimes poor hair regrowth and, less frequently, risk of developing myelodysplastic syndromes, whose incidence depends on the length of the disease before the autologous transplantation, number of vaso-occlusive episodes (VOEs), dosage and duration of hydroxyurea treatment, and finally, the use on this background of busulfan for the conditioning regimen.

For nonmalignant disorders in which an antitumoral effect is not required, a strong rationale does exist for developing minimally toxic conditioning regimens. Recent examples are the use of antibodies, such as anti-CD45 and anti–c-kit, but more clinical studies are necessary to determine whether their use is sufficient to guarantee a curative level of chimerism.[13,14]

HSPC Dose and Transduction Modalities

Regarding dosing, it is generally acknowledged that 2 to 3 × 10^6 CD34$^+$ HSPCs/kg of body weight are required for a successful outcome in the autologous HSCT setting. Considering that between 50% and 80% of CD34 cells can be corrected by gene therapy and that the culture conditions themselves decrease the engraftment capacity of the graft and the yield

after thawing, a minimum harvest of 1 × 10^7 CD34$^+$ cells/kg would be required at the beginning of the procedure.

Indeed, a growing body of experimental evidence has shown that cultured HSPCs progressively lose their engraftment capacity as a result of recruitment into the cell cycle. The HSPC shed adhesion molecules during growth and culture (which impedes their homing to the appropriate niches) and show greater lineage commitment and differentiation.

The ex vivo cell culture time is correlated with the level of transcriptional modifications and the engraftment capacity of the cells, both of which were much lower when the culture time was extended from 24 to 48 hours.[15,16] Loss of engraftment capacity is particularly problematic in inflammatory contexts such as in patients with HbSS disease or chronic granulomatous disease. Moreover, HSPCs react to high doses of viral vectors by activating innate immune sensors and antiviral factors that target the retroviral integration process.[17] Transduction of HSPCs with a lentiviral vector reportedly activates the p53 signaling pathway, which leads to an elevation in apoptosis, delayed proliferation (which correlated with the VCN), and decreased engraftment capacity.[15] All of these data have to be considered in order to optimize the transduction process, shorten the culture period, and inhibit the inflammatory response elicited by the detection of the vector by adding new reagents. Over the past 5 years, numerous cell culture supplements have been tested for their ability to increase vector transduction and optimize the yield of cell products, such as cyclosporin and rapamycin or prostaglandin E2,[18,19] among others.

Finally, critical to a successful outcome is the level of damage to the microenvironment associated with systemic endothelial dysfunction within complex dyserythropoietic BM. Erythroid hyperplasia, abnormally low reticulocyte responses, the presence of hemoglobin S polymers in reticulocytes, sickling of nucleated erythroblasts, and extensive marrow erythrophagocytosis result in the abnormally elevated apoptotic activity that characterizes the dyserythropoiesis in HbSS patients. Corrected donor cells are not susceptible to this pathology and, therefore, have a significant selective advantage that is even more pronounced than the advantage observed in thalassemic patients.

The selective advantage of healthy erythroid precursors cells in the allogeneic transplantation setting in the presence of mixed hematopoietic chimerism strongly supports the hypothesis that ineffective erythropoiesis is an important disease mechanism in SCD. The exact definition of all these parameters (ie, source, dose, transduction, conditioning regimen) is essential for a successful gene therapy approach, both for gene addition and gene editing.

Integrative Lentiviral Approaches for Treating SCD

The introduction of HIV-derived lentiviral (LV) vectors constituted a major breakthrough thanks to the LV's capacity to accommodate complex transcriptional units and efficiently transduce HSPCs. Furthermore, the use of self-inactivating vectors lacking the enhancer/promoter region in the long terminal repeat has eliminated the risk of transactivation of the adjacent cellular genes by the viral cis-regulatory elements.

Preclinical studies showed the potential of LV-based gene therapy in correcting the SCD phenotype. The vectors used in these studies used globin promoter/locus control region (LCR) expression cassette combinations that allowed the targeted expression of globins with the potential to interfere with HbS polymerization, such as the βT87Q,[20] fetal γ-globin,[21,22] or the βAS3 mutants.[23-25]

Gene Addition of Antisickling Hemoglobin

As discussed earlier, the experience with allogeneic transplantation enables investigators to predict the minimal level of corrected HSPCs necessary to achieve clinical benefit in SCD patients. Stable mixed chimeras with donor AA HSPC levels of 30% provide significant hematologic and clinical improvement.[26-28] These data, combined with the evidence from individuals with SCD plus hereditary persistence of fetal hemoglobin (HPFH), predict that engraftment of 30% to 50% of autologous HSPC-producing RBCs with >30% antisickling hemoglobin levels could improve symptoms and abrogate the need for transfusions.

Clinical development of gene therapy for SCD started with the first patient treated in France with transplantation of CD34+ HSPCs transduced with the BB305 replication-defective, self-inactivating LV vector encoding an engineered form of human β-globin gene, β-A-T87Q (bT87Q), where the threonine at position 87 has been substituted with glutamine. The transplanted dose of 5×10^6 cells/kg led to an average copy number of 1 after a full dose of busulfan used as single agent to achieve myeloablation. Reconstitution of all hematopoietic lineages was sustained and complete at 3 months after transplantation, and no adverse events were see after >3 years of follow-up. The patient achieved a level of therapeutic HbA^T87Q globin of around 50% and transfusion independence, with a clinical and biologic picture similar to that of an HbS carrier.[29]

Integration site analysis showed polyclonal hematopoietic reconstitution and no clonal abnormality. The results obtained in this first patient encouraged the treatment of additional severe SCD patients in the context of 2 ongoing clinical trials in France and the United States. However, the interim report of the first 7 adult patients treated in the multicenter US trial demonstrated that treatment failed to achieve a level of correction comparable to that observed in the first patient. Patients received a median dose of 2×10^6 CD34+ HSPCs obtained from at least 2 BM harvests with a median VCN of 0.6. Two years after the treatment, the VCN in peripheral blood was around 0.1, and HbA^T78Q levels were <1 g/dL. HbA^T87Q accounted for <10% of the total hemoglobin.

A second group of 2 patients received preharvest RBC transfusions (as in the HB-205 trial) and a cell dose of 2.2 and 3.2×10^6/kg.[30] The drug product manufacturing process and the myeloablation regimen were optimized. Both patients showed a higher VCN (1.4 and 5), higher percentages of total and therapeutic hemoglobin, and lower levels of hemolysis markers (relative to the first group of 7 patients). Finally, in a third group of 14 patients, the use of plerixafor to

safely harvest a large number of autologous HSPCs was a key improvement. The first 6 treated patients received a mean dose of 7.1×10^6 CD34+ cells/kg with a high VCN, and the preliminary results are promising.[31] Taken as a whole, these data show that the optimization of the drug manufacturing process, patient conditioning, cell dose, and HSC source can lead to therapeutically relevant outcomes in gene therapy by gene addition for SCD.

In the United States, 2 other phase I/II protocols have been initiated. Malik et al[32] used an LV encoding a modified γ-globin transgene to treat 2 HbS/β⁰ patients after reduced-intensity conditioning. The early results appear promising with excellent safety and LV-derived fetal hemoglobin (HbF) expression accounting for about 20% of the total hemoglobin.[32] The patient with the longest follow-up (1 year) showed an improvement in anemia, less chronic pain, and no acute VOEs. In the second clinical trial, the vector contained a β-globin gene with 3 antisickling mutations.[24]

Gene Addition Aiming to Produce or Increase the HbF Level

Another promising LV-based approach has been designed to increase levels of endogenous HbF. Deng et al[33] generated an LV encoding a fusion protein between a zinc-finger domain (which binds to the γ-globin promoters) and LDB1 (a looping factor involved in the LCR/β-like promoter interactions) (Figure 29-2). This approach led to HbF reactivation in vitro via forced looping between the LCR and the γ-globin promoters in primary erythroblasts derived from SCD patients with HbF accounting for up to approximately 50% of the total hemoglobin and correction of the SCD phenotype with a low VCN per cell.[33,34] Recently, this approach was tested in vitro in nonhuman primate HSPCs. Upon differentiation toward the erythroid lineage, the progeny of genetically modified HSPCs produced elevated levels of HbF.[34]

The BCL11A transcriptional repressor is another potential target for reactivating HbF expression. Given that BCL11A knockdown has a negative impact in HSPCs and B cells,[35-37] investigators developed an LV that expresses a microRNA-adapted shRNA targeting BCL11A under the control of erythroid-restricted β-globin promoter/LCR HS2 and HS3 elements[38] (Figure 29-3). HbF upregulation was observed in vitro in human primary erythroblasts and in vivo in a sickle mouse model.[35,39] Based on these results, a phase I clinical trial for SCD was initiated in May 2018 (Table 29-1). An optimized transduction protocol led to a VCN of 3 to 5 in the drug product. Three months after transplantation, an SCD patient treated with plerixafor-mobilized, transduced HSPCs showed good levels of HbF (accounting for 23% of total hemoglobin), and 60% of the RBCs expressed HbF.[40]

Gene Therapy by Gene Editing

Gene editing strategies for SCD can be categorized into 2 major groups: (1) modifications designed to upregulate HbF and (2) modifications designed to correct the sickle mutation (GTG

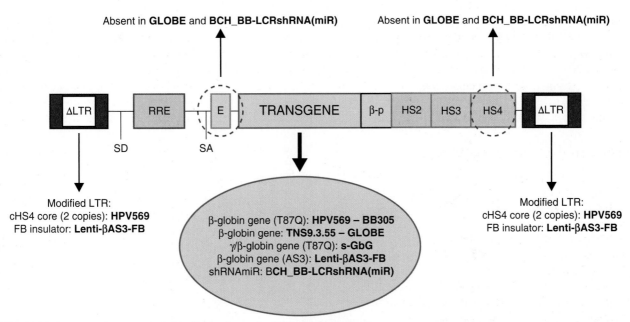

FIGURE 29-2 **The structure of lentiviral (LV) vectors used in clinical trials for β-hemoglobinopathies.** The LV names are given in bold type. β-p, β-globin promoter; E, β-globin gene enhancer; HS2, HS3, HS4, hypersensitive sites from the locus control region (LCR); ΔLTR, self-inactivating long terminal repeat; RRE, Rev-responsive element; SA and SD, splicing acceptor and donor. Magrin E, Miccio A, Cavazzana M. Lentiviral and genome-editing strategies for the treatment of β-hemoglobinopathies. *Blood*. 2019 Oct 10;134(15):1203-1213.

to GAG) or to insert an antisickling β-globin cDNA (β^AS3) at the β-globin gene translational start site. These general strategies and the specific subdivisions of these approaches will be described in the following sections.

Gene Editing Strategies to Reactivate HbF

- Deletion of the *BCL11a* gene erythroid-specific enhancer[41-45]
- Deletion of the BCL11a binding site in the γ-globin gene promoter[46-49]
- Hypomorphic mutation of the *KLF1* gene[50-53]
- Deletion of the LRF binding site in the γ-globin gene promoter[47,54,55]

- Creation of a TAL1 binding site in the γ-globin gene promoter[56]
- Creation of a KLF1 binding site in the γ-globin gene promoter[57]
- Creation of a GATA1 binding site in the γ-globin gene promoter[58]
- Deletion of a 13.6-kb DNA fragment encompassing the δ- and β^S-globin genes[59,60]
- Deletion of *HBBP1* in the β-globin locus[61,62]
- Hypomorphic mutation of the *POGZ* gene[63]
- Hypomorphic mutations of the *Mi2β*[64] or *MBD2* genes[65]
- Hypomorphic mutations of the *LSD1*[66] or *BAP1* genes[67]

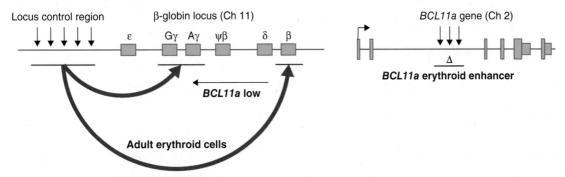

FIGURE 29-3 **Schematic diagram of the β-like globin locus on chromosome (Ch) 11 and the *BCL11a* gene on chromosome 2.** β-Like globin gene switching during the first year of life is regulated by competition between γ- and β-globin genes for interactions with the locus control region (LCR; marked by 5 DNase I hypersensitive sites).[73-75] The switch from γ- to β-globin gene expression is controlled by upregulation of KLF1 and, consequently, upregulation of BCL11a during development.[50,51] Deletion (Δ) of a small region of the BCL11a erythroid-specific enhancer (marked by 3 DNase I hypersensitive sites) in hematopoietic stem and progenitor cells reduces BCL11a levels and relieves γ-globin gene repression in adult erythroid cells.[41-45]

TABLE 29-1 Gene therapy clinical trials for TDT and SCD patients

	Trial identification no.	Phase	Sponsor	Site	Start date/recruitment status	No. of patients	Vector and transgene/nuclease and DP name	Cell source	Conditioning	DP administration	References
β Thalassemia	LG001	I/II	bluebird bio	France	September 2006; completed	2	HPV569 (β^{A-T87Q}-globin)	G-CSF mPBC or BM	Myeloablative (busulfan)	IV	Cavazzana et al, *Nature*, 2010
	NCT01639690	I	Memorial Sloan Kettering Cancer Center	US	July 2012; active not recruiting	4	TNS9.3.55 (β^{A}-globin)	G-CSF mPBC	Nonmyeloablative (busulfan 8 mg/kg)	IV	Mansilla-Soto et al, *Human Gene Therapy*, 2016
	NCT02151526 (HGB205)	I/II	bluebird bio	France	July 2013; active, not recruiting	4	BB305 (β^{A-T87Q}-globin)	G-CSF + plerixafor mPBC	Myeloablative (busulfan)	IV	Thompson et al, *NEJM*, 2018
	NCT01745120 (HGB204)	I/II	bluebird bio	US, Australia, Thailand	August 2013; completed	18	BB305 (β^{A-T87Q}-globin)	G-CSF + plerixafor mPBC	Myeloablative (busulfan)	IV	Thompson et al, *NEJM*, 2018
	NCT02453477	I/II	IRCCS San Raffaele	Italy	May 2015; active, not recruiting	10	GLOBE (βA-globin)	G-CSF + plerixafor mPBC	Myeloablative (thiotepa + treosulfan)	IO	Marktel et al, *Nature Medicine*, 2019
	NCT02906202 (HGB207)	III	bluebird bio	US, France, Germany, Greece, Italy, UK	July 2016; recruiting	23 estimated patients	BB305 (β^{A-T87Q}-globin)	G-CSF + plerixafor mPBC	Myeloablative (busulfan)	IV	Locatelli et al, 61st ASH meeting, 2018, oral presentation
	NCT02906202 (HGB212)	III	bluebird bio	USA, France, Germany, Greece, Italy, UK	June 2017; recruiting	15 estimated patients	BB305 (β^{A-T87Q}-globin)	G-CSF + plerixafor mPBC	Myeloablative (busulfan)	IV	Locatelli et al, 61st ASH meeting, 2018, oral presentation
	NCT03432364	I/II	Sangamo Therapeutics and Bioverativ Therapeutics Inc.	US	February 2018; recruiting	6	ZFN (DP: ST-400)	mPBC	Myeloablative (busulfan)	IV	NA

	NCT number	Phase	Sponsor	Country	Start date; status	No. of patients	DP (drug product)	Cell source	Conditioning	Route	Reference
SCD	NCT03655678	I/II	Vertex Pharmaceuticals Incorporated and CRISPR Therapeutics	Germany, UK	September 2018; recruiting	12 estimated patients (may be expanded to 45 patients)	CRISPR/Cas9 (DP: CTX001)	NA	Myeloablative (busulfan)	IV	NA
	NCT02151526 (HGB205)	I/II	bluebird bio	France	July 2013; active, not recruiting	3	BB305 (β^{A-T87Q}_globin)	BM	Myeloablative (busulfan)	IV	Ribeil et al, *NEJM*, 2017
	NCT02186418	I/II	Children's Hospital Medical Center, Cincinnati	US, Jamaica	July 2014; recruiting	10	sGbG (γ-globin)	BM and plerixafor mPBC	Reduced-intensity conditioning (melphalan 140 mg/m^2 BSA)	IV	Malik et al, 61st ASH meeting, 2018, oral presentation
	NCT02247843	I	University of California Children's Hospital, Los Angeles	US	July 2014; recruiting	6	βAS3-FB (β^{A63}-globin)	BM	Myeloablative (busulfan)	IV	NA
	NCT02140554 (HGB206)	I	bluebird bio	US	August 2014; recruiting	3 groups (A, B, C): 50 estimated patients	BB305 (β^{A-T87Q}_globin)	BM (A and B) plerixafor mPBC (C)	Myeloablative (busulfan)	IV	Tisdale et al, 61st ASH meeting, 2018, oral presentation
	NCT03282656	I	David Williams Boston Children's Hospital	US	February 2018; recruiting	7	BCH_BB-LCRsh-RNA(miR) shRNAmiR	Plerixafor mPBC	Myeloablative (busulfan)	IV	Esrick et al, 61st ASH meeting, 2018, oral presentation
	NCT03745287	I/II	Vertex Pharmaceuticals Incorporated and CRISPR Therapeutics	US	November 2018; recruiting	12 estimated patients (may be expanded to 45 patients)	CRISPR/Cas9 (DP: CTX001)	NA	Myeloablative (busulfan)	IV	NA

Abbreviations: ASH, American Society of Hematology; BM, bone marrow; BSA, body surface area; DP, drug product; G-CSF, granulocyte colony-stimulating factor; IO, intraosseously; IRCCS, Istituto di Ricovero e Cura a Carattere Scientifico; IV, intravenous; mPBC, mobilized peripheral blood cells; NA, not available; *NEJM*, *New England Journal of Medicine*; SCD, sickle cell disease; TDT, transfusion-dependent β thalassemia; UK, United Kingdom; US, United States.

- Hypomorphic mutation of the *HR1* kinase gene[68]
- Hypomorphic mutation of the CHD4 CHDCT2 domain[69]

Deletion of the BCL11a Gene Erythroid-Specific Enhancer

The most advanced gene editing solution for the treatment of SCD is based on the ground-breaking discoveries of Dr. Stuart Orkin and colleagues at Boston Children's Hospital. Dr. Orkin performed a genome-wide association study of individuals with HPFH and identified a region of human chromosome 2 that was associated with high HbF levels in adults.[70] This finding confirmed and narrowed a region originally identified by Dr. Swee Lay Thein at King's College Hospital, London.[71] Subsequently, in a tour de force,[41-44] Dr. Orkin and colleagues discovered that the *BCL11a* gene in this region of chromosome 2 encoded a repressor of γ-globin gene expression in adult erythroid cells, defined an erythroid-specific enhancer of BCL11a, and demonstrated that deletion of a small region of this enhancer resulted in dramatic upregulation of HbF (Figure 29-3). Dr. Daniel Bauer and colleagues subsequently demonstrated that deletion of the BCL11a erythroid enhancer in HSPC from SCD patients results in HbF levels that inhibit RBC sickling.[45] These studies form the foundation for a phase I/II clinical trial by CRISPR Therapeutics and Vertex Pharmaceuticals (ClinicalTrials.gov identifier: NCT03745287). This is a beautiful example of the way in which discoveries from basic science studies can lead to new therapeutic strategies that, hopefully, will cure patients.

Deletion of BCL11a Binding Site in the γ-Globin Gene Promoter

Upregulation of γ-globin gene expression can also be accomplished by the deletion of the BCL11a binding site in the γ-globin gene promoter. The laboratories of Drs. Merlin Crossley and Stuart Orkin[46,47] independently demonstrated that sequence variations around –115, which result in HPFH, inhibit binding of the repressor. The Crossley lab[47] used exquisite gel shift assays to demonstrate that BCL11a binds directly to the –115 region of the γ-globin gene promoter. Subsequently, these investigators created a single nucleotide substitution at –117, which is found in some individuals with HPFH (TGACCA to TAACCA), and demonstrated convincingly that this change inhibited binding of BCL11a and resulted in dramatic upregulation of γ-globin gene expression in adult erythroid cells. The Orkin lab[46] used a novel method developed by Dr. Steve Henikoff's group[72] designated CUT&RUN to define the BCL11a binding site in the γ-globin gene promoter (–118 TGACCA –113) and to demonstrate that BCL11a binds to this site in adult erythroid cells. They also convincingly demonstrated that mutation of this sequence resulted in looping of the LCR to the γ-globin gene promoter and in dramatic upregulation of γ-globin gene expression in adult erythroid cells. Finally, Traxler et al[48] and Humbert et al[49] used CRISPR/Cas9 to create a 13-bp deletion that encompassed the BCL11a site in the γ-globin gene promoter in CD34+ HSPCs from humans

and nonhuman primates and demonstrated significant upregulation of HbF in vitro and in vivo, respectively. The 13-bp deletion was designed to mimic a naturally occurring HPFH variant that dramatically upregulates HbF in humans. All of these results confirm that the BCL11a binding site in the γ-globin gene promoter (–118 TGACCA –113) is an important target for editing in SCD patient HSPCs.

Hypomorphic Mutation of the KLF1 Gene

In 1990, 2 groups demonstrated that human fetal to adult globin gene switching results from competition of the γ- and β-globin genes for interaction with the powerful LCR.[73-75] Subsequently, 2 groups demonstrated that the level of Kruppel-like factor 1 (KLF1) controls the switch by differential binding of KLF1 to the γ- and β-globin gene CACCC boxes (see supplemental Figures 3 and 4 in Zhou et al[51]) and by directly regulating *BCL11a* gene expression.[50,51] KLF1 levels increase 3-fold in erythroid progenitors between fetal and adult development,[76,77] and this increase results in a switch of KLF1 binding from the γ- to β-globin gene promoter CACCC box (–90 CACCC –86).[51] The increased level of KLF1 also directly activates *BCL11a* gene expression in adult erythroid cells by binding to the BCL11a promoter CACCC box (–371 CACCC –367).[77] Interestingly, deletion of the distal enhancer of the *KLF1* gene in the mouse reduces KLF1 levels and, consequently, BCL11a levels and activates fetal globin gene expression in adult erythroid cells without inhibiting erythroid cell maturation.[77] These results suggest that editing of *KLF1* regulatory sequences in adult SCD patient HSPCs will upregulate HbF in differentiated erythroid cells. In addition, Borg et al[50] and Liu et al[78] have demonstrated that inactivation of 1 of the 2 *KLF1* genes can result in significant HPFH (also see commentary by Manwani and Bieker[79]). Therefore, creation in SCD patient HSPCs of *KLF1* inactivating, hypomorphic, or regulatory mutations, which are guided by HPFH discoveries in various human populations, should result in high levels of HbF in adult erythroid cells and should ameliorate symptoms in SCD patients.

Deletion of the LRF/ZBTB7A Binding Site in the γ-Globin Gene Promoter

Recently, 2 groups demonstrated that the LRF/ZBTB7A repressor, which like BCL11a recruits the nucleosome remodeling and deacetylase (NuRD) repressor complex, binds specifically to the –200 region of the γ-globin gene promoter in adult erythroid cells.[47,54] Specific sequence variations in this region (–204 CCCTTCCCC –194) are associated with HPFH. Masuda et al[54] and Martyn et al[47] demonstrated that (1) LRF/ZBTB7A binds directly to the –200 region, (2) HPFH sequence variations in the region inhibit LRF/ZBTB7A binding, and (3) editing of the LRF/ZBTB7A binding site results in reactivation of the γ-globin gene in adult erythroid cells. These results establish LRF/ZBTB7A as a major γ-globin gene repressor. Therefore, editing of the –200 region in SCD HSPCs followed by transplantation should result in high levels of HbF in adult erythroid cells. Interestingly, Norton et al[55] recently demonstrated that KLF1 binds directly to the LRF/ZBTB7A gene promoter and upregulates expression in adult erythroid cells. These results suggest that the KLF1 modifications discussed in the previous sections may result in extremely high levels of HbF in adult erythroid cells by inhibiting expression of both of these independent γ-globin gene repressors.

Creation of TAL1, KLF1, or GATA1 Binding Sites in the γ-Globin Gene Promoter

Merlin Crossley's group[56-58] has also demonstrated that CRISPR/Cas9 creation of single base substitutions, which create specific transcription factor binding sites in the γ-globin gene promoter, significantly upregulate γ-globin gene expression. These single base substitutions mimic HPFH variants. The −175T>C transition produces a TAL1/SCL binding site, the −198T>C transition produces a KLF1 binding site, and the −113A>G transition produces a GATA1 binding site, which does not alter the binding of BCL11a. Editing to create these base substitutions individually or in combination in SCD patient HSPCs is predicted to increase HbF to levels that ameliorate the disease.

Deletion of the ψβ-Globin Gene (HBBP1) and/or the δ- and βˢ-Globin Genes

In 2017, Dr. Gerd Blobel and colleagues demonstrated that the *HBBP1* gene forms differential chromatin contacts in the β-globin locus during fetal and adult stages of development.[62] In the fetal stage, HBBP1 interacts with 2 DNaseI-sensitive regions that flank the locus and are bound by CTCF. The authors suggest that in this configuration, the γ-globin genes can interact with the LCR, but β-globin genes are excluded. In the adult stage, HBBP1 interacts with the ε-globin gene in a configuration that presumably excludes the γ-globin genes from interacting with the LCR and enables preferential access of the δ- and β-globin genes to the LCR. These results suggested a role for the *HBBP1* gene in the fetal to adult hemoglobin switch. Therefore, this group used CRISPR/Cas9 to delete a 2.3-kb DNA fragment containing HBBP1 in adult hematopoietic progenitors and demonstrated a significant increase in γ-globin gene expression. These results suggest that deletion of the *HBBP1* gene in SCD patient HSPCs will increase HbF to levels that ameliorate the disease.

Other investigators have recently demonstrated that CRISPR/Cas9 deletion of a 13.6-kb DNA fragment encompassing the δ- and β-globin genes in adult hematopoietic progenitors increases the interaction of γ-globin genes with the LCR and significantly upregulates γ-globin gene expression in adult erythroid cells.[59,60] This deletion mimics a natural deletion found in some individuals with deletional HPFH. These results suggest that large deletions encompassing the adult globin genes result in upregulation of the remaining γ-globin genes in adult erythroid cells by loss of competition with adult genes even in the presence of multiple γ-globin gene repressor binding sites.[73,75]

Hypomorphic Mutation of the POGZ Gene

Gudmundsdottir et al[63] recently demonstrated that the zinc-finger transcription factor POGZ plays a role in BCL11a expression. Knockdown of *POGZ* gene expression in adult CD34⁺ HSPCs followed by differentiation into mature erythroid cells results in a significant downregulation of BCL11a and, consequently, upregulation of HbF production. Approximately 25% of total hemoglobin in *POGZ* knockdown erythroid cells is HbF. These results suggest that deletion or hypomorphic mutation of *POGZ* in HSPCs of SCD patients will increase HbF to levels that ameliorate the disease. Interestingly, Gudmundsdottir et al[63] also report that *POGZ* gene expression in adult erythroid cells is regulated by KLF1. These results again suggest that KLF1 downregulation or hypomorphic mutation could be an excellent strategy for HbF upregulation.

Hypomorphic Mutation of the MBD2 Gene

Yu et al[65] have recently demonstrated that CRISPR/Cas9 deletion of the *MBD2* gene, which encodes a member of the methyl-CpG binding domain protein family, upregulates HbF levels in adult erythroid cells at levels similar to those achieved by inactivation of the *BCL11a* and *LRF* genes. *MBD2* recruits specific proteins of the NuRD corepressor complex, which is also recruited by *BCL11a* and *LRF*. Although the specific mechanism by which *MBD2* recruits the NuRD complex to the γ-globin genes is not known, deletion or hypomorphic mutation of the *MBD2* gene in SCD patient HSPCs should increase HbF to levels that ameliorate the disease.

Hypomorphic Mutation of the LSD1 and BAP1 Genes

Engel and colleagues have published convincing evidence that the nuclear receptors TR2 and TR4 bind to the γ-globin gene promoters in adult erythroid progenitors and recruit the corepressor *LSD1*.[66,80] Knockdown of *LSD1* results in significant upregulation of HbF production. Recently, these groups have also demonstrated that TR4 recruits the nuclear corepressor 1 (NCoR1) and *BAP1*, which regulates NCoR1 stability, to γ-globin gene promoters in adult erythroid progenitors. Knockdown or CRISPR/Cas deletion of *BAP1* results in upregulation of HbF in adult erythroid progenitors.[67] These results establish *LSD1* and *BAP1* as therapeutic targets for upregulation of HbF.

Hypomorphic Mutation of the HR1 Kinase Gene

Blobel and colleagues have recently performed an ingenious CRISPR/Cas9 screen to identify novel genes that regulate HbF production.[68] This screen revealed the heme-regulated inhibitor HR1 as a major inhibitor of γ-globin gene expression in adult erythroid cells. Depletion of HR1 resulted in a dramatic decrease in expression of BCL11a and consequent upregulation of HbF, and knockdown of HR1 in human sickle patient CD34⁺ cells dramatically decreased the number of sickled erythroid cells after 15 days of differentiation. Interestingly, HR1 appears to regulate BCL11a transcription, rather than translation. This is surprising because HR1 is an erythroid-specific kinase that is known to phosphorylate the translation factor eIF2a, which regulates globin mRNA translation in response to heme levels. Nevertheless, the data powerfully establish HR1 as a target for therapeutic upregulation of HbF in adult erythroid cells. Deletion or hypomorphic mutation of the *HR1* gene in SCD patient HSPCs should increase HbF to levels that ameliorate the disease.

Hypomorphic Mutation of the CHD4 CHDCT2 Domain

Bauer and colleagues recently performed an elegant CRISPR/Cas9 mutagenesis screen of components of the NuRD complex and demonstrated that a single domain (CHDCT2) of the CHD4 protein is essential for repression of γ-globin gene expression in human adult erythroid progenitors.[69] Specific mutations of this domain in human HSPCs inhibited interaction of CHD4 with the NuRD complex after differentiation of the HSPCs into erythroid progenitors and significantly enhanced γ-globin gene expression. These experiments establish a general approach to define important interactions of components in epigenetic complexes and specifically identify a new target for hypomorphic mutation for the treatment of SCD.

Gene Editing Strategies to Produce Hemoglobin A

- Insertion of β^{AS3}-globin cDNA into the β^{S}-globin gene[81-83]
- Correction of the sickle mutation (GTG to GAG)
  - In HSCs (Ding, Sun, Li, et al, unpublished data)[84-88]
  - In induced pluripotent stem cells (iPSCs)[89-91]

Insertion of β^{AS3}-Globin cDNA Into the β^{S}-Globin Gene

In 2016 and 2018, Porteus and colleagues[81,82] published landmark papers demonstrating efficient, CRISPR/Cas9-mediated knockin of a powerful antisickling globin sequence (β^{AS3})[23,92,93] downstream of the β^{S}-globin gene translational start site in human patient HSPCs (Figure 29-4). Site-specific insertion of this cDNA resulted in high-level, erythroid-specific expression of β^{AS3} driven by the endogenous LCR and β-globin promoter elements. The β^{AS3} cDNA and sequences responsible for homology-directed repair (HDR) were delivered with a recombinant adeno-associated virus (rAAV) vector. The investigators electroporated a gRNA/Cas9 RNP (ribonucleoprotein complex) into human SCD patient CD34^{+} cells and then transduced the cells with the rAAV vector. Interestingly, the vector also contained a truncated nerve growth factor receptor (tNGFR) cDNA driven by a eukaryotic promoter. This design enabled the investigators to select HSPCs in which the tNGFR sequence and, consequently, the β^{AS3} cDNA had been incorporated site specifically into the genome. When this enriched population of cells was transplanted into genetically immunodeficient NSG mice and analyzed after 16 weeks, both lymphoid and myeloid cell lineages contained correctly inserted β^{AS3} sequences. These results strongly suggest that long-term HSCs were correctly modified. The authors also differentiated targeted HSPCs into erythroid cells in culture and demonstrated that >50% of total hemoglobin was hemoglobin A (HbA). Another strength of this approach is that both SCD and the majority of β thalassemias could be corrected with the same gRNA/Cas9 complex plus AAV vector. In the case of β thalassemias, the inserted β^{AS3}-globin (or β^{A}-globin) cDNA should result in the production of sufficient β-globin polypeptide to ameliorate or cure all patients with coding region and splicing mutations. Only β thalassemias caused by deletions encompassing the β-globin gene translational start site or LCR mutations would require new guide RNAs (gRNAs) and rAAV construct designs.

Correction of the Sickle Mutation (GTG to GAG) in HSPCs

A number of groups have successfully corrected the HbS mutation in SCD patient HSPCs (Ding, Sun, Li, et al, unpublished data).[84-88] In most cases, the primary strategy of these investigators is to electroporate CD34^{+} cells derived from BM, plerixafor-mobilized blood, or cord blood with a gRNA/Cas9 ribonuclear protein plus a single-stranded oligodeoxynucleotide (ssODN; ~100 nucleotides) correction template. The gRNA contains the HbS mutation in order to direct the nuclease to a position near the mutation. Figure 29-5 illustrates a typical cut site located 1 bp downstream of the mutation. The double strand cut is repaired by 2 mechanisms. The most efficient mechanism is nonhomologous end joining (NHEJ) in which the ends are usually trimmed by exonucleases and subsequently religated. The second mechanism is HDR in which the mutation is corrected by sequences derived from the

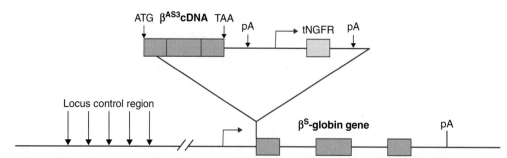

FIGURE 29-4 Schematic representation of CRISPR/Cas9-mediated knockin of an antisickling globin gene. In 2016 and 2018, Dever et al[81] and Vakulskas et al[82] published landmark papers demonstrating efficient, CRISPR/Cas9-mediated knockin of a powerful antisickling globin sequence (β^{AS3})[23,92,93] downstream of the β^{S}-globin gene translational start site in human patient hematopoietic stem and progenitor cells.

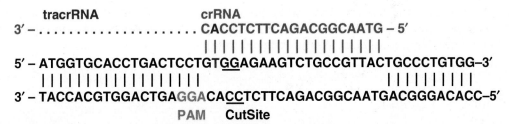

FIGURE 29-5 Schematic of CRISPR guide RNA annealing to the human β^S-globin gene sequence containing the sickle muta-tion (GTG). Typically, the transCRISPR RNA (tracrRNA) is linked to CRISPR RNA (crRNA) to form a single-guide RNA (sgRNA). This sgRNA is complexed with CAS9 to form am ribonucleoprotein (RNP), which is electroporated into sickle cell disease (SCD) patient CD34+ hematopoietic stem and progenitor cells (HSPCs) with a single-stranded oligodeoxynucleotide (ssODN) of approximately 100 nucleotides. This correction template contains β^A-globin sequence and several wobble site changes that inhibit retargeting. The cut site is 1 bp downstream of the sickle mutation (Ding, Sun, Li, et al, unpublished data). PAM is the protospacer adjacent region.[105] The tracerRNA is not homologous to β-globin sequences and is depicted as illustrated earlier for simplicity.[105]

ssODN. Cells in which a single, corrective base change (GTG to GAG) has occurred cannot be selected from the popula-tion; therefore, methods that enhance the ratio of HDR:NHEJ must be used. Before electroporation, Jennifer Doudna and colleagues[94] synchronized cells in the S phase of the cell cycle in which HDR is more active, and 2 groups[95,96] have used com-pounds that inhibit enzymes involved in NHEJ. Interestingly, Jacob Corn and colleagues[97] have suggested that HDR in the presence of high concentrations of ssODN uses a mechanism for repair involving enzymes identified in basic research on Fanconi anemia. These enzymes are apparently capable of HDR even in quiescent cells.

Ding et al (unpublished data) have taken a different approach to enhancing the HDR:NHEJ ratio. We modified Cas9 (mCas9) by adding various protein domains to the carboxy-terminal region of the protein. Although the precise mechanism responsible for enhancing the ratio of HDR to NHEJ is not known, the extraneous domain(s) slows the rate of enzymatic activity as much as 60-fold without inhibiting the overall level of HDR. One hypothesis for the increase in HDR:NHEJ is that access of the CRISPR/mCas9-cleaved ends to exonucleases is inhibited by the extraneous domain and, therefore, a higher number of cleaved sites can be religated without resulting in deletions.

An example of the data from Ding et al (unpublished data) is described here. These data are indicative of results obtained from Sanger sequencing of 96 individual BFU-E and GEMM colonies picked 2 weeks after electroporated, cord blood HSPCs are plated in methylcellulose. Each colony contains hundreds of cells; however, the colonies are derived from single cells. Therefore, this is a single-cell assay in which both alleles can be examined. Cells with at least one corrected S allele (GTG to GAG) produce erythroid cells that do not sickle. In a typi-cal assay of HbSS cord blood CD34+ cells electroporated with wild-type Cas9 RNP plus ssODN, cells with at least one cor-rected allele represent 56% of the total population. This level of correction should provide enough corrected cells to cure the disease. Unfortunately, the proportion of cells containing 2 deleted alleles is also high (40%). If transplanted, these HSPCs would occupy niches in the BM and produce β⁰ thalassemic erythroid cells. Finally, most of the cells that appear to contain

2 corrected alleles (AA) actually contain only 1 corrected S allele and a large deletion[98] of the other S allele. Therefore, most of the corrected HSPCs produce erythroid cells that syn-thesize only 50% of the normal level of hemoglobin. In con-trast, when the same SS cord blood HSPCs are electroporated with carboxy-terminally modified Cas9 RNP plus ssODN, only 10% of the cells contain 2 deleted alleles. Cells containing at least one corrected allele are 46% of the total, and most of the cells that contain one corrected allele also contain an intact S allele. Therefore, erythroid cells derived from these HSPCs in the BM after transplantation will produce hemoglobin at a level that approximates normal (29 pg per cell). This retention of the HbS alleles is important because total hemoglobin levels of 8 to 10 g/dL are required for sufficient oxygen delivery and, therefore, to render a patient transfusion independent.

Table 29-2 illustrates the same principle as the previous data with mCas9; however, in this case, corrected S alleles and remaining S alleles are measured at 16 weeks after transplan-tation of electroporated AS (sickle carrier) cord blood HSPCs into immunodeficient (NSG) mice by intrafemoral injection. S alleles are corrected to A^W (A^{WOBBLE}) to distinguish these alleles from A. Results from 4 separate cord blood CD34+ samples treated with mrCas9 RNP plus ssODN are listed; both high levels of S correction to A and high levels of S allele reten-tion are observed. These results suggest that the enhanced HDR:NHEJ ratios observed in BFU-E and GEMM progeni-tors with the terminally modified Cas9 also occur in long-term HSCs. Again, this is important because the remaining S alleles produce HbS protein levels that are critical for normal oxygen-carrying capacity of RBCs.

Additional basic research is certain to provide novel insights into additional means of enhancing HDR:NHEJ ratios in HSCs. Large-scale screens of chemical compounds that enhance HDR and/or inhibit NHEJ may provide even higher HDR:NHEJ ratios that produce higher correction efficiencies and further decrease deletions resulting from NHEJ.

Finally, Figure 29-6A demonstrates that treatment of SCD patient HSPCs with wild-type Cas9 RNP plus ssODN results in significant off-target modification of a genomic site des-ignated OT-5, which contains 3 base pairs of mismatch with the gRNA. However, this site is not altered with carboxy-

TABLE 29-2 Percentage of S allele correction and S allele retention measured at 16 weeks after transplantation of electroporated AS (sickle carrier) cord blood CD34+ cells into immunodeficient (NSG) mice by intrafemoral injection (Ding, Sun, Li, et al, unpublished data)

Cord blood	% Human chimerism	% S allele correction			% S allele retention		
		HSC CD34+	Myeloid CD33+	Lymphoid CD19+	HSC CD34+	Myeloid CD33+	Lymphoid CD19+
CB-1	25%	41%	45%	45%	30%	42%	35%
CB-2	14%	32%	29%	11%	59%	64%	79%
CB-3	33%	54%	33%	37%	46%	52%	58%
CB-4	28%	77%	72%	82%	7%	22%	3%

Note. DNA from fluorescent activated cell sorted CD34+, CD33+, and CD19+ cells was analyzed by droplet digital polymerase chain reaction to determine percent S allele correction and percent S allele retention.[80] S alleles were corrected to A[W] (A[WOBBLE]) to distinguish these alleles from A. Percent S alleles corrected and retained were normalized to the endogenous CCR5 gene. Results from 4 independent cord blood CD34+ samples treated with our mrCas9 ribonucleoprotein plus single-stranded oligodeoxynucleotide are listed. Twenty-five percent of S alleles corrected corresponds to 50% of cells with one S allele corrected. Matched sibling donor transplants have demonstrated that 50% AS cells are sufficient to cure the disease. Both high levels of gene correction and high levels of S allele retention are observed. Retention of S alleles that are not corrected is essential for the production of total hemoglobin levels of approximately 29 pg per red blood cell. Unless correction is extremely high, as in CB-4, deletion of S alleles that are not corrected is predicted to result in low levels of total hemoglobin per cell and, consequently, β thalassemia.

Abbreviations: HSC, hematopoietic stem cells; NSG, NOD scid gamma.

Magrin E, Miccio A, Cavazzana M. Lentiviral and genome-editing strategies for the treatment of β-hemoglobinopathies. *Blood.* 2019 Oct 10;134(15):1203-1213.

terminally modified Cas9 RNP plus ssODN. Another off-target site, which was defined independently by CIRCLE-seq (Ding, Sun, Li, et al, unpublished data)[99] and GUIDE-seq[87] assays, was also examined (Figure 29-6B); this site is the most abundant off-target site cleaved in CD34+ HSPCs by the gRNA in Figure 29-5 complexed with wild-type Cas9. The level of cleavage at this site is 5.38% with wild-type Cas9 and only 0.51% with mrCas9. This off-target sequence is not located in a gene or any known regulatory element and is embedded in a genomic region rich in odorant receptor genes that are not expressed in hematopoietic cells.

Correction of the Sickle Mutation (GTG to GAG) in iPSCs

Several groups have corrected the HbS mutation in human iPSCs derived from patient skin fibroblasts, skin keratinocytes, peripheral blood mononuclear cells, or BM HSPCs.[89-91] In 2015, Huang et al[89] corrected the SCD mutation by electroporating iPSCs with a gRNA, a Cas9 eukaryotic expression vector, and a double-stranded DNA correction vector containing a selectable marker. RBCs derived from these iPSCs produced normal HbA. In 2016, Li et al[90] demonstrated that human SCD patient iPSCs

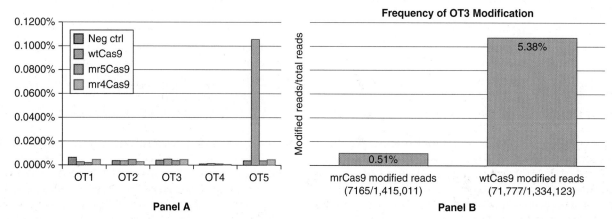

FIGURE 29-6 **A.** Deep-sequencing of 5 off-target (OT) sites after electroporation of human sickle cell disease (SCD) patient CD34+ cells with wild-type Cas9 (wtCas9) ribonucleoprotein (RNP) plus single-stranded oligodeoxynucleotide (ssODN) complex or with 2 different versions of terminally modified Cas9 RNP plus ssODN (Ding, Sun, Li, et al, unpublished data). **B.** Another off-target site, which was defined independently by CIRCLE-seq (Ding, Sun, Li, et al, unpublished data)[99] and GUIDE-seq[87] assays, was also examined; this site is the most abundant off-target site cleaved in CD34+ hematopoietic stem and progenitor cells (HSPCs) by the guide RNA (gRNA) in Figure 29-5 complexed with wtCas9. The level of cleavage at this site is 5.38% with wtCas9 and only 0.51% with mrCas9. This off-target sequence is not located in a gene or any known regulatory element and is embedded in a genomic region rich in odorant receptor genes that are not expressed in hematopoietic cells. Neg Ctrl, negative control.

could be corrected by delivering CRISPR/Cas9 with a helper-dependent adenoviral vector followed by nucleoporation with a 70-nt ssODN. Correction efficiencies of up to 68% were obtained, and whole-genome sequencing of corrected iPSC lines demonstrated no off-target modifications in 1467 potential sites and no modifications in tumor suppressor genes or other genes associated with pathology. Finally, in 2019, Martin et al[91] reported HbS gene correction efficiencies in human patient iPSCs of 63% after electroporation of gRNA/Cas9 RNP followed by transduction with an AAV correction vector. When corrected iPSCs were differentiated into erythroid cells and analyzed for β^S- and β^A-globin mRNA, β^S mRNA was virtually eliminated and β^A mRNA was expressed at high levels.

Although high HbS gene correction efficiencies can be obtained in iPSCs, the therapeutic potential of these corrected cells is diminished because differentiation into HSPCs is extremely difficult. However, some progress has been made in recent years,[100-103] and further basic studies may provide a foundation for a safe and effective treatment derived from iPSCs.[104]

Conclusion

Almost 20 years after correction of mouse models of SCD by gene addition therapy, LV delivery of globin genes has cured a number of patients, and the future appears bright for expanding treatment to hundreds of patients. Gene editing to reactivate HbF is also progressing rapidly. Clinical trials have been initiated, and early results are promising. Finally, gene editing of the β^S-globin gene by β^{AS3}-globin gene insertion or by simply correcting the sickle mutation (GTG to GAG) is not far behind. Clinical trials of all of these approaches are essential to provide therapies that maximize safety, clinical efficacy, and cost-effectiveness. Perhaps the different therapeutic approaches discussed in this chapter will be necessary to treat patients at different ages or different stages of disease severity. Of course, correction of the disease in newborns before tissue or organ damage has occurred is the goal of the future. The next few years will be truly revolutionary for SCD patients and their families and will hopefully reverse this debilitating disorder that was first described in the literature >100 years ago.

High-Yield Facts

- ◆ Results from recent clinical trials demonstrate that gene therapy for sickle cell disease can be curative.
- ◆ For gene addition therapy, recent optimizations of the vector manufacturing process, patient conditioning, cell dose, and hematopoietic stem cell source have provided the foundation for excellent outcomes.
- ◆ For gene editing therapy, deletion of an erythroid-specific regulatory sequence in the *BCL11A* gene reactivates HbF synthesis and results in therapeutic outcomes.
- ◆ Preclinical data demonstrate that gene editing of additional targets can reactivate HbF and that correction of the specific nucleotide base that causes the disease is effective in humanized sickle mice and in human hematopoietic stem and progenitor cells; therefore, human clinical trials of these approaches may be initiated soon.
- ◆ Safe and effective gene addition and gene editing therapies during the first year of life before irreversible tissue and organ damage have occurred remain important long-term goals.

References

1. Sundd P, Gladwin MT, Novelli EM. Pathophysiology of sickle cell disease. *Annu Rev Pathol.* 2019;14:263-292.
2. Ford AL, Ragan DK, Fellah S, et al. Silent infarcts in sickle cell disease occur in the border zone region and are associated with low cerebral blood flow. *Blood.* 2018;132(16):1714-1723.
3. Gluckman E, Cappelli B, Bernaudin F, et al. Sickle cell disease: an international survey of results of HLA-identical sibling hematopoietic stem cell transplantation. *Blood.* 2017;129(11):1548-1556.
4. Abboud M, Laver J, Blau CA. Granulocytosis causing sickle-cell crisis. *Lancet.* 1998;351(9107):959.
5. Adler BK, Salzman DE, Carabasi MH, Vaughan WP, Reddy VV, Prchal JT. Fatal sickle cell crisis after granulocyte colony-stimulating factor administration. *Blood.* 2001;97(10):3313-3314.
6. Grigg AP. Granulocyte colony-stimulating factor-induced sickle cell crisis and multiorgan dysfunction in a patient with compound heterozygous sickle cell/beta+ thalassemia. *Blood.* 2001;97(12):3998-3999.
7. Lagresle-Peyrou C, Lefrere F, Magrin E, et al. Plerixafor enables safe, rapid, efficient mobilization of hematopoietic stem cells in sickle cell disease patients after exchange transfusion. *Haematologica.* 2018;103(5):778-786.
8. Boulad F, Shore T, van Besien K, et al. Safety and efficacy of plerixafor dose escalation for the mobilization of CD34(+) hematopoietic progenitor cells in patients with sickle cell disease: interim results. *Haematologica.* 2018;103(5):770-777.
9. Esrick EB, Manis JP, Daley H, et al. Successful hematopoietic stem cell mobilization and apheresis collection using plerixafor alone in sickle cell patients. *Blood Adv.* 2018;2(19):2505-2512.
10. Booth C, Gaspar HB, Thrasher AJ. Treating immunodeficiency through HSC gene therapy. *Trends Mol Med.* 2016;22(4):317-327.

11. Magnani A, Pondarré C, Bouazza N, et al. Extensive multilineage analysis in patients with mixed chimerism after allogeneic transplantation for sickle cell disease: insight into hematopoiesis and engraftment thresholds for gene therapy. *Haematologica.* 2020 May;105(5):1240-1247.

12. Weber L, Poletti V, Magrin E, et al. An optimized lentiviral vector efficiently corrects the human sickle cell disease phenotype. *Mol Ther Methods Clin Dev.* 2018;10:268-280.

13. Palchaudhuri R, Saez B, Hoggatt J, et al. Non-genotoxic conditioning for hematopoietic stem cell transplantation using a hematopoietic-cell-specific internalizing immunotoxin. *Nat Biotechnol.* 2016;34(7):738-745.

14. Arai Y, Choi U, Corsino CI, et al. Myeloid conditioning with c-kit-targeted CAR-T cells enables donor stem cell engraftment. *Mol Ther.* 2018;26(5):1181-1197.

15. Piras F, Riba M, Petrillo C, et al. Lentiviral vectors escape innate sensing but trigger p53 in human hematopoietic stem and progenitor cells. *EMBO Mol Med.* 2017;9(9):1198-1211.

16. Zonari E, Desantis G, Petrillo C, et al. Efficient ex vivo engineering and expansion of highly purified human hematopoietic stem and progenitor cell populations for gene therapy. *Stem Cell Rep.* 2017;8(4):977-990.

17. Kajaste-Rudnitski A, Naldini L. Cellular innate immunity and restriction of viral infection: implications for lentiviral gene therapy in human hematopoietic cells. *Hum Gene Ther.* 2015;26(4):201-209.

18. Heffner GC, Bonner M, Christiansen L, et al. Prostaglandin E2 increases lentiviral vector transduction efficiency of adult human hematopoietic stem and progenitor cells. *Mol Ther.* 2018;26(1):320-328.

19. Petrillo C, Cesana D, Piras F, et al. Cyclosporin A and rapamycin relieve distinct lentiviral restriction blocks in hematopoietic stem and progenitor cells. *Mol Ther.* 2015;23(2):352-362.

20. Pawliuk R, Westerman KA, Fabry ME, et al. Correction of sickle cell disease in transgenic mouse models by gene therapy. *Science.* 2001;294(5550):2368-2371.

21. Pestina TI, Hargrove PW, Jay D, Gray JT, Boyd KM, Persons DA. Correction of murine sickle cell disease using gamma-globin lentiviral vectors to mediate high-level expression of fetal hemoglobin. *Mol Ther.* 2009;17(2):245-252.

22. Perumbeti A, Higashimoto T, Urbinati F, et al. A novel human gamma-globin gene vector for genetic correction of sickle cell anemia in a humanized sickle mouse model: critical determinants for successful correction. *Blood.* 2009;114(6):1174-1185.

23. Levasseur DN, Ryan TM, Pawlik KM, Townes TM. Correction of a mouse model of sickle cell disease: lentiviral/antisickling beta-globin gene transduction of unmobilized, purified hematopoietic stem cells. *Blood.* 2003;102(13):4312-4319.

24. Romero Z, Urbinati F, Geiger S, et al. beta-globin gene transfer to human bone marrow for sickle cell disease. *J Clin Invest.* 2013;123(8):3317-3330.

25. Urbinati F, Hargrove PW, Geiger S, et al. Potentially therapeutic levels of anti-sickling globin gene expression following lentivirus-mediated gene transfer in sickle cell disease bone marrow CD34+ cells. *Exp Hematol.* 2015;43(5):346-351.

26. Andreani M, Testi M, Gaziev J, et al. Quantitatively different red cell/nucleated cell chimerism in patients with long-term, persistent hematopoietic mixed chimerism after bone marrow transplantation for thalassemia major or sickle cell disease. *Haematologica.* 2011;96(1):128-133.

27. Walters MC, Patience M, Leisenring W, et al. Stable mixed hematopoietic chimerism after bone marrow transplantation for sickle cell anemia. *Biol Blood Marrow Transplant.* 2001; 7(12):665-673.

28. Wu CJ, Gladwin M, Tisdale J, et al. Mixed haematopoietic chimerism for sickle cell disease prevents intravascular haemolysis. *Br J Haematol.* 2007;139(3):504-507.

29. Ribeil JA, Hacein-Bey-Abina S, Payen E, et al. Gene therapy in a patient with sickle cell disease. *N Engl J Med.* 2017;376(9):848-855.

30. Kanter J, Tisdale JF, Kwiatkowski JL, et al. Outcomes for initial patient cohorts with up to 33 months of follow-up in the Hgb-206 phase 1 trial. *Blood.* 2018;132:1080.

31. Tisdale JF, Kanter J, Mapara MY, et al. Current results of lentiglobin gene therapy in patients with severe sickle cell disease treated under a refined protocol in the phase 1 Hgb-206 study. *Blood.* 2018;132:1026.

32. Malik P, Grimley M, Quinn CT, et al. Gene therapy for sickle cell anemia using a modified gamma globin lentivirus vector and reduced intensity conditioning transplant shows promising correction of the disease phenotype. *Blood.* 2018;132:1021.

33. Deng W, Rupon JW, Krivega I, et al. Reactivation of developmentally silenced globin genes by forced chromatin looping. *Cell.* 2014;158(4):849-860.

34. Demirci S, Bhardwaj SK, Uchida N, et al. Robust erythroid differentiation system for rhesus hematopoietic progenitor cells allowing preclinical screening of genetic treatment strategies for the hemoglobinopathies. *Cytotherapy.* 2018;20(10): 1278-1287.

35. Brendel C, Guda S, Renella R, et al. Lineage-specific BCL11A knockdown circumvents toxicities and reverses sickle phenotype. *J Clin Invest.* 2016;126(10):3868-3878.

36. Luc S, Huang J, McEldoon JL, et al. Bcl11a deficiency leads to hematopoietic stem cell defects with an aging-like phenotype. *Cell Rep.* 2016;16(12):3181-3194.

37. Tsang JC, Yu Y, Burke S, et al. Single-cell transcriptomic reconstruction reveals cell cycle and multi-lineage differentiation defects in Bcl11a-deficient hematopoietic stem cells. *Genome Biol.* 2015;16:178.

38. Miccio A, Cesari R, Lotti F, et al. In vivo selection of genetically modified erythroblastic progenitors leads to long-term correction of beta-thalassemia. *Proc Natl Acad Sci U S A.* 2008;105(30):10547-10552.

39. Guda S, Brendel C, Renella R, et al. miRNA-embedded shRNAs for lineage-specific BCL11A knockdown and hemoglobin F induction. *Mol Ther.* 2015;23(9):1465-1474.

40. Esrick EB, Brendel C, Manis JP, et al. Flipping the switch: initial results of genetic targeting of the fetal to adult globin switch in sickle cell patients. *Blood.* 2018;132(suppl 1):1023.

41. Sankaran VG, Menne TF, Xu J, et al. Human fetal hemoglobin expression is regulated by the developmental stage-specific repressor BCL11A. *Science.* 2008;322(5909):1839-1842.

42. Bauer DE, Kamran SC, Lessard S, et al. An erythroid enhancer of BCL11A subject to genetic variation determines fetal hemoglobin level. *Science.* 2013;342(6155):253-257.

43. Xu J, Peng C, Sankaran VG, et al. Correction of sickle cell disease in adult mice by interference with fetal hemoglobin silencing. *Science.* 2011;334(6058):993-996.

44. Canver MC, Smith EC, Sher F, et al. BCL11A enhancer dissection by Cas9-mediated in situ saturating mutagenesis. *Nature.* 2015;527(7577):192-197.

45. Wu Y, Zeng J, Roscoe BP, et al. Highly efficient therapeutic gene editing of human hematopoietic stem cells. *Nat Med.* 2019;25(5):776-783.

46. Liu N, Hargreaves VV, Zhu Q, et al. Direct promoter repression by BCL11A controls the fetal to adult hemoglobin switch. *Cell.* 2018;173(2):430-442.e417.

47. Martyn GE, Wienert B, Yang L, et al. Natural regulatory mutations elevate the fetal globin gene via disruption of BCL11A or ZBTB7A binding. *Nat Genet.* 2018;50(4):498-503.

48. Traxler EA, Yao Y, Wang YD, et al. A genome-editing strategy to treat beta-hemoglobinopathies that recapitulates a mutation associated with a benign genetic condition. *Nat Med.* 2016;22(9):987-990.

49. Humbert O, Radtke S, Samuelson C, et al. Therapeutically relevant engraftment of a CRISPR-Cas9-edited HSC-enriched population with HbF reactivation in nonhuman primates. *Sci Transl Med.* 2019;11(503):eaaw3768.

50. Borg J, Papadopoulos P, Georgitsi M, et al. Haploinsufficiency for the erythroid transcription factor KLF1 causes hereditary persistence of fetal hemoglobin. *Nat Genet.* 2010;42(9):801-805.

51. Zhou D, Liu K, Sun CW, Pawlik KM, Townes TM. KLF1 regulates BCL11A expression and gamma- to beta-globin gene switching. *Nat Genet.* 2010;42(9):742-744.

52. Perkins A, Xu X, Higgs DR, et al. Krüppeling erythropoiesis: an unexpected broad spectrum of human red blood cell disorders due to KLF1 variants. *Blood.* 2016;127(15):1856-1862.

53. Gnanapragasam MN, Crispino JD, Ali AM, et al. Survey and evaluation of mutations in the human KLF1 transcription unit. *Sci Rep.* 2018;8(1):6587.

54. Masuda T, Wang X, Maeda M, et al. Transcription factors LRF and BCL11A independently repress expression of fetal hemoglobin. *Science.* 2016;351(6270):285-289.

55. Norton LJ, Funnell APW, Burdach J, et al. KLF1 directly activates expression of the novel fetal globin repressor ZBTB7A/LRF in erythroid cells. *Blood Adv.* 2017;1(11):685-692.

56. Wienert B, Funnell AP, Norton LJ, et al. Editing the genome to introduce a beneficial naturally occurring mutation associated with increased fetal globin. *Nat Commun.* 2015;6:7085.

57. Wienert B, Martyn GE, Kurita R, Nakamura Y, Quinlan KGR, Crossley M. KLF1 drives the expression of fetal hemoglobin in British HPFH. *Blood.* 2017;130(6):803-807.

58. Martyn GE, Wienert B, Kurita R, Nakamura Y, Quinlan KGR, Crossley M. A natural regulatory mutation in the proximal promoter elevates fetal globin expression by creating a de novo GATA1 site. *Blood.* 2019;133(8):852-856.

59. Antoniani C, Meneghini V, Lattanzi A, et al. Induction of fetal hemoglobin synthesis by CRISPR/Cas9-mediated editing of the human beta-globin locus. *Blood.* 2018;131(17):1960-1973.

60. Lattanzi A, Meneghini V, Pavani G, et al. Optimization of CRISPR/Cas9 delivery to human hematopoietic stem and progenitor cells for therapeutic genomic rearrangements. *Mol Ther.* 2019;27(1):137-150.

61. Blobel GA, Crossley M. Charting a noncoding gene for gamma-globin activation. *Blood.* 2018;132(18):1865-1867.

62. Huang P, Keller CA, Giardine B, et al. Comparative analysis of three-dimensional chromosomal architecture identifies a novel fetal hemoglobin regulatory element. *Genes Dev.* 2017;31(16):1704-1713.

63. Gudmundsdottir B, Gudmundsson KO, Klarmann KD, et al. POGZ is required for silencing mouse embryonic beta-like hemoglobin and human fetal hemoglobin expression. *Cell Rep.* 2018;23(11):3236-3248.

64. Amaya M, Desai M, Gnanapragasam MN, et al. Mi2beta-mediated silencing of the fetal gamma-globin gene in adult erythroid cells. *Blood.* 2013;121(17):3493-3501.

65. Yu X, Azzo A, Bilinovich SM, et al. Disruption of the MBD2-NuRD complex but not MBD3-NuRD induces high level HbF expression in human erythroid cells. *Haematologica.* 2019;104(12):2361-2371.

66. Shi L, Cui S, Engel JD, Tanabe O. Lysine-specific demethylase 1 is a therapeutic target for fetal hemoglobin induction. *Nat Med.* 2013;19(3):291-294.

67. Yu L, Jearawiriyapaisarn N, Lee MP, et al. BAP1 regulation of the key adaptor protein NCoR1 is critical for gamma-globin gene repression. *Genes Dev.* 2018;32(23-24):1537-1549.

68. Grevet JD, Lan X, Hamagami N, et al. Domain-focused CRISPR screen identifies HRI as a fetal hemoglobin regulator in human erythroid cells. *Science.* 2018;361(6399):285-290.

69. Sher F, Hossain M, Seruggia D, et al. Rational targeting of a NuRD subcomplex guided by comprehensive in situ mutagenesis. *Nat Genet.* 2019;51:1149-1159.

70. Uda M, Galanello R, Sanna S, et al. Genome-wide association study shows BCL11A associated with persistent fetal hemoglobin and amelioration of the phenotype of beta-thalassemia. *Proc Natl Acad Sci U S A.* 2008;105(5):1620-1625.

71. Menzel S, Garner C, Gut I, et al. A QTL influencing F cell production maps to a gene encoding a zinc-finger protein on chromosome 2p15. *Nat Genet.* 2007;39(10):1197-1199.

72. Skene PJ, Henikoff S. An efficient targeted nuclease strategy for high-resolution mapping of DNA binding sites. *Elife.* 2017;6:e21856.

73. Behringer RR, Ryan TM, Palmiter RD, Brinster RL, Townes TM. Human gamma- to beta-globin gene switching in transgenic mice. *Genes Dev.* 1990;4(3):380-389.

74. Enver T, Raich N, Ebens AJ, Papayannopoulou T, Costantini F, Stamatoyannopoulos G. Developmental regulation of human fetal-to-adult globin gene switching in transgenic mice. *Nature.* 1990;344(6264):309-313.

75. Townes TM, Behringer RR. Human globin locus activation region (LAR): role in temporal control. *Trends Genet.* 1990;6(7):219-223.

76. Donze D, Townes TM, Bieker JJ. Role of erythroid Kruppel-like factor in human gamma- to beta-globin gene switching. *J Biol Chem.* 1995;270(4):1955-1959.

77. Zhou D, Pawlik KM, Ren J, Sun CW, Townes TM. Differential binding of erythroid Krupple-like factor to embryonic/fetal globin gene promoters during development. *J Biol Chem.* 2006;281(23):16052-16057.

78. Liu D, Zhang X, Yu L, et al. KLF1 mutations are relatively more common in a thalassemia endemic region and ameliorate the severity of beta-thalassemia. *Blood.* 2014;124(5):803-811.

79. Manwani D, Bieker JJ. KLF1: when less is more. *Blood.* 2014;124(5):672-673.

80. Cui S, Kolodziej KE, Obara N, et al. Nuclear receptors TR2 and TR4 recruit multiple epigenetic transcriptional corepressors that associate specifically with the embryonic beta-type globin promoters in differentiated adult erythroid cells. *Mol Cell Biol.* 2011;31(16):3298-3311.

81. Dever DP, Bak RO, Reinisch A, et al. CRISPR/Cas9 beta-globin gene targeting in human haematopoietic stem cells. *Nature.* 2016;539(7629):384-389.

82. Vakulskas CA, Dever DP, Rettig GR, et al. A high-fidelity Cas9 mutant delivered as a ribonucleoprotein complex enables efficient gene editing in human hematopoietic stem and progenitor cells. *Nat Med.* 2018;24(8):1216-1224.

83. Charlesworth CT, Camarena J, Cromer MK, et al. Priming human repopulating hematopoietic stem and progenitor

cells for Cas9/sgRNA gene targeting. *Mol Ther Nucleic Acids.* 2018;12:89-104.

84. DeWitt MA, Magis W, Bray NL, et al. Selection-free genome editing of the sickle mutation in human adult hematopoietic stem/progenitor cells. *Sci Transl Med.* 2016;8(360): 360ra134.

85. Hoban MD, Cost GJ, Mendel MC, et al. Correction of the sickle cell disease mutation in human hematopoietic stem/progenitor cells. *Blood.* 2015;125(17):2597-2604.

86. Hoban MD, Lumaquin D, Kuo CY, et al. CRISPR/Cas9-Mediated Correction of the Sickle Mutation in Human CD34+ cells. *Mol Ther.* 2016;24(9):1561-1569.

87. Park SH, Lee CM, Dever DP, et al. Highly efficient editing of the beta-globin gene in patient-derived hematopoietic stem and progenitor cells to treat sickle cell disease. *Nucleic Acids Res.* 2019;47(15):7955-7972.

88. Romero Z, Lomova A, Said S, et al. Editing the sickle cell disease mutation in human hematopoietic stem cells: comparison of endonucleases and homologous donor templates. *Mol Ther.* 2019;27(8):1389-1406.

89. Huang X, Wang Y, Yan W, et al. Production of gene-corrected adult beta globin protein in human erythrocytes differentiated from patient iPSCs after genome editing of the sickle point mutation. *Stem Cells.* 2015;33(5):1470-1479.

90. Li C, Ding L, Sun CW, et al. Novel HDAd/EBV reprogramming vector and highly efficient Ad/CRISPR-Cas sickle cell disease gene correction. *Sci Rep.* 2016;6:30422.

91. Martin RM, Ikeda K, Cromer MK, et al. Highly efficient and marker-free genome editing of human pluripotent stem cells by CRISPR-Cas9 RNP and AAV6 donor-mediated homologous recombination. *Cell Stem Cell.* 2019;24(5):821-828.e825.

92. Levasseur DN, Ryan TM, Reilly MP, McCune SL, Asakura T, Townes TM. A recombinant human hemoglobin with anti-sickling properties greater than fetal hemoglobin. *J Biol Chem.* 2004;279(26):27518-27524.

93. McCune SL, Reilly MP, Chomo MJ, Asakura T, Townes TM. Recombinant human hemoglobins designed for gene therapy of sickle cell disease. *Proc Natl Acad Sci U S A.* 1994;91(21): 9852-9856.

94. Lin S, Staahl BT, Alla RK, Doudna JA. Enhanced homology-directed human genome engineering by controlled timing of CRISPR/Cas9 delivery. *Elife.* 2014;3:e04766.

95. Chu VT, Weber T, Wefers B, et al. Increasing the efficiency of homology-directed repair for CRISPR-Cas9-induced precise gene editing in mammalian cells. *Nat Biotechnol.* 2015;33(5): 543-548.

96. Maruyama T, Dougan SK, Truttmann MC, Bilate AM, Ingram JR, Ploegh HL. Increasing the efficiency of precise genome editing with CRISPR-Cas9 by inhibition of nonhomologous end joining. *Nat Biotechnol.* 2015;33(5):538-542.

97. Richardson CD, Kazane KR, Feng SJ, et al. CRISPR-Cas9 genome editing in human cells occurs via the Fanconi anemia pathway. *Nat Genet.* 2018;50(8):1132-1139.

98. Kosicki M, Tomberg K, Bradley A. Repair of double-strand breaks induced by CRISPR-Cas9 leads to large deletions and complex rearrangements. *Nat Biotechnol.* 2018;36(8):765-771.

99. Tsai SQ, Nguyen NT, Malagon-Lopez J, Topkar VV, Aryee MJ, Joung JK. CIRCLE-seq: a highly sensitive in vitro screen for genome-wide CRISPR-Cas9 nuclease off-targets. *Nat Methods.* 2017;14(6):607-614.

100. Doulatov S, Vo LT, Chou SS, et al. Induction of multipotential hematopoietic progenitors from human pluripotent stem cells via respecification of lineage-restricted precursors. *Cell Stem Cell.* 2013;13(4):459-470.

101. Gori JL, Butler JM, Chan YY, et al. Vascular niche promotes hematopoietic multipotent progenitor formation from pluripotent stem cells. *J Clin Invest.* 2015;125(3):1243-1254.

102. Sandler VM, Lis R, Liu Y, et al. Reprogramming human endothelial cells to haematopoietic cells requires vascular induction. *Nature.* 2014;511(7509):312-318.

103. Sugimura R, Jha DK, Han A, et al. Haematopoietic stem and progenitor cells from human pluripotent stem cells. *Nature.* 2017;545(7655):432-438.

104. Blau HM, Daley GQ. Stem cells in the treatment of disease. *N Engl J Med.* 2019;380(18):1748-1760.

105. Sternberg SH, Redding S, Jinek M, Greene EC, Doudna JA. DNA interrogation by the CRISPR RNA-guided endonuclease Cas9. *Nature.* 2014;507(7490):62-67.

Hydroxyurea and Sickle Cell Disease

Authors: *Winfred C. Wang, Russell E. Ware*

Chapter Outline

Overview

Mechanisms of Action

Efficacy

Vaso-occlusive Events

Organ Function

Mortality

Hydroxyurea Dosing

Variation in Dose Amount

Individualized Dosing

Toxicity and Safety

Hydroxyurea Trials in Africa

Combination Treatment With Hydroxyurea

Adherence

Health Literacy

Decision Making and Treatment Initiation

Conclusion

Case Studies

Overview

Landmark natural history studies, including the Cooperative Study of Sickle Cell Disease[1] and the Jamaican Cohort Study,[2] generated the seminal observations that fetal hemoglobin (HbF) is a critically important laboratory parameter for individuals with sickle cell anemia (SCA). Higher HbF levels are associated with better clinical outcomes including reduced mortality,[3-5] and if present at sufficient levels with pancellular distribution, higher HbF levels can lead to a benign condition.[6]

Because HbF declines rapidly in the postnatal period, it should theoretically be possible to inhibit or reverse the physiologic suppression of HbF production. The search for pharmacologic modifiers to boost HbF began in the early 1980s with the recognition that γ-globin genes were likely silenced due to methylation of the promoter sequences. Initial treatment with the demethylating agent 5-azacytidine was found to increase HbF production in a patient with SCA, but was predictably toxic.[7] In studies by Nathan and colleagues, hydroxyurea was tested as an S-phase–specific cytotoxic/cytostatic agent that does not influence DNA methylation and, unexpectedly, was found to boost F-cells dramatically, first in anemic monkeys[8] and then in human patients.[9]

Since these initial proof-of-principle publications in 1984, hundreds of articles have been published, which collectively have firmly established hydroxyurea as the first and best disease-modifying treatment of SCA. As illustrated in Figure 30-1, a large number of phase I/II and III trials

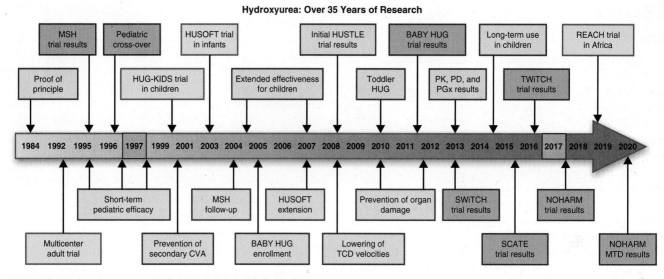

FIGURE 30-1 **Hydroxyurea clinical trials over the past 35 years.** From the initial 1984 proof-of-principle study in 2 adults to the randomized double-blind NOHARM MTD trial in Africa that found increased benefit from escalated hydroxyurea dosing, hydroxyurea has been carefully investigated in many settings and study designs. Green shading indicates phase I/II trials, whereas red shading indicates phase III trials. The purple boxes indicate the years in which hydroxyurea was US Food and Drug Administration approved for adults (1997) and then for children (2017). CVA, cerebrovascular accident; MTD, maximum-tolerated dose; PD, pharmacodynamics; PGx, pharmacogenomics; PK, pharmacokinetics; TCD, transcranial Doppler. See text for trial acronyms.

have been conducted in adults, children, and even infants that together document the safety and efficacy of hydroxyurea. Over the past decade, trials have focused on the use of hydroxyurea in specific clinical settings, including the long-term effects on organ function and preservation in babies and young children; the prevention or stabilization of established cerebrovascular disease such as conditional or abnormal transcranial Doppler ultrasound (TCD) velocities; and the safety and feasibility of treatment for patients living in low-resource settings including sub-Saharan Africa. The cumulative data provide compelling evidence for hydroxyurea, leading to evidence-based recommendations for treatment across the life span.[10]

Mechanisms of Action

The primary disease-modifying mechanism of hydroxyurea occurs via the induction of HbF, which interferes with HbS polymerization. Hydroxyurea is a potent ribonucleotide reductase (RR) inhibitor that has been used to treat myeloproliferative disorders and chronic myelogenous leukemia since the 1960s.[11] However, the exact mechanisms by which hydroxyurea induces HbF production are not fully understood. Cytotoxic effects of hydroxyurea through RR inhibition

on the bone marrow erythroblasts produce stress erythropoiesis with increased HbF production.[12] In vitro studies using K562 erythroleukemia cells and human erythroid progenitor cells have demonstrated that hydroxyurea nitrosylates (nitric oxide [NO] binding to ferrous heme) and activates soluble guanylate cyclase (sGC) with subsequent increased expression of cyclic guanosine monophosphate (cGMP)-dependent protein kinase.[13,14] The NO-sGC-cGMP pathways are thought to play a role in induced expression of γ-globin. Hydroxyurea-induced increases in percent HbF will invariably be associated with increased cellular distribution, with HbF levels >30% approaching pancellular distribution[15,16] with full protection against sickling.

Hydroxyurea has numerous beneficial effects beyond induction of HbF, including decreased neutrophil and reticulocyte counts caused by marrow cytotoxicity, reduced expression of adhesion molecules on neutrophils and red blood cells (RBCs), increased erythrocyte hydration and deformability with subsequent reduction in hemolysis, and local release of NO, potentially resulting in vasodilatation.[17-20] Hydroxyurea also reduces oxidative stress within sickle erythrocytes, possibly through modulating the NO synthase signaling pathway and direct binding to βCys93.[21,22] A specific anti-inflammatory mechanism was suggested from a study of hydroxyurea in sickle cell mice, in which their survival from pneumococcal pneumonia was improved through reduction in E-selection expression.[23] A reduction in adenosine activity in hydroxyurea-treated patients whose monocytes express CD26 may also be beneficial.[24] Hydroxyurea may have immediate benefits after dosing, by altering endothelial cell adhesion molecule expression and reducing leukocyte recruitment to the microvasculature.[25]

Efficacy

Vaso-occlusive Events

The efficacy of hydroxyurea in the reduction of vaso-occlusive events (pain, acute chest syndrome) has been established through randomized, placebo-controlled trials and numerous observational studies in adults and children.[26,27]

A phase I/II trial in adults with SCA investigating hydroxyurea at doses from 10 to 35 mg/kg/d found that the drug was well tolerated and led to increases in HbF, hemoglobin level, and mean corpuscular volume (MCV).[28] This was followed by a landmark double-blinded phase III trial that led to US Food and Drug Administration approval of the drug for adults with clinically severe SCA. In this trial, the Multicenter Study of Hydroxyurea (MSH), 299 patients were randomized to receive hydroxyurea or placebo.[26] The study was halted early due to a statistically significant increase in time to first painful vaso-occlusive event in the hydroxyurea arm. Persons randomized to this arm also had 40% to 50% reductions in secondary study end points, including the incidence of painful events, acute chest syndrome, transfusions, and hospitalizations.

The largest of several nonrandomized studies in children with SCA in the United States was the Hydroxyurea Group KIDS (HUG-KIDS) trial, a phase I/II trial in 84 school-age children with SCA,[15] which showed similar hematologic responses to those seen in adults, including increases in HbF, MCV, and hemoglobin levels and decreases in white blood cell (WBC) and absolute neutrophil counts. This led to the phase III, double-blind, multicenter BABY Hydroxyurea Group (BABY HUG) trial,[27] which involved 193 infants between 9 and 18 months of age who were randomized to receive hydroxyurea at a fixed dose of 20 mg/kg/d or placebo for a 2-year period, with the primary objective of demonstrating better preservation of organ function in the spleen (based on uptake on technetium-99 [99Tc] liver-spleen scans) and kidneys (based on glomerular filtration rate measured by 99Tc-diethylenetriaminepentaacetic acid [DTPA] renal clearance). Although the primary end points were not achieved, the study demonstrated that the hydroxyurea group had significantly fewer episodes of pain, dactylitis, acute chest syndrome, hospitalizations, and transfusions, along with higher levels of hemoglobin, HbF, and MCV and decreased WBC, neutrophil, and reticulocyte counts. Administering daily hydroxyurea in a liquid formulation was feasible and well tolerated with no significant toxicity, except for the expected mild to moderate neutropenia, which was not associated with increased risk for invasive infection. Most patients from the BABY HUG trial continued in a follow-up study, which will be important for identifying long-term benefits and risks.

Organ Function

End-organ impairment is now the primary or secondary cause of mortality in 45% of adults with sickle cell disease (SCD).[29] Better understanding of the value of hydroxyurea in the prevention, stabilization, or reversal of organ dysfunction in SCD is needed to guide its use. In Table 30-1, we summarize recent studies of organ function in patients receiving hydroxyurea.

Splenic and renal function are affected early in life in SCA, and these 2 organs have been the focus of several studies.[30,31] A primary end point of the BABY HUG trial was a comparison of splenic function at study exit (after 2 years of hydroxyurea or placebo) with that at entry.[27] Splenic uptake on nuclear scan was classified as normal, decreased, or absent. Using these criteria, 27% of patients on hydroxyurea had a decrease in spleen function compared with 38% of those receiving placebo; this difference was not statistically significant. However, secondary measures, including quantitation of splenic uptake and enumeration of pitted RBCs and Howell-Jolly bodies, showed significantly worse splenic function among those receiving placebo compared to those on hydroxyurea.[31] In addition, there have been observational reports involving small cohorts of sickle cell patients, mostly school-age children at single institutions, suggesting improved splenic function on hydroxyurea. For example, spleen scans in 40 children with a mean age of 9.1 years demonstrated splenic uptake in a relatively high proportion (33%) after 3 years of hydroxyurea treatment.[32]

Renal function assessed by glomerular filtration rate (GFR) measured by 99Tc-DTPA clearance was a co-primary end point of the BABY HUG study; no significant lessening of the elevated GFR in the hydroxyurea group was observed.[27] However, several key secondary renal end points were achieved in hydroxyurea-treated patients, including higher urine osmolality and urine specific gravity after overnight fasting and lower total kidney volume measured by ultrasound scanning.[33] In a small retrospective series of 3 pediatric patients with nephrotic-range proteinuria, the addition of hydroxyurea to enalapril therapy significantly reduced and eventually normalized protein excretion.[34] In the prospective Hydroxyurea Study of Long-Term Effects (HUSTLE) trial, hydroxyurea treatment of school-age children for 3 years did not reduce microalbuminuria but was associated with significantly decreased GFR.[35] Over a longer treatment period, however, one-third of children enrolled in HUSTLE with albuminuria had resolution, especially with lower levels of baseline proteinuria and earlier treatment initiation.[36] In another cohort, the median albumin-to-creatinine ratio in school-age children who had baseline microalbuminuria decreased from 96 to 25 mg/g after 2 years of treatment.[37] Finally, in a cross-sectional study of 149 adults with SCD, the prevalence of albuminuria was lower among patients on hydroxyurea (35% vs 55%), and multivariate analysis found an odds ratio of 0.28 for the likelihood of albuminuria while taking hydroxyurea.[38]

Recent exploration of the effects of hydroxyurea on the central nervous system (CNS) has included multicenter randomized trials that examined both primary and secondary stroke prevention in comparison with chronic transfusion. Standard management for *primary* stroke prophylaxis has been based on the landmark Stroke Prevention in Sickle Cell Anemia (STOP) trial, which demonstrated that chronic transfusion in children

TABLE 30-1 Hydroxyurea and organ function

Organ	Type of study	Patient population	No. of patients	Evaluation	Effect of HU	Reference
Spleen	Rand. (BABY HUG)	9-18 months	91[a]	Spleen scan	No difference	Wang et al,[27] 2011
				Pit cells	↓	
				HJB	↓	
				Spleen volume	No difference	
	Observ	10 years	43	Spleen scan	14% recovery	Hankins et al,[155] 2008
		3-22 years	21	Spleen scan	↑ 10, ↓ 3, stable 8	Santos et al,[156] 2002
		12.3 years	12	Pit cells	No difference	Olivieri and Vichinsky,[126] 1998
		—	—	HJB	↑	Harrod et al,[157] 2007
		9.1 years	40	Spleen scan	33% with uptake	Nottage et al,[32] 2014
Kidneys	Rand. (BABY HUG)	9-18 months	91[a]	DTPA GFR	No difference	Wang et al,[27] 2011
				Urine osmolality	↑	Alvarez et al,[33] 2012
				Urine specific gravity	↑	
				Total kidney volume	↓	
	Observ	Adults	26	Microalbuminuria	↓	Thompson et al,[158] 2007
	Observ	Children	9	Microalbuminuria	↓	McKie et al,[159] 2007
	Observ	35 months	14	DTPA GFR	Stable	Thornburg et al,[68] 2008
	Observ	8 years	3	Proteinuria	↓ (also on enalapril)	Fitzhugh et al,[34] 2005
	Observ	7.5 years	23	GFR	↓	Aygun et al,[35] 2013
				Microalbuminuria	No difference	
	Observ	Adults	149	Albumin: creatinine ratio/ proteinuria	↓	Laurin et al,[38] 2014
	Observ	7-18 years	63	Albumin: creatinine ratio	↓	Tehseen et al,[37] 2017
	Observ	2-18 years	88	Albumin: creatinine ratio	↓	Zahr et al,[36] 2018
Brain						
1° stroke proph	Rand. (BABY HUG)	0-18 months	91[a]	TCD velocity	No difference	Wang et al,[27] 2011

(continued)

TABLE 30-1 Hydroxyurea and organ function (Continued)

Organ	Type of study	Patient population	No. of patients	Evaluation	Effect of HU	Reference
	Rand. (TWiTCH)	Chronic transfusion for abnormal TCD	60	TCD velocity	Not inferior to chronic transfusion ↓ velocity	Ware et al,[44] 2016 Zimmerman et al,[43] 2007
	Rand. (SCATE)	Conditional TCD (5.4 years)	22	TCD velocity	Abnormal TCD: 9% on HU 47% on Observ	Hankins et al,[45] 2015
	Observ	Abnormal TCD (5.5 years)	23	Clinical course, TCD velocity	No CVA/84 patient-years ↓ abnormal velocity	Lefevre et al,[42] 2008
		Initiation of HU	24	TCD velocity	↓ velocity by 13 cm/s	Kratovil et al,[160] 2006
		Abnormal TCD	34	Clinical course, TCD velocity	1 CVA/96 patient-years	Gulbis et al,[40] 2005
		Elevated TCD velocity	104	Clinical course, TCD velocity	Mean TCD velocity 198→169	Lagunju et al,[108] 2019
		Abnormal TCD	29	Feasibility	Good adherence, no strokes	Galadanci et al,[107] 2017
2° stroke proph	Rand. (SWiTCH)	Children with primary stroke, mean treatment history = 7 years	66 standard treatment 67 HU + phlebotomy	Overt CVA; iron overload status	HU: 7 strokes CTX: 0 strokes	Ware et al,[46] 2013
	Observ	Children with primary stroke	35	Overt CVA	4.6 events/100 patient-years	Greenway et al,[48] 2011
		Children with primary stroke	5	Overt CVA	0 events/34 patient-years	Sumoza et al,[49] 2002
		Children with primary stroke	6	Overt CVA	2 strokes	de Montalembert et al,[47] 2008
		Children with primary stroke	8	Overt CVA	1 stroke/44 patient-years	Gulbis et al,[40] 2005
		Children with primary stroke	10/33	Overt CVA	1/10 on HU (2/100 patient-years) 20/33 not on HU (20/100 patient-years)	Ali et al,[50] 2011
SCIs	Rand. (SIT)	10 years (not on HU)	196	SCI, CVA over 3 years (CTX vs Observ)	SCI/CVA ↑ in Observ group; HU begun in 14% (vs 3% CTX)	DeBaun et al,[51] 2014

(continued)

TABLE 30-1 Hydroxyurea and organ function (Continued)

Organ	Type of study	Patient population	No. of patients	Evaluation	Effect of HU	Reference
	Observ	Paris cohort (6.4 years)	54 nl TCD and MRA → HU	Observ	2 abnl TCD/225 patient-years on HU	Bernaudin et al,[161] 2011
			13 abnl TCD/nl MRA → CTX → HU	Observ	3/13 recurrent abnl TCD on HU	
	Observ	SCA children (9.4 years)	50	MRI/MRA at 0, 3, 6 years	SCI present in 38%, 41%, and 41%	Nottage et al,[52] 2016
	Observ	Alabama cohort (10.9 years)	27	MRI at ≤3 years	3/27 new SCIs	Rushton et al,[162] 2018
	Observ	Italian cohort	86	MRI	SCI 17% → 59%	Rigano et al,[53] 2018
Neuropsychological	Observ	SCD children	15 on HU 50 not on HU	Neuropsychological battery	HU → better verbal comprehension, general cognition	Puffer et al,[54] 2007
	Rand. (BABY HUG)	9-18 months	91[a]	Bayley exam	No difference FSIQ HU vs placebo	Wang et al,[27] 2011
Cardiopulmonary	Observ	Male school children	41	HR, time on treadmill	↑ exercise tolerance	Wali and Moheeb,[57] 2011
	Observ	Children	152 HU; 247 not on HU	Echocardiogram	No difference in TRJ velocity	Gordeuk et al,[55] 2009
	Observ	Children with recurrent ACS	3	Oxygen saturation	Resolution of hypoxemia	Singh et al,[163] 2008
	Observ	SCA 5-21 years	11	Oxygen saturation	Oxygen saturation 95→98%	Pashankar et al,[164] 2015
	Review	10 studies		PH/TRJ velocity	Inconsistent effect	Buckner and Ataga,[165] 2014
	Review	2 studies		PH/right heart catheter	No effect	Parent et al,[166] 2011
	Observ	MSH F/U		17.5 years F/U	24% pulmonary mortality; 87% <5 years HU treatment	Steinberg et al,[56] 2010
	Observ	LaSHS F/U		5-8 years F/U	No ↓ in PH mortality	Voskaridou et al,[66] 2010

(continued)

TABLE 30-1 Hydroxyurea and organ function (Continued)

Organ	Type of study	Patient population	No. of patients	Evaluation	Effect of HU	Reference
	Observ	Children with OSA, seen in Toronto sleep lab	37 on HU; 104 not on HU	Polysomnography	OSA in 38% on HU and 52% not on HU (P = .14)	Narang et al,[58] 2015
Growth	Observ	HbSS, 5-16 years	68	Serial height and weight	Girls: no difference from historical cohorts; boys: ↑ height and weight	Wang et al,[59] 2002
	Rand. (BABY HUG)	HbSS, 9-18 months	91[a]	Serial height, weight, HC measures	No difference HU vs placebo	Rana et al,[60] 2014
Priapism	Observ	Adult men	5	Clinical course	4/5 benefited	Saad et al,[65] 2004
	Observ	16-year-old male	1	Clinical course	Correction of ED	Anele et al,[167] 2014
Retinopathy	Observ	HbSS, 10-18 years	123	Ophthalmologic exam	HbF < 15% → 7-fold ↑ in retinopathy; HU helpful	Estepp et al,[62] 2013
Infection	Observ	HbSS/Sβ	120	Clinical course of HPV	↓ transfusions, ↑ Hb, ↑ asymptomatic infection	Hankins et al,[64] 2016
AVN	Observ	HbSS/Sβ° 10-21 years in NYC	182	Plain films of hips	AVN positive, 69% on HU AVN negative, 42% on HU	Mahadeo et al[168] 2011
	Retros	SCD children and adults in California	6237	ICD-9 code for AVN	IR pre-HU = 2.37/100 person-years IR post-HU = 1.52/100 person-years	Adesina et al,[169] 2017
	Observ	SCD children in Kuwait	40	Serial MRIs of hips before and on HU	↓ frequency and progression of AVN compared with previous experience	Adekile et al,[63] 2019

[a]Similar number of subjects received placebo.

Abbreviations: 1° stroke proph, Primary stroke prophylaxis; 2° stroke proph, secondary stroke prophylaxis; abnl, abnormal; ACS, acute chest syndrome; AVN, avascular necrosis of the hip; CVA, cerebrovascular accident; CTX, chronic transfusion; DTPA FSIQ, full-scale intelligence quotient; ED, erectile dysfunction; F/U, follow-up; GFR, diethylenetriaminepentaacetic acid glomerular filtration rate; Hb, hemoglobin; HbF, fetal hemoglobin; HC, head circumference; HJB, Howell-Jolly bodies; HR, heart rate; HPV, human papillomavirus; HU, hydroxyurea; nl, normal; ICD-9, International Classification of Diseases, Ninth Edition; IR, incidence rate; MRA, magnetic resonance angiography; MRI, magnetic resonance imaging; NYC, New York City; Observ, observational; OSA, obstructive sleep apnea; PH, pulmonary hypertension; Rand, randomize; Retros, retrospective; SCA, sickle cell anemia; SCD, sickle cell disease; SCI, silent cerebral infarct; TCD, transcranial Doppler ultrasound velocity; TRJ, tricuspid regurgitant jet (velocity).

with abnormally elevated TCD velocities in the internal carotid and middle cerebral arteries was 92% effective for the prevention of primary strokes.[39] In addition, several reports involving children with SCA, including some who had velocities in the abnormal range but were not candidates for chronic transfusion, described decreased TCD velocities after starting hydroxyurea, indicating a reduced risk for stroke.[40-43] These findings led to the multicenter randomized TCD With Transfusions Changing to Hydroxyurea (TWiTCH) trial in which patients with abnormal TCD velocities who had received chronic transfusion for at least 1 year and who did not have severe stenosis on magnetic resonance angiography (MRA) were randomized to continue chronic transfusion or substitute hydroxyurea for transfusion.[44] This trial was halted early due to observed noninferiority of the hydroxyurea group and demonstrated that properly managed hydroxyurea treatment can substitute for chronic transfusion to maintain lower TCD velocities and prevent primary stroke. In the international randomized Sparing Conversion to Abnormal TCD Elevation (SCATE) trial, fewer children with conditional TCD velocities had conversion to abnormal velocities on hydroxyurea than on observation alone.[45] In the BABY HUG study, there was no significant difference in the mean TCD velocities of the hydroxyurea and placebo arms at the trial's conclusion, but the age-related increase in velocity between entry and exit was significantly worse in the placebo arm.[27]

The role of hydroxyurea in *secondary* stroke prophylaxis was examined in the multicenter, randomized Stroke With Transfusions Changing to Hydroxyurea (SWiTCH) trial.[46] Standard management for sickle cell patients who have suffered an overt ischemic stroke has been chronic transfusion, despite its attendant toxicities of iron overload and alloantibody induction. This intervention is effective in reducing the stroke reoccurrence rate from approximately 60% to 70% to 15%, but transfusion must be continued indefinitely. In the SWiTCH trial, standard management with continued chronic transfusion (plus iron chelation) was compared with hydroxyurea treatment (plus phlebotomy for reduction of iron overload). The study was halted due to lack of superior iron unloading in the phlebotomy group compared to chelation, which was a co-primary end point; at the time of study termination, there were 7 recurrent strokes in the hydroxyurea group (10%) versus none in the chronic transfusion group, which was within the study-accepted noninferiority margin of <20%.[46] Other studies have evaluated smaller cohorts of patients receiving hydroxyurea for secondary stroke prevention, but results have been mixed.[40,47-49] For example, a Jamaican study found that hydroxyurea was more efficacious for secondary stroke prevention than no treatment at all.[50] Overall, hydroxyurea cannot be recommended for secondary stroke prevention if safe chronic transfusion is available, but it has an important role in common clinical settings such as multiple erythrocyte alloantibodies, massive iron overload, religious objection to blood, and low-resource settings (see later section titled "Hydroxyurea Trials in Africa").

The role of hydroxyurea in the prevention or management of silent cerebral infarcts (SCIs), which may occur in up to 38%

of children and >50% of adults with HbSS, is unclear. In the recent Silent Cerebral Infarct Trial (SIT), chronic transfusion reduced the frequency of new overt/silent infarcts in children with SCA who had SCI on magnetic resonance imaging (MRI) screening compared to observation alone, but patients receiving hydroxyurea were excluded from the study.[51] In a single-institution prospective trial, children with SCA had a 38% prevalence of SCI at baseline and, subsequently, a similar prevalence (41%) after 3 and 6 years of hydroxyurea at maximum-tolerated dose (MTD).[52] In contrast, frequent new SCIs occurred on hydroxyurea in a recent report of Italian patients with SCD, particularly in those with previous infarcts and those with HbS-β thalassemia.[53] Based on these limited data, hydroxyurea appears to have a beneficial role for early cerebrovascular disease (exemplified by conditional TCD velocity), but transfusions are likely superior for patients with advanced anatomic/structural disease.

The effects of hydroxyurea on psychometric performance in children with SCD have not been fully established. In a single-institution study comparing 15 children with SCD on hydroxyurea with 50 SCD children not on hydroxyurea, the former had better verbal comprehension and general cognition.[54] In the BABY HUG trial, infants with SCA who were randomized to receive hydroxyurea for 2 years had no difference in the Bayley Mental Development Index (MDI) score at study exit compared with those receiving placebo, but 5 children in the placebo group had an MDI <70 compared with no children in the hydroxyurea group.[27]

The effects of hydroxyurea on cardiopulmonary function have been examined in several observational studies. In a review of 10 studies that evaluated subjects with elevated tricuspid valve regurgitant jet velocity (a biomarker associated with increased risk of pulmonary hypertension), the effects of hydroxyurea therapy were inconsistent.[55] For example, in a cross-sectional comparison of 152 children on hydroxyurea with 247 children who were not receiving hydroxyurea, there was no difference in the prevalence of increased tricuspid valve regurgitant jet velocity.[55] In the Laikon Study of Hydroxyurea in Sickle Cell Syndromes (LaSHS), a prospective phase II adult study, hydroxyurea was not associated with decreased mortality from pulmonary hypertension.[53] In the 2 studies in which pulmonary hypertension was measured directly by right heart catheterization, no effect from hydroxyurea was seen.[54,55] However, after 17.5 years of follow-up of the MSH cohort, there was substantial mortality (24%) due to pulmonary causes, the vast majority of which (87%) occurred in patients who had received limited hydroxyurea treatment.[56]

Although the previously discussed evidence suggests that hydroxyurea may not be effective for proven pulmonary hypertension in SCD, a study of 41 male school children from Oman found that exercise tolerance was increased on hydroxyurea.[57] Furthermore, in a retrospective study generated by a sleep laboratory in Toronto, it was found that although obstructive sleep apnea was not significantly less in children with SCD on hydroxyurea compared with those not on hydroxyurea (38% vs 52%, respectively), those on hydroxyurea had higher median oxygen saturation levels both awake (98.6% vs 96.1%, respectively; $P < .001$) and asleep (91.4% vs 85.0%, respectively; $P = .0002$).[58]

Growth in children with SCD does not appear to be adversely affected by hydroxyurea and, if anything, may be improved. In 2 multicenter trials of 5- to 16-year-old children (HUG-KIDS[59]) and 9- to 18-month-old infants (BABY HUG[60]), as well as a large single-institution cohort[61] with long-term follow-up, hydroxyurea was associated with expected increases in both weight and height, plus normal sexual development.

Studies of other organs affected by SCD have generated several reports related to possible positive effects of hydroxyurea. Children with HbSS were found to have a 7-fold greater likelihood of developing retinopathy if their HbF level was <15%; hydroxyurea-related HbF induction was likely beneficial.[62] In a prospective study of children in Kuwait, the frequency and rate of progression of avascular necrosis of the femoral head were less than those previously reported for patients not treated with hydroxyurea.[63] A retrospective review of 120 cases of aplastic "crises" due to parvovirus B19 infection found that children with HbSS-Sβ[0] thalassemia required fewer transfusions and had less severe hemoglobin concentration nadirs if they were receiving hydroxyurea.[64] Finally, 4 of 5 adult men with recurrent priapism benefited from hydroxyurea.[65]

Mortality (Table 30-2)

Hydroxyurea has a beneficial effect on mortality in adults with SCA. In a 17.5-year follow-up of the MSH, mortality was significantly reduced in individuals with long-term hydroxyurea exposure.[56] In the LaSHS study of 330 adult Greek patients with HbSS, Sβ[0], or Sβ[+] thalassemia, significant reductions occurred in pain, acute chest syndrome, transfusion, hospitalization, stroke, and overall mortality (10-year survival, 86% in the hydroxyurea-treated group vs 65% in the untreated group).[66] In adults followed at the National Institutes of Health in the

TABLE 30-2 Hydroxyurea and mortality

Author/location	Patient population/ study design	Genotype/ inclusion criteria	No. of patients	Follow-up period, mean/ median (range)	Mortality
Steinberg et al,[56] 2010 (MSH)/ North America	Adults/ prospective	SCA; MSH cohort; analysis by HU use, not original trial assignment	129/299 of original cohort deceased	Up to 17.5 years	HU for at least 5 years had ↓ mortality (compared with <5 years)
Voskaridou et al,[66] 2010 (LaSHS)/ Greece	Adults/ prospective	HbSS 34, HbS-β[0] thalassemia 131, HbS-β[+] thalassemia 165; ≥3 VOCs in previous year; CVA or ACS in past 5 years	330 (HU: 131 [SS/Sβ[0]: 87; Sβ[+] thalassemia: 44])	HU: 8 years (0.1-17) No HU: 5 years (0.1-18)	10-year survival: 86% for HU; 65% for non-HU; $P = .001$
Fitzhugh et al,[67] 2015/United States	Adults/ retrospective	HbSS	383 (HU 66%, recommended-dose HU 44%)	2.6 years (0.1-11.7)	↓ mortality on HU (HR, 0.58); greater ↓ if on recommended dose HU (HR, 0.36)
Karacaoglu et al,[170] 2016/ Turkey (Eti-Turks)	Adults/ retrospective	SCD	735	5.5 years	↓ mortality on HU
Lobo et al,[69] 2013/ Brazil	Children/ retrospective	SCD; indications for HU: recurrent VOC; >1 ACS; Hb <6 g/dL; CVA	1760 (HU: 267)	7 years (3-17) HU: 2 years (0.1-6.5)	↓ mortality; 1 death in HU group; 37 deaths in no-HU group
Le et al,[70] 2015/ Belgium	Lifetime cohort/ retrospective/ prospective	SCD	469 (HU: 185)	HU 10.3 years	↓ mortality on HU compared to HSCT and no treatment (0.14, 0.36, 0.38/100 patient-years)

Abbreviations: ACS, acute chest syndrome; CVA, cerebrovascular accident; HR, hazard ratio; HSCT, hematopoietic stem cell transplantation; HU, hydroxyurea; LaSHS, Laikon Study of Hydroxyurea in Sickle Cell Syndromes; MSH, Multicenter Study of Hydroxyurea; SCA, sickle cell anemia; VOC, vaso-occlusive crisis.

United States, decreased mortality was seen in those receiving hydroxyurea, particularly if they were on recommended dosing (15-35 mg/kg/d).[67] Similar results were seen in an Eti-Turk population.[68]

Two studies have evaluated mortality in children with SCD. In Rio de Janeiro, Brazil, among 1760 children, 267 were treated with hydroxyurea because of clinical severity for a median of 2 years.[69] Although this was not a randomized trial, the sicker hydroxyurea-treated children had significant reductions in hospitalizations, transfusions, and, most notably, mortality due to fewer deaths from acute chest syndrome and infection (99.5% vs 94.5% survival in children treated with hydroxyurea vs those not treated, respectively; $P = .01$). A report from the Belgian Registry, which included both children and adults, found significantly decreased mortality in those treated with hydroxyurea compared to those receiving hematopoietic stem cell transplantation or no treatment and similar mortality between those on hydroxyurea versus on chronic transfusion.[70]

Hydroxyurea Dosing

Variation in Dose Amount

In the early years of its use, "standard" hydroxyurea treatment was often initiated at a dose of 15 to 20 mg/kg given once daily by mouth. However, the benefits and risks of gradually escalating the dose to the MTD (defined as a daily dose that leads to mild marrow suppression without toxicities) versus maintenance at a fixed dose have been a controversial topic. In a 2010 review article, it was noted that hematologists in Europe tended to use a fixed dose, whereas those in North America typically escalated dosing to MTD[20] (Tables 30-3 and 30-4). The review also noted that escalation to >25 mg/kg/d typically achieved laboratory thresholds of hemoglobin >9 g/dL, MCV >100 fL, and HbF approximately 20%, which are all greater than the levels reached on a fixed dose of 15 to 20 mg/kg/d. In the 2014 Evidence-Based Management of Sickle Cell Disease Expert Panel Report published by the US National Heart, Lung, and Blood Institute (NHLBI), starting doses of 15 and 20 mg/kg/d were recommended in adults and children, respectively, and dose escalation by increments of 5 mg/kg/d every 8 weeks was recommended "if dose escalation is warranted."[71] In 2018, the "Guidelines for the Use of Hydroxycarbamide (Hydroxyurea) in Children and Adults With Sickle Cell Disease" were published by the British Society for Haematology.[72] These guidelines recommended the same dosing approach as that of the NHLBI, but added that if the drug is given to children with SCD for replacement of chronic transfusion for primary stroke prevention or if it is for management of conditional TCD velocities, it should be escalated to MTD. Figure 30-2 illustrates a clinical protocol that features serial dose escalation with the goal of reaching MTD.

It should be noted that numerous reports have described the benefit of higher HbF levels in SCD.[5,73] The hypothetical threshold of 20% HbF was supported by a study of children with SCA (n = 230) treated with hydroxyurea to MTD.[74] With all HUSTLE study participants receiving dose escalation using a standardized approach, when the MTD HbF values were ≤20%, children had twice the odds of hospitalization for reasons including vaso-occlusive pain and acute chest syndrome and 4 times the odds of admission for fever. In a recent phase I/II trial (Realizing Effectiveness of Hydroxyurea Across Continents [REACH]) from 4 countries in sub-Saharan Africa (n = 606), hydroxyurea administration in children with SCA was escalated after an initial 6 months of fixed dosing at a mean dose of 17.5 mg/kg/d. The mean HbF level was 19.3% at 6 months, but after dose escalation to MTD, the mean HbF level was further increased to 23.4% at 12 months.[75]

TABLE 30-3 Hematologic response to hydroxyurea at fixed dose

Year	Author	No. of patients	Average age, years	Average dose, mg/kg/d	Treatment duration, years	Hb, g/dL	MCV, fL	HbF, %	ANC, × 10⁹/L
1996	Ferster et al[171]	22	8	~20	0.5	8.5	96	15.3	
2001	Wang et al[172]	21	1.3	~20	2.0	8.8	90	20.3	4.2
2001	Ferster et al[173]	22	7	~20	5	8.7	97	12.9	4.0
2005	Gulbis et al[40]	32	6	~20	6	8.8	92	12.5	4.6
2010	Voskaridou et al[66]	131[a]	33	~20		9.5	97	17.4	9.0
2011	Wang et al[27]	91	1.1	20	2.0	9.1	92	22.4	4.5
2017	Galadanci et al[107]	29	6.8	19	2.1		96	14.3	
2017	Opoka et al[106]	104	2.2	20	1.0	8.7	88	22.9	5.2

[a]Includes SS, Sβ⁰, and Sβ⁺.

Abbreviations: ANC, absolute neutrophil count; Hb, hemoglobin; HbF, hemoglobin F; MCV, mean corpuscular volume.

Adapted from Ware RE. How I use hydroxyurea to treat young patients with sickle cell anemia. *Blood*. 2010;115(26):5300-5311.

TABLE 30-4 Hematologic response to hydroxyurea at maximum-tolerated dose

Year	Author	No. of patients	Average age, years	Average dose, mg/kg/d	Treatment duration, years	Hb, g/dL	MCV, fL	HbF, %	ANC, × 10⁹/L
1995	Charache et al[26]	32	27.6	21.3	0.8	9.7	117	15	4.6
1999	Kinney et al[15]	71	9.8	25.6	1.5	9.1	102	16.3	4.4
2004	Zimmerman et al[61]	106	10.3	25.9	3.8	9.5	107	19.7	3.6
2005	Hankins et al[174]	11	3.4	30.0	6	9.0	96	23.3	NA
2007	Zimmerman et al[43]	37	6.8	27.9	0.8	9.4	104	22.7	NA
2009	Thornburg et al[68]	14	3.9	28	2.1	9.5	99	25.9	3.0
2009	Ware et al[175]	111	7.6	26.7	3.2	9.7	107	23.2	3.8
2017	Estepp et al[74]	92	7.7	26.7	4	9.2	108	21.5	3.3
2019	Tshilolo et al[75]	535	1-10	22.5	3	8.3	91	21.2	4.3
2019	McGann et al[87]	50	0.9	27.7	1.5	10.1	92	33.3	3.3

Abbreviations: ANC, absolute neutrophil count; Hb, hemoglobin; HbF, hemoglobin F; MCV, mean corpuscular volume; NA, not available.

However, randomized trials directly comparing fixed versus MTD dosing with respect to efficacy in reducing clinical symptoms and maximizing HbF levels have been limited. Currently, a pilot study in 4 US institutions is comparing fixed dosing (20 mg/kg/d) versus escalation to MTD in 9- to 36-month-old infants with SCA, who are followed for 12 months after randomization, with end points of feasibility, toxicity, and HbF levels (NCT03020615). Reported in the last year, the Novel Use of Hydroxyurea in an African Region with Malaria (NOHARM) MTD randomized double-blind trial in Uganda compared fixed dosing at 20 mg/kg/d with escalated dosing to an average of 30 mg/kg/d and found, over 18 months, significantly greater HbF (30% vs 20%) and fewer vaso-occlusive pain crises, cases of acute chest syndrome, transfusions, and hospitalizations in the higher dose group, without an increase in toxicity (NCT03128515).[75a]

In contrast to the previously discussed considerations, some recent reports have suggested that fixed low-dose hydroxyurea (~10 mg/kg/d) might yield efficacy comparable to that of higher doses, but with the advantages of less frequent monitoring, better adherence, and lower cost due to savings in lab, clinic visit, and drug expenses (Table 30-5).[76-80] Most of these reports come from India, with one each from the Caribbean, Oman, and Nigeria; therefore, many of the patients are of the Arab-Indian haplotype with higher baseline HbF levels. In general, low-dose treatment was associated with marked decreases in vaso-occlusive pain, acute chest syndrome, and hospitalization and some increases in hemoglobin level and MCV, but only modest increases in HbF (3.5%-6%). In Ibadan, Nigeria, a fixed low dose of 500 mg/d (~10 mg/kg/d) was given to 48 adults for 24 weeks, leading to lab and clinical responses similar to those seen in the MSH study using MTD dosing.[81] At present, a randomized, prospective, phase III trial of moderate-dose (20 mg/kg/d) versus low-dose (10 mg/kg/d) hydroxyurea is ongoing in Kano, Nigeria, to determine the effectiveness of this treatment for secondary stroke prevention in children with SCA who have had an acute overt stroke (NCT02675790).

Individualized Dosing

In the early trials of hydroxyurea for adults with SCA, including both the original multicenter phase I/II trial[28] and the subsequent phase III MSH trial,[26] substantial variation was noted in the hydroxyurea treatment effects. Laboratory responses, especially the percent HbF induction, as well as clinical responses in reduction of acute vaso-occlusive events, demonstrated impressive interpatient variation. Similar phenotypic variation in treatment responses was noted in hydroxyurea trials involving children with SCA.[15,47,61]

Part of the observed variation can be explained by differences in hydroxyurea pharmacokinetics (PK); the drug half-life is 1 to 4 hours in most patients,[82,83] with shorter time frames for children, thus affecting the drug exposure based on area under the curve (AUC) calculations. Most of the drug is excreted unchanged in the urine; hence, patients with renal impairment and reduced GFRs will have longer drug exposure and require lower milligram per kilogram doses to avoid toxicity.[84] Efforts to identify genetic influences on hydroxyurea PK and, specifically, single nucleotide polymorphisms that affect the absorption, distribution, metabolism, or excretion of hydroxyurea have identified several candidates.[85,86] To date, however, no genetic assays have moved into clinical practice for predicting either dosing or treatment responses.

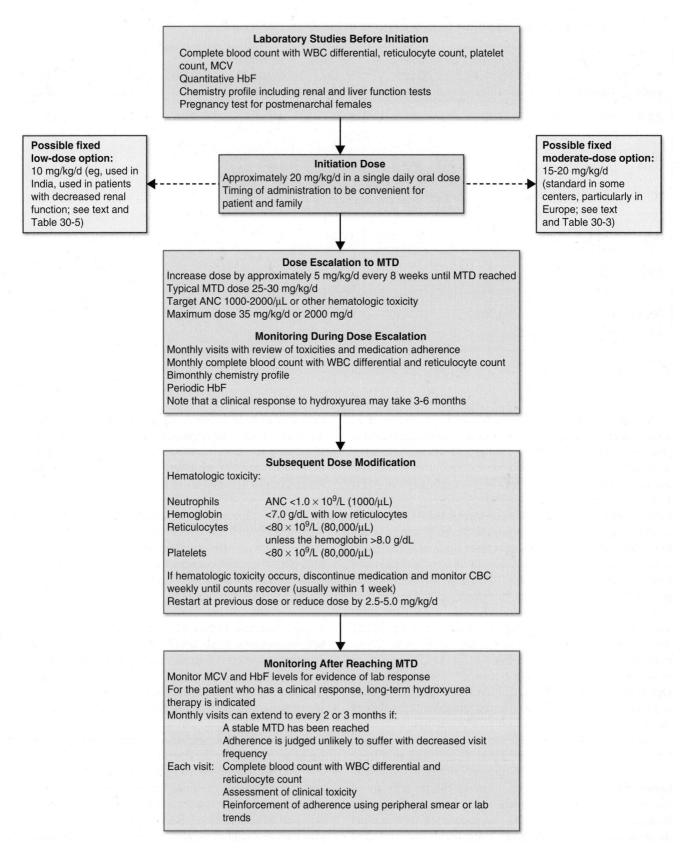

FIGURE 30-2 Hydroxyurea treatment initiation and monitoring. Guidelines for treatment to maximum-tolerated dose (MTD) are shown in the central portion of the figure. Alternative dosing options for fixed low-dose and moderate-dose approaches are also indicated. ANC, absolute neutrophil count; CBC, complete blood count; HbF, fetal hemoglobin; MCV, mean corpuscular volume; WBC, white blood cell.

TABLE 30-5 Hematologic response to hydroxyurea at fixed low dose

Year	Author	Location	No. of patients	Average age, years	Average dose, mg/kg/d	Treatment duration, years	Hb, g/dL	MCV, fL	HbF, %	WBC, × 10⁹/L
2006	Svarch et al[80]	Caribbean	51	4-18	15	2.0	8.5	—	12.4	9.8
2012	Patel et al[77]	Odisha, India	118	Pediatric/ adult	10	2.0	10.1	86	22.5	7.9
2013	Jain et al[76]	Nagpur, India	144	3.5-18	10	2.0	9.7	88	22.0	8.8
2013	Sharef et al[79]	Oman	44	8 (5-16)	10-16	3.9 (1)	9.8	70	15.2	3.0[a]
2018	Sethy et al[78]	Cuttack, India	128	>18	10	1	9.8	91	21.7	8.5
2019	Akingbola et al[81]	Ibadan, Nigeria	48	Adults	~10	0.5	8.3	96	8.9	9.2

[a]Absolute neutrophil count.
Abbreviations: Hb, hemoglobin; HbF, hemoglobin F; MCV, mean corpuscular volume.

To help explain the observed variation in hydroxyurea treatment effects, a careful analysis of first-dose and MTD PK and pharmacodynamics yielded a sparse sampling strategy with Bayesian estimation of the optimal dose. This PK-guided dosing model incorporates 3 patient-specific measurements at 15 to 20, 60, and 180 minutes after an initial test dose of 20 mg/kg/d. A software algorithm then determines the dose necessary to achieve the optimal drug exposure based on AUC calculations. This individualized dosing strategy was recently tested in a single-institution prospective trial, the Therapeutic Response Evaluation and Adherence Trial (TREAT, NCT02286154), which prospectively evaluated this approach in children with time to MTD as the primary study end point. Fifty children started hydroxyurea at an average dose of 27.7 mg/kg/d, and >80% did not require a subsequent mg/kg/d dose change before MTD was independently declared.[87] Excellent treatment responses were observed with few drug-related toxicities. The Hydroxyurea Optimization Through Precision Study (HOPS, NCT03789591) is a follow-up multicenter randomized trial that will compare this PK-guided dosing strategy with traditional dose escalation.

Toxicity and Safety

Short-term toxicities of hydroxyurea treatment primarily involve dose-dependent, transient myelosuppression resulting in decreased absolute neutrophil count, which has been readily manageable and not associated with invasive infection.[88,89] Moderate thrombocytopenia and significantly worsened anemia accompanied by reticulocytopenia are seen infrequently and may require dose adjustment. The short-term safety profile was further illustrated by a case report of a 2-year-old child with SCA who ingested a 35-fold overdose but had

only transient mild myelosuppression with no long-term sequelae.[90] Over time, significant splenomegaly with cytopenias from hypersplenism has been reported in a few cases, primarily in adults.[91] Melanonychia and skin hyperpigmentation occur in a small proportion of patients but are solely cosmetic and do not portend any cutaneous disorders.[92] There is no evidence of immune suppression due to hydroxyurea; evaluation of immune function in the BABY HUG trial showed that hydroxyurea was associated with "normalization" of lymphocyte subpopulations and appropriate immune responses to both pneumococcal and measles vaccinations.[93]

Patient cohorts have now been followed for >15 to 20 years without clinically apparent long-term toxicity.[45,56] However, concerns have been raised because hydroxyurea in high doses acts as a mutagen, carcinogen, and teratogen in animals and in vitro.[94-96] In the BABY HUG study, chromosomal karyotype, VDJ recombination events, and reticulocyte micronuclei were evaluated as measures of genotoxicity; no differences were found between hydroxyurea and placebo subjects.[97] Other studies that evaluated RBC micronuclei and chromosomal damage did not show increased risk in hydroxyurea-treated patients.[98,99] However, a recent Brazilian report indicated that hydroxyurea was associated with an increased DNA damage index and WBC micronuclei in adult patients.[100] The clinical risk of carcinogenesis from hydroxyurea has been hard to evaluate. Although there have been at least 6 cases of leukemia (mostly acute myelogenous leukemia [AML]) reported in sickle cell patients taking the drug, the total number of persons at risk is unknown but likely >100,000 persons, especially when considered on a global scale. Recently, a report using health insurance claims databases found no increased risk for AML with hydroxyurea treatment.[101] Another report using administrative data noted an increased risk of leukemia among SCD patients in California, but no increased risk after 1998, which is the time when hydroxyurea was approved.[102] Together, the available data over 20 to 30 years of clinical experience do not support a carcinogenic risk of hydroxyurea for persons with SCD, although ongoing surveillance should continue, especially for younger patients.

Deleterious effects on fertility from hydroxyurea therapy have been postulated, as well as possible teratogenic effects, that have led to the drug being listed as contraindicated during pregnancy. However, a review of reproductive issues in SCD advocated more research on the teratogenic risks of hydroxyurea before abandoning its use during pregnancy.[103] In an analysis of 94 pregnancy outcomes involving both males and females who participated in the MSH trial, exposure of the fetus to hydroxyurea was not teratogenic in those pregnancies that resulted in live births.[104] An ongoing concern is the possible effects of hydroxyurea on spermatogenesis. This has been poorly defined, in part because untreated SCD itself, presumably through repeated infarction and priapism, adversely affects both sperm count and function. A recent report evaluated spermatogenesis in 35 men before and after 6 months of treatment with hydroxyurea.[105] Before treatment, 40% had an abnormally low total sperm count, whereas on treatment, the mean sperm count decreased from 130 million to 24 million and the proportion of cryptospermic or azoospermic participants increased from 3% to 31%. Semen volume was unchanged, and sperm function was not reported, nor was the fertility of the men before or after treatment, although all study participants were offered sperm banking. Unanswered questions include whether the observed reduction in total sperm count is reversible, the effects of initiating hydroxyurea in boys, and whether there is any deleterious impact on male fertility. Current evidence, however, suggests that both male and female adults receiving hydroxyurea remain fertile, based on data in the MSH follow-up report[104] and from widespread clinical experience.

Hydroxyurea Trials in Africa

A remarkable development over the past decade has been the initiation of numerous clinical trials of hydroxyurea in sub-Saharan Africa (Table 30-6). Three informative recently published studies have been the NOHARM trial (Kampala, Uganda),[106] the REACH trial (Angola, Democratic Republic of Congo, Kenya, Uganda),[75] and the Stroke Prevention in Nigeria (SPIN) trial (Kano, Nigeria).[107] The NOHARM study was a randomized, double-blind trial in children with SCA in malaria-endemic Uganda that compared moderate-dose hydroxyurea to placebo over a 12-month period. Hydroxyurea did not increase the incidence or severity of malaria events but did provide significant clinical and laboratory benefits, suggesting it will be safe and effective in malarial regions of Africa. The REACH study enrolled children 1 to 10 years of age with SCA in 4 sub-Saharan countries. Children received hydroxyurea at 15 to 20 mg/kg/d for 6 months, followed by

dose escalation. Hydroxyurea treatment was feasible and safe and reduced the incidence of vaso-occlusive events, malaria, other infections, transfusions, and death, supporting the need for wider access to treatment in sub-Saharan Africa. A recent feasibility trial in Kano, Nigeria (SPIN trial), examined the use of moderate-dose hydroxyurea as the initial intervention for stroke prevention in patients with abnormal TCDs (because safe chronic transfusion was not available).[107] There was excellent adherence with hydroxyurea treatment, and no strokes occurred among the 25 patients enrolled and followed for a median of 2.1 years. In addition, in Ibadan, Nigeria, 104 children with conditional or abnormal TCD velocities were treated with hydroxyurea up to the MTD and followed over a mean of 3.6 years.[108] Mean TCD velocities declined significantly from 198 to 169 cm/s, and only 1 overt stroke occurred in the cohort (incidence of 0.27/100 person-years).

The successful conduct of the previously discussed studies and ongoing research in India, the Middle East, and Latin America are driving expanded investigation of hydroxyurea treatment in those areas of the globe where the vast majority of the sickle cell population lives. Efforts are needed to coordinate future drug supply with the projected increased demand, emphasizing the need for medication affordability in low-resource settings.

Combination Treatment With Hydroxyurea

An area that has been mostly unexplored is the use of combination pharmacotherapy for SCD, in which a well-studied effective drug (hydroxyurea) is combined with a relatively experimental and/or underutilized agent.[109] Ideally, the drugs used in combination should have different mechanisms of action, nonoverlapping and relatively limited toxicities, ease of administration, and nonprohibitive costs. Early studies of erythropoietin (EPO) added to hydroxyurea showed additionally increased HbF if iron was also provided.[110,111] It was later speculated that EPO may allow higher hydroxyurea dosing in the face of renal dysfunction.[112] A more recent trial tested the combination of hydroxyurea and magnesium pidolate (cation transport blocker to promote erythrocyte hydration) in HbSC disease, but the lack of biologic response to magnesium has dampened enthusiasm for this agent.[113] Concurrent use of hydroxyurea with poloxamer 188 (surfactant),[114] arginine (NO precursor),[115] sildenafil (phosphodiesterase inhibitor),[115] senicapoc (Gardos channel blocker),[116] prasugrel (platelet function inhibitor),[117] rivipansel/GMI-1070 (pan-selectin inhibitor),[118] regadenoson (adenosine A2A receptor agonist),[119] crizanlizumab (anti–P-selectin),[38] L-glutamine (NADH enhancer),[120] and voxelotor (oxygen-binding enhancer)[121] has been reported from trials focused on the novel agent. Typically, these trials allowed patients who had been receiving a stable dose of hydroxyurea (generally for several months) to be enrolled and to continue hydroxyurea. The reports are listed in Table 30-7, in which the effect of the experimental antisickling agent by

TABLE 30-6 Hydroxyurea trials in sub-Saharan Africa[a]

Clinical trial	ClinicalTrials.gov identifier	Performance site	Hydroxyurea intervention	No. of participants	Primary study end points	Status
Sickle Cell Disease – Stroke Prevention in Nigeria Trial (SPIN)	NCT01801423	Kano, Nigeria	~20 mg/kg/d	60	Adherence, acceptability	Active, not recruiting
Realizing Effectiveness of Hydroxyurea Across Continents (REACH)	NCT01966731	Luanda, Angola; Kinshasa, DRC; Kilifi, Kenya; Mbale, Uganda	~17.5 mg/kg/d for 6 months, then escalation to MTD	606	Adherence, toxicity, dosing	Active, not recruiting
Risk Clinical Stratification of Sickle Cell Disease in Nigeria: Assessment of Efficacy/Safety of Hydroxyurea Treatment	NCT02149537	Ibadan, Nigeria	~10 mg/kg/d for 6 months versus no treatment, with crossover design	53	Cytopenia	Active, not recruiting
Primary Prevention of Stroke in Children With Sickle Cell Disease in Sub-Saharan Africa II (SPRING)	NCT02560935	Kano, Nigeria	~10 mg/kg/d versus ~20 mg/kg/d	440	Clinical stroke or TIA	Active, not recruiting
Low-Dose Hydroxyurea for Secondary Stroke Prevention in Children With Sickle Cell Disease in Sub-Saharan Africa (SPRINT)	NCT02675790	Kano, Nigeria	~10 mg/kg/d versus ~20 mg/kg/d	120	Stroke recurrence, TIA, or death	Recruiting
Optimizing Hydroxyurea Therapy in Children With Sickle Cell Anemia in Malaria Endemic Areas (NOHARM-MTD)	NCT03128515	Kampala, Uganda	~20 mg/kg/d versus MTD (~30 mg/kg/d)	180	Hb ≥9.0 g/dL or HbF ≥20%	Greater HbF, fewer clinical complications in MTD arm
Management of Severe Acute Malnutrition in Sickle Cell Disease, in Northern Nigeria	NCT03634488	Kano, Nigeria	~20 mg/kg/d for 12 weeks	100	Adherence, acceptability	Not yet recruiting
Stroke Prevention with Hydroxyurea Enabled Through Research and Education (SPHERE)	NCT03948867	Mwanza, Tanzania	~20 mg/kg/d for 6 months, then escalation to MTD	200	TCD velocity	Recruiting

[a]Current prospective research trials using hydroxyurea treatment for patients with sickle cell anemia living in sub-Saharan Africa. The ClinicalTrials.gov website was last accessed July 6, 2019.

Abbreviations: DRC, Democratic Republic of Congo; Hb, hemoglobin; HbF, hemoglobin F; MTD, maximum-tolerated dose; TCD, transcranial Doppler; TIA, transient ischemic attack.

TABLE 30-7 Combination treatment including hydroxyurea

Year	Author	Combination	No. of patients on study drug	Effects of study drug alone	No. of patients on study drug + HU	Effects of study drug + HU	Comments
1990	Goldberg et al[110]	HU + EPO	5	No ↑ HbF from EPO	3	HU + EPO = HU alone	HU → ↑ HbF
1993	Rodgers et al[111]	HU + EPO + Fe			4	HU + EPO + Fe → ↑ HbF	Effect more than HU alone
2001	Orringer et al[114]	Poloxamer 188 + HU	28	Crisis resolution in 4/28 (14%)	26	Crisis resolution in 12/26 (46%) ($P = .02$)	Overall pain duration not less on poloxamer
2009	Little et al[115]	HU + arginine

HU + sildenafil | | | | HU + arginine → no effect

HU + sildenafil → ↑ 6-minute walk distance, ↑ HbF | |
2011	Ataga et al[116]	Senicapoc ± HU[a]	61	Pain crisis rate = 0.37/month	84	Pain crisis rate = 0.39/month	Senicapoc not better than PL
2015	Telen et al[118]	Rivipansel (GMI-1070) ± HU[a]	21		22		Trend toward faster VOC resolution from rivipansel compared to PL (?)
2016	Heeney et al[117]	Prasugrel ± HU[a]	94	Events/year = 1.98	77	Events/year = 2.61	Children 2-17 years old; prasugrel not better than PL
2017	Field et al[119]	Regadenoson ± HU[a]	38		15		Regadenoson infusion during VOC not better than PL in reducing iNKT
2017	Ataga et al[176]	Crizanlizumab (high dose) ± HU[a]	25	Median crisis rate = 1.00/year	42	Median crisis rate = 2.43/year	High-dose crizanlizumab better than PL
2018	Niihara et al[120]	L-Glutamine ± HU[a]	~34	Pain crisis rate ratio = 0.78	~67	Pain crisis rate ratio = 0.77	Median pain crises: glutamine, 3.0; PL, 4.0 ($P = .00$); two-thirds of patients on HU
2019	Vichinsky et al[177]	Voxelotor (1500 mg) ± HU[a]	30	Mean ↑ in Hb = 1.2 g/dL	51	Mean ↑ in Hb = 1.0 g/dL	Median ↑ in Hb ~1 g/dL regardless of whether patient on HU

[a]In these trials, main comparison was between study drug (± HU) versus placebo (± HU); data shown here are from study drug with HU compared to study drug without HU.
Abbreviations: EPO, erythropoietin; Fe, iron; Hb, hemoglobin; HbF, hemoglobin F; HU, hydroxyurea; iNKT, invariant natural killer T cells; PL, placebo; VOC, vaso-occlusive crisis.

itself is compared with the effect of that agent plus hydroxyurea (when such data are available). In most reports, there was neither significant influence from hydroxyurea on primary end point efficacy nor any additive toxicity, although these studies were not designed to compare single versus combination therapy. There was also no obvious influence of the pharmacologic mechanisms of action of the drugs on outcomes. However, there were examples of possible additive effects, as seen in the study of poloxamer 188, in which there was a higher proportion of subjects with crisis resolution in patients who were also receiving hydroxyurea,[114] and in the recent phase III trial of voxelotor, in which the addition of this agent was associated with a further increase in hemoglobin level in patients who had already been receiving hydroxyurea.[121]

Adherence

Although numerous studies have clearly demonstrated the efficacy of hydroxyurea in reducing the morbidity and mortality of SCD, a major barrier to its effectiveness has been adherence with taking this daily oral medication. Two recent systematic review articles have summarized problems with adherence among pediatric patients with SCD.[122,123] The first review covered 23 articles on adherence with antibiotic prophylaxis, iron chelation, or hydroxyurea; adherence rates ranged from 16% to 89%, with most studies reporting "moderate" adherence. Nonadherence with hydroxyurea was associated with more vaso-occlusive crises and hospitalizations. The second review included 13 studies that specifically addressed hydroxyurea treatment with reported adherence rates ranging from 12% to 100% (mean, 74%; median, 80%). The broad range in results was attributed in part to the variability in assessment strategies and unclear definitions of adherence. Those authors recommended the following: evidence-based adherence assessment tools; evaluating barriers to the medication regimen; use of biomarkers for associations with adherence; evaluating socioenvironmental factors that contribute to poor adherence; improved examination of the association between adherence and health outcomes; assessing adherence over time; and describing interventions to improve adherence.[122] Diminished treatment adherence has been linked to poor health-related quality of life (HRQOL).[124] As might be expected, discrimination experienced by patients within the health care system has been associated with greater likelihood of nonadherence to physician recommendations. Trust in medical professionals has been found to mediate the discrimination-nonadherence relationship.[125]

Methodology for measuring adherence has advanced. Approximately 20 years ago, the use of computerized pill bottle caps containing microprocessors that monitor the frequency of bottle openings was described.[126] In 17 children, compliance with hydroxyurea was estimated to be 96% and was associated with an increase in HbF from 7.7% to 16.7%. Contemporary studies have taken advantage of the ubiquity of cell phone ownership among parents and older children.[127] In one study, patients with SCA younger than 19 years old who were receiving hydroxyurea at MTD were offered automated daily text message reminders. Subsequently, they were found to have higher MCV, hemoglobin, and HbF levels, thereby reversing waning medication compliance prior to initiation of text messaging. Another study involving cell phone apps surveyed preferences for app features, which were (in order) (1) daily medication reminders, (2) education about SCD, (3) adherence text prompts, (4) education about SCD medications, and (5) a medication log.[128] Recently, an innovative approach has used electronic "directly observed therapy," in which participants submitted daily videos of themselves taking their hydroxyurea associated with electronic reminder alerts, personalized feedback, and incentives to encourage adherence.[129] Using this methodology, participants' use of hydroxyurea, reported as the medication possession ratio (MPR; defined as the ratio of days with medication from a pharmacy divided by the total number of days), improved from 0.75 to 0.91, and the median hydroxyurea adherence was 93%, with increases in both median MCV and HbF.

An "intensive training program" approach to improving adherence has used a mobile health intervention to promote disease knowledge, adherence, and patient-provider communication.[130] The 90-day program involved 3 education modules and tracked adherence through self-reported videos. This resulted in a significantly increased MPR and improved disease knowledge. Still another recent approach has been the use of community health workers who perform support primarily through home visits augmented by daily text message reminders.[131] Preliminary data showed better HbF levels and improved hydroxyurea usage according to pharmacy records.

Two of the programs described earlier have now been associated with improved HRQOL.[132,133] In the first, participants with better adherence perceived more benefits from hydroxyurea, which was positively correlated with HbF and MCV values, in contrast to participants with more negative perceptions, who perceived fewer hydroxyurea benefits and reported worse fatigue, pain, anxiety, and depression.[132] In the second program, subjects evaluated after 6 months of intervention were found to have improved overall HRQOL scores along with better subscale scores for worry, emotions, and communication.[133]

Obviously, monitoring of hydroxyurea treatment requires adherence with clinic appointments, but this may be compromised by socioenvironmental factors.[134] Improved hydroxyurea adherence has been linked to better health care utilization. Good adherence with hydroxyurea, as indicated by an MPR ≥80%, was associated with no readmissions within 30 days of a hospitalization.[135] In contrast, low adherence (along with worse HRQOL scores) was associated with increased health care utilization and more frequent hospitalizations and emergency department visits.[136] Although most data come from pediatric studies, a recent evaluation of adults in 2 large hospital programs found a 62% adherence rate with hydroxyurea usage, indicating a need for interventions to improve preventative care in this population.[137]

In an effort to improve understanding of patients' views regarding hydroxyurea, the Beliefs About Medicine

Questionnaire was used to examine the relationship between beliefs, hydroxyurea adherence, and HRQOL.[138] In 34 adolescents with SCD, concerns about hydroxyurea and the overall harm of medications correlated with anxiety and depression and inversely correlated with peer relationships. Fifty percent of participants reported low hydroxyurea adherence, and this was worse in adolescents with greater concerns about hydroxyurea. Less well studied have been the perspectives of adults with SCD.[139] Patients 18 to 30 years old were more likely to be receiving hydroxyurea than those aged 31 to 67 years (65% vs 41%, respectively; P = .01). The younger patients on hydroxyurea indicated that the decision to start was often made by a parent; they expressed trust in the efficacy of hydroxyurea as well as trust that their physician had adequately shared risks and benefits of the medication. Among the older patients who were not taking hydroxyurea, there was concern that all the risks and benefits of hydroxyurea were not known, that the efficacy of hydroxyurea was not proven, and that they were not receiving complete information about its side effects. It was concluded that age-related differences in adult sickle cell patients' attitudes toward hydroxyurea should inform shared decision making. Of note, a unique report described 36 interviews with physicians who care for patients with SCD.[140] Two possible approaches for treatment-related decision making were described: (1) a "collaborative" approach emphasizing the need to discuss all possible treatment options, and (2) a "proponent" approach characterized by strongly advocating a predetermined treatment plan with the objective of convincing the patient to accept the treatment. These findings point to the potential value of developing systems that foster patient engagement and facilitate shared decision making.

Health Literacy

Health literacy is defined as "the degree to which individuals have the capacity to obtain, process, and understand basic health information and services needed to make appropriate health decisions."[141] Health literacy and numeracy (ability to use numbers and mathematical concepts) are associated with higher levels of health knowledge, more positive health behaviors, and improved clinical outcomes in adults. The Newest Vital Sign self-literacy instrument, when given to adolescents with SCD, takes approximately 5 minutes to administer and was found to be a rapid and reliable snapshot of health literacy levels.[142] Scores were substantially lower in these subjects compared to the scores of healthy adolescents. When parents of children with SCD were asked to assess hypothetical risks associated with hydroxyurea, visual depiction (pie charts, histograms) was superior to abstract numerical material.[143] In a study that assessed "functional health literacy" and disease-specific knowledge of caregivers of children with SCD, those with higher scores had children who had greater annual emergency department utilization and hospitalization, suggesting that knowledgeable caregivers may be better able to recognize illness and more apt to seek professional help.[144] A recent report addressed children with SCA who were not receiving hydroxyurea and who were seen in the emergency department for pain or acute chest syndrome.[145] They were referred to a quick start hydroxyurea initiation program that they attended within a few days. This program included a hematologist-led discussion of hydroxyurea, a video, and an offer to start hydroxyurea immediately. Fifty-five percent of the subjects started hydroxyurea, and 83% of those who started were still receiving hydroxyurea at a median follow-up time of 49 weeks. Overall, the children whose parents attended the quick start program were much more likely to start hydroxyurea than those who did not (53% vs 20%, respectively). A Cochrane review of interventions to improve knowledge of SCD reported an overall slight increase in patient knowledge and a decrease in depression based on 5 trials.[146] Two good examples of available information for lay persons are booklets (both entitled "Hydroxyurea for Sickle Cell Disease") from the American Society of Hematology[147] and from the Children's National Medical Center.

Decision Making and Treatment Initiation

Assessment of the associated risk is a factor in the decisions of parents of children with SCD to use a particular intervention.[148] In a study involving patients with severe SCA, parents received brochures describing the risks and benefits of hydroxyurea, chronic transfusion, and hematopoietic stem cell transplantation (HSCT) and had a face-to-face discussion of those interventions with a nurse educator and then indicated their treatment preferences.[147] Among 40 parents, hydroxyurea was preferred by 70%, chronic transfusion by 17%, and HSCT by 10%, with 3% undecided, reflecting the frequency of interventions in the sickle cell program of the institution. "Efficacy" and "safety of treatment" were the most commonly cited factors in the parents' treatment decisions.[147] In a study of parents of 58 children with SCD regarding acceptable risks associated with hydroxyurea treatment, 50% were unwilling to take any risk at all of hydroxyurea causing cancer and 50% also would not be willing to take any risk of birth defects.[149] Fortunately, these theoretical risks have not been realized. Recently, caregivers of children with clinically severe SCD who had been offered hydroxyurea previously were interviewed.[150] Caregivers who chose hydroxyurea (n = 9) reported their children had severe SCD symptoms; hence, they sought information about hydroxyurea and accepted hydroxyurea as a preventative therapy. In contrast, caregivers who did not choose hydroxyurea (n = 10) did not perceive their children as having severe SCD and did not ask their child's provider about hydroxyurea.

In the 2014 NHLBI clinical guidelines, it was recommended that hydroxyurea be offered to young patients, regardless of clinical severity, through shared decision making between providers and caregivers.[71] To accomplish this, aids that help patients and parents feel empowered to make this decision and help providers feel comfortable in discussing hydroxyurea as a preventive treatment have been developed to facilitate shared discussions between families and providers.[151] Six strategies for providers have been recommended: (1) ask the family to invite all persons involved in the decision to attend a clinic appointment; (2) provide the family education about hydroxyurea use in SCA and/or refer parents to trustworthy internet resources; (3) address safety concerns including an explanation of the package inserts that contain warnings about hydroxyurea usage; (4) mention hydroxyurea as a possible preventive treatment during the child's initial visit with the goal of offering it as a treatment option once the child is 9 months of age or older; (5) plan multiple follow-up conversations about hydroxyurea with parents; and (6) develop a hydroxyurea treatment protocol that includes labs to monitor toxicity and adherence, lab draw intervals, and methods for promoting hydroxyurea adherence. The same authors have developed a hydroxyurea decision aid for parents that provides useful talking points to address their concerns.[152] Despite these recommendations, a recent survey of experienced sickle cell clinicians found that adherence with hydroxyurea counseling was only 72%, most commonly related to a lack of provider agreement with the recommendations or inadequate support staff or time.[153]

The benefits of early treatment initiation through shared decision making have been recently reported. A total of 65 patients were started on hydroxyurea at <5 years of age, with the youngest cohort of 35 started at a mean age of 7.2 months.[154] A remarkably robust response (with no excess toxicity) was seen in the youngest cohort after a mean duration of 31 months of treatment; mean HbF level was 29.9%, and subjects had fewer hospitalizations, pain crises, and transfusions than the slightly older cohorts. Further information regarding initiation of hydroxyurea very early in life is pending from the BABY HUG long-term follow-up studies, the TREAT cohort, and the ongoing multicenter trial of fixed versus MTD dosing of hydroxyurea. Effective strategies for discussing the benefits of hydroxyurea initiation and adherence are needed to address potential barriers and ensure wider usage.

Conclusion

Hydroxyurea is the best-studied, clinically proven, disease-modifying therapy for SCA. Hydroxyurea has been tested in propsective research studies for 35 years, and the overwhelming and compelling body of evidence suggests it is a safe and effective treatment option for both acute and chronic disease complications. The primary mechanism of action is the induction of HbF, which inhibits intracellular sickling, but hydroxyurea has numerous other salutary effects for erythrocytes, leukocytes, inflammatory pathways, and endothelial cells. When used at a daily dose that provides mild marrow supression but without hematologic toxicity, commonly referred to as the MTD, hydroxyurea leads to significant laboratory and clinical improvements. Greater amounts of percent HbF lead to higher F-cell distrubtion and are associated with better outcomes, including prolonged survival. Randomized controlled trials have demonstrated signficiant benefits of hydroxyurea for reduction of acute vaso-occlusive events such as pain crisis and acute chest syndrome, decreases in hospitalizations and transfusions, and management of cerebrovascular disease. Long-term use is safe and effective, with prolonged survival documented in several cohorts. Future research is needed to define the risks and benefits of hydroxyurea for individuals with non-HbSS genotypes, as well as for women during pregnancy and breastfeeding. Early treatment initiation, along with early PK-guided dosing, may offer the opportunity to achieve optimal HbF responses and help prevent chronic organ damage. Improved methods of monitoring and encouraging adherence are needed to reach this goal. The use of hydroxyurea in combination with recently developed antisickling agents warrants further study. Most importantly, hydroxyurea has enormous potential for treatment of SCA in low-resource settings including sub-Saharan Africa, which has the greatest burden of disease.

Case Studies

Case Study 1

A 10-year-old African American boy with HbSS was seen in the sickle cell hematology clinic following a 9-month period of failure to keep clinic appointments. His previous history was remarkable for multiple episodes of acute chest syndrome, 2 of which were severe enough to require intensive care unit admission, intubation, chest tubes, and exchange transfusion. Between ages 6.5 and 9 years, treatment with hydroxyurea at 2 other institutions had been unsuccessful, primarily because of poor adherence with taking the medication. Associated with this was an unstable environment, including a large number of family members in the home, multiple relocations, and school truancy problems.

At the clinic visit, the patient's physical examination was unremarkable except for scleral icterus (related in part to Gilbert syndrome). Laboratory assessment included the following: hemoglobin of 7.9 g/dL; MCV of 84 fL; absolute neutrophil count of 5690/μL; HbF of 9.5%; serum creatinine of 0.33 mg/dL; and, most concerning, a urine microalbumin-to-creatinine ratio (MCR) of 580 mg/g (normal <30 mg/g). At the visit, a nurse practitioner and social worker met with the mother and stepfather and discussed at length the long-term complications of SCD, particularly addressing the patient's risk of chronic damage to the kidneys, lungs, and heart. Following this discussion, the patient was restarted on hydroxyurea at a dose of 23 mg/kg/d with a plan for close follow-up.

On subsequent visits, the patient had the following laboratory results: after 2 months, hemoglobin of 8.7 g/dL, MCV of 89 fL, HbF of 12.7%, and urine MCR of 171 mg/g; after 4 months, hemoglobin of 10.1 g/dL, MCV of 97 fL, HbF of 21.2%,

Case Studies: Continued

and urine MCR of 133 mg/g; and after 6 months, hemoglobin of 9.7 g/dL, MCV of 106 fL, HbF of 23.7%, serum creatinine of 0.33 mg/dL, and urine MCR of 104 mg/g. During this period, the dose of hydroxyurea was increased to 26 mg/kg/d and then 29 mg/kg/d without laboratory toxicity. The patient was also evaluated regularly by a pediatric nephrologist, who recommended addition of an acetylcholinesterase inhibitor if the MCR did not continue to decrease and reach the normal range.

Comments

Poor adherence with hydroxyurea treatment is often a barrier to clinical efficacy, but adherence may be improved by an effective educational approach, as in this patient (see section on adherence). Renal dysfunction is a major cause of morbidity and mortality in the adult with SCD, but it is often heralded in childhood by increased urine MCR; hydroxyurea may be effective in stabilizing or reversing an elevated MCR, particularly in younger patients.[36]

Case Study 2

At age 3 years, an African American girl with HbSS was found to have an abnormal TCD velocity (202 cm/s, right middle cerebral artery) and, after confirmation, was begun on monthly RBC transfusions. After 18 months of good adherence with transfusions, she was enrolled in the TWiTCH study comparing transfusion/iron chelation with hydroxyurea/phlebotomy. She was randomized to the hydroxyurea/phlebotomy arm and received hydroxyurea, beginning at 20 mg/kg/d, with MTD determined to be 25 mg/kg/d after 4 months. Transfusions were gradually tapered and discontinued 6 months after randomization. Therapeutic phlebotomy was initiated at 5 mL/kg and increased 4 weeks later to 10 mL/kg monthly. Hydroxyurea was continued with an eventual dose of 22 mg/kg/d.

During and subsequent to the conversion from chronic transfusion to hydroxyurea, the patient was monitored for iron overload and CNS status. Liver iron content, measured by FerriScan or T2* MRI, gradually decreased from 11.2 mg of iron/g liver tissue to 3.5 mg of iron/g over the course of phlebotomy, which totaled 4700 mL in 3.7 years. Phlebotomy was then discontinued. Initial MRI of the brain did not show evidence of SCIs or stroke, and no new lesions appeared over the course of 6 years of serial monitoring. MRA initially showed mild narrowing of posterior cerebral artery segments, but despite bilateral tortuosity, no significant stenosis developed in any vessels. TCD velocities showed gradual improvement with velocities declining into the high conditional, low conditional, and, most recently, normal range. Neuropsychological assessment revealed mild developmental delay dating back to screening tests at age 3 years. Influential factors may have been "mental disability" in the patient's biologic mother and a history of meconium aspiration at birth. Recent neuropsychological testing showed a full-scale IQ of 68 with impairment in reading and mathematics.

Comment

At present, by far the most common reason for initiating chronic transfusion in children with SCA is the finding of an abnormal velocity on TCD examination, indicating greatly increased risk for stroke. Standard management has been chronic transfusion for an indefinite period, coupled with chelation to limit iron accumulation. However, as this case illustrates, a less burdensome alternative in appropriate patients who have received initial chronic transfusion is the long-term use of hydroxyurea along with a temporary period of iron chelation or phlebotomy.[44] Hydroxyurea may also be valuable in the prevention of worsening of moderately elevated TCD velocities and, when chronic transfusion is not feasible, in the prevention of secondary stroke.[45,50,107]

High-Yield Facts

- ◆ The National Institutes of Health, the American Society of Hematology, and the British Society of Haematology have published evidence-based guidelines recommending the use of hydroxyurea for individuals with SCA.
- ◆ Hydroxyurea should be prescribed to adults with SCA in the following situations:
  - Moderate to severe painful crises
  - Sickle cell–associated pain that interferes with daily activities and quality of life
  - Severe or recurrent acute chest syndrome
  - Severe symptomatic chronic anemia that interferes with daily activities and quality of life
  - Chronic renal disease and taking EPO

High-Yield Facts (Cont.)

◆ Hydroxyurea should be offered to children with SCA after age 9 months to reduce the clinical severity of SCA, regardless of clinical symptoms.

◆ Hydroxyurea should be prescribed with escalation to MTD to optimize daily dosing while minimizing toxicities.

◆ Hydroxyurea has unproven benefits for individuals for non-HbSS genotypes (eg, HbSC and HbS-β⁺ thalassemia) but can be used on a case-by-case basis until prospective randomized controlled trials are conducted.

◆ Hydroxyurea has unproven risks for normal neonates and thus should be discontinued in pregnant or lactating women until more data are collected.

◆ Hydroxyurea has great potential for use in low-resource settings such as sub-Saharan Africa, where transfusions or other treatment options are not safe or readily available.

References

1. Gaston M, Rosse WF. The cooperative study of sickle cell disease: review of study design and objectives. *Am J Pediatr Hematol Oncol.* 1982;4(2):197-201.

2. Mason KP, Grandison Y, Hayes RJ, et al. Post-natal decline of fetal haemoglobin in homozygous sickle cell disease: relationship to parenteral Hb F levels. *Br J Haematol.* 1982;52(3):455-463.

3. Bailey K, Morris JS, Thomas P, Serjeant GR. Fetal haemoglobin and early manifestations of homozygous sickle cell disease. *Arch Dis Child.* 1992;67(4):517-520.

4. Platt OS, Brambilla DJ, Rosse WF, et al. Mortality in sickle cell disease. Life expectancy and risk factors for early death. *N Engl J Med.* 1994;330(23):1639-1644.

5. Platt OS, Thorington BD, Brambilla DJ, et al. Pain in sickle cell disease. Rates and risk factors. *N Engl J Med.* 1991;325(1):11-16.

6. Murray N, Serjeant BE, Serjeant GR. Sickle cell-hereditary persistence of fetal haemoglobin and its differentiation from other sickle cell syndromes. *Br J Haematol.* 1988;69(1):89-92.

7. Dover GJ, Charache SH, Boyer SH, Talbot CC Jr, Smith KD. 5-Azacytidine increases fetal hemoglobin production in a patient with sickle cell disease. *Prog Clin Biol Res.* 1983;134:475-488.

8. Letvin NL, Linch DC, Beardsley GP, McIntyre KW, Nathan DG. Augmentation of fetal-hemoglobin production in anemic monkeys by hydroxyurea. *N Engl J Med.* 1984;310(14):869-873.

9. Platt OS, Orkin SH, Dover G, Beardsley GP, Miller B, Nathan DG. Hydroxyurea enhances fetal hemoglobin production in sickle cell anemia. *J Clin Invest.* 1984;74(2):652-656.

10. Yawn BP, Buchanan GR, Afenyi-Annan AN, et al. Management of sickle cell disease: summary of the 2014 evidence-based report by expert panel members. *JAMA.* 2014;312(10):1033-1048.

11. Kennedy BJ, Yarbro JW. Metabolic and therapeutic effects of hydroxyurea in chronic myeloid leukemia. *JAMA.* 1966;195(12):1038-1043.

12. Mabaera R, West RJ, Conine SJ, et al. A cell stress signaling model of fetal hemoglobin induction: what doesn't kill red blood cells may make them stronger. *Exp Hematol.* 2008;36(9):1057-1072.

13. Cokic VP, Smith RD, Beleslin-Cokic BB, et al. Hydroxyurea induces fetal hemoglobin by the nitric oxide-dependent activation of soluble guanylyl cyclase. *J Clin Invest.* 2003;111(2):231-239.

14. Ikuta T, Ausenda S, Cappellini MD. Mechanism for fetal globin gene expression: role of the soluble guanylate cyclase-cGMP-dependent protein kinase pathway. *Proc Natl Acad Sci U S A.* 2001;98(4):1847-1852.

15. Kinney TR, Helms RW, O'Branski EE, et al. Safety of hydroxyurea in children with sickle cell anemia: results of the HUG-KIDS study, a phase I/II trial. Pediatric Hydroxyurea Group. *Blood.* 1999;94(5):1550-1554.

16. Marcus SJ, Kinney TR, Schultz WH, O'Branski EE, Ware RE. Quantitative analysis of erythrocytes containing fetal hemoglobin (F cells) in children with sickle cell disease. *Am J Hematol.* 1997;54(1):40-46.

17. Gladwin MT, Shelhamer JH, Ognibene FP, et al. Nitric oxide donor properties of hydroxyurea in patients with sickle cell disease. *Br J Haematol.* 2002;116(2):436-444.

18. Lou TF, Singh M, Mackie A, Li W, Pace BS. Hydroxyurea generates nitric oxide in human erythroid cells: mechanisms for gamma-globin gene activation. *Exp Biol Med (Maywood).* 2009;234(11):1374-1382.

19. Odievre MH, Bony V, Benkerrou M, et al. Modulation of erythroid adhesion receptor expression by hydroxyurea in children with sickle cell disease. *Haematologica.* 2008;93(4):502-510.

20. Ware RE. How I use hydroxyurea to treat young patients with sickle cell anemia. *Blood.* 2010;115(26):5300-5311.

21. Kassa T, Wood F, Strader MB, Alayash AI. Antisickling drugs targeting betaCys93 reduce iron oxidation and oxidative changes in sickle cell hemoglobin. *Front Physiol.* 2019;10:931.

22. Nader E, Grau M, Fort R, et al. Hydroxyurea therapy modulates sickle cell anemia red blood cell physiology: impact on RBC deformability, oxidative stress, nitrite levels and nitric oxide synthase signalling pathway. *Nitric Oxide.* 2018;81:28-35.

23. Lebensburger JD, Howard T, Hu Y, et al. Hydroxyurea therapy of a murine model of sickle cell anemia inhibits the progression of pneumococcal disease by down-modulating E-selectin. *Blood.* 2012;119(8):1915-1921.

24. Silva-Pinto AC, Dias-Carlos C, Saldanha-Araujo F, et al. Hydroxycarbamide modulates components involved in the regulation of adenosine levels in blood cells from sickle-cell anemia patients. *Ann Hematol.* 2014;93(9):1457-1465.

25. Almeida CB, Scheiermann C, Jang JE, et al. Hydroxyurea and a cGMP-amplifying agent have immediate benefits on acute vaso-occlusive events in sickle cell disease mice. *Blood.* 2012;120(14):2879-2888.

26. Charache S, Terrin ML, Moore RD, et al. Effect of hydroxyurea on the frequency of painful crises in sickle cell anemia. Investigators of the Multicenter Study of Hydroxyurea in Sickle Cell Anemia. *N Engl J Med.* 1995;332(20):1317-1322.

27. Wang WC, Ware RE, Miller ST, et al. Hydroxycarbamide in very young children with sickle-cell anaemia: a multicentre, randomised, controlled trial (BABY HUG). *Lancet*. 2011;377(9778): 1663-1672.

28. Charache S, Dover GJ, Moore RD, et al. Hydroxyurea: effects on hemoglobin F production in patients with sickle cell anemia. *Blood*. 1992;79(10):2555-2565.

29. Chaturvedi S, Ghafuri DL, Jordan N, Kassim A, Rodeghier M, DeBaun MR. Clustering of end-organ disease and earlier mortality in adults with sickle cell disease: a retrospective-prospective cohort study. *Am J Hematol*. 2018;93(9):1153-1160.

30. Ware RE, Rees RC, Sarnaik SA, et al. Renal function in infants with sickle cell anemia: baseline data from the BABY HUG trial. *J Pediatr*. 2010;156(1):66-70.e61.

31. Rogers ZR, Wang WC, Luo Z, et al. Biomarkers of splenic function in infants with sickle cell anemia: baseline data from the BABY HUG Trial. *Blood*. 2011;117(9):2614-2617.

32. Nottage KA, Ware RE, Winter B, et al. Predictors of splenic function preservation in children with sickle cell anemia treated with hydroxyurea. *Eur J Haematol*. 2014;93(5):377-383.

33. Alvarez O, Miller ST, Wang WC, et al. Effect of hydroxyurea treatment on renal function parameters: results from the multi-center placebo-controlled BABY HUG clinical trial for infants with sickle cell anemia. *Pediatr Blood Cancer*. 2012;59(4):668-674.

34. Fitzhugh CD, Wigfall DR, Ware RE. Enalapril and hydroxyurea therapy for children with sickle nephropathy. *Pediatr Blood Cancer*. 2005;45(7):982-985.

35. Aygun B, Mortier NA, Smeltzer MP, Shulkin BL, Hankins JS, Ware RE. Hydroxyurea treatment decreases glomerular hyperfiltration in children with sickle cell anemia. *Am J Hematol*. 2013;88(2):116-119.

36. Zahr RS, Hankins JS, Kang G, et al. Hydroxyurea prevents onset and progression of albuminuria in children with sickle cell anemia. *Am J Hematol*. 2019;94(1):E27-E29.

37. Tehseen S, Joiner CH, Lane PA, Yee ME. Changes in urine albumin to creatinine ratio with the initiation of hydroxyurea therapy among children and adolescents with sickle cell disease. *Pediatr Blood Cancer*. 2017;64:12.

38. Laurin LP, Nachman PH, Desai PC, Ataga KI, Derebail VK. Hydroxyurea is associated with lower prevalence of albuminuria in adults with sickle cell disease. *Nephrol Dial Transplant*. 2014;29(6):1211-1218.

39. Adams RJ, McKie VC, Hsu L, et al. Prevention of a first stroke by transfusions in children with sickle cell anemia and abnormal results on transcranial Doppler ultrasonography. *N Engl J Med*. 1998;339(1):5-11.

40. Gulbis B, Haberman D, Dufour D, et al. Hydroxyurea for sickle cell disease in children and for prevention of cerebrovascular events: the Belgian experience. *Blood*. 2005;105(7):2685-2690.

41. Lagunju I, Brown BJ, Sodeinde O. Hydroxyurea lowers transcranial Doppler flow velocities in children with sickle cell anaemia in a Nigerian cohort. *Pediatr Blood Cancer*. 2015;62(9):1587-1591.

42. Lefevre N, Dufour D, Gulbis B, Le PQ, Heijmans C, Ferster A. Use of hydroxyurea in prevention of stroke in children with sickle cell disease. *Blood*. 2008;111(2):963-964; author reply 964.

43. Zimmerman SA, Schultz WH, Burgett S, Mortier NA, Ware RE. Hydroxyurea therapy lowers transcranial Doppler flow velocities in children with sickle cell anemia. *Blood*. 2007; 110(3):1043-1047.

44. Ware RE, Davis BR, Schultz WH, et al. Hydroxycarbamide versus chronic transfusion for maintenance of transcranial

Doppler flow velocities in children with sickle cell anaemia—TCD With Transfusions Changing to Hydroxyurea (TWiTCH): a multicentre, open-label, phase 3, non-inferiority trial. *Lancet*. 2016;387(10019):661-670.

45. Hankins JS, McCarville MB, Rankine-Mullings A, et al. Prevention of conversion to abnormal transcranial Doppler with hydroxyurea in sickle cell anemia: a phase III international randomized clinical trial. *Am J Hematol*. 2015;90(12):1099-1105.

46. Ware RE, Helms RW, SWiTCH Investigators. Stroke With Transfusions Changing to Hydroxyurea (SWiTCH). *Blood*. 2012;119(17):3925-3932.

47. de Montalembert M, Brousse V, Elie C, et al. Long-term hydroxyurea treatment in children with sickle cell disease: tolerance and clinical outcomes. *Haematologica*. 2006;91(1):125-128.

48. Greenway A, Ware RE, Thornburg CD. Long-term results using hydroxyurea/phlebotomy for reducing secondary stroke risk in children with sickle cell anemia and iron overload. *Am J Hematol*. 2011;86(4):357-361.

49. Sumoza A, de Bisotti R, Sumoza D, Fairbanks V. Hydroxyurea (HU) for prevention of recurrent stroke in sickle cell anemia (SCA). *Am J Hematol*. 2002;71(3):161-165.

50. Ali SB, Moosang M, King L, Knight-Madden J, Reid M. Stroke recurrence in children with sickle cell disease treated with hydroxyurea following first clinical stroke. *Am J Hematol*. 2011; 86(10):846-850.

51. DeBaun MR, Gordon M, McKinstry RC, et al. Controlled trial of transfusions for silent cerebral infarcts in sickle cell anemia. *N Engl J Med*. 2014;371(8):699-710.

52. Nottage KA, Ware RE, Aygun B, et al. Hydroxycarbamide treatment and brain MRI/MRA findings in children with sickle cell anaemia. *Br J Haematol*. 2016;175(2):331-338.

53. Rigano P, De Franceschi L, Sainati L, et al. Real-life experience with hydroxyurea in sickle cell disease: a multicenter study in a cohort of patients with heterogeneous descent. *Blood Cells Mol Dis*. 2018;69:82-89.

54. Puffer E, Schatz J, Roberts CW. The association of oral hydroxyurea therapy with improved cognitive functioning in sickle cell disease. *Child Neuropsychol*. 2007;13(2):142-154.

55. Gordeuk VR, Campbell A, Rana S, et al. Relationship of erythropoietin, fetal hemoglobin, and hydroxyurea treatment to tricuspid regurgitation velocity in children with sickle cell disease. *Blood*. 2009;114(21):4639-4644.

56. Steinberg MH, McCarthy WF, Castro O, et al. The risks and benefits of long-term use of hydroxyurea in sickle cell anemia: a 17.5 year follow-up. *Am J Hematol*. 2010;85(6):403-408.

57. Wali YA, Moheeb H. Effect of hydroxyurea on physical fitness indices in children with sickle cell anemia. *Pediatr Hematol Oncol*. 2011;28(1):43-50.

58. Narang I, Kadmon G, Lai D, et al. Higher nocturnal and awake oxygen saturations in children with sickle cell disease receiving hydroxyurea therapy. *Ann Am Thorac Soc*. 2015;12(7):1044-1049.

59. Wang WC, Helms RW, Lynn HS, et al. Effect of hydroxyurea on growth in children with sickle cell anemia: results of the HUG-KIDS Study. *J Pediatr*. 2002;140(2):225-229.

60. Rana S, Houston PE, Wang WC, et al. Hydroxyurea and growth in young children with sickle cell disease. *Pediatrics*. 2014;134(3):465-472.

61. Zimmerman SA, Schultz WH, Davis JS, et al. Sustained long-term hematologic efficacy of hydroxyurea at maximum tolerated dose in children with sickle cell disease. *Blood*. 2004;103(6): 2039-2045.

62. Estepp JH, Smeltzer MP, Wang WC, Hoehn ME, Hankins JS, Aygun B. Protection from sickle cell retinopathy is associated with elevated HbF levels and hydroxycarbamide use in children. *Br J Haematol.* 2013;161(3):402-405.

63. Adekile AD, Gupta R, Al-Khayat A, Mohammed A, Atyani S, Thomas D. Risk of avascular necrosis of the femoral head in children with sickle cell disease on hydroxyurea: MRI evaluation. *Pediatr Blood Cancer.* 2019;66(2):e27503.

64. Hankins JS, Penkert RR, Lavoie P, Tang L, Sun Y, Hurwitz JL. Original research: parvovirus B19 infection in children with sickle cell disease in the hydroxyurea era. *Exp Biol Med (Maywood).* 2016;241(7):749-754.

65. Saad ST, Lajolo C, Gilli S, et al. Follow-up of sickle cell disease patients with priapism treated by hydroxyurea. *Am J Hematol.* 2004;77(1):45-49.

66. Voskaridou E, Christoulas D, Bilalis A, et al. The effect of prolonged administration of hydroxyurea on morbidity and mortality in adult patients with sickle cell syndromes: results of a 17-year, single-center trial (LaSHS). *Blood.* 2010;115(12):2354-2363.

67. Fitzhugh CD, Hsieh MM, Allen D, et al. Hydroxyurea-increased fetal hemoglobin is associated with less organ damage and longer survival in adults with sickle cell anemia. *PLoS One.* 2015;10(11):e0141706.

68. Thornburg CD, Dixon N, Burgett S, et al. A pilot study of hydroxyurea to prevent chronic organ damage in young children with sickle cell anemia. *Pediatr Blood Cancer.* 2009;52(5):609-615.

69. Lobo CL, Pinto JF, Nascimento EM, Moura PG, Cardoso GP, Hankins JS. The effect of hydroxcarbamide therapy on survival of children with sickle cell disease. *Br J Haematol.* 2013;161(6):852-860.

70. Le PQ, Gulbis B, Dedeken L, et al. Survival among children and adults with sickle cell disease in Belgium: benefit from hydroxyurea treatment. *Pediatr Blood Cancer.* 2015;62(11):1956-1961.

71. National Institutes of Health. Expert Panel Report. Evidence-based management of sickle cell disease. US Department of Health and Human Services, National Institutes of Health. 2014. https://www.nhlbi.nih.gov/sites/default/files/media/docs/sickle-cell-disease-report%20020816_0.pdf. Accessed July 29, 2020.

72. Qureshi A, Kaya B, Pancham S, et al. Guidelines for the use of hydroxycarbamide in children and adults with sickle cell disease: a British Society for Haematology guideline. *Br J Haematol.* 2018;181(4):460-475.

73. Powars DR, Weiss JN, Chan LS, Schroeder WA. Is there a threshold level of fetal hemoglobin that ameliorates morbidity in sickle cell anemia? *Blood.* 1984;63(4):921-926.

74. Estepp JH, Smeltzer MP, Kang G, et al. A clinically meaningful fetal hemoglobin threshold for children with sickle cell anemia during hydroxyurea therapy. *Am J Hematol.* 2017;92(12):1333-1339.

75. Tshilolo L, Tomlinson G, Williams TN, et al. Hydroxyurea for children with sickle cell anemia in sub-Saharan Africa. *N Engl J Med.* 2019;380(2):121-131.

75a. John CC, Opoka RO, Latham TS, et al. Hydroxyurea dose escalation for sickle cell anemia in Sub-Saharan Africa. *N Engl J Med.* 2020;382(26):2524-2533.

76. Jain DL, Apte M, Colah R, et al. Efficacy of fixed low dose hydroxyurea in Indian children with sickle cell anemia: a single centre experience. *Indian Pediatr.* 2013;50(10):929-933.

77. Patel DK, Mashon RS, Patel S, Das BS, Purohit P, Bishwal SC. Low dose hydroxyurea is effective in reducing the incidence of painful crisis and frequency of blood transfusion in sickle cell anemia patients from eastern India. *Hemoglobin.* 2012;36(5):409-420.

78. Sethy S, Panda T, Jena RK. Beneficial effect of low fixed dose of hydroxyurea in vaso-occlusive crisis and transfusion requirements in adult HbSS patients: a prospective study in a tertiary care center. *Indian J Hematol Blood Transfus.* 2018;34(2):294-298.

79. Sharef SW, Al-Hajri M, Beshlawi I, et al. Optimizing hydroxyurea use in children with sickle cell disease: low dose regimen is effective. *Eur J Haematol.* 2013;90(6):519-524.

80. Svarch E, Machin S, Nieves RM, Mancia de Reyes AG, Navarrete M, Rodriguez H. Hydroxyurea treatment in children with sickle cell anemia in Central America and the Caribbean countries. *Pediatr Blood Cancer.* 2006;47(1):111-112.

81. Akingbola TS, Tayo BO, Ezekekwu CA, et al. "Maximum tolerated dose" vs "fixed low-dose" hydroxyurea for treatment of adults with sickle cell anemia. *Am J Hematol.* 2019;94(4):E112-E115.

82. de Montalembert M, Bachir D, Hulin A, et al. Pharmacokinetics of hydroxyurea 1,000 mg coated breakable tablets and 500 mg capsules in pediatric and adult patients with sickle cell disease. *Haematologica.* 2006;91(12):1685-1688.

83. Rodriguez GI, Kuhn JG, Weiss GR, et al. A bioavailability and pharmacokinetic study of oral and intravenous hydroxyurea. *Blood.* 1998;91(5):1533-1541.

84. Yan JH, Ataga K, Kaul S, et al. The influence of renal function on hydroxyurea pharmacokinetics in adults with sickle cell disease. *J Clin Pharmacol.* 2005;45(4):434-445.

85. Ma Q, Wyszynski DF, Farrell JJ, et al. Fetal hemoglobin in sickle cell anemia: genetic determinants of response to hydroxyurea. *Pharmacogenomics J.* 2007;7(6):386-394.

86. Ware RE, Despotovic JM, Mortier NA, et al. Pharmacokinetics, pharmacodynamics, and pharmacogenetics of hydroxyurea treatment for children with sickle cell anemia. *Blood.* 2011;118(18):4985-4991.

87. McGann PT, Niss O, Dong M, et al. Robust clinical and laboratory response to hydroxyurea using pharmacokinetically guided dosing for young children with sickle cell anemia. *Am J Hematol.* 2019;94(8):871-879.

88. DeSimone J, Heller P, Hall L, Zwiers D. 5-Azacytidine stimulates fetal hemoglobin synthesis in anemic baboons. *Proc Natl Acad Sci U S A.* 1982;79(14):4428-4431.

89. Lettre G, Sankaran VG, Bezerra MA, et al. DNA polymorphisms at the BCL11A, HBS1L-MYB, and beta-globin loci associate with fetal hemoglobin levels and pain crises in sickle cell disease. *Proc Natl Acad Sci U S A.* 2008;105(33):11869-11874.

90. Miller ST, Rey K, He J, et al. Massive accidental overdose of hydroxyurea in a young child with sickle cell anemia. *Pediatr Blood Cancer.* 2012;59(1):170-172.

91. Claster S, Vichinsky E. First report of reversal of organ dysfunction in sickle cell anemia by the use of hydroxyurea: splenic regeneration. *Blood.* 1996;88(6):1951-1953.

92. O'Branski EE, Ware RE, Prose NS, Kinney TR. Skin and nail changes in children with sickle cell anemia receiving hydroxyurea therapy. *J Am Acad Dermatol.* 2001;44(5):859-861.

93. Lederman HM, Connolly MA, Kalpatthi R, et al. Immunologic effects of hydroxyurea in sickle cell anemia. *Pediatrics.* 2014;134(4):686-695.

94. Murphy ML, Chaube S. Preliminary survey of hydroxyurea (Nsc-32065) as a teratogen. *Cancer Chemother Rep.* 1964;40:1-7.

95. Sakano K, Oikawa S, Hasegawa K, Kawanishi S. Hydroxyurea induces site-specific DNA damage via formation of hydrogen peroxide and nitric oxide. *Jpn J Cancer Res.* 2001;92.

96. Ziegler-Skylakakis K, Schwarz LR, Andrae U. Microsome- and hepatocyte-mediated mutagenicity of hydroxyurea and related aliphatic hydroxamic acids in V79 Chinese hamster cells. *Mutat Res.* 1985;152(2-3):225-231.

97. McGann PT, Flanagan JM, Howard TA, et al. Genotoxicity associated with hydroxyurea exposure in infants with sickle cell anemia: results from the BABY-HUG phase III clinical trial. *Pediatr Blood Cancer.* 2012;59(2):254-257.

98. Flanagan JM, Howard TA, Mortier N, et al. Assessment of genotoxicity associated with hydroxyurea therapy in children with sickle cell anemia. *Mutat Res.* 2010;698(1-2):38-42.

99. McGann PT, Howard TA, Flanagan JM, Lahti JM, Ware RE. Chromosome damage and repair in children with sickle cell anaemia and long-term hydroxycarbamide exposure. *Br J Haematol.* 2011;154(1):134-140.

100. Maia Filho PA, Pereira JF, Almeida Filho TP, Cavalcanti BC, Sousa JC, Lemes RPG. Is chronic use of hydroxyurea safe for patients with sickle cell anemia? An account of genotoxicity and mutagenicity. *Environ Mol Mutagen.* 2019;60(3):302-304.

101. Castro O, Nouraie M, Oneal P. Hydroxycarbamide treatment in sickle cell disease: estimates of possible leukaemia risk and of hospitalization survival benefit. *Br J Haematol.* 2014;167(5):687-691.

102. Brunson A, Keegan THM, Bang H, Mahajan A, Paulukonis S, Wun T. Increased risk of leukemia among sickle cell disease patients in California. *Blood.* 2017;130(13):1597-1599.

103. Smith-Whitley K. Reproductive issues in sickle cell disease. *Blood.* 2014;124(24):3538-3543.

104. Ballas SK, McCarthy WF, Guo N, et al. Exposure to hydroxyurea and pregnancy outcomes in patients with sickle cell anemia. *J Natl Med Assoc.* 2009;101(10):1046-1051.

105. Berthaut I, Bachir D, Kotti S, et al. Adverse effect of hydroxyurea on spermatogenesis in patients with sickle cell anemia after 6 months of treatment. *Blood.* 2017;130(21):2354-2356.

106. Opoka RO, Ndugwa CM, Latham TS, et al. Novel use of hydroxyurea in an African region with malaria (NOHARM): a trial for children with sickle cell anemia. *Blood.* 2017;130(24):2585-2593.

107. Galadanci NA, Umar Abdullahi S, Vance LD, et al. Feasibility trial for primary stroke prevention in children with sickle cell anemia in Nigeria (SPIN trial). *Am J Hematol.* 2017;92(8):780-788.

108. Lagunju I, Brown BJ, Oyinlade AO, et al. Annual stroke incidence in Nigerian children with sickle cell disease and elevated TCD velocities treated with hydroxyurea. *Pediatr Blood Cancer.* 2019;66(3):e27252.

109. Steinberg MH. Clinical trials in sickle cell disease: adopting the combination chemotherapy paradigm. *Am J Hematol.* 2008;83(1):1-3.

110. Goldberg MA, Brugnara C, Dover GJ, Schapira L, Charache S, Bunn HF. Treatment of sickle cell anemia with hydroxyurea and erythropoietin. *N Engl J Med.* 1990;323(6):366-372.

111. Rodgers GP, Dover GJ, Uyesaka N, Noguchi CT, Schechter AN, Nienhuis AW. Augmentation by erythropoietin of the fetal-hemoglobin response to hydroxyurea in sickle cell disease. *N Engl J Med.* 1993;328(2):73-80.

112. Little JA, McGowan VR, Kato GJ, et al. Combination erythropoietin-hydroxyurea therapy in sickle cell disease: experience from the National Institutes of Health and a literature review. *Haematologica.* 2006;91(8):1076-1083.

113. Wang W, Brugnara C, Snyder C, et al. The effects of hydroxycarbamide and magnesium on haemoglobin SC disease: results of the multi-centre CHAMPS trial. *Br J Haematol.* 2011;152(6):771-776.

114. Orringer EP, Casella JF, Ataga KI, et al. Purified poloxamer 188 for treatment of acute vaso-occlusive crisis of sickle cell disease: a randomized controlled trial. *JAMA.* 2001;286(17):2099-2106.

115. Little JA, Hauser KP, Martyr SE, et al. Hematologic, biochemical, and cardiopulmonary effects of L-arginine supplementation or phosphodiesterase 5 inhibition in patients with sickle cell disease who are on hydroxyurea therapy. *Eur J Haematol.* 2009;82(4):315-321.

116. Ataga KI, Reid M, Ballas SK, et al. Improvements in haemolysis and indicators of erythrocyte survival do not correlate with acute vaso-occlusive crises in patients with sickle cell disease: a phase III randomized, placebo-controlled, double-blind study of the Gardos channel blocker senicapoc (ICA-17043). *Br J Haematol.* 2011;153(1):92-104.

117. Heeney MM, Hoppe CC, Abboud MR, et al. A multinational trial of prasugrel for sickle cell vaso-occlusive events. *N Engl J Med.* 2016;374(7):625-635.

118. Telen MJ, Wun T, McCavit TL, et al. Randomized phase 2 study of GMI-1070 in SCD: reduction in time to resolution of vaso-occlusive events and decreased opioid use. *Blood.* 2015;125(17):2656-2664.

119. Field JJ, Majerus E, Gordeuk VR, et al. Randomized phase 2 trial of regadenoson for treatment of acute vaso-occlusive crises in sickle cell disease. *Blood Adv.* 2017;1(20):1645-1649.

120. Niihara Y, Miller ST, Kanter J, et al. A phase 3 trial of l-glutamine in sickle cell disease. *N Engl J Med.* 2018;379(3):226-235.

121. Howard J, Hemmaway CJ, Telfer P, et al. A phase 1/2 ascending dose study and open-label extension study of voxelotor in patients with sickle cell disease. *Blood.* 2019;133(17):1865-1875.

122. Loiselle K, Lee JL, Szulczewski L, Drake S, Crosby LE, Pai AL. Systematic and meta-analytic review: medication adherence among pediatric patients with sickle cell disease. *J Pediatr Psychol.* 2016;41(4):406-418.

123. Walsh KE, Cutrona SL, Kavanagh PL, et al. Medication adherence among pediatric patients with sickle cell disease: a systematic review. *Pediatrics.* 2014;134(6):1175-1183.

124. Fisak B, Belkin MH, von Lehe AC, Bansal MM. The relation between health-related quality of life, treatment adherence and disease severity in a paediatric sickle cell disease sample. *Child Care Health Dev.* 2012;38(2):204-210.

125. Haywood C Jr, Lanzkron S, Bediako S, et al. Perceived discrimination, patient trust, and adherence to medical recommendations among persons with sickle cell disease. *J Gen Intern Med.* 2014;29(12):1657-1662.

126. Olivieri NF, Vichinsky EP. Hydroxyurea in children with sickle cell disease: impact on splenic function and compliance with therapy. *J Pediatr Hematol Oncol.* 1998;20(1):26-31.

127. Estepp JH, Winter B, Johnson M, Smeltzer MP, Howard SC, Hankins JS. Improved hydroxyurea effect with the use of text messaging in children with sickle cell anemia. *Pediatr Blood Cancer.* 2014;61(11):2031-2036.

128. Badawy SM, Thompson AA, Liem RI. Technology access and smartphone app preferences for medication adherence in adolescents and young adults with sickle cell disease. *Pediatr Blood Cancer.* 2016;63(5):848-852.

129. Creary SE, Gladwin MT, Byrne M, Hildesheim M, Krishnamurti L. A pilot study of electronic directly observed therapy to improve hydroxyurea adherence in pediatric patients with sickle-cell disease. *Pediatr Blood Cancer.* 2014;61(6):1068-1073.

130. Anderson LM, Leonard S, Jonassaint J, Lunyera J, Bonner M, Shah N. Mobile health intervention for youth with sickle cell disease: impact on adherence, disease knowledge, and quality of life. *Pediatr Blood Cancer.* 2018;65(8):e27081.

131. Green NS, Manwani D, Matos S, et al. Randomized feasibility trial to improve hydroxyurea adherence in youth ages 10-18 years through community health workers: the HABIT study. *Pediatr Blood Cancer.* 2017;64(12):10.1002/pbc.26689.

132. Badawy SM, Thompson AA, Lai JS, Penedo FJ, Rychlik K, Liem RI. Adherence to hydroxyurea, health-related quality of life domains, and patients' perceptions of sickle cell disease and hydroxyurea: a cross-sectional study in adolescents and young adults. *Health Qual Life Outcomes.* 2017;15(1):136.

133. Smaldone A, Findley S, Manwani D, Jia H, Green NS. HABIT, a randomized feasibility trial to increase hydroxyurea adherence, suggests improved health-related quality of life in youths with sickle cell disease. *J Pediatr.* 2018;197:177-185.e172.

134. Ingerski LM, Arnold TL, Banks G, Porter JS, Wang WC. Clinic attendance of youth with sickle cell disease on hydroxyurea treatment. *J Pediatr Hematol Oncol.* 2017;39(5):345-349.

135. Zhou J, Han J, Nutescu EA, Gordeuk VR, Saraf SL, Calip GS. Hydroxycarbamide adherence and cumulative dose associated with hospital readmission in sickle cell disease: a 6-year population-based cohort study. *Br J Haematol.* 2018;182(2):259-270.

136. Badawy SM, Thompson AA, Holl JL, Penedo FJ, Liem RI. Healthcare utilization and hydroxyurea adherence in youth with sickle cell disease. *Pediatr Hematol Oncol.* 2018;35(5-6):297-308.

137. Ter-Minassian M, Lanzkron S, Derus A, Brown E, Horberg MA. Quality metrics and health care utilization for adult patients with sickle cell disease. *J Natl Med Assoc.* 2019;111(1):54-61.

138. Badawy SM, Thompson AA, Liem RI. Beliefs about hydroxyurea in youth with sickle cell disease. *Hematol Oncol Stem Cell Ther.* 2018;11(3):142-148.

139. Sinha CB, Bakshi N, Ross D, Krishnamurti L. From trust to skepticism: an in-depth analysis across age groups of adults with sickle cell disease on their perspectives regarding hydroxyurea. *PLoS One.* 2018;13(6):e0199375.

140. Bakshi N, Sinha CB, Ross D, Khemani K, Loewenstein G, Krishnamurti L. Proponent or collaborative: Physician perspectives and approaches to disease modifying therapies in sickle cell disease. *PLoS One.* 2017;12(7):e0178413.

141. Perry EL, Carter PA, Becker HA, Garcia AA, Mackert M, Johnson KE. Health literacy in adolescents with sickle cell disease. *J Pediatr Nurs.* 2017;36:191-196.

142. Caldwell EP, Carter P, Becker H, Mackert M. The use of the newest vital sign health literacy instrument in adolescents with sickle cell disease. *J Pediatr Oncol Nurs.* 2018;35(5):361-367.

143. Patterson CA, Barakat LP, Henderson PK, et al. Comparing abstract numerical and visual depictions of risk in survey of parental assessment of risk in sickle hydroxyurea treatment. *J Pediatr Hematol Oncol.* 2011;33(1):4-9.

144. Carden MA, Newlin J, Smith W, Sisler I. Health literacy and disease-specific knowledge of caregivers for children with sickle cell disease. *Pediatr Hematol Oncol.* 2016;33(2):121-133.

145. Pecker LH, Kappa S, Greenfest A, Darbari DS, Nickel RS. Targeted hydroxyurea education after an emergency department visit increases hydroxyurea use in children with sickle cell anemia. *J Pediatr.* 2018;201:221-228.e216.

146. Asnani MR, Quimby KR, Bennett NR, Francis DK. Interventions for patients and caregivers to improve knowledge of sickle cell disease and recognition of its related complications. *Cochrane Database Syst Rev.* 2016;10:CD011175.

147. American Society of Hematology. Hydroxyurea for sickle cell disease. Treatment information from the American Society of Hematology. https://www.in.gov/isdh/files/con_SCD_ASH_Hydroxyurea.pdf. Accessed July 29, 2020.

148. Hankins J, Hinds P, Day S, et al. Therapy preference and decision-making among patients with severe sickle cell anemia and their families. *Pediatr Blood Cancer.* 2007;48(7):705-710.

149. Meyappan JD, Lampl M, Hsu LL. Parents' assessment of risk in sickle cell disease treatment with hydroxyurea. *J Pediatr Hematol Oncol.* 2005;27(12):644-650.

150. Creary S, Zickmund S, Ross D, Krishnamurti L, Bogen DL. Hydroxyurea therapy for children with sickle cell disease: describing how caregivers make this decision. *BMC Res Notes.* 2015;8:372.

151. Crosby LE, Shook LM, Ware RE, Brinkman WB. Shared decision making for hydroxyurea treatment initiation in children with sickle cell anemia. *Pediatr Blood Cancer.* 2015;62(2):184-185.

152. Crosby LE, Walton A, Shook LM, et al. Development of a hydroxyurea decision aid for parents of children with sickle cell anemia. *J Pediatr Hematol Oncol.* 2019;41(1):56-63.

153. Cabana MD, Kanter J, Marsh AM, et al. Barriers to pediatric sickle cell disease guideline recommendations. *Glob Pediatr Health.* 2019;6:2333794X19847026.

154. Schuchard SB, Lissick JR, Nickel A, et al. Hydroxyurea use in young infants with sickle cell disease. *Pediatr Blood Cancer.* 2019;66(7):e27650.

155. Hankins JS, Helton KJ, McCarville MB, Li CS, Wang WC, Ware RE. Preservation of spleen and brain function in children with sickle cell anemia treated with hydroxyurea. *Pediatr Blood Cancer.* 2008;50(2):293-297.

156. Santos A, Pinheiro V, Anjos C, et al. Scintigraphic follow-up of the effects of therapy with hydroxyurea on splenic function in patients with sickle cell disease. *Eur J Nucl Med Mol Imaging.* 2002;29(4):536-541.

157. Harrod VL, Howard TA, Zimmerman SA, Dertinger SD, Ware RE. Quantitative analysis of Howell-Jolly bodies in children with sickle cell disease. *Exp Hematol.* 2007;35(2):179-183.

158. Thompson J, Reid M, Hambleton I, Serjeant GR. Albuminuria and renal function in homozygous sickle cell disease: observations from a cohort study. *Arch Intern Med.* 2007;167(7):701-708.

159. McKie KT, Hanevold CD, Hernandez C, Waller JL, Ortiz L, McKie KM. Prevalence, prevention, and treatment of microalbuminuria and proteinuria in children with sickle cell disease. *J Pediatr Hematol Oncol.* 2007;29(3):140-144.

160. Kratovil T, Bulas D, Driscoll MC, Speller-Brown B, McCarter R, Minniti CP. Hydroxyurea therapy lowers TCD velocities in children with sickle cell disease. *Pediatr Blood Cancer.* 2006;47(7):894-900.

161. Bernaudin F, Verlhac S, Arnaud C, et al. Impact of early transcranial Doppler screening and intensive therapy on cerebral vasculopathy outcome in a newborn sickle cell anemia cohort. *Blood.* 2011;117(4):1130-1140; quiz 1436.

162. Rushton T, Aban I, Young D, Howard T, Hilliard L, Lebensburger J. Hydroxycarbamide for patients with silent cerebral infarcts: outcomes and patient preference. *Br J Haematol.* 2018;181(1):145-148.

163. Singh SA, Koumbourlis AC, Aygun B. Resolution of chronic hypoxemia in pediatric sickle cell patients after treatment with hydroxyurea. *Pediatr Blood Cancer.* 2008;50(6):1258-1260.

164. Pashankar FD, Manwani D, Lee MT, Green NS. Hydroxyurea improves oxygen saturation in children with sickle cell disease. *J Pediatr Hematol Oncol.* 2015;37(3):242-243.

165. Buckner TW, Ataga KI. Does hydroxyurea prevent pulmonary complications of sickle cell disease? *Hematology Am Soc Hematol Educ Program.* 2014;2014(1):432-437.

166. Parent F, Bachir D, Inamo J, et al. A hemodynamic study of pulmonary hypertension in sickle cell disease. *N Engl J Med.* 2011;365(1):44-53.

167. Anele UA, Mack AK, Resar LMS, Burnett AL. Hydroxyurea therapy for priapism prevention and erectile function recovery in sickle cell disease: a case report and review of the literature. *Int Urol Nephrol.* 2014;46(9):1733-1736.

168. Mahadeo KM, Oyeku S, Taragin B, et al. Increased prevalence of osteonecrosis of the femoral head in children and adolescents with sickle-cell disease. *Am J Hematol.* 2011;86(9):806-808.

169. Adesina O, Brunson A, Keegan THM, Wun T. Osteonecrosis of the femoral head in sickle cell disease: prevalence, comorbidities, and surgical outcomes in California. *Blood Adv.* 2017;1(16):1287-1295.

170. Karacaoglu PK, Asma S, Korur A, et al. East Mediterranean region sickle cell disease mortality trial: retrospective multicenter cohort analysis of 735 patients. *Ann Hematol.* 2016;95(6):993-1000.

171. Ferster A, Vermylen C, Cornu G, et al. Hydroxyurea for treatment of severe sickle cell anemia: a pediatric clinical trial. *Blood.* 1996;88(6):1960-1964.

172. Wang WC, Wynn LW, Rogers ZR, Scott JP, Lane PA, Ware RE. A two-year pilot trial of hydroxyurea in very young children with sickle-cell anemia. *J Pediatr.* 2001;139(6):790-796.

173. Ferster A, Tahriri P, Vermylen C, et al. Five years of experience with hydroxyurea in children and young adults with sickle cell disease. *Blood.* 2001;97(11):3628-3632.

174. Hankins JS, Ware RE, Rogers ZR, et al. Long-term hydroxyurea therapy for infants with sickle cell anemia: the HUSOFT extension study. *Blood.* 2005;106(7):2269-2275.

175. Ware RE, Aygun B. Advances in the use of hydroxyurea. *Hematology Am Soc Hematol Educ Program.* 2009:62-69.

176. Ataga KI, Kutlar A, Kanter J, et al. Crizanlizumab for the prevention of pain crises in sickle cell disease. *N Engl J Med.* 2017;376(5):429-439.

177. Vichinsky E, Hoppe CC, Ataga KI, et al. A phase 3 randomized trial of voxelotor in sickle cell disease. *N Engl J Med.* 2019;381(6):509-519.

The Burden of the Sickle Cell Gene in India

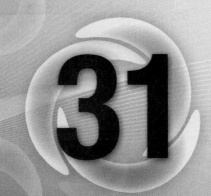

Authors: *Yazdi Italia, Dipty Jain, Roshan Colah,*
Khushnooma Italia

Chapter Outline

Overview

The burden of sickle cell disease (SCD) in India is high. SCD is widespread not only among the indigenous populations but also among the scheduled castes and other backward classes. The sickle gene is linked to the Asian haplotype with high fetal hemoglobin (HbF) levels, but SCD patients have an extremely diverse clinical presentation in different regions of the country. The frequency of associated α thalassemia is variable in different populations, and this also modulates the severity of the disease. The main causes of morbidity are acute or chronic painful events, infections, and anemia. The spectrum of bacterial infections in Indian SCD patients is different from African cohorts; *Staphylococcus aureus*, *Salmonella*, *Klebsiella*, and *Escherichia coli* are more commonly seen. Fixed low-dose hydroxyurea therapy has been effective in Indian patients; however, compliance, availability of the drug, and accessibility are some of the constraints. The Gujarat SCD control program has served as a model for community screening using solubility test and high-performance liquid chromatography (HPLC) analysis followed by counseling and prenatal diagnosis in different states. Some challenges include limited awareness and late registration in antenatal clinics. Newborn screening programs have been introduced relatively recently in a few states, and follow-up of birth cohorts will help to understand the natural history of SCD in India. Curative options such as hematopoietic stem cell transplantation are not easily available to these economically disadvantaged populations due to the high cost and lack of suitable donors. Different government initiatives are also supporting care and control programs, and these should lead to a national registry of SCD patients in India.

Introduction

In India, the sickle cell gene was first reported among the hill tribes of northern Tamil Nadu in 1952.[1] There followed a debate as to whether there had been a single origin of the sickle cell mutation with subsequent migration into Equatorial Africa, Saudi Arabia, and India or whether there had been several independent occurrences of the sickle cell gene. Analyzing polymorphisms on the β-globin gene cluster surrounding the sickle hemoglobin (HbS) gene locus has discerned patterns believed to represent ancestral DNA structures upon which the HbS mutation has occurred relatively recently. These patterns are referred to as β-globin haplotypes, and there are at least 3 African haplotypes named after the areas where they were first described—the Benin, Senegal, and Bantu (or Central African Republic) haplotypes.[2] The β-globin gene flanking the HbS locus in eastern Saudi Arabia and in India has a different structure not seen in African populations and is believed to represent a fourth independent occurrence of the HbS mutation, the Arab-Indian or Asian haplotype.[3] However, the most recent evidence using whole-genome sequencing data points to a single origin of the sickle allele approximately 7300 years ago during the Holocene Wet Phase or Green Sahara.[4] The Asian haplotype associated with higher fetal hemoglobin levels and variable disease severity is now recognized to account for the majority of the cases of the disease in India and also the Eastern Province of Saudi Arabia.[5]

Extent of the Burden

The fact that the first report of the HbS gene in India was among tribal people led to the misconception that the HbS gene was confined to indigenous populations. However, later experience has indicated that the gene is also widespread among other economically disadvantaged groups, the scheduled castes, and other backward classes. Approximately 300 population groups have been screened, and the prevalence of sickle cell carriers

(HbAS) varies from 1% to 35%[6-16] (Figure 31-1). The highest predicted frequencies of sickle homozygous (HbSS) cases are in central India.[16]

Apart from the HbS gene, India houses many other structural hemoglobin variants such as HbE, HbD Punjab, HbD Iran, HbQ India, Hb Lepore, and HbJ, along with thalassemias such as β thalassemia, α thalassemia, δβ thalassemia, and hereditary persistence of fetal hemoglobin. The prevalence of β thalassemia is around 3% to 17% in different caste groups.[17] Thus, the prevalence of double heterozygotes for HbS-β thalassemia is high in some regions.[18]

Clinical Presentation of the Disease in India

SCD patients in India have a diverse clinical presentation, and severity of SCD varies by region. The possibility that some individuals with severe disease may have died before diagnosis or reaching a health care facility cannot be ruled out. However, many patients, particularly among the tribal groups from Orissa in the east, the Nilgiris in the south, and Gujarat in the west, have an unusually mild clinical presentation similar to that described earlier in the Eastern Province of Saudi Arabia.[5,8,19-21] Often, children are diagnosed with SCD when they present with severe complications. After diagnosis, many are lost to follow-up due to illiteracy and poverty and commonly present to emergency medical services. Furthermore, basic facilities including drugs for management are not readily available at many Indian centers, adding to the challenge faced by those living with the disease.[22]

Clinical Heterogenicity

Even though the genotype is the same, there is considerable diversity in manifestations of SCD, leading to extremely diverse clinical features. The presence of the Arab-Indian haplotype with higher HbF levels and co-inheritance of α thalassemia are known to modulate the clinical severity of the disease. Generally, painful events, infections, and anemia are the 3 most common causes of morbidity in SCD patients in India.[22]

Acute Painful Episodes

Pain is the hallmark clinical feature of SCD and presents as acute, chronic, or neuropathic. An acute episode in infants presents as dactylitis, and both children and adults have pain affecting bones in the extremities, chest, and back. Nonsteroidal anti-inflammatory drugs provide relief during acute episodes. Currently, there is a shift from treating pain to preventing pain episodes by early and rapid treatment. Twenty-five percent of patients will have chronic pain, with avascular necrosis of the bone being the main underlying pathology. Neuropathic pain is seen in around 30% of adults and presents as tingling, numbness, pins-and-needle sensation, and hyperalgesia. The latter is treated with drugs such as gabapentin.[23]

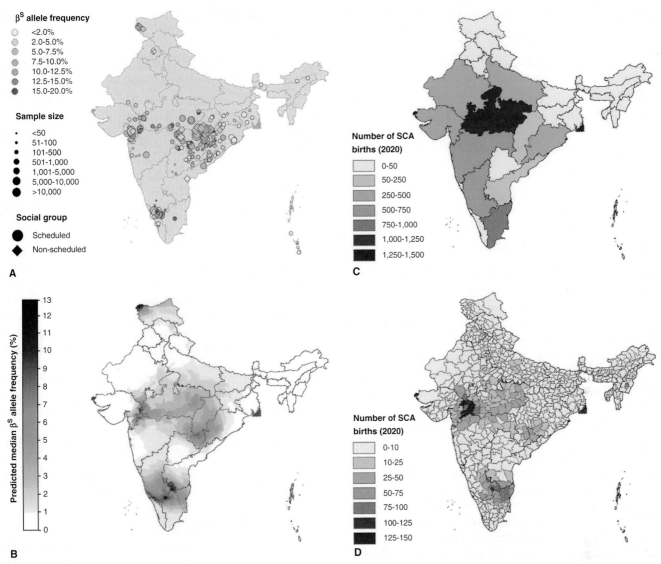

FIGURE 31-1 A map of the sickle-cell surveys included in our database (n = 249). Data points are colored according to the β^S allele frequency reported in the study sample. The size of the data points relates to their sample size. A spatial jitter of up to 0.3° latitude and longitude decimal degrees coordinates was applied to improve visualisation of the data (**A**). Map of median predicted β^S allele frequency estimates at a resolution of 10 km x 10 km (**B**). State boundaries are displayed in dark gray. Map of the estimated number of scheduled newborns born with SCA in India by state (**C**) and by district (**D**), in 2020. The medians of the predictive probability distribution of the areal estimates are displayed. The district shaded gray in Tamil Nadu in (**D**) is where the 95% CI was very large (>1000). State boundaries are displayed in dark gray and district boundaries in light gray.

Dactylitis

Dactylitis, or hand-foot syndrome, is often the first manifestation of SCD and manifests as symmetric or unilateral swelling of the hands and/or feet. Although in a Jamaican and Guadeloupe cohort, 50% of children had dactylitis by 2 years, the prevalence is highly variable in India, being lowest in Gujarat (1 of 32 patients by 1.5-5 years), moderate in Nagpur in Maharashtra (8.8 per 100 person-years), and highest in Chhattisgarh (up to 25%; personal communication by P.K. Patra).[22]

Bacterial Infections

SCD with fever in a child is an emergency suggesting infection and can happen as early as 6 months of age due to splenic dysfunction. Infections are one of the most common causes of hospitalization in children with SCD in India. The spectrum of bacterial infections is different in Indian cohorts and African cohorts. The most common infections in the Indian cohort include *S aureus* (60%), *Salmonella* (18%), *Klebsiella* (10%), and *E coli* (5%). Both the implementation of regular penicillin prophylaxis and other local factors such as climatic conditions, socioeconomic status, nutritional status, and pollution may influence the observed bacterial pattern in the Indian subcontinent. In addition, resistance to β-lactams is highly prevalent among both gram-positive and gram-negative bacteria, which can be attributed to the irrational use of antibiotics in children with SCD. There is also a significant correlation between seasonal variation and incidence of hospitalization. The peak incidence is during the monsoon season, which could be due to the high prevalence of waterborne infections during this season.[22] Interestingly, the peak for all crises in SCD is also during the monsoon months.

Anemia

Unlike in Western countries, anemia in Indian children with SCD is multifactorial. Additional contributory factors, such as nutrition, infections, and parasitic infestations, should be considered. Deficiency of essential micronutrients (eg, vitamin A, iron, and iodine) and macronutrients from malnutrition is common in children with SCD and aggravates the magnitude of anemia and overall disease status. A significant number of patients from different tribes in India were found to be iron deficient. Identifying the treatable causes of anemia is of utmost importance in a developing country such as India due to the unavailability of and safety issues concerned with blood transfusions.[24] However, aplastic crisis is less common in Indian children with SCD. HbS-β thalassemia and HbSD disease, which are common in many regions of India, are often associated with severe anemia requiring more frequent blood transfusions. Chronic hypersplenism presents with marked anemia, gross splenomegaly, and growth retardation due to red blood cell sequestration in the spleen. It usually occurs between 5 and 15 years of age and is associated with a gradual lowering of hemoglobin below the steady-state levels over a period of a few months.

Acute Chest Syndrome

There are variable reports on the prevalence (0-23 cases per 100 person-years) of acute chest syndrome (ACS) in Indian SCD patients. These data are usually confounded by the high prevalence of lower respiratory tract infections, especially in young children. Most patients do not have a single identifiable cause of ACS, and hence, the recommended treatment is also multimodal. Prophylactic use of a spirometer has helped in preventing ACS.[22]

Stroke

There is a varied presentation of neurologic complications in SCD ranging from overt stroke to silent infarcts. It is not uncommon to diagnose SCD after an episode of stroke in India.[1] Almost 5% of children with SCD suffer from stroke in central India, an incidence similar to that reported in African cohorts. However, certain parts of western India, such as Gujarat, have a lower prevalence of stroke. A pilot study in central India showed the feasibility of transcranial Doppler (TCD) screening in the Indian population; one-fourth of the patients were found to have abnormal TCD results.[25]

Priapism and Leg Ulcers

Priapism and leg ulcers are rare in SCD patients from Maharashtra, Odisha, and Gujarat. However, they are common in Chhattisgarh, where around 15% of patients have at least 1 episode of priapism by 20 years of age and 15% have leg ulcers by young adulthood.[22]

Avascular Necrosis

Avascular necrosis (AVN) occurs in approximately 10% of SCD children by the second decade and is a source of both acute and chronic pain. Most often, the femoral head is affected, but the humeral head and mandible can also be involved. The burden of AVN is significant in young adults from Odisha. In the Indian setting, hip pain is often misattributed to a simple painful event; thus, investigations are often delayed, leading to complications of AVN.[22]

Splenomegaly

In patients with SCD from India, the spleen is larger and preserved for a longer duration. Even during the second decade of life, a total of 71.4% of patients continue to have splenomegaly. This is more common in HbS-β thalassemia (82.6%) than in sickle cell anemia (SCA) patients (68.8%). This partly explains the higher transfusion rates in patients with HbS-β thalassemia, who can have acute splenic sequestration events throughout adolescence and adulthood.[22] Although most parents of children with SCD in India are from a low socioeconomic status with low literacy levels, parental education in regular measurements of the spleen and detection of pallor may be an effective way to detect sequestration early in their children.

Renal Involvement

Renal disease in SCD is a major comorbid condition leading to premature death. It may present with hematuria, proteinuria, renal insufficiency, concentrating defects, and hypertension. In a large prospective study from central India, renal function was assessed in 616 patients with SCD (507 with SCA and 109 with HbS-β thalassemia). This study revealed glomerular hyperfiltration in 16% of SCA patients and 10.1% of HbS-β thalassemia patients.[22] Screening for microalbuminuria is important in patients with SCD for early identification and intervention to prevent rapid progression to renal disease. In an ongoing study at Government Medical College, Nagpur, screening of 150 patients with SCD age 5 to 20 years was performed and revealed a 15.3% prevalence of microalbuminuria and 2% prevalence of macroalbuminuria.

Pregnancy Outcome

A community-based hospital study on pregnancy outcomes in a tribal block of Gujarat found that among SCD admissions, 9.9% had stillbirths, compared to 4.4% in sickle cell trait pregnancies and 3.6% in non-SCD pregnancies. The odds ratio of low birth weight and preterm delivery was 3 times higher in SCD than in non-SCD pregnancies.[26]

Adoption of Hydroxyurea in India

Hydroxyurea (HU) was the first and only disease-modifying agent in SCD patients for decades. A safety and feasibility trial in children with SCA showed that HU was safe and well tolerated in children >5 years of age. Current recommendations are that all children with SCA should be offered HU beginning at 9 months of age. HU has been effective in decreasing painful episodes, blood transfusion requirements, and rate of hospitalizations. No clinical adverse effects were identified, and the primary toxicity related to myelosuppression reversed on cessation of the drug. The long-term toxicity of HU in very young children has not yet been established. However, significant obstacles, such as adherence, availability, and accessibility of the drug, follow-up, and monitoring, were encountered. Five studies from India have reported that a fixed low dose of HU (10-15 mg/kg/d) without dose escalation is as effective as the recommended schedule.[22] Fixed low-dose HU may be advantageous in low-resource settings because of lower toxicity with less need for monitoring.[27] Because India is a diverse country with different states following different protocols, a universally acceptable protocol has also been designed and is under study. According to this protocol, HU is started at 10 mg/kg/d for 6 weeks, and then patients' clinical outcome and toxicities are monitored. If there is 75% improvement in the patient's clinical outcome, the same dose of HU is continued. However, if no improvement is noted, the dose can be escalated by 5 mg/kg/d and monitored every 6 months until a maximum dose of 30 mg/kg/d.[22] Unfortunately, there are barriers to the adoption of HU, including physician concerns about long-term mutagenic effects and lack of familiarity of primary care providers with the use of chemotherapeutic agents. Despite these hurdles, HU is frequently used for patients with SCD in India, and it has been incorporated in the National Health Mission (NHM) guidelines as part of management of severe SCD cases[28]; many patients are on HU with regular follow-up and no adverse side effects.[29]

Regional Heterogeneity of SCD in India

In a study conducted by Italia et al[30] on 77 clinically severe patients from the Mahar, Nav Buddha, and Kunbi caste groups (nontribal) residing in Maharashtra and Madhya Pradesh, where the disease manifestations are most severe, all patients had severe vaso-occlusive episodes (3-12 episodes per year), and 80% needed hospitalization due to severe pain from 1 to >5 times per year. Fifty-three percent of patients (42 of 77 patients) had been occasionally transfused, whereas 19.5% required 3 to 5 transfusions per year to maintain hemoglobin levels of >7.0 g/dL, and one patient was transfusion dependent. Almost 6.5% of patients reported ACS once in their lifetime, whereas 15.6% of patients had stroke and 9.1% had AVN of the femoral head. Splenomegaly, diagnosed as a palpable spleen between 3 and 7 cm below the costal margin, was seen in 44% of patients. Many patients had more than one type of complication during their lifetime, of which vaso-occlusive episode was the most common.[30] Other commonly seen clinical conditions were hand-foot syndrome and infections in children <5 years of age. Mortality was reported in 2 patients.

Jain et al[31] reported on 144 clinically severe patients from Nagpur, Maharashtra. Of these patients, 78.5% had severe vaso-occlusive episodes >3 times per year, whereas 5% of them had both vaso-occlusive episodes and transfusion requirements due to severe anemia. Almost 8% of patients had an episode of stroke along with vaso-occlusive episode. ACS was reported among 4% of the patients, and 6.5% had splenic sequestration crisis. Blood transfusion requirements were common in 11.7% of patients and were required >3 times per year. Stroke was observed in 1.3% of patients, whereas leg ulcers and priapism were rarely seen.[31]

Sethy et al[32] reported on the clinical presentation of patients from Cuttack, Odisha, where of the 128 clinically severe patients, 64% presented with repeat vaso-occlusive episodes, 13% had regular transfusion requirements, and 23% presented with both of these complications.

In Gujarat, the most common clinical findings in SCD patients are frequent vaso-occlusive episodes, infection, severe anemia leading to blood transfusion requirements, stroke, ACS, AVN, hand-foot syndrome, and, in children <5 years old, frequent infections. Chronic renal failure is rarely observed. The symptoms less commonly seen are leg ulcers and priapism. Nearly 20% of pregnancies are complicated by severe preeclampsia, eclampsia, intrauterine growth retardation, intrauterine fetal death, anemia, ACS, and painful crisis.[29] Retarded growth is seen in 60% to 70% of patients, as shown in Figure 31-2, where a child with HbSS can be seen to be much shorter than his dizygotic twin sister with HbAA.

A Case Study: The Gujarat Experience

The state of Gujarat, with a population of approximately 60 million people, is in western India. Negi[33] reported the incidence of HbS in the tribal belt of the Gujarat-Maharashtra border areas in 1972. However, the first patient, a tribal individual from the south Gujarat area, was diagnosed with SCD in 1978 and is still alive in 2019 with overall good health (Figure 31-3).

The Sickle Cell Anemia Control Program was initiated in fiscal year 2005-2006 in southern Gujarat (because of the high prevalence of the gene in this area) with the aims to improve the health status of SCD patients and to reduce morbidity and mortality. The initial goals of the program were to organize screening programs, create infrastructure for early diagnosis including molecular analysis, initiate genetic counseling services, and prevent the birth of children with SCD by marriage counseling and prenatal diagnosis. Later, the program was extended to all tribal areas of Gujarat. The program was established as a public-private partnership joint collaborative work. The Gujarat model is designed as an integrated part of the existing health system. Common medicines such as folic acid, analgesics, and penicillin prophylaxis are provided at the doorstep by multipurpose health workers. Adherence is monitored on a monthly basis by determining the medication possession ratio. Sickle cell counselors are appointed in each district and are constantly in touch with all individuals living with SCD.

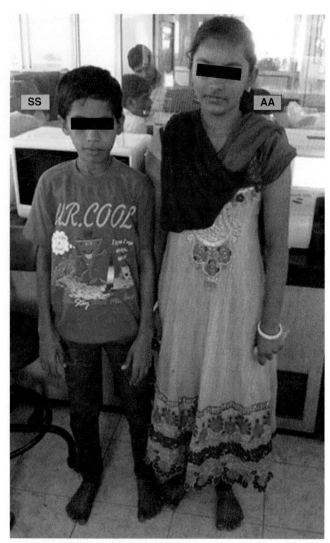

FIGURE 31-2 Dizygotic twins in a family show retarded growth; a child with HbSS can be seen to be much shorter than his dizygotic twin sister with HbAA.

A Novel Approach to Mass Sickle Cell Screening

Various screening programs in India have been conducted by multiple entities, including the Indian Council of Medical Research, state governments, various nongovernmental organizations, and the Indian Red Cross Society (especially in Gujarat). During 2013 to 2017, 95% of the tribal populations of Gujarat were screened for the sickle cell gene in 14 tribal districts. The dithionate tube turbidity (DTT) test, based on the insolubility of HbS when combined with dithionate, was used for the initial screening, and HPLC on the Variant II Hemoglobin Testing System (Biorad Laboratories, Hercules, CA) was used for confirmation of all DTT-positive and doubtful cases. The results of the test were used for genetic and premarital counseling; unions between positive individuals were discouraged and couples at risk were encouraged to opt for prenatal diagnosis (Figure 31-4).

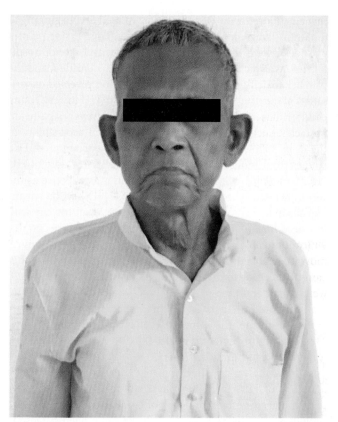

FIGURE 31-3 In 1978, a tribal male from the South Gujarat area was diagnosed with sickle cell disease and treated and is still alive in 2020.

The results of mass sickle cell screening showed 28,862 sickle homozygous cases (0.28%), 1,022 HbS-β thalassemia cases (0.01%), and 728,421 individuals with sickle cell trait (7.13%) among 10,217,862 tribal individuals screened.

Antenatal Screening and Prenatal Diagnosis

All high-risk couples underwent prenatal diagnosis (PND) after genetic counseling before 20 weeks of pregnancy. There were many challenges for PND programs such as the late registration of pregnancies and the dilemma for many families of whether to terminate the pregnancy. Some families opted to continue the pregnancy due to having prior children with SCD who were relatively asymptomatic, pressure from family members, or religious reasons. Because only the DTT technique was used for initial screening, many cases of β thalassemia went undiagnosed.

Many other states in India where the sickle gene is prevalent have ongoing programs for antenatal screening and PND. Chorionic villus sampling at 10 to 12 weeks of gestation and DNA analysis by reverse dot blot hybridization or allele-specific polymerase chain reaction are the methods of choice for PND, similar to in other countries. Besides the sickle gene, 2 β thalassemia mutations (IVS1-5[G>C] and codon 15[G>A]) are common among tribal groups, accounting for

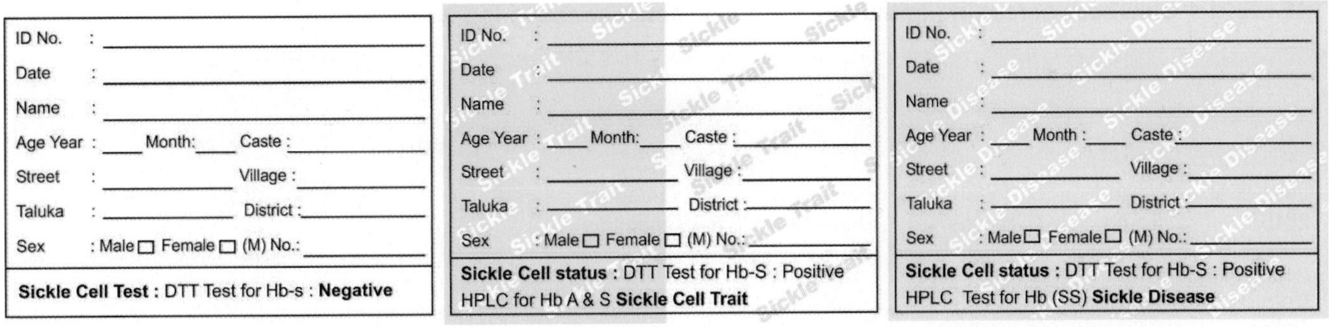

ID No. :
Date :
Name :
Age Year : Month: Caste :
Street : Village :
Taluka : District :
Sex : Male ☐ Female ☐ (M) No.:
Sickle Cell Test : DTT Test for Hb-s : **Negative**

ID No. :
Date :
Name :
Age Year : Month: Caste :
Street : Village :
Taluka : District :
Sex : Male ☐ Female ☐ (M) No.:
Sickle Cell status : DTT Test for Hb-S : Positive
HPLC for Hb A & S **Sickle Cell Trait**

ID No. :
Date :
Name :
Age Year : Month : Caste :
Street : Village :
Taluka : District :
Sex : Male ☐ Female ☐ (M) No.:
Sickle Cell status : DTT Test for Hb-S : Positive
HPLC Test for Hb (SS) **Sickle Disease**

Normal hemoglobin card | Sickle cell trait | Sickle cell disease

FIGURE 31-4 Color-coded laminated identification cards.

90% of the β thalassemia alleles. This made PND simpler and more cost-effective in tribal populations. For couples who came late, cordocentesis and fetal blood analysis by HPLC were done.[34]

Newborn Screening

There is ample evidence worldwide that newborn screening and comprehensive care, including early interventions for SCD, dramatically reduce morbidity and mortality in the first 5 years of life. Newborn screening programs have been initiated relatively recently in Gujarat, Maharashtra, Chhattisgarh, Odisha, Madhya Pradesh, and Tripura. These are summarized in Table 31-1. Both indigenous and nontribal populations have been screened; however, follow-up of babies and comprehensive care have been reported only in a few of these studies in Gujarat and Maharashtra.[33-42]

The feasibility of newborn screening in the tribal areas of Southern Gujarat was demonstrated by Italia et al[35] as part of an Indo-US collaborative pilot study. A total of 5467 newborn babies were screened over 2 years by HPLC (Variant NBS Newborn Screening System, Biorad Laboratories), along with molecular analysis. Forty-six babies with SCD were followed clinically and hematologically up to age 5 years to describe the course of the disease. The families of babies who screened positive were given mobile phones and were followed by telemedicine. Thirty-three babies (0.60%) were sickle homozygous, 13 (0.23%) had sickle β thalassemia, 687 (12.5%) had HbAS, and the rest were unaffected. The parents of SCD babies were educated and counseled about home care. Seven babies (21.8%) presented with severe clinical complications, whereas 18 (56.2%) were asymptomatic until the second follow-up. Variable clinical presentations were seen because of ameliorating factors, such as high HbF, presence of Xmn-I polymorphism, and co-inheritance of α thalassemia.[35]

In Nagpur (Maharashtra), 113 babies with SCD were diagnosed. In this cohort, 73% of babies were followed for 3 to 8 years. Penicillin prophylaxis was given to the babies who came regularly to the center. As compared to the cohort in Gujarat, many babies presented earlier, and 45% of them required hospitalization between 3 months and 2 years of age for painful events, infections, and severe anemia. Eight babies had sepsis, and 6 patients died during the observation period.[36]

Role of the National Health Mission

The NHM (previously known as National Rural Health Mission) is India's government-funded health program to ensure achievement of basic health indicators. Gujarat was the first state to introduce the Sickle Cell Anemia Control Program as a state-specific innovative program through NHM funding in 2010. Comprehensive Guidelines for Control and Management of Hemoglobinopathies have been prepared by NHM and sent to the states to initiate the prevention and management of hemoglobinopathies in their residents.

Recently, the government of India has introduced Ayushman Bharat, a National Health Protection Scheme that will cover >100 million low-income and vulnerable families (approximately 500 million individual beneficiaries) providing coverage of 0.5 million Indian rupees (equivalent to US$6800 per family per year at September 2020 exchange rate) for secondary and tertiary care hospitalizations. Major complications of SCD are covered under this scheme.

The Future of the Sickle Cell Anemia Control Program in India

Extrapolating from the results of the mass sickle cell screening in Gujarat, the estimated burden of the HbS gene in India will be 8.2 million individuals with sickle trait and 0.34 million patients with SCD. This is a very high burden for any country in the world. Because the disease is most common among low-income groups, the majority of patients depend on government health services, and therefore, their management results in a high financial burden to the health care system. Considering the decadal growth of 17.64%, a burden of approximately 1.65 million new sickle cell trait cases and 60,600 new cases of SCD will be added per year in India.

TABLE 31-1 Newborn screening initiatives for sickle cell disease in India

Study	District/state	Newborn babies	Blood sample	Methodology	No. screened	SCD, No. (%)	Sickle trait, No. (%)	Follow-up period
Italia et al, 2015[35]	Valsad/South Gujarat	Tribal babies	Heel prick; dried blood spot	HPLC-Variant NBS machine	5467	46 (0.8%)	687 (12.5%)	5-6 years
Unpublished	Valsad and Bharuch/South Gujarat	Tribal babies	Heel prick; dried blood spot	HPLC-Variant NBS machine	2944	76 (2.6%)	649 (22.0%)	2 years
Upadhye et al, 2016[36]	Nagpur/Maharashtra	Mainly nontribal babies of sickle trait mothers	Cord blood/heel prick	HPLC-Variant Hb Testing System	2134	113 (5.3%)	978 (45.8%)	3-8 years
Unpublished	Jabalpur/Madhya Pradesh	Tribal babies of sickle trait mothers	Cord blood/heel prick	HPLC-Variant Hb Testing System	461	6 (1.3%)	36 (7.8%)	1 year
Panigrahi et al, 2012[37]	Raipur/Chhattisgarh	Tribal and nontribal babies	Heel prick; dried blood spot	HPLC-Variant NBS machine	1158	6 (0.5%)	61 (5.3%)	Not reported
Mohanty et al, 2010[38]	Kalahandi/Odisha	Tribal and nontribal babies	Heel prick; dried blood spot	HPLC-Variant Hb Testing System	1668	34 (2.0%)	293 (17.6%)	Not reported
Dixit et al, 2015[39]	Kalahandi/Odisha	Tribal babies	Cord blood	HPLC-Variant Hb Testing System	761	13 (1.7%)	112 (14.7%)	Not reported
Upadhye et al, 2018[40]	Agartala/Tripura	Tribal and nontribal babies	Cord blood	HPLC-Variant Hb Testing System	2400	0 (0.0%)	15 (0.6%)	Not reported
Unpublished	Chandrapur/Maharashtra	Tribal and nontribal babies	Cord blood/heel prick	HPLC-Variant Hb Testing System	1010	4 (0.4%)	83 (8.4%)	Not reported
Mukherjee et al, 2020[41]	Valsad and Bharuch/South Gujarat; Nagpur and Chandrapur/Maharashtra	Tribal and nontribal babies	Heel prick; Hemo Type SC blood sampling device and dried blood spot	Point-of-care Hemo Type SC and Variant NBS machine	980	6 (0.6%)	99 (10.1%)	Not reported

Abbreviations: HPLC, high-performance liquid chromatography; SCD, sickle cell disease.
Adapted from Colah RB, Mehta P, Mukherjee MB. Newborn screening for sickle cell disease: Indian experience. *Int J Neonatal Screen*. 2018;4:31.

Inclusion of the Gujarat model for prevention and control of hemoglobinopathies in India by NHM in 2015 and inclusion of hemoglobinopathies in the 2016 Rights of Persons with Disabilities Bill by the Indian parliament have boosted the provision of services to individuals living with SCD. This bill will bring Indian law in line with the UN Convention on the Rights of Persons with Disabilities, to which India is a signatory. In addition, it will provide an effective mechanism for ensuring the empowerment and true inclusion of individuals with SCD into the society in a respectable manner. All of these efforts have definitely reduced morbidity and mortality in patients with SCD and will help India reduce the overall burden of SCD.

Future Strategies

Progress in the following areas can lead to better diagnosis and management of patients with SCD in India:

1. There is a need for better clinical documentation of SCD, both during crisis and when stable.

2. Neonatal screening programs should be encouraged at the hospital and community level in areas with high SCD prevalence.

3. A national registry of SCD in India should be generated by collating data from different parts of India. This can lead to larger genomic studies in patients from different geographical regions, which would help to identify the genetic modifiers accounting for the vast phenotypic variability.

4. Strategies, including new technologies, should be employed to promote patient compliance and adherence to HU.

5. The adoption of established and emerging curative therapies should be encouraged, including hematopoietic stem cell transplantation and gene therapy.

6. Community-based care and grassroots efforts to raise awareness in SCD are essential.

7. Building political consensus on the urgency to provide comprehensive care programs for SCD patients will also be critical.[43]

Conclusion

SCD poses a huge burden in India. The clinical presentation is extremely diverse and not uniformly mild, as believed earlier. Better clinical documentation is required in different states. More studies on genetic modifiers are needed to understand the phenotypic diversity. Fixed low-dose HU therapy has been effectively used. Newborn screening programs must be expanded to other regions, ensuring a better follow-up of newborn cohorts. Curative options are expensive and beyond the reach of most families, although some government support is now available.

High-Yield Facts

- SCD is prevalent among the indigenous populations, scheduled castes, and other backward classes in India.
- The HbS gene is linked to the Asian haplotype with high HbF levels.
- The clinical presentation is extremely diverse, being more severe in central India.
- Painful events, infections, and anemia are the main causes of morbidity.
- Fixed low-dose HU has been effective in Indian patients in different regions.
- Screening and prenatal diagnosis are available in different states to reduce the burden of the disease.
- Newborn screening programs have been initiated in a few states, and follow-up of these cohorts will aid in understanding the natural history of the disease.

References

1. Lehmann H, Cutbush M. Sickle-cell trait in Southern India. *Br Med J.* 1952;1:404-405.

2. Pagnier J, Mears JG, Belkhodja OD, et al. Evidence for the multicentric origin of the sickle cell hemoglobin gene in Africa. *Proc Natl Acad Sci USA.* 1984;81:1771-1773.

3. Kulozik AE, Wainscoat JS, Serjeant GR, et al. Geographical survey of β^S-globin gene haplotypes: evidence for an independent Asian origin of the sickle-cell mutation. *Am J Hum Genet.* 1986;39:239-244.

4. Shriner D, Rotinni CN. Whole genome sequence based haplotypes reveal single origin of the sickle allele during the Holocene Wet Phase. *Am J Hum Genet.* 2018;102:547-556.

5. Kar BC, Satapathy RK, Kulozik AE, et al. Sickle cell disease in Orissa State, India. *Lancet.* 1986;2(8517):1198-1201.

6. Rao VR. Genetics and epidemiology of sickle cell anemia in India. *ICMR Bull.* 1988;9:87-90.

7. Kaur M, Das GP, Verma IC. Sickle cell trait and disease among tribal communities in Orissa, Madhya Pradesh and Kerala. *Indian J Med Res.* 1997;55:104-109.

8. Mohanty D, Mukherjee MB. Sickle cell disease in India. *Curr Opin Hematol.* 2002;9:117-122.

9. Patra PK, Chauhan VS, Khodiar PK, et al. Screening for the sickle cell gene in Chhattisgarh state, India: an approach to a major public health problem. *J Community Genet.* 2011;2:147-151.

10. Patel AP, Naik MR, Shah NM, Sharma NP, Parmar PH. Prevalence of common hemoglobinopathies in Gujarat: an analysis of a large population screening programme. *Nat J Community Med.* 2012;3:112-116.

11. Patel J, Patel B, Gamit N, Serjeant GR. Screening for the sickle cell gene in Gujarat India: a village based model. *J Community Genet.* 2013;4:43-47.

12. Kaur M, Dani CBS, Singh M, Singh H, Kapoor S. Burden of sickle cell disease among tribes of India: a burning problem. *Int Res J Pharm Appl Sci.* 2013;3:60-80.

13. Mohanty D, Mukherjee MB, Colah RB, et al. Spectrum of hemoglobinopathies among the primitive tribes: a multicentric study in India. *Asia Pac J Public Health.* 2015;27(2):NP562-NP571.

14. Urade BP. Incidence of sickle cell anemia and thalassemia in central India. *Open J Blood Dis.* 2012;2:71-80.

15. Colah R, Mukherjee M, Ghosh K. Sickle cell disease in India. *Curr Opin Hematol.* 2014;21(3):215-223.

16. Hocham C, Bhatt S, Colah R, et al. The spacial epidemiology of sickle cell anemia in India. *Sci Rep.* 2018;8(1):17685.

17. Colah R, Italia K, Gorakshakar A. Burden of thalassemia in India: the roadmap for control. *Pediatr Hematol Oncol J.* 2017;2(4):79-84.

18. Jain D, Warthe V, Dayama P, et al. Sickle cell disease in central India: a potentially severe syndrome. *Indian J Pediatr.* 2016;83:1071-1076.

19. Brittenham G, Lozoff B, Harris JW, et al. Sickle cell anemia and trait in Southern India: further studies. *Am J Hematol.* 1979;6:107-123.

20. Perrine RP, Brown MJ, Clegg JB, Weatherall DJ, May A. Benign sickle-cell anaemia. *Lancet.* 1972;2:1163-1167.

21. Mukherjee MB, Lu CY, Ducrocq R, et al. Effect of α-thalassemia on sickle-cell anemia linked to the Arab–Indian haplotype in India. *Am J Hematol.* 1997;55:104-109.

22. Jain D, Mohanty D. Clinical manifestations of sickle cell disease in India: misconceptions and reality. *Curr Opin Hematol.* 2018;25:171-176.

23. Jain D, Dani V, Colah R, Tirpude B. Sickle cell disease. In: Gupta P, Menon PSN, Ramji S, Lodha R, eds. *Textbook of Pediatrics. Volume 1: General Pediatrics and Neonatology,* ed 2. New Delhi, India: Jaypee Brothers; 2018:1860-1867.

24. Mohanty D, Mukherjee MB, Colah RB. et al. Iron deficiency anaemia in sickle cell disorders in India. *Indian J Med Res.* 2008; 127:366-369.

25. Jain D, Ganesan K, Sahota S, Darbari DS. Transcranial Doppler screening in children with sickle cell anemia is feasible in central India and reveals high risk of stroke. *Blood.* 2019;134(suppl 1):2279.

26. Desai G, Anand A, Shah P, et al. Sickle cell disease and pregnancy outcomes: a study of a community-based hospital in a tribal block of Gujarat, India. *J Health Popul Nutr.* 2017;36:3.

27. Jain D, Sarathi V, Desai S. Low fixed dose hydroxyurea in severely affected Indian children with sickle cell disease. *Hemoglobin.* 2012;36:323-332.

28. Ministry of Health and Family Welfare, Government of India: Prevention and Control of Hemoglobinopathies in India–Thalassemias, Sickle Cell Disease and Other Variant Hemoglobins. National Health Mission Guidelines on Hemoglobinopathies in India, 2016. https://nhm.gov.in/images/pdf/programmes/RBSK/Resource_Documents/Guidelines_on_Hemoglobinopathies_in%20India.pdf. Accessed September 25, 2020.

29. Jain D, Atmapoojia P, Colah R, Lodha P. Sickle cell disease and pregnancy. *Med J Hematol Infect Dis.* 2019;11:e2019040.

30. Italia K, Jain D, Gattani S, et al. Hydroxyurea in sickle cell disease: a study of clinico-pharmacological efficacy in the Indian haplotype. *Blood Cells Mol Dis.* 2009;42:25-31.

31. Jain DL, Apte M, Colah R, et al. Efficacy of fixed low dose hydroxyurea in Indian children with sickle cell anemia: a single centre experience. *Indian Pediatr.* 2013;50:929-933.

32. Sethy S, Panda T, Jena RK. Beneficial effect of low fixed dose of hydroxyurea in vaso-occlusive crisis and transfusion requirements in adult HbSS patients: a prospective study in a tertiary care center. *Indian J Hematol Blood Transfus.* 2018;34:294-298.

33. Negi RS. Sickle cell trait in India. A review of known distribution. *Bull Anthropol Surv India.* 1972;17:439-449.

34. Colah RB, Mukherjee MB, Martin S, Ghosh K. Sickle cell disease in tribal populations in India. *Indian J Med Res.* 2015;141(5): 509-515.

35. Italia Y, Krishnamurti L, Mehta V, et al. Feasibility of a newborn screening and follow-up programme for sickle cell disease among South Gujarat (India) tribal populations. *J Med Screen.* 2015;22:1-7.

36. Upadhye DS, Jain DL, Trivedi YI, et al. Neonatal screening and the clinical outcome in children with sickle cell disease in central India. *PLoS One.* 2016;11:e0147081.

37. Panigrahi S, Patra PK, Khodiar PK. Neonatal screening of sickle cell disease: a preliminary report. *Indian J Pediatr.* 2012;79: 747-750.

38. Mohanty D, Das K, Mishra K. Newborn screening for sickle cell disease and congenital hypothyroidism in western Orissa. In Proceedings of the 4th International Congress on Sickle Cell Disease, Raipur, India, November 22-27, 2010, pp 29-30.

39. Dixit S, Sahu P, Kar SK, Negi S. Identification of a hotspot area for sickle cell disease using cord blood screening at a district hospital: an Indian perspective. *J Community Genet.* 2015;6:383-387.

40. Upadhye D, Das R, Ray J, et al. Newborn screening for hemoglobinopathies and red cell enzymopathies in Tripura state: a malaria endemic state in Northeast India. *Hemoglobin.* 2018;42:43-46.

41. Mukherjee MB, Colah RB, Mehta PR, et al. Multicentre evaluation of hemotype SC as a point-of-care sickle cell disease rapid diagnostic test for newborns and adults across India. *Am J Clin Pathol.* 2020;153:82-87.

42. Colah RB, Mehta P, Mukherjee MB. Newborn screening for sickle cell disease: Indian experience. *Int J Neonatal Screen.* 2018;4:31.

43. Jain D, Lothe A, Colah R. Sickle cell disease: current challenges *J Hematol Thromb Dis.* 2015;3(6):224.

Sickle Cell Disease in Jamaica: Observations From a Small Island

Authors: Graham Serjeant, Beryl Serjeant

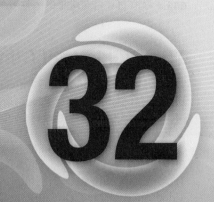

Chapter Outline

Overview

Jamaica is an island in the Caribbean approximately 140 km south of Cuba. Maximum dimensions are 235 km long and 84 km wide, with a land mass of 10,911 km^2 and an estimated population of 2.9 million in 2018. The people are predominantly of West African origin, with smaller groups from India, China, the Mediterranean, and northern Europe, especially the United Kingdom. This diversity results in a population where 10% have the sickle cell trait, 3.5% have the HbC trait, and 0.9% have the β thalassemia trait. Although Jamaica is in many ways a developing society, it has excellent public health and medical facilities and is malaria free. Furthermore, some sophistication results from its closeness geographically to the United States and culturally to the United Kingdom, which also means that these countries are home to a large Jamaican diaspora. Within Jamaica, despite a shift of the population toward urban centers, nearly half the people reside in rural areas where they maintain stable households. This population structure is invaluable for long-term follow-up of patients and, hence, ideal for studies of the natural history of disease generally and has provided a unique "island laboratory" for studies of sickle cell disease.

The Sickle Cell Clinic in Jamaica

The Sickle Cell Clinic at the University Hospital of the West Indies was started by Dr. Paul Milner in 1965 and gradually increased in size until it served 5500 patients with sickle cell disease by 1999. Supported by the British Medical Research Council from 1972, the staff grew from 2 to 28, and with further support from a locally based charity, the Sickle Cell Trust, the facilities steadily improved, with the opening of a dedicated Sickle Cell Clinic in 1988. In addition, due to a bequest from the local cable and wireless facilities, an Education Centre for Sickle Cell Disease opened in 1994. Clinics were conducted 5-and-a-half days per week, and an electronic patient management system allowed real-time collection of clinical, hematologic, and other data, which were immediately available for patient management and research.

Early Challenges

In 1966, there was a striking discrepancy between the mild clinical features of many patients in the recently formed Sickle Cell Clinics and the almost uniformly severe disease described in the contemporary textbooks, suggesting that there may have been a symptomatic bias in the medical experience of the disease. This hypothesis was tested by seeking to trace 50 patients with SS disease then aged >30 years who had not been seen by the clinics at the University Hospital for >10 years. The natural assumption was that these patients had died. Funded by the Wellcome Trust, a mobile clinical unit (Figure 32-1) traced patients to their homes, where 5 were found to have emigrated, 5 had died, 17 were untraceable, and 23 were located and well. When questioned, most stated that their symptoms

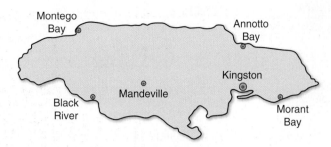

FIGURE 32-2 Map of Jamaica showing peripheral hospitals at which sickle cell clinics were initiated.

had ameliorated with age and they no longer needed medical attention. This realization that some features of the disease improved with age was the background to more serious attempts to reduce this potential bias by taking the clinics to the patients, and 5 sickle cell clinics were operated attached to country hospitals (Figure 32-2) so that no patient had to travel >30 miles, transport costs were reimbursed where necessary, and the mobile clinical unit traced continually defaulting patients. Although reduced, the symptomatic bias persisted, as illustrated in a home visit in western Jamaica to a symptomatic patient with sickle cell–β^0 thalassemia. Aged 13 years, she was photographed alongside her supposedly unaffected healthy sibling who was 2 years younger (Figure 32-3) to illustrate the effect of severe sickle cell disease on growth, but blood tests showed that the sister had the same disease. The realization that bias persisted was the background to the Jamaican Cohort Study of Sickle Cell Disease, which was initiated to define and follow-up a group of patients diagnosed at birth. The problem was that, in 1973, it was widely considered impossible to diagnose the disease at birth because of the high levels of fetal hemoglobin.

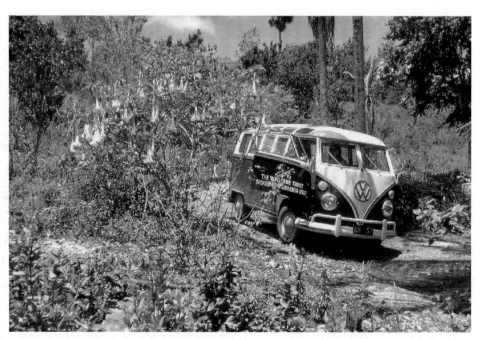

FIGURE 32-1 Mobile clinical unit in St. Elizabeth (southwestern Jamaica) used for domestic outreach.

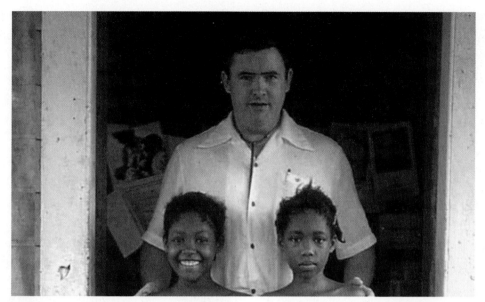

FIGURE 32-3 Siblings in Western Jamaica. A 13-year-old severely affected patient with HbS-β⁰ thalassemia (right) alongside her 11-year-old asymptomatic sibling who was found to have the same condition.

Jamaican Cohort Study of Sickle Cell Disease

In 1973, the main government maternity hospital (Victoria Jubilee) in Kingston (Figure 32-4) delivered 15,000 babies annually, and from June 25, a program was set up to screen 100,000 consecutive nonoperative deliveries (Figure 32-5). The technology for the diagnosis modified existing agar gel techniques,[1,2] and over the next 8.5 years, 311 babies with SS disease, 173 with sickle cell–hemoglobin C (SC) disease, 35 with HbS-β⁺ thalassemia, and 13 with HbS-β⁰ thalassemia

were recruited. The first 125 babies with an SS phenotype were each matched by age and gender with 2 babies with an AA phenotype as controls, and the total of 782 subjects has been followed from birth, with the oldest now being 45 years old. This cohort has been a major asset for working on sickle cell disease on the island, but also important are the extended family system, the ability to trace defaulted patients through their friends and relatives, and the overall cooperation of Jamaican families. These advantages have enabled many contributions to the understanding of the disease and its natural history. Most of these contributions are based on the cohort, but where

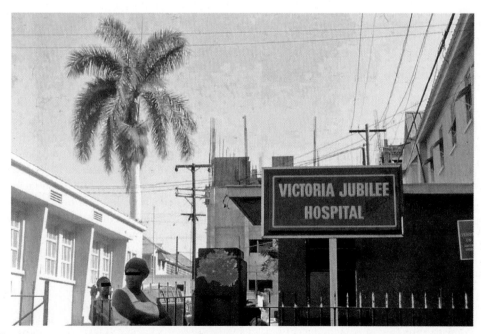

FIGURE 32-4 Maternity ward at Victoria Jubilee Hospital. The old hospital is behind the building on left, and a new hospital is under construction in the background.

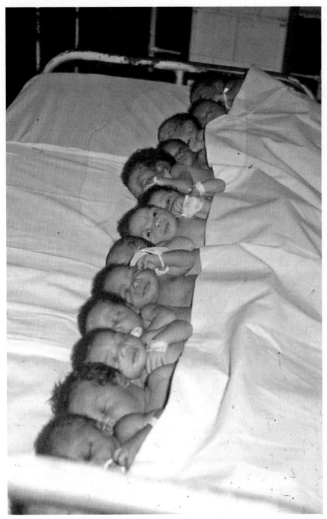

FIGURE 32-5 Result of one night's work in 1 of 2 labor wards in the old Victoria Jubilee Hospital.

necessary, these have been supplemented by children from the pediatric clinic. Pneumococcal septicemia and acute splenic sequestration were important causes of early death, but as the cohort has aged, other contributions have been possible and are briefly described.

Pneumococcal Prophylaxis

Prevention of invasive pneumococcal disease was assessed in a randomized trial of 242 children aged 6 months to 3 years at entry allocated to 4 groups receiving the 14-valent pneumococcal vaccine and penicillin, 14-valent vaccine alone, *Haemophilus influenzae* type B vaccine and penicillin, and *H influenzae* type B vaccine alone. To avoid problems of compliance, penicillin was given as a monthly depot injection usually at home (Figure 32-6), so these transiently painful injections were not associated with clinic attendance. Penicillin was stopped at the age of 3 years because this was past the high-risk period defined from pretrial data. Infection rates were lowest in the group receiving penicillin and vaccine, but because of the relatively small numbers of patients and the

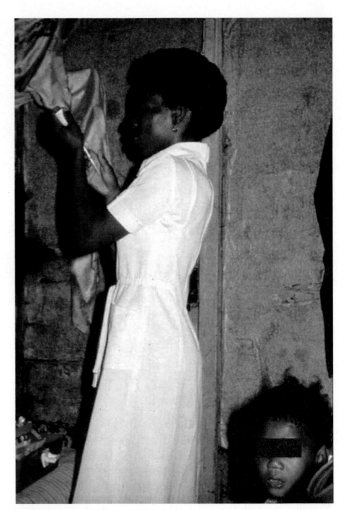

FIGURE 32-6 Nurse preparing to give injection of depot penicillin at patient's home.

infrequency of pneumococcal isolations, the results did not reach significance at the 5% level.[3] The protective effect of penicillin and vaccine was later confirmed in a larger group from a cooperative study in the United States.[4]

Acute Splenic Sequestration

In the cohort, acute splenic sequestration occurred as early as 3 months of age, and the cumulative probability was 0.297 by the age of 3 years. Thirteen children died, usually before transfusion could be implemented, and of the 78 children who survived the first attack, 47% developed recurrences, often within 6 months, and further attacks occurred at shorter intervals, which has led to a policy of prophylactic splenectomy after 2 attacks. For the first attack, teaching mothers to detect acute splenic sequestration (Figure 32-7) doubled the apparent incidence of this complication, but the death rate fell by 90%.[5]

Aplastic Crisis

In Jamaica, episodes of acute anemia (usually 3-5 g/dL) associated with virtual absence of reticulocytes from the

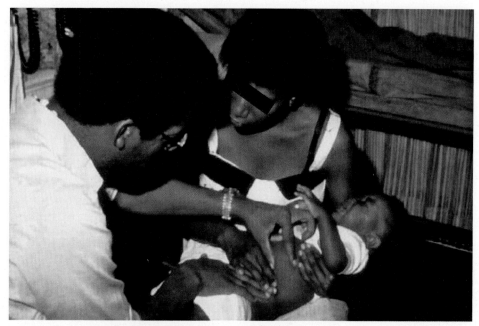

FIGURE 32-7 A pediatrician showing a mother how to feel for the spleen.

peripheral blood occur in epidemics at approximately 4-year intervals. Collaboration with colleagues revealed that virtually all clinically defined aplasias were associated with infection by parvovirus B19.[6] This organism was shown to be highly infective, with susceptible siblings being affected in about 80% of cases, either simultaneously or within 3 weeks. If oxygen carriage is maintained by transfusion, the outcome is benign, and most Jamaican patients are treated as outpatients, with assessment 3 to 4 days later to ensure that the reticulocytosis of the recovery phase has occurred. Predominantly a pediatric problem, >60% of patients seroconvert by the age of 15 years and 70% by the age of 20 years, and recurrent parvovirus-induced aplastic crisis has never been reported.

Folate Deficiency

Bone marrow expansion as a result of the increased hemolysis in SS disease leads to greater demand for energy and hematinics. Folate requirements are increased, and folate supplementation has become routine in the management of children with SS disease. Folic acid is cheap and harmless, but signs of folate dependency in Jamaica led to a double-blind controlled trial in patients aged 2 to 9 years. All patients received a little yellow tablet, but only half of those tablets contained folic acid. At the end of a 1-year trial, there was no difference in hematological indices or growth between the groups, but those receiving folate were more prone to dactylitis.[7] Although folate deficiency can lead to megaloblastic change, most cases in the literature are from West Africa where the dietary availability of folate is low. The Jamaican diet contains fresh fruit and vegetables, and thus, folate deficiency is rarely seen, although it was seen after Hurricane Gilbert when these foods were difficult to obtain.[8]

Gallstones

The increased bilirubin excretion due to the rapid hemolysis in SS disease results in gallstones, so the prevalence and natural history of gallstones were studied by annual gallbladder ultrasounds in the cohort. These examinations commenced at 5 years, when already 7% of the SS patients had gallstones (Figure 32-8), and the prevalence increased steadily to 50% by the age of 25 years.[9] However, the clinical features of the 96 patients with gallstones showed few differences from those without gallstones, and at that time, only 8 subjects developed symptoms requiring cholecystectomy.

Chronic Hypersplenism

Sustained splenomegaly, often ≥6 cm below the left costal margin, associated with markedly shortened red blood cell survival, a new hematologic equilibrium of hemoglobin >3 g, and reticulocytes that were markedly increased compared to previous steady-state values, occurred in about 5% of cohort patients. The etiology was largely unknown, and some cases resolved spontaneously, but others had morbidity associated with frequent hospital admissions and blood transfusions and some mortality associated with coincident acute splenic sequestration or parvovirus-induced aplasia. All patients with hypersplenism should be monitored closely with monthly assessments of hemoglobin and reticulocytes and height and weight. If there is no evidence of spontaneous resolution after 6 months, or earlier if height crosses growth percentiles, then splenectomy is performed. The excessive red blood cell destruction and associated bone marrow expansion have high-energy costs, and whole-body protein turnover, resting metabolic rate, and impaired growth are reversed after splenectomy.[10,11]

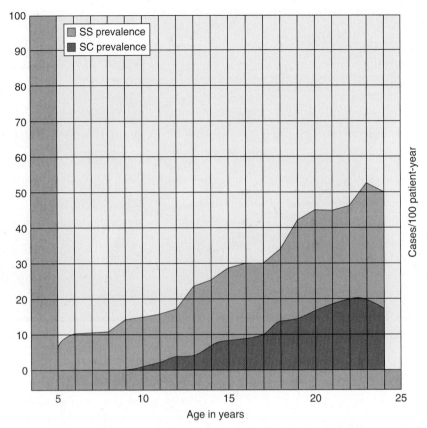

FIGURE 32-8 Prevalence of gallstones from annual ultrasound examinations in the cohort.

Bone Marrow Necrosis

Necrosis of active bone marrow is believed to be a common feature of dactylitis (hand-foot syndrome), bone pain crisis, rib involvement, and avascular necrosis of the femoral head. Bone pain crisis is a major determinant of morbidity and hospital admission in most settings. Approaches to relief and prevention are dictated by local cultural and medical practices, but Jamaica pioneered models of day care for this condition. With >5000 patients, 10 to 15 patients are seen daily with bone pain deemed of sufficient severity to required opiate-based analgesia. Previously, these patients languished on trolleys in emergency departments awaiting hospital admission, but with the advent of day care, patients were monitored and given fluids and pain relief, and at the end of the afternoon, >90% of patients chose to return home with the same analgesia in oral form.[12] The day care facility in the dedicated sickle cell clinic was increased from 4 to 8 beds and has been an invaluable resource for patients.

Menarche and Pregnancy

Prospective follow-up of patients and controls by the same observers has provided the most accurate estimates of menarche and demonstrates a delay of menarche in SS subjects of 2.4 years.[13] Pregnancy in cohort SS patients is associated with a significantly lower rate of successful outcome (57.1% vs 88.8% of non-SS individuals; χ^2, 18.7; P <.001), higher rate of spontaneous abortion, significantly lower birth weight, lower gestational age,[14] greater retained placenta,[15] and greater maternal mortality (Lewis 2018, unpublished data).

Priapism

Priapism, a painful involuntary penile erection unassociated with sex, is usually underestimated in sickle cell disease, partly because of patient embarrassment but also because patients do not realize that this complication is related to sickle cell disease. The practice of routine enquiry of all males in the clinic has revealed that priapism occurs in 33% of males overall; this rate increases to 60% by age 40 years. In 4 of 52 patients, priapism led to impotence.[16]

Chronic Leg Ulceration

Defined as a duration of ≥6 months, chronic leg ulceration is a major cause of morbidity. It affected 75% of Jamaican SS patients in earlier studies, but this rate decreased to 30% in the cohort study.[17] Improved healing on complete bed rest led to the hypothesis of venous incompetence, which was confirmed by studies using handheld Doppler,[18] and led to the recommendation of firm supportive elastic bandages.

Renal Function

Impaired renal function is common among older patients with SS disease. Studies in the cohort patients aged 18 to

23 years determined revised upper limits of normal for glomerular filtration rates in SS patients of 80 μmol/L in males and 68 μmol/L in females.[19] Values declined by 3.2 μmol/L annually over a 13-year period.[20]

Overall Survival

Estimates of survival are difficult to determine and are influenced by ascertainment of the study group and changing interventions. With these reservations, median estimates of survival in SS disease were 42 years for males and 48 years for females in a cooperative study in the United States[21] and 53 years for males and 58.5 years for females in a clinic-based study in Jamaica.[22] In the Jamaican cohort, 55.5% of patients survived to 40 years, and median survival time was 40.2 years for males and not yet been reached for females by September 2016.[23]

Manchester Project

The Manchester Project is named after the parish of Manchester in central Jamaica. After an island-wide education program on sickle cell disease and its genetics delivered to secondary schools between 2001 and 2007, the information

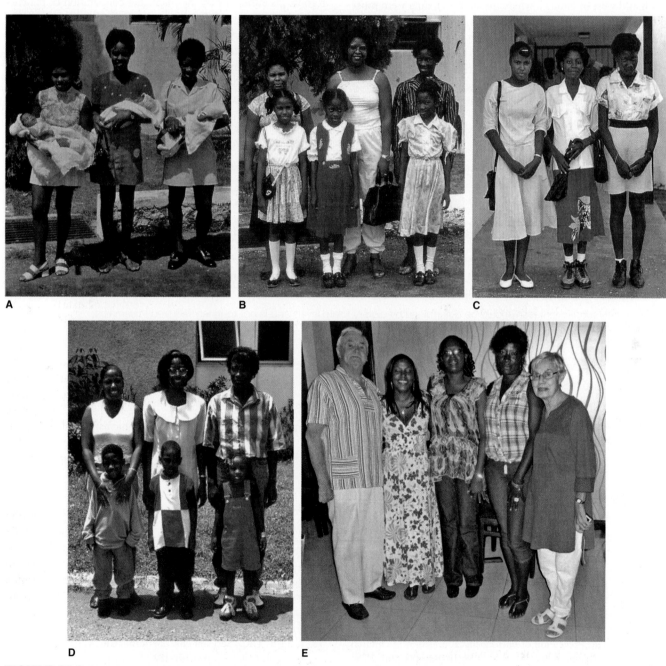

FIGURE 32-9 Images of a single cohort (cohort 10), the SS patient at the center flanked by her normal controls at 9 days (A), 9 years (B), 15 years (C), 26 years (D), and with the authors at 39 years (E).

most required by students was knowledge of their hemoglobin genotype. In collaboration with the Ministry of Health, screening was offered to the senior classes, mostly aged 15 to 19 years, at 14 secondary schools in the parish over a 6-year period (2007-2013). Compliance with voluntary screening conducted in the schools increased from 55% to 92% during this period, and among 16,612 students, the sickle cell trait occurred in 9.6% and the HbC trait in 3.5%.[24] All students were given laminated cards with their genotypes, and those with abnormal genotypes were offered counseling. To determine the effects of this intervention on subsequent pregnancies, newborn screening was set up in 12 hospitals throughout the south and west of Jamaica where these participants were most likely to have their deliveries. Analysis of 2442 live deliveries to females screened at the school found that of the 216 first deliveries among mothers with the sickle cell trait, there were 5 babies with SS disease compared with 5.5 babies predicted from random mating; thus, knowledge of genotype had not influenced pregnancy outcome in Jamaica at that time.[25]

Conclusion

The island of Jamaica is small, but because it is geographically limited, it has proved a superb resource for long-term studies of disease. This is illustrated by the fact that 45 years after initiation of the Jamaican Cohort Study of Sickle Cell Disease, not one of the 311 subjects admitted to the study has been lost to follow-up. Deaths have been documented (and often the cause of death), emigrations have been recorded, and those still alive and resident in Jamaica are readily located. A great deal has been learned, for which we are indebted to our patients, and images of a token cohort are provided in Figure 32-9 to illustrate this. This resource is enhanced by the intelligent cooperation of patients and their families and their understanding of the importance of assisting research programs. Although there may be limitations in the sophistication of locally available technology, these have been overcome by collaboration with laboratories elsewhere, and there are likely few societies in which patient follow-up over 45 years remains at close to 100%.

High-Yield Facts

- In the mid-1960s, the literature on sickle cell disease was heavily biased by clinic and hospital data, and the ability to reach long-defaulted patients in Jamaica showed that many patients older than age 30 years were alive and well.
- The Jamaican Cohort Study based on newborn screening was designed to reduce this symptomatic bias.
- Mothers were successfully taught splenic palpation, and this reduced the death rate from this complication by 90%.
- Aplastic crisis was shown to be caused by parvovirus B19.
- Folate supplementation should be determined by dietary folate levels and is not routinely required in Jamaica.
- Gallstones were observed in patients as early as 5 years of age, and their prevalence in SS disease increased to 50% by 25 years.
- Day care can play a major role in the treatment of the bone pain crisis.
- Excessive red blood cell destruction associated with hypersplenism may impair growth.
- A history of stuttering priapism should be routinely sought because direct questioning elicits a prevalence of >30%.
- Renal failure in SS disease requires a different definition, and chronic renal failure is common, especially among older adults.
- Jamaica presents an "island laboratory" that is superb for long-term studies of disease.

References

1. Schneider RG. Developments in laboratory diagnosis. In: Abramson H, Bertles JF, Wethers DL, eds. *Sickle Cell Disease, Diagnosis, Management, Education, and Research.* CV Mosby Co.; 1973:230.
2. Serjeant BE, Forbes M, Williams LL, Serjeant GR. Screening cord bloods for detection of sickle cell disease in Jamaica. *Clin Chem.* 1974;20:666-669.
3. John AB, Ramlal A, Jackson H, Maude GH, Waight-Sharma A, Serjeant GR. Prevention of pneumococcal infection in children with homozygous sickle cell disease. *Br Med J.* 1984;288:1567-1570.
4. Gaston MH, Verter JI, Woods G, et al. Prophylaxis with oral penicillin in children with sickle cell anemia. A randomized trial. *N Engl J Med.* 1986;314:1593-1599.
5. Emond AM, Collis R, Darvill D, Higgs DR, Maude GH, Serjeant GR. Acute splenic sequestration in homozygous sickle cell disease: natural history and management. *J Pediatr.* 1985;107:201-206.
6. Serjeant GR, Serjeant BE, Thomas P, Anderson MJ, Patou G, Pattison JR. Human parvovirus infection in homozygous sickle cell disease. *Lancet.* 1993;341:1237-1240.
7. Rabb LM, Grandison Y, Mason K, Hayes RJ, Serjeant BE, Serjeant GR. A trial of folate supplementation in children with homozygous sickle cell disease. *Br J Haematol.* 1983;54:589.
8. Readett DRJ, Serjeant BE, Serjeant GR. Hurricane Gilbert anaemia. *Lancet.* 1989;2:101-102.
9. Walker TM, Hambleton IR, Serjeant GR. Gallstones in sickle cell disease: observations from the Jamaican Cohort Study. *J Pediatr.* 2000;136:80-85.

10. Badaloo AV, Singhal A, Forrester TE, Serjeant GR, Jackson AA. The effect of splenectomy for hypersplenism on whole body protein turnover, resting metabolic rate and growth in sickle cell disease. *Eur J Clin Nutr.* 1996;50:672-675.

11. Singhal A, Thomas P, Kearney T, Venugopal S, Serjeant G. Acceleration in linear growth after splenectomy for hypersplenism in homozygous sickle cell disease. *Arch Dis Child.* 1995;72:227-229.

12. Ware ME, Hambleton I, Ochaya I, Serjeant GR. Sickle cell painful crises in Jamaica: a day care approach to management. *Br J Haematol.* 1999;105:93-96.

13. Serjeant GR, Singhal A, Hambleton IR. Sickle cell disease and age at menarche in Jamaican girls: observations from a cohort study. *Arch Dis Child.* 2001;85:375-378.

14. Serjeant GR, Look Loy L, Crowther M, Hambleton IR, Thame M. The outcome of pregnancy in homozygous sickle cell disease. *Obstet Gynecol.* 2004;103:1278-1285.

15. Simms-Stewart D, Thame M, Hemans-Keens A, Hambleton I, Serjeant GR. Retained placenta in homozygous sickle cell disease. *Obstet Gynecol.* 2009;114:825-828.

16. Serjeant GR, Hambleton I. Priapism in homozygous sickle cell disease: a 40 year study of the natural history. *West Indian Med J.* 2015;64:175-180.

17. Cumming V, King L, Fraser R, Serjeant G, Reid M. Venous incompetence, poverty and lactate dehydrogenase in Jamaica are important predictors of leg ulceration in sickle cell anaemia. *Br J Haematol.* 2008;142:119-125.

18. Clare A, FitzHenley M, Harris J, Hambleton I, Serjeant GR. Chronic leg ulceration in homozygous sickle cell disease: a role of venous incompetence. *Br J Haematol.* 2002;119:567-571.

19. Thompson J, Hambleton IR, Reid M, Serjeant GR. Albuminuria and renal function in homozygous sickle cell disease: observations from a cohort study. *Arch Intern Med.* 2007;167:701-708.

20. Asnani M, Serjeant G, Reid M. Renal function in the Jamaican cohort with homozygous sickle cell disease: longitudinal observations. *Br J Haematol.* 2016;173:461-468.

21. Platt OS, Brambilla DJ, Rosse WF, et al. Mortality in sickle cell disease. Life expectancy and risk factors for early death. *N Engl J Med.* 1994;330:1639-1644.

22. Wierenga KJ, Hambleton IR, Lewis NA. Survival estimates for patients with homozygous sickle-cell disease in Jamaica: a clinic-based population study. *Lancet.* 2001;357:680-683.

23. Serjeant GR, Chin N, Asnani MR, et al. Causes of death and early life determinants of survival in homozygous sickle cell disease: the Jamaican cohort study from birth. *PLoS One.* 2018;13:e0192710.

24. Mason K, Gibson F, Higgs D, et al. Haemoglobin variant screening in Jamaica: meeting student's request. *Br J Haematol.* 2016;172:634-636.

25. Serjeant GR, Serjeant BE, Mason KP, et al. Voluntary premarital screening to prevent sickle cell disease in Jamaica: does it work? *J Commun Genet.* 2017;8:133-139.

Sickle Cell Disease in Brazil

Author: Fernando Ferreira Costa

Chapter Outline

Overview

Brazil is a continental country with a very heterogeneous population in regard to ethnic origin. Although most of the Native American (ie, Indian) population is extinct today, their genomic inheritance has contributed to the ethnic mix of the current Brazilian population. The country was colonized by the Portuguese, but from the 16th to 19th centuries, it received about 4 million slaves from Africa. From the 19th century to the middle of 20th century, a very important contingent of immigrants from several countries, including Italy (1.5 million), Spain (0.6 million), Japan, Germany, and Lebanon, arrived and integrated into the Brazilian genetic pool. Several studies have shown that these different ethnic groups are continuously in a process of admixture, which indicates that Brazil has an extremely unique population regarding genetic diseases and, specifically, regarding hemoglobinopathies. In addition, it is important to emphasize that the population is heterogeneously distributed within its different geographical regions. Hence, patients with sickle cell disease (SCD) in Brazil constitute a very singular admixture-rich ethnic population. Studies that have compared the genetic makeup of SCD patient cohorts from Brazil and the United States have revealed high levels of divergence among cases, with a higher European genomic background in Brazil. Moreover, in some region of the country, patients with HbS/β thalassemia compose almost 30% of all SCD patients. Almost all patients with SCD in the country are treated within the Public Healthcare System *(Sistema Único de Saúde* [SUS]), which provides universal care and covers all health-related costs. To provide care to patients with SCD, the system is organized by government-funded special hematology centers affiliated with state or federal medical institutions, and these are named *hemocentros* (hemocenters). In each of the 26 Brazilian states, at least 1 of these centers is responsible for the diagnosis and treatment of SCD patients.

In this chapter, we describe the origin and genetic background of the Brazilian population, how they impact the prevalence of SCD, and several clinical and laboratory characteristics of these patients. In addition, we present a description of how the public health system is organized for taking care of SCD patients and outline future challenges related to probable budget reductions in the universal public health system in the country.

Introduction to Brazil

Brazil is one of the largest countries in the world, with approximately 8.5 million km^2 of land and an estimated population of 208 million inhabitants in 2018. The population presents a very heterogeneous ethnic origin, which has contributed to the distinguishing characteristics of the Brazilian people who self-classify according to their skin color as White (43.6%), Black (8.2%), Brown (46.8%), and Asiatic or Amerindian (0.9%). It should also be emphasized that the ethnic origin of the population is very diverse in different regions of the country.[1]

The genesis of the present Brazilian population is complex and still not completely studied.[2-6] A high proportion of the Native Indian population is probably extinct today, although they have evidently contributed significantly to the formation of the Brazilian population.[2,5,6] The Portuguese were the first colonists to settle in the country, at the beginning of the 16th century, and from the beginning of colonization until the 19th century, the country received approximately 4 million slaves as a result of forced immigration from Africa. In addition, particularly in the 19th and 20th centuries, Brazil also admitted immigrants from several countries, including Italians (1.5 million), Portuguese (1.4 million), Spanish (0.6 million), Germans, Japanese, Lebanese, and other Middle Easterners.[3]

There is considerable evidence to indicate that all of these different ethnic groups are continuously in a process of admixture.[2,4-6] Most of the population (~70%) resides in urban areas. Thus, as expected, the distribution of the hereditary abnormalities of hemoglobin in Brazil is different in each region of the country, reflecting the ethnic composition of the local population. It is important to mention that several studies have not found any significant abnormalities concerning hemoglobinopathies, particularly HbS, in the Brazilian indigenous population.[2,3,7,8]

History of SCD in Brazil

Reports on sickle cell anemia (SCA) have been published in the Brazilian medical literature since the middle of the 20th century. Indeed, the first description of an accurate genetic transmission of the disease was published in 1947 by Accioly, a physician from the state of Bahia. Unfortunately, it was written in Portuguese and published in a small regional medical journal and remained unheard of for a long time.[9]

The first studies employing reliable technical procedures for diagnosing hemoglobin disorders were carried out in the late 1960s and, in general, were done with the objective of estimating the prevalence of hemoglobinopathies HbS and HbC. As expected, these values showed a significant variability according to the region of the country where the analysis was conducted. Reports indicated frequencies of HbS heterozygotes ranging from 5.9% to 6.8% among African Brazilians and 1.2% to 2.8% in the general population of individuals from the southern region of the country. In contrast, in a survey carried out in a general population of individuals from the northeastern region, where most of the population is classified as African Brazilian, the percentage of heterozygotes was 7.6%.[3] Taken together, the most recent available data suggest that there are approximately 30,000 to 50,000 patients with SCD in the entire country. In addition, the prevalence of the β^s allele ranges from 1.2% to 10.9% according to the region of the country, whereas the prevalence of β^c alleles is estimated to be between 0.15% and 7.4%.[10]

Newborn Screening in Brazil

In Brazil, the newborn screening program was implanted as a nationwide program in 1990 but included only screening for phenylketonuria and congenital hypothyroidism. Although a few states initiated sickle hemoglobin (HbS) screening earlier, the federal government only started the National Neonatal Screening Program, which includes testing for HbS, in 2001. In the same year, the Ministry of Health published a comprehensive review concerning almost all aspects of SCD, including the diagnosis and treatment of the disease, written by Brazilian experts in the field.[10,11]

Presently, the program is available in all 26 states of the country. However, the coverage is variable in the different states. In the south and southeast, most of the hospitals are included in the program, in contrast to the north and northeast, where the coverage is lower. Again, given the ethnic heterogeneity of the Brazilian population, it is expected that the incidence of SCD detected by newborn screening is significantly different among the regions of the country. Thus, the incidence of SCD is about 1 in every 650 newborns screened in Salvador in the state of

Frequency of the S gene in Brazil

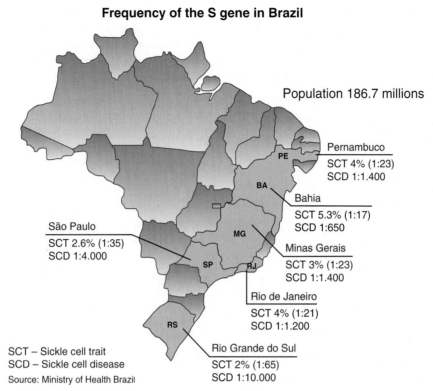

Population 186.7 millions

Pernambuco
SCT 4% (1:23)
SCD 1:1.400

Bahia
SCT 5.3% (1:17)
SCD 1:650

São Paulo
SCT 2.6% (1:35)
SCD 1:4.000

Minas Gerais
SCT 3% (1:23)
SCD 1:1.400

Rio de Janeiro
SCT 4% (1:21)
SCD 1:1.200

SCT – Sickle cell trait
SCD – Sickle cell disease
Source: Ministry of Health Brazil

Rio Grande do Sul
SCT 2% (1:65)
SCD 1:10.000

FIGURE 33-1 A simplified vision of the frequency of the gene for hemoglobin S in Brazil. The incidence of sickle cell disease is about 1 in every 650 newborns screened in Salvador, in the state of Bahia (northeast), 1 in 1400 newborns in Minas Gerais (southeast), and 1 in 10,000 newborns in Rio Grande do Sul (south). From Cancado RD, Jesus JA. Sickle cell disease in Brazil. *Rev Bras Hematol Hemoter*. 2007;29(3):203-204, and cited in Kato GJ, Piel FB, Reid CD, et al. Sickle cell disease. *Nat Rev Dis Primers*. 2018;4:18010.

Bahia (northeast), 1 in 1400 in Minas Gerais (southeast), and 1 in 10,000 in Rio Grande do Sul (south) (Figure 33-1). For the whole country, the Ministry of Health estimates that there were 1071 newborns with SCD and 60,418 heterozygotes for hemoglobin S in 2016.[10,12]

Despite the heterogeneity of coverage among the states and also problems regarding follow-up programs in some states, the newborn screening program resulted in better knowledge of the number of children with SCD and probably increased their survival, although the number of deaths is still high when compared to the United States and Europe. There have been at least 2 major studies concerning the survival of children with SCD in Brazil after neonatal screening was initiated. The most organized program, in the state of Minas Gerais, achieved screening of 3,617,912 newborns from March 1998 to February 2012, and 2576 children with SCD were detected. During this period, the mortality rate was 7.4% (193 deaths). The major cause of death was infection (45%), followed by acute splenic sequestration (14%).[13] Another important study, which included 1,217,893 newborns in the state of Rio de Janeiro, found 912 patients with SCD. During a period of 10 years, the number of deaths was 38 (4.1%), and the most frequent causes of death were acute chest syndrome (36.8%), sepsis (31.6%), and splenic sequestration (21.1%).[14] The program also enabled studies in a large cohort of newborns with SCD focusing on several

aspects of the disease. As an example, the study of 461 newborns with HbSC hemoglobinopathy was able to strongly suggest that the co-inheritance of α thalassemia significantly reduced the risk of splenic sequestration in these patients.[15]

Early Clinical and Genetic Studies in Brazil

The first studies using dependable methods to analyze clinical and genetic aspects of SCD in Brazil showed interesting and peculiar results. In the state of São Paulo (southeast), a detailed analysis of 40 patients with SCD showed that 14 of them were HbS-β^0 thalassemia, suggesting a high incidence of β^0 thalassemia in some regions of Brazil. In addition, clinical analysis indicated that both groups (SS and S/β^0 thalassemia) were equally affected with regard to the severity of the disease.[16] These findings were further confirmed in a larger cohort of SCD patients (Table 33-1).[3] Other investigators described clinical and laboratory data in 409 patients aged 6 months to 54 years in the city of Rio de Janeiro. The severity of the clinical course of patients was apparently similar to that described in a population from the United States.[17] In other publications, the same authors described other interesting findings, including a very high degree of fetal

TABLE 33-1 Table showing the hematologic data of one of the first studies of sickle cell disease in Brazil (n = 156)

Table II—Hematological data (mean ± 1SD) of 156 patients with sickle-cell diseases (Zago *et al.*, 1983b)			
	SS (92 cases)	**S/β⁰-thal (32 cases)**	**S/β⁺-thal (6 cases)**	**HbS/HbC (26 cases)**
Hb (g/dl)	7.7 ± 1.5	8.0 ± 1.7	10.0 ± 0.7	11.0 ± 1.5
R.B.C. ($\times 10^{12}$/l)	2.6 ± 0.5	3.5 ± 0.8	4.7 ± 0.5	3.8 ± 0.6
M.C.V. (fl)*	95.3 ± 10.9	75.3 ± 10.8	66.2 ± 4.9	87.2 ± 11.4
M.C.H. (pg)**	30.2 ± 4.1	22.9 ± 2.5	21.5 ± 2.3	29.1 ± 3.2
HbA$_2$ (%)	2.5 ± 0.4	4.3 ± 1.0	4.3 ± 0.8	—
HbF (%)	7.4 ± 6.7	11.6 ± 7.3	9.8 ± 8.6	2.8 ± 2.8

*Mean corpuscular volume
**Mean corpuscular haemoglobin
Note. It is interesting to note the high proportion of S/β⁰ thalassemia patients. Values are means ± 1SD.
Abbreviations: Hb, hemoglobin; HbF, fetal hemoglobin; RBC, red blood cell; SD, standard deviation.
Reproduced with permission from Zago MA, Costa FF. Hereditary haemoglobin disorders in Brazil. *Trans R Soc Trop Med Hyg.* 1985;79:385-388.

loss (48% in 67 pregnancies) and the correlation of higher levels of fetal hemoglobin (HbF) with a more benign clinical course.[17-19]

β^S Haplotypes and α Thalassemia in Brazil

The Bantu haplotype is predominant among SCA patients in almost all regions of Brazil, with the exception of the state of Bahia, where there is a slightly higher proportion of the Benin haplotype.[20-25] This distribution is in agreement with the historical Portuguese Atlantic slave trade from Africa to Brazil. Records show that most of the slaves were probably brought to Brazil from Angola, Congo, and Mozambique (with β^s Bantu predominance), but Bahia also received slaves from West Africa and the Bay of Benin (where Benin haplotypes are prevalent). The Senegal and Cameroon haplotypes are seldom seen in Brazilian patients.[22,25] In a study in Southeast Brazil, we found 34% of patients to be homozygotes for the Bantu haplotype, 45% to have Bantu/Benin haplotype, and 11% to be homozygotes for the Benin haplotype.[21] The data from this report also suggested that HbF levels were higher and the prevalence of leg ulcers was lower in patients who were homozygotes for the Benin haplotype compared to the other 2 groups. α Thalassemia (3.7 deletion) was present in 17.5% of the patients, and the data suggested higher hemoglobin levels in this group and probably protection against stroke.

In a more recent study, 2 SCA cohorts from Brazil and the United States were analyzed at genome-wide and chromosomal levels by single nucleotide polymorphism array. As expected, patients from Brazil showed significantly more admixture and had a higher European background.[26,27]

Specialized Centers for the Diagnosis and Treatment of SCD in Brazil

Special centers for the diagnosis and treatment of SCD with the support of the Ministry of Health and the Public Healthcare System (SUS) were developed in several states of Brazil to provide clinical care for patients. Most of these centers were created at public university hospitals or public centers for blood transfusions and hematology, called hemocenters (*hemocentros*). In fact, multidisciplinary units that care for patients with SCD can be found all over Brazil, for example, in Rio de Janeiro (HemoRio), São Paulo (Hemocentros USP and UNIFESP), Campinas (Hemocentro Unicamp), Ribeirão Preto (Hemocentro Ribeirão Preto), Pernambuco (HemoPe), Bahia (HemoBa), and Amazonas (HemoAm), among others. In addition to providing free medical care, blood transfusion, penicillin prophylaxis, immunization including pneumococcal vaccination, and hydroxyurea and others drugs to the patients, some of these centers, with funds from federal or state research agencies, also develop a number of research projects concerning several clinical and laboratory aspects of SCD. An overview of some of the most important studies carried out in these centers is described in the following sections.

Genomic Polymorphisms and Possible Implications for Clinical Diversity

One of the first studies that suggested that the UDP-glucuronosyltransferase 1 gene promoter polymorphism is associated with increased serum bilirubin levels and cholecystectomy in SCD was carried out in Brazil.[28] In addition, a report suggesting the low clinical impact of inherited hypercoagulability risks factors, such as the prothrombin mutation (allele 20210A), factor V Leiden mutation, and homozygosity for transition 677C→T in the methylenetetrahydrofolate reductase gene, in SCD was carried out in Brazil.[29] Brazilian laboratories, in collaboration with international investigators, have also participated in identifying DNA polymorphisms at the *BCL11A* and *HMIP2* loci and their association with fetal hemoglobin levels and influence on some clinical complications of the disease.[30,31]

An extensive list of polymorphisms presenting possible associations with clinical aspects of the disease have been studied in Brazilian patients with SCD, including the following[32]: G463A myeloperoxidase gene polymorphism and infection,[33] interleukin *IL6 G-174C* and stroke,[34] *HMOX1* gene and levels of HbF,[35] haptoglobin genotypes,[36] platelet antigen 5 system and risk of vaso-occlusion,[37] *SOD2* (*Val16Ala*) and acute splenic sequestration,[38] *MBL2* gene and vaso-occlusive events,[39] *IL.1B* and *IL.6* and pulmonary hypertension,[40] and tumor necrosis factor *TNFα* (−308G>A) and *VCAM1* (c.1238G>C) and cerebrovascular disease.[41] In addition, a more recent study using whole-exome analysis showed possible linkage between leg ulcers and a polymorphism in the *FLG2* gene.[42]

Pregnancy in SCD Patients in Brazil

Several reports from different regions of the country suggest a very high occurrence of complications in SCD patients during pregnancy in Brazil. In one study, the authors described an intrauterine death rate of 15% in patients with SCD[43]; in another cohort, 30% of patients had near misses with a 4.8% fetal death rate[44]; and in a third publication, spontaneous abortions were found in 26% of cases and 29% of the patients presented with acute chest syndrome.[45] Some analyses suggest that prophylactic transfusion reduced the frequency of complications; however, the number of patients was too small to draw definitive conclusions.[46] Two recent reports also indicated inflammatory alterations in placentas from patients with SCD during pregnancy.[47,48]

Priapism in SCD Patients in Brazil

Priapism has been described in several reports. A 5.6% prevalence of priapism in male children and adolescents with SCD was found in a cohort of 599 patients.[49] Another careful study showed an association of priapism with sleep hypoxia,[50] and another investigation suggested a possible improvement in patients treated with hydroxyurea.[51]

In addition, a considerable number of studies aiming to investigate the mechanisms and treatment of priapism in SCD animal models have been carried out in the country. The central mechanism of priapism in SCD seems to be alterations of the nitric oxide (NO)–cyclic guanosine monophosphate (cGMP)–phosphodiesterase 5 (PDE5) signaling pathway. Berkeley and Townes transgenic sickle cell mice display a priapism phenotype that is associated with an amplified corpus cavernosum relaxation response mediated by the NO-cGMP signaling pathway.[52,53] Exaggerated erectile responses are associated with low NO bioavailability, which leads to downregulation of PDE5 expression in the penis.[54] In Berkeley SCD mice, treatment with a new NO donor, a hybrid derived from thalidomide and hydroxyurea, upregulated PDE5 expression in the penis and reversed the phenotype.[53]

Hydroxyurea, Vaso-occlusion, and Inflammation

In the past decade, there has been a significant increase in the number of patients, including children, receiving hydroxyurea (HU) in Brazil, probably due to the fact that the medication is provided free of cost by the SUS and most hematologists are aware of its efficacy. A study in a cohort of children with SCA in Rio de Janeiro suggested that HU may reduce morbidity and decrease mortality.[55] Aspects of the complex molecular mechanisms associated with increased production of HbF in bone marrow cells associated with HU therapy in SCA were described in a patient.[56] In fact, several factors linked to vaso-occlusion have been studied in patients or in animal models of the disease. In addition to studies confirming the role of neutrophils in SCD pathophysiology,[57-59] the importance of the interaction of platelets in leukocyte–red blood cell (RBC) heterocellular aggregates that trigger vaso-occlusion is becoming clearer.[60] Numerous intracellular signaling pathways, including NO-cGMP–dependent pathways and transcription factor activation pathways, prompt the recruitment of cells to the blood vessel walls,[61,62] and agents that can elevate intracellular cGMP, such as phosphodiesterase 9 (PDE9) inhibitors and soluble guanylate cyclase (sGC) stimulators, may be able to counter some of these effects.[63-66] More recently, it was shown that HU, which has NO-donating/sGC-stimulating properties, has acute and immediate effects on leukocyte recruitment and vaso-occlusive mechanisms and is able to increase the survival of mice with SCD subjected to models of inflammatory vaso-occlusion.[63] Furthermore, HU may potentially be used in hemolytic disorders in general, because a single administration of this drug is able to prevent the extensive vascular inflammation that is triggered by hemolysis via a cGMP-dependent mechanism.[63]

The chronic inflammatory state is an important factor in SCD. In addition to elevated white blood cell counts, patients with SCD have alterations in the gene expression and production of some pro- and anti-inflammatory mediators.[67] The augmentation of the adhesive properties of sickle RBCs,[68] eosinophils,[69] and neutrophils and their augmented chemotactic capacity[63,70,71] may contribute to the vaso-occlusive process. HU has beneficial effects on neutrophil function[63] and reduces the adhesion of eosinophils[72] and sickle erythrocytes.[68]

Transfusion and Alloimmunization

Transfusion is also available free of cost to all patients with SCD through the SUS. The main public blood banks (part of the *hemocentros*) have standardized protocols for transfusion according to recent recommendations. For example, at the Hemocentro Unicamp, transfusion units are submitted to leukoreduction, are HbS negative, and are phenotypically matched for ABO, Rh (D, C, c, E, e), K, Fy^a/ Fy^b, JK^a/JK^b, S, and Die antigens. Genotyping for RBC antigens is also carried out in a few major university hospitals.[73,74] However, it is important to point out that it is not uncommon for patients to be transfused in regional, smaller hospitals, without a general standard procedure for transfusion in patients with SCD. The percentage of alloimmunization varies among different reports. A study performed in São Paulo found 12.5% alloimmunization,[75] whereas another study carried out in Bahia reported 51% alloimmunization[76] and a third one in the city of Campinas found 41% alloimmunization.[77] In all studies, most of the cases were secondary to alloimmunization by the antigens in the Rhesus and Kell systems.[76,77-80]

Brazil's Contribution to the Search for New Drugs to Treat SCD

The search to uncover a substance that could prevent or reduce the polymerization of HbS dates from the 1970s in Brazil. Several drugs, including piracetam and iodoacetamide, were tested without a detectable antisickling action in vitro and in vitro in animal models.[81] In addition, a small clinical trial with aspirin in SCD did not show any improvement in the frequency of vaso-occlusive episodes compared with placebo.[82]

More recently, new compounds have been developed to be tested as a possible treatment for SCD.[83] A novel hybrid compound family has been synthesized that displays the pharmacophoric properties of thalidomide plus the NO-donor properties of HU. The most effective compound displays analgesic activity, anti-inflammatory activity, and NO-donor properties.[83] In supernatants of monocyte cultures from transgenic SCD mice, this compound decreased TNF-α, IL-1β, IL-6, and keratinocyte chemoattractant (KC) levels, whereas HU does not show this kind of activity.[83,84] Two months of therapy with the compound also increased HbF production in transgenic SCD mice.[84] New NO-donor phenylsulfonylfuroxan derivates have emerged as γ-globin inducers that function via histone H3 and H4 acetylation in K562 cells.[85] These compounds demonstrated the capacity to decrease TNF-α levels in mice monocyte cultures and inhibit adenosine diphosphate–induced platelet aggregation.[85]

Important Clinical Aspects of SCD in Brazil

As previously described, the support from the SUS, although sometimes heterogeneous among the different states, has allowed the operation of several centers of excellence for SCD care. As a consequence, a substantial number of careful clinical reports have been carried out in different regions of the country, as detailed here. One very interesting study compared clinical and hematologic characteristics among children with SCD from São Paulo (southeast) and Salvador, Bahia (northeast). Despite the small number of patients, a significant finding was the observation of a possible milder phenotype among patients in Salvador, possibly due to genetic, environmental, and socioeconomic factors.[86]

A study of 155 adult patients with HbSC disease in São Paulo showed that the most common complications were painful crises (38.3%), retinopathy (33.8%), cholelithiasis (30.3%), osteonecrosis (24.8%), and sensorineural hearing disorders (9.7%). This last phenomenon seems to be an independent predictor for mortality.[87] Others analyses of patients with HbSC disease have been carried out in Minas Gerais, Bahia, and Campinas.[25,88-90]

Transcranial Doppler flow velocity screenings are performed in most specialized pediatric SCD centers and are covered by the SUS. There are at least 2 studies of transcranial Doppler screening in SCD; one study in São Paulo suggested that the procedure may be useful even in adult patients,[91] and another report from Bahia showed abnormal transcranial Doppler results in patients with HbSC.[89]

Leg ulcers seem to be a common complication of SCA in Brazil. In a cohort of 680 adult patients from Pernambuco (Bezerra M, personal communication), 22.8% presented with leg ulcers. In addition, in a group of 220 adults with SCD in Campinas, we found leg ulcers in 15%. The severity of many of the cases is high, with some cases requiring amputation.[92]

Pulmonary hypertension was investigated by right heart catheterization in 80 patients with SCA by researchers from São Paulo. They found that 40% of patients had elevated tricuspid regurgitant jet velocity but were able to confirm hypertension by catheterization in 10% of these patients using a mean of 25 mm Hg to diagnose pulmonary hypertension. This study suggests that echocardiography is useful as a screening procedure for pulmonary hypertension, but for confirmation of the diagnosis, right heart catheterization should be performed.[93]

Abnormalities of conjunctival and retinal vessels have been the subject of several studies in Brazil. A study from Ribeirão Preto in São Paulo reported conjunctive vessel alteration in 97.9% of patients with SCA, 76% of HbS/β⁰ thalassemia patients, and 75% of HbSC patients.[94] Another report from Campinas, also in São Paulo state, described retinopathy in 36% of HbSS and 47% of HbSC adult patients.[95] Data also indicated that lower hemoglobin levels is a risk factor for retinopathy in HbSS patients and that higher levels of HbF are protective in HbSC patients. Occurrence of retinopathy was described as associated with increased circulating pigment epithelium-derived factor (PEDF) and low soluble intercellular adhesion molecule 1 (ICAM1)[96] and also with abnormalities in the angiogenic process.[97]

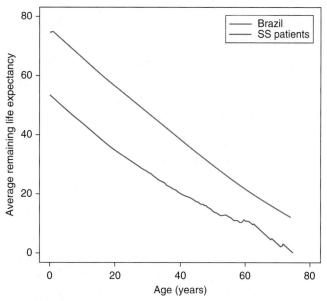

FIGURE 33-2 Mortality data in Rio de Janeiro showing the life expectancy for the general population compared with sickle cell anemia (SS) patients. Used with permission from Lobo CLC, Nascimento EM, Jesus LJC, et al. Mortality in children, adolescents and adults with sickle cell anemia in Rio de Janeiro, Brazil. *Hematol Transfus Cell Ther.* 2018;40(1):37-42.

An interesting study investigated the mortality rate among 1676 children, adolescents, and adults with SCD followed at a single institution in Rio de Janeiro for 15 years (1998-2012). The authors found an 18.87% mortality rate for adults and a 16.72% mortality rate when including all patients. These data suggest that the survival of patients with SCD is 21.3 years less than the life expectancy of the general Brazilian population (Figure 33-2).[98] The most frequent causes of death were acute chest syndrome, infection, stroke, chronic organ damage and death during crises.[99]

There are also reports of cognitive profiles in children with SCA,[100] elevated hypercoagulability markers in hemoglobin SC disease,[101] albuminuria and treatment with enalapril,[102] and abnormalities of iron metabolism in SCA.[103]

Bone marrow transplantation is also supported by the SUS, with some restrictions and well-defined indications, and there is at least one center with strong expertise in transplantation.[104] A recent review estimated that in a cohort of 2064 Brazilian patients with SCA, at least 16% of the children and 26% of the adults had at least one indication for hematopoietic stem cell transplantation.[105]

Recently, a panel of experts from the Brazilian Association of Hematology and Hemotherapy (ABHH) published a comprehensive guideline on neonatal screening, diagnosis, and treatment in SCD, aimed specifically at patients in Brazil.[106]

Future challenges for the management of SCD in Brazil depend on maintaining and increasing the budget from the federal government to the SUS, despite the economic crisis in the country. This is particularly important because patients are surviving for longer and taking care of older adult patients who present with high morbidity is increasingly expensive.

Conclusion

Although the ethnic origins of the Brazilian population are unique, the clinical and laboratory characteristics of SCD are not that different when compared to cases described in United States and Europe. The care of patients is fully covered by the Public Healthcare System and may be a model for other countries with similar economic and social problems of Brazil. It should be mentioned that the newborn screening program, called the National Neonatal Screening Program (Program Nacional de Teste Neonatal [PNTN]) is funded by the Ministry of Health for all states, as is the free distribution of HU for management of SCD.

High-Yield Facts

◆ Brazil is the largest country in South America, with an estimated population of 208 million inhabitants (2018). The population has a very heterogeneous ethnic origin and is diverse in different regions of the country.

◆ The National Neonatal Screening Program (PNTN) is a universal program funded by the Ministry of Health for all states since 2001. The rate of HbS heterozygotes is estimated at 5.9% to 8% among African Brazilians, 1.2% to 2.8% in the general mixed-ethnicity population in southern Brazil, and 7.6% in some populations in the northeastern region. The number of patients with SCD at any given time is between 30,000 and 50,000 in the whole country.

◆ Two large studies in 2 different states (Rio de Janeiro and Minas Gerais) measured the survival of children with SCD in Brazil after neonatal screening was initiated and found a high mortality rate (4.1% and 7.4%, respectively). The majority of deaths were caused by infections.

◆ The Public Healthcare System (Sistema Único de Saúde [SUS]) covers all the costs of diagnosis and treatment of SCD in Brazil. Special centers in public-funded institutions were created to provide care for the diagnosis and treatment of SCD (called *hemocentros*). In each state, at least one of these centers is in charge of health care for SCD patients.

◆ These centers are, in general, very well organized and have contributed to an important increase in the quality of care for SCD in Brazil. In addition, they allow for a significant number of clinical and translational studies related to the myriad of clinical and laboratory manifestations of SCD.

References

1. Brazilian Institute of Geography and Statistic. Brazilian population projection. https://ibge.gov.br/apps/populacao/projecao/. Accessed July 30, 2020.

2. Krieger H, Norton NE, Mi MP, Azevedo E, Freire-Maia A, Yasuda N. Racial admixture in north-eastern Brazil. *Ann Hum Genet.* 1965;29:113-125.

3. Zago MA, Costa FF. Hereditary haemoglobin disorders in Brazil. *Trans R Soc Trop Med Hyg.* 1985;79:385-388.

4. Azevedo ES, Silva KMC, Silva MCBO, Lima AMVM, Fortuna CMM, Santos MG. Genetic and anthropological studies in the island of Itaparica, Bahia, Brazil. *Hum Hered.* 1981;31: 353-357.

5. Pena SD, Bastos-Rodrigues L, Pimenta JR, Bydlowski SP. DNA tests probe the genomic ancestry of Brazilians. *Braz J Med Biol Res.* 2009;42(10):870-876.

6. Pimenta JR, Zuccherato LW, Debes AA, et al. Color and genomic ancestry in Brazilians: a study with forensic microsatellites. *Hum Hered.* 2006;62(4):190-195.

7. Neel JV. Rare variants, private polymorphisms, and locus heterozygosity in Amerindian populations. *Am J Hum Genet.* 1978;30:465-490.

8. Salzano FM, Tondo CV. Hemoglobin types in Brazilian populations. *Hemoglobin.* 1983;6:85-97.

9. Azevêdo E. Historical note on in inheritance of sickle cell anemia. *Am Hum Genet.* 1973;25:457-458.

10. Kato GJ, Piel FB, Reid CD, et al. Sickle cell disease. *Nat Rev Dis Primers.* 2018;4:18010.

11. Brazilian National Health Surveillance Agency. Manual of diagnosis and treatment of sickle disease, 2001 [Portuguese]. Manual de Diagnóstico e tratamento de Doenças Falciformes, edited by ANVISA (Brazilian National Health Surveillance Agency). Brasília, 2001.

12. Ministry of Health Brazil. Sickle cell disease: what you should know about genetic inheritance. http://bvsms.saude.gov.br/bvs/publicacoes/doenca_falciforme_deve_saber_sobre_heranca.pdf. Accessed July 30, 2020.

13. Sabarense AP, Lima GO, Silva LML, et al. Survival of children with sickle cell disease in the comprehensive newborn screening programme in Minas Gerais, Brazil. *Paediatr Int Child Health.* 2015;35(4):329-332.

14. Lobo CLC, Ballas SK, Domingos AD, et al. Newborn screening program for hemoglobinopathies in Rio de Janeiro, Brazil. *Pediatr Blood Cancer.* 2014;61(1):34-39.

15. Rezende PV, Belisário AR, Oliveira EL, et al. Co-inheritance of alpha thalassemia dramatically decreases the risk of acute splenic sequestration in a large cohort of newborns with hemoglobin SC. *Haematologica.* 2019;104(7):e281-e283.

16. Zago MA, Costa FF, Freitas TC, Bottura C. Clinical, hematological and genetic features of sickle cell anemia and sickle cell-β thalassemia in a Brazilian population. *Clin Genet.* 1980;18: 58-64.

17. Hutz MH, Salzano FM. Sickle cell anemia in Rio de Janeiro, Brazil: demographic, clinical and laboratory data. *Braz J Med Biol Res.* 1983;16(3):219-226.

18. Hutz MH, Salzano FM, Adams J, et al. Hb F levels, longevity of homozygotes and clinical course of sickle cell anemia in Brazil. *Am J Med Genet.* 1983;14(4):669-676.

19. Salzano FM. Incidence, effects, and management of sickle cell disease in Brazil. *Am J Pediatr Hematol Oncol.* 1985;7(3):240-244.

20. Zago MA, Figueiredo MS, Ogo SH. Bantu βˢ cluster haplotype predominates among Brazilian blacks. *Am J Phys Anthropol.* 1992;88(3):295-298.

21. Figueiredo MS, Kerbauy J, Gonçalves MS, et al. Effect of alpha-thalassemia and beta-globin gene cluster haplotypes on the hematological and clinical features of sickle-cell anemia in Brazil. *Am J Hematol.* 1996;53(2):72-76.

22. Gonçalves MS, Nechtman JF, Figueiredo MS, et al. Sickle cell disease in a Brazilian population from Sao Paulo: a study of the βˢ haplotypes. *Hum Hered.* 1994;44(6):322-327.

23. Costa FF, Arruda VR, Gonçalves MG, et al. Beta S-gene-cluster haplotypes in sickle cell anemia patients from two regions of Brazil. *Am J Hematol.* 1994;45(1):96-97.

24. Gonçalves MS, Bomfim GC, Maciel E, et al. βˢ-Haplotypes in sickle cell anemia patients from Salvador, Bahia, Northeastern Brazil. *Braz J Med Biol Res.* 2003;36(10):1283-1288.

25. Aleluia MM, Fonseca TCC, Souza RQ, et al. Comparative study of sickle cell anaemia and hemoglobin SC disease: clinical characterization, laboratory biomarkers and genetic profiles. *BMC Hematol.* 2017;17:15.

26. Cruz, PRS, Ananina, G, Gil-da-Silva-Lopes, VL, et al. Genetic comparison of sickle cell anaemia cohorts from Brazil and the United States reveals high levels of divergence. *Sci Rep.* 9, 10896, 2019.

27. Silva MC, Zuccherato LW, Lucena FC, et al. Extensive admixture in Brazilian sickle cell patients: implication for the mapping of genetic modifiers. *Blood.* 2011;118:4493-4494.

28. Fertrin KY, Melo MB, Assis AM, Saad ST, Costa FF. UDP-glucuronosyltransferase 1 gene promoter polymorphism is associated with increased serum bilirubin levels and cholecystectomy in patients with sickle cell anemia. *Clin Genet.* 2003;64:160-162.

29. Andrade FL, Annichino-Bizzacchi JM, Saad ST, Costa FF, Arruda VR. Prothrombin mutant, factor V Leiden, and thermolabile variant of methylenetetrahydrofolate reductase among patients with sickle cell disease in Brazil. *Am J Hematol.* 1998;59(1): 46-50.

30. Lettre G, Sankaran VG, Bezerra MA. DNA polymorphisms at the BCL11A, HBS1L-MYB, and beta-globin loci associate with fetal hemoglobin levels and pain crises in sickle cell disease. *Proc Natl Acad Sci USA.* 2008;105(33):11869-11874.

31. Leonardo FC, Brugnerotto AF, Domingos IF. Reduced rate of sickle-related complications in Brazilian patients carrying HbF-promoting alleles at the BCL11A and HMIP-2 loci. *Br J Haematol.* 2016;173(3):456-460.

32. Fertrin KY, Costa FF. Genomic polymorphisms in sickle cell disease: implications for clinical diversity and treatment. *Exp Rev Hematol.* 2010;3(4):443-458.

33. Costa RN, Conran N, Albuquerque DM, Soares PH, Saad ST, Costa FF. Association of the G-463A myeloperoxidase polymorphism with infection in sickle cell anemia. *Haematologica.* 2005;90(7):977-979.

34. Domingos IF, Pereira-Martins DA, Coelho-Silva JL, et al. Interleukin-6 G-174C polymorphism predicts higher risk of stroke in sickle cell anaemia. *Br J Haematol.* 2018;182:276-307.

35. Gil GP, Ananina G, Oliveira MB, et al. Polymorphism in the HMOX1 gene is associated with high levels of fetal hemoglobin in Brazilian patients with sickle cell anemia. *Hemoglobin.* 2013;37(4):315-324.

36. Santos MN, Bezerra MA, Domingues BL, et al. Haptoglobin genotypes in sickle-cell disease. *Genet Test Mol Biomarkers.* 2011;15(10):709-713.

37. Castro V, Alberto FL, Costa RNP, et al. Polymorphism of the human platelet antigen-5 system is a risk factor for occlusive vascular complications in patients with sickle cell anemia. *Vox Sang.* 2004;87(2):118-123.

38. Farias ICC, Mendonça-Belmont TF, daSilva AS, et al. Association of the *SOD2* polymorphism (Val16Ala) and SOD activity with vaso-occlusive crisis and acute splenic sequestration in children with sickle cell anemia. *Mediterr J Hematol Infect Dis.* 2018;10(1):e2018012.

39. Medeiros FA, Mendonça TF, Lopes KAM, et al. Combined genotypes of the *MBL2* gene related to low mannose-binding lectin levels are associated with vaso-occlusive events in children with sickle cell anemia. *Genet Mol Biol.* 2017;40(3):600-603.

40. Vicari P, Adegoke SA, Mazzotti DR, Nagutti MA, Figueiredo MS. Interleukin-1 beta and interleukin-6 gene polymorphisms are associated with modifications of sickle cell anemia. *Blood Cells Mol.* 2015;54:244-249.

41. Belisario AR, Nogueira FZ, Rodrigues RS, et al. Association of alpha-thalassemia, TNF-alpha (-308G>A) and VCAM-1 (c.1238G>C) gene polymorphisms with cerebrovascular disease in a newborn cohort of 411 children with sickle cell anemia. *Blood Cells Mol.* 2015;54:44-50.

42. de Carvalho-Siqueira GQ, Ananina G, de Souza BB. Whole-exome sequencing indicates FLG2 variant associated with leg ulcers in Brazilian sickle cell anemia patients. *Exp Biol Med (Maywood).* 2019;244(11):932-939.

43. Silva FAC, Ferreira ALCG, Hazin-Costa MF, et al. Adverse clinical and obstetric outcomes among pregnant women with different sickle cell disease genotypes. *Int J Gynaecol Obstet.* 2018;143(1):89-93.

44. Resende Cardoso PS, Lopes Pessoa de Aguiar RA, Viana MB. Clinical complications in pregnant women with sickle cell disease: prospective study of factors predicting maternal death or near miss. *Rev Bras Hematol Hemoter.* 2014;36(4):256-263.

45. Silva-Pinto AC, de Oliveira Domigues Ladeira S, Brunetta DM, et al. Sickle cell disease and pregnancy: analysis of 34 patients followed at the Regional Blood Center of Ribeirão Preto, Brazil. *Rev Bras Hematol Hemoter.* 2014;36(5):329-333.

46. Gilli SC, De Paula EV, Biscaro FP, et al. Third-trimester erythrocytapheresis in pregnant patients with sickle cell disease. *Int J Gynaecol Obstet.* 2006;96(1):8-11.

47. Baptista LC, Costa ML, Ferreira R, et al. Abnormal expression of inflammatory genes in placentas of women sickle cell anemia and sickle hemoglobin C disease. *Ann Hematol.* 2016;95(11):1859-1867.

48. Baptista LC, Figueira CO, Souza BB, et al. Highlight article: different morphological and gene expression profile in placentas of the same sickle cell anemia patient in pregnancies of opposite outcomes. *Exp Biol Med.* 2019;244(5):395-403.

49. Furtado PS, Costa MP, Ribeiro do Prado Valladares F. The prevalence of priapism in children and adolescents with sickle cell disease in Brazil. *Int J Hematol.* 2012;95(6):648-651.

50. Roizenblatt M, Figueiredo MS, Cançado RD, et al. Priapism is associated with sleep hypoxemia in sickle cell disease. *J Urol.* 2012;188(4):1245-1251.

51. Saad STO, Lajolo C, Gilli S, et al. Follow-up of sickle cell disease patients with priapism treated by hydroxyurea. *Am J Hematol.* 2004;77(1):45-49.

52. Claudino MA, Franco-Penteado CF, Corat MA, et al. Increased cavernosal relaxations in sickle cell mice priapism are associated with alterations in the NO-cGMP signaling pathway. *J Sex Med.* 2009;6(8):2187-2196.

53. Silva FH, Claudino MA, Calmasini FB, et al. Sympathetic hyperactivity, increased tyrosine hydroxylase and exaggerated corpus cavernosum relaxations associated with oxidative stress plays a major role in the penis dysfunction in Townes sickle cell mouse. *PLoS One.* 2016;11:e0166291.

54. Silva FH, Alexandre EC, Calmasini FB, Calixto MC, Antunes E. Treatment with metformin improves erectile dysfunction in a murine model of obesity associated with insulin resistance. *Urology.* 2015;86(2):423.e1-6.

55. Lobo CLC, Pinto JFC, Nascimento EM, et al. The effect of hydroxcarbamide therapy on survival of children with sickle cell disease. *Br J Haematol.* 2013;161:852-860.

56. Costa FC, da Cunha AF, Fattori A, et al. Gene expression profiles of erythroid precursors characterise several mechanisms of the action of hydroxycarbamide in sickle cell anaemia. *Br J Haematol.* 2007;136(2):333-342.

57. Canalli AA, Proença RF, Franco-Penteado CF, et al. Participation of Mac-1, LFA-1 and VLA-4 integrins in the in vitro adhesion of sickle cell disease neutrophils to endothelial layers, and reversal of adhesion by simvastatin. *Haematologica.* 2011;96(4):526-533.

58. Dominical VM, Vital DM, Garrido VT, et al. Interactions of sickle red blood cells with neutrophils are stabilized on endothelial cell layers. *Blood Cells Mol Dis.* 2016;56(1):38-40.

59. Dominical VM, Vital DM, O'Dowd F, Saad ST, Costa FF, Conran N. In vitro microfluidic model for the study of vaso-occlusive processes. *Exp Hematol.* 2015;43(3):223-228.

60. Dominical VM, Samsel L, Nichols JS, et al. Prominent role of platelets in the formation of circulating neutrophil-red cell heterocellular aggregates in sickle cell anemia. *Haematologica.* 2014;99(11):e214-e217.

61. Silveira AAA, Dominical VM, Almeida CB, et al. TNF induces neutrophil adhesion via formin-dependent cytoskeletal reorganization and activation of β-integrin function. *J Leukoc Biol.* 2018;103(1):87-98.

62. Canalli AA, Franco-Penteado CF, Saad ST, Conran N, Costa FF. Increased adhesive properties of neutrophils in sickle cell disease may be reversed by pharmacological nitric oxide donation. *Haematologica.* 2008;93(4):605-609.

63. Almeida CB, Scheiermann C, Jang JE, et al. Hydroxyurea and a cGMP-amplifying agent have immediate benefits on acute vaso-occlusive events in sickle cell disease mice. *Blood.* 2012;120(14):2879-2888.

64. Almeida CB, Traina F, Lanaro C, et al. High expression of the cGMP-specific phosphodiesterase, PDE9A, in sickle cell disease (SCD) and the effects of its inhibition in erythroid cells and SCD neutrophils. *Br J Haematol.* 2008;142(5):836-844.

65. Conran N, Torres L. cGMP modulation therapeutics for sickle cell disease. *Exp Biol Med (Maywood).* 2019;244(2):132-146.

66. Miguel LI, Almeida CB, Traina F, et al. Inhibition of phosphodiesterase 9A reduces cytokine-stimulated in vitro adhesion of neutrophils from sickle cell anemia individuals. *Inflamm Res.* 2011;60(7):633-642.

67. Lanaro C, Franco-Penteado CF, Albuqueque DM, Saad ST, Conran N, Costa FF. Altered levels of cytokines and inflammatory mediators in plasma and leukocytes of sickle cell anemia patients and effects of hydroxyurea therapy. *J Leukoc Biol.* 2009;85(2):235-242.

68. Gambero S, Canalli AA, Traina F, et al. Therapy with hydroxyurea is associated with reduced adhesion molecule gene and protein

expression in sickle red cells with a concomitant reduction in adhesive properties. *Eur J Haematol.* 2007;78(2):144-151.

69. Canalli AA, Conran N, Fattori A, Saad ST, Costa FF. Increased adhesive properties of eosinophils in sickle cell disease. *Exp Hematol.* 2004;32(8):728-734.

70. Assis A, Conran N, Canalli AA, Lorand-Metze I, Saad ST, Costa FF. Effect of cytokines and chemokines on sickle neutrophil adhesion to fibronectin. *Acta Haematol.* 2005;113(2): 130-136.

71. Canalli AA, Franco-Penteado CF, Traina F, Saad ST, Costa FF, Conran N. Role for cAMP-protein kinase A signalling in augmented neutrophil adhesion and chemotaxis in sickle cell disease. *Eur J Haematol.* 2007;79(4):330-337.

72. Pallis FR, Conran N, Fertrin KY, Olalla Saad ST, Costa FF, Franco-Penteado CF. Hydroxycarbamide reduces eosinophil adhesion and degranulation in sickle cell anaemia patients. *Br J Haematol.* 2014;164(2):286-295.

73. Castilho L, Rios M, Bianco C, et al. DNA-based typing of blood groups for the management of multiply-transfused sickle cell disease patients. *Transfusion.* 2002;42(2):232-238.

74. Ribeiro KR, Guarnieri MH, Costa DC, et al. DNA array analysis for red blood cell antigens facilitates the transfusion support with antigen-matched blood in patients with sickle cell disease. *Vox Sang.* 2009;97(2):147-152.

75. Moreira Júniro G, Bordin JO, Kuroda A, Kerbauy J. Red blood cell alloimmunization in sickle cell disease: the influence of racial and antigenic pattern differences between donors and recipients in Brazil. *Am J Hematol.* 1996;52(3):197-200.

76. Dias Zenette AM, Souza Gonçalves M, Vilasboas Schettini L, et al. Alloimmunization and clinical profile of sickle cell disease patients from Salvador-Brazil. *Ethn Dis.* 2010;20(2):136-141.

77. Sippert EA, Visentainer JE, Alves HV, et al. Red blood cell alloimmunization in patients with sickle cell disease: correlation with HLA and cytokine gene polymorphisms. *Transfusion.* 2017;57(2):379-389.

78. Castilho L, Rios M, Rodrigues A, et al. High frequency of partial *DIIIa* and *DAR* alleles found in sickle cell disease patients suggests increased risk of alloimmunization to RhD. *Transfus Med.* 2005;15(1):49-55.

79. Cruz BR, de Souza Silva TC, de Souza Castro B, et al. Molecular matching for patients with haematological diseases expressing altered *RHD-RHCE* genotypes. *Vox Sang.* 2019;114(6):605-615.

80. Rodrigues C, Sell AM, Guelsin GAS, et al. HLA polymorphisms and risk of red blood cell alloimmunisation in polytransfused patients with sickle cell anaemia. *Transfus Med.* 2017;27(6):437-443.

81. Costa FF, Zago MA, Bottura C. Effects of piracetam and iodocetamide on erythrocyte sickling. *Lancet.* 1979;2(8155):1302.

82. Zago MA, Costa FF, Ismael SJ, et al. Treatment of sickle cell disease with aspirin. *Acta Haematologica.* 1984;72:61-64.

83. dos Santos JL, Lanaro C, Lima LM, et al. Design, synthesis, and pharmacological evaluation of novel hybrid compounds to treat sickle cell disease symptoms. *J Med Chem.* 2011;54(16):5811-5819.

84. Lanaro C, Franco-Penteado CF, Silva FH, et al. A thalidomide-hydroxyurea hybrid increases HbF production in sickle cell mice and reduces the release of proinflammatory cytokines in cultured monocytes. *Exp Hematol.* 2018;58:35-38.

85. Melo TRF, Kumkhaek C, Fernandes GFDS, et al. Discovery of phenylsulfonylfuroxan derivatives as gamma globin inducers by histone acetylation. *Eur J Med Chem.* 2018;154:341-353.

86. Lyra IM, Gonçalves MS, Braga JA, et al. Clinical, hematological, and molecular characterization of sickle cell anemia pediatric patients from two different cities in Brazil. *Cad Saude Publica.* 2005;21(4):1287-1290.

87. Gualandro SF, Fonseca GHH, Yokomizo IK, et al. Cohort study of adult patients with haemoglobin SC disease: clinical characteristics and predictors of mortality. *Br J Haematol.* 2015;171:631-637.

88. Rezende PV, Santos MV, Campos GF, et al. Clinical and hematological profile in a newborn cohort with hemoglobin SC. *J Pediatr (Rio J).* 2018;94(6):666-672.

89. Vieira C, Oliveira CN, Figueiredo LA, et al. Transcranial Doppler in hemoglobin SC disease. *Pediatr Blood Cancer.* 2017; 64(5):10.1002/pbc.26342.

90. Conran N, Costa FF. *Sickle Cell Anemia: From Basic Science to Clinical Practice.* Springer International Publishing; 2016.

91. Rodrigues DLG, Adegoke SA, Campos RSM, et al. Patients with sickle cell disease are frequently excluded from the benefits of transcranial Doppler screening for the risk of stroke despite extensive and compelling evidence. *Arq Nuero-Psiquiatr.* 2017;75(1):15-19.

92. Maximo C, Olalla Saad ST, Thome E, et al. Amputations in sickle cell disease: case series and literature review. *Hemoglobin.* 2016;40(3):150-155.

93. Fonseca GH, Souza R, Salemi VM, et al. Pulmonary hypertension diagnosed by right heart catheterisation in sickle cell disease. *Eur Respir J.* 2012;39(1):112-118.

94. Siqueira WC, Figueiredo MS, Cruz AA, Costa FF, Zago MA. Conjunctival vessel abnormalities in sickle cell diseases: the influence of age and genotype. *Acta Ophthalmol.* 1990;68(5): 515-518.

95. Lima CS, Rocha EM, Silva NM, Sonati MF, Costa FF, Saad ST. Risk factors for conjunctival and retinal vessel alterations in sickle cell disease. *Acta Ophthalmol Scand.* 2006;84(2):234-241.

96. Cruz PR, Lira RP, Prereira Filho SA, et al. Increased circulating PEDF and low sICAM-1 are associated with sickle cell retinopathy. *Blood Cells Mol Dis.* 2015;54(1):33-37.

97. Lopes FC, Traina F, Almeida CB, et al. Key endothelial cell angiogenic mechanisms are stimulated by the circulating milieu in sickle cell disease and attenuated by hydroxyurea. *Haematologica.* 2015;100(6):730-739.

98. Lobo CLC, Nascimento EM, Jesus LJC, et al. Mortality in children, adolescents and adults with sickle cell anemia in Rio de Janeiro, Brazil. *Hematol Transfus Cell Ther.* 2018;40(1):37-42.

99. Nascimento EM, Lobo CL, Pereira BB, Ballas S. Survival probability in patients with Sickle cell anemia using the cognitive risk statistical model. *Mediterr J Hematol Infect Dis.* 2019;11(1):e2019022.

100. Castro IPS, Viana MB. Cognitive profile of children with sickle cell anemia compared to healthy controls. *J Pediatr.* 2019;4:451-457.

101. Colella MP, de Paula EV, Machado-Neto JA, et al. Elevated hypercoagulability markers in hemoglobin SC disease. *Haematologica.* 2015;100:466-471.

102. Aoki RY, Saad ST. Enalapril reduces the albuminuria of patients with sickle cell disease. *Am J Med.* 1995;98(5):432-435.

103. Fertrin KY, Lanaro C, Franco-Penteado C, et al. Erythropoiesis-driven regulation of hepcidin in human red cell disorders is better reflected through concentrations of soluble transferrin receptor rather than growth differentiation factor 15. *Am J Hematol.* 2014;89(4):385-390.

104. Gluckman E, Cappelli B, Bernaudin F. Sickle cell disease: an international survey of results of HLA-identical sibling hematopoietic stem cell transplantation. *Blood.* 2016;129(11):1548-1556.

105. Flor-Park MV, Kelly S, Preiss L, et al. Identification and characterization of hematopoietic stem cell transplant candidates in a sickle cell disease cohort. *Biol Blood Marrow Transplant.* 2019;25(10):2103-2109.

106. Braga JA, Verissimo MP, Saad ST, Cançado RD, Loggetto SR. Guidelines on neonatal screening and painful vaso-occlusive crisis in sickle cell disease: Associação Brasileira de Hematologia, Hemoterapia e Terapia Celular: Project guidelines: Associação Médica Brasileira–2016. *Rev Bras Hematol Hemoter.* 2016;38(2):147-157.

Sickle Cell Disease in Africa

Authors: *Amma Twumwa Owusu-Ansah, Julie Makani, Kwaku Ohene-Frempong*

Chapter Outline

Overview

Africa is the second largest region of the world ranked by population, after Asia. It occupies a land mass of 11, 447, 338 square miles. Its current population according to latest estimates by the United Nations is 1,349, 886, 357, making up 16.72% of the world's population. Its population is young, with a median age of 19.7 years. 43.8% of Africa's population is urban. Most of the world's sickle cell disease (SCD) births occur in Africa. In light of these facts, no program or strategy to advance disease-modifying or curative therapies will have major or lasting impact without involving Africa or consideration from an African perspective.

Researchers using whole-genome sequencing data from 156 individuals with sickle cell trait (1 copy of the β^s mutation Glu6Val, rs334) out of 2932 individuals from the 1000 Genomes Project, the African Genome Variation Project, and Qatar have posited that the initial β^s mutation arose in Africa, possibly in the Green Sahara and Western Central Africa approximately 7300 years ago.[1] The hemoglobin C mutation (β6Glu-Lys) is assumed to have arisen from a unique origin in West Africa (highest prevalence in Northern Ghana and Burkina Faso and rarely found in western Nigeria)[2-5] and perhaps independently in Southeast Asia.[6,7]

Centuries before the first description of sickle cell disease (SCD) in the medical literature in 1910 by Dr. James Herrick in the United States, in Africa, SCD was recognized as a disorder that clustered in families, referred to by local dialects (referred to as *chwechweechwe* in Ga, *nwiiwii* in Fante, and *ahotutuo* in Twi), and was described with enough accuracy to permit tracing to several generations in a family in Ghana as early as 1670 AD.[8] Evidence of SCD was found from studies of 6 predynastic Egyptian mummies dating back to 3200 BC.[9]

The β^s mutation is an oft-cited example of balanced polymorphism where the heterozygous state confers a survival advantage over either homozygote. Studies in children from areas where malaria was hyperendemic show significantly less malarial parasitemia in those with sickle cell trait compared to those without it and demonstrated the similar distribution of sickle cell trait and hyperendemic malaria.[10-12] Hemoglobin C trait and homozygous CC are also associated with a 29% and 93% risk reduction of clinical malaria, respectively.[2,13]

Historically, SCD was almost exclusively a disease of childhood, due to the high mortality rate, but with the early identification of individuals through screening programs (beginning in the mid-1970s), comprehensive care and disease-modifying therapies, as well as epidemiologic transition, a new chapter in the history of SCD is being written.

Environmental and Cultural Features Influencing SCD in Africa

The geographic distribution of the β^s allele and therefore SCD within Africa is not homogenous and is influenced indirectly by factors such as altitude, rainfall, and survival of the *Anopheles* mosquito, and directly by selection pressure from malaria. Although large areas have >9% frequency of the β^s allele, it is largely absent from countries in the Horn of Africa, South Africa, Morocco, and Algeria.[14,15] In East Africa, the frequency of the β^s allele was 20% around the coastal communities and <1% in the highlands.[11]

Societal attitudes toward those living with SCD impact their quality of life. In Africa, cultural, traditional, and religious beliefs or practices significantly shape society's attitudes toward SCD, while also shaping the general or health-seeking behavior of those with SCD.[16] A classic case in point is the cultural myth of the *malevolent ogbanje* among the Igbo people of Nigeria. *Malevolent ogbanje* are believed to be vengeful, chronically ill individuals who go through repeated cycles of birth, death, and reincarnation to torment parents. These children may have distinctive, unpleasant names to discourage their behavior. A similar concept exists in some parts of Ghana.[17] A study of 100 individuals identified as *malevolent ogbanje* showed a 70% prevalence of SCD, and many of them had death-themed names.[18] Universal newborn screening with comprehensive care would educate families about the nature of their children's condition, but awareness of prevalent beliefs in the community is important to inform one's approach to program implementation. Stigma associated with SCD in Africa is prevalent and may present a significant obstacle to seeking and delivering medical care. The stigma may deny the individual with SCD basic opportunities to which they would be otherwise entitled (eg, a good education). This stigma may be directed at people with SCD for various reasons, including appearance (eg, persistent jaundice, growth delay) and anticipation of early death,[19] or at their mothers, who are blamed for their child's illness and may have their child's paternity questioned.[20] Certain SCD clinical syndromes have secondary complications that are independently associated with stigma with devastating consequences in Africa (eg, priapism causing erectile dysfunction, an emasculating condition, particularly in patriarchal societies where masculinity is cherished and must be proven).[21,22] The prevalence of erectile dysfunction in SCD ranges from 21% to 35%,[23-25] and its occurrence increases with delayed treatment of priapism, which is a common occurrence.[26]

Conversely, cultural background may positively influence pain-coping skills. In a study that compared SCD patients in the United Kingdom and Nigeria, the former reported significantly more pain episodes, pain episodes of longer duration, and more health care utilization, and the latter applied more active psychological techniques to deal with their pain outside of the health care system.[27] Other factors, such as personal cost of seeking care, probably contribute to this difference. Studies have described the important role of parents and the family environment on coping skills in children with SCD.[28] Spirituality also impacts disease self-management, with some individuals with SCD using prayer as a coping mechanism.[29]

Any program designed to identify and provide care to SCD individuals must have built in counseling, as for other genetic disorders, as well as strategies to provide rapid access to care and to combat stigma.

Differences in SCD Epidemiology in Africa Versus Western Countries

Contribution of Africa to Global Burden of SCD

Currently, it is estimated that >300,000 people are born with SCD each year worldwide, approximately 75% of whom are born in Africa.[30,31] Three countries account for half of the world's SCD births, 2 of them African—Nigeria and Democratic Republic of Congo (Figure 34-1).[15,32] The number of babies born annually with SCD worldwide is predicted to exceed 400,000 by the year 2050.[33,34] Models predict that

Nigeria, which in 2010 had an estimated 91,000 newborns with SCD (95% confidence interval [CI], 77,900-106,100), will have an estimated 140,800 babies born with SCD in the year 2050 (95% CI, 95,500-200,600), and that the Democratic Republic of the Congo, which had an estimated 39,700 babies born with SCD in 2010 (95% CI, 32,600-48,800), will have an estimated 44,700 born in 2050 (95% CI, 27,100-70,500).[33]

Even though no sub-Saharan African country has universal newborn screening programs in place,[34] several pilot programs have been successfully completed in several countries (eg, Ghana, Tanzania, Liberia, Benin, Angola, and Burkina Faso) that provide specific data on birth prevalence of SCD (Table 34-1).[35-40]

With epidemiologic transition, Africa's attendant reduced mortality from infectious disease and malnutrition, migration to

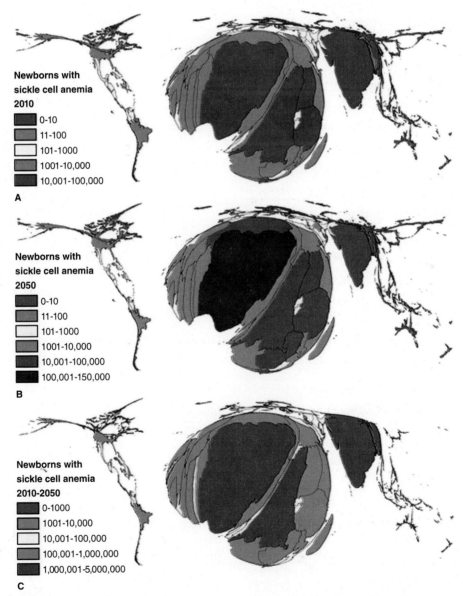

FIGURE 34-1 **Cartograms of the estimated number of newborns with SCA per country.** Piel FB, Hay SI, Gupta S, Weatherall DJ, Williams TN (2013) Global Burden of Sickle Cell Anaemia in Children under Five, 2010–2050: Modelling Based on Demographics, Excess Mortality, and Interventions. PLOS Medicine 10(7): e1001484. https://doi.org/10.1371/journal.pmed.1001484.

TABLE 34-1 Pilot newborn screening programs in sub-Saharan Africa, with estimates of birth prevalence, incidence of SCD, proportion or number of newborns with SCD, and outcome of screening

Starting date or date range	Country	First author	Screened for SCD (no.)	Estimate	Outcome
May 1993-April 1996	Republic of Benin	Rahimy et al[39]	1189	135 positive	85% enrolled in comprehensive care 80% retained at 5 years of follow-up 10-fold reduction in infant mortality rate in SCD vs national rate
February 1995-December 2005	Ghana	Ohene-Frempong et al[35]	202,244	1.9% birth prevalence 1.04% FS 0.83% FSC	Enrolled in KATH Sickle Cell Clinic Some transitioned to adult care
June 2000-September 2000	Nigeria	Odunvbun[44a]	644	3% birth prevalence 2.8% FS 0.2% FSC	99.7% acceptability of NBS to parent
2000-2004 2006	Burkina Faso	Kafando et al[40]	2341 53	1 in 57 6 in 53	Pediatrician follow-up arranged; some lost to follow-up
July 2011-March 2013	Angola	McGann et al[38]	36,453	1.51% FS 0.019% FSC	Enrolled in pediatric clinic for SCD comprehensive care 96.6% compliance with visits Comparable SCD infant mortality rate to national rate
January 2015-November 2016	Tanzania	Nkya[36]	3981	Birth prevalence 0.8%	90.3% enrolled in comprehensive care
N/A	DRC	Tshilolo[44b]	31,304	1.4%	Confirmatory testing at 6 months, PCN at 3 months 60% follow-up at 6 months
N/A	Liberia	Tubman et al[37]	2785	Incidence 1.2%	76% received care

Abbreviations: DRC, Democratic Republic of Congo; N/A, not available; NBS, newborn screening; PCN, penicillin; SCD, sickle cell disease.

highly resourced countries with excellent access to comprehensive care, and improved survival rates of individuals with SCD in certain parts of Africa with comprehensive care programs, the prevalence and burden of SCD are set to increase (Table 34-1).[32]

Clinical Presentations That Differ in Africa

No sub-Saharan country has implemented universal newborn screening, which means individuals with a mild course are diagnosed later in life (eg, acute chest syndrome in pregnancy as an initial clinical presentation of SCD).[41] Health providers must, therefore, maintain a high index of suspicion for SCD when caring for patients of any age, not only in Africa but also in the West, given the easy movement of people across borders. Health providers must listen for, notice, and ask further questions about subtle cues (eg, the individual with a history of "rheumatism" or who gets mild body pain whenever it rains or the weather turns cold; the persistently jaundiced individual; the person with a thin body habitus and short stature, frontal bossing, or increased prominence of the maxilla from marrow expansion [sickle cell gnathopathy]; the infant who appears fussy, will not bear weight for no apparent reason, has a high white blood cell count, or whose parents casually remark that both their "blood groups" are AS; or rarely, the individual with multiple longitudinal scarification marks along the thighs and over the left upper quadrant[42] made by a traditional healer[43]). For these patients, it may be their first opportunity to be diagnosed with SCD and receive appropriate medical care. Data from an SCD registry in Germany, which does not have a universal newborn screening program, showed that children were presenting with complications of SCD prior to being diagnosed.[44]

Although there are many similarities in clinical presentation of SCD between the West and Africa, significant differences exist in certain circumstances, influenced by physical environment, malaria, socioeconomic status, nutrition, and availability (or otherwise) of early identification and comprehensive care. SCD is independently described in diverse communities across Africa with names that strikingly convey the same or similar meaning, such as pain likened to "body biting," "gnawing," and "fever or illness of the bones."[16,20] Studies show that similar bacterial species cause invasive infections in SCD in sub-Saharan Africa and the West; the incidence of pneumococcal bacteremia in sub-Saharan Africa is in the same range (1.5 to 11.6/100 patient-years)[44c] as what it was in the West prior to the introduction of penicillin prophylaxis and pneumococcal vaccines. Likewise, other complications have similar prevalence, including splenic sequestration, acute chest syndrome, avascular necrosis, and gallstone disease. Several clinical scenarios, however, differ significantly and deserve special mention.

Malaria and Splenomegaly

Falciparum malaria is endemic to sub-Saharan Africa. Although the β^s mutation confers protection from malaria in the heterozygous state, this does not apply to SCD. A 10-year retrospective study found that 63.3% of 108 SCD individuals hospitalized had clinical malaria.[45] Although individuals with SCD have a lower malaria parasite load and suffer from clinical malaria less than those without SCD, they have a much higher mortality.[46-48] The excess mortality is likely due to interaction between SCD and malaria through multiple mechanisms including increased hemolysis with severe anemia (hemoglobin ≤5 g/dL), which is independently associated with increased risk of mortality[48] and a heightened risk of bacteremia complicating malaria.[49,50]

The spleen is one of the first organs to be impacted early in SCD. Splenomegaly develops early in life and can be associated with potentially fatal splenic sequestration episodes[51] and hypersplenism. With repeated episodes of infarction, the spleen undergoes atrophy (particularly in homozygous SCD), or it may remain enlarged but with diminished function (functional asplenia or hyposplenia).[52,53] This typical course has been noted in the West,[54] as has delay or reversal with interventions such as hydroxyurea[55,56] and chronic transfusion therapy.[57] Although most would not expect to find a palpable spleen in an individual with homozygous SCD, this is not unusual in children, adolescents, and young adults in sub-Saharan Africa.[48,58] The persistence of splenomegaly in this area is thought to be related to malaria; SCD patients from Nigeria with splenomegaly had greater parasitemia than those without splenomegaly,[59] and malarial immunoglobulin G antibody titers positively correlated with spleen size in another study.[58,60]

Stroke

Unmodified SCD is associated with a high risk of stroke. Data from the Cooperative Study of Sickle Cell Disease showed an 11% risk of having a stroke by age 20 in those homozygous for β^s and a 2% risk for individuals who are compound heterozygous for hemoglobin S and C.[61] With the Stroke Prevention Trial in Sickle Cell Anemia Trial showing that chronic transfusions to lower HbS to <30% are associated with a 90% reduction in stroke risk,[62] overt stroke in childhood is now a rare occurrence in the West. A systematic review and meta-analysis of overt stroke in children with SCD in sub-Saharan Africa found a variable stroke prevalence ranging from 2.9% to 16.9% from clinic-based data from 7 countries (Figure 34-2). Using pediatric mortality data and country-specific β^s gene frequencies, the pooled estimate of overt stroke prevalence was 2.9% (95% CI, 2.49%-3.31%) by fixed-effect analysis and 5.82% (95% CI, 3.60%-8.03%) by random-effect analysis.[62] This translates to approximately 60,000 children affected by overt stroke in sub-Saharan Africa, a conservative estimate given that available data were skewed toward those who survived and those able to seek hospital-based care.[63] The BRAIN SAFE study of 265 children investigated for neurologic abnormalities showed that 5.7% had a prior stroke; 2% had an abnormal transcranial Doppler ultrasound (TCD), which is associated with an increased risk of stroke; and 15.1% had a conditional TCD.[64]

Outcomes That Differ in Africa, Including Newborn and Lifetime Mortality Rate

SCD is associated with high mortality in sub-Saharan Africa, with peaks in children <5 years of age, adolescents, and pregnant women; however, there is lack of up-to-date mortality data for the region. It is estimated that SCD is responsible for 5% to 16% of deaths in some parts of sub-Saharan Africa.[65,66] The earliest data on SCD mortality came from a study done in the Garki District of Nigeria, which showed a cumulative excess mortality rate of 92% from birth to age 15 years. A review of published and unpublished mortality data provided an estimated mortality rate between 50% and 90%.[66,67] The probability of early death in SCD approaches 90% in rural areas with no or poor access to health care and 50% for areas with better access.[66] In contrast, survival analysis predicted a cumulative overall survival in SCD at age 18 to be 85.6% in the United States.[68] In a London-based childhood SCD cohort with 2158 person-years of observation, estimated survival of children with homozygous SCD at age 16 years was 99% (95% CI, 93.2%-99.9%).[69]

The feasibility and life-saving effects of newborn screening for SCD and close follow-up for comprehensive care in sub-Saharan Africa have been demonstrated in several cohorts.

A pilot newborn screening program in the Republic of Benin that enrolled and followed 85% of newborns who tested positive for SCD was still following 80% of them at 5 years and detected an under-age-5 mortality rate decrease in that period to 15.5 per 10,000, which was 10 times lower than the under-age-5 mortality rate in the general pediatric population.[39] Another study in Lusaka, Zambia, saw a decrease

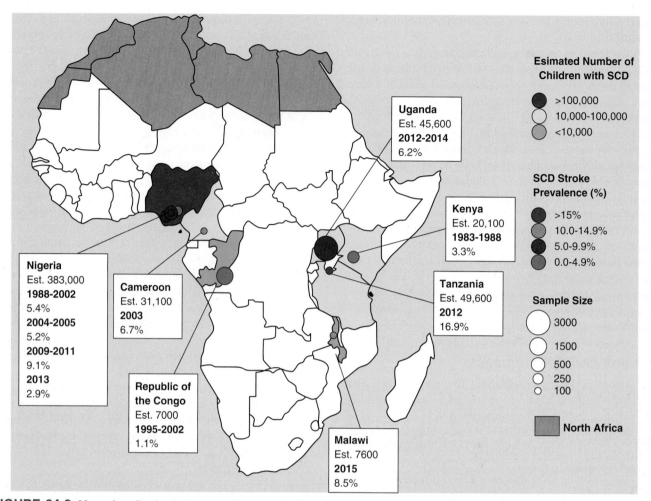

FIGURE 34-2 **Map of pediatric stroke prevalence in sickle cell disease (SCD) in sub-Saharan Africa.** Countries with published studies are shown. Countries are color-coded based on number of children estimated to have sickle cell disease, with the estimate listed under each country. Study years of each published study are shown, along with reported prevalence of stroke. Reproduced, with permission, from Marks LJ, Munube D, Kasirye P, et al. Stroke prevalence in children with sickle cell disease in sub-Saharan Africa: a systematic review and meta-analysis. *Glob Pediatr Health.* 2018;5:2333794X18774970.

in case fatality rates of homozygous SCD children admitted to one institution from 18.6% in 1970 to 6.6% between 1987 and 1989, likely reflecting improved public health measures and medical care.[67] In the Muhimbili National Hospital cohort in which 1564 SCD individuals contributed 4482 person-years of observation, the overall mortality rate was 1.9%.[70]

In adolescents and young adults with SCD, acute chest syndrome appeared to be the leading cause of death in sub-Saharan Africa. A retrospective study of 52 autopsies performed on 52 patients with SCD whose mean age of death was 21 years found evidence of fatal pulmonary thromboembolic events (37%) and infection (78%) and peak mortality in the second and third decades of life.[71] Autopsies performed on adolescents aged 10 to 19 years in Ghana showed SCD to be the leading cause of death among noncommunicable diseases.[72]

Maternal mortality in SCD is approximately 10%.[73,74] Pregnancy increased the risk of mortality >20-fold in women with SCD compared to those without it in a study in Ghana. Acute chest syndrome was the cause of death in 86% of maternal deaths in SCD over the period from 2010 to 2016.[75] A feasibility

study of an intervention consisting of outpatient and inpatient care and monitoring by a multidisciplinary team that included obstetricians and hematologists, fetal surveillance, and institution of management protocols for acute chest syndrome and painful vaso-occlusive episodes demonstrated an 89.1% reduction in maternal mortality risk.[76] Follow-up studies showed that maternal and perinatal mortality rates decreased to the same levels as for non-SCD individuals in Ghana.[73]

Standard of Care Management and Therapy

Diagnostic Screening

A new era is slowly dawning across sub-Saharan Africa and bringing change with it. The current top priority of management is the identification of SCD individuals through newborn screening and the institution of a comprehensive care package that is accessible and affordable to individuals with SCD.[77] A cost-effectiveness analysis in 43 sub-Saharan African countries found newborn screening and preventive care to be highly cost-effective where there was a 0.2% to 0.3% incidence of SCD; 34 countries sub-Saharan Africa fall in this category.[77,78] Ghana Health Services, for instance, has planned to establish a nationwide SCD program based on the life-saving impact of the Pilot Newborn Screening Program carried out in Kumasi and Tikrom, Ghana.[35] In anticipation of and planning for universal newborn screening in sub-Saharan Africa, several point-of-care tests (POCT) to screen for SCD have been field tested in some areas of sub-Saharan Africa (eg, Nigeria and Uganda; Table 34-2). These tests can provide results in minutes and are cheaper than standard methods of detection. A total of 1121 babies were screened for SCD using the HemoTypeSC POCT (Silver Lake Research, Azusa, CA) in Nigeria in a multicenter study. The HemoTypeSC demonstrated 93.4% sensitivity and 99.9% specificity for homozygous SCD and correctly identified all individuals with hemoglobin C trait.[79] The same device demonstrated >99% accuracy in detection of hemoglobins A, S, and C in a blinded prospective diagnostic accuracy trial in southeastern Uganda.[80] SickleScan (BioMedomics, Morrisville, NC), another POCT, was field tested for diagnostic accuracy in a case-control study (the DREPATEST study) in 2 sub-Saharan Africa countries, Mali and Togo. Subjects were in the following categories (known cases of SCD [HbSS, HbSC] or sickle trait [HbAS] or HbC heterozygotes [HbAC] or homozygotes [HbCC]). The trial demonstrated 100% sensitivity and specificity in identifying HbAA and HbCC. In samples from individuals in Togo, sensitivity was 97.7%, 97.6%, 95.6%, and 94.9% for HbSC, HbSS, HbAS, and HbAC, respectively. In Mali, 100% sensitivity and specificity for cases and controls were reported.[81] Both POCTs operate based on lateral flow

immunoassay using antibodies to visually detect the various types of hemoglobin.[82] HemeChip, also known by its trademarked name Gazelle (Hemex Health, Portland, OR), is the first single-use, cartridge-based, microchip electrophoresis-based hemoglobin screening POCT. It was validated in 248 individuals—20 adults from Cleveland, Ohio, and 228 children aged 1 to 5 years from Kano, Nigeria. High-performance liquid chromatography (HPLC) was the standard against which it was tested. It had 100% sensitivity for all hemoglobin types tested, whereas specificity was 96.4% for HbSS versus HbAA, 98.2% for HbSS versus HbAS, 100% for HbSC versus HbAS, and 100% for HbAS versus HbAA.[83] Once individuals are identified through newborn screening, a comprehensive care package consisting of the following interventions is implemented.

Antibiotic and Malaria Prophylaxis

Penicillin V prophylaxis, when introduced into the care of SCD children <5 years, dramatically reduced childhood mortality in the West.[84-86] Penicillin V is on the World Health Organization (WHO) Essential Medicines list[77] and is generally affordable. Some countries have a national health insurance scheme or policy that may cover SCD-related prescriptions and care at no additional cost to patients; however, support services, either formal or informal (family support schemes), are key to continued engagement of the SCD individual and family.[87] Patients who are allergic to penicillin receive macrolide antibiotics.

WHO recommends using malaria prophylaxis, but no specific recommendations have been provided.[34] Monthly prophylaxis with sulfadoxine-pyrimethamine during the season for peak transmission of malaria was well tolerated in a small

TABLE 34-2 Results from validation of several POCT designed to screen for SCD

POCT	Country	No. screened	Sensitivity (%)	Specificity (%)	PPV (%)	NPV (%)	Standard	Authors
HemoTypeSC	Nigeria	1121	93.4 (SS)	99.9 (SS)	100 (SS)	100 (SS)	HPLC	Nnodu et al[79]
	Uganda	1000	100 (SS)	100 (SS)	100 (SS)	100 (SS)	CZE	Nankanja et al[80]
SickleScan	Togo	295	97.6 (SS) 97.7 (SC)	99.6 (SS) 99.6 (SC)	Not reported	Not reported	CE	Segbena et al[81]
	Mali	240	100	100	Not reported	Not reported	HPLC	
	Nigeria	57	100	98.2	Not reported	Not reported	HPLC	Nwegbu et al[82a]
HemeChip	Nigeria United States	228 20	100 100	100 (SC) 96.4-98.2 (SS)			HPLC HPLC	Hasan et al[83]

Note. The POCTs were tested against the following standards: HPLC, CZE, and CE.

Abbreviations: CE, capillary electrophoresis; CZE, capillary zone electrophoresis; HPLC, high-performance liquid chromatography; NPV, negative predictive value; POCT, point-of-care test; PPV, positive predictive value; SCD, sickle cell disease.

placebo-controlled study; there was no clinical malaria on the treatment arm, whereas the placebo group had 6.6% prevalence of malaria.[88] Proguanil was more effective than pyrimethamine in lowering parasitemia in another study of seasonal malaria prophylaxis.[89] A systematic review and meta-analysis of the safety and efficacy of 7 different antimalarial preparations showed that antimalarial prophylaxis in SCD is effective and there was no difference in the occurrence of adverse events between groups. A randomized controlled trial of malaria prophylaxis in children with SCD (EPITOMISE) is currently underway (see later discussion). The use of insecticide-impregnated bed nets as a general measure has reduced malaria mortality in sub-Saharan Africa by 60%, benefiting SCD individuals as well.[34]

Immunizations

Per the recommendation of the Advisory Committee on Immunization Practices (ACIP), SCD children should receive the full complement of PCV-13 pneumococcal vaccines followed by the PCV-23 vaccine, with the first dose at age 2 years and a second dose at age 5, and vaccines for *Haemophilus influenzae* type B (HIB).[90] PCV-13 and HIB are available through the Expanded Program on Immunization (EPI). The EPI is supported by GAVI, the Vaccine Alliance, in low-income countries but not middle-income countries.[34] Therefore, affordability may be a barrier to receiving PCV-13 in middle-income countries with SCD individuals (eg, Angola). PCV-13 vaccination is available in 34 African countries,[91] but the PCV-23 vaccine is not universally or easily available.

Prompt Treatment of Infections and Febrile Illness

Per WHO guidelines, the febrile SCD patient should be treated with both antibiotics and antimalarials. In Ghana, this has been done with 2 doses of ceftriaxone and 3 days of antimalarial therapy.[87] Similar practices exist where there are established cohorts of SCD children receiving comprehensive care.

Hydroxyurea

This SCD-modifying therapy reduces the rate of painful vaso-occlusive episodes, acute chest syndrome, and severe anemia by 50% and improves survival. Hydroxyurea's safety, feasibility, and benefits have been evaluated in sub-Saharan Africa in several studies (eg, the SPIN, NOHARM, and REACH trials).[92-94] Hydroxyurea has become more available in sub-Saharan Africa, is now on the WHO Essential Medicines list, and is becoming more affordable through local production (eg, partnerships with pharmaceutical companies). For instance, Novartis has provided free hydroxyurea doses for all SCD patients to the Ghana Health Service and is supporting development of guidelines and capacity-building efforts. Hydroxyurea used in the Stroke Prevention in Children With SCA in Nigeria (SPIN) trial was locally produced at the cost of $0.13 per daily dose.[77] Tanzania is also producing hydroxyurea locally.[95]

Blood Transfusion

Blood transfusions for acute complications and stroke prevention are used as per indication. Exchange transfusion has been used for acute SCD complications including acute chest syndrome.[96,97] Currently, the substantial financial toll associated with chronic transfusions may reduce the feasibility of their widespread application. Hydroxyurea has been used for primary stroke prevention in certain instances. TCD screening is available in some tertiary health institutions.

Hematopoietic Stem Cell Transplantation

Hematopoietic stem cell transplantation, the definitive cure for SCD, is not available to most SCD individuals within sub-Saharan Africa. A case report of the first successful transplant in 2011 of a 7-year-old child with SCD and previous stroke in Nigeria was published in 2014.[98] There was an attempt to set up an HSCT unit or service in Ghana that was not successful. A large investment in infrastructure and buy-in from multiple stakeholders are needed for this to be successfully implemented.[99]

Gene Therapy

Gene therapy is still in the experimental phase in the United States for SCD. Tanzania has developed a strategy to integrate curative therapies into SCD care, including gene therapy, leveraging the genomics research that is currently occurring in sub-Saharan Africa.[95]

Transition From Pediatric to Adult Care

The transition from pediatric to adult care in sub-Saharan Africa tends to occur much earlier than in the West. A few studies are have begun to explore this in sub-Saharan Africa.[100,101] It will gain increasing relevance as all of the strategies discussed earlier become more available and increasing numbers of individuals survive to adulthood.

Future Research and Clinical Directions

H3Africa

Human Health and Heredity Africa (H3Africa) is a consortium established to build African research capacity in genomics and its application to human health and disease. Cardiovascular events are prevalent in sub-Saharan Africa and are poorly understood. H3Africa has funded 20-plus projects to study cardiovascular disease (eg, stroke) and kidney disease in African countries where SCD also happens to be prevalent.[102] These projects provided the opportunity for a network of SCD researchers in Cameroon, Ghana, Nigeria, South Africa, and Tanzania to conduct multicenter studies based in sub-Saharan Africa to better understand the genomics of SCD. An H3Africa-funded project in Ghana, Cameroon, and Tanzania was implemented to study attitudes toward implementation of genomic research and to "assess perceptions about public health interventions to increase awareness, early detection and prevention of SCD-related complications." Another project embarked on by the H3Africa SCD Investigators is to build a repository of genomic and clinical data from their countries to enable the translation of these data into improved health outcomes for SCD patients.[103]

SickleGenAfrica

"The SickleGenAfrica Network is made up of African scientists and international collaborators studying 7000 children and adults with SCD in Africa to identify genetic markers associated with the development of organ damage, with a special emphasis on the body's defense against molecules released from damaged red blood cells that cause tissue injury. The long-term goal of the network is to develop strategies to predict, prevent and treat organ damage in SCD."[104]

Three projects are being carried out under the auspices of SickleGenAfrica:

1. Determine variation in levels of cytoprotective proteins involved in the response to hemolysis, catalog associated genome-wide variants, and determine the prevalence of acute organ damage in a cohort of 7000 individuals in Ghana, Nigeria, and Tanzania.

2. Determine the prevalence of malaria and its severe complications including anemia, cerebral malaria, and acute respiratory distress syndrome, and catalog genome-wide variants associated with these complications in a longitudinal cohort of 7000 patients.

3. Phenotype major echocardiograph-based biomarkers in 2000 adults with SCD from West and East Africa and catalog the genetic variants associated with the phenotypes.

REACH Trial

The "Realizing Effectiveness Across Continents With Hydroxyurea" (REACH) Trial is an international, prospective, phase I/II, open-label dose-escalation study of hydroxyurea that successfully enrolled 635 children age 1 to 10 years with SCD in 4 sub-Saharan African countries (Angola, Democratic Republic of Congo, Kenya, and Uganda). Six hundred six participants completed screening and were followed for 3 years. The primary study end point was severe hematologic toxicities that would occur during the fixed-dose treatment phase. The rationale for this study was the recognized urgent need for disease-modifying therapy for SCD in sub-Saharan Africa and the gap in knowledge of the effect of coexistent malaria and malnutrition on feasibility and safety of hydroxyurea in SCD. Participants were started on a fixed dose of 15 to 20 mg/kg for 6 months with monitoring, followed by dose escalation. Hydroxyurea was found to be safe and feasible in children with SCD living in sub-Saharan Africa and significantly reduced the incidence of painful vaso-occlusive events, infections including malaria, need for blood transfusion, and death.[94,105]

EPiTOMISE Trial

The EPiTOMISE Trial is a randomized, 3-arm, open-label trial of malaria chemoprevention in children with sickle cell anemia (SCA) at a single site in Homa Bay, Kenya. The objectives of this trial are to compare the efficacy of 3 malaria chemoprevention regimens to reduce the incidence of malaria and the incidence of severe complications of SCA. The goal for enrollment is 246 children aged <10 years. Participants will be randomized in a 1:1:1 ratio to 1 of 3 arms of malaria chemoprevention: proguanil oral tablet, sulfadoxine/pyrimethamine-amodiaquine, or dihydroartemisinic-piperaquine. They will be followed monthly for 12 months. The primary end point is incidence of malaria over 12 months. The study is ongoing, and no results are yet available (ClinicalTrials.gov identifier: NCT03178643).

Conclusion

In conclusion, the history, burden, and challenges posed by SCD in sub-Saharan Africa have been reviewed, as well as several distinguishing features. Pilot studies have shown that early identification of SCD through newborn screening can significantly reduce SCD morbidity and mortality. Hydroxyurea is safe and effective in reducing not only painful vaso-occlusive events, need for blood transfusions, and death, but also malaria infection. Efforts are ongoing to facilitate early diagnosis of SCD and improve access to hydroxyurea, including through the African Newborn Screening and Early Intervention Consortium established by the American Society of Hematology,[34] validation and dissemination of POCT devices, recognition of hydroxyurea as a WHO-listed essential medication, local production of hydroxyurea, and partnerships with pharmaceutical companies. Going forward, there needs to be buy-in and commitment from various governments and stakeholders in sub-Saharan Africa to provide the technical support needed for the diagnosis and treatment of SCD and its complication; training programs for health providers, families, and the general public on SCD to ensure excellent comprehensive care and eliminate stigma; and finally, investment in the infrastructure required to make clinical trials and curative therapies universally available.

Case Study

A 3-month-old female was brought by her parents to a comprehensive pediatric sickle cell clinic located within a teaching hospital in West Africa. The reason for her visit was confirmation testing and genetic counseling for an abnormal newborn screen result that read "FSC," which indicates compound heterozygosity for hemoglobin S and C. The infant was well-appearing with normal growth parameters, and the physical exam was completely normal. However, her parents were visibly upset; her father was particularly beside himself and was questioning the test results. Both parents had undergone premarital testing for SCD and sickle cell trait; the mother had sickle cell trait, but because the father's testing was apparently normal, they were reassured about starting a family with no concerns for having children with SCD.

Confirmatory testing was performed using HPLC, which showed hemoglobin F, S, and C. The parents were offered testing. The mother had sickle cell trait, and the father had hemoglobin C trait. Appropriate genetic counseling was done, thoroughly explaining to the parents the 25% probability of having a child with genotype AA, AC, AS, or SC with each birth. Their infant was enrolled in the pediatric comprehensive sickle cell clinic for care.

The initial screening method used in the premarital testing of the parents was a hemoglobin solubility test (either based on sodium hyposulfite or sodium metabisulfite [common in many resource-limited countries]). Sodium hyposulfite and metabisulfite are reducing agents that deoxygenate hemoglobin. In tests based on the former (Sickledex), a positive test is indicated by increased turbidity of a solution containing the blood sample, phosphate buffer, and sodium hyposulfite, making it difficult to read a card with black lines held behind the tube. The latter test is dependent on a solution of 2% sodium metabisulfite that has to be freshly prepared on a daily basis, mixed with a drop of blood on a coverslip that is inverted on a slide, and viewed under a microscope for evidence of sickled erythrocytes.[106,107] Both tests have limited sensitivity and specificity, are operator dependent, and do not detect hemoglobin C.

Relatively inexpensive, easily operated point-of-care hemoglobinopathy testing devices are being validated. Widespread use is anticipated in sub-Saharan Africa,[108] hopefully eliminating such unfortunate clinical scenarios.

High-Yield Facts

◆ SCD was recognized as a global public health problem by the WHO in 2006.

◆ The global burden of SCD is increasing and will continue to rise significantly in the next few decades.

◆ Sub-Saharan Africa bears the greatest disease burden with the highest number of SCD births and highest mortality.

◆ No implementation strategy or program to prevent and comprehensively manage SCD is complete without examining the clinical, socioeconomic, and environmental challenges as well as potential opportunities in this field from an African perspective.

References

1. Shriner D, Rotimi CN. Whole-genome-sequence-based haplotypes reveal single origin of the sickle allele during the holocene wet phase. *Am J Hum Genet.* 2018;102(4):547-556.
2. Piel FB, Howes RE, Patil AP, et al. The distribution of haemoglobin C and its prevalence in newborns in Africa. *Sci Rep.* 2013; 3:1671.
3. Talacki CA, Rappaport E, Schwartz E, Surrey S, Ballas SK. Beta-globin gene cluster haplotypes in Hb C heterozygotes. *Hemoglobin.* 1990;14(3):229-240.
4. Boehm CD, Dowling CE, Antonarakis SE, Honig GR, Kazazian HH Jr. Evidence supporting a single origin of the beta(C)-globin gene in blacks. *Am J Hum Genet.* 1985;37(4):771-777.
5. Kan YW, Dozy AM. Evolution of the hemoglobin S and C genes in world populations. *Science.* 1980;209(4454):388-391.
6. Siriboon W, Srisomsap C, Winichagoon P, Fucharoen S, Svasti J. Identification of Hb C [beta 6(A3)Glu-->Lys] in a Thai male. *Hemoglobin.* 1993;17(5):419-425.
7. Sanchaisuriya K, Fucharoen G, Sae-ung N, Siriratmanawong N, Surapot S, Fucharoen S. Molecular characterization of hemoglobin C in Thailand. *Am J Hematol.* 2001;67(3):189-193.
8. Konotey-Ahulu FI. The sickle cell diseases. Clinical manifestations including the "sickle crisis." *Arch Intern Med.* 1974;133(4): 611-619.
9. Marin A, Cerutti N, Massa ER. Use of the amplification refractory mutation system (ARMS) in the study of HbS in predynastic Egyptian remains. *Boll Soc Ital Biol Sper.* 1999;75(5-6):27-30.
10. Allison AC. Protection afforded by sickle-cell trait against subtertian malareal infection. *Br Med J.* 1954;1(4857):290-294.

11. Allison AC. The distribution of the sickle-cell trait in East Africa and elsewhere, and its apparent relationship to the incidence of subtertian malaria. *Trans R Soc Trop Med Hyg.* 1954;48(4): 312-318.

12. Allison AC. The discovery of resistance to malaria of sickle-cell heterozygotes. *Biochem Mol Biol Educ.* 2002;30(5):279-287.

13. Modiano D, Luoni G, Sirima BS, et al. Haemoglobin C protects against clinical Plasmodium falciparum malaria. *Nature.* 2001;414(6861):305-308.

14. Piel FB, Patil AP, Howes RE, et al. Global distribution of the sickle cell gene and geographical confirmation of the malaria hypothesis. *Nat Commun.* 2010;1:104.

15. Piel FB, Patil AP, Howes RE, et al. Global epidemiology of sickle haemoglobin in neonates: a contemporary geostatistical model-based map and population estimates. *Lancet.* 2013;381(9861):142-151.

16. Anie KA, Egunjobi FE, Akinyanju OO. Psychosocial impact of sickle cell disorder: perspectives from a Nigerian setting. *Global Health.* 2010;6:2.

17. Allotey P, Reidpath D. Establishing the causes of childhood mortality in Ghana: the "spirit child." *Soc Sci Med.* 2001;52(7): 1007-1012.

18. Nzewi E. Malevolent ogbanje: recurrent reincarnation or sickle cell disease? *Soc Sci Med.* 2001;52(9):1403-1416.

19. Dennis-Antwi JA, Culley L, Hiles DR, Dyson SM. "I can die today, I can die tomorrow": lay perceptions of sickle cell disease in Kumasi, Ghana at a point of transition. *Ethn Health.* 2011; 16(4-5):465-481.

20. Marsh VM, Kamuya DM, Molyneux SS. "All her children are born that way": gendered experiences of stigma in families affected by sickle cell disorder in rural Kenya. *Ethn Health.* 2011;16(4-5):343-359.

21. Adinkrah M. Better dead than dishonored: masculinity and male suicidal behavior in contemporary Ghana. *Soc Sci Med.* 2012;74(4):474-481.

22. Moyo S. Indigenous knowledge systems and attitudes towards male infertility in Mhondoro-Ngezi, Zimbabwe. *Cult Health Sex.* 2013;15(6):667-679.

23. Smith-Whitley K. Reproductive issues in sickle cell disease. *Blood.* 2014;124(24):3538-3543.

24. Adeyoju AB, Olujohungbe AB, Morris J, et al. Priapism in sickle-cell disease; incidence, risk factors and complications: an international multicentre study. *BJU Int.* 2002;90(9):898-902.

25. Gbadoe AD, Dogba A, Segbena AY, et al. Priapism in sickle cell anemia in Togo: prevalence and knowledge of this complication. *Hemoglobin.* 2001;25(4):355-361.

26. Ugwumba F, Ekwedigwe H, Echetabu K, Okoh A, Nnabugwu I, Ugwuidu E. Ischemic priapism in South-East Nigeria: presentation, management challenges, and aftermath issues. *Niger J Clin Pract.* 2016;19(2):207-211.

27. Anie KA, Dasgupta T, Ezenduka P, Anarado A, Emodi I. A cross-cultural study of psychosocial aspects of sickle cell disease in the UK and Nigeria. *Psychol Health Med.* 2007;12(3): 299-304.

28. Kliewer W, Lewis H. Family influences on coping processes in children and adolescents with sickle cell disease. *J Pediatr Psychol.* 1995;20(4):511-525.

29. Ohaeri JU, Shokunbi WA, Akinlade KS, Dare LO. The psychosocial problems of sickle cell disease sufferers and their methods of coping. *Soc Sci Med.* 1995;40(7):955-960.

30. Weatherall DJ, Clegg JB. Inherited haemoglobin disorders: an increasing global health problem. *Bull World Health Org.* 2001;79(8):704-712.

31. Makani J, Ofori-Acquah SF, Nnodu O, Wonkam A, Ohene-Frempong K. Sickle cell disease: new opportunities and challenges in Africa. *ScientificWorldJournal.* 2013;2013:193252.

32. Williams TN. Sickle cell disease in sub-Saharan Africa. *Hematol Oncol Clin North Am.* 2016;30(2):343-358.

33. Piel FB, Hay SI, Gupta S, Weatherall DJ, Williams TN. Global burden of sickle cell anaemia in children under five, 2010-2050: modelling based on demographics, excess mortality, and interventions. *PLoS Med.* 2013;10(7):e1001484.

34. Mburu J, Odame I. Sickle cell disease: reducing the global disease burden. *Int J Lab Hematol.* 2019;41(S1):82-88.

35. Ohene-Frempong K, Oduro J, Tetteh H, Nkrumah F. Screening newborns for sickle cell disease in Ghana. *Pediatrics.* 2008;121(suppl 2):S120-S121.

36. Nkya S, Mtei L, Soka D, et al. Newborn screening for sickle cell disease: an innovative pilot program to improve child survival in Dar es Salaam, Tanzania. *Int Health.* 2019;11(6):589-595.

37. Tubman VN, Marshall R, Jallah W, et al. Newborn screening for sickle cell disease in Liberia: a pilot study. *Pediatr Blood Cancer.* 2016;63(4):671-676.

38. McGann PT, Ferris MG, Ramamurthy U, et al. A prospective newborn screening and treatment program for sickle cell anemia in Luanda, Angola. *Am J Hematol.* 2013;88(12):984-989.

39. Rahimy MC, Gangbo A, Ahouignan G, Alihonou E. Newborn screening for sickle cell disease in the Republic of Benin. *J Clin Pathol.* 2009;62(1):46-48.

40. Kafando E, Nacoulma E, Ouattara Y, et al. Neonatal haemoglobinopathy screening in Burkina Faso. *J Clin Pathol.* 2009;62(1):39-41.

41. Campbell K, Ali U, Bahtiyar M. Acute chest syndrome during pregnancy as initial presentation of sickle cell disease: a case report. *Am J Perinatol.* 2008;25(9):547-549.

42. Ibadin OM, Ofili AN, Airauhi LU, Ozolua EI, Umoru AB. Splenic enlargement and abdominal scarification in childhood malaria. Beliefs, practices and their possible roles in management in Benin City, Nigeria. *Niger Postgrad Med J.* 2008;15(4):229-233.

43. Emechebe G, Emodi I, Ikefuna A, et al. Demographic and sociocultural characteristics of sickle anaemia children with positive hepatitis B surface antigenaemia in a tertiary health facility in Enugu. *Niger J Clin Pract.* 2010;13(3):317-320.

44. Kunz JB, Lobitz S, Grosse R, et al. Sickle cell disease in Germany: results from a national registry. *Pediatr Blood Cancer.* 2020;67(4): e28130.

44a. Odunvbun ME, Okolo AA, Rahimy CM. Newborn screening for sickle cell disease in a Nigerian hospital. *Public Health.* 2008 Oct;122(10):1111-1116.

44b. Tshilolo L, Aissi LM, Lukusa D, Kinsiama C, et al. Neonatal screening for sickle cell anaemia in the Democratic Republic of the Congo: experience from a pioneer project on 31 204 newborns. *J Clin Pathol.* 2009 Jan;62(1):35-38.

44c. Williams TN, Uyoga S, Macharia A, Ndila C, McAuley CF, Opi DH, Mwarumba S, Makani J, Komba A, Ndiritu MN, Sharif SK, Marsh K, Berkley JA, Scott JA. Bacteraemia in Kenyan children with sickle-cell anaemia: a retrospective cohort and case-control study. *Lancet.* 2009 Oct 17;374(9698):1364-1370.

45. Aloni MN, Tshimanga BK, Ekulu PM, Ehungu JLG, Ngiyulu RM. Malaria, clinical features and acute crisis in children

suffering from sickle cell disease in resource-limited settings: a retrospective description of 90 cases. *Pathog Glob Health.* 2013;107(4):198-201.

46. Williams TN, Obaro SK. Sickle cell disease and malaria morbidity: a tale with two tails. *Trends Parasitol.* 2011;27(7):315-320.

47. Komba AN, Makani J, Sadarangani M, et al. Malaria as a cause of morbidity and mortality in children with homozygous sickle cell disease on the coast of Kenya. *Clin Infect Dis.* 2009;49(2):216-222.

48. Makani J, Komba AN, Cox SE, et al. Malaria in patients with sickle cell anemia: burden, risk factors, and outcome at the outpatient clinic and during hospitalization. *Blood.* 2010;115(2):215-220.

49. Berkley J, Mwarumba S, Bramham K, Lowe B, Marsh K. Bacteraemia complicating severe malaria in children. *Trans R Soc Trop Med Hyg.* 1999;93(3):283-286.

50. Scott JA, Berkley JA, Mwangi I, et al. Relation between falciparum malaria and bacteraemia in Kenyan children: a population-based, case-control study and a longitudinal study. *Lancet.* 2011;378(9799):1316-1323.

51. Gill FM, Sleeper LA, Weiner SJ, et al. Clinical events in the first decade in a cohort of infants with sickle cell disease. Cooperative Study of Sickle Cell Disease. *Blood.* 1995;86(2):776-783.

52. Pearson HA, Spencer RP, Cornelius EA. Functional asplenia in sickle-cell anemia. *N Engl J Med.* 1969;281(17):923-926.

53. Brousse V, Buffet P, Rees D. The spleen and sickle cell disease: the sick(led) spleen. *Br J Haematol.* 2014;166(2):165-176.

54. Rogers ZR, Wang WC, Luo Z, et al. Biomarkers of splenic function in infants with sickle cell anemia: baseline data from the BABY HUG Trial. *Blood.* 2011;117(9):2614-2617.

55. Wang WC, Wynn LW, Rogers ZR, Scott JP, Lane PA, Ware RE. A two-year pilot trial of hydroxyurea in very young children with sickle-cell anemia. *J Pediatr.* 2001;139(6):790-796.

56. Hankins JS, Helton KJ, McCarville MB, Li CS, Wang WC, Ware RE. Preservation of spleen and brain function in children with sickle cell anemia treated with hydroxyurea. *Pediatr Blood Cancer.* 2008;50(2):293-297.

57. Pearson HA, Cornelius EA, Schwartz AD, Zelson JH, Wolfson SL, Spencer RP. Transfusion-reversible functional asplenia in young children with sickle-cell anemia. *N Engl J Med.* 1970; 283(7):334-337.

58. Tubman VN, Makani J. Turf wars: exploring splenomegaly in sickle cell disease in malaria-endemic regions. *Br J Haematol.* 2017;177(6):938-946.

59. Awotua-Efebo O, Alikor EA, Nkanginieme KE. Malaria parasite density and splenic status by ultrasonography in stable sickle-cell anaemia (HbSS) children. *Niger J Med.* 2004;13(1):40-43.

60. Adekile AD, McKie KM, Adeodu OO, et al. Spleen in sickle cell anemia: comparative studies of Nigerian and U.S. patients. *Am J Haematol.* 1993;42(3):316-321.

61. Ohene-Frempong K, Weiner SJ, Sleeper LA, et al. Cerebrovascular accidents in sickle cell disease: rates and risk factors. *Blood.* 1998;91(1):288-294.

62. Adams RJ. Lessons from the Stroke Prevention Trial in Sickle Cell Anemia (STOP) study. *J Child Neurol.* 2000;15(5): 344-349.

63. Marks LJ, Munube D, Kasirye P, et al. Stroke prevalence in children with sickle cell disease in sub-Saharan Africa: a systematic review and meta-analysis. *Glob Pediatr Health.* 2018;5:2333794X18774970-2333794X.

64. Green NS, Munube D, Bangirana P, et al. Burden of neurological and neurocognitive impairment in pediatric sickle cell anemia

in Uganda (BRAIN SAFE): a cross-sectional study. *BMC Pediatr.* 2019;19(1):381.

65. World Health Organization. Management of birth defects and haemoglobin disorders: report of a joint WHO-March of Dimes meeting, Geneva, Switzerland, May 17-19, 2006.

66. Grosse SD, Odame I, Atrash HK, Amendah DD, Piel FB, Williams TN. Sickle cell disease in Africa: a neglected cause of early childhood mortality. *Am J Prev Med.* 2011;41(6 suppl 4): S398-S405.

67. Athale UH, Chintu C. Clinical analysis of mortality in hospitalized Zambian children with sickle cell anaemia. *East Afr Med J.* 1994;71(6):388-391.

68. Quinn CT, Rogers ZR, Buchanan GR. Survival of children with sickle cell disease. *Blood.* 2004;103(11):4023-4027.

69. Telfer P, Coen P, Chakravorty S, et al. Clinical outcomes in children with sickle cell disease living in England: a neonatal cohort in East London. *Haematologica.* 2007;92(7):905-912.

70. Makani J, Cox SE, Soka D, et al. Mortality in sickle cell anemia in Africa: a prospective cohort study in Tanzania. *PLoS One.* 2011;6(2):e14699.

71. Ogun GO, Ebili H, Kotila TR. Autopsy findings and pattern of mortality in Nigerian sickle cell disease patients. *Pan Afr Med J.* 2014;18:30.

72. Ohene S-A, Tettey Y, Kumoji R. Cause of death among Ghanaian adolescents in Accra using autopsy data. *BMC Res Notes.* 2011; 4:353.

73. Oppong SA, Asare EV, Olayemi E, et al. Multidisciplinary care results in similar maternal and perinatal mortality rates for women with and without SCD in a low-resource setting. *Am J Hematol.* 2019;94(2):223-230.

74. Muganyizi PS, Kidanto H. Sickle cell disease in pregnancy: trend and pregnancy outcomes at a tertiary hospital in Tanzania. *PLoS One.* 2013;8(2):e56541.

75. Asare EV, Olayemi E, Boafor T, et al. A case series describing causes of death in pregnant women with sickle cell disease in a low-resource setting. *Am J Hematol.* 2018;93(7):E167-E170.

76. Asare EV, Olayemi E, Boafor T, et al. Implementation of multidisciplinary care reduces maternal mortality in women with sickle cell disease living in low-resource setting. *Am J Hematol.* 2017;92(9):872-878.

77. Oron AP, Chao DL, Ezeanolue EE, et al. Caring for Africa's sickle cell children: will we rise to the challenge? *BMC Med.* 2020;18(1):92.

78. Kuznik A, Habib AG, Munube D, Lamorde M. Newborn screening and prophylactic interventions for sickle cell disease in 47 countries in sub-Saharan Africa: a cost-effectiveness analysis. *BMC Health Serv Res.* 2016;16:304.

79. Nnodu O, Isa H, Nwegbu M, et al. HemoTypeSC, a low-cost point-of-care testing device for sickle cell disease: promises and challenges. *Blood Cells Mol Dis.* 2019;78:22-28.

80. Nankanja R, Kadhumbula S, Tagoola A, Geisberg M, Serrao E, Balyegyusa S. HemoTypeSC demonstrates >99% field accuracy in a sickle cell disease screening initiative in children of southeastern Uganda. *Am J Hematol.* 2019;94(6):E164-E166.

81. Segbena AY, Guindo A, Buono R, et al. Diagnostic accuracy in field conditions of the sickle SCAN(R) rapid test for sickle cell disease among children and adults in two West African settings: the DREPATEST study. *BMC Hematol.* 2018;18:26.

82. Alapan Y, Fraiwan A, Kucukal E, et al. Emerging point-of-care technologies for sickle cell disease screening and monitoring. *Exp Rev Med Dev.* 2016;13(12):1073-1093.

82a. Nwegbu MM, Isa HA, Nwankwo BB, et al. Preliminary Evaluation of a Point-of-Care Testing Device (SickleSCAN™) in Screening for Sickle Cell Disease. *Hemoglobin*. 2017 Mar;41(2):77-82.

83. Hasan MN, Fraiwan A, Thota P, et al. Clinical testing of Hemechip in Nigeria for point-of-care screening of sickle cell disease. *Blood*. 2018;132(suppl 1):1095.

84. Gaston MH, Verter JI, Woods G, et al. Prophylaxis with oral penicillin in children with sickle cell anemia. A randomized trial. *N Engl J Med*. 1986;314(25):1593-1599.

85. Telfer P, Coen P, Chakravorty S, et al. Clinical outcomes in children with sickle cell disease living in England: a neonatal cohort in East London. *Haematologica*. 2007;92(7):905-912.

86. Leikin SL, Gallagher D, Kinney TR, Sloane D, Klug P, Rida W. Mortality in children and adolescents with sickle cell disease. *Pediatrics*. 1989;84(3):500-508.

87. Dennis-Antwi J, Dyson S, Ohene-Frempong K. Healthcare provision for sickle cell disease in Ghana: challenges for the African context. *Div Health Soc Care*. 2008;5:241-254.

88. Diop S, Soudre F, Seck M, et al. Sickle-cell disease and malaria: evaluation of seasonal intermittent preventive treatment with sulfadoxine-pyrimethamine in Senegalese patients-a randomized placebo-controlled trial. *Ann Hematol*. 2011;90(1):23-27.

89. Eke FU, Anochie I. Effects of pyrimethamine versus proguanil in malarial chemoprophylaxis in children with sickle cell disease: a randomized, placebo-controlled, open-label study. *Curr Ther Res Clin Exp*. 2003;64(8):616-625.

90. Ahmed F, Temte JL, Campos-Outcalt D, Schunemann HJ. Methods for developing evidence-based recommendations by the Advisory Committee on Immunization Practices (ACIP) of the U.S. Centers for Disease Control and Prevention (CDC). *Vaccine*. 2011;29(49):9171-9176.

91. Kalata NL, Nyazika TK, Swarthout TD, et al. Pneumococcal pneumonia and carriage in Africa before and after introduction of pneumococcal conjugate vaccines, 2000-2019: protocol for systematic review. *BMJ Open*. 2019;9(11):e030981.

92. Galadanci NA, Umar Abdullahi S, Vance LD, et al. Feasibility trial for primary stroke prevention in children with sickle cell anemia in Nigeria (SPIN trial). *Am J Hematol*. 2017;92(8):780-788.

93. Opoka RO, Ndugwa CM, Latham TS, et al. Novel use Of Hydroxyurea in an African Region with Malaria (NOHARM): a trial for children with sickle cell anemia. *Blood*. 2017;130(24):2585-2593.

94. Tshilolo L, Tomlinson G, Williams TN, et al. Hydroxyurea for children with sickle cell anemia in sub-Saharan Africa. *N Engl J Med*. 2019;380(2):121-131.

95. Makani J, Sickle Cell Programme, Muhimbili University of Health and Allied Sciences. Curative options for sickle cell disease in Africa: approach in Tanzania. *Hematol Oncol Stem Cell Ther*. 2020;13(2):66-70.

96. Boma Muteb P, Kaluila Mamba JFJ, Muhau Pfutila P, Bilo V, Panda Mulefu JD, Diallo DA. Effectiveness, safety, and cost of partial exchange transfusions in patients with sickle-cell anemia at a sickle cell disease center in sub-Saharan Africa. *Med Sante Trop*. 2017;27(4):387-391.

97. Chamba C, Iddy H, Tebuka E, et al. Limited exchange transfusion can be very beneficial in sickle cell anemia with acute chest syndrome: a case report from Tanzania. *Case Rep Hematol*. 2018;2018:5253625.

98. Bazuaye N, Nwogoh B, Ikponmwen D, et al. First successful allogeneic hematopoietic stem cell transplantation for a sickle cell disease patient in a low resource country (Nigeria): a case report. *Ann Transplant*. 2014;19:210-213.

99. Faulkner L. How to setup a successful transplant program for hemoglobinopathies in developing countries: the Cure2-Children approach. *Hematol Oncol Stem Cell Ther*. 2020;13(2):71-75.

100. Kwarteng-Siaw M, Paintsil V, Toboh CK, Owusu-Ansah A, Green NS. Assessment of transition readiness in adolescents with sickle cell disease and their caretakers: a single institution experience. *Int J Hematol Res*. 2017;3(1):171-179.

101. Inusa BPD, Stewart CE, Mathurin-Charles S, et al. Paediatric to adult transition care for patients with sickle cell disease: a global perspective. *Lancet Haematol*. 2020;7(4):e329-e341.

102. Consortium HA, Rotimi C, Abayomi A, et al. Research capacity. Enabling the genomic revolution in Africa. *Science*. 2014;344(6190):1346-1348.

103. Wonkam A, Makani J, Ofori-Aquah S, et al. Sickle cell disease and H3Africa: enhancing genomic research on cardiovascular diseases in African patients. *Cardiovasc J Afr*. 2015;26(2 suppl 1):S50-S55.

104. West African Genetic Medicine Centre. Sickle cell disease projects. https://wagmc.org/research/sickle-cell-disease/sicklegenafrica/projects-cores.php. Accessed August 2, 2020.

105. McGann PT, Tshilolo L, Santos B, et al. Hydroxyurea therapy for children with sickle cell anemia in sub-Saharan Africa: rationale and design of the REACH trial. *Pediatr Blood Cancer*. 2016;63(1):98-104.

106. Schneider RG, Alperin JB, Lehmann H. Sickling tests. Pitfalls in performance and interpretation. *JAMA*. 1967;202(5):419-421.

107. Tubman VN, Field JJ. Sickle solubility test to screen for sickle cell trait: what's the harm? *Hematology*. 2015;2015(1):433-435.

108. McGann PT, Hernandez AG, Ware RE. Sickle cell anemia in sub-Saharan Africa: advancing the clinical paradigm through partnerships and research. *Blood*. 2017;129(2):155-161.

The letter *b*, *f*, or *t* following a page number indicates a box, figure, or table, respectively.